milk matters

Also by Maureen Minchin

*Revolutions and Rosewater: the Victorian Nursing Council 1923-1973* (VNC 1976)

*Food for Thought: a parent's guide to food intolerance* (1982, multiple editions including Allen & Unwin, and Oxford University Press; latest 1992 by Alma Publications 1992)

*Breastfeeding Matters: what we need to know about infant feeding.* (1985; various editions by Allen & Unwin and Alma Publications, latest edition 1996.)

Other publications include journal articles and multiple leaflets and pamphlets such as

*Artificial feeding: risky for any baby?* (various editions from 1994)

*Towards Safer Bottle Feeding* (circulated to global BFHI meeting in London 2001);

*From Collaboration to Control: BFHI in Australia 1991-2001* (limited edition available at libraries of record)

*AIDS and Infant Feeding: what are the choices?* (1987)

*Breast or Bottle: what will you choose?*

*Is your baby sleeping safely?*

Background briefing reports such as

*Vitamin K and infant feeding* (for WHO Geneva)

*Breastmilk expression in developing countries* (for USAID/Wellstart)

*NUK advertising claims* (for the Australian Trades Practices Commission)

# milk matters

## Infant feeding
## and
## immune disorder

# maureen minchin

Disclaimer
This book assumes that sensible parents consult appropriate health professionals about the suitability of advice for their individual situation and child, and that growth monitoring of children is routine. While it encourages parents to take responsibility for their children's health, this is to be done within a supportive healthcare system. (And if parents do not find it supportive, they are encouraged to improve it by honest feedback, not abandon it for unorthodox alternatives.)

Cover design and typeset by BookPOD Pty Ltd

Cover image © iStockphoto

National Library of Australia Cataloguing-in-Publication entry

Creator:  Minchin, Maureen K. (Maureen Kathryn), 1945- author.

Title:  Milk matters : infant feeding and immune disorder / Maureen Minchin.

ISBN:  9780959318319 (hardback)

Notes:  Includes bibliographical references and index.

Subjects:  Breastfeeding--Health aspects.
Breast milk--Health aspects.
Infant formulas.
Infants--Nutrition.
Immunologic diseases.
Child development.

Dewey Number:  649.33

# Contents

# BOOK 2
# Creating a 'perfect' breastmilk substitute: reality and myths .....195

## Chapter 3

# BOOK 3

## Chapter 4

## Chapter 5

## Chapter 6

# Chapter 7

# Chapter 8

# Appendix 1

# Appendix 2

# Appendix 3

# List of Figures

# Preface

A reviewer of *Breastfeeding Matters* way back in 1988 stated that 'it is arguable whether politics, science and practical advice should be so inextricably mingled'. While that reviewer concurred with Professor David Baum (and Dr Bill Silverman and Dr Frank Oski and others) that the book was important, even 'a milestone in breastfeeding history and a good read', she failed to see that the book was that milestone precisely *because* it mixed science, politics and practical advice – as every book does to some degree – though from what felt to her like an uncomfortably unorthodox position. Orthodoxy about infant feeding has changed since the 1980s, a process to which both *Food for Thought* and *Breastfeeding Matters* have contributed. But not enough. Too many scientists do not know either the real history or the clinical problems of infant feeding, just as too few historians know the science, and parents are kept ignorant of the past and present realities, left to struggle with the intergenerational consequences without understanding why having a baby is so distressing in too many cases.

So I am again mixing science, politics, and practical advice, on an even grander scale. Those whose equally personal mix differs from mine may not like it ... but historians are bound to tell the truth as they see it. To quote Eric Hobsbawm, 'Every historian has his or her lifetime, a private perch from which to survey the world[1], and from my perch, politics, science and practical advice are all, and always, inextricably linked. The personal is indeed political. Understanding someone's writing is facilitated by awareness of their personal history, so I feel obliged to be open about the platform of my life to date. Read Appendix 3 if you want to know what has shaped and drives me.

I also know that some of what I say in this book will prove to be outdated and some inaccurate, though not for want of effort, time or care. As Professor Geoffrey Blainey said in a review of a book about mining,

> The book must carry at the very least about 20,000 facts and snippets of evidence, and anyone who has written on large themes knows only too well that in such books a sprinkling of errors seems unavoidable. (*Saturday Age* 19 October 2013)

That comment from a former mentor is reassuring, and I hope it is only a sprinkling! Please advise me of any errors or omissions that you spot, along with references to support your criticism. Infant formula industry scientists and historians with specialised knowledge of some aspects are particularly welcome to make such suggestions. They will be treated no differently from suggestions from other respondents: taken at face value, the evidence assessed, any assumptions questioned, and a decision made about appropriate action. For I am well aware that industry knows more about its products than is ever published, and I may have got some things wrong. For that reason, I have deliberately created a short run first

---

1    EJ Hobsbawm, The Present as History: Writing the History of One's Own Times. 1993 Creighton lecture.

edition, in order to be able to make any needed important corrections before the book is made more widely available. Since a short print run increases not only unit cost but also long-term value, a hardback seemed the appropriate choice. Send all suggestions for amendment (and any other comments you'd like to make) by email to: womensmilkmatters@gmail.com.

Some of this book will be made freely available on my website-to-be, infantfeedingmatters. com, and updated as necessary. These first hardbacks may be the only versions of the book to include all sections and addenda as written in 2014. I would be very happy to collaborate with someone wanting to write a short popular version of what the book is saying, referring to the original as validation for what might seem extreme statements if not fully referenced.

There are many people who know that these views are not extreme. I thank all those who have contributed to making this book better than it might have been. Many colleagues and friends have helped me formulate my thoughts over decades. Some have provided hospitality that allowed me to recover from a decade spent caring for elderly parents, and to write undisturbed. Others have challenged me and extended my knowledge, or shared their experiences as professional, parent, patient or all three. Among those I am grateful to be able to include, in random order, Phil Minchin, Roger Short, Tony Williams, James Akre, Brandon Menzies, Vicki von Witt, Pat Lewis, Barb Glare, Julie Smith, Lisa Amir, Joy Anderson, Heather Harris, Kathy Dettwyler, Chloe Fisher, Mary Renfrew, Denise Drane, Mike Weisenberger, Rhonda Hillis, illustrators Catherine Horsfall, Sarah Garner and John Van Loon, and perhaps above all, my excellent structural editor, Nan McNab, along with Sylvie Blair of Bookpod – and Jenny and the staff at the Cats Bistro, my second office. All have made the book and my life richer. None is responsible for its deficiencies or errors, of fact, expression, or judgment.

Above all, I thank my three children, who have changed my life in so many ways, and who are responsible for my going down the path of infant feeding research, with the support of their father, Jim Minchin. My choice to do so, and to help parents gratis, rather than say, return to academia and paid employment, has inevitably meant some relative hardship for my family, but they have always supported me and still do. They have each had a variety of inputs into all my work, including this. And their children give me added reasons to want to improve the society bottle-feeding has helped create. Philip especially deserves thanks for dealing well with his allergies, and for major work on this book.

Of all the work that I have done, mothering was and is the most rewarding, and responsive breastfeeding taught me what it takes to be a mother. So I also thank my own mother, Moya Hillis, who was one of only 10 per cent of women in her local area breastfeeding after I was born: had she 'chosen' to bottle-feed (or been able to afford to do so) in the 1940s, my life, and my children's, would have been very different. Her death some months ago at the age of 97 means that she will not see this book, but her small legacy has made publishing it possible. Similarly, I express my abiding gratitude for the life of Dr Mavis Gunther, whose rational approach to infant feeding in the benighted 1970s was a beacon of hope, and so helped create *Breastfeeding matters* and the changes it has wrought. It was a great joy to meet her in 1983 and subsequently, and to ensure that the ILCA Board honoured her with the inaugural Cicely Williams Award in 1991. Women and writers will always have debts to those who went before, and should acknowledge those debts publicly, as we live and work in an interconnected web of life and thought.

I would also like to acknowledge my debt to Professor Roger Short, who is an under-recognised but crucial figure in the resurgence of breastfeeding worldwide. When in 1983, in some trepidation, I outlined the then-heretical *Breastfeeding matters*, Roger encouraged me and gave me valuable introductions to UK paediatric luminaries, who might not otherwise have engaged in discussion. (Peter Howie was one – see the footnote on page 435.) Roger's enthusiasm for this book has been an enormous help in keeping me on track. He has similarly encouraged and supported many students, and influenced many scientists and doctors and international organisations (even the Vatican!) to see the importance of breastfeeding to responsible birth spacing and human health. And above all, he introduced me to Mary Renfrew, a former student of his and now a professor in Dundee and major luminary in UK public health, who has been a friend and colleague for almost thirty years. My debts to her and to Roger are incalculable. I also thank all the frontline healthworkers, breastfeeding counsellors and lactation consultants, GPs, pharmacists and others, who have taught or been taught by me over the decades. I can honestly say that I have learned from my students, and enjoyed the process of teaching so many good caring people. I have also learned a great deal from many brave families: those I have met directly, those who have written honestly of their experiences, those who have set up support groups despite coping with major difficulties. May your children be to you the lifelong joy that mine are to me, and may your sacrifices for them be rewarded as mine have been.

I know of the sterling work of not only breastfeeding mothers' support groups, but also many parent groups concerned about allergy, autism, infant distress, and much more. The burgeoning fields of nutrition and biomedicine are involving even conventional professionals. All such groups may find much that supports them in a book that is about confronting unpleasant realities, finding answers, creating hope and motivating change. I know it does the first, I hope it does the latter.

In advance I thank my readers, who will decide whether this message reaches people who need to hear it. Each of you is important in the lives of others, and through you, families can be helped. I particularly acknowledge and thank the thousands of selfless breastfeeding mother volunteers and supporters worldwide, often viciously denigrated by people who do far less to help another family. You are doing more than you can ever know to create a healthy future society and environment. Read this book, and be proud of your work. Every baby who is breastfed or bottle-fed more lovingly because of you will be different, and will raise their children differently than if you had not helped their mother. Women are denied any real choice about infant feeding in almost every society, and all those who work to make that choice more possible need to stay strong, work together, and value one another. People created this problem. People can fix it.

Maureen Minchin
Geelong, Australia 2014

## How to read this trilogy

First of all, scan the Table of Contents as a guide to work your way through the books whenever you can. It will give you an idea of the massive scope of what I am trying to address, and how the three books connect together.

## New parents with a crying baby

If you are looking for practical advice on dealing with a distressed infant, go straight to Book 3 and read Chapters 4 and 5. Once you have done that, Book 1 explains the reasoning behind this advice in more detail if you want to understand the underlying logic. Book 2 will be of interest once things have begun to settle down, and you want to understand how this all came about.

## Parents wondering about growth or introducing foods other than milk

If you are looking for advice on these subjects, begin in Book 3 with Chapters 6 and 7.

## Pregnant parents

If you are preparing for the birth of a child, do the questionnaire at the start of Book 3 before you start reading. Then read Book 1, so you understand the importance of pregnancy and birth to having a calm and settled baby. Book 2 will help you understand more about alternatives some people may urge you to consider, or discuss as a "choice." Skim Book 3, Parts 4-5 in case you need them (which, with luck and the right support, you won't, until after 5-6 months of happy exclusive breastfeeding, when Chapter 7 will be very relevant).

## Health professionals

If you are a health professional, in most cases you should read the whole book in sequence. I hope it will persuade you to consider more critically both the advertising you see and the advice about infant feeding that you give. If you are dealing with parents of a crying breastfed baby, try out the practical strategies in Book 3.

## Researchers and scientists

If you are a scientist or researcher, Books 1 and 2 will be of the most interest. I hope that as Professor David Baum said in his introduction to my earlier book, *Breastfeeding Matters* in 1985, you will find a research topic on every page! And learning from the clinical experience outlined in Book 3 would be a good idea, especially if you are an allergy researcher.

## General readers

If you are interested public or private health, read the three books in sequence. Book 3 is about real-world problems in young infants and might not seem to be relevant, but you were once a baby; take a personal allergy check via the questionnaire. If you presently believe you have no allergy problems, there might be some surprises for you. If you are an historian or a sociologist or feminist I hope these inconvenient truths will influence your perspectives, as they have mine. And I hope all readers will become more aware of their underlying assumptions about infant feeding, and see the need for more critical thinking and better research in future.

**BOOK ONE**

# The milk hypothesis, immune disorder and allergy epidemics

Since causes are never manifest, the only way of proceeding is to propose a plausible theory and then test its explanatory power against further evidence, and in comparison with the power of rival theories. Since most theories prove to be untenable, advancing them is a hazardous business and requires a courage Darwin never lacked.

Bowlby 1991

# Foreword

As author of *Breastfeeding Matters*, Maureen Minchin gave health professionals much to think about thirty years ago. In this book she puts a lifetime of scholarship into a very practical context from her perspective as an historian, an experienced lactation counselor and mother. She succeeds in explaining eloquently just why "milk matters" so much, challenges us, and sets out intriguing questions that deserve answers.

The success of the human species has led us to forget that we are mammals, organisms distinguished by lactation, a reproductive strategy older than placentation, that assures safe transition of the offspring through the stresses of early life. Many humans today consider it little more than a lifestyle choice. But how well-informed is such choice? In this lively and readable exploration of the published and unpublished literature Minchin leads us through the gamut of biological, psychosocial, clinical and economic reasons to believe that the options are in fact unbalanced. She reveals the numerous consequences of disrupting adaptation to life outside the womb.

Of course many will find her views extreme, perhaps even heretical. After all, aren't the majority of infants in industrialised societies now artificially fed, or breastfed only for short periods? And aren't we healthier now than ever?  Here Minchin challenges us again to question what we mean by "normal" in the face of a "...*population scale experiment of artificial feeding*" that has now been experienced by several generations.  She asks astutely whether it just coincidence that "developed" societies now find themselves exposed to the burden of so-called non-communicable disease. Building on the increasing evidence that later adult health is influenced not only by the offspring's own environment, but also that of previous generations of offspring, Minchin points out the potential for disrupted adaptation to amplify through epigenetic mechanisms. In other words the diseases that characterize the new "normal" are in her words *"vertically communicable"* through the generations. You may not be just what you ate as a baby but what your mother and grandmother ate as  babies as well!

Minchin's "milk hypothesis" uniquely brings together a lifetime of learning and practical experience. As she correctly observes, *"There are many forms of evidence other than the scientific"* so testing the hypothesis will require the cooperation of many conventional disciplines.  It is to be hoped all those involved with infant feeding, whether as politicians, scientists, health professionals or parents, will give it serious consideration. Reading this book will no doubt be the starting point for fascinating research, but above all should stimulate greater global commitment to protect, promote and support human lactation and breastfeeding. Milk clearly does matter; the question is, just how much?

Anthony F. Williams
Formerly Consultant in Neonatal Paediatrics and Reader in Child Nutrition, St George's, University of London; Chair, Sub-group on Maternal and Child Nutrition, Scientific Advisory Committee on Nutrition, UK.
January 2015.

# CHAPTER 1

# The allergy epidemic and
# the milk hypothesis

It is time to re-evaluate the allergy paradigm and implement new kinds
of actions, when allergic individuals are becoming a majority of Western
populations and their numbers are increasing worldwide.

Finnish Allergy Group 2012

From birth to death, what we humans take into our bodies affects the development and functioning of our immune system. We thrive best with an immune system that is neither under-active nor over-reactive, selective rather than scattergun. We need an immune system that can remember and rapidly activate to repel or control multiplying invaders, clear away dead cells, direct tissue healing, and much more. We also want one that rapidly scales down to standby after doing its job, because the inflammation created as an initial step in the immune response pathway can make us very ill if not switched off.

Inflammation can destroy threats to our health, and it can damage us in doing so. It is increasingly seen as responsible for many adult ills, and may be responsible for much of the harms of the so-called non-communicable diseases (NCDs) such as cancers, cardiovascular problems, diabetes, chronic respiratory disease, mental health problems such as depression and autism, and other metabolic and autoimmune disorders, even dementia. All have become or are becoming endemic in Western nations since modernisation and industrialisation. All involve the presence of inappropriate inflammatory responses – too much, too little, wrongly directed. The NCDs share common risk factors: tobacco use and other chemical exposure, physical inactivity, alcohol abuse, hormonal disturbance, and unhealthy diets, which begin at birth in many cases. This is the context in which the allergy epidemic has emerged. Allergy is immune disorder manifest in many ways, communicated not as infections, but as inheritances dependent on environmental conditions. And above all dependent on infant feeding.

**Simply stated, the milk hypothesis is that** milk is *the necessary bridge* between the womb and the world; a species-specific way by which young mammals are helped to adapt to extra-uterine life and so thrive in their differing environments.

Implicit in this hypothesis is that

- feeding infants artificial substitutes for their natural diet has damaged both individuals and populations;
- the damage includes immediate and long-term harms, as well as epigenetic (see below) and heritable distortion, accumulating inter-generationally;
- effects emerge and interact in unexpected ways, modulated by genomes and microbiomes, and can range from slight to serious;
- any recovery from acquired damage – in individuals and populations – will be incremental and slow;
- recovery requires exclusive human milk feeding of infants for at least the first months, preferably six months or more, preferably with continued breastfeeding for longer than is now usual in industrialised nations;
- efforts to eradicate early exposure to any food other than breastmilk – and any other unnecessary microbiomic distortion – must be international, strenuous, and structural.

The milk hypothesis asserts that the artificial feeding of infants is the *single greatest avoidable negative input* into normal human development and health. As I first said in 1985, it is the largest uncontrolled in vivo experiment in human history, and the scale on which it has occurred has made its effects appear normal – to those blind to history, culture and the broad spectrum of ill health and 'dis-ease'.

To me, western epidemics of allergy and autoimmune disease are the inevitable and predictable result of generations of infant dysnutrition, compounded by other environmental factors. Subtle as well as serious harms of artificial feeding echo and amplify through generations in unpredictable ways, due to both genetic and epigenetic influences. (Epigenetic influences are influences that change not which genes are in our DNA, but how the body uses the options the DNA gives it – genes can effectively be 'switched on' or 'shut down' by epigenetic influences.)

- Genes influence bodily development.
- Genes influence how we utilise nutrients.
- Nutrition can alter how genes are expressed. Some of these changes will persist and be passed on to the next generation, whether in the form of a modified genome or as a result of gestation in an altered body, or both.

Diet also alters the infant's microbiome, the multiple ecosystems of living microbes that affect immediate and lifelong health. By doing so, it affects the infant's developing immune system and neurochemistry, since our microbes work symbiotically with our bodies.

Many disorders could have a causal link to infant feeding, including the

- immunological and nutritional;
- endocrine and neurological (through the influence of nutrition on biochemistry);
- neuropsychological[2] and behavioural (through the influence of the gut, the brain and hormones on behaviour and mood).

Each of these steps makes the causality less direct and more conditional, but the interactive and iterative processes that drive the human body means that some harms are compounding through generations. The egg that produces any child is formed in the body of that child's maternal grandmother. Infant girls are born with their full complement of eggs already in their ovaries, so both the grandmother's body and the mother's body influence any individual. The milk that mothers make today is influenced by both genetic and epigenetic factors, including the allergy caused by their feeding as infants.

Obviously infant formula is not always the only, or sometimes even the primary, cause of adult medical ills, even those where feeding methods could reasonably be involved. For instance, the rise in non-communicable diseases such as heart disease and diabetes is **also** obviously due to sedentary lives, calorific foods once rare, and the rapid and profit-driven industrialisation of agriculture and food production.

Yet even with these diseases, there is still a definite causal link to early infant feeding method, which programs metabolism and control of inflammation, as well as to infant formula ingredients that have directly increased risks and levels of inflammation, and dramatically re-shaped the human infant microbiome. The same is true of that other obvious link, to our wider environment: how and where we live after childhood are critical factors in health, but how we are fed as infants helps determine how bodies deal with those environmental challenges.

So while the use of substitutes for breastfeeding is not the sole cause of all modern ailments, the milk hypothesis asserts that is it *a fundamental and increasingly serious cause that is not being properly investigated*, despite the fact that this is one of the few areas where radical and universal change is possible in each person in each generation.

In summary, the milk hypothesis states that the shift from natural mammalian milk to artificial substitutes as the default method of infant feeding has substantially changed both individuals and societies.

---

2    Rook GA, Raison CL, Lowry CA. Microbiota, immunoregulatory old friends and psychiatric disorders. (PMID:24997041) *Advances in Experimental Medicine and Biology* 2014, 817:319-356. DOI: 10.1007/978-1-4939-0897-4_15

Further, that this change has been very much for the worse, and is responsible for many disorders of growth, development, and social relationships, some on an epidemic scale.

Lastly, that this damage is compounding inter-generationally[3] and cannot be reversed in one generation, but can be ameliorated, and perhaps eventually negated, by breastfeeding. Ideally, that breastfeeding will be for the two years or more recommended by the World Health Organization. After all, world allergy experts have concluded that "Probably a more or less continuous stimulation of innate immunity is needed to build up and maintain tolerance, not only intervention of 6 months."[4] When a body such as the World Allergy Organisation can recognise that fact, surely they can acknowledge the importance of the whole WHO recommendation of around six months' exclusive breastfeeding and continued breastfeeding into the second year and beyond. Breastfeeding is the natural human way of providing exactly that continuous stimulation to the child's developing microbiome and immune system. Partial breastfeeding continued through the first year would ensure a greater likelihood of tolerance, ending the pointless but confusing wrangle over four versus six months as the better age for introduction to other foods. Strong medical advocacy in support of the WHO goal might just be enough to generate the societal re-structuring that would be needed for such breastfeeding to become possible for more than advantaged minorities.

A mother's own milk, fed from her own body, has been the physiological norm since mammals evolved millions of years ago. The milk of each species has evolved to perfectly suit that species and no other, and individual mothers of that species produce milk tailored both for that child and for the environment in which they and their infant live. No substitute can ever support truly normal physiological development, and the harms done by such breastmilk substitutes to date are only now beginning to be calculated, a century after they began to influence the health of whole populations. Infant formula harms radiate into society, as well as more directly into the global environment. Although this book is focussed principally on the harm to children through generations, infant formula's collateral damage is immense (page 184).

As Australia's remarkable first woman prime minister, Julia Gillard, famously said of misogyny, artificial feeding 'does not explain everything; it does not explain nothing. It explains some things.' In this, as in her case, I think it explains a great deal. Read on and see if you agree with me about how much milk matters. But first, what do I mean by allergy? And what does allergy mean to sufferers?

---

3   A typical scenario of such compounding harms is described in Appendix 1.
4   Haahtela T, Holgate S, Pawankar R, Akdis CA et al, WAO Special Committee on Climate Change and Biodiversity: The biodiversity hypothesis and allergic disease: world allergy organization position statement. *World Allergy Organ J* 2013, 6(1):3. 10.1186/1939-4551-6-3. It is typical, however, that this realisation was generated in relation to the effects of probotics, not breastmilk. Most medical groups are so entrenched in the societal status quo that they  accept a situation where the ideal is not possible, then look for expensive pharmaceutical palliatives for the problems that status quo creates. They happily stand at the bottom of the cliff treating victims kindly, while not trying to stop those pushing them off the cliff in the first place. Their organisations often see themselves as "apolitical' and reject any role as lobbyists for societal change, while also feeling free to reject  WHO guidelines about infant feeding as irrelevant because impractical in their social context. That is a political stance which supports the creation and expansion  of illness. There is no such thing as an apolitical organisation. To do nothing is to act, to support the status quo.

# 1.1   What does 'allergy' mean?

Allergy means different things to different people. It might be as simple (and tiresome) as fits of sneezing and a runny nose in hayfever season. It might be as dramatic as struggling to breathe, when your airway swells in anaphylaxis. It might be chronic headaches, painful joints, itchy hives, gut pain, flaky skin, incontinence, a gradual or sudden inability to breathe, or dozens of other physical symptoms. It can affect any and every part of the body. It can mean impaired health and growth, mental confusion or irritation at crucial moments, a fundamental distrust of one's own body, and complications when dealing with other health problems.

When you know what triggers these symptoms, it can also mean the embarrassment of having to make a fuss about things others take for granted: leaving the room if a heavily scented person or smoker comes in, asking your friends not to eat strong-smelling foods in your presence, or interrogating the staff at a restaurant, while never being sure that you won't be ambushed by an allergen anyway, if the staff make a mistake, or decide you're being fussy or neurotic, or the food supplied to the restaurant has been badly labelled or contaminated. It might mean awkward moments in a budding relationship as you have to refuse hospitality. It can mean anaphylaxis if you kiss someone who has been exposed to your allergens. It may mean major rows with grandparents who insist that just a little of a forbidden allergen can't do any harm to your child.

You might have grown up as the class weirdo, developing a reflexively apologetic or self-deprecating manner to reassure people that you're not the kind of person who makes any unnecessary fuss. At work, you may have had to choose between being excluded, and being seen as a nuisance whenever catering has to be arranged. In a more hostile environment, your allergy might occasion outright mockery and bullying,[5] and a higher price for standing out in other ways (such as being too bright, or challenging groupthink, or taking a leadership role). None of these negative outcomes are reasonable consequences of a condition that is a punishment in its own right, but any allergic person will recognise them as part of the allergy problem they live with.

If you don't know what causes your galaxy of allergy symptoms, it means doctor visits, pills and treatments, and of course all the accompanying bills. Perhaps even worse, it often means accepting a poor quality of life as simply normal: never knowing why you are visited with unreliable moods, erratic concentration, unsightly rashes, chronic aches and sudden pains, and embarrassing bodily malfunctions ... and perhaps coming to the conclusion that you are simply defective in some fundamental way. It isn't unknown for allergy sufferers to question whether they have the right to inflict their 'defects' on a child. Not seeing any end to their symptoms, some even question whether it's worth living. (If, like many before you, you are at

---

5   A survey presented at the 2010 annual meeting of the American Academy of Allergy, Asthma and Immunology (AAAAI) found that nearly 50 per cent of food-allergic children over the age of 10 reported being bullied because of their allergy. AAAAI Press release, 26/08/2013. So serious is this problems that AAAAI has produced a video, online at http://aaaai.execinc.com/videos/conditions-and-treatments/Food-Allergy-Videos/food-allergies-asthma-and-bullying.asp

this point, get both emotional support, and thoroughly investigate allergy as a possible cause of your chronic problems. An end to symptoms can be swift with the right help.)

For societies, the rise in allergic and other immune disorders means a reduction in the available productive capacity, as individuals lose their ability to contribute to their fullest, both physically and mentally. At the same time, it means diverting resources to the production of remedies and crutches to help people deal with their symptoms. To the extent that allergy increases individuals' emotional and social problems, on a mass scale it also erodes the bonds that make a society function as a coherent whole. If, as the evidence increasingly suggests, allergy (and other immune disorder) is also linked to more drastic mental and psychological dysfunctions, this goes so far as to result in higher levels of violent crime and incarceration than would otherwise be the case.

Allergy is not the only cause of such problems, either on the individual or social level. But it is affecting considerable numbers of people, and contributing to social problems. Whatever the size of that contribution, if we can reduce it – and it is my aim to show that we could – we have a duty to take the attempt seriously.

In this book, I will be discussing allergy in its original, broader sense, still the popular understanding of the term: basically, any adverse bodily reaction to something that others tolerate without adverse symptoms. In other words, both 'allergy' and 'intolerance' without distinguishing between causes.

(There is another current collective medical term for both allergies and intolerances: 'hypersensitivity'. However, in common parlance that implies an emotional component, or even personal fault. Those blaming overtones can, and sometimes do, bleed over into medical practitioners' dealings with the 'hypersensitive'. I would prefer hyper-reactivity – as opposed to tolerance – myself. But both are mouthfuls, and the word allergy is understood by more people.)

Of course I know, and my readers will, that many professional allergists, such as Canadian pioneer John Gerrard, early distinguished between 'true' allergy, where the immune system could be shown to be directly involved in the reaction, and intolerance or hypersensitivity, where the mechanism causing the symptom is not initially an immune reaction, even though the response will also involve the immune system.

Others went further and considered just one variety of immune reaction, mediated by IgE, a specific type of immune cell, to be true allergy.[6]

Such distinctions are useful for research into causes, and treatments. But it's not helpful to be told 'you're not allergic', when you know from repeated bitter experience that some food reliably causes you misery.

---

6    The chapter by Freed, 'The Immunology of Allergy', in Rees AR, Purcell HJ (eds). *Disease and the Environment.* (John Wiley & Sons 1982) charted the changes in meaning over time from von Pirquet's 1906 definition until the inaugural conference of the first Society for Environmental Therapy, a pioneering group seen as radical in 1982, whose ideas are now largely accepted.

So 'allergy', for the purposes of this book, means adverse physical reactions involving inflammation and immune dysfunction in any area of the body, including the brain; over-reactions to substances other people tolerate without such symptoms. The initial response might be due to a defective enzyme reaction, or an increased uptake from a damaged mucosal surface, but will result in inflammation and immune activation on a disproportionate scale.

The Finnish national allergy plan has adopted an overarching umbrella perspective, seeing allergy in all its hideous variety as a single issue of long-term immune dysfunction requiring concerted action. (See figure below.[7])

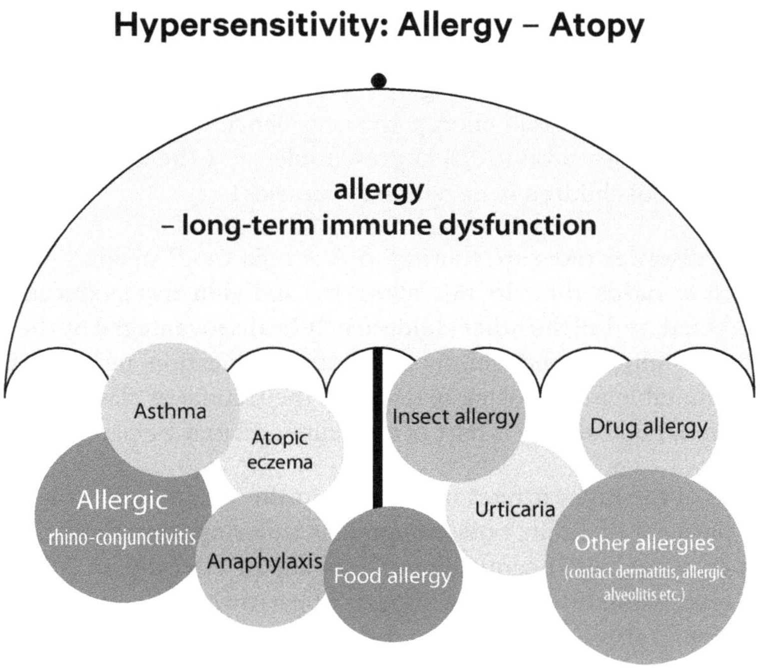

## Hypersensitivity: Allergy – Atopy

Figure 1-1-1 The broad range of allergy, with circle size relative to incidence[8] (Haahtela 2012)

How much of a problem is allergy? Huge. Even limiting consideration to the top end of a wide spectrum, medically diagnosed immune-related reactions, allergy is exploding worldwide. Since 1990, UK hospital admissions for anaphylaxis have increased by 700 per cent, for food allergy by 500 per cent, for urticaria (hives) by 100 per cent, and for angio-oedema by 40 per cent. Prescriptions issued for all types of allergy have increased

7    Haahtela T, Valovirta E, Kauppi P, Tommila E et al. The Finnish Allergy Programme 2008-2018 - scientific rationale and practical implementation. (PMID:23130334) Free full text article *Asia Pac Allergy* 2012, 2(4):275-279. DOI: 10.5415/apallergy.2012.2.4.275.  2012. License  found at http://creativecommons.org/licenses/by/4.0/legalcode.
8    Haahtela T, Holgate S, Pawankar R, Akdis CA et al, WAO Special Committee on Climate Change and Biodiversity: The biodiversity hypothesis and allergic disease: World Allergy Organization position statement. *World Allergy Organ J* 2013, 6(1):3. 10.1186/1939-4551-6-3 DOI: 10.1186/1939-4551-6-3

dramatically since 1991.[9] Diagnosed coeliac disease in the UK has increased fourfold since 1990.[10]

One in eight US children has asthma, at an annual cost of US$18 billion; the incidence has doubled since 1980. One in ten US children has a learning disability, creating over $77 billion in special educational costs each year. One in 68 is actually diagnosed as being on the autism spectrum (linked by parent groups with food reactivity). No one knows how many remain undiagnosed.[11] Following the Finnish example, countries are considering and funding national allergy plans. Infant feeding is not a major focus in some plans, despite this being a contributory factor more readily changed than, say, chemical exposure, and one with major cost-savings.

As for Asia ... 'In large and rapidly emerging societies of Asia, such as China, where there are documented increases in food allergy, the prevalence of clinical (oral food challenge proven) food allergy is now around 7% in preschoolers.'[12] (The authors claim it is already 10 per cent in preschool children in developed countries).

Childhood brain disorder rates are soaring in Australia too,[13] making huge demands on teachers with class ratios that do not allow for individualised education. Classroom dynamics are affected, and all the other children may be disadvantaged by the teacher having to deal with such children's needs. In my home state, education authorities have recently been judged accountable for exposing teachers to the trauma of classes of disordered and ineducable children. Food allergy is part of the cause and may be part of the solution.

Australia has one of the highest rates of allergies in the world, with at least 5 per cent of children and 1 per cent of adults now accepted as suffering from food allergies. The rate of allergies is increasing, with peanut allergy doubling in a decade. In 2011, the Australian Broadcasting Commission reported the impacts of narrowly defined allergy in Australia as being $8 billion a year, affecting 40 per cent of the population, 10 per cent of children.[14] And they reported comments such as 'no one could have foreseen this rapid growth in 'allergy', and its persistence later in life than ever before'.

That's not true. Some parents did. Although often ignored by our local doctors, some of us saw allergy blooming in the 1980s. And many of us with allergic children saw artificial infant feeding – a shape-shifting, unregulated (and largely unmonitored) experiment on whole populations – as one extremely likely source of such an exponential growth of immune

9    Gupta R, Sheikh A, Strachan DP, Anderson HR. Time trends in allergic disorders in the UK. (PMID:16950836) *Thorax* 2007, 62(1):91–96.
10   Gibbons L. Diagnosed coeliac cases rising at a staggering rate. *Food Manufacture UK*, 12 May 2014 Online at http://www.foodmanufacture.co.uk/People/Diagnosed-coeliac-cases-rising-at-a-staggering-rate
11   Steingraber, S. *Raising Elijah*. (da Capo Press, 2011) p. xiv. I have since seen the figure of 1 in 88.
12   Prescott SL, Pawankar R, Allen KJ, Campbell DE. et al. op. cit.
13   http://aww.ninemsn.com.au/news/inthemag/8522914/the-autism-generation-why-are-so-many-children-born-autistic
14   http://www.abc.net.au/news/2011-04-06/australia-holds-record-for-food-allergies/2627836

disorder.[15] We even found solutions for some of our children, in many cases despite being scoffed at by those who should have been helping. To us, it was obvious that food was, and is, a critical factor in creating allergy in our children, since it is the stuff of which our bodies are constructed. And those bodies must create the next generation. Yet while inhalant allergy was widely recognised, our children's allergy to common foods was seen as something we parents imagined – though we live with our children and know far more about them than any medical test will reveal.

We therefore saw allergy's potential for an even greater expansion in each coming generation, and in every region foolish enough to adopt Western infant feeding practices.[16] Parents set up support groups like HACSG (Hyperactive Children's Support Group) and AIA (Allergy Induced Autism) and AESSRA (Allergy and Environmental Sensitivity Support and Research Association). Parents – including some open-minded doctors – lobbied and watched as our children grew and the prevalence and manifestations of allergy increased. We noted the constant links to foods used for a century of artificial feeding, like cows' milk, corn, wheat, soy and peanuts. Breastfeeding counsellors and mothers were well aware in the 1970s that babies reacted to maternal diet, even when told by medical authorities that this was not likely. (It is.)

It is my contention that

- infant nutrition has been and is the single largest underlying factor in the development of this epidemic of allergy and immune disorder in any society where breastfeeding has been displaced by synthetic substitutes, and that

- the effects extend beyond the badly fed infant, to the next generations, so that we are looking at intergenerationally communicated diseases –IGCDs, not NCDs, or perhaps VCDs: vertically communicated. Or even an acquired immuno-reactive syndrome –AIRS, as opposed to AIDS.

A great deal of research is underway to explain precisely which genes are linked to which diseases, what affects genes and how they are inherited. That science is advancing rapidly but much of it is outside the scope of this book.[17] We know now that infant feeding affects how genes are expressed. In fact, breastfeeding modulates the immune system that each child is born with,[18] an immune system already affected by the mother's body during

---

15  My book, *Food for Thought: a parent's guide to food intolerance*, based on such parental experience, was first published in 1982, and was published in the UK by OUP and in Japan in the 1980s, remaining in print till 1995.

16  Prescott SL, Pawankar R, Allen KJ, Campbell DE. et al. A global survey of changing patterns of food allergy burden in children. *World Allergy Org J* 2013; 6(1):21. DOI: 10.1186/1939-4551-6-21 (PMCID:PMC3879010) Will researchers continue to overlook the massive growth in artificial feeding in China, then express surprise at auto-immune disease rates in another thirty years' time?

17   Those interested in knowing more about the basic science will need to read the scientific literature, or look for reliable reviews. Dr Susan Prescott's book, *The Allergy Epidemic* (University of Western Australia Press 2011) is an excellent starting place for parents, and she has a new book coming out in 2015. She summarises things clearly from the perspective of the hospital-based scientist. The field is advancing so rapidly that all books (including this one) can be a bit out of date before they are published.

18  Hanson LA. The mother-offspring dyad and the immune system. *Acta Paediatr* 2000, 89(3):252–58. (PMID:10772267)

gestation. Why would we be surprised that some maternal and infant immune systems are dysfunctional when so many babies have not been breastfed for generations?

For milk plays a key role both in gene expression and in getting an efficient immune system established, as it does in every other area of normal human development. Immune reactions naturally vary over a lifetime as bodies change; but it seems that the potential for hyper-reactivity persists once created, and can be passed on to our children. It is universally accepted that having allergic parents or siblings increases the risk of allergy in any child. This was once assumed to be due to an inherited genetic defect, and certainly there are genes linked to disease: but the hypersensitivity itself, the adverse reactions, are not inherited. It is the interplay between genes, the rest of the body, and the environment (including but not limited to nutrition) that will determine how inherited genes are expressed, and whether tolerance or hypersensitivity results from our exposures.

Our immune system is the central regulator that will determine the outcome for each individual. It can be seen as the shield or umbrella that copes with the onslaught of potentially damaging challenges. Allergy rates, and rates of so-called non-communicable diseases like obesity, brain disorder including autism, and other health problems are increasing as that shield is disrupted. That disruption has much to do with infant feeding, or so my milk hypothesis will argue.

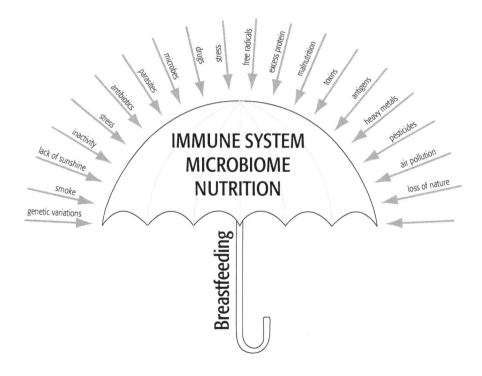

Figure 1-1-2 Breastfeeding supports our immune shield

# Intergenerational links

- Half of every baby starts out as an egg in grandma's womb.

- Girls are born with all the eggs they will ever have, which means those eggs that will become her children are formed (as her own body forms) in her mother's womb, inside their grandmother.

- After the egg that formed in grandma's womb is fertilised, the baby is then gestated in her mother's womb, before being born and exposed to nutritional influences on development, and especially through milk. Studies have shown that pregnant women's blood carries cells from their own mothers. The number of these cells from the foetus's grandmother increases as pregnancy progresses.[19] What is more, researchers 'think the mother's cells shape the ability of the developing immune system to learn tolerance', and 'wonder if the grandmother's cells are continuing that education process in some way'.

- So whatever affected grandma's genetic expression can affect not only her daughter, but also even her granddaughter.

- And nutrition affects each generation's genetic expression. Everyone accepts that serious maternal malnutrition in pregnancy can have negative consequences for the infant, and that this affects expression of the infant's genes.

- Infant nutrition has an additional and heritable effect.

- So milks matter!

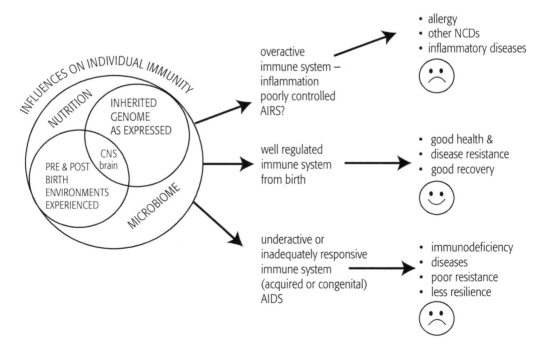

Figure 1-1-3 Influences on individual immunity

---

19    Gammill HS, Adams Waldorf KM, Aydelotte TM, Lucas J et al. Pregnancy, microchimerism, and the maternal grandmother. (PMID:21912617) *PLoS one* 2011, 6(8):e24101. DOI: 10.1371/journal.pone.0024101

**CHAPTER 2**

# How milk shapes humans

## 2.1 Allergy epidemics and infant feeding: context

The rapid twentieth-century increase in allergies and disease has had many suggested explanations, almost all linked to large and recent changes in the human environment. Chemical toxins and contaminants, multiple vaccine exposure, industrial agriculture: some of these are discussed later in this book. The 'hygiene hypothesis' of causation first advanced by John W Gerrard rapidly became a dominant explanation. It proposed that babies were not developing tolerance of substances harmless to others, because their world has become too 'clean' (see page 71) This frames allergy as a price of progress and, as popularised, makes little or no reference to artificial feeding, much less to the details of that feeding. Yet Professor Gerrard himself was a lifelong staunch advocate of exclusive breastfeeding for the prevention of allergic disease. When staying with us in the 1980s, he assured me that he too found that this worked for many families. But how are babies being fed?

The Growing Up in Australia report,[20] funded by the Australian Government, makes for depressing reading on the state of breastfeeding in Australia. Amongst the infant cohort in 2004 there was a sharp decline in both full and any breastfeeding with each month post birth:

- 92 per cent of women began breastfeeding
- after one week only 80 per cent of infants were fully breastfed with a steady decline each month
- at most, only 56 per cent of infants were fully breastfed at three months
- only 14 per cent were fully breastfed at six months, and
- the rate of any breastfeeding at six months was only 56 per cent

Dismal figures, frankly, as this doesn't include any detail about infant exposure to other foods soon after birth. The bottom line: only half Australia's children are fully breastfed

---

20   http://www.growingupinaustralia.gov.au/pubs/ar/ar200607/breastfeeding.html

at 3 months, only one in seven at 6 months. No wonder formula sales are increasing and breastfeeding mothers are being targetted!

But US and UK figures are even more depressing: only 77 per cent of US and 74 per cent of UK infants[21] are even initially breastfed, and the figure for what was dubiously called exclusive breastfeeding[22] at three months is just 38 per cent in the US.[23] In the UK, the solely-breastfeeding rate drops to 45 per cent by four weeks, and only a third are still breastfeeding at all at six months, possibly only one per cent exclusively.[24] Rising initiation rates since 2000 tell us that parents are hearing that breastfeeding is important. The breastfeeding duration rates tell us that many find it impossible to sustain this basic physiological process (for which their bodies are perfectly well-equipped) in their society. The vast majority of infants in all three countries are not fed optimally, and that creates serious negative consequences, sometimes fatal, for mother and child, and across whole populations in the short and long term. Imagine the concern if such rates of bodily dysfunction characterised any other physiological process in normal adults, and could be shown to result from social structures!

This drop in natural feeding is global and important. Infant feeding is accepted as significant for both immune function and the human microbiome in infancy and throughout later life. This is because, among other things,

> Breast milk stimulates the proliferation of a well balanced and diverse microbiota which initially influences a switch from an intrauterine Th2 predominant to aTh1/Th2 balanced response and with activation of T-regulatory cells by breast milk-stimulated specific organisms … The breast milk influence on initial intestinal microbiota also prevents expression of immune-mediated diseases (asthma, IBD, type 1 diabetes) later in life through a balanced initial immune response, underscoring the necessity of breast feeding as the first source of nutrition.[25]

The factors influencing the milk microbiome and the potential impact of microbes on infant health are only recently being uncovered.[26] Breast milk is increasingly recognised as the 'single most important postpartum element in neonatal metabolic and immunologic programming,'[27] a concept discussed later in this book.

---

21 Both the UK and the US now collect data on breastfeeding. For the latest UK figures see http://www.england.nhs.uk/statistics/wp-content/uploads/sites/2/2014/03/Breastfeeding-1314Q3.pdf

22 Many of this group would have been formula-exposed in the early days of lactation, even if they self-report that at 3 months they are giving only breastmilk and no other foods. Any exposure means they are not 'exclusively breastfed' by accepted global standards.

23 US CDC Breastfeeding Report Card 2013. Online at http://www.cdc.gov/breastfeeding/pdf/2013breastfeedingreportcard.pdf; Infant Feeding Survey 2005: a commentary on infant feeding practices in the UK, Position Statement by the Scientific Advisory Committee on Nutrition. (TSO London 2008) The 2010 Survey report shows further rises:see

24 Another useful source is the UK BFI site: see http://www.unicef.org.uk/babyfriendly/about-baby-friendly/breastfeeding-in-the-uk/uk-breastfeeding-rates/

25 Walker WA, Shuba Iyengar R. Breastmilk, Microbiota and Intestinal Immune Homeostasis. (PMID:25310762) *Pediatr Res* 2014. DOI:10.1038/pr.2014.160.

26 Cabrera-Rubio R, Collado MC, Laitinen K, Salminen S, et al. The human milk microbiome changes over lactation and is shaped by maternal weight and mode of delivery. *Am J Clin Nutr,* 2012; 96 (3): 544 . DOI: 10.3945/ajcn.112.037382.

27 Cabrera-Rubio R, Collado MC, Laitinen K, Salminen S, et al. The human milk microbiome changes over lactation and is shaped by maternal weight and mode of delivery. *Am J Clin Nutr,* 2012; 96 (3): 544 . DOI: 10.3945/

Any deviation from normal physiological processes creates risk. The more fundamental the process, the younger the person, and the greater the deviation, the greater the risk of both immediate and ongoing harm. That's not controversial, just common sense. So before going further, let's put the problem of allergy into the bigger context of infant feeding, where, since mammals evolved millions of years ago, the physiological norm has always been the mother's own milk fed from her own body.

> We do not call ourselves mammals without good reason; the breast has evolved as the umbilical cord of the newborn, and throughout our evolutionary history successful lactation has been the sine qua non of survival.[28]

## Mammalian evolution and milk

Mammals are defined by their ability to produce milk. Mammalian milk is a species-specific food that allows infant mammals to grow normally until they are old enough to consume other foods in their environment safely. But that is not all that milk does.

> The constant evolutionary pressure on milk as the sole source of nourishment for mammalian infants has resulted in a remarkable model for how diet affects all aspects of development and health. Maternal investment, specifically the composition of breast milk, has been shaped by natural selection acting on both the infant and the mother, maximizing infant survival, growth, and activity while minimising the costs of lactation for the mother (5). One of the most remarkable apparent functions of breast milk is the selective colonisation and support of a protective microbiota. How milk has been able to attain the goal of guiding the evolutionary emergence of specific strains of bacteria in infants for their mutual health benefit is precisely the kind of question that science needs to understand to achieve similar successes for a wide range of human/microbial interactions.[29]

Mammalian milk seems to have emerged initially not as a food, but as a protective strategy,[30] co-operating with and feeding a vast microbial population dedicated to its own and its host's survival. Milk evolved into being the first and best convenience food,[31] reducing placental gestation periods, with all their risks, while allowing for optimal growth after birth. 'Lactation has evolved to minimise the energy cost to the mother while maximising the utilisation of energy and nutrients by her offspring'[32] – it improves both infant and maternal survival. Had

ajcn.112.037382.

28　Short RV, in *Breastfeeding and the Mother* (Ciba Symposium 45, Elsevier 1976) p. 73

29　Zivkovic AM, German JB, Lebrilla CB, Mills DA. Human milk glycobiome and its impact on the infant gastrointestinal microbiota. (PMID:20679197) *Proc Nat Acad Sci* 2011, 108 Suppl 1:4653-4658. The numbers in parentheses are his references – do read the original article.

30　Goldman AS. Evolution of immune finctions of the mammary gland and protection of the infant. *Breastfeed Med* 2012; 7(3): 132–42.

31　Hale and Hartmann's *Textbook of Human Lactation* (Hale Publishing 2007) summarises what is known for anyone interested in human lactation. Peter Hartmann's chapter 1, *Mammary Gland: Past Present and Future*, and Ch. 10, Lars Hanson's *The Role of Breastfeeding in the Defence of the Infant*, go into much greater depth on these topics. Additionally, evolutionary medicine texts by McKenna, anthropological work by Trevathan and Blaffer Hrdy, together with a modern text on milk such as Park & Haenlein's *Milk and Dairy Products in Human Nutrition*, are required reading: see the bibliography.

32　Hernell O. Human milk versus cows' milk and the evolution of infant formulas. In Clemens RA, Hernell O, Michaelsen KF (eds) *Milk and Milk Products in Human Nutrition*. Nestle Nutr Inst Workshop Ser Paediatr

milk-making been a huge burden that undermined maternal health, it is unlikely to have been a successful survival strategy. Lactation both compelled and enabled mothers to stay close to their infants and recover from birth, by minimising the work of providing suitable food. Others could assist the mother by bringing her food from the wider range suitable for an adult body. She could provide what the baby needed without foraging effort.

So lactation evolved to protect the infant, but also the mother, by increasing her metabolic efficiency, suppressing her fertility, improving her memory, as well as minimising her workload, and increasing her chance of successful infant rearing. Lactation maximises mother-infant closeness emotionally and physically amongst humans;[33] lactating mother and child function as a single unit, or dyad. Literally: what a mother eats, her baby tastes in her milk, and ideally develops tolerance to. If a mother breathes, swallows or contacts anything that might do harm, her adult body responds to it – and then, via her milk, she shares the protection she has created with her infant.

In fact milk samples the mother's diet and environment, exposing the infant to small doses of everything, good and bad.[34] It provides multiple bioactive immune factors to enable the infant to deal with environmental components, creating appropriate tolerance or reaction within the baby's body.[35] The first milk – colostrum – and the weaning phase – regression milk – both provide concentrated versions of the massive daily dose of immune factors a mother-fed offspring enjoys. Not until five to seven months does the human infant begin to develop any significant independent adaptive immunity, just the age at which contaminated food and water pose new threats to an exploring omnivorous baby. Fortunate babies still being breastfed have two immune systems to help deal with those threats: mother's via her milk, and their own, constructed by breastfeeding.

No wonder survival is so much better in children still being breastfed through gradual weaning.[36] No wonder immune responses to vaccinations (which the body treats as a threat) can be noticeably different when babies are being breastfed. No wonder allergists are virtually unanimous in seeing possible advantages in continued breastfeeding throughout the period of novel food introduction,[37] even though some fail to realise that continued breastfeeding

---

Program, Vol 67. p. 19. (Karger/Nestec 2011) Available online.

33　In some other mammalian species, constant closeness is neither necessary nor desirable, and feeds can be a day apart: the milk is then more concentrated and has higher protein content.

34　Florence Williams' *Breasts: a natural and unnatural history* (WW Norton Co NY 2012) superbly outlines the bad (and some of the good) without critically examining the safety of alternatives to breastmilk. I interpret the facts differently because I cannot share her assumption of safety. In fact I believe that the harms done by artificial feeding in previous generations account for much of what she fears may be due to breastmilk contamination. Babies are born from women's bodies as well as fed by their milk. By contrast, Steingraber's work (see bibliography) gets the assumptions right: breastmilk is essential and pollution must be reduced.

35　Newburg DS, Walker WA. Protection of the neonate by the innate immune system of developing gut and of human milk. *Pediatr Res* 2007, 61(1):2–8. PMID:17211132)

36　Kwashiorkhor, or protein-caloric malnutrition, has killed millions of children abruptly weaned when a new pregnancy causes a mother's milk supply to drop. Toddlers in many societies rely on breastmilk as a source of high-quality protein and calories, as well as immune factors. In many contexts, without breastmilk, survival is endangered and malnutrition damages children. See Austin CR, Short RV. *Manipulating Reproduction.* (Cambridge Uni Press 1986} pp. 67–8.

37　Krawinkel MB. Benefits from longer breastfeeding: do we need to revise the recommendations? (PMID:21939907) *Curr Probl Pediatr Adolesc Health Care* 2011, 41(9):240–43.

can encompass the first year or longer – not just the first four to six months of life! – and preferably well past the first year.[38] No wonder one of the world's foremost gastroenterologists has written of 'the *necessity* of breastfeeding as the first source of nutrition.'[39] But we have grown a long way from the lifestyle in which this immune interaction and interdependence evolved. In the past, in hunter-gatherer and other traditional communities, a fertile woman would be a healthy breastfed survivor of innumerable childhood challenges – less-healthy girl children died. She would be culturally adapted to her traditional, varied, omnivore diet; adapted to scarcity, with important hormone-mediated metabolic adaptive capacity in pregnancy and lactation, to make the most of any food available.[40] Her diet – by comparison with affluent modern diets – was usually relatively low in animal protein, with high vegetable intake; meat and fat were a coveted treat where it was scarce.

Such a woman enjoyed variety and moderation of seasonally varied foods, even during pregnancy and lactation. Her milk reflected her diet, even the air she breathed,[41] and her multiple daily exposures to pathogens. Her body made milk that – via the gastrointestinal tract or gut and its organisms – created tolerance to the foods and environmental agents, and defence against potential pathogens. The sampling mechanisms and response routes are now well-documented: both the enteromammary (gut to breast) and bronchomammary (airways to breast) circulation, which both result in specialised antibodies being excreted in breastmilk, the enteromammary in response to those ingested, the bronchomammary, those inhaled.[42] It has been shown that

> Even a low level of exposure of the mucosa (eg, by inhalant allergens) can induce antibody secretion into the milk, both in allergic and non-allergic mothers.[43]

Thus all lactating women provide their babies with the protection against disease that scientists labour for months or years to create via vaccinations. If the child becomes sick, the content of the milk changes:

> During active infection in nursing infants, the total number of white blood cells, specifically the number of macrophages, and TNFα levels increase in their mothers' breast milk. These

---

38 Dettwyler KA. The hominid blueprint for the natural age of weaning in modern human populations. In Stuart-Macadam P, Dettwyler KA (eds) *Breastfeeding: Biocultural Perspectives*. (Aldine de Gruyter NY 1995). Biocultural and anthropological and primate studies are all of great relevance to what in the past have been seen as narrowly medical or nutritional concerns. *Splash! Milk science update*, the monthly newsletter of the International Milk Genomics Consortium, is well worth subscribing too, and the work of women like Kathy Dettwyler, Sarah Blaffer Hrdy and Wenda Trevathan should be on everyone's reading list. Narrow medical and nursing perspectives have done a great deal of harm.

39 Walker WA, Shuba Iyengar R. op. cit.

40 For example, women's metabolic efficiency of calcium absorption doubles in pregnancy and triples in lactation, so that the same amount of food yields more nutrients.

41 Casas R, Böttcher MF, Duchén K, Björkstén B. Detection of IgA antibodies to cat, beta-lactoglobulin, and ovalbumin allergens in human milk. (PMID:10856160) *J Allergy Clin Immunol* 2000; 105(6 pt 1):1236–40.

42 Brandtzaeg P. The mucosal immune system and its integration with the mammary glands. *J Peds* 2010; 156(2) S8-S15 DOI: 10/1016/lpeds.2009.11.2014; Hanson LA. *Immunobiology of Human Milk: How Breastfeeding Protects Babies*. (Hale Publishing 2004); Hanson LÅ, Telemo E, Wiedermann U, et al. Immunological mechanisms of the gut. *Pediatr Allergy Immunol*. 1995;6(Suppl 8):7–12

43 Casas R op. cit.

results may support the dynamic nature of the immune defense provided by breastfeeding sick infants.[44]

And breastfed babies inherit a unique immune repertoire created by their mother's past experience, as well as benefit promptly from her present responses to current threats.[45] As one recent review said, 'breast-feeding represents an ingenious immunologic integration of mother and child.'[46] The mother's nasal and gut associated lymphoid tissue (NALT and GALT) detect and respond to environmental antigens and pathogens. Whether the environment is a day-care centre or a mud hut, breastmilk will provide significant protection, keeping babies and their families healthier.[47]

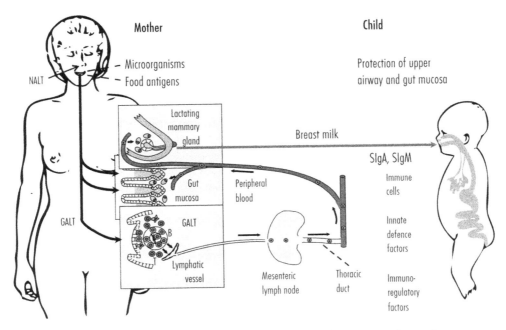

Figure 2-1-1 Integration of secretory immunity between mother and child[48] (© Wageningen Academic Publishers 2013)

Even the formula industry now concedes in its advertising that breastmilk is very different from formula when it comes to antibodies and immunity. But breastmilk offers more protection than just specific immunity via antibodies. Breastmilk and breastfeeding both provide an

44    Riskin A, Almog M, Peri R, Halasz K et al. Changes in immunomodulatory constituents of human milk in response to active infection in the nursing infant. (PMID:22258136) *Pediatr Res* 2012, 71(2):220–225

45    Hamosh M Breastfeeding: Unraveling the Mysteries of Mother's Milk. (PMID:9746642) *Medscape Women's Health* 1996; 1(9):4–7. www.ncbi.nlm.nih.gov/pubmed/9746642 We've learned a lot since then, but this shows where we were in 1996 -and not many parents heard about it.

46    Brandtzaeg P. The Mucosal Immune System and Its Integration with the Mammary Glands *J Pediatr* 2010; 156(2) Suppl. pp. S8–S15.

47    Cohen R, Mrtek MB, Mrtek RG. Comparison of maternal absenteeism and infant illness rates among breast-feeding and formula-feeding women in two corporations. (PMID:10160049) *Am J Health Promot 1995,* 10(2):148–153.

48    Figure from Brandtzaeg P. *Immune aspects of breast milk: an overview.* In Zibadi S, Watson RR, Preedy VR (eds) *Handbook of dietary and nutritional aspects of human breast milk.* (Wageningen Academic Press 2013) p. 67 © Wageningen Academic Publishers 2013

enormous, complex array of general and specific immune defences. The ingredients of human milk, and their biological activity, have been well reviewed in specialist books and articles.[49] There are thousands of ingredients that interact positively to affect the health and growth of the suckling child,[50] while also protecting the mother.[51] A fascinating historical review makes it clear that many immune properties of colostrum and milk have been known – and their importance often ignored or denied – since the nineteenth century.[52]

In the human evolutionary context, mother's milk is the necessary bridge between the largely protected womb[53] and the risky world – a post-birth umbilical cord, as eminent physiologist Professor Roger Short called it in the epigraph to this chapter. Initially the mother's body is the infant's environment; her body and her milk are the highly evolved means of safely introducing the infant to the broader environment it must adapt to. Skin contact and above all, breastmilk, are the means of creating a whole body microbiome that results both in active defence against threats, and in tolerance of foods and useful microbes. The creation of a diverse and healthy gut microbiome is critical to both nutrition and immunity: antigen handling by the gut determines the development of tolerance to foods, and good nutrition is the foundation of health in later life. These new stimuli in the newborn gut should trigger many responses, including inflammation, which multiple components of breastmilk reduce,[54] preventing damage and allowing friendly bacteria to thrive and process the breastmilk nutrients needed for growth, immunity and optimal gene expression. Milk is central to all these processes. In fact, milk is necessary to normal development.

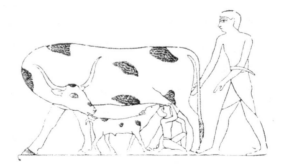

Figure 2-1-2 Cow feeding calf and boy. Image from Ploss H, Bartels M. *Woman: an historical, gynaecological and anthropological compendium.* Vol 3 p. 210.

49    Serpero LD, Frigiola A, Gazzolo D. Human milk and formulae: neurotrophic and new biological factors. (PMID:22261291) *Early Human Development* 2012, 88 Suppl 1:S9–12. DOI: 10.1016/j.earlhumdev.2011.12.021

50    For a quick but incomplete visual overview which makes a strong point, check out the poster at http://bcbabyfriendly.ca/whatsinbreastmilkposter.pdf

51    Ip S, Chung M, Raman G, Chew P, Magila N, DeVine D et al. *Breastfeeding and maternal and infant health outcomes in developed countries.* AHRQ Publication No. 07-E007. Rockville, MD: Agency for Healthcare Research and Quality, 2007; Horta BL, Bahl R, Martines JC, Victora CG. *Evidence on the long-term effects of breastfeeding: systematic reviews and meta-analyses.* Geneva: World Health Organization, 2007.

52    Wheeler RT, Hodgkinson AJ, Prosser CP, Davis CR. Immune Components of Colostrum and Milk – A Historical Perspective. *J Mammary Gland Biol Neoplasia* 2007; 12 (4): 237–47. DOI: 10.1007/s10911-007-9051-7

53    The related issue of the role of pregnancy and intra-uterine sensitisation is discussed elsewhere in the next chapter 2.2.

54    Walker A. Breastmilk as the gold standard for protective nutrients. *J Pediatrics* 2010; 156, I56 (2), Supplement, S3–S7 http://dx.doi.org/10.1016/j.jpeds.2009.11.021

## 2.2  Milks: mammalian or ersatz, and their impacts

Before going further, let's be clear: all milk, including cows' milk, is a useful and valuable food – but only for those animals, humans included, who can tolerate it.[55] Some communities rely on it and always have, developing ways to reduce its inherent risks. Acidification, fermentation, cheese-making and cooking have all rendered milk a useful staple in communities without access to refrigeration and sanitation.[56]

But one of the basic realities of life is that any substance capable of doing you good is also capable of doing you harm – in excess, or even in small quantities if you cannot process it. Salt is essential, but excess is damaging. Amino acids from protein are crucial to development, but for those unable to properly process them, they can destroy intelligence: which is why phenylketonurics, who lack the enzyme to break down phenylalanine, have to avoid aspartame.[57] Even water can kill you if you drink too much! Cows' milk per se is probably not the problem, even though it is an immunologically active food designed for calves. There would always have been some people who reacted adversely; as Morrow Brown wrote,

> That milk can cause illness is by no means a recent discovery. In 460 BC Hippocrates recorded that milk could cause gastric upsets and hives ... by 1905 the first reports of allergic reactions to milk were published in American medical journals, but not until 1944 in the UK ... In adults many diverse diseases can be due to milk at any age, even over 70.[58]

This book will argue throughout that two uniquely twentieth-century practices seem likely to have increased the numbers of the intolerant: exposing infants to other species' milk and other foods soon after birth, and urging women to consume vast amounts of milk when pregnant or lactating. The fact that for much of the first century of infant formula, early exposure to cows' milk formulas also meant exposure to gluten would have affected reactivity rates as well, as we now know that exposure to gluten under three months of age is linked to the pattern of gut damage known as coeliac disease (see page 609).

Again, this is not to point the finger at cows' milk as uniquely damaging in itself. Any mammalian milk, or soy milk, or any food, used in the same ways would have caused, or will cause, similar problems. And the fact is that Western society has come to depend on bovine products for protein and calcium. To the newly diagnosed allergic, it can seem impossible to have a healthy diet without them. But of course it is perfectly possible. Milk's nutrients can be found in many other sources, and most humans on the planet have thrived without relying on animal milks. No one food source is essential. Humans are intelligent omnivores.

---

55   Oski FA, Paige DM. *Cow's milk is a good food for some and a poor choice for others: eliminating the hyperbole.* (PMID:8143001) *Arch Pediatr Adolesc Med* 1994, 148(1):104–07.

56    Schmid R. *The Untold Story of Milk* (New Trends Publishing, 2009)

57   A task made much harder by the diet food industry, which uses aspartame/Nutra-sweet in everything from chewing gum to drinks. Even normal individuals can consume enough to cause cerebral symptoms if they are not careful to limit their intake.

58    H. Morrow Brown, The Health Hazards of Milk, in *Milk: Beyond the Dairy.* (ed) Harlan Walker. (Prospect Books, 2000) p. 259–60. The chapter records many unusual but convincing case histories.

Few food sources are as *convenient* in Western diet as milk, but this convenience is not accidental: it resulted from the early-twentieth-century effort by governments and agricultural interests to industrialise dairy production, combined with heavily endorsed marketing campaigns in Anglophone countries, focussed on child health and pregnant women. Milk was provided free in schools to all children regardless of income; pregnant women were urged to drink more milk for its calcium content, for fear of losing their teeth and having weak bones; hospitals provided postpartum women with powdered milk drinks. While other agricultural production was also being industrialised with government subsidies, those foods were not so directly promoted to parents as critical in pregnancy and lactation.

This recent reliance on dairy in Western diet is not without its critics. Others writing about human consumption of animal milk are convinced of its unique harmfulness, and time may prove them to be right. Dr Frank Oski's *Don't Drink Your Milk!*[59] was only one of many books to warn against the consumption of bovine milk; a current title is *Milk: The Deadly Poison*,[60] which discusses many valid concerns arising from industrialised agriculture, such as the use of recombinant (genetically modified) growth hormone to increase milk yield.

Yet even without such modern biotechnology concerns, milk is powerful stuff. We are coming to understand the power and bioactivity of any mammalian milk, and to respect its unique role in creating normal offspring of that species. The more we learn, the more certain scientists become that normal young cannot be produced if they are fed non-species-specific milk when their basic metabolic processes are developing.

This is true even when dealing with very closely related species. Studies in marsupials provide scientific evidence of the dramatic impact of foreign milks on growth and development of the young.[61] Marsupials in general have very short gestation lengths and longer lactation lengths, so that the majority of development occurs after birth (as is true of the human infant brain) fed by milk. The composition of marsupial milk changes dramatically through lactation to meet the changing developmental needs of the young. Scientists have experimented with cross-fostering, taking the newborn pouch young from one species, like the Tammar wallaby, and placing it in the pouch of another species of similar size, like the Parma wallaby. Remarkably, even though these species are quite closely related, their growth can be dramatically affected by the milk which the foster mother provides. 'Tammars cross-fostered into the pouches of Parmas grew at a similar rate to naturally reared Tammar young and had developmental milestones at a similar age. However, Parma young cross-fostered between the day of birth and fifteen days post-partum into Tammars that were carrying young of equivalent developmental stages did not grow normally and were lost from the pouch. Parma young cross-fostered at thirty days survived, but had significantly reduced growth rates and their developmental milestones were delayed compared with normally reared Parma young.'[62]

59  Oski FA. *Don't Drink Your Milk!* (Wyden Books, Chicago 1977)
60  Cohen R. *Milk the Deadly Poison*. (Argus Publishing, New Jersey 1997)
61  Menzies BR, Shaw G, Fletcher TP, Renfree MB. Perturbed growth and development in marsupial young after reciprocal cross-fostering between species. (PMID:18076830) *Reprod Fertil Dev* 2007, 19(8):976–83.
62  ibid.

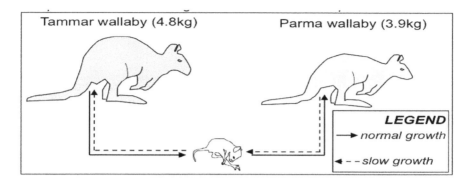

Figure 2-2-1 Inter-species cross-fostering between Tammar and Parma wallabies (Menzies et al 2007)

The results of these wallaby studies 'suggest that maternal milk regulates the timing of development of each species, and a mismatch in the time that each young receives critical milk components can have a marked effect on their growth and development.' [63]

Wallabies can also be 'fostered-forward' in development by transferring them to the pouches of females at a later stage of lactation, where the mums are producing a higher volume and higher energy milk. In this situation, pouch young wallabies experience accelerated development and may become overweight, because at this stage of development they will grow in proportion to the amount of energy they receive. The effects on later adult health of growing too slowly or too quickly are only now being investigated.[64]

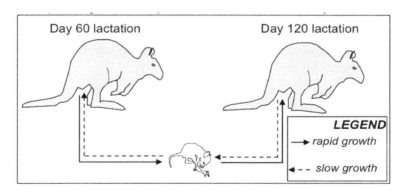

Figure 2-2-2 Intra-species growth manipulation in the Tammar wallaby (© Brandon Menzies)

As Professor Roger Short rather colourfully commented:

> Putting the newborn pouch young of one species onto the teat of another species is the most dramatic example of the lifelong effects of milk on the development, health and growth of the fostered species. It is living proof of DOHaD! *[Developmental Origins of Health and Disease, an*

---

63  ibid.
64  Findlay L, Renfree MB. Growth, development and secretion of the mammary gland of macropodid marsupials. *Symp Zool Soc Lond* 1984; **51**: 403–32; Trott JF, Simpson KJ, Moyle RL, Hearn CM, Shaw G, Nicholas KR, Renfree MB. Maternal regulation of milk composition, milk production, and pouch young development in the Tammar wallaby (*Macropus eugenii*). *Biology of Reproduction* 2003; *68:929*–36.

*important acronym in public health. MM]* ... Any Human Ethics Committee that was aware of these facts would regard it as criminally insane to foster human infants onto the milk of cows.[65]

And zoologist author Brandon Menzies added:

Animals have very specific nutritional requirements for placentation and lactation that have been honed over millions of years of evolution. We would never dream of growing a human in a cow's uterus, so why would we feed a human infant cows' milk?[66]

Of course, nobody knew about this when our current human dependence on cows' milk for infants began. Other mammal milk, such as camel or donkey, is only now being researched.[67] But the more we know, the more likely it seems that harm must come from not giving the right milk to a young mammal whose metabolic processes are developing. Each uniquely wrong milk given undoubtedly causes harms that may differ somewhat from each other. However altered, cows' milk is the basis of most infant formulas, and the survival of humans even on largely unaltered cows' milk mixes has been used to assert the safety of artificial feeding by many. ('I was bottle fed and I'm normal.') Where this quasi-cross fostering of humans to cows[68] has been done over whole populations, and for generations, any harms done will have become common, and thus appear 'normal', rather than being rare.

That has certainly been my experience. Within a few weeks, my mother's middle-aged carer, a doctor friend, a close relative, and many mothers (and babies) have discovered milk allergy to be the cause of very diverse symptoms, from headaches to eczema to gut problems – and not all at my suggestion, as you might reasonably suspect! None has been formally diagnosed, but all are limiting or avoiding milk and finding their symptoms greatly or even completely relieved. This is far more common than allergists and public health specialists would ever know from official data. Look into any supermarket and see the alternative products multiplying!

## Species-specific milk and allergies

Research in the 1980s suggested that high intakes of immunologically active animal milks during pregnancy might greatly amplify the antigen exposure of the infant. Cows' milk naturally contains both the antigens from the cows' environment (grasses, moulds, fungi, stockfeed, and so on) and the antibodies to those antigens.[69] As we have discussed, this seems to be a function of milk, to sample the environment and present it to the young – by smell and taste and physical reality – in buffered ways that make for familiarity, acceptance and tolerance rather than reactivity.

---

65  Correspondence on file June 2013.
66  Correspondence on file June 2013.
67   Park YW, Haenlein GFW (eds) *Milk and Dairy Products in Human Nutrition: Production, Composition and Health* (Wiley Blackwell 2013.)
68  In a NZ dairy research institute, I saw a poster claiming the cow to be 'the foster-mother of the human race.'
69  Collins AM. *Xenogeneic antibodies and atopic disease.* (PMID:2895263) *Lancet* 1988; 1(8588):734–37; Collins AM, Roberton DM, Hosking CS, Flannery GR Bovine milk, including pasteurised milk, contains antibodies directed against allergens of clinical importance to man. (PMID:1809694) *Int arch all app imm* 1991; 96(4):362–7

But mammalian milks did not develop to be suitable for cross-species consumption by adults. Imagine the competition there might be in animal families if older siblings did not lose their interest in and desire for the teat at some point, developing a preference for other foods: younger offspring would have a difficult time getting enough food to survive. The emergence of lactose intolerance in childhood around three to four years might well be a natural way of encouraging older offspring to wean. So too might be the changes in milk taste during a new pregnancy[70] – the decrease in sweetness and increase in saltiness – which could serve to protect the gestating female from excessive nutritional demands.

In some parts of the planet, humans have been living on cows' or goats' or sheep or camels' milk for thousands of years with no apparent ill effects, having domesticated the animals and developed multiple ways of processing their milk to reduce its risks and increase its tolerability. But humans are doing something biologically unusual in consuming fresh immunologically active non-species-specific milk as adults, and even more so when gestating and feeding their own young. The pregnant cow is not fed horse milk. Horse, cow or human mothers sample their specific environment and supply their foetuses and infants with manageable doses of antigens and antibodies via blood and milk to prepare their young for life as a horse, cow or human.

Human pregnancy and lactation involve the transfer of antigens and antibodies to the child. A pregnant woman drinking cows' milk will make antibodies to the antigens in that milk. She will also make antibodies to the antibodies that the cow has made and put in that milk: these latter are called anti-antibodies. As when you take a cast of a key and get a key-shaped empty space, and then fill that cast to copy the original key, anti-antibodies mimic the shape of the original antigen. Both maternal antibodies and anti-antibodies circulate through the blood, and may affect the unborn child. The child is thus effectively exposed to a double dose of antigen, which can result in sensitisation before birth, and an irritable-from-birth, hard-to-console baby.

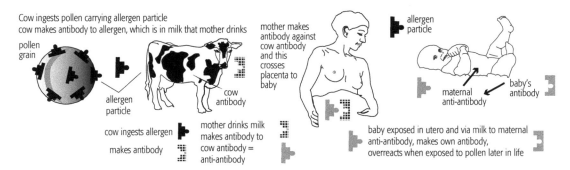

Figure 2-2-3 Bovine milk in pregnancy and the formation of antibodies and anti-antibodies[71]

From clinical experience I would say that this is especially likely if the mother herself had been sensitised by formula exposure as a child, and was milk-reactive. These mothers often

---

70    Progesterone inhibits lactose synthesis, and as milk volume drops the mineral content rises. Many children will stop breastfeeding around 2–3 months into the mother's next pregnancy; if old enough, some will say it is because the milk tastes different.

71    Re-drawn from *The Age* March 1992 with Fairfax Media consent. Image by John van Loon.

have very reactive foetuses, as evidenced by kicking and incessant hiccuping in response to certain foods. This may be an important factor in the process of intergenerational amplification of immune problems, or progressive degeneration of inherited immune systems. That this is true is part of the milk hypothesis.

There is also plenty of evidence that allergenic bovine proteins such as beta-lactoglobulin are present in women's milk, and cause reactions in some children, including colic,[72] gut and skin symptoms, enuresis (inability to control urine), cerebral symptoms,[73] and failure to thrive. This will be discussed further on in Book 3. But excessive milk exposure over the twentieth century may have made some women's milk more like formula, containing excesses of animal allergens..

Thus avoiding dairy products in pregnancy could be good for one mother-to-be with a family history of allergy – and not for another. Food avoidance might prevent the normal development of tolerance – or it might prevent the development of milk allergy. Such avoidance clearly works in some allergic families: I have known milk-allergic women who previously have had hyperactive foetuses and miserable babies, who avoided milk during pregnancy and lactation, and produced a much less allergy-affected infant. And I have also known women who avoided milk as best they could during pregnancy, and yet had infants who reacted to milk they drank while lactating.

At present there seems to be no single right advice for all mothers, no matter how much allergy authorities create one-size-fits-all recommendations. We are a long way from understanding the determining immune mechanisms. Many doctors really don't know, or can't afford the time, to individualise advice, so they opt for 'eat normally', whatever that means for the mother. Without a great many more studies that monitor the appropriate variables, advice to pregnant women about their milk consumption is based on little more than faith or prejudice, along with awareness of both the valuable nutrients milk can supply, and the growing rates of milk allergy. I consider each mother a unique experiment, and understanding her own history is presently the best clue to the likely best course of action for her.

What is best or safest in relation to pregnancy milk intake is unknown, and the answer will doubtless vary between individuals. However, given that we have reason to believe that there is some adverse effect in an unknown number of cases, the safest forms of milk for pregnant and lactating women need to be defined. In practical terms, it has long been thought that the more denatured the milk, the less intact antigen survives (heat denatures protein). So custard may be less problematic than a glass of fresh milk.

But note that these effects can only alter risks, not eliminate them. A UK study showed that for the same basic SMA formula, different heat-treatment (to produce powder, concentrate

---

72   One of the earliest post WWII reports was Jakobsson I, Lindberg T. Cow's milk as a cause of infantile colic in breast-fed infants. (PMID:79803) *Lancet* 1978, 2(8087):437–39.

73   Jakobsson I. Unusual presentation of adverse reactions to cow's milk proteins. (PMID:4046494) *Klin Padiatr* 1985; 197(4):360–62. See also Bibliography – Dr Doris Rapp successfully treated such symptoms by diet quite commonly in US children.

and ready-to-feed products) resulted in different degrees of allergenicity.[74] Powder (spray-dried) was more sensitising than liquids heated to 121°C for 4.6 minutes (ready to feed), or 122°C for 5.6 minutes (concentrate). When I asked a renowned UK dairy scientist whether denatured heat-treated milk could be non-allergenic, he replied 'You could boil milk till it was black, and there would still be enough intact protein to cause reactions.'[75]

A recent review makes it clear that there is no simple answer to how processing affects allergenicity:

> The persistence of allergenicity in heat-treated milk is clinically confirmed by the fact that in some children CMA [cows' milk allergy] develops after the ingestion of heat-treated milk. Furthermore, heating processes can only modify conformational epitopes [antibody attachment points on an antigen], which might lose their binding capacity to specific IgE antibody, while sequential epitopes maintain their allergenic potential even after heating (Fig. 4–2).[40] Milk proteins contain both types of epitopes and, even though a slight reduction of antigenicity can be observed with whey proteins, insignificant alterations in binding properties are reported with caseins. To complicate the picture, vigorous heating (such as that used for certain sterilisation processes [121°C for 20 minutes]) but also the less drastic pasteurisation process, have also been shown to enhance some allergenic characteristics.[41] Furthermore, milk proteins can be oxidised during industrial treatment, resulting in the formation of modified/oxidised amino acid residues, particularly in BLG [beta-lactoglobulin], which may be responsible for the development of new immunologically reactive structures.[76]

Great news, heating milk can in fact either reduce, or increase, allergenicity – or even create brand new allergens! It's possible that the milk from different types of cows may produce different outcomes, though of course formula is made from the mixed milk of thousands of cows of varying breeds.[77] (Which is why I use the plural term, cows' milk, throughout this book.) If genuinely low-allergy formulas are possible, and can be made palatable for adults, perhaps well-organised research into the milk intake of pregnant and lactating women, and its connection with allergy in infants would be useful. Combined with some genetic investigations, it might reveal the possibly genetic basis for individual mothers' differences in response to milk ingestion, and allow for better advice to be developed about which allergic mothers would be best to drink small quantities of milk throughout pregnancy, and who would be better to avoid it altogether. Not that such investigation will have any public health benefit until gene sequencing has become globally affordable!

---

74  McLauchlan P, Coombs RRA. Experimental studies on sensitisation to cows' milk. In Freed DLJ. (ed) *The Health Hazards of Milk.* (Bailliere Tindall 1984) p. 129. That too may be relevant to national differences in allergy prevalence.

75   Malcolm Peaker (conversation in Reading, England, October 1983).

76  World Allergy Organization (WAO) Diagnosis and Rationale for Action against Cow's Milk Allergy (DRACMA) Guidelines. *World Allergy Organ J.* 2010; 3(4): 57–161. PMCID: PMC3488907. DOI: 10.1097/WOX.0b013e3181defeb9 Published online 2010 April 23.

77  Which is why I use the plural term cows' milk, not the singular.

A pint or two daily?

We should record for posterity some of the unbelievably silly excesses of twentieth-century industry – and marketing-driven advice to drink milk.

Readers may have clear memories, as I have, of being urged to drink at least a litre or more of milk a day while pregnant, or risk losing teeth and having bones crumble. After the birth, women were not only urged to drink milk, it was milk fortified with added patent dried milk powders, 'tonic foods' such as Lactagol, or chocolate powders like Akta-Vite, full of milk protein, cereal grains and sugar. 'Drink milk to make milk', we were told – though no other mammal does!

That milk intake was in addition to cheese and yoghurt and other bovine protein sources, and in a diet where animal protein was more than adequate. This amount of milk is no longer suggested as necessary for health in any age group.

Warm milk was also suggested at bedtime: not irrational given the tryptophan dose this provided. The neurotransmitter dose in milk made it addictive for some, who produced such distressed babies that they tracked me down to ask for help (and a milk-free diet worked wonders).

One such mother told me that she had disliked the taste of milk but made herself eat cheese for the baby's sake, and gradually her intake increased. In the third trimester, she was waking at 2 am each night, putting half a pint of milk in a saucepan, grating in 'a packet' – usually 200–250 g or around 8 ounces – of cheese, and drinking all this 'cheese soup' before going back to bed to sleep soundly. Her weight gain had been excessive; when she took all milk out of her diet on my advice, she lost weight and the baby stopped crying. I would love to be able to follow that family into the next generation! (If you are reading this, please do get back in touch.)

## Allergies and pregnancy diet

There is good evidence that infants are exposed prenatally[78] to many antigens, with long-lasting consequences. Intra-uterine sensitisation explains some cases of severe food allergy, including lower gastrointestinal bleeding, in the neonatal period,since it takes at least 10 days after the first exposure to generate an immune reaction, [79] and cord blood cells are already reactive to food proteins.

Infant prenatal exposure to high levels of antibodies against wheat (which suggests high maternal wheat intake) is linked to a higher risk of non-affective psychosis by one study.[80]

78   Szépfalusi Z, Nentwich I, Gerstmayr M, Jost E et al. Prenatal allergen contact with milk proteins. (PMID:9117877) *Clin Exper Allergy* 1997; 27(1):28–35. DOI: 10.1046/j.1365-2222.1997.d01-417.x

79   Mizuno M, Masaki H, Yoshinare R, et al. Hematochezia before the first feeding in a newborn with food protein-induced enterocolitis syndrome. *AJP Rep* 2011; 1:53–58.

80   Karlsson H, Blomström A, Wicks S, Yang S et al. Maternal antibodies to dietary antigens and risk for nonaffective psychosis in offspring. (MED:22535227) *American J Psychiatr* 2012; 169(6):625–32.

Infant prenatal exposure to parasites is also reflected in later infant health: routine de-worming medications resulted in a higher risk of eczema and wheeze in infancy,[81] possibly due to gut damage by the medication and higher antigen uptake, not necessarily the absence of worms! (Then again, it may have been the absence of worms which allowed allergy to develop, because the immune system would almost certainly prioritise worm control ahead of reacting to less invasive foods, and only so many antibodies can be generated without using nutrients needed for basic metabolic purposes.)

Studies are indicating that immune development during pregnancy is indeed related to maternal diet, and influences the emergence of allergic symptoms. For example, when a trial of maternal egg avoidance in pregnancy was done:

> Serum-specific IgG to OVA [ovalbumin, a notable egg allergen], but not the unrelated allergen, cow's milk beta-lactoglobulin, decreased over pregnancy in egg-avoiding women only (P<0.001). Cord OVA IgG concentration correlated with maternal IgG at delivery (r=0.944; P<0.001), and for infants born to atopic women, cord concentration was higher than that of their mother's (P<0.001) ... Serum OVA IgG concentration reflects egg consumption, thereby indicating dietary allergen doses to which the developing immune system might be exposed. Trans-placental maternal IgG must be considered among early life factors that regulate infant atopic programming.[82]

And in plain English the result in this study was: young babies with both very high or very low levels of IgG in their cord blood were less likely to show symptoms of allergy.

This could be due to two different mechanisms – a level of egg antigen too low to cause reactions, or a level high enough to stimulate the immune system to switch them off. Or it may be due to other immune factors in maternal blood, infant blood, and probably above all maternal milk, which regulate the expression of symptoms after this initial pregnancy exposure. There is still a lot we do not know; after all, even the discovery of pluripotent stem cells in breastmilk is quite recent.

We are carrying our mothers' and grandmothers' cells, and perhaps even our siblings' cells.[83] Whether or how that might influence particular allergic manifestations will be varied, and until we know a lot more about the genetics and immunology involved, probably unpredictable. But as I said earlier, whether allergy/hypersensitivity is bred or fed into a family line, or triggered by some environmental adjuvants, it will not suddenly disappear, even if symptoms remit completely for decades. Symptoms will re-emerge if and when the body's capacity to cope is overstretched (see Figure 4-6-1 on page 610). Observant families notice these associations between symptoms and stress, but often consider the stress as the

---

81  Mpairwe H, Webb EL, Muhangi L, Ndibazza J wt al. Anthelminthic treatment during pregnancy is associated with increased risk of infantile eczema: randomised-controlled trial results. (PMCID:PMC3130136) *Paed Allergy Immunol* 2011; 22(3):305–12. DOI: 10.1111/j.1399-3038.2010.01122.x

82  Vance GH, Grimshaw KE, Briggs R, Lewis SA et al. Serum ovalbumin-specific immunoglobulin G responses during pregnancy reflect maternal intake of dietary egg and relate to the development of allergy in early infancy. (PMID:15663559) *Clin Exp Allergy* 2004; 34(12):1855–61.

83  Dierselhuis MP, Blokland EC, Pool J, Schrama E, et al Transmaternal cell flow leads to antigen-experienced cord blood. PMID:22627770) *Blood* 2012; 120(3):505–10.

cause, rather than a precipitant, or trigger factor. Pregnancy itself may be such a stress, and some symptoms that emerge in pregnancy may in fact be due to food sensitivies now emerging. Anecdotally, severe nausea and vomiting in pregnancy have dramatically abated with maternal diet changes, even hyperemesis of the kind that the Duchess of Cambridge famously experienced. Others may test whether this was coincidence or a true association.

From an evolutionary perspective, it is useful for women to be more sensitive to potentially damaging foods when gestating a baby, and for their bodies to reject such foods; but it is counterproductive for pregnant women to be wasting food when their nutrient needs have increased. On that basis some greater tendency to reject 'bad' foods seems helpful (women 'go off' alcoholic or strongly caffeinated drinks, for example) but the extremes of hyperemesis (frequent vomiting) are dangerous to survival, and so must be pathological, a response to something harmful, or the result of a deranged immune response.

## Allergies and postnatal maternal diet

Maternal diet in pregnancy[84] is clearly one part of the cumulative and interactive process that shapes an infant's immune system and general health. So too is maternal diet during lactation.

| Factors involved in oral tolerance induction | Breast milk factors possibly affecting tolerance induction in infants |
|---|---|
| antigen | antigen present in breast milk: dietary antigens, self antigens, maternal allogeneic antigens, respiratory antigens |
| | antigen transfer across neonate gut barrier |
| | antigen presentation by neonate antigen presenting cells |
| tolerogenic molecules | tolerogenic molecules: TGF-β, IL-10, n-3 fatty acids,... |
| | inflammatory molecules: TNF-a, IL-6, IL-1, IFN-g, IL-4, Il-5, IL-13 |
| | • the balance between the tolerogenic and inflammatory mediators in milk will influence breastfed child immune response to the transferred antigen |
| gut microbiota | maternal IgA, lysozyme, lactoferrin, oligosaccharide, nucleotides, soluble CD14, soluble TLR2, bacteria in maternal milk |
| | • the exposure of the infant to environmental bacteria and to maternal milk bacterial growth factor and anti-microbial molecules will shape infant microbiota and thereby immune system maturation |
| gut permeability | growth factors: EGF, erythropoetin, insulin like growth factor, hepatocyte growth factor, basic fibroblast growth |
| | healing factors: EGF, TGF-β, soluble TLR2 |
| | • milk gut growth factors and healing factors will stimulate infant gut maturation and barrier integrity which will affect antigen transfer across the gut barrier |

Figure 2-2-4 Breastmilk factors possibly involved in inducing tolerance[86] (© Wageningen Academic Publishers 2013.)

---

84   Polte T, Hennig C, Hansen G. Allergy prevention starts before conception: maternofetal transfer of tolerance protects against the development of asthma. (PMID:19000583) *J Allergy Clin Immunol* 2008, 122(5):1022–30.e5

Animal studies support the milk hypothesis by indicating that 'oral tolerance induced by breast milk-mediated transfer of dietary antigens along with their specific immunoglobulins to offspring [during lactation] leads to antigen-specific protection from food allergy.'[85] This is not a simple process: many factors may be involved, as the previous table[86] makes clear.

Interestingly, the animal studies mentioned were in mice made allergic during lactation, i.e. first-generation allergic mother mice, which had no apparent food sensitivities before or during their infants' gestation. Outcomes could be different if the mother mice had been deprived of mouse milk as infants, and forced to survive and grow on mouse formula/chow from birth, before this experiment was repeated. And for the parallel to be more accurate, we need to follow them for whole mouse lifetimes, not sacrifice them young. So we need two or three generations of mice studied, with the groups randomised to mouse milk and infant mouse formula(!)[87] in each generation, to test the effects of artificial feeding. After all, it is possible that in the artificially fed or badly breastfed human generations who are now lactating and feeding their own children, there will be some adverse consequences of their childhood diet. Yet when dealing with lactating women, too rarely is attention given to their individual lifetime diet history or their current diet.

Many mothers suspect that their breastfed child's symptoms are related to the food that they themselves are eating and passing through to the child in their milk, some with good reason (see Figure 5-3-1 on page 662). Not many health professionals are as useless as the dietician who flippantly answered a mother's well-founded concern about the effects of her diet on her baby with, 'You'll be fine so long as you avoid cyanide'.[88]

Even so, all too often the solution offered to such mothers is a formula, rather than help to identify and eliminate problem foods and chemicals affecting her baby. Some symptoms may initially improve on switching to artificial feeding, especially in the crying baby who was simply underfed and hungry, or the baby who was reacting to allergens in breastmilk not present in the formula. But normal immune function will be compromised, with a greater risk of inflammation and infection – and there are better ways to resolve both those problems. (Feed the hungry baby; fix the mother's diet. See page 586).

Hypersensitivity bred or fed into a family line, or triggered by some environmental adjuvants or stressors, will not suddenly disappear, even if symptoms ease. How family genes are expressed matters for a lifetime, not just in the first months. On first principles, it seems likely to be a bad idea to add other distortions to normal development by swapping babies

---

85   Yamamoto T, Tsubota Y, Kodama T, Kageyama-Yahara N et al. Oral tolerance induced by transfer of food antigens via breast milk of allergic mothers prevents offspring from developing allergic symptoms in a mouse food allergy model. *Clin Dev Immunol.* 2012; 2012: 721085. Published online 27/3/2012. DOI: *10.1155/2012/721085* PMCID:PMC3310277)

86   Macchiaverni P, Tulic MK Verhasselt V. *Antigens in breastmilk: possible impact on immune system education.* in Zibadi S, Watson RR, Preedy VR (eds) op. cit. p. 450. © Wageningen Academic Publishers 2013.

87   A major difficulty with animal studies is that without any mother's milk, many offspring die or fail to reproduce. Not all animals have human omnivore capacity.

88   In fact the mother who ate cyanide needn't worry about her breastmilk, as she would be dead. This was reported to me by a reliable witness in 2012. While extreme, it is not totally atypical.

off the breast on to industrial milks, however much they might – or more often might not – reduce some immediate symptoms. This is discussed further on page 638.

## Genes and the wrong milk, or lack of the right milk

Does the wrong milk, or lack of the right milk, affect our genes? Short answer: yes. Milks are species-specific, and designed to create normal growth at the cellular level as well as in more easily measurable ways. Cancer results from cellular dysfunction. Cancer researchers are now investigating the mutagenic (gene-changing) effects of not breastfeeding; that is, of formula-feeding. They began to do so because it would be one plausible explanation for the documented higher cancer rates in children who are not breastfed.[89] (The absence of those cancer-killing agents recently found in breastmilk[90] is of course another possible explanation: breastmilk component HAMLET – human α-lactalbumin made lethal to tumour cells – kills cancer cells while stimulating an innate immune response in surrounding healthy tissue.[91])

Unfortunately, there are not many studies of diet-induced DNA damage yet, but those that exist are disturbing. One group of cancer researchers has shown in a small study that rates of actual chromosomal damage are significantly higher in artificially fed children as young as nine to twelve months. Their paper begins: 'There are many advantages of human milk for infants, including protection against cancer development.' These cancer researchers conclude that the 'molecular mechanism of DNA damage caused by the absence of human milk needs to be investigated.'[92]

Indeed it does. And we should always keep in mind that it is not just the absence of breastmilk's anti-cancer agents that may be doing the damage. Where there is no breastmilk, there will be instead one of the wide variety of formulas or artificial foods. Artificial feeding may be more or less damaging in itself, depending on the artificial substance being fed, which could help explain differing results sometimes seen in studies of anonymous 'formulas'.

Looking at very low birth weight (VLBW) infants, another research group found that 'oxidative DNA damage is considerably more suppressed in breastfed VLBW infants than in formula-fed VLBW infants'.[93] (If breastfeeding were regarded as the human norm, this statement would read: 'formula-fed VLBW infants exhibit considerably more oxidative DNA damage than breastfed VLBW infants' – the same basic information, but what a difference to the human mind that reads it!)

89    Ortega-García JA, Ferrís-Tortajada J, Torres-Cantero AM, Soldin OP et al. Full breastfeeding and paediatric cancer. *J Paediatr Child Health* 2008; 44:10–13. (PMID:17999666)
90    See Davanzo R, Zauli G, Monasta L, Vecchi Brumatti L et al. Human colostrum and breastmilk contain high levels of TNF-related apoptosis-inducing ligand (TRAIL). (PMID:22529245) *J Hum Lact* 2013, 29(1):23–25.
91    Storm P, Klausen TK, Trulsson M, Ho C S J, et al. A unifying mechanism for cancer cell death through ion channel activation by HAMLET.(PMID:23505537) *PLoS* One 2013, 8(3):e58578. Free full text article.
92    Dündaröz R, Aydin HI, Ulucan H, Baltaci V, Denli M, Gökçay E (Preliminary study on DNA damage in non breast-fed infants. *Pediatrics International* (2002) 44 (2): 127–30.) PMID:11896867); Dündaröz R, Ulucan H, Aydin HI, Güngör T, Baltaci V, Denli M, Sanisoğlu Y. Analysis of DNA damage using the comet assay in infants fed cow's milk. (PMID:12907847) *Biol Neonate* 2003, 84(2):135–41.
93    Shoji H, Shimizu T, Shinohara K, Oguchi S, et al. Suppressive effects of breast milk on oxidative DNA damage in very low birthweight infants. (2004). *Disease in Childhood Fetal and Neonatal Edition* 89:F13

Blurred definitions once again affect outcomes. The infants in that study were defined as formula-fed if formula was 90 per cent or more of the diet, and breastfed if breastmilk was 90 per cent or more of the diet. This means that the difference could be more marked than this study shows, as it is unlikely that many breastfed infants didn't get a little bit of formula, and vice versa.)

So not being breastfed – or being formula-fed, or both – does increase genetic damage. It also alters the expression of genes in unknown ways, at least in the few cases studied to date. One recent study showed that breast milk contains high expression levels of acid-stable micro-RNAs (miRNAs) indicating that breast milk transfers this genetic material to infants.[94] These are small regulatory RNA molecules that modulate immune activity and have other roles in a wide range of bodily processes. If such material is being passed to the next generation not just in the process of fertilisation but also by breastmilk, further research should be a matter of urgency – and not just to see if these molecules can be synthesised and added to infant formula![95]

Obviously all preventive health researchers should make infant feeding a factor they consider in every study looking for causes of disease, from cancer to kidneys. Does breastmilk's repair work decrease the risk for infants of smoking parents? Does formula interact synergistically with smoking to increase cancer risk, as it does the risk of hospitalisation for respiratory disease?[96] Japanese researchers have shown that even at one month of age, breastfed infants have lower levels of a chemical marker of DNA damage, a fact they ascribe to the many antioxidants in breastmilk. As they say, 'During the perinatal period, oxidative stress is intimately involved in pathologic processes of serious diseases … Our data suggest that breast milk, not artificial formula, acts as an antioxidant during infancy.'[97] Or, to rephrase that to reflect the proper biological default, formulas act as additional oxidative stresses for already stressed infants. This effect on their DNA may help to explain why formula-fed babies are less healthy, even lifelong. Free radicals were discovered in the 1950s, and since then it has been 'difficult to find pathological phenomena not associated with reactive oxygen species (ROS)'.[98] Industry is trying to reduce these in infant formula.

# Hormones, physical development, and the wrong milk

Does the wrong milk, or lack of the right milk, affect physical development? Short answer again: absolutely yes. How can it not? Look at what milk contains.

---

94    Kosaka N, Izumi H, Sekine K, Ochiya T. MicroRNA as a new immune-regulatory agent in breast milk. (PMCID:PMC2847997) Free full text article *Silence* 2010; 1(1):7

95    As an aside, it seems that our diet may contribute such genetic material to us lifelong. See Jabr F. Eating greens alters genes. *New Scientist* 2011; 2832: 10–11.

96    Chen Y. Synergistic effect of passive smoking and artificial feeding on hospitalisation for respiratory illness in early childhood.(PMID:2785023) *Chest* 1989, 95(5):1004–07.

97    Shoji H, Oguchi S, Shimizu T, Yamashiro Y. Effect of human breast milk on urinary 8-hydroxy-2'-deoxyguanosine excretion in infants. *Pediatric Research* 2003, 53(5):850-852. (PMID:12621121)

98    Tsukahara H. Redox modulatory factors of human breast milk. In Zibadi et al. op. cit.

| Bombesin | Epidermal growth factor | Gastric inhibitory peptide |
|---|---|---|
| Cortisol | Insulin-like growth factors | Gastrin-releasing peptide |
| Oxytocin | Mammotrope differentiating peptide | Parathyroid hormone-related peptide |
| Prolactin | Nerve growth factor | Vasoactive intestinal polypeptide |
| Relaxin | Fibroblast growth factor | Endorphins |
| Oestrogen | Gonadotropin releasing hormone | Transforming growth factor |
| Thyroxin | Somastatin | Bradykinin |
| Resistin | Ghrelin | Motilin |
| Leptin | And many more ... | Osteoprotegerin |

Figure 2-2-5 Some of the many hormones and other bioactive factors in milk

As Natalie Angier said in her impressive overview,[99] both blood and milk are 'rivers of life whose depths scientists have yet to fathom.' All mammalian milk is loaded with a huge variety of hormones and growth factors, different for each species. That has been known for decades. It was sometimes asserted or assumed that these bioactive ingredients were there simply as bystanders, by-products of lactation, accumulated from blood, perhaps mildly useful for mothers and the health of the breast, but not making much difference to baby. Not until the 1990s was it realised that neural growth factors and important hormones like GnRH were being made by the breast itself.

Common-sense observers have always thought that any factor normally found in breastmilk was likely to have some positive effect. But while scientists did not know how these factors worked, or have the tools to test this, the generally accepted position was that any effects of hormones and growth factors on the infant had to be proved beyond doubt before this could be publicly stated – and through such statements, suggest to every intelligent parent that infant formula was deeply inferior. We now know enough to state categorically that all these agents do indeed affect infant development. In fact,

> Human milk may be a medium whereby the hormonal milieu (in response to internal factors and the environment) of the mother can be used to communicate with the breast-fed infant to modify infant metabolic processes. Transmission of information from mother to infant through milk may allow adaptation to fluctuating environmental conditions.[100]

In short, breastmilk modulates the baby's response to its environment. There are dozens of breastmilk hormones, and each can have multiple functions. Here I will simply mention

---

99  Angier N. Woman (Houghton Mifflin 1999 ) A wonderful book everyone should read.
100 Newburg DS, Woo JG, Morrow AL. Characteristics and potential functions of human milk adiponectin. http://dx.doi.org/10.1016/j.jpeds.2009.11.020 In Makrides M, Ochoa J, Szajewska H (eds). *The Importance of Immunonutrition* NNI Workshop Series vol 77, 2013. Online at http://www.nestlenutrition-institute.org/ Resources/Library/Free/workshop/NNIW77/Pages/The-Importance-of-Immunonutrition.aspx

a few of the many linked to growth regulation, and absent from infant formulas: insulin, leptin, grehlin, and adiponectin.

Insulin is known for its role in carbohydrate metabolism. It affects gut maturation and mucosal enzyme expression, increasing lactase activity and influencing intestinal permeability, along with other indirect systemic effects. It has been shown in preterm infants to decrease the time it takes for them to tolerate full feeds. One result of this finding, of course, is that it is being considered for inclusion in infant formula:

> If the addition of insulin to preterm infant formulas results in better growth and accelerated intestinal maturation, future studies will need to address insulin supplementation in term infants and assess the efficacy of such supplementation in enhancing gut maturation and preventing non-communicable diseases such as allergy, autoimmune diseases and obesity.[101]

That's a trial they had better monitor very carefully!

Similarly, leptin has been widely talked about in relation to appetite control and weight loss. Among other things, it is thought to influence the amount of adipose tissue in the body and promote the synthesis of an appetite suppressant.[102] In mice, leptin influences the formation of neural circuits that regulate both lifelong food intake and amount of body fat.[103] One study has found that low infant serum levels of leptin are associated with higher BMI and suggested this as a potential indicator of later obesity.[104] While some might decry this as unproven, industry is already investigating the possibility of adding leptin to infant formula, to permanently alter the infant brain as neural circuits develop. But others think this science fiction, or 'so scary that it would mean a whole new approach about how such treatments can be tested and approved for use.'[105] Yes.

Adiponectin is a hormone that is produced by adipose tissue. There is more of it than leptin in breastmilk. Those researching it write that it enhances insulin sensitivity, metabolic control, and suppresses inflammation:

> An inverse relationship between adiponectin levels in milk and adiposity (weight-for-height) of the breast-fed infant was observed and could be due to modulation of infant metabolism by milk adiponectin and may be related to the observed protection against obesity by breast-feeding.[106]

---

101  Shamir R, Shehadeh N. Insulin in human milk and the use of hormones in infant formula, ibid.
102  Hassiotou F, Geddes DT. Programming of appetite control during breastfeeding as a preventative strategy against the obesity epidemic. (PMID:24646683) *J Hum Lact* 2014, 30(2):136–142
103  Bronsky J, Mitrova K. Adiponectin, adipocyte fatty-acid binding protein and leptin in human breast milk and impact in the infant. In Zibadi et al, p. 393,
104  Savino F, Liguori SA, Benetti S, Sorrenti M et al. High serum leptin levels in infancy can potentially predict obesity in childhood, especially in formula-fed infants. (PMID:23844562) *Acta Paediatr* 2013; 102(10):e455-9] DOI: 10.1111/apa.12354
105  Curtis P. Scientists working on formula milk that prevents child obesity. *The Guardian*, 23 April 2007; reporting on attempts, led by Prof MA Cawthorne of the University of Buckingham in the UK, to add leptin to infant formula recorded in Chemistry and Industry 2007. http://www.theguardian.com/science/2007/apr/23/medicalresearch.ethicsofscience
106  Newburg DS, Woo JG, Morrow AL. op. cit.

Industry may well be considering how to substitute these three hormones, and others, in formulas. And I could write their advertising campaigns now, full of suggestions of proven benefit, implied through weasel words and images of babies not necessarily even fed their products. But every mammalian milk contains hormones which work together with many other factors to influence infant development. In fact, researchers studying our monkey cousins suggest that some of the hormones in milk are in fact signals that will affect infant feeding behaviour, temperament, and growth.[107] Milk is remarkably sophisticated indeed, as one commentator said. That is, of course, fresh mothers' milk.

Heavy-duty industrial processing alters these components of cows' milk, which in any case are meant to develop a calf appropriately, not a child. Whatever is left in formula of the bovine analogues cannot possibly have the same effects on infant metabolism and development as fresh breastmilk. We know that as soon as small amounts of oral feeding start in very low birthweight infants, blood biochemical profiles are different if the baby is fed formula.[108] And we know, and do not need to prove, that a few industrially produced and processed analogues cannot possibly have the same effect as the multiplicity of interactions between hormones and other ingredients in fresh human milk. Does this matter when infants survive without them? Common sense says it does. Those who think it doesn't need to prove that.

I repeat, before industry (or any doctor or parent or formula advocate) suggests that the formula-fed baby's altered blood chemistry, or lack of key human hormones, or lesser brain growth, makes no difference, *they* need to prove that. I do not have to prove anything. A priori, if human hormones are in breastmilk, an infant deprived of them is disadvantaged. That makes this an issue of formula safety as well as adequacy: how dare formula makers claim to provide all necessary nutritional support for the immune system, when they don't include ingredients that affect both nutrition and immunity?

## Is this relevant to obesity?

The extent of this breastmilk support and the ways it affects normal physical development seem to me to be more likely to be under-estimated than exaggerated. Consider infant obesity, one form of dysnutrition, as an example.

A recent 'systematic review and meta-analysis of risk factors for childhood overweight identifiable during infancy'[109] compared 'ever breastfed' UK children with 'never breastfed' ones from a wide range of studies. Such a study should result in little or no difference

---

107 Hinde K, Skibiel KL, Foster AB, Del Rosso L et al. Cortisol in mother's milk across lactation reflects maternal life history and predicts infant temperament. *Behavioural Ecology* 2014; DOI: 10.1093/beheco/aru186. Published online 31 Oct 2014. Report in *NY Times* 6 Nov 2014. http://www.nytimes.com/2014/11/06/science/in-a-mothers-milk-nutrients-and-a-message-too.html

108 Verd S, García M, Gutiérrez A, Moliner E et al. Blood biochemical profile of very preterm infants before and after trophic feeding with exclusive human milk or with formula milk. (PMID:24576499) *Clin Biochem* 2014, 47(7–8):584–87

109 Weng SF, Redsell SA, Swift JA, Yang M, Glazebrook CP. Systematic review and meta-analysis of risk factors for childhood overweight identifiable during infancy. (PMID:23109090) *Arch Dis Child* 2012, 97(12):1019-1026. DOI: 10.1136/archdischild-2012-302263

being shown, because so many children in any UK 'ever breastfed group' would have been formula-feeding within days or weeks. Despite this, there was an almost 18% increased odds ratio for overweight in those 'never breastfed'.

The findings were further minimised by taking the exclusively formula-fed as the scientific norm and so stating that 'ever' breastfeeding decreased the odds ratio by 15 per cent. The review's conclusion – 'A moderate protective effect of ever breastfeeding on subsequent development of child overweight' – can be misunderstood as meaning that short durations of breastfeeding are good enough. Comparing ever – versus never – breastfed data may be concealing the fact that the protective effect of breastfeeding against obesity may be almost non-existent for very short periods, like a week, and massive for longer periods. Or may depend on exclusive breastfeeding at a critical developmental stage.

Weng et al quoted one study that 'found a significant decrease in the odds of overweight at 2 years of age for infants breastfed for more than 6 months compared with those breastfed for less than 3 months.'[110] (Again, the figure would have been greater were the breastfed the scientific norm: formula increases risks, breastfeeding does not decrease them.) But what we need – and do not have – are studies of solely formula-fed children versus children breastfed exclusively and then partially for differing periods of time. Basic science suggests there may be greater risks of obesity in children according to the mode of breastfeeding as well as the composition of the infant formula.

Why? We know that there are many other ways in which artificial feeding may create obesity: not only the products fed, but also the ways they are fed. Studies show that direct breastfeeding results in better appetite control, for example, when compared with bottle-feeding – regardless of the content of the bottle.[111] Relevant sections in Chapter 3 outline plausible mechanisms for the obesogenic effect of too much protein and the wrong fats over time in two or three generations. And of course the insulin and other hormones and enzymes and growth factors in breastmilk may well play a part in programming infant carbohydrate metabolism for life. Regardless, the existence of effects is indisputable: one meta-analysis of nine studies with more than 69,000 participants showed that breastfeeding reduced the risk of obesity in childhood significantly: or rather, that being formula-fed increased the risk by 25 per cent.[112]

Of course when obese women breastfeed, after birthing heavier babies, the impact of their lifelong obesity will affect comparative risk in the next generation, as both higher birthweight *and* maternal obesity increase the risk of infant obesity. The rate of obesity among breastfed

---

110 Weyermann M, Rothenbacher D, Brenner H. Duration of breastfeeding and risk of overweight in childhood: a prospective birth cohort study from Germany. *Int J Obes* 2006;**30**:1281–7.

111 Li R, Fein SB, and Grummer-Strawn LM (2010) Do infants fed from bottles lack self-regulation of milk intake compared with directly breastfed infants? *Pediatrics* 2010; 125(6): e1386–93.Also Di Santis KI, Collins BN, Fisher Jo, Davey A. Do infants fed directly from the breast have improved appetite regulation and slower growth during early childhood compared with infants fed from a bottle? *Int J Behav Nutr Phys Act* 2011; 8:89. See also Li R, Magadia J, Fein SB, Grummer-Strawn LM. Risk of bottle-feeding for rapid weight gain during the first year of life. (PMID:22566543) *Arch Pediatr Adolesc Med* 2012;166(5):431–36.

112 Arenz S, Rückerl R, Koletzko B, von Kries R. Breast-feeding and childhood obesity – a systematic review. *Int J Obes Relat Metab Disord.* 2004; 28(10):1247–56.

children will rise. Rates of obesity among the artificially fed should decrease a little with the latest lowering of formula protein levels and changes in fat blends. (Although differences in body composition will remain.) Thus differences in infant obesity by mode of feeding may be reduced, while the baseline population risk remains elevated from what it would have been without formula feeding in either generation. But the mother's obesity may be due to her own infant feeding history. *Bottle feeding in the previous generation may have made the next breastfed generation more like the bottle-fed.* Clearly, breast or bottle-feeding has measurable impacts on usual bodily development. When industry claims outcomes closer to a breastfed norm, we need to know that the norm has not been distorted by bottle feeding *past and present*.

But there is other evidence of small but disturbing bodily differences between children who are breastfed and those who are formula-fed, whether the formula is milk- or soy-based. The most publicised concerns – but not necessarily the greatest concerns – relate to soy formulas.

## Soy formulas and infant development

Soy formulas contain plant-based substances that mimic the natural hormone oestrogen (referred to as phyto-oestrogens or isoflavones). Concern about possible effects on child reproductive development and thyroid function has caused them to fall from favour with paediatric groups. But is soy formula any worse than cows' milk formula?

Millions of acres in America are devoted to growing soy beans, and almost every processed food in America contains some soy product. They are a hugely important and cheap food source. Perhaps for this reason, researchers from the Arkansas Children's Nutrition Center, working for the United States Department of Agriculture (USDA) Agricultural Research Service based in Arkansas (a major soy producer) would seem to have a vested interest in finding that soy formulas are not inferior to (i.e., no worse than) bovine milk formulas. Certainly they conducted, and are continuing, some extensive research into the question; their articles[113] indicate that they found soy and bovine formula to have roughly comparable (if slightly different) effects.

But along with groups of infants fed on soy- and cows' milk formula, they included a partially breastfed control group, unlike some prominent industry researchers who argue that new formulas should only be compared with older formulas, not with breastmilk.[114] I

---

113 Gilchrist JM, Moore MB, Andres A, Estroff JA, Badger TM. Ultrasonographic patterns of reproductive organs in infants fed soy formula: comparisons to infants fed breast milk and milk formula. *J Pediatr*. 2010 Feb;156(2):215–20; Badger TM, Gilchrist JM, Pivik RT, Andres A et al. The health implications of soy infant formula. *Am J Clin Nutr*. 2009; 89 (5):1668S–1672S; Jing H, Gilchrist JM, et al. A longitudinal study of differences in electroencephalographic activity among breastfed, milk formula-fed, and soy formula-fed infants during the first year of life. *Early Hum Dev*. 2010 Feb;86(2):119–25

114 Transcripts of the November 18–19 2002 meeting of the USDA Food Advisory Committee on Infant Formula make enlightening reading. Go to http://www.fda.gov/ohrms/dockets/ac/cfsan02.htm to download these. One speaker stated that 'if you want to study a new formula, you should study it in comparison with old formulas, and not with some group that we think might represent ideal growth.' Another thought that 'fifty years of formula experience ... with reasonable [sic] good outcomes' meant that comparison with breastfed infants was unnecessary. Do parents want reasonably good, or the best possible, outcomes?

find their results deeply disturbing, even if the numbers in each group, and the reported outcome effects, are small. In fact, their articles could have been summarised as: 'Both cows'-milk formulas and soy formulas are clearly inferior to breastmilk.'

These researchers began by asserting accurately that 'The extent to which adequate nutrition from infant diets differentially influences developmental outcomes in healthy infants has not been determined.'[115] In English: we don't know yet how different types of formulas affect normal healthy babies. *Note that well: after one hundred and fifty years – fifty of 'modern' whey-dominant formula – we still don't know.* Cognitive and reproductive development was never measured when formulas were being assessed for safety and efficacy in the past. Which makes it hard to know if nutrition is indeed 'adequate' except in the simplest terms of 'enough nutrients to keep babies alive and gaining weight'.

Back to the Arkansas studies. In one, the researchers used ultrasound to assess the development of breast buds, uterus, ovaries, prostate, and testicular volumes in forty breastfed (BF), forty-one milk-fed (MF) and thirty-nine soy-fed (SF) four-month-old infants. And this study found that:

> Among girls, there were no feeding group differences in breast bud or uterine volume. MF infants had greater mean ovarian volume and greater numbers of ovarian cysts per ovary than did BF infants ... [Among boys] there were no feeding group differences in prostate or breast bud volumes. Mean testicular volume did not differ between SF and MF boys, but both formula-fed groups had lower testicular volumes than BF infants.[116]

I found that alarming. Differences in ovarian and testicular development evident at four months of age? What might be the effects by the time these children reach puberty, if they are being programmed already to develop differently? Do they reach puberty earlier than breastfed children? It is astonishing how many popular discussions[117] of the reality of premature puberty omit any discussion of infant feeding as a likely influence, despite all that is now accepted about the programming effect of early nutrition, its effects on other bodily growth, and the higher prevalence and earlier onset of early puberty in those groups.

In fact, in America the age of onset of puberty has been dropping steadily through the bottle-feeding twentieth century. 'Boys now reach puberty up to two years earlier than experts had believed,' says the New York Times, reporting on a major study just released by the American Academy of Pediatrics.[118] That is two years earlier than the generally accepted age of eleven and a half years. Meanwhile, one in ten Caucasian-American girls and one in five African-American girls are now beginning breast development before the age of

---

115 Gilchrist JM, et al., op. cit.

116 ibid.

117 e.g., Christopher L. Girl, you'll be a woman soon. *The Saturday Age, Good Weekend* magazine, September 7, 2013, pp.12–15.

118 Herman-Giddens ME, Steffes J, Harris D, Slora E, et al. Secondary sexual characteristics in boys: data from the pediatric research in office settings network. (PMID:23085608) *Pediatrics* 2012, 130(5):e1058–68.

eight![119] (African-American communities have low breastfeeding rates.[120]) Is this linked to differences in early breast development associated with soy?[121]

Early puberty increases cancer risk, and has been associated with depression.[122] What might be the effects by the time these children are seeking to have their own children, perhaps thirty years on? Could this contribute to Western epidemics of infertility, polycystic ovary syndrome and low sperm counts? Does it contribute to the development of insufficient mammary gland tissue? Is it part of the reason for the rise in increasingly early and aggressive reproductive cancers? Are these Arkansas children – and their children – to be followed up for the next sixty years? You'd hope so. Did their parents even know the results for each child? What effect does that have on the family? What ongoing support is in place?

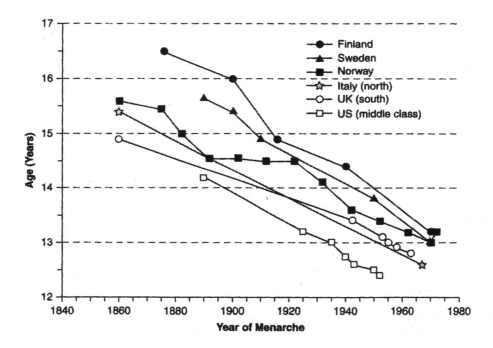

Figure 2-2-6 Declining age of puberty 1840–1980[123] © Wenda Trevathan

119 Steingraber, op. cit. p. xv.
120 AAP. *Pediatric Nutrition Handbook* 5th edition May 2012. p. 87; Currie D. Breastfeeding rates for black US women increase, but lag overall: Continuing disparity raises concerns. *The Nation's Health* 2013; 43 (3): 1–20. http://thenationshealth.aphapublications.org/content/43/3/1.3.full?sid=fd5bf00f-a218-43b0-9490-a40921f3b011
121 Zung A, Glaser T, Kerem Z, Zadik Z. Breast development in the first 2 years of life: an association with soy-based infant formulas. *J Pediatr Gastroenterol Nutr.* 2008; 46(2):191–5
122 Whittle S, Yücel M, Lorenzetti V, Byrne ML et al. Pituitary volume mediates the relationship between pubertal timing and depressive symptoms during adolescence. (PMID:22071452) *Psychoneuroendocrinology* 2012, 37(7):881–91.
123 Trevathan W. *Ancient Bodies, Modern Lives. How Evolution has shaped women's health.* (OUP 2010) p. 24. Used with permission.

Any study of forty children is too small to enable population conclusions to be drawn. Perhaps it is true, as the soy researchers clearly believe, that we needn't worry more about soy formulas than we should about bovine formula.

In 2001 a study was published[124] which also asserted that the outcomes of feeding soy and cows milk to infants in the period 1965–78 were similar in young adults, although there were some differences in menstrual bleeding and discomfort among those fed soy, which the (male) researchers thought of little importance. The adolescents involved might not agree. Because 'Exposure to soy formula does not appear to lead to different general health or reproductive outcomes than exposure to cow milk formula' the researchers felt that 'our findings are reassuring about the safety of infant soy formula.' This was yet another study with no exclusively breastfed controls. So because cows' milk is safe, so is soy? Logical? Only if you live in a society that depends on artificial feeding.

That cows milk and soy outcomes may be similar means little, if both deviate from the biological norm! Both formulas lack GnRH (gonadotropin releasing hormone) made by the breast and fed in milk, and known to suppress ovarian function.[125] I agree with these researchers that 'the few positive findings [the differences in menstruation] should be explored in future studies,' and suggest that they try to find a set of normal controls! For after all, bovine milk can contain significant amounts of more-bioactive oestrogen analogues derived from pasture and stock feed (which can include soy). Do the cows supplying milk for infant formula eat soy?

Despite the similarities in outcomes, soy formula use is actively discouraged by paediatricians, on the basis of quite reasonable speculation about possible effects, while bovine milk formula remains under investigated and assumed to be safe, without such public speculation about likely, possible and known effects. These studies indicate such effects do exist, as much for bovine milk as for soy. The Australian National Health and Medical Research Council (NHMRC) 2013 *Infant Feeding Guidelines* are typical of the current medical consensus and double talk:

> A number of concerns have been raised about soy-based infant formulas, on the basis of possible physiological effects of isoflavone compounds on the infant's developing neuroendocrine system. [True. We can't recommend them because we don't want to be responsible for any harm.] There is no clear clinical or scientific evidence to support the position that these compounds are harmful [so if you've used them don't worry] although no long-term studies have conclusively documented the product's safety in infants.[126] [So perhaps you shouldn't use them.]

This is having one's cake and eating it too, trying to keep everyone happy. Until the major companies move out of soy, the position will be 'hazard unproven'. If and when industry

124  Strom BL, Schinnar R, Ziegler EE, Barnhart KT et al. Exposure to soy-based formula in infancy and endocrinological and reproductive outcomes in young adulthood. (PMID:11497534) *JAMA* 2001;286(7):807–14 DOI: 10.1001/jama.286.7.807

125  Angier N. Mother's Milk Found to Be Potent Cocktail Of Hormones *New York Times* May 24, 1994. http://www.nytimes.com/1994/05/24/science/mother-s-milk-found-to-be-potent-cocktail-of-hormones.html

126  NHMRC. *Infant Feeding Guidelines for Healthworkers.* 2013. p.81.

does, which will be when some other cheap alternative has emerged, soy-based formula may be denounced as a bad idea, not to be discussed, a mistake like gluten in infant formula, or beef hearts, or peanut oil. But soy is still necessary at present, because many children react badly to bovine formula, so industry and US paediatricians[127] won't let it go just yet. Australia's NHMRC agrees:

> It is appropriate to use soy infant formula in the management of galactosaemia. Its use may also be appropriate for infants who cannot consume dairy-based products for cultural or religious reasons.[128]

Oh, and has anyone seen long-term studies showing no proof of harm from bovine formula? I'd say both soy and bovine rely on the same long-term 'evidence': 'look at the survivors (not too closely, mind), they were fed brand X and they are all 'normal' in a society where reproductive dysfunction, allergy, heart disease, obesity and so on are normal.'

So far as I can see, and I have looked, there is as much (which is to say as little) evidence of the long-term safety of cows' milk formulas as there is of soy, if one wears historical glasses. Without the Arkansas agricultural scientists' defence of soy, we would not have evidence that by as young as four months some aspects of infant reproductive development are already affected by bovine milk formulas as well as soy. I look forward to the long-term studies on these children who by four months of age were deviating from the (poorly defined and not exclusively) breastfed norm of reproductive tissue development at that early age. Think about this in relation to the concept of programming, the fact that early small changes can set development off on a different path (see page 62).

The Arkansas scientists concluded:

> Our data do not support major diet-related differences in reproductive organ size as measured by ultrasound in infants at age 4 months, although there is some evidence that ovarian development may be advanced in MF-fed infants and that testicular development may be slower in both MF and SF infants as compared with BF. There was no evidence that feeding SF exerts any estrogenic effects on reproductive organs studied.[129] *[Other possible effects and organs were not studied.]*

To me, this is a classic example of putting the best gloss on bad news. Who decides what differences at four months of age are major and minor? *Any* change in reproductive development, including advanced ovarian and delayed testicular development, sounds pretty major to most parents. They might prefer to read a clearer conclusion, such as:

> Both milk- and soy-formula-fed infants are already deviating slightly from the more-normal reproductive development of partially breastfed infants by as young as four months of age, although at that age, in these forty children, the deviations were not considered

---

127  Cohen S. *What to Feed Your Baby: cost-conscious nutrition for your infant.* (Rowman and Littlefield 2013). Cohen makes it clear that questions of cost make soy indispensable in WIC programmes, through which almost half of America's infant formula is distributed.

128  ibid,

129  Gilchrist JM et al. op. cit.

major. However, there is some evidence that ovarian development may be advanced in MF-fed infants and that testicular development may be slower in both MF and SF infants as compared with partially BF infants, which would be of concern to parents, as any deviation from normal growth parameters can be progressive over time. We did not have data from a group of exclusively breastfed infants for comparison, hence we have not mapped normal reproductive growth rates. Further research over the lifespan must be a priority. Meanwhile breastfeeding should be encouraged for these as for many other reasons.

The precautionary principle always suggests that until we know for certain that formula is safe it should be used only when there is no better alternative. (But there always could be, if women's milk was valued as it should be.)

One other thing struck me. The Arkansas soy researchers wrote that 'there were no significant feeding group effects in anthropometric or body composition'. But there should have been such differences by four months,[130] as breastfed infants typically grow along different parameters to babies fed infant formula. Breastfed babies are fatter at three months, and leaner at twelve months, than formula-fed ones. That's why growth charts have been altered.[131] And why industry has dropped the level of protein in formula lately. (See page 263.)

But no such effect was detected in these groups. Was the sample size too small to detect growth differences? Or was it the fact that none of these three groups was clearly defined? How much formula did the breastfed consume?

Reading the study carefully, it is clear that the breastfed infants may have been comp-fed, changing gut flora and with it, growth. Only 23 per cent of infants in the soy-formula-fed group had actually been fed soy formula from birth; 45 per cent switched to soy feeding within four weeks, and 32 per cent between four and eight weeks. Only 54 per cent of the bovine-formula-fed were so from birth; 41 per cent switched from breastmilk to cows' milk formula within four weeks, and 5 per cent switched between four and eight weeks. So many of those soy- and cow-milk-fed babies were breastfed as well as formula-fed, and the soy-fed might have got some cows' milk as well.[132]

What a muddle. It seems possible that all three groups included some infants who had been breastfed for a month (but none exclusively)! Perhaps growth differences would have shown up in properly defined groups.

That in turn would raise the question of whether much greater differences in reproductive tissue (as well as growth) might have been evident had the control group been completely breastfed from birth and the formula-fed never breastfed, or the sample size larger. An

130 Gale C, Logan KM, Santhakumaran S, Parkinson JR, Hyde MJ, Modi N. Effect of breastfeeding compared with formula-feeding on infant body composition: a systematic review and meta-analysis. *Am J Clin Nutr* 2012; 95(3):656–9.

131 de Onis M. Update on the Implementation of the WHO Child Growth Standards. *World Rev Nutr Diet* 2013; 106:75–82. (PMID:23428684)

132 How many stopped breastfeeding because free formula was on offer, I wonder? Will they regret doing so?

optimist would hope that a larger sample might cause the differences to become non-significant, that perhaps these were an aberrant or atypical sample of susceptible infants. Working from basic science and first principles, I would say the opposite would be more likely: the differences would be greater. Perhaps even 'major'.

Pilot studies are underway,[133] half a century after soy became a commonplace formula. A larger study was funded, but without many other large, totally independent, studies involving exclusively breastfed infants as controls, we won't know. Who will fund those studies? And if they're not funded, do we assume formula is safe, or warn parents of the possible risks? Even the word 'risk' is inflammatory when linked with infant feeding. (But not with any other avoidable risk our babies face.[134])

## So is soy worse than cows' milk?

At this stage of the debate, as with reproductive development, there seems to be little evidence that soy formula is uniquely worse than cows' milk formula, just plenty of evidence that both are inferior to women's milk. One expert US panel[135] that examined this concluded that 'there is minimal concern for adverse effects on development in infants who consume soy infant formula'. All the same, reading the full report on which this conclusion was based makes for great unease. As they say:

> Infants fed soy infant formula are reported to consume as much as 6.2 mg/kg bw/day of total genistein, thus a 5 kg infant would consume ~30 mg/day of total genistein. Blood levels of total genistein in infants fed a soy infant formula diet can exceed those reported in young rats or mice treated with genistein during development at dose levels that produced adverse effects, i.e., early onset of sexual maturation, altered estrous cyclicity and decreased litter size.[136]

The Report of the National Toxicology Program (NTP) goes on to note that other oestrogen analogues can indeed be found in babies fed on cows' milk formulas:

> The finding of equol being more readily detected in infants fed a cow milk-based formula [compared with infants fed soy or breastmilk] is not unexpected given that cows can

133 Bernbaum JC, Umbach DM, Ragan NB, Ballard JL, Archer JI, Schmidt-Davis H, Rogan WJ. Pilot studies of estrogen-related physical findings in infants. *Environ Health Perspect.* 2008 Mar;116(3):416–20.

134 Smith JP, Dunstone MD, Elliott-Rudde ME. 'Voldemort' And Health Professional Knowledge Of Breastfeeding – Do Journal Titles And Abstracts Accurately Convey Findings On Differential Health Outcomes For Formula Fed Infants? ACERH Working Paper Number 4 December 2008. Accessible online .acerh.edu.au/publications/ACERH_WP4.pdf See also Appendix 2.

135 McCarver G, Bhatia J, Chambers C, Bernbaum JC, Umbach DM, Ragan NB, Ballard JL, Archer JI, Schmidt-Davis H, Rogan WJ. Pilot studies of estrogen-related physical findings in infants. Environ Health Perspect. 2008 Mar;116(3):416–20. Clarke R et al. NTP-CERHR expert panel report on the developmental toxicity of soy infant formula. (PMID:21948615) *Birth Defects Research. Part B, Developmental and Reproductive Toxicology* 2011, 92(5):421–68. Can be downloaded from http://ntp.niehs.nih.gov/ntp/ohat/genistein-soy/soyformula/Soy-report-final.pdf

136 *NTP Brief on Soy Formula,* Sept 16, 2010. p. 41. Available at: http://ntp.niehs.nih.gov/ntp/ohat/genistein-soy/SoyFormulaUpdt/FinalNTPBriefSoyFormula_9_20_2010.pdf

produce equol from either the formononetin found in red clover or daidzein found in soy (King et al. 1998). [137]

The stated reason why the National Toxicology Program's official concern level is 'minimal' is simply because no scientific evidence exists:

> While these types of adverse effects have not been reported in humans during 60 years of soy infant formula usage, adequate studies of the reproductive system have also not been conducted on girls or women following use of soy infant formula during infancy. Thus, the data in humans are not sufficient to dismiss the possibility of subtle or long-term adverse health effects in these infants. [138]

Not sufficient indeed, especially in America, where (as we have seen) the age of puberty onset has been dropping, along with rising rates of uterine dysfunction and falling sperm counts, all in concert with babies exposed to both formula-feeding and petrochemical pollution. I strongly recommend, indeed urge, all my readers to buy a copy of *Raising Elijah: protecting our children in an age of environmental crisis,* by Sandra Steingraber. [139] As she makes clear, small changes can be significant. I did not find it surprising that two of the NTP's expert panel wanted to raise the level of stated risk above 'minimal.' Nor that with industry representation on the panel, they could not do so.

But, like concern about many other formula ingredients, the concern about soy is not what happens immediately, but what may be the results of such early tiny changes over a lifetime. There may be an association between being fed soy formula as a baby and prolonged more painful menstruation, [140] for example, and uterine changes such as fibroids. [141] I have not seen studies of endometriosis that looked at early childhood feeding patterns, but would be interested to see if that recent plague is more common in those soy-exposed as children.

## Soy researchers ask about infant brains

These same Arkansas scientists decided to 'compare the effects of the major infant diets on the development of brain electrical activity' during periods of quiet wakefulness at three, six, nine, and twelve months. Three groups of forty infants, who had been fed soy or cow formulas, or breastmilk, for six months, with other foods added after that, were studied.

Their conclusion opens up serious questions about the safety of all artificial feeding for neurological development:

> The development of brain electrical activity during infancy differs between those who are breastfed compared with those fed either milk or soy formula, but is generally similar for formula-fed groups. These variations in EEG activity reflect diet-related influences

---

137   ibid p. 38.
138   ibid p. 41.
139   Steingraber S. op. cit.
140   Strom BL, Schinnar R, Ziegler EE, Barnhart KT et al. op. cit.
141   D'Aloisio AA, Baird DD, DeRoo LA, Sandler DP. Association of intrauterine and early-life exposures with diagnosis of uterine leiomyomata by 35 years of age in the sister study. *Environ Health Perspect.* 2010 Mar;118(3):375–81. Erratum in: Environ Health Perspect. 2010 Mar;118(3):380

on the development of brain structure and function *that could put infants on different neurodevelopmental trajectories along which cognitive and brain function development will proceed.*[142]

A remarkably brave and honest statement. Both soy and bovine formula make for different brain development. Yet when asked about this research, one of the leading authors replied by email, 'I think parents who feed their children formulas, whether soy or milk, should not worry about any adverse effects.'[143] Neat evasion, even if I agree with him that there is little point in such families *worrying* about what cannot now be changed for their children! But did anyone think they heard him saying 'There is nothing to worry about, there are no adverse effects of soy formula.'? He didn't. And the journalist didn't press him to. Thus community ignorance of the impact of formulas on brain development is maintained.

Other researchers have pointed out that 'The primary concern of the ACNC (Arkansas Children's Nutrition Centre) would appear to have been the alleged health dangers arising from the isoflavone content of the soy protein isolate used in soy formula' and then gone on to say that 'in none of their reports to date has the ACNC acknowledged the potential problem associated with the [high] Manganese content of soy formula.'[144]

Should we be concerned, not about those already using formula, but about those yet to do so? The last trimester of pregnancy and the first two years of life are crucial for brain development. As Belfort et al summarised,

> During that time, the brain develops rapidly through the processes of neurogenesis, axonal and dendritic growth, synaptogenesis, cell death, synaptic pruning, myelination, and gliogenesis. These developmental processes build on each other over time so that a small disruption in any of the processes may have wide and long-lasting effects on brain structure and function.[145]

There is ample evidence that breastfed babies' brains develop differently from those of formula-fed babies, as we have already seen. These Arkansas researchers have themselves recently published a study[146] showing that the brains of breastfed babies at three and six months respond differently to speech compared to the brains of formula-fed babies. (Again, this is despite feeding being defined in ways that would tend to minimise the visible effect.

142 Jing H, Gilchrist JM, et al. A longitudinal study of differences in electroencephalographic activity among breastfed, milk formula-fed, and soy formula-fed infants during the first year of life. *Early Hum Dev.* 2010 Feb;86(2):119–25.

143 Badger: see http://www.reuters.com/article/2012/06/01/us-babies-soy-formula-idUSBRE8501BZ20120601 I agree that there is no point in parents worrying if already feeding soy. But other parents will choose soy needlessly if scientists make soothing noises whenever disturbing news is reported. Whoever suppresses truth is responsible for the consequences.

144 Schuck SEB, Emmerson N, Abdullah M, Crinella FM. Soy-based infant formula associated with increased risk for ADHD. In Preedy VR, Watson RR, Zibardi S (eds), op. cit. (Wageningen Academic Publishers 2014) p. 638

145 Belfort MB, Rifas-Shiman SL, Kleinman KP, Guthrie LB et al. Infant feeding and childhood cognition at ages 3 and 7 years: Effects of breastfeeding duration and exclusivity. (PMID:23896931) *JAMA Pediatr* 2013, 167(9):836–44.

146 Pivik RT, Andres A, Badger TM Effects of diet on early stage cortical perception and discrimination of syllables differing in voice-onset time: a longitudinal ERP study in 3 and 6-month-old infants. *Brain and Language* 2012, 120(1):27–41. DOI: 10.1016/j.bandl.2011.08.004

And despite the groups excluding all but healthy term infants, on whom the effects should be less than for preterm or sick infants.) The researchers concluded that 'the observed processing differences among diet groups may indicate that infants are on unique diet-associated paths of neurodevelopment.' Where do those paths lead? Another study has produced evidence that with soy formula there are effects on gender-role play in children at the age of forty-two months.[147]

Ongoing studies have shown other effects even in middle childhood.[148] Autism researchers suggest a relationship between soy-based infant formulas, manganese neurotoxicity and symptoms of ADHD,[149] while others are concerned about the impact of neurotoxins produced by gut bacteria which are not found in exclusively breastfed children (for more on autism see page 444). The different sleep patterns of breastfed and artificially fed infants[150] will result in developmental differences. The legacy of lead solder in infant formula cans and water supplies may affect a new generation. The absence of breastmilk's many hormones will certainly affect brain development. A huge range of differences between formulas could have differing effects on brain development. A finding that breastfeeding possibly 'protects against' the development of ADHD[151] needs to be re-investigated to ascertain which formulas most commonly produce it, and why. Especially when researchers have concluded that

> The most likely scenario is that infant ingestion of soy-based formula would not, in itself, precipitate full-blown (i.e., diagnosable) ADHD; however, the work reviewed here suggests that over-absorption of Mn could act to lower the threshold for the expression of ADHD symptoms in individuals who may be vulnerable, based on genetic and/or epigenetic influences.[152]

I could go on endlessly here, but the picture is clear: formula-fed kids are not going to develop as they would have if they had been breastfed.[153] And no one can predict how important will be the deviation from the normal expression of their genome, whether major or minor. It seems to me that there is little reason to be over-optimistic about the outcomes, when the US Centers for Disease Control and Prevention (CDC) reports that

147  Adgent MA, Daniels JL, Edwards LJ, Siega-Riz AM, Rogan WJ. Early-life Soy Exposure and Gender-role Play Behavior in Children. *Environ Health Perspect.* 2011;119(12):1811–16.

148  *Whitehouse AJ, Robinson M, Li J, Oddy WH.* Duration of breast feeding and language ability in middle childhood. (PMID:21133968) *Paediatric and Perinatal Epidemiology* 2011, 25(1):44–52.

149  Crinella FM Does soy-based infant formula cause ADHD? Update and public policy considerations. (PMID:22449212) *Expert Review of Neurotherapeutics* 2012, 12(4):395–407.

150  A topic which is a book in itself: I suggest reading anything by Dr James McKenna or Dr Helen Ball. See bibliography.

151  Mimouni-Bloch A, Kachevanskaya A, Mimouni FB, Shuper A et al. Breastfeeding May Protect from Developing Attention-Deficit/Hyperactivity Disorder. (PMID:23560473) *Breastfeed* Med 2013; 8(2): DOI:10.1089/bfm.2012.0145. Available at http://online.liebertpub.com/doi/full/10.1089/bfm.2012.0145

152  Schuck SEB, Emmerson N, Abdullah M et al. Soy-based infant formula associated with increased risk for ADHD. In Preedy V, Watson RR, Zibadi S (eds), op. cit. (Wageningen Academic Publishers 2014) p. 639

153  Oddy WH, Li J, Robinson M, Whitehouse AJO. The Long-Term Effects of Breastfeeding on Development in *Özdemir* O (ed), *Contemporary Pediatrics* 2012. ISBN 978-953-51-0154-3 DOI: 10.5772/34422 Open access. Available at http://www.intechopen.com/books/contemporary-pediatrics/the-long-term-effects-of-breastfeeding-on-development

between 13 and 20 per cent of US children 'experience a mental disorder in a given year and an estimated $247 billion is spent each year on childhood mental disorders'.[154]

There has long been stiff resistance to the idea that formula affects children's cerebral and cognitive development, and reassurances that children develop within normal limits with maybe just a small advantage to the breastfed. Few people have questioned how much those 'normal limits' have been influenced by past formula feeding. But by 2012 the fact that infant formula reduces potential is accepted by those studying the question in any scientific way. Some of that information is reviewed later (see 2.7.6) To cite just one source: the UK Millennium Cohort has produced a number of studies confirming that breastfeeding is associated with improved cognitive development, particularly in children born preterm;[155] that longer duration of breastfeeding, at all or exclusively, is associated with better educational achievement at age five;[156] and that longer duration of breastfeeding is associated with fewer parent-rated behavioural problems in children aged five years.[157] That's in a country where only 1 per cent of infants are solely breastfed to 6 months of age.

Despite the dearth of exclusively breastfed babies in most studies reviewed, and the failure to compare them with exclusively formula-fed babies, there is clearly an effect on brain development (which of course affects everything else). We simply don't know how big the effect is. Nor do we understand all the influences and mechanisms involved.

## Gold Formula for intelligence?

Industry marketing is already way out of sync with this science. From conversations with mothers, I am sure that global marketing has convinced many parents that infant formula with oils from genetically engineered fungi and algae, or other sources of DHA and ARA (long-chain fatty acids in breastmilk), will make their children just as smart, maybe even smarter, than breastfed babies of mothers whose diet is low in these essential fatty acids. Disadvantaged women, so little valued by society that many feel they have no reason to value their own body's product, and many who know their diet is less than perfect, may be tempted to choose the so-called 'Gold' formula which promises greater health and intelligence for their child.[158]

Yet, despite the expense, there is in fact very little evidence that these Gold formulas make any such difference. Follow-up even of preterm 'Gold' babies has shown no positive effect of supplements of long-chain polyunsaturated fatty acids (LCPUFAs) ten years later, unlike follow-up of breastfed children. The hypothesis had been that consumption of infant

---

154  The Report can be accessed online: see http://www.cdc.gov/features/childrensmentalhealth/

155  Quigley MA, Hockley C, Carson C, Kelly Y, Renfrew MJ, Sacker A. Breastfeeding is associated with improved child cognitive development: a population-based cohort study. (PMID:21839469) *The Journal of Pediatrics* 2012, 160(1):25–32.

156  Heikkilä K, Kelly Y, Renfrew MJ, Sacker A, Quigley MA. Breastfeeding and educational achievement at age 5. (PMID:22462489) *Maternal & Child Nutrition* 2012.DOI: 10.1111/j.1740-8709.2012.00402.x

157  Heikkilä K, Sacker A, Kelly Y, Renfrew MJ, Quigley MA. Breast feeding and child behaviour in the Millennium Cohort Study. (PMID:21555784) *Archives of Disease in Childhood* 2011, 96(7):635–42.

158  The explosion in sales of these products despite their high cost relative to unsupplemented formulas is proof of the success of this marketing campaign.

formulas containing LCPUFAs by preterm infants would favourably influence growth, body composition and blood pressure (BP) at ten years of age. The reality proved to be that

> Girls born preterm and randomised to LCPUFA-supplemented formula showed increased weight, adiposity and BP at nine to eleven years, which might have adverse consequences for later health. No effects were seen in boys. Long-term follow-up of other LCPUFA supplementation trials is required to further investigate this finding.[159]

A larger European study also found no positive benefit to such supplementation.[160] Those girls will gestate the next generation. Yet for almost twenty years now parents have been reading marketing aimed at them (talking of 'your baby') stating that what industry *acknowledges as the better brain and nervous system development of breastfed babies* 'are due to the presence of LCPs in breast milk.'[161] Well, some of that was factual, and only some misleading. But infant and child cognitive development is affected by much more than the fats in milk: see Figure 2-2-8 on page 53 and Figure 2-2-9 on page 54.

But fats are important, which is why, no matter what the breastfeeding mother's diet, her milk always includes some of the essential fatty acids DHA and ARA. Levels of these fatty acids in milk do increase with supplements or fish intake, but not all breastmilk fats are derived from diet: body stores contribute, and some are manufactured de novo by every breastfeeding woman. And only some babies seem to benefit from increased levels in breastmilk of these fats.[162] However, increasing the level is worth considering in allergic families.[163]

Even in the extreme case of donated low-fat 'drip milk' – breastmilk collected by spontaneous leakage into breast shells, a method which results in abnormally low fat content in that milk[164] – we know that giving some such milk to formula-fed infants can produce positive results (even when it is pasteurised before use,[165] not fresh, as women's donated milk has been in Norway since 1920.)

159  Kennedy K, Ross S, Isaacs EB, Weaver LT et al. The 10-year follow-up of a randomised trial of long-chain polyunsaturated fatty acid supplementation in preterm infants: effects on growth and blood pressure. (PMID:20515959) *Archives of Disease in Childhood* 2010, 95(8):588–95.

160  Beyerlein A, Hadders-Algra M, Kennedy K, Fewtrell M et al. Infant formula supplementation with long-chain polyunsaturated fatty acids has no effect on Bayley developmental scores at 18 months of age – IPD meta-analysis of 4 large clinical trials.. (PMID:19881391) *J Pediatr Gastroent Nutrition* 2010, 50(1):79–84.

161  Nutricia Australia material collected 1998, complete with cute bear with building blocks and statement that 'if your child is to reach their full genetic potential it is important that these nutrients [LCPs, described as building blocks for the brain] are supplied.'

162  Makrides M. DHA supplementation during the perinatal period and neurodevelopment: do some babies benefit more than others? (PMID:22698951) *Prostaglandins Leukot Essent Fatty Acids* 2013, 88(1):87–90.

163  Linnamaa P, Nieminen K, Koulu L, Tuomasjukka S, et al. Black currant seed oil supplementation of mothers enhances IFN-γ and suppresses IL-4 production in breast milk. (PMID:23980846) *Pediatr Allergy Immunol* 2013; 24(6):562–66.

164  Daly SEJ, Kent JC, Atwood CS, Warner BJ et al. Breastmilk fat content increases with the degree of breast emptying. (AGR:FNI93002536) *Proceedings – Nutrition Society of Australia.* 1991; 16:126.

165  Lucas A, Morley R, Cole TJ, Gore SM. A randomised multicentre study of human milk versus formula and later development in preterm infants. (PMID:8154907) *Arch Dis Child* 1994; 70(2):F141–6.

The study is worth looking at in detail. Of 300 mothers of preterm infants, 210 expressed a desire to breastfeed and 90 to formula-feed. In fact, only 193 provided some breastmilk, and only 35 of those were breastfeeding at discharge, so that 265 of the 300 were fully formula-fed as they went home. No details of post-discharge feeding was given, some mothers may have managed to re-lactate and breastfeed, but this would have been exceptional in 1980s UK. Yet at seven years of age, there were significant differences between the groups: the IQ advantage to the 193 defined as breastfed, over the 107 solely formula fed, was 8.3 points, and maternal choice made no difference to outcomes.[166]

What was not widely discussed about this IQ study is interesting. Sadly, the authors noted that 'before the start of the study in 1982, all infants in the three centres were fed on human milk (banked, or mother's own, or a combination.')[167] That would soon end. How dreadful the breastfeeding rates became in major UK neonatal units in the 1980s. Consider:

- Only 193 of 300 babies were breastmilk-fed at all, although 210 mothers had made the choice to breastfeed. Already 17 disappointed mothers.

- Then, only 35 of 193 breastmilk-fed babies were discharged home breastfeeding at all (not having breastmilk exclusively from birth).

- So another 158 disappointed mothers. 158+17 = 175 of 210 mothers who wanted to breastfeed, but went home with a bottle-fed baby.

- The overall IQ advantage for the 193 who got some breastmilk was 8.3 points.

- Interestingly, after the results for 35 breastfed at discharge babies were deducted, the overall IQ advantage in the remaining breastmilk-fed group of 158 dropped to 7.5 points.

- For that to be the case (if my maths are right) those 35 breastfed babies' average IQ advantage was 12.5 points! (193x8.3) – (158x7.5) = 436.9 divided by 35 = 12.48.

- Those 35 babies were not necessarily exclusively breastmilk fed, they were just the lucky few whose mothers managed to take them home breastfeeding. How long they continued to breastfeed after discharge into the hostile UK environment is not reported. How many were exclusively breastfed after discharge? For how long? How many exclusively breastfed until 6 months adjusted age? What was the *range* of advantage in that group and how did it correlate with breastfeeding duration? (The number is too small to be more than suggestive.)

- Perhaps that more than twelve point IQ advantage of the breastfed-at-discharge babies was the outcome of determined assertive mothers, who did their very best for the baby in other ways as well.

- Perhaps those 35 mothers were empowered and motivated by the effect on their mothering of lactation and breastfeeding.

---

166  Morley R, Cole TJ, Powell R, Lucas A. Mother's choice to provide breast milk and developmental outcome. (PMID:3202647) Free full text article *Arch Dis Child* 1988; 63(11):1382–85

167  Lucas A, Morley R, Cole TJ, Gore SM et al. Early diet in preterm babies and developmental status in infancy. *Arch Dis Child* 1989; 64: 1570–78.

- Or perhaps it was the breastmilk they supplied for so much longer, which programmed children for very different brain development?

- Either way, 175 mothers who began to breastfeed (and 175 former prems) seem to me to have reason to be angry: breastfeeding was not both respected and facilitated in units capable of conducting good research, but not capable of good clinical practice in breastfeeding support before and after discharge. And were there sound reasons why 17/210 mothers who wanted to breastfeed did not even begin?

- Altogether 265 of 300 mothers of premature babies never breastfed them at home, a shocking statistic.

These results are summarised below.

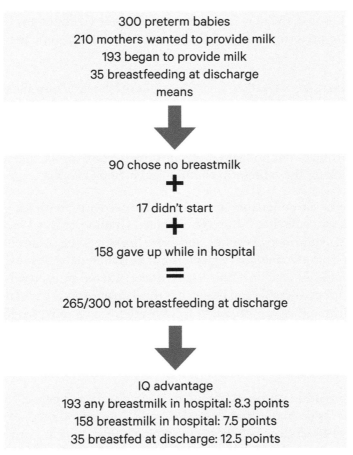

Figure 2-2-7 Preterm babies and IQ difference

The same group did a comparative study of the effects of infant formulas. One 1982-1985 cohort of low-birth-weight infants was widely reported as showing better cognitive outcomes for those fed a newly developed preterm formula.[168] Boys fed solely term formula

---

168  Lucas A, Morley R, Cole TJ. Randomised trial of early diet in preterm babies and later intelligence quotient. (PMID:9831573) *BMJ* 1998, 317(7171):1481–87.

(or solely low-calorie banked drip breastmilk) were significantly disadvantaged, more so than girls, both at eighteen months,[169] and

> At 7½–8 years boys previously fed standard versus preterm formula **as sole diet** had a 12.2-point disadvantage (95% confidence interval 3.7 to 20.6; P<0.01) in verbal IQ. In those with highest intakes of trial diets corresponding figures were 9.5-point disadvantage and 14.4-point disadvantage in overall IQ (1.2 to 17.7; P<0.05) and verbal IQ (5.7 to 23.2; P<0.01).[170]

Yet few noticed that receiving a little donated breastmilk of uncertain quality obliterated those significant differences in neurodevelopmental outcomes between the two groups of artificially-fed babies. Dr Michael Wooldridge drew this to my attention. That fact is not commented on. Instead, the difference in outcomes between those fed solely standard term infant formula and solely the new Farley preterm formula (without any breastmilk) led to a rapid adoption of preterm formula globally, and presumably, some benefit to the patent holders.[171]

Interestingly, while there was talk of the advantages of breastmilk over standard formula in the earlier study, the reporting here is of the *disadvantage* standard formula created. Had the first study been reported differently, emphasising a twelve point disadvantage created by standard formula, it may have sparked renewed global interest in using breastmilk, rather than expensive formulas. It is not hard to obtain donated breastmilk, and just a month or so of donor breastmilk for these preterm children had lifelong effects.

Personally, I have never understood how any major paediatric research group could have used low-fat milk as a sole diet for preterm infants. Granted, it was 1982 when this study began, but every dairy farmer, every vet, and every breastfeeding counsellor was aware that milk which leaks from the mammary gland is not as rich in fat as that expressed by infant mouth, human hands, or machine. The disadvantage suffered by preterms fed only banked breastmilk was both predictable and tragic; it is the damage done by under-nutrition. Heat-treated banked drip milk is very different from mother's own milk, freshly fed. I can only see this multi-centre study as a marker for medical ignorance of lactation at the time. Its results will continue to emerge over time as the children are followed up. The damage may be no more than would have been done by infant formula, but it was still avoidable.

There are numerous other studies about infant feeding and intelligence. None suggests that artificially fed infants do better than breastfed ones. Though the method of delivering the milk may also have effects, the benefit of consuming human milk at critical developmental moments, does not depend on the method of delivery, as Lucas et al have shown.

---

169  Lucas A, Morley R, Cole TJ, Gore SM et al. Early diet in preterm babies and developmental status in infancy. *Arch Dis Child* 1989; 64: 1570–78.

170  Lucas A, Morley R, Cole TJ, Lister G et al. Breast milk and subsequent intelligence quotient in children born preterm.(PMID:1346280) *Lancet* 1992; 339(8788):261-264. **DOI:** 10.1016/0140-6736(92)91329–7 ;

171  It is free to search patent databases such as http://patft.uspto.gov and discover the names of those patenting the formula.

Children who had consumed mother's milk in the early weeks of life had a significantly higher IQ at 7 1/2–8 years than did those who received no maternal milk. An 8.3 point advantage (over half a standard deviation) in IQ remained even after adjustment for differences between groups in mother's education and social class (p less than 0.0001). This advantage was associated with being fed mother's milk *by tube rather than with the process of breastfeeding.*[172]

By comparison with women's milk and breastfeeding, artificial formula (regular or Gold) and bottle feeding reduces infants' cognitive potential. It can do so through many pathways. It is not controversial that nutrition and mode of feeding affects infant nutritional status, immune response, and oro-facial structure, as well as maternal behaviour. Some of the links between just these four factors these and cognitive outcomes are summarised in the following confuseagram..

## Some infant feeding factors with wider effects

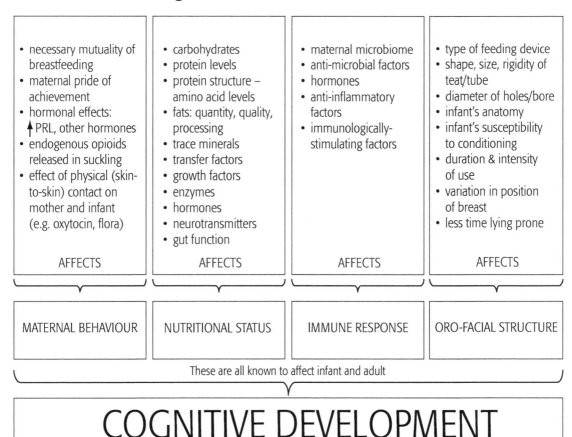

Figure 2-2-8 Some infant feeding factors with wider effects

172  Lucas A, Morley R, Cole TJ, Lister G et al.. Breast milk and subsequent intelligence quotient in children born preterm. (PMID:1346280) *Lancet* 1992, 339(8788):261-264] DOI: 10.1016/0140-6736(92)91329-7.

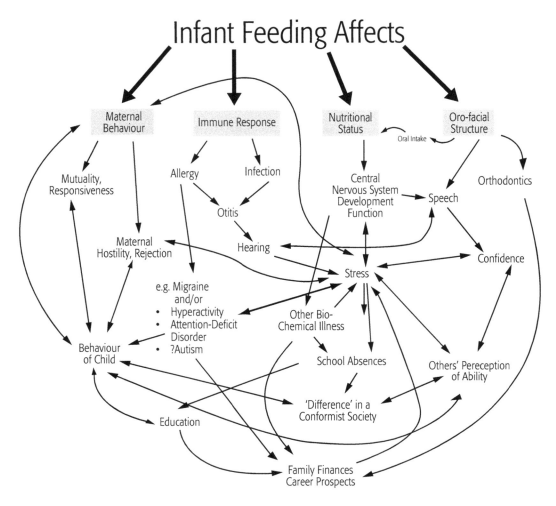

# Infant Feeding Affects

Figure 2-2-9 Pathways for feeding effects on child development

The effects of each of these details is both direct and indirect, greater in infants with poorer immune systems created by the absence of breastmilk and the presence of higher allergen loads via formula. Yet all too often child intelligence is discussed, formula's role is downplayed and the other factors implicated, in order to spare the feelings of parents who have not breastfed. Many healthworkers who downplay the effects were themselves or have themselves formula fed, of course: it was educated women who took up bottle feeding in the first half of the twentieth century, remember.

The most that modern formula advocates can do is to claim that the differences measured are not all that big – or if they are, allege that they are the result of other unmeasured confounding factors. And if that doesn't work, they simply impugn the motives of those measuring. Some formula fantasists claim that the newest formulas have addressed this problem by adding those fungal and algal oils, even though – as noted elsewhere – there is no proof of benefit from such additives. Instead, as Dr Robert Lawrence says, 'The constant frenzy of formula companies including one more additive in their formula ... to make it better than the rest and more like breast milk is one more proof that breast milk remains the gold standard for infant feeding.'[173]

## Cognition and genetic difference

Cognitive development effects may also be linked to genetic differences. Indications are emerging, such as a variation in fatty acid metabolism (see page 139).[174] (But did feeding influence maternal or infant gene expression?) We need vast amounts of data about how genes are expressed, and how brains function, and bodies grow, comparing infants who are fully breastfed with infants who are not,[175] ascertaining if the mothers with unfavourable genetic differences were themselves formula fed as children. Will any of this be a priority for research funding? If the formula corporations fund such studies, will the results be published if they are likely to damage sales? There is no obligation on industry to publish, and a great deal of company research is simply cited as 'data on file.' (Trust us, we're the good guys.)

Some claim that it is the mother's education which makes the difference, not her milk. Before accepting that, we also need studies assessing how the process of lactation and feeding affects women's gene expression, their cerebral structures, and their ongoing cognitive and maternal development. Like pregnancy, lactation seems likely to grow the mother-brain (see page 17).

## An intelligent perspective

It is true, however, that all this discussion of intelligence and cognitive development needs to be kept in perspective. Firstly, as one previewer of this book wrote to me,

> It is also good to point out that despite all the avoidable problems from bottle-feeding, people have never lived so long! ... [My bottle-fed mother] got a first class degree and lived to 93.

That mother, born in 1914, was not fed modern industrial milks, but would have been bottle-fed diluted cows' milk, perhaps with lactose, cod-liver oil, and the rest of the regime usual in the early years of the twentieth century. Today, health authorities would see this infant's diet as deficient in many ways, utter dire warnings to any parents following such guides, and in America probably have the child taken into care if parents persisted in feeding it. Yet infant adaptability is such that provided they get enough clean food and water, some

---

173  Lawrence RA, Pane CA op. cit., p. 17.
174  Caspi A, Williams B, Kim-Cohen J et al (2007). 'Moderation of breastfeeding effects on the IQ by genetic variation in fatty acid metabolism' *Proceedings of the National Academy of Sciences* 104 (47): 18860–5. PMC 2141867. PMID 17984066. DOI:10.1073/pnas.0704292104. ^ N. W. Martin, B. Benyamin, N. K. Hansell, G. W. Montgomery et al. Cognitive function in adolescence: testing for interactions between breast-feeding and FADS2 polymorphisms. *J Am Acad Child Adolesc Psychiatr*, 2011; 50, 55-62 e4. 10.1016/j.jaac.2010.10.010 ^ Steer CD, Davey Smith G, Emmett PM, Hibbeln JR et al. 'FADS2 polymorphisms modify the effect of breastfeeding on child IQ'. *PLoS ONE* 2010; 5 (7): e11570. DOI:10.1371/journal.pone.0011570. PMC 2903485. PMID 20644632.
175  Baby's IQ Raised by Breastmilk and Genes Source: http://today.duke.edu/2007/11/breastIQ.html

babies can adapt to any diet and thrive, as Iceland's centuries of disastrous artificial feeding proved. Icelandic babies were fed raw milk, raw cream, fish and chewed meat. The infant mortality rate was appalling; most died before twelve months; interbirth intervals were short. Of a typical fifteen children, two or three survived. 'Only among the poorest would the infants survive, because they could not afford cows' milk' (and so were breastfed!)[176] The observed facts did not alter the cultural prejudice that richer foods would be better than women's milk.

About that bottle-fed grandmother, born in 1914, who lived to 93. Her daughter, a doctor, added:

> But she did have horrible migraines and severe short sight. Two of her children had obvious allergy problems, two have ended up with diabetes, and all three with various degrees of obesity. I am 4 inches shorter than my mother and both my grandmothers. I was bottle fed in the 1940s. The first two years of my life I vomited frequently, was diagnosed with 'acidosis,' and failed to gain much weight; later suffered from eczema and bronchitis and was diagnosed as allergic to fur, dust mite and feathers (no test for milk) by the age of eight. In my teens I developed sinus problems, which became chronic, but have finally improved – so long as I totally avoid all cow's milk products. I am OK with sheep and goat yoghurt and cheese.
>
> I breast fed my son for six months, but he had been comp fed (supposedly to help his very mild neonatal jaundice) after induced delivery (for no good reason) at term. Five weeks later he developed encephalitis for which he was hospitalized, and again fed artificially by nasogastric tube for a week. I was surprised how quickly my breast milk production recovered when he revived and sucked well; he remained well until weaning foods were given from 6 months, when he started to become miserable, failed to thrive, and had chronic diarrhoea, which all resolved when he was taken off all cow's milk products aged 8 months.
>
> I have a daughter now in her forties, who has developed some recurring respiratory symptoms and is obese, but never seemed to be intolerant of cow's milk. I drank much less milk while pregnant with my daughter as I was on a weight watchers diet. I breast fed my daughter fully for 3 months and partially to 6 months. My daughter now has my first grandchild, who has been fully breastfed for 6 months and partially until the present, when he is 14 months. He has had a few infections of the gastrointestinal and respiratory tract, no doubt picked up from other families they mix with, but appears to be fundamentally healthy and well able to tolerate a wide variety of foods.

The life force is strong, and survival the priority. As Icelandic babies proved, the weakest and worst-fed may go to their grave, others may be less than they might have been, but *some babies will survive and grow on any food in any environment.* And their parents will believe

---

176  See Hastrup K, A question of reason: breast-feeding patterns in 17th and 18th century Iceland. In Maher V (ed.) *The Anthropology of Breastfeeding: Natural Law or Social Contract*? (Berg Publishers Oxford 1992); also Gardarsdottir O . The dramatic decline of infant mortality in Iceland 1770–1930. http://www.rhd.uit.no/kvinnforsk/papers/Olof_Gardarsdottir.pdf

that this is because of the food, not despite it. Formula is widely credited with lowering infant mortality. In fact, the biggest drop in infant mortality came before antibiotics and vaccines and modern formulas. Basic sanitation, communal hygiene measures, pasteurisation of milk, adequate nutrition and female education were the keys. Those were the factors that first improved western life expectancy rates: if they survived the first ten years of childhood, nineteenth-century men lived on average to seventy-one and women to seventy-seven. They are the factors still missing in too much of the globe, and in their absence infant formula will be more often lethal.

Secondly, many bottle-fed babies will be just fine cognitively, as this woman clearly was (despite not being fed a 'Gold' formula!) But that doesn't mean that there are no adverse consequences. The family history shows how immune disorder – probably connected to infant diet – resonates through this woman's descendants. There is talk now of this generation outliving its children thanks to the NCDs. Which infant feeding influences.

## The societal impact

So of course some bottle fed babies are smart. But it should be emphasised that, as Needleman said about lead, average figures ('means' in statistics) for IQ or verbal skill losses don't tell the whole story.

> This four to seven point difference in means [between lead-exposed and non-exposed children] has been taken by some as a small effect. This is deceptive ... A shift in the curve resulting in a difference in medians of 6 points results in a fourfold increase in the rate of severe deficit (IQ<80). In addition, the same shift in distribution truncates the upper end of the curve, where superior function is displayed, by 16 points. This means that 5% of lead-exposed children are prevented from achieving truly superior function (IQ>125). The costs of this effect at the high end of the distribution have received no attention. They may be extraordinarily important to our society.[177]

As Anderson et al said in the conclusion to their meta-analysis,

> An IQ increase of 3 points (one-fifth of a standard deviation) from 100 to 103 would elevate an individual from the 50th to the 58th percentile of the population and would potentially be associated with higher educational achievement, occupational achievement, and social adjustment.[178]

Just imagine what a difference over 12 IQ points makes to the population distribution and to those individuals at the ends of the range especially. The following diagram makes the point:

---

177  Needleman HL. The persistent threat of lead: a singular opportunity.(PMID:2650573). *Am J Public Hlth* 1989; 79: 643-5. Free online.

178  Anderson JW, Johnstone BM, Remley DT. Breastfeeding and cognitive development: a meta-analysis. *Am J Clin Nutr* 1999; 70: 525–35.

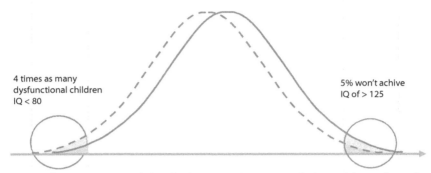

| **Low IQ Individuals** | **Bulk of population** | **High IQ Individuals** |
|---|---|---|
| Small shift in the curve results in large **increase** of individuals with lower IQ than is required to function day to day. | IQ drop of a few points is real, but not discernible on day to day basis; other inputs may compensate. | Small shift in the curve results in large reduction of "gifted" individuals within a population |

4 times as many
dysfunctional children
IQ < 80

5% won't achive
IQ of > 125

Intelligence conforms to a normal distribution curve in any population, with small numbers at the top and bottom of the range. When the IQ of the whole population is affected by any external factor, whether lead or infant formula, these areas are the most affected. The effect can also be extreme in individuals with genetic susceptibilities to the factor involved.

Figure 2-2-10 Normal distribution curve and the effects of a
loss of IQ points [Image by Catherine Horsfall]

The loss of an average few IQ points might not make much difference to the child of average intelligence, who is well cared for by articulate bottle feeding mothers with high incomes, who goes to a good school and has many social opportunities.

For poorer families, that same loss of just a few points can mean no access to a scholarship that might have changed a child's whole future and his family's, as it did mine.

At the population level, shifting that bell curve just a little means a large jump in the number of people with costly intellectual disabilities and heartbreak for their families, along with a substantial drop in the number of geniuses.

Needleman argued that the loss of potential (due to lead) at both ends of the curve was hugely costly to society. Rutter commented that

> The cognitive deficits which have been found are usually in the order of 3–5 points, and it has been argued that a 5-point difference is so trivial in its effects that it can be safely ignored. That is a totally fallacious argument. A drop of 5 points in mean IQ for any population must necessarily result in a more than two-fold increase in the percentage of individuals with an IQ below 70, that is, a doubling of the number of mentally retarded children.[179]

---

179   Wilson D. *The Lead Scandal.* (Heinemann 1983) p. 24.

Whether due to lead or to infant formula, that is horrendous. At the family level, just one damaged child requiring special education and care over a lifetime can be utterly devastating, even for those with abundant financial resources. I find it deeply distasteful that any educated middle class mother – or doctor, or academic – could argue against intensive, effective, emotion-stirring marketing, and social re-structuring and rewards to enable breastfeeding, just because such social marketing makes currently-bottle-feeding mothers feel bad. Future lives are at stake: other people's children stand to lose far more than theirs from ignorance and lack of support. Parents *are* ignorant: the 'breast is best' mantra conveys nothing of the risks of not breastfeeding. And parents *do* lack support, and they will for so long as formula is thought to be safe enough. And because in large numbers formula feeders do so publicly, so will aspiring parents in communities where to do so is often lethal, and remediation of damage difficult.

The population-wide impact of artificial feeding on cognitive development does not mean that any parent will necessarily see clear impacts on individual intelligence and cognition. There will still be many smart formula-fed children – which proves nothing. Thanks to brain plasticity (the ability of the brain to grow new connections), a positive learning environment can help make up any cognitive deficits – unless serious structural damage has been done, deranging essential neurological development. Obviously social disadvantage and lack of access to such an environment are part of the reason for worse outcomes for some children. And who can tell when any child could have been a genius, but is now only clever – because not breastfed? Or was going to be of average intelligence, and instead is a bit slow to learn – because not breastfed? Just as some children inherit a greater risk for allergy, others for metabolic disorders, so some children will inherit a greater risk for obvious neurological or cognitive defects. That some others are not *obviously* harmed does not mean that invisible harms, caused directly or potentiated by artificial feeding, are not real in the population at large. Just as with lead exposure, or serious pesticide contamination, talk of average losses obscures the reality of serious damage to some. Only the self-interested or stupid fail to acknowledge this obvious point.

What is more, on top of any inherent damage from the composition or contaminants of 'properly used' formula, needless further damage to the infant brain may occur, due to over-concentration or dilution of feeds, or to 'progressing/advancing' very young babies on to what in the past have been higher-protein follow-on formulas. Industry politely warns against these things, saying 'improper preparation' is hazardous, but never so plainly as to raise concerns about the utter impossibility of exact formulation. The nature of the product, the widespread lack of parental education about infant formula, and financial constraints, make such problems inevitable. Yet if a child is found to have been harmed, society judges – often harshly – that *the parents* are culpable, not the industry which did not highlight problems to all its customers, the semi-literate, illiterate, non-native speaking, and intellectually challenged, as well as to the careful, educated label-reader. (This is an industry which sometimes even sells products labelled in a foreign language in contexts where illiteracy is high!)

Harm can also come from not diversifying the artificially-fed diet appropriately, so that babies go on being fed a virtual cows' milk diet for a year or even longer, trusting the 'nutritional insurance' of follow-on and then toddler formula, and not bothering too much about the quality of other foods offered. Industry is to blame here when the recommended amounts of such mixtures, up to 1.2 L per day in one case, reduce infant appetite for other food. As noted elsewhere, every month of formula-feeding and delay in widening the diet of formula-fed infants seems to be associated with higher levels of childhood leukaemia:[180] Is it also associated with brain injury? Does the difference in brain white matter development noted in children who become autistic start with their feeding habits?[181] And does the base protein matter: for instance, is soy formula uniquely dangerous to brain development, or are cows' milk formulas just as dangerous in the same, or different, ways? The many possibilities in infant formula protein and the effects of processing add up to a reality in which commercial infant formulas can fall within the (necessarily?) wide limits of regulated composition, while varying greatly in quality. Differences are not limited to soy versus cows' milk, and there is a lot more research to be done.

## It's not just breastmilk or breastfeeding, it's also the formula!

The intelligence discussion in the past has centred on breastfeeding as beneficial, and tried to ascertain if it is the milk itself, the handling and contact that breastfeeding entails, or simply the characteristics of the women who breastfeed that makes the difference. Because these are enmeshed factors, it's impossible to know exactly how much each contributes. But as the percipient Dr Jerome L Sullivan said,

> There is a third class of possible explanations ... Some property of infant formula may diminish developmental potential. This alternative explanation raises the possibility that breastfed children represent a normal reference population and that formula-fed children are harmed in some way in comparison with the breastfed group. The findings appear equally compatible with either an improved outcome from breastfeeding or, alternatively, a deficit conferred by some property of infant formula.[182]

Until recently many did not accept that breastfed children represent a normal reference population, and instead used formula-fed children as that reference. Such cognitive deficit and subtle distortion seems to me inevitable while formulas continue to expose babies to high levels or different balances of amino acids (brain neurotransmitters) and minerals such as cadmium, aluminium and manganese,[183] a particular problem for soy formulas and the more heavily processed formulas, such as those for preterm infants or children with metabolic disorders, even in 2010.[184] Then there was twenty to one hundred times as

---

180  http://www.medicaldaily.com/articles/12766/20121018/longer-period-infant-formula-feeding-increase-leukemia.htm#iEBzCokEBoU3wCUW.99

181  Wolff JJ, Gu H, Gerig G, Elison JT et al. IBIS Network. Differences in white matter fiber tract development present from 6 to 24 months in infants with autism. (PMID:22362397) *Am J Psychiatry* 2012, 169(6):589-600. See also Deoni SC, Dean DC 3rd, Piryatinksy I, O'Muircheartaigh J et al. Breastfeeding and early white matter development. (PMID: 23721722) *Neuroimage*, 2013. DOI: 10.1016/j.neuroimage.2013.05.090;

182  Sullivan JL. Cognitive Development: Breast-Milk Benefit vs Infant Formula Hazard. *Arch Gen Psychiatry* 2008; 65 (12): 1456. Downloaded from www.archgenpsychiatry.com April 24, 2012

183  Lönnerdal B. Nutritional aspects of soy formula. *Acta Paediatr* 1994, 402:105-108; Erikson KM, Thompson K, Aschner J, Aschner M. Manganese neurotoxicity: a focus on the neonate. *Pharmacol Ther* 2007; 113 (2):369–77.

184  Burrell SA, Exley C. There is (still) too much aluminium in infant formulas. (MED:20807425) *BMC Pediatrics* 2010, 10:63. DOI: 10.1186/1471-2431-10-63.

much chromium in Belgian formula-fed children,[185] eighty to one hundred times as much fluoride ...[186] And doubtless they still do when this book is published: no company has yet trumpeted that they can consistently provide a formula with lower levels of heavy metals than those in the past. Industry has always marketed even small changes: that would be a game changer! Not, however, one I think likely to be used as a marketing tool ... Later chapters of this book provide more information about such relevant, though inadvertent, infant formula ingredients.

Effects on intelligence in children will vary. We can never know ahead of time exactly which children are the most vulnerable, or the best protected, against such damage by artificial feeding. As a group, preterm babies are known to be at greater risk of cognitive damage, as are intra-uterine growth restricted infants. And, almost certainly, children of allergic families. In western communities, that is a very large and ever-increasing number of higher-risk children, in whom cerebral effects are often overlooked or wrongly ascribed to parental care. It has been interesting to hear from adults now conscious of definite and immediate mood and emotion swings in response to unexpected allergen exposure, with the allergen identified after the mood swing raised suspicion about exposure. (See page 652)

There is less in this book about the effects of infant feeding and later diet on temperament and relationships and pyschological development and such intangibles than I would like. Concentrating on more readily-measurable physical markers is not an indication that I think such 'mental' issues less important, or styles of parenting not to have marked effects on child development. Responsive caregiving can probably help make up IQ lost to early dysnutrition, in all but those unlucky enough to have been brain-injured at a critical time of development. Anyone who doubts the importance of consistent and responsive caregiving should read the writings of Alison Fleming and Oliver James and Margot Sunderland, to which I will refer later. But of course there are mutual feedback loops set in train along the right paths for most humans, by the experiences of birth and breastfeeding.

---

185  Deelstra H et al. Daily chromium intake of infants in Belgium. *Acta Paediatr Scand* 1988; 77: 402–7.
186  Ekstrand J, Boreus LO, de Chateau P. No evidence of transfer of fluoride from plasma to breast milk. (PMCID:PMC1506856) Free full text article B*r Med J* (Clin Res Ed) 1981; 283(6294):761–62

## 2.3 Programming babies

Discussions of 'programming' in infancy took off after the CIBA Foundation's 1991 Symposium presentations,[187] in which many speakers discussed the idea. 'Programming' describes the reality that small early changes in physical and neurological development in pregnancy and after birth may take a baby's tissue and organ growth subtly or grossly off track, with long-term consequences. As Lucas said in that symposium, 'a stimulus or insult at a critical stage of development has lasting or lifelong significance.' The deviation from the (solely breastfed) norm may be small initially, but it can result in major differences later after tissues develop along different trajectories than they would have done without that initial tiny distortion. The differences can be imperceptible or seemingly slight at a few months of age, like those reproductive tissue differences Arkansas scientists observed. Only later will the results emerge, and then only be seen if looked for. The first drop of mineral-laden water in a cave is unseen, yet over time drops of water build rock formations, stalactites and stalagmites. A constant tiny breeze in one area of the cave means one formation grows at an angle, while without that tiny breeze another stays vertical. Changes in growth trajectories are often unnoticeable at the beginning, but result in different outcomes over time.

That rocky metaphor is limited. Growing a body is infinitely more complex, with so many organs and tissues all needing to develop into their optimal shape, interact, and work well. Small things at critical moments can derail complex developments. How much the difference matters can be hard to assess until it is too late to fix ('For the want of a nail ...'). Differences in areas of the brain controlling behaviours like speech, for example, might begin before or after birth. But they will not become obvious until the normal age of speech development, and as the range of normal can be wide, delays in diagnosis of problems are common. 'Adequate nutrition' may allow for normal visible external growth, but no one can begin to assess subtle deficiencies and problems until they have emerged. By then it is too late for prevention, and even remediation may be difficult unless some awareness of contributing factors emerges.

Each baby is an unrepeatable one-off experiment. Even a cloned animal grows in a different environment from its original; and among identical twins raised in the same household differences can and do arise, and can compound over time to become substantial. And *some* of the similar health problems in twins raised separately may be due to the greater likelihood of multiples not having been breastfed at all, much less for the same length of time, and the effect of that artificial feeding on their genome and microbiome. This is rarely mentioned in studies of adult twins.

Likewise, as this book argues, seemingly small changes arising from formula-feeding may be linked to Western epidemics of ADHD and autism, as well as obesity and 'allergy' and diabetes and the rest. Other environmental exposures can also have such effects, but unlike some of these, artificial feeding is almost always avoidable. Do we just accept that infant formula may have such impacts on human development, and rationalise its results as 'normal' just because they are usual? Do we accept a society in which a growing

---

187 CIBA Foundation Symposium 156. *The Childhood Environment and Adult Disease.* (John Wiley & Sons, 1991)

underclass of women are forced to return to low-paid work early by policies and economic systems that disregard women's important biological role of breastfeeding, thereby further disadvantaging their babies? Do we reward the wealthy by policies that allow only privileged educated mothers to breastfeed? If we do, we are programming our society away from what I see as fundamental Australian norms of democratic equality of opportunity – as well as our babies away from their mammalian blueprint. Both biologically and culturally, changes such as these are serious and cumulative, affecting more than the exposed generation.[188]

## Programming the allergy-to-autoimmune-disease march?

Stockbreeders are well aware of the phenomenon of inter-generational amplification of immune problems, seen in the progressive degeneration of animal health. They don't breed from unhealthy animals, but cull them – just as some deplorable eugenicists of the early twentieth century wished to do with the 'lower classes' from which some of us are descended. But this concept of amplifying intergenerational harms by infant feeding isn't discussed in standard allergy textbooks, despite the clear evidence of parental history affecting children's risks.

Clinicians naturally focus on the patient and the immediate issues, and patients do grow out of some symptoms over time, or learn instinctively or consciously to avoid the dietary or airborne allergens causing symptoms. There may seem little point in trying to identify inherited risks and when they arose. I think doing so is important for both psychological and practical reasons, as the chapters to come explain. And when you look for ongoing allergy through life in people who outgrew some classic identified symptom like eczema, you find it, in quite large numbers of people, as those Finnish researchers did with their cohort of seventeen-year-olds (see page 72).

Of course, people also grow into other symptoms that cannot be ignored, so the very limited concept of the 'allergic march' (eczema to asthma, for example) is now accepted. But in my experience, that allergic march – or more accurately 'slide', as it's mostly helplessly downhill – continues to the grave. I know many people who have grown out of some symptoms, or learned to tolerate small amounts of foods that once caused them great distress. Over decades of dealing with this, I know no one who has completely grown out of established hypersensitivity or allergy. I know many people who have grown out of specific symptoms when exposed to allergenic foods, had years of better health, then found symptoms emerging unpredictably in later years, usually in times of stress or immune overload (see Figure 4-6-1 on page 610). And the new symptoms can be far more varied (and far more easily overlooked, ignored or denied) than eczema, asthma and hayfever, the classic trio doctors accept as allergic in origin. In fact, children who showed no sign of any cerebral or mental effects such as hyperactivity, aggression or depression can manifest these in adulthood. Inflammatory diseases of many kinds emerge, including autoimmune disease. The march continues, the band plays on, and the tunes are idiosyncratic by the time people reach middle age.

---

188   For parents who want to understand more of the epigenetic mechanisms, I cannot recommend too highly Susan Prescott's simple outline of what is involved. And the bibliography will serve as a reading guide!

Every human being is a unique composition, and so the manifestations of immune-related dysfunction can be surprising. When a follow up of four-year-old children who had 'grown out of' what their doctors described as colic was undertaken, the colic survivors 'displayed more negative emotions according to the temperament scale. There were also more negative moods during meals, and more reported stomach-ache.' From which the researchers concluded that 'the findings point toward a possible temperamental contribution to the pathogenesis of the infantile colic syndrome.' Really? The reverse is also possible: that having had such painful bodily disturbances when little, they were still experiencing problems, and it made them feel rather negative, especially around food, which still gave them stomach aches (or head aches),[189] though perhaps not so acutely. The burden of coping with this form of ill-health, often being misunderstood or blamed or accused of malingering, and badgered about eating, can leave its own emotional scars and shape relationships and personalities – influencing lifelong 'temperaments'.[190]

Parents often see things that way, and ask me intelligent questions about the allergic march and its heritability. My realisation that the allergic band plays on into the next generation was initially the result of conversations with involved grandmothers. Very often, these women would remark on the fact that at the same age as their daughters now were, they had had all the symptoms that their daughters had just lost after changing diet – at my suggestion – to solve their breastfed baby's colic problems. Now realising that these problems might be related to immune dysfunction, and immune dysfunction to food, they would ask whether their now diagnosed autoimmune diseases (Crohn's disease, lupus, MS, etc.) could be related to those earlier problems.

Grandma would tell me that daughter had been just such another crying 'difficult' baby, that daughter had developed allergic symptoms as a child, that daughter's health was so much better now that she was on a diet that made her breastfed baby happy ... and that grandma's own life mirrored that of her daughter's. Two questions were raised: would daughter also progress to autoimmune disease, if she went back to her old diet after weaning the baby? Would grandmother's autoimmune disease improve if she tried the dietary changes that had helped her daughter?[191]

---

189  The idea that colic may be associated with parental migraine seems to be gaining strength, so that a new theory is defining infant colic as being infant migraine or headache. The association is there, but the question is what triggers both, and adults already know that food can cause both gut and head pain. Treating young infants with analgesics for weeks at a stretch will almost certainly be the result of the definition; many parents already know that using paracetamol does nothing to soothe serious colic. (The phenomenal rise in the use of this drug for children has not lowered colic rates!) Colic as head pain is of course a very convenient explanation which the food industry can be relied on to popularise! For more on this see on page 579.

190  Canivet C, Jakobsson I, Hagander B. Infantile colic. Follow-up at four years of age: still more 'emotional'. PMID:10677050) *Acta Paed* 2000, 89(1):13–17 DOI: 10.1080/080352500750028988

191  My response has always been, I don't know, but it seems plausible, and only you can find out. As long as you're careful about nutrition there is no harm in trying. I know it has helped some people with whom I have ongoing contact. Some wrote later that their health had improved. Others, I have no idea. Over the years I have heard from no one disappointed or angry over advice I have given them, even though it involved them in major life changes, never easy. Many were initially sceptical because they had been told dogmatically that such ideas were nonsense. But after years of treatment misery, they were prepared to try anything. When it works, they ask me why no one told them all this before: what can I answer?

Later in the book, studies of complementary feeding and allergy are discussed (see page 89 on Comp-feeding).[192, 193] One revealed that perhaps 25 per cent of the five-year-old Dutch children in the study were allergic; by now those children are adults. Their own children are at greater risk of atopy, having been conceived and gestated by atopic parents. And so the prevalence rates will rise, even with some breastfeeding ... as they have been doing everywhere.

Allergy snowballs: as the number in the high risk for atopy group increases in one generation, so the number in the next generation will increase exponentially. The next generation's infant feeding mixes will undoubtedly be different, perhaps even less allergenic for those exposed to them de novo, if industry can achieve this profitably. But despite this, the next generation of allergic children may still be even more sensitive than the last, if they are being gestated by allergic mothers, and if their mothers' milk provides less biodiversity and fewer bioactive ingredients.

Bottle fed children of this generation may tolerate some ingredients in a formula without obvious identified harms, but be sensitised and pass on that sensitivity to their children. I suspect this occurs when I hear of formulas that seemed to suit the allergic children of one generation now causing problems in the next. Of course the formulas change, but so do their recipients' sensitivities.

As I wrote this I had a phone call from a lactation consultant about an apparent increase in breastfed babies reacting with vomiting, shock, even anaphylaxis to infant formula. Why did lactation consultants so rarely see this extreme reaction even twenty years ago? I asked her to record her experience, and her note is below.

> I have received telephone calls from two breastfeeding mothers in the past year in relation to their babies having severe reactions to infant formula. Both mothers had intended to gradually wean their babies onto formula after four months.
>
> Mother 1 explained that her baby had a small amount of formula at about 4 weeks of age, and vomited some of it afterwards. At 4 months the infant was given a bottle of formula. The reaction included severe vomiting and collapse, requiring ambulance transfer to hospital.
>
> Mother 2 attempted to give her 4-month-old infant a bottle of formula; but the baby refused to take it, possibly swallowing about one mouthful of milk. The infant was put into bed; but was unusually restless and crying intermittently for about 20 minutes. When he was checked he was found to have a rash and to be 'swollen all over', so was taken to hospital immediately. (The only other time this infant had formula was 24 hours after birth whilst in Special Care Nursery).

---

192  Høst A. Importance of the first meal on the development of cow's milk allergy and intolerance. (PMID:1936970) *Allergy Proceedings* 1991, 12(4):227–32.; Høst A, Husby S, Osterballe O. A prospective study of cow's milk allergy in exclusively breast-fed infants. Incidence, pathogenetic role of early inadvertent exposure to cow's milk formula, and characterisation of bovine milk protein in human milk. (PMID:3201972) *Acta Paed Scand* 1988; 77(5):663–70.

193  de Jong MH, Scharp-van der Linden VTM, Aalberse RC. Randomised controlled trial of brief neonatal exposure to cows' milk on the development of atopy. *Arch Dis Child* 1998;79:126–30.

The mothers and infants were linked with an allergy clinic and recommended to continue breastfeeding. Both mothers contacted me as they wanted some further information about maintaining a good milk supply. Have you had any other reports of reactions to artificial baby milks becoming more severe and/or more common?

The harms of formula feeding in one generation echo in the next. As an allergic population, Americans are probably a couple of generations ahead of the rest of the world (thanks to industry/government promotion and supply of infant formula, chemical pollution, and industrial agriculture and food production[194]) but the rest of the world is catching up – in allergy and auto-immune disease rates, and in rates of related problems such as childhood obesity[195] and diabetes. And the extent of the problem in America has probably been concealed by the lack of access to affordable medical care endured by many of its citizens.[196] You won't be diagnosed if you can't afford to get to a doctor, or if cultural prejudice provides a psychosocial label that attributes your ills to some aspect of your character or identity.

## The hygiene hypothesis and the allergy epidemic

The role of mammalian milk in infant immune regulation and development is so elegant and economical that it has astonished me to find it largely omitted from the widespread popular and scientific discussion of the Hygiene Hypothesis. This attractive no-fault hypothesis explains the rise in allergies in terms of the absence of 'dirt' and the microbes and other threats to the infant immune system that it contains. The infant's world has become too 'clean', so to speak. This suggests that it is biologically useful to expose infants to unregulated doses of antigens, pathogens and parasites, the very threats that injure and kill children in poverty. One hears this everywhere, in far less sophisticated terms than advanced by its originator, John Gerrard.

However, there are some very obvious problems with this theory. People in crowded urban centres around the world, including in high-income countries, are still getting plenty of exposure to pathogens and parasites, much more than they'd prefer for good health. People expose other people to pathogens in crowded and unsanitary living conditions, in communal gatherings and pools, in schools and childcare and on public transport. Yet more of those who survive these pathogens are also becoming allergic in childhood: allergy rates rise with urbanisation. (The full extent of that rise may be underestimated: where poverty and premature death prevent people accessing doctors and allergy medication, allergy is unlikely to be diagnosed.)

The urban poor generally have higher levels of allergy than people in the poor rural areas they migrated from. Where the increase in allergy among the urban poor is acknowledged,

---

194   Some postulate that chemical exposure itself pre-disposes to allergy: see McFadden JP, White JM, Basketter DA, Kimber I. Does hapten exposure predispose to atopic disease? The hapten-atopy hypothesis. *Trends in Immunology* 2009, 30(2):67–74. (PMID:19138566)

195   Scott J. The relationship between breastfeeding and weight status in a national sample of Australian children and adolescents.(PMID:22314050) *BMC Public Health* 2012, 12:107.

196   I am still shocked when I remember reading of about a hospital refusing to help a desperate mother who had given birth to a preterm baby on Christmas Day. Mike Moore's film *Sicko* says it all about US healthcare policy. Google where to watch it now.

it has sometimes been attributed to such things as bedding changes and increases in dustmite exposure or traffic, which may well contribute – where they exist. It is not clear that the urban poor will always have more bedding or clothes than the rural poor or those in traditional communities, or be less exposed to dangerous chemicals – though again, that assumption is implicit in this explanation.

So survivors in poor quality living conditions, still heavily exposed to organisms and allergens, develop allergy. Their neighbours in cleaner suburbs and homes develop allergy, despite clean floors and bedding, and clean water supplies and toilets. The hygiene standards and rates of parasitism may vary greatly, but the immune disorders don't: though of course a higher infant mortality wherever sanitation is lacking will later influence allergy prevalence figures. You can't be an allergy statistic if poverty has killed you.

For example, at least in Caracas, the endemic parasite Giardia lamblia does not protect slum children from allergy; rather the reverse – the damage the parasite does is thought to be responsible for a higher rate of allergy to cows' milk: '22% of the children belonging to the low socioeconomic level demonstrated the presence of significant levels of specific IgE against this antigen [bovine milk]; of these 40 per cent were infected with G. lamblia.'[197]

What also happens when rural folk move into urban slums (though allergy commentators rarely note it) is that breastfeeding becomes much more difficult and less compatible with the work needed for survival. And at the same time, infant formula becomes more visible and available, sometimes being provided to the poor by well-meaning charities or authorities.

Infant feeding is rarely discussed in depth by those who argue that dirt and germs are protective, which is how many in the community understand the hygiene hypothesis. But they are right to see that the timing of exposure to pathogens is important (though wrong to ignore the medium of exposure!) The infant's adaptive immune system does need to be programmed after birth to deal with the environment it will grow up in, and that environment will influence allergy outcomes.[198] Babies are meant to be exposed to constant small but manageable doses of the common foods and non-invasive microbes their bodies must learn to tolerate, or even incorporate. Their bodies must also learn to identify and defeat common pathogens. And mother's milk is able to programme the infant both for tolerance of the helpful, and effective control of the harmful.

To me, a milk hypothesis makes much more sense than an uncontrolled exposure/ contamination/hygiene hypothesis, which suggests that exposing infants to unregulated doses of antigens, pathogens and parasites – the very threats that injure and kill children in poverty – may protect against allergies. By contrast, mother's milk and her body – the breastfed baby's environment – educates the infant immune system about those same nasties, but via priming doses in very restricted quantities that generate immediate helpful responses. (Immunotherapy for peanut allergy tries to do just that, with greater risks

197   Di Prisco MC, Hagel I, Lynch NR, Barrios RM, Alvarez N, López R Possible relationship between allergic disease and infection by Giardia lamblia. (PMID:8452315) *Annals of Allergy* [1993, 70(3):210–3.

198   von Mutius E. The environmental predictors of allergic disease. *J Allergy Clin Immunol.* 2000;105:9–19

but some success.) And milk presents these potential threats only after they have been processed by, and filtered through, an adult body, and then fed to the infant along with thousands of helpful anti-infective, anti-inflammatory, metabolically supportive and stress-reducing factors. Just look at this table of *some of* the activities of defence factors found in breastmilk by the 1990s,[199] unknown when those early formulas boasted of containing "everything that is in breastmilk". The list grows longer as work continues.

| | Representative function |
|---|---|
| Anti-infectious agent | |
| Oligosaccharides–glycoconjugates | Inhibit binding of bacterial pathogens and toxins to epithelium |
| Lactoferrin | Decrease multiplication of siderophilic bacteria/fungi by $Fe^{3+}$ chelation |
| Lysozyme | Disrupts peptidoglycans of cell walls on susceptible bacteria |
| Secretory IgA | Antibodies inhibit adherence of pathogens to epithelium; neutralize toxins |
| Mucin | Inhibits rotavirus |
| Lipids | Disrupt enveloped viruses |
| Anti-inflammatory agents | |
| Uric acid, ascorbate, α-tocopherol, β-carotene | Antioxidants |
| Prostaglandins | Cytoprotective |
| Cortisol, lactoferrin, EGF | Epithelial growth factors |
| Platelet-activating factor— acetylhydrolase | Degrades PAF |
| Immunomodulators | |
| Interleukin-1β | Activates T cells/monocytes |
| Interleukin-6 | Aids terminal differentiation of IgA-producing cells |
| Tumor necrosis factor-α | Upregulates production of secretory component. |
| | Activates T cells/monocytes |

Figure 2-3-1 Some of the activities of defence factors found in breastmilk by the 1990s[199] © Elsevier Ltd. Used with permission obtained through Copyright Clearance Center.

Small wonder that fully breastfed babies everywhere in the world can be such pictures of robust health. Industry is now tinkering with patented genetically-modified microbes and nutrients in an attempt to emulate this marvel (see page 517).

---

199 Goldman AS, Goldblum RM. Defense agents in human milk. In Jensen RG. *Handbook of Milk Composition*, p. 68 (Academic Press Inc, San Diego 1995) © Elsevier Ltd.

Thus it didn't surprise me that an allergy researcher presented a paper entitled: 'The hygiene hypothesis: do we still believe in it?'[200] As Bjorksten says,

> Epidemiological, clinical and animal studies taken together suggest that broad exposure to a wealth of commensal, non-pathogenic microorganisms early in life are associated with protection, not only against IgE-mediated allergies, but also conceivably against type-1 diabetes and inflammatory bowel disease. This has little relationship with 'hygiene' in the usual meaning of the word. The term 'hygiene hypothesis' is unfortunate, as it is misleading. No one would seriously question the enormous gains in public health by improved hygiene and nobody would argue for severe childhood infections merely to reduce the incidence of hay fever.

Splendid, just what I would hope to hear from more scientists. But what does Bjorksten suggest to replace the term, and why?

> A better term would therefore be 'microbial deprivation hypothesis' as this would point towards the possibility of preventing, or perhaps even treating, several immunologically mediated diseases with cocktails of nonpathogenic, probiotic microorganisms and antigen mixtures derived from them.[201]

How important language is in framing these discussions, and how important underlying assumptions are to the choice of language! If the problem is 'microbial deprivation', all the expensive corporate-funded research on genetically modified laboratory-grown bugs is justified, despite its risks and difficulties. Only people in affluent circumstances will be able to access and afford these, once proven 'safe'. Industry could then demand taxpayer subsidies to make these 'probiotics' ('microbes' or 'bacteria' sound too off-putting) available to poor families, as they have for the still unproved algal and fungal oils in formula (see page 315). The result: massive profits, as infant formula has provided for a century; and scientists will enjoy lifetimes of interesting work, paid for by industry and recouped from industry profits worldwide, an unseen tax on every family that buys their brands. What a useful term 'microbial deprivation' will be for those already advantaged in the world artificial feeding has created.

But are children really 'microbially deprived' nowadays? Certainly not. All environments and all humans are inevitably colonised with a wide array of microbial life, and all babies are soon colonised by what they are exposed to. Western infants were once born at home and lived in family surrounds. They have possibly never been exposed so young to such a huge variety of non-familial pathogens, by being born in hospitals, fed infant formulas and antibiotics, and brought together in non-familial care centres. (Which, by the way, do not result in lower allergy rates, despite resulting in much greater exposure to microbes, as evidenced in higher illness rates.) A study of eczema (also known as atopic dermatitis, or

---

200  Bjorksten B. in Per Brandtzaeg P, Isolauri E, Prescott SL (eds). *Microbial Host-Interaction: Tolerance versus Allergy.* Nestlé Nutrition Institute Workshop Series Pediatric Program Volume 64, 2008. Proceedings online at http://www.nestlenutrition-institute.org/Resources/Library/Free/workshop/NNIWBook64/
201  ibid.

'AD') found that 'Factors related to the hygiene hypothesis like day-care attendance and number of older siblings were not associated with a decreased risk of AD.'[202]

Hospital births, artificial feeding, child care and antibiotics do not result in microbial deprivation, but they do result in distortion of both the child's metabolism, their immune system, and their microbiome, the unique microbial bodily ecosystem that is essential to – and to some degree regulates – health and nutrition. Selectively, some children are indeed deprived: deprived of the immune system and the microbiome they would have had if they had been fully breastfed from birth after being born naturally. They will develop hundreds of different microbial species in their gut, but these will not be the same species, in the same balance, that they would have developed had they been vaginally born and breastfed.

> Upon birth, the intestinal tract of the infant begins to be colonised, ultimately creating a rich and diverse microenvironment. The microbiota is first acquired in the birth canal during delivery and then through breast milk. *[This was published before the discovery of the placental microbiome.]* Fecal microbial profiles of infants show a striking similarity to maternal vaginal and breast milk bacterial profiles.[203]

So let's call the problem what it is: 'microbiomic and immune distortion due to breastmilk deprivation and artificial formula exposure through generations' or simply 'due to artificial feeding', together perhaps with 'the use of antibiotics during often needlessly interventionist birthing.'[204]

That language would justify far more investment by public health authorities in enabling, not just verbally encouraging, good births and exclusive breastfeeding. And yes, that involves political re-working of societies that in the past and at present actively prevent women from birthing optimally, and from breastfeeding their babies into toddlerhood. This would be the only truly just, democratic and egalitarian strategy. Like Elisabet Helsing and the Norwegian feminist movement, I have 'never seen a contradiction between women's liberation and their breastfeeding. If society hinders optimal feeding of infants by mothers, then it is society that has to change, not breastfeeding.'[205] Those who believe in the best possible start for all human beings, regardless of background (or gender!), would agree with this basic assertion – just as we would also agree that society's response ought not be to dump all the costs of the necessary changes onto women, as is currently the case.

The 'microbial deprivation hypothesis' as described in the literature is the hygiene hypothesis renamed, similarly failing to mention the importance of early and exclusive breastfeeding to normal infant development. As outlined in that citation earlier, it supports unjust societies

---

202  Zutavern A, Hirsch T, Leupold W, Weiland S, Keil U, von Mutius E Atopic dermatitis, extrinsic atopic dermatitis and the hygiene hypothesis: results from a cross-sectional study. *Clin Exp Allergy* 2005, 35(10):1301–08.DOI: 10.1111/j.1365-2222.2005.02350.x

203  Agata Korecka and Velmurugesan Arulampalam. The gut microbiome: scourge, sentinel or spectator? *J Oral Microbiol.* 2012; 4: 10.3402/jom.v4i0.9367. Published online 2012 February 21. DOI: 10.3402/jom.v4i0.9367

204  Exclusive breastfeeding may help infant guts recover from antibiotic trauma, so this is a secondary issue.

205  Helsing E. Women's liberation and breastfeeding. *J Trop Paediatr Envir Child Health* 1975; 21 (5) 290–4.

that unwittingly impose immune dysfunction on infants and their descendants,[206] and then sell a privileged minority a variety of treatments for the problems created, with preventive strategies based on commercial products which the elite have helped to develop and profit from. No wonder that hypothesis is acceptable to those who profit from those societies and their illnesses, and those who feel they have no responsibility for the health of future generations or the Earth itself. They help create the problems, then sell the unsatisfactory solutions. Deprive a child of breastmilk and the mother will need contraception and maybe lactation suppressants and anti-depressants and more medication and health services later in life; the child too will need more frequent and expensive special food and medications.

By contrast, elites and giant multinational vested interests lose wherever breastmilk is universally available – as it can be wherever breastfeeding is valued. Action to support maternal breastfeeding reduces social inequity, and makes for healthier women, children and grandchildren across all classes and income ranges. Even if it were proved eventually to have little effect on allergy in a world lacking biodiversity (see below), it would thus still be worth any outlays involved.

## The biodiversity theory and reality

The next (and very current) theory proposed as an explanation for rising allergy rates is in fact the biodiversity hypothesis, a refinement of the hygiene and microbial deprivation hypotheses. Population growth and urbanization leads to loss of environmental biodiversity including the microbiota; this in turn impoverishes the human microbiome creating dysbiosis, which results in immune dysfunction, inappropriate inflammatory responses, and finally symptoms and clinical disease. The biodiversity pyramid from an open access editorial in the journal, *Pediatric Allergy and Immunology*,[207] illustrates the theory well.

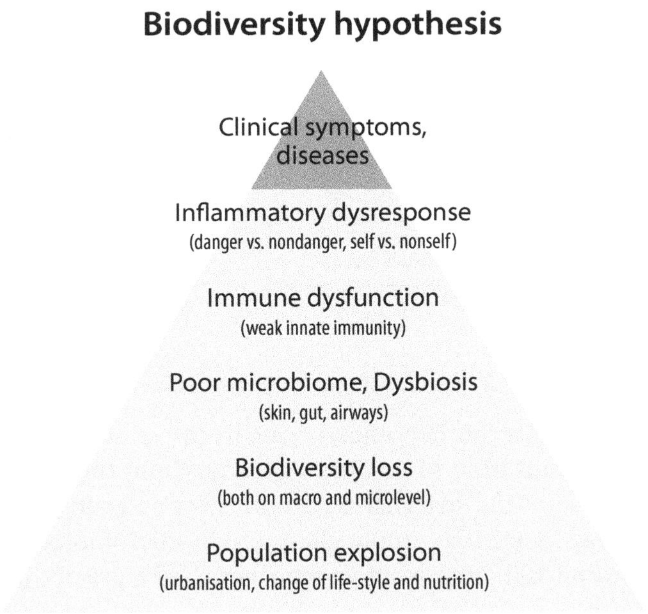

### Biodiversity hypothesis

Clinical symptoms, diseases

Inflammatory dysresponse
(danger vs. nondanger, self vs. nonself)

Immune dysfunction
(weak innate immunity)

Poor microbiome, Dysbiosis
(skin, gut, airways)

Biodiversity loss
(both on macro and microlevel)

Population explosion
(urbanisation, change of life-style and nutrition)

Figure 2-3-2 The biodiversity theory illustrated (Haahtela 2014). © John Wiley and Sons Inc, permission via Rightslink. Free online.

206  Boswell-Penc M. *Tainted Milk: breastmilk, feminisms, and the politics of environmental degradation*. (State University of New York, 2006) contains an interesting analysis of the degree to which American feminism has ignored or distorted breastfeeding issues.

207  Haahtela T. What is needed for allergic children? *Pediatr Allergy Immunol* 2014: 25: 21–24.DOI:10.1111/pai.12189 © John Wiley & Sons.

There are now innumerable publications discussing the missing microbes, among them an excellent book with that title.[208] This hypothesis is widely acceptable, perhaps because loss of biodiversity is another cost of progress, so no one vested interest can be held accountable for the rise in allergy. But as this book argues, this theory lacks real awareness of the contribution and complexities of both birth and infant feeding issues. Its proponents rightly argue that:

> Adaptation to modern urban life is a challenge to immune development and mismatched immunologic mechanisms lead to symptoms and disease. Contact with natural environments rich in species seems to be strongly related to immunotolerance via the presence of beneficial microbes of the skin, gut and airways. These microbes create a living interface between the human body and the environment and extend deeper into the tissue than known before.[209]

All true. But why is there so little acknowledgment[210] of the contribution of infant feeding at every level of this pyramid?

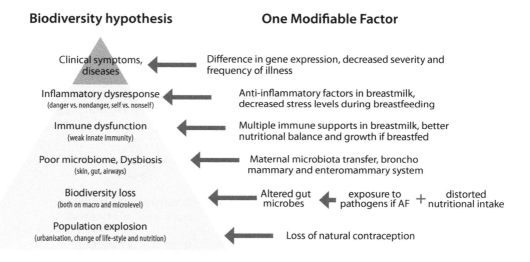

Figure 2-3-3 The Biodiversity theory and infant feeding: a neglected reality.

Support for this hypothesis came from a study in northeast Finland. Teenagers were tested for sensitisation to common allergens, and the composition of their skin microbiota was analysed. The external environment was analysed for plant species and land use, and it was found that atopic allergy, skin microbiome, and environmental biodiversity were interrelated. Non-reactive teenagers had a greater diversity of certain bacteria (including

---

208 Blaser MJ. *Missing Microbes: how the use of antibiotics is fueling our modern plagues.* (Henry Holt, 2014) Again, a wonderful exposition, very readable, which even discusses birth and antibiotics – but largely omits the potential and real harms of artificial feeding.

209 Nakatsuji T, Chiang H-I, Jiang SB, Nagarajan H, Zengler K, Gallo RL. The microbiome extends to subepidermal compartments of normal skin. *Nat Commun* 2013: 4: 1431.

210 See Haahtela T, Holgate ST, Pawankar R, et al. The biodiversity hypothesis and allergic disease: World Allergy Organization position statement. *World Allergy Organ J* 2013: 6: 3. Why is there more discussion of the effects of infant exposure to antibiotics than of infant formula? © John Wiley & Sons.

gammaproteobacteria) on their skin, and had higher blood levels of an anti-inflammatory chemical, interleukin-10. The researchers stated:

> The results suggested that contact with biodiverse natural environment with abundant bacteria and probably with other microbes can protect people from becoming sensitised to allergens, by building up the immune system.[211]

True, they do suggest that. Equally, they might suggest that an immune system well-built from birth permits colonisation and persistence to adolescence of favourable bacteria related to those acquired in infancy, since the authors note that the location of gammaproteobacteria in humans is the armpit and breastmilk. The reports give no information about the infant feeding of the teenagers sampled, and there is no discussion about typical flora and immune factors in women's milk in both regions. A follow up study could be useful, even though time has elapsed and so changes may have occurred, especially if free infant formula samples have invaded Russian healthcare systems, or rates of surgical birth and antibiotic use have changed. A comparative study of the milk of Swedish and Estonian women did show significant differences in levels of immune factors, no doubt in response to different environmental challenges[212] and factors such as disinfection of water supplies, use of fluoride, etc.

Of course we can expect that in reducing the biodiversity children are exposed to, the development of their immune system will be affected. But what are the most fundamental primary sources of that biodiversity for human infants? Not directly the backyard or garden or farm or nearby forest or the number of native flowering plants. That all comes later, and has its own hazards: nature is not always benign.

The fundamental source of biodiversity for infants is the mother's body, with all its diverse flora in their niche environments: the wetlands of her vagina, the damp forests of her armpits, the clear plains or grasslands of her breasts and skin, the caverns of her mouth and respiratory tree, and the rivers of her milk, where hundreds of species flourish.[213] Biodiversity for the newborn begins with biodiversity in the mother, and continues to develop from that provided it is not rudely interrupted. And if the mother's biodiversity is the problem, the causes may be her feeding as a child, as well as her birth and home environment.

In short, the biodiversity theory could well be the milk hypothesis in disguise. This is important, because urbanites cannot re-afforest the city, but they could potentially repopulate their babies' bodies by breastfeeding! Increasing sensitisation and greater reactivity in succeeding generations is predicted by the milk hypothesis – and is occurring;[214] this makes action urgent, as Finland has realised.

---

211 Hanski I, von Hertzen L, Fyhrquistc N, et al. Environmental biodiversity, human microbiota, and allergy are interrelated. *Proc Natl Acad Sci* USA 2012: 109: 8334–9. PMCID:PMC3361383 doi: 10.1073/pnas.1205624109

212 Tomicić S, Johansson G, Voor T, Björkstén B, et al. Breast milk cytokine and IgA composition differ in Estonian and Swedish mothers – relationship to microbial pressure and infant allergy.(PMID:20581738) *Pediatr Research* 2010, 68(4):330–34.

213 Cabrera-Rubio R, Collado MC, Laitinen K, Salminen S, et al. op. cit.

214 von Hertzen l, Mäkelä MJ, Petäys T, Jousilahti P et al. Growing disparities in atopy between Finns and Russians: A comparison of 2 generations. *J Allergy Clin Immunol* 2006; 117(1): 151–57, DOI: 10.1016/j.jaci.2005.07.028

# Biodiversity: genes and microbes and microbiomes

Recently there has been a flood of new research and writing about the importance of both our genome (our unique mix of genes, and how they are expressed) and our microbiome (the unique mix of microbes inhabiting us). The two are inextricably linked, since microbes are an essential working part of the organism they inhabit, and influence not only immediate functioning, but also even the evolution of the organism in response to its changing environment – including its diet. So important and prolific[215] are they that someone commented that rather than say that they are our microbes, we could say that we are their body, providing food to sustain them! As Daphne Chung wrote ten years ago, 'The interactions between all these bacteria are so complex that researchers view the community as an ecosystem.'[216] And the bacterial community is interlocked with fungi and viruses and any other life forms present. Since we humans cannot live without our bugs, some writers go so far as to see the human being as a chimera, a single organism composed of genetically distinct cells. That chimera evolved with breastmilk as its food for millions of years.

And food is what grows us. There is considerable support for the idea that nutrition directly affects both metabolism and immune system in multiple ways, creating inflammation, and with it, the resulting array of western diseases of affluence. The research in this field is coming from the perspective of addressing and perhaps reversing adult disease, both physical and mental, and prolonging life, and seems very promising. Adults can reduce inflammatory processes by changing their diet, and maintain improvement by continuing with high fibre, high omega 3 and anti-oxidant intake, and all the other aspects of good diet. This is thought to be important in cardiovascular, auto-immune, and neurological disorders such as autism, and perhaps even schizophrenia. Research has uncovered the impact of specific aspects of nutrition on the adult microbiota and its production of metabolites such as short chain fatty acids, which have been shown to be protective in a variety of animal studies. The mechanisms of action are being spelt out, and were well-described in the 85th Nestle Nutrition Institute conference, Preventive Aspects of Early Nutrition.[217] Professor Susan Prescott opens with a global and societal overview of the whole issue; while Dr Charles Mackay spells out links between the diet, the microbiome and its metabolites, and the metabolic and immune systems. The latter presentation, although seemingly not conscious of its direct relevance to the question of early milk feeds, supports my milk hypothesis, offering as it does technical explanations for how nutrition makes such a difference.

What is often missing from industry-supported talks is a strong awareness of the possibility that what is seen in adults is the result of programming in the very early days of infancy when food is first consumed orally and the gut microbiome develops; and a recognition that the acknowledged connections with maternal obesity and pregnancy may also be an unacknowledged legacy of the previous generations' infant diet. Perhaps not surprisingly given the widespread ignorance about lactation, and the focus on adult disease, there

---

215 There are many more microbes than human cells in any body. It is in their interests to keep us alive to serve them, and to repel invaders that would destroy us. But living organisms can change, if they pick up other characteristics from competitors.

216 Chung D. It's a jungle in there. *New Scientist* 2004; 182 (2444):43–45.

217 November 2014; videos will doubtless be on the NNI website in due course..

seems to be little awareness of the unique characteristics of women's milk and its incredible bioactivity, its anti-inflammatory and immune properties. Nor does there seem to be any awareness of the particular and peculiar hazards of industrial milks, and their inevitable advanced glycation products (see page 251), their deficiencies and excesses, and so on and on. These are the scientists I most want to read this book and apply their in-depth immune knowledge to uncover just what happens when we feed young humans extensively heat-treated artificial formulas instead of fresh breastmilk, distorting normal metabolic processes, creating dysbiosis, and skewing the immune system towards reactivity rather than tolerance.

We have learned from other ecosystems than any one change can have unpredictable consequences. What alters our microbiome alters us, and the human microbiome has been considerably altered in cosmopolitan areas in the last hundred years.[218] Infant feeding is one absolutely fundamental part of creating and maintaining our microbiome.

If mother's milk is an evolutionary bridge between the largely protected womb[219] and the risky world, and her armpits and milk the location of the gammaproteobacteria[220] that Finnish researchers think are important contributors to immune development, common sense says breastfeeding will matter – *and the burden of proof rests with those who assume that it is possible to interfere in long-established highly evolved mechanisms without harmful consequences.*

Why would anyone assume that early exposure to alien foods in past and present generations could do no damage to the vulnerable neonate? It is for formula advocates to prove safe even the slightest amount of formula exposure, not for breastfeeding advocates to prove it risky. Responsibility for proving safety lies with those advocating deviation from a physiological norm. Those adhering to such norms do not need to prove deviation a risk: it self-evidently is. As Dr Cuthbert Garza, playing devil's advocate, asked in the FDA meeting on Infant Formula in 2002:

> Is there any other circumstance in medicine where a significant deviation from perceived normal physiology would be interpreted by default as acceptable without proving that, in fact, there were no problems; where the absence of information is sufficient, rather than the presence of information?[221]

No, there isn't. If gestation, skin contact and breastmilk are the means of creating a microbiome that results both in active defence against threats, tolerance of foods, and optimal gene expression, then surely limiting skin contact, and interference with exclusive breastfeeding in pathogen-laden hospital environments matters hugely. Interfering with these highly evolved defences must have consequences. A normal immune system is the basis of lifelong health, and the gift we pass on to our children with that healthy microbiome we hope they inherit from us.

---

218  Tito RY, Knights D, Metcalfe J, Obregon-Tito AJ et al. Insights from characterising extinct human gut microbiomes. *PloS One* 2012; 7: e51146.
219  The related issue of the role of pregnancy and intra-uterine sensitisation is discussed elsewhere. See page 582.
220  Hanski et al op. cit.
221  Transcript, November 19 2002 meeting of the USDA Food Advisory Committee, op. cit. November 19.

# 2.4 Where does our immune system come from?

Our immune system is a complex multi-generational inheritance. Each of us begins as an egg in our mother's body, created while she was developing in our grandmother's body. Once fertilised, the egg that will produce us, develops inside our mother's body. So what will become you began in your maternal grandmother's womb. If no eggs had formed there, or it had been a hostile environment, you would never have existed.

That egg combines with sperm that has developed in an adult male body, and which provides a second set of genes along with traces of whatever has influenced that male body. Both sets of genes (as they have been expressed) shape the development of our individual innate immune system during pregnancy; the contribution of fathers is now attracting more research attention. So influences on our development are complex, long before we are born.

After eighteen weeks' gestation, maternal immune cells are transferred across the placenta, providing a boost to our developing immune system via direct transfer in utero from our mother's adult body. The infant immune system begins to develop from around then. So a term baby is born with some ability to recognise, and deal with, threats the mother's body has previously dealt with during her life, just as her body was given such protection by her own mother's body in utero. In addition, very recent research indicates that the placenta itself is the site of a unique microbial population, whose importance is yet to be fully understood.[222] However, the placental microbiome is more akin to the mother's oral, and the infant gut microbiomes, than either is to the vaginal microbiome before birth and the passage of the placenta.

That is a particularly interesting finding, which perhaps suggests maternal oral health and microbiomes could be considered in future research. It makes sense that the oral microbiota matters, given that food digestion begins in the mouth. But why the difference from maternal vaginal flora, when surely that is the most usual source of infant gut colonisation during normal birth? Does the placental microbiome colonise the vagina during and after birth, and is this related to postpartum infection rates? Or does a healthy vagina resist colonisation with placental species, and is not influenced by the passage of amniotic fluid and the child? That seems unlikely, but there are many more questions raised by this recent finding. (Among them the question of whether there is in fact greater synchrony between oral and vaginal flora in women of communities not using antibacterial and fluoridated toothpastes and mouthwashes known to alter oral flora,[223] indeed, designed to do so.)

Traces of related bacterial DNA have also been found in the amniotic fluid, all suggesting that the process of infant gut colonisation begins before birth, and is dependent on the

---

222 Aagaard K, Jun M, Antony KM, Radhika G et al. The Placenta Harbors a Unique Microbiome. *Sci Transl Med* 2014; 6:237. DOI: 10.1126/scitranslmed.3008599. Discussed online at http://www.nytimes.com/2014/05/22/health/study-sees-bigger-role-for-placenta-in-newborns-health.html?hp&_r=1
223 Kary T. Colgate Total Ingredient Linked to Hormones, Cancer Spotlights FDA Process. *Bloomberg News 12* Aug 2014. http://www.bloomberg.com/news/2014-08-11/in-35-pages-buried-at-fda-worries-over-colgate-s-total.html

mother's microbiome, before being established by breastmilk. The old idea that babies are born sterile has been disproved. This will surely lead to a great deal of re-thinking. Among that re-thinking, investigations of the maternal skin and milk microbiome need to be included, as breastfeeding a baby involves the passage of microbes from both sources. Bottle feeding also provides multiple microbial exposures, less likely to be helpful ones. Recent research indicates that although more hygienic care might nowadays be taken of bottles and teats, oral objects can indeed be the source of pathogens which can colonise the child's mouth.

> Researchers report that they found a wide range of disease-causing bacteria, fungus and mold on pacifiers that young children had been using. They added that pacifiers can often grow a slimy coating of bacteria – called a biofilm – that actually alters the normal bacteria in a baby or toddler's mouth. That biofilm can spur inflammation and potentially increase the risk of developing gastrointestinal problems such as colic or even ear infections.[224]

Birth itself matters greatly when it comes to our immune system. A recent Canadian study,[225] which used modern techniques to 'provide new evidence for the effects of delivery mode and infant diet as determinants of this essential microbial community in early life.' Both Caesarean-section (especially elective surgery) and lack of breastmilk resulted in marked microbiome differences between groups of infants at four months of life. Both the lack of exposure to maternal vaginal flora and the use of antibiotics in pregnancy and surgical births were flagged as possible influences. A more recent study showed that caesarean sections result in epigenetic differences.[226] Other studies have confirmed the importance of the mode of delivery, but not investigated either placental differences or followed up the mode of infant feeding in detail.[227] For example, there is a study which notes that metabolic disease in mid-life is more common in those born by Caesarean section without factoring in postnatal nutrition.[228] But whatever a baby's innate immunity, microbiome, and metabolome before and during birth, all will be modulated, shaped, even determined, by what happens after the birth. And that we can control more readily than placental colonisation or the need for surgery!

---

224 Gray, BB. Dirty pacifiers may make infants sick. http://health.usnews.com/health-news/news/articles/2012/11/02/dirty-pacifiers-may-make-infants-sick-study

225 Azad MB, Konya T, Maughan H, Guttman DS et al Gut microbiota of healthy Canadian infants: profiles by mode of delivery and infant diet at 4 months. *CMAJ* February 11, 2013 cmaj.121189, DOI: 10.1503. Available online. Oddly, the terms richness and diversity are used when describing the gut microbiota. Diversity is a neutral term, but richness (for density, intensity, variety, or total population of microbes) is unfortunately loaded, almost always implying benefit in the English language. The formula fed babies had a richer population of microbes ... so the breastfed babies a poorer one? How will that be understood if this term is used to the public? I urge scientists to think about – and take responsibility for – their use of language.

226 Almgren M, Schlinzig T, Gomez-Cabrero D, Gunnar A et al. Cesarean section and hematopoietic stem cell epigenetics in the newborn infant – implications for future health? *Am J Obstet Gynecol* online 1 July 2014, DOI: http://dx.doi.org/10.1016/j.ajog.2014.05.014

227 http://europepmc.org/articles/PMC3602254 Biasucci G, Rubini M, Riboni S, Morelli L, et al. Mode of delivery affects the bacterial community in the newborn gut. PMID:20133091) *Early Hum Dev* 2010; 86 (Suppl 1):13–15.

228 Bouhanick B, Ehlinger V, Delpierre C et al. Mode of delivery at birth and the metabolic syndrome in midlife: the role of the birth environment in a prospective birth cohort study. *BMJ Open.* 2014;4(5):e005031. DOI: 10.1136/bmjopen-2014-005031.This was deliberate; the assumption was that feeding might be a mediating factoe, but not a causative one, and no useful feeding dats was collected. (Email on file 28/11/2014)

# The immune system, infant feeding and postpartum care practices

Our extraordinary immune system is not just a birthright we inherit. It develops as an ongoing adaptive response to our environment, in tandem with maternal support. Maternal transplacental IgG may persist for up to three months, and while our adaptive immune system begins to develop, our mother supports us, initially by providing colostrum, and then milk.

Colostrum is in fact a sort of super-concentrated, low-volume, high-impact milk. It contains essential proteins, growth factors, white blood cells, vitamins, enzymes, hormones, anti-oxidants, and a variety of antibodies, some of which travel via the blood to reach other mucosal surfaces such as the bladder. It also supplies dozens of other immune factors, and friendly bacteria, just as breastmilk does. The concentration of anti-oxidants, protein and minerals is higher, and fat and carbohydrates lower, than in the milk that will soon follow. That package of nutrients and medications comes in a highly concentrated small dose, so as not to require the baby to take in large amounts of fluid (see Figure 2-4-1 below).1 It is precisely what newborn babies' bodies have evolved to rely on as support. And only breastfed babies get human colostrum.[229]

Figure 2-4-1 What meconium is known to contain. [230]

- epithelial cells
- secretions of intestinal glands
- gut constituents (proteins, fatty acids, steroids)
- components of amniotic fluid
- vernix caseosa
- bile acids (unconjugated and conjugated bile species)
- minerals and trace elements
- proinflammatory substances (IL-1, IL-6, IL-8)
- antimicrobial peptides (defensins, cathelicidins, calprotectin)
- aerobic bacteria (*Escherichia coli* and Streptococci)

In utero, the infant's gut has been protected by meconium, a complex substance. Meconium is the black and tarry first faeces that the mother's naturally laxative colostrum will cause the baby's gut to expel, while colonising that infant gut with a flourishing ecosystem of hundreds of different species of 'friendly' microbes derived from the mother's body and her milk. Meconium was once thought to be sterile, but is now known to contain bacteria such as E coli and Streptococci, presumably ingested via amniotic fluid.[231] (Obviously this relates to the very recent findings about placental colonisation with maternal microbes: see page 76) It might prove to be critically important for meconium and colostrum to interact in creating the infant

---

229  Although of course other mammals also make such a first feed, and heat-damaged and inappropriate bovine colostrum has been fashionable among athletes, and even trialled as prophylaxis against rotavirus infection. See Davidson GP, Whyte PB, Daniels E, Franklin K, et al. Passive immunisation of children with bovine colostrum containing antibodies to human rotavirus. (PMID:2570959) *Lancet* 1989, 2(8665):709–12.

230  Baldassarre ME, Formula feeds and meconium. In Preedy Watson Zibadi, op. cit., p. 344. © Wageningen Academic Publishers 2013.

231  Jiménez E, Marín ML. Martín R, Odriozola J et al. Is meconium from healthy newborns actually sterile? *Research in Microbiology* 2008; 159 (3):187–93. http://dx.doi.org/10.1016/j.resmic.2007.12.007; Madan JC, Salari RC, Saxena D, Davidson L, et al. Gut microbial colonisation in premature neonates predicts neonatal sepsis. (PMID:22562869) *Arch Dis Child Fetal Neonatal E*d 2012; 97(6):f456–62.

microbiome, as meconium also contains antimicrobial peptides, as well as minerals and trace elements, bile acids, and much more.

And perhaps that special mix also depends on the breakdown products of the extra blood volume babies needed in utero. Levels of bilirubin in the newborn's blood naturally increase after birth as the baby's extra red blood cells are broken down. Blood and stools will both contain bilirubin, a powerful antioxidant. Antioxidants protect body cells from oxidation, damaging changes due to the exposure to oxygen.[232] Anti-oxidants help maintain a healthy immune system and reduce the risk of diseases such as cancer. Birth and the period immediately after it are times of oxidative stress, as the baby begins to breathe, cry, move, feed, and respond to temperature changes and sensory stimulation. It is also a time of low dietary antioxidant intake, making bilirubin crucial to the health of the newborn and their immune system. And as noted before (see p. 42) by a month of age breastfed infants have lower levels of DNA damage, which those Japanese researchers ascribed to their higher intakes of antioxidants – despite the high levels put into infant formulas.

Only small quantities of high-protein colostrum are taken in on the first day. The normal process of colostrum clearing meconium from the gut allows some bilirubin to be excreted, while some is recirculated in the infant's body, until the volume of milk intake increases. As milk intake increases, so do levels of other antioxidants, and the protein needed to bind bilirubin and excrete it. Extremely high levels of bilirubin may cause jaundice and other problems,[233] but babies are well adapted to the normal, limited recirculation of bilirubin found in healthy breastfed babies. Like everything else we consume, some bilirubin can be useful, and huge excesses hazardous.

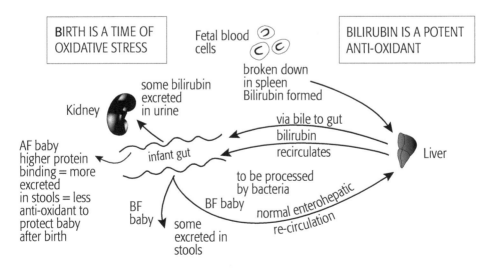

Figure 2-4-2 The bilirubin cycle and infant feeding image by Sarah Garner.

---

232 Rust on metals, or rancidity in butter, are perhaps the best known forms of oxidation.
233 An excellent clinical protocol and patient materials for dealing with elevated neonatal bilirubin levels can be found online at the UK NICE (National Institute of Clinical Excellence) website, http://www.nice.org.uk/CG98. Were this followed, infant exposure to formula would drop.

The average colostrum feed size is around a teaspoon, and TOTAL colostrum intake on day one is on average 15–20 ml. This will double on the second day, and then rapidly increase as lactation gets underway.[234] Which it will do, from 20–48 hours onwards, as pregnancy-associated high progesterone levels in the mother drop,[235] provided there are no overriding hormonal complications to suppress this automatic progress. (Retained placental fragments can inhibit this process.)

Lactation is an inbuilt survival mechanism, which is on autopilot after the birth. It takes serious interference in its governing mechanisms to prevent milk being produced just as baby needs it to be. Regrettably, many twentieth-century Western hospital practices could have been designed precisely to create such serious interference!

## Fluid intake postpartum

Though babies can take in much larger quantities of breastmilk if it is provided, newborns are well-adapted to small quantities of liquid intake in the first days after birth, and usually blurt back the excess. If proof were needed, the survival and later normal development of forty newborns buried for days, some up to a week, under the rubble of the 1981 Mexican earthquake should have supplied it.[236] Despite this, longstanding and ill-informed concern has persisted about the neonatal need for a greater volume of fluid than most breastfeeding women will supply. In traditional communities babies may indeed have taken in more milk from other women without problems; even preterm babies can cope with larger volumes of breastmilk. But even in countries where breastfeeding is encouraged, other liquids have been routinely given to most infants, interfering with normal post-birth developments. (Some babies are restless until they get more than colostrum - almost never, however, if they are kept skin to skin with a familiar body. If what babies are given is breastmilk, there is little reason for concern.)

| DAY | Physiologic Stomach capacity | Breastmilk feed volume (average) | Breastmilk 24 hour intake average and range |
|---|---|---|---|
| 1 | 7 ml | 7 ml | 37 ml (7–123) |
| 2 | 13 ml | 14 ml | 84 ml (44–335) |
| 3 | 27 ml | 38 ml | 408 ml (98–775) |
| 4 | 46 ml | 56 ml | 625 ml (378–876) |
| 7 | 68 ml | 65 ml | 576 ml (200–1013) |

Figure 2-4-3 Infant of 2–4 kg; stomach capacity and milk intake

The initial small doses of colostrum not only act as an effective laxative to remove meconium; they also begin to establish a normal, protective microbiome, providing whole-body immune protection. High doses of secretory IgA (an

234 Saint L, Smith M, Hartmann PE. The yield and nutrient content of colostrum and milk of women from giving birth to 1 month post-partum. (PMID:6743645) *Br J Nutr* 1984; 52(1):87–95; Casey CE, Neifert MR, Seacat JM, Neville MC Nutrient intake by breast-fed infants during the first five days after birth. (PMID:3740001) *Am J Dis Child* 1986;140(9):933–36.

235 The pregnancy hormone progesterone inhibits prolactin, preventing lactose synthesis; lactose drives milk secretion. See Hale and Hartmann op. cit. for any needed understanding of lactation processes.

236 http://www.nytimes.com/1985/10/16/world/mexico-s-entombed-babies-win-the-fight-for-life.html. I remember reading in the 1980s that UNICEF had followed up these babies to assess outcomes, and threw a birthday party for them at twelve months, when all survivors had developed normally.

antibody unique to milk which acts as a protective coating on the gut mucosal surfaces, from mouth to anus) and other immune factors in breastmilk are fed every day, including immunoglobulins tailored to the environment the child must survive in – provided mother and baby are not separated. This fact makes it a serious matter indeed to send a breastfeeding mother home from hospital when she wishes to stay. Lack of this 'antiseptic *[and anti-inflammatory]* paint which coats the bowel wall'[237] can be the cause of devastating infection or antigen penetration. Such mucosal protection is also provided to the baby's respiratory passages by the nature of breastfeeding: many babies inhale aerosols of breastmilk and even aspirate milk without incident other than spluttering. The sight of breastmilk flowing from little noses is not uncommon. The position at the back of the throat of the infant's eustachian tubes (which lead into the ears, and when blocked by inflammation allow otitis media to develop) probably allows exposure to protective breastmilk. The respiratory tree and the gut are both dosed daily with secretory IgA and the rest.

Unfortunate babies not being breastfed are less protected and more immediately stressed. The amounts of allergenic formula poured into them at arbitrary intervals within hours of birth are huge by contrast with colostrum doses; such high doses from birth have no easily discernible scientific justification, and interfere with normal interaction between mother and child.

Human infants have evolved to thrive on the amounts and types of nutrients available to them in breastmilk immediately after birth, while their kidneys, liver and digestive tract are all beginning to function for the first time outside the womb. They have not evolved to cope with the large amounts of liquid and high levels of protein in formula, both of which must stress their immature kidneys, which by three months are measurably larger in the formula-fed infant than the breastfed.[238] This is surely part of the reason for the incredible increase in renal (kidney) disease in Australia and elsewhere, affecting indigenous and First Nations peoples disproportionately, and creating huge costs financially and socially. Bathing the back of the infant throat in reactive formula ingredients almost certainly helps produce the middle ear infections so common in artificially fed infants, while aspiration of such alien foods can cause pneumonia. Early colonisation with the wrong bacteria (dysbiosis) can lead to a greater incidence of bronchiolitis and pneumonia in the early years of life,[239] especially in disadvantaged groups.

Bovine protein in the many formula mixes based on cows' milk binds the baby's beneficial bilirubin, preventing its normal levels of re-circulation, and so reducing the baby's natural antioxidant protection. Formula supplies synthetic antioxidants that are not as protective (see page 145 for DNA effects). The alien formula proteins are broken down into amino acids that circulate in the blood and reach the brain. There they can distort normal neurotransmitter balances, some reaching levels high enough to cause anxiety about brain

---

237  Bentley D, Aubrey S, Bentley M. *Infant Feeding and Nutrition for Primary Care.* (Radcliffe Publishing Ltd, Oxford 2004). p. 2

238  Schmidt IM, Damgaard In, Boisen KA, Mau C et al. Increased kidney growth in formula-fed versus breastfed infants. *Pediatr. Nephrol* 2004; 19: 1137–44.

239  Vissing NH, Chawes BL, Bisgaard H. Increased risk of pneumonia and bronchiolitis after bacterial colonization of the airways as neonates.(PMID:24090102) *Am J Respir Crit Care Med* 2013; 188(10):1246–52

insult.[240] Inevitably with artificial feeding, waste products are unnatural in both consistency and amount. These must be expelled from the infant gut, forcing the gastrointestinal tract to work unnaturally, and affecting the critical processes of gut development, and microbial colonisation. (And having long-lasting effects on, for example, gall bladder function.[241] Which will in turn affect gut bacteria and function, as bile affects digestion.)

## The neonatal gut microbiome and infant formula

Over the millennia of human evolution, newborns received only women's milk, from mothers and others whose bodies and breasts were sampling the natural environment of which they were part. (Those societies which did give ritual, usually token, pre-lacteal feeds of valued foods no doubt contributed to their higher infant mortality rates.) Babies' guts have not evolved to cope well with strange mixtures of many processed foodstuffs, some containing pathogens such as Enterobacter[242, 243] and Salmonella.[244] In fact infant formula can be the vehicle[245] that introduces some very unfriendly microbes (pathogens) into the newborn gut. It only took a tiny hole in the inner lining of a factory spray drier for Salmonella Ealing to become a problem.[246] One such bacterial contamination incident bankrupted UK formula-maker Farley's,[247] owned by Glaxo, which then sold Farley's and its products (Ostermilk and Oster Feed etc.) to Boots. Ironically around that time Farley's was advertising 'All baby milks come close [to breastmilk]. Only OsterFeed gets it right.' Both statements were patently untrue, as the costly recall indicated.

This makes a nonsense of the fear campaigns that drive formula use, themes like 'Because a mother's instinct is protection.' Formula advertising, with its perennial claims of purity and protection, has often been untruthful – or at best misleading. Parents generally did not know that powdered formula is not sterile.[248] Some have been incredulous on hearing the fact, after decades of advertising stating the purity and safety of the product. Even if formula does not itself introduce the pathogens, it creates the wrong environment for friendly bacteria, and favours instead the growth of pathogens omnipresent in hospital

240  Neumann CG, Jelliffe EFP. Effects of Infant Feeding. In Jelliffe D. *Adverse Effects of Foods* (Plenum Press 1982) p. 544.

241  Formula has longlasting effects on bile acid secretion: Mott GE, Lewis DS, McGill HC Jr. Programming of cholesterol metabolism by breast or formula feeding. *Ciba Foundation Symposium* 1991, 156:56–66; discussion 66–76. (PMID:1855416)

242  Cetinkaya E, Joseph S, Ayhan K, Forsythe SJ. Comparison of methods for the microbiological identification and profiling of Cronobacter species from ingredients used in the preparation of infant formula. (PMID:23089182) *Molecular and Cellular Probes* 2013; 27(1):60–64.

243  Yan QQ, Condell O, Power K, Butler F, Tall BD, Fanning S. Cronobacter species (formerly known as Enterobacter sakazakii) in powdered infant formula: a review of our current understanding of the biology of this bacterium. (PMID:22420458) *J Appl Microbiol* [2012, 113(1):1–15.

244  Cahill SM, Wachsmuth IK, Costarrica Mde L, Ben Embarek PK. Powdered infant formula as a source of Salmonella infection in infants.(PMID:18171262) *Clin Infect Dis* 2008, 46(2):268–73.

245  Muytjens HL, Roelofs-Willemse H, Jaspar GH. Quality of powdered substitutes for breast milk with regard to members of the family Enterobacteriaceae. *J Clin Microbiol* 1988; 26(4):743–46. (PMID:3284901)

246  Rowe et al *Lancet* 1988; ii: 900–03.

247  This is discussed in Book 2, Infant Feeding Past present and Future, see page 252.

248  Jason J. Prevention of invasive Cronobacter infections in young infants fed powdered infant formulas. *Pediatrics* [2012, 130(5):e1076–84. (PMID:23045556)

and home environments, for which the mother's immune system cannot prepare the baby (unless she works in that environment).

The human gut is not a single environment, but a complex series of environments, affected by all its inputs. (Just as a river varies from source to sea, depending on what feeds into it and how that interacts with its physical structures.) The gut needs both to absorb and to exclude, to foster and to discourage, to allow the passage of nutrients and prevent the passage of harmful substances. The cells that line the gut are critical to gut performance, and initially in the neonatal gut rely on breast milk to assist them.

> The intestinal barrier is both tightly regulated and highly dynamic, with the ability to adapt to endogenous stimuli, such as hormones and neuromediators. It is also highly influenced by luminal stimuli, including the gut microbiota and nutrients. The neonatal period provides an evolution of luminal content diversity by the colonisation of commensal bacteria and is also the period of gut immune cell education, reacting towards this evolving external milieu.

As Boudry and Hamilton go on to say very graphically,

> Intestinal epithelia cells play the role of a music conductor that orchestrates, organises, and achieves immediate, but also long-term, gut homeostasis. The diverse mechanisms leading to gut homeostasis during the neonatal period *rely on breast milk* providing passive immune protection of the host.[249]

The newborn gut has evolved to be uniquely receptive to, and dependent upon, both breastmilk and microbial colonisation. The complex structure of a neonate's intestinal tract grows exponentially in the first days and weeks, protected by that coating of secretory IgA while the microbiome gets working to establish itself. The multiplicity of colonising organisms – viruses, fungi, as well as bacteria – communicate with one another[250] and with gut cells, orchestrating how the gut develops, in complex ways that not only ensure their own preservation, proliferation and evolution, but also block out rival bugs.[251] Similarly, the gut cells induce changes in the microbes, allowing them to develop effectively. This is true symbiosis, different life forms living closely together for mutual benefit. The gut bacteria

> ... form biofilms, interconnected microbial communities that can resist the forces that threaten to dislodge them ... Individual bacteria utilise different genes and acquire new properties when they become part of a biofilm. These genes are induced by the gut epithelia and mucus, allowing the bacteria to adhere together and to change their nutrient intake.[252]

---

249 Boudry G, Hamilton MK. Milk formula and intestinal barrier function. In Preedy VR, Watson RR, Zibadi A, op. cit., p. 569
250 Gobbetti M, Di Cagno R. *Bacterial Communication in Foods* (Springer 2013.)
251 Macfarlane GT, Macfarlane S. Human colonic microbes: ecology, physiology and metabolic potential of intestinal bacteria. In Isolauri E, Walker WA (eds): *Allergic Diseases and the Environment*. Nestlé Nutrition Workshops Series Paediatric Program vol. 53, pp. 179–98. Karger Switzerland/Nestec 2004.
252 Gilbert SF, Epel D. *Ecological Developmental Biology: integrating epigenetics, medicine and evolution* (Sinauer Associates 2009) pp. 98–100.

Gut mucus varies in thickness and composition, and so different bacteria form biofilms in different regions of the gut.[253] Bacteria break down different food components into nutrients that can be absorbed by the baby's gut and/or used as nutrients by different bacteria further downstream. Newly-discovered viruses[254] may be acting as control mechanisms. It's a complex ecosystem, with, some think, the appendix acting as a reserve store of the gut microbiota, enabling rapid re-inoculation should the balance be destroyed by diarrhoeal disease or toxins, or indeed, antibiotics.[255]

As the authors of a recent study said,

> The gut microbiota has profound effects on the health and wellness of the host [i.e. the baby]. For example, studies in germ-free piglets clearly illustrate altered intestinal growth, digestive enzyme activity and development of the gut-associated lymphoid tissue. Molecular-level studies, enabled by metagenomic, metatranscriptomic and metaproteomic analytical techniques, are reshaping our understanding of how the gut microbiome modulates gastrointestinal morphological, immune development, gene expression, and the biology of the host in general.[256]

This study demonstrated that diet affected gut bacteria, which affected gene expression in babies, and that this differed between those breastfed and those not breastfed. It looked not only at the effect of diet on the infant microbiota, but – by examining cells shed from the babies' gut lining and retrieved from faeces – also the infant's own genome, and the transcriptome-level cross-talk between the developing infant gut and its colonising microbiota. (The transcriptome is the complete set of messenger RNA molecules. RNA is present in all cells, and carries instructions from DNA. The idea that human gut cells and bacteria can communicate would once have seemed as unlikely as humans talking to aliens!) So the food we give our babies affects their genes.

The non-human proteins in formula trigger immune responses that can include alterations in gut transit time and dangerous inflammation, which the baby lacking breastmilk is not well-equipped to bring under control. The non-human fats in formula break down into free fatty acids that can be toxic to intestinal cells, directly causing gut inflammation.[257] Assaulting the normal infant stomach and gut with unnecessarily large volumes of formula produces larger volumes of waste, which support gut bacteria of different kinds. Pathogens like Clostridia[258] are more likely to thrive and become entrenched, and infection can

253 Bollinger RR, Barbas AS, Bush EL, Lin SS, Parker W. Biofilms in the normal human large bowel: fact rather than fiction. *Gut* 2007, 56(10):1481–82. (PMID:17872584) Free full text article

254 Ghoraysi A. The super-abundant virus controlling our gut. *New Scientist* 2 August 2014, p. 15.

255 Bollinger RR, Barbas AS, Bush EL, Lin SS, Parker W. Biofilms in the large bowel suggest an apparent function of the human vermiform appendix. (PMID:17936308) *J Theor Biol* 2007; 249(4):826–31.

256 Schwartz S, Friedberg I, Ivanov IV, Davidson LA et al. A metagenomic study of diet-dependent interaction between gut microbiota and host in infants reveals differences in immune response *Genome Biology* 2012, 13:r32 DOI:10.1186/gb-2012-13-4-r32

257 Penn AH, Altshuler AE, Small JW, Taylor SF et al. Digested formula but not digested fresh human milk causes death of intestinal cells *in vitro*: implications for necrotising enterocolitis. *Pediatric Research* 2012; 72: 560–67 DOI:10.1038/pr.2012.125

258 This spore-forming highly resistant bug has been linked with late onset autism. Finegold SM *Therapy and epidemiology of autism – clostridial spores as key elements.* (PMID:17904761) *Med Hypoth* 2008, 70(3):508–11.

sometimes spread from the gut to deep within the body, causing sepsis[259] and osteomyelitis (bone disease). Animals as well as humans are vulnerable to this.[260]

Clostridium perfringens type B has also been recently suggested as a suspect for triggering multiple sclerosis[261] thanks to its ability to affect blood brain barrier permeability and allow bacterial toxins to affect the brain. Many other diseases, including meningitis are now suspected of arising from such gut problems.

Yet many studies fail to look for the effects of quantity and type of formula, even when it would seem relevant to their aims. To the Canadian authors referred to earlier (see page 77) the daily diet of the newborn infant seemed a taboo topic. There was no discussion of maternal flora at birth and four months, little detail about early exposure of the breastfed infants to formula in hospital (much less microbiological testing of that formula), and nothing at all about the actual formulas infants were consuming at four months. So even this (very small) Canadian study failed dismally to compare the outcomes of true exclusive breastfeeding from birth to the time of the study, with outcomes in infants fed different specific infant formulas, as by then the sample would be. Similarly, even in recent studies of biodiversity in older children, no investigation of birthing or feeding methods was involved. Were those fully breastfed in Russia and Finland more likely to foster the helpful microbes from their environment? More likely to deal effectively with the higher bacterial loads in the water supply in Russia?[262] The studies don't say. The realisation decades ago that infant formula altered the infant's faecal flora should have been reason enough to advise against all artificial feeding – had doctors then understood how central to health are our bugs.

Despite that, the commercially motivated sales pitches persuading people to eat this or that strain of 'probiotic' (live bacteria, remember, with the specific strain not always named), or to feed probiotics to their babies, are proceeding apace without much obvious critical independent scrutiny, much less regulation,[263] of such products and their long-term effects. Does this matter?

It takes time to create a stable healthy microbiome, and many factors influence it, not least the use of foods other than breastmilk. To appreciate the complexity of the processes involved, it is worth reading about the even more complex evolution of our genetic blueprint in conjunction with bacteria and viruses over three billion years, in Le Page's article, 'A brief history of the genome' in New Scientist of 15 September 2012.[264] He makes

---

259  Hanson LA. *Immunobiology of Human Milk.* op. cit., p. 16.
260  Steinwender G, Schimpl G, Sixl B, Wenzl HH Gut-derived bone infection in the neonatal rat. (PMID:11726738) *Pediatric Research* 2001; 50(6):767–71.
261  Rumah KR, Linden J, Fischetti VA, Vartanian T (2013) Isolation of Clostridium perfringens Type B in an Individual at First Clinical Presentation of Multiple Sclerosis Provides Clues for Environmental Triggers of the Disease. *PLoS ONE* 8(10): e76359. DOI:10.1371/journal.pone.0076359
262  Von Hertzen L, Laatikainen T, Pitkänen T, Vlasoff T et al. Microbial content of drinking water in Finnish and Russian Karelia – implications for atopy prevalence. (PMID:17298346) *Allergy* 2007, 62(3):288–92. DOI: 10.1111/j.1398-9995.2006.01281.x
263  Dr. Martin Blaser comments that 'It's the Wild West: the field is almost completely unregulated.' op. cit., p. 210. He's head of the Human Microbiology Project at NYU. Read his book.
264  Le Page M. A brief history of the genome. *New Scientist* 2012; 215 (2882); 30–35.

the point that we are all still evolving: 'You have around 100 mutations in your genome that are not present in your mother or father, ranging from one or two letter changes to the loss or gain of huge chunks of DNA.'

Generally, it has become accepted that, as Zivkovic summarises it,

> The interaction of humans with microorganisms remains one of the most important relationships to both acute survival and long-term health. Humans emerged into a microbial world, and the microbial world continues to shape human evolutionary progress ... Understanding how to manage microbial biology in the future will require more sophisticated tools aimed at modifying microbial populations and functions toward human health benefits other than simply preventing pathogenic infection. Insights into how to guide human/ microbial interactions to be net favorable for both are needed. The connection between human breast milk and infants' growth, development, and health exemplifies this link. Human milk is the culmination of 200 million years of Darwinian pressure on mammalian lactation as the source of early infant immunoprotection and nourishment. Human milk components not only nourish the infant, they provide myriad bioactive compounds for the offspring that influence the growth, stimulation, and modulation of the immune system, cognitive development, protection from toxins and pathogenic diseases, and perhaps most remarkably, the establishment of the intestinal microbiota (1–3). Considerable efforts made to understand the biology of human milk and its effects on the infant (4) are beginning to elucidate the structure/function properties and benefits that milk provides.[265]

As Zivkovic flags, mothers' milk provides many growth factors and specific nutrients for friendly bacteria that accelerate and assist normal gut development. Animal research has shown that within a few days of birth the gut of a colostrum-fed piglet has developed more complex structures, compared with an artificially fed piglet of identical bodyweight.[266] Any gut developed by pathogens will harbour those pathogens longer, and thus behave differently, than a gut developed by the friendly commensals that breastmilk fosters and the breastfeeding mother's body supplies.

The high protein level, different fats, and many other ingredients in formula all affect the postnatal development of gut microbiota, the epithelial barrier and immune function in piglets and alter gut responses to inflammatory mediators later in life.[267] All those much higher-protein formulas of the 1950s to 1980s have almost certainly been involved in Western gut disorders of epidemic proportions. Though they have dropped considerably over time, levels of protein in formula are still high (13–19 g/L) by comparison with breastmilk (9 g/L). But while the higher protein levels feed these altered biomes, the solution isn't as simple as reducing the amount of protein in formula. Compared to breastmilk's natural proteins, the proteins that formula

---

265   Zivkovic AM, et al.
266   Reinhart GA, Simmen FA, Mahan DC, White ME, Roehrig KL. Intestinal development and fatty acid binding protein activity of newborn pigs fed colostrum or milk. *Biol Neonate* 1992; 62(2–3):155–63. (PMID:1420614); Wang T, Xu RJ. Effects of colostrum feeding on intestinal development in newborn pigs. *Biol Neonate* 1996, 70(6):339–48. (PMID:9001695)
267   Chatelais L, Jamin A, Gras-Le Guen C, Lallès J-P et al. The level of protein in milk formula modifies ileal sensitivity to LPS later in life in a piglet model. (PMCID:PMC3090415) *PLoS One*. 2011; 6(5): e19594. DOI: *10.1371/journal.pone.0019594*

companies use are less bioavailable, i.e. less easily absorbed by the baby, and deficiency diseases could result from lowering formula protein levels to those of breastmilk.

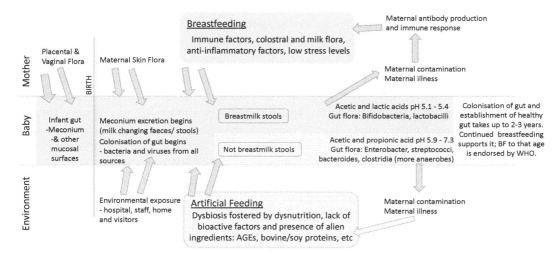

Figure 2-4-4 Developing the gut microbiome  Diagram by Catherine HorsfallL

Of course there are those who would say that animal evidence is irrelevant. Yet such animal studies are routinely used as the basis of safety studies for infant formula. And pigs are seen as the best model to use for researching gut issues, as mammals that have digestive systems akin to ours.[268] It is obviously impossible to conduct any studies on human babies that involve the sacrifice and dissection of the subject! So animal studies are as close as we can get before industry tests the product in the real world, on small numbers of babies, usually in countries where parents are less likely to sue companies than in America. Learning from that live-baby testing has driven and will always drive infant formula development. Industry publications now say clearly that

> There is good experimental evidence that the intestinal microbiota is a main driver of the development of the mucosal immune system, with a critical phase during initial colonization after birth ... Therefore, it is easily understandable that perturbations/changes of the colonization process may cause health problems with short- and eventually long-term consequences. Examples of diseases resulting from a disturbed microbial-host interaction are numerous, such as allergic diseases or dysimmune disorders, particularly those involving the intestinal tract, such as inflammatory bowel diseases.[269]

We have known for decades that both formulas[270] and antibiotics drastically affect the infant's developing microbiome or ecosystem. There is widespread agreement about those facts. Studies in germ-free mice suggest that having been given antibiotics may increase the risk

---

268 Guilloteau P, Zabielski R, Hammon HM, Metges CC. Nutritional programming of gastrointestinal tract development. Is the pig a good model for man? *Nutr Res Rev* 2010, 23(1):4–22. PMID:20500926

269 Ruemmle F, Garnier-Lengliné H. Transforming Growth Factor and Intestinal Inflammation: The Role of Nutrition. Nestle Nutr Inst Workshop Ser 2013, 77:91–98

270 Bullen CL, Tearle PV, Willis AT. Bifidobacteria in the intestinal tract of infants: an in-vivo study. *J Med Microbiol* 1976, 9(3):325–33. (PMID:8646)

of allergy, as well.[271] We know that it can be weeks before the infant microbiome returns to normal after such insults, if it ever does, in the fully breastfed infant. In a study of the levels of beneficial Lactobacilli species (which inhibit the growth of Streptococci bacteria) in the oral microbiota of three-month-old children, none was found in formula-fed infants. Those helpful bacteria were found in the oral microbiota of breastfed infants, but not all of them, possibly due to antibiotic use.[272] Does this documented difference in mouth bacteria help explain the bottle-fed infant's greater susceptibility to respiratory disease, ear infection and perhaps dental caries? New questions about the risks of artificial feeding seem endless. A mouth or gut blitzed by either perinatal antibiotics or infant formula may be at risk of subsequent invasion and colonisation by the hardiest microbes, which may not be the healthiest. Western society has attacked all of the fundamental pillars of our immune system.

Which raises the controversial question of the dangers of 'complementary feeding' of infant formula, usually the earliest exposure of infants to a wide variety of foods other than breastmilk. This next section about such feeds is both longer and shorter than I would like, as it is hard to do justice to the many aspects of this issue. There is additional material in Book 3, Chapter 6. And to understand the underlying science, I recommend a review of 'early-life nutrition, its effects on the microbiota and the consequences of diet-induced perturbation of the structure of the microbial community on mucosal immunity and disease susceptibility'[273] discovered just as this book is going to press. It (Figure 2-12-2 on page 194) sums up much that I have been laboriously putting into words on the topic of the developing microbiome. But I need to point out a small but serious inconsistency in that diagram, one which I did not expect to see from authors so aware of breastmilk's effects.

---

271  Rodriguez B, Prioult G, Bibiloni R, Nicolis I et al. Germ-free status and altered caecal subdominant microbiota are associated with a high susceptibility to cow's milk allergy in mice. *FEMS Microbiology Ecology* [2011, 76(1):133–44. DOI: 10.1111/j.1574-6941.2010.01035.

272  Holgerson PL, Vestman NR, Claesson R, Ohman C, et al. Oral microbial profile discriminates breast-fed from formula-fed infants. *J Pediatr Gastroenterol Nutr* 2013, 56(2):127–36. (PMID:22955450)

273  Jain N, Walker WA. Diet and host-microbial crosstalk in postnatal intestinal immune homeostasis. (PMID:25201040) *Nat Rev Gastroenterol Hepatol* 2015; 12: 14-25 DOI: 10.1038/nrgastro.2014.153

# 2.5 Complementary feeds given to breastfed babies

Before going any further, terms need to be clarified. Back in the 1960s and 1970s there were solemn discussions of the difference between 'complementary' and 'supplementary' feeds given to breastfed babies. 'Complementary' feeds were supposed to simply top up baby without affecting lactation (they 'complemented' lactation), while 'supplementary' feeds were supposedly needed to supplement a poor milk supply, otherwise baby would starve. Both were supplements, in the more generally accepted usage of the word, or additives to the breastfed baby's diet. Indeed Abbott/Ross is now marketing a version of Similac targeting breastfed babies who are supposedly in need of supplements.[274] Which of course means in reality, encouraging mixed feeding and so early weaning, as their website clearly demonstrates to anyone knowledgeable about lactation. (See page 513)

Like many 1970s mothers, I could see no logical difference between comps and supps: they were both feeding babies, so how could anyone be sure that lactation was not affected?[275] 'Prelacteal feeds' (given before the first breastfeed) were simply not talked about. Now the language has changed. 'Pre-lacteal' is increasingly used to mean feeds before milk volume increases after childbirth. This illogical and inaccurate description implies that the feeds are pre- (before) lactation, and yet lactation is already well underway, just in its early deliberately low-volume phase. Meanwhile, amusingly, in the new Guidelines from Australia's National Health and Medical Research Council (NHMRC) the old usage has now been completely reversed:

> In Australia there is no clear differentiation between the terms 'supplementary feeding' and 'complementary feeding'. In these Guidelines, supplementary feeding is defined as 'additional liquids given to the infant during the first 7 days after birth, including glucose solutions, water, and commercial infant formula'. Complementary feeding is defined as the process starting when breast milk alone is no longer sufficient to meet the nutritional requirements of infants, and therefore other foods and liquids are needed, along with breast milk.[276]

So in that set of Guidelines 'complementary feeding' means the widening of the infant diet at six months or so. And supplementary feeding is what I will discuss as 'comp feeds'. The NHMRC definitions make sense, though I can see no logical reason to limit the definition of 'supplementary' feeds to seven days after birth, especially when companies are now aggressively marketing infant formula products as supplements to breastfeeding. But I'd better make it clear that in this book, when I refer to 'comp feeds', I mean any liquids or foods given in hospital or after discharge to young breastfed babies while the mother's

---

274  Whatever Abbott's avowed intentions, the formula seems no different from any of their other versions of the same brand. And they are protecting their products from proof of inadequacy, not protecting babies, by mixing these feeds.

275  Once I understood that each breast can rapidly and independently adjust its initial overproduction down to making just what the infant drinks, it was obvious that giving anything would, over time, reduce the amount of milk made. Supply responds to demand via elegant and powerful feedback mechanisms.

276  NHMRC 2013. *Infant Feeding Guidelines for Healthworkers*, p. 71.

milk supply and the baby's gut microbiome are both being established. That's the term that was usual among 1970s nursing staff, and may be recognised by readers: 'baby needed a comp feed'. And it's ironically appropriate: these feeds often were '**compli**mentary' (free of charge) thanks to industry gifts to hospitals, and they were not **comple**mentary at all, but **comp**etitive with, lactation. Competitive feeds decrease the amount the baby takes from the breast, and so depress milk synthesis rates, which are faster when breasts are emptier. Yet such exposures to infant formula are still very common in 2013. Official statements like those *NHMRC Guidelines for Healthworkers*[277] do little to discourage the giving of what they now call supplements, not even mentioning their inevitable distorting impact on the microbiome, while urging that 'the mother's agreement' be secured: i.e., protecting the institution, but not the infant or family.

## Comp-feeding – why did the practice arise?

The underlying medical assumption that enabled unrestricted comp-feeding from the 1930s onwards was that for many children, food other than the mother's own milk was necessary to avoid catastrophic harms due to hypoglycaemia (low blood sugar) or severe jaundice or even dehydration.[278] This assumption arose from ignorance of the normal course of lactation and the importance of limited volumes of fluid to the newborn. It was never proven before being widely accepted.

In fact, hospital policies based on artificial feeding and limited knowledge of lactation had been *causing* both starvation jaundice (by limiting feed times and making milk transfer difficult) and hypoglycaemia (by not allowing babies breast access for hours after birth, and giving water or sugar solutions.) Restricting skin-to-skin contact, breast access and breastfeeding had been routine. Until the 1980s, no one had measured usual breastmilk intake in the first days of life, and cadaver studies had been used to determine infant stomach volumes – and stomachs are distensible! The fact that a stomach can be over-filled is not a reason to do so. Live babies simply blurt back a lot of it, but that can be traumatic.

Even though studies showed low intakes were normal,[279] and unrestricted breastfeeding was shown to prevent both hypoglycaemia and jaundice, some staff refused to take in the knowledge or change their practice. The tiny quantities of colostrum and milk produced in the first couple of days certainly were not enough to stop the baby feeding more often than every three or four hours, and frequent feeding meant more staff were needed to assist mothers. Routine weighing showed how little babies were getting from the breast: 'You've

---

277  ibid. References to increased morbidity and mortality in China will not discourage use in countries like Australia. Discussion of dysbiosis might.

278  Dehydration with disastrous consequences is indeed on record in breastfed babies sent home unable to breastfeed well (usually thanks to poor breast attachment) from mothers whose milk supply is not well-established and who are unsupported and poorly educated about infant needs and growth. The problem is not breastmilk,or breastfeeding, or the mother, but starvation thanks to poor management of such mothers. Every hospital which records such cases in its postpartum women needs to take responsibility for the consequences, and initiate preventive strategies.

279  Average feed size: day 1: 7 ml; day 2: 14 ml; day 3: 38 ml; day 4: 58 ml. Average total daily intake: day 1: 15 ml; day 2: 37 ml; day 3: 84 ml.

only given him 10 ml, Mrs Jones, he'll need a top-up to last till his next feed.' That was within hours of birth, when in fact 10 ml is a substantial amount for any one feed.

Hospital management was organised, and still is, around the availability of staff, not around the needs of babies or their mothers. Scheduled feeds had no scientific justification, but were convenient for staff who kept babies in distant nurseries, to be wheeled out only at specified, predictable times. Infant formula 'top-ups' (or comp feeds) were a way of stretching out breastfeeds to the four hours seen as desirable or practical in many hospitals. (Formula makers Abbott-Ross provided free architectural 'services to hospitals for planning and layout',[280] 'building bottle-feeding into the facility by physically separating mother and infant to make bottle-feeding more convenient than breastfeeding for hospital staff.'[281] And of course, industry supplied all that was needed for bottle-feeding: throwaway bottles and teats and single serve formulas in some places. Artificial feeding rapidly became the norm (see Book 2).

A Swedish study[282] which compared three cohorts from the years 1970, 1973 and 1976, from the same hospital in an industrial town, illustrates how rapidly commercial infant formula could replace breastmilk. Overall, in the period 1970–76, 33 per cent of 736 infants were fed mothers' milk plus formula. This was mostly in 1976, when in fact 68 per cent, or 162/239 infants, were comp fed formula. Just two of 282 (0.7 per cent) had been fed infant formula in 1970. This was in a hospital where fresh unpasteurised donor human milk was freely available and had been routinely used, during hospital stays of six to eight days postpartum. So the practice of giving extra milk was entrenched, and then formula was made available and assumed to be safe. As a result, from 1970–76 formula use increased almost a hundredfold. The duration of breastfeeding was only 3–4 months, and very few (18/754) children were formula-fed *before* being breastfed, with none *solely* breastfed from birth. In this largely breastfed and early-weaned population, the formula-fed from birth, the formula-fed before breastfeeding, and those solely breastfed for 6 months, are the groups that might have different allergy outcomes from the norm, but there are simply too few in each of those groups to generalise from. Same country, same hospital, and in just six years the feeding patterns were revolutionised by commercial forces.

In some countries like the US it is difficult to enrol exclusively breastfed children for research purposes; in Scandinavian countries[283] it can be hard now to find exclusively formula-fed children! (That has not always been the case: Dr Gro Nylander asserts that 'for several decades up to about 1975 formula was routinely given to all babies in Norwegian maternity wards ... After that, sugar water was given instead.'[284])

---

280  Abbott/Ross Annual Report 1972, cited in ICCR *The Corporate Examiner* 1982; issue 7–8, p. 3.

281  ibid.

282  Gustafsson D, Lowhagen T, Andersson K. Risk of developing atopic disease after early feeding with cows' milk-based formula. *Arch Dis Child* 1992; 67: 1008–10.

283  In the past all these countries have had extremely low rates of breastfeeding, and so those now breastfeeding may have been affected by artificial feeding via their parents.

284  Nylander G. *Becoming a Mother: birth to 6 months.* (Celestial Arts Press, 2002) p. 154. In epic quantities. Her study showed that they averaged 20 ounces of sugar water in the first 3 days, in bodyweight terms 'the equivalent of more than 40 bottles of soft drink' by adults. p. 155.

It is said that a similar process happened in traditional communities in which acceptance of the child into the family involved the paternal grandmother putting the child to breast. Once infant formula was marketed, for family acceptance it became necessary for the grandmother to feed the child some formula. A harmless and helpful custom became a damaging one because of the assumption that formula was the same as breastmilk – or better, since it cost more.

## Effects of the odd hospital bottle

Does that early exposure matter? How harmless are a couple of hospital bottles? There has been considerable discussion of this issue in the medical literature. Most of what has been written is unreliable because feeding has not been clearly researched and documented. But those studies have been widely publicised, so that many wrongly think the question resolved. Almost any study that talks about 'exclusively breastfed' children born in the mid-1970s must have been finding children born in hospitals unknown to the infant formula companies of the day! And when any study does not document either the exclusivity, or the duration of exclusive breastfeeding, any conclusions about health outcomes in infancy or adulthood are deeply suspect.

So let's start not from limited and limiting studies, or reviews of those studies, but from first principles, from the basic science of normal gastrointestinal and immune development.' Giving any bioactive substance other than breastmilk is disruptive to the normal development of the gut, and so has the potential to affect the development of tolerance to foods being sampled in breastmilk. That's a fact. Anything given to a newborn needs to be proven safe beyond reasonable doubt. 'First do no harm' is the guiding principle of medicine. So there must be a major body of literature showing that 'comp feeds' do no harm, do not change the infant microbiome, do not increase allergy rather than create tolerance, do not interfere with lactation, do not stress infant kidneys – or comp feeds would not be happening. Right?

Wrong. There is no such reassuring proof. Research has for decades[285] shown very different gut flora in breastfed and artificially fed babies. Newer developments in infant formula and the exposure of breastfeeding women to antibiotics have brought changes, but there are still, and always will be, major differences between breastfed and formula-fed children. Gut flora is influenced by the mother's milk, skin and vaginal flora,[286] and these in turn will be influenced by her environment, diet and exposure to her infant and partner and other children as well. This is a feedback loop, and formula in hospital may have direct and indirect effects.

285  Willis AT, Bullen CL, Williams K, Fagg CG, et al. *Breast milk substitute: a bacteriological study*. (PMID:4583181) *Br Med J* 1973, 4(5884):67–72; Bullen CL, Tearle PV, Stewart MG The effect of 'humanised' milks and supplemented breast feeding on the faecal flora of infants. (PMID:21296) *J Med Microbiol* 1977; 10(4):403–13

286  Jost T, Lacroix C, Braegger CP, Rochat F et al. Vertical mother-neonate transmission of maternal gut bacteria via breast-feeding. *Envir Microbiol.* 2013; DOI: 10.1111.1462-2920.12238 ; Jost T, Lacroix C, Braegger CP, Chassard C. New insights in gut microbiota establishment in healthy breast fed neonates. (PMID:22957008) Free full text article *PLoS One* 2012; 7(8):e44595. DOI:10.1371/journal.p one.04495

As noted earlier Infant formula companies are actively experimenting with what they call supplementation of the breastfed infant, and I call competitive mixed feeding. But as yet there have been few detailed long-term studies to ascertain in full the microbial and immune outcomes of comp-feeding, even that ubiquitous 'just one bottle'.[287] A recent Canadian study found persistent microbial differences at four months[288]. Another study of children who were solely breastfed for varying times after the first three days, found that

> Exposure to cow's milk (formula) during the first three days of life stimulated IgG antibody production to cow's milk proteins and this was still obvious at two years of age, while feeding with a casein hydrolysate (formula) during the first three days of life was associated with low levels of IgG antibodies to cow's milk proteins.[289]

They claimed (others disagree) that high IgG levels can be a marker of reactivity.[290] The effects, whatever their consequences, were most marked in babies solely breastfed for less than two months after this initial exposure. I'll refer back to this when discussing genetic polymorphism[291] a bit further on.

In fact, it would take a lot of money and techniques only recently developed – or still unavailable – to log the long-term effects of formula use on gut flora and gut development. The gut bugs we currently can identify are possibly only about 10 per cent of the total microbiome. We still know very little about interactions even between known microbes.

As for research into long-term immunological outcomes, where would the money come from? Hospital comp-feeding has been around for decades; it became almost universal. (Such wide reach is the prerequisite for creating widespread immune distortion.) In Finland in a consecutive series of 6209 infants in 1994–95, 5385 babies 'required supplementary milk at hospital because of insufficient secretion of breastmilk.'[292] It is still happening in many Australian hospitals, just with mothers persuaded that they authorised it by signing a bit of paper. Everyone 'knows' it is perfectly safe, or 'they wouldn't do it, would they?' Is this another assumption, akin to the one that resulted in the blinding of preterm infants when doctors 'knew' that oxygen was safe to administer? Or 'knew' (and told parents)

287  See Walker M. Supplementation of the breastfed baby. Just one bottle won't hurt: or will it? Online at http://www.naba-breastfeeding.org/images/Just%20One%20Bottle.pdf or www.health-e-learning.com/articles/JustOneBottle.pdf

288  Biasucci G, Rubini M, Riboni S, Morelli L, et al. Mode of delivery affects the bacterial community in the newborn gut. PMID:20133091) *Early Human Development* 2010; 86 Suppl 1:13–15.

289  Juvonen P, Månsson M, Kjellman NI, Björkstén B, Jakobsson I. Development of immunoglobulin G and immunoglobulin E antibodies to cow's milk proteins and ovalbumin after a temporary neonatal exposure to hydrolyzed and whole cow's milk proteins. (PMID:10565560) *Pediatr Allergy Immunol* 1999, 10(3):191–98.

290  Eysink PE, De Jong MH, Bindels PJ, Scharp-Van Der Linden VT et al. Relation between IgG antibodies to foods and IgE antibodies to milk, egg, cat, dog and/or mite in a cross-sectional study. *Clinical and Experimental Allergy* 1999; 29(5):604–10.

291  Poly – many; morph – form; polymorphism is used to describe the different forms of a single gene that can exist in a person or a group. An example of genetic polymorphism is different blood groups in humans. Polymorphism is when multiple genetic varieties exist in any population, whereas a mutation is a change in a gene in one individual.

292  Saarinen KM et al (1999) op. cit. It is simply impossible that lactation has failed so badly in such a short time that 87 per cent of Finnish women cannot produce enough milk for the first few day of an infant's life. This is proof of poor hospital practice and medical lack of understanding of lactation..

that laying refluxing babies down to sleep prone made for better sleep? Eternal sleep was not what parents had in mind! Many (un)informed consent forms used by hospitals are a precaution designed to protect the facility, not the infant.

So should we continue to assume that such feeds are safe? That 'the great majority of healthy infants tolerate these supplements with no deleterious effect'?[293] Or should we recognise that the effects of gut un-ease, even disease, and infant crying have become so common that they characterise the 'great majority' and are therefore accepted as normal behaviour?

That comp feeds mess up the microbiome has been known for over half a century, long before scientists realised how central that microbiome is to infant and adult metabolism and programming of growth. Even without any evidence about long term programming, or genetic damage, or effects on lactation, or other deleterious effects, I would assume that the single fact of dysbiosis (the wrong microbiome) means such comp feeds are risky, because they alter a normal process of development. They alter the normal processes, and instead lead to sensitisation and later reaction.

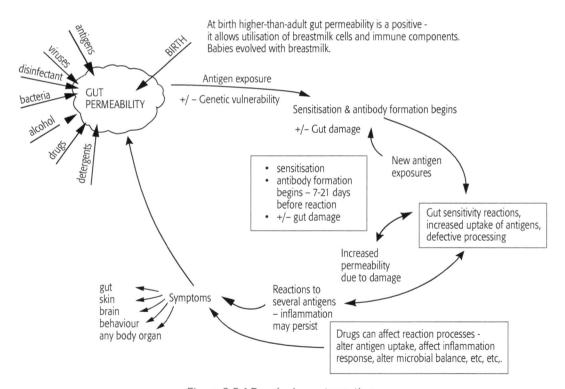

Figure 2-5-1 Developing gut reactions

How dangerous are they? Until we have a great deal more research, we can't catalogue all the harmful outcomes, though we know some, like the connection between shorter

293 ibid.

breastfeeding duration[294] and higher risks of necrotising enterocolitis especially, but not only, in preterm infants. There are many possible effects, from infection to nutritional intakes to gut function. Most of the colicky babies I have known go on to have ongoing gut unease and disease. (And their childhood and adult symptoms are usually responsive to diet changes.)

But do we need proof of universal harm before we outlaw the practice of comp-feeding babies with alien milks? Why would we, when they are both unnecessary and on first principles risky? Along with the World Health Organization (WHO), UNICEF, and other authoritative bodies, the US Joint Commission, which accredits hospitals, has decided actively to promote exclusive breastfeeding: they are all convinced that such formula feeds may do harm to at least *some* children, and *any* is too many.

Yet some healthworkers are reluctant to change. Perhaps this is because they have been giving such foreign feeds, and issuing such unwarranted and dogmatic opinions, for so long. Perhaps it is because of the tacit approval in official statements written by health professionals unwilling to spell out the science and criticise their colleagues' practices. In the case of parents, perhaps they have a damaged child and want to believe that the damage is solely genetic in origin.

Even the Finnish Allergy Group, despite their concern about microbiomes and environments, have not made it clear that human milk feeding needs to be exclusive from birth, and formula feeding in hospitals should be treated as seriously as any other medical intervention affecting gut colonisation and infant metabolism, with needless use penalised! Their Plan says more about restricting antibiotics than about restricting infant formula, though both inevitably distort development of the infant microbiome. Perhaps infant formula is considered more necessary than antibiotics? (Yet as noted earlier, Professor Allan Walker now talks of the *necessity* of breastmilk.) See page 15.

It can be very hard to face up to the possibility that something we allowed, or perhaps even requested, may have harmed children. What we don't face, we don't fix.

## Comp feeds and allergy

Both for lactation to become problematic for 90 per cent of women, and for allergy to explode within populations, the causes have to be ubiquitous, population-wide. The widespread use of comp feeds certainly undermine women's confidence in their ability to provide milk for their babies, and interferes with the normal onset of lactation. But were comp feeds on this population-wide scale also increasing rates of allergic disease? My clinical and personal experience says yes, but what about the studies I referred to?

There are studies that show that exclusive breastfeeding (no comps from birth) reduces the risk of allergic disease. One of the few early long-term studies available looking at this shows

294 Chantry CJ, Dewey KG, Peerson JM, Wagner EA et al. *In-hospital formula use increases early breastfeeding cessation among first-time mothers intending to exclusively breastfeed. J Pediatr* 2014, 164(6):1339-45.e5 PMID:24529621. DOI: 10.1016/j.jpeds.2013.12.035

clear and enduring benefit in relation to allergy.[295] In Finland they 'followed up healthy infants during their first year, and then at one, three, five, ten, and seventeen years to determine the effect on atopic disease of breastfeeding.' Children were classified into three groups as regards breastfeeding duration: less than one month (little or no breastfeeding), one to six months (short breastfeeding), and more than six months (prolonged breastfeeding – which WHO would define as normal these days). Of the initial 236 children, 150 completed the seventeen-year follow-up, 'involving history-taking, physical examination, and laboratory tests for allergy'.

Manifest allergy throughout follow-up was highest in the group who had little or no breastfeeding. Eczema at one and three years was lowest in those breastfed beyond six months; food allergy was highest in the little or no breastfeeding group at one to three years. Respiratory allergy (asthma, rhinoconjunctivitis) prevalence had risen to 65 per cent (two-thirds!) in the little or no breastfeeding group by seventeen years of age. Prevalence of severe atopy generally at age seventeen in the prolonged, short, and little or no breastfeeding groups was 8 per cent, 23 per cent, and 54 per cent. The Finnish researchers concluded that 'breastfeeding is prophylactic against atopic disease – including atopic eczema, food allergy, and respiratory allergy – throughout childhood and adolescence.' I would add, 'in that generation, whose mothers were birthed in the postwar period of austerity in Europe'. The children of allergic Finnish families in 2014 (whose mothers, as noted earlier, were very likely exposed to formula neonatally in the 1980s) may have more problems, though exclusive breastfeeding is still the only safe initial option.

Similarly in Australia a decade later, a careful prospective birth cohort study found that delayed introduction of milk other than breastmilk[296] was associated with a reduction in the risk of asthma and allergy at age six, and with a significant delay in the age at onset of wheezing and medically diagnosed asthma.[297] But one Dutch study did find that breastfeeding to nine months reduced eczema risk,[298] an outcome not widely reported perhaps due to the sense that this was exceptional, an abnormal duration of breastfeeding. Yet only a generation back, breastfeeding to nine months was seen as normal.

By the mid-1980s, infant formula was accepted in most hospitals. One centre in Denmark set up a study of allergy that provides information about comp feeds. It was a prospective study of 1749 newborns. In this 1985 Danish cohort, none of 210 children who were truly exclusively breastfed in hospital developed cows' milk allergy under twelve months, and all of the thirty-nine partially breastfed children who did develop allergy under twelve months had been comp-fed 'significantly more often in the first month of life' than others in the study. The full study also revealed that only nine of that thirty-nine developed symptoms while still solely breastfed after discharge: in the other thirty, symptoms emerged after

295 Saarinen UM, Kajosaari M. Breastfeeding as prophylaxis against atopic disease: prospective follow-up study until 17 years. (PMID:7564787) *Lancet* 1995, 346(8982):1065–69 DOI: 10.1016/S0140-6736(95)91742-X
296 Until at least four months of age, not six weeks, as in a Dutch study I'll discuss later.
297 Oddy WH, Holt PG, Sly PD, et al. Association between breast feeding and asthma in 6 year old children: findings of a prospective birth cohort study. *BMJ* 1999;319:815–19.
298 Sicherer SH. The natural history of IgE-mediated cow's milk allergy. *Pediatrics* 2008; 122: S186; doi:10.1542/peds.2008-2139X citing Snijders

other foods were introduced. And scandalously, only one of those nine mothers was aware that her child had been comp fed in hospital. The amount fed in hospital ranged from 40 to 830 ml, or eight teaspoons to most of a litre, which makes it hard to posit any safe or beneficial level of exposure! [299]

However, note that even here, only 210 of 1749 babies escaped hospital without being exposed to cows' milk protein, i.e., were probably exclusively breastfed from birth. Thankfully, only thirty-nine of the 1539 breastfed infants exposed to bovine milk in the first month went on to develop the particular symptoms that in this study defined allergy, a low rate compared with later studies, perhaps because of the intergenerational effects of their mother's feeding. Thirty of the thirty-nine developed allergy only after foods other than breastmilk were fed. But it is physiologically certain that the other 1500 who did not develop certified allergy or intolerance did develop an altered microbiome, and may have had other health problems to deal with as a result. No one assessed the timing of onset or severity of colic, or reflux, or abnormal behaviour, or otitis media, or unexpected infant death, for example.

And what of the other long-term health outcomes, like irritable bowel disease[300] or diabetes (more common in those exposed to cows' milk in formula at a young age),[301] which seem to emerge in Australian families I have worked with over the decades? There is a very plausible case for diabetes risk being increased by early exposure and antibody reaction to bovine insulin, causing later auto-immune beta-cell destruction. For human and bovine insulin there is only a difference of three amino acids, located in the immunogenic areas of the insulin molecule.[1] If diabetes researchers had asked those Danish mothers about neonatal cows' milk exposure, there were at least eight mothers who wrongly believed that their babies had not been so exposed early in life. How many mothers access national Freedom of Information Acts to access public hospital records and see what is written on the feeding charts? (I did; in those days it was affordable.)

A number of recent studies have looked at the issue of whether exposing newborn infants to the many antigens in infant formula is helpful or harmful in relation to allergic disease. The results are as varied as the generations, populations, doses, brands, procedures, and timing of the experiments, and no firm conclusions have emerged. An Italian study says harmful,[302] an Israeli study says helpful.[303] Animal studies suggest that giving sporadic doses almost

---

299  Høst A. Importance of the first meal on the development of cow's milk allergy and intolerance. (PMID:1936970) *Allergy Proceedings* 1991, 12(4):227–32.; Høst A, Husby S, Osterballe O. A prospective study of cow's milk allergy in exclusively breast-fed infants. Incidence, pathogenetic role of early inadvertent exposure to cow's milk formula, and characterisation of bovine milk protein in human milk. (PMID:3201972) *Acta Paed Scand* 1988; 77(5):663–70.

300  Glassman MS, Newman LJ, Berezin S, Gryboski JD. Cow's milk protein sensitivity during infancy in patients with inflammatory bowel disease. (PMID:2371984) *Am J Gastroenterol* 1990; 85(7):838–40.

301  Gottlieb S. Early exposure to cows' milk raises risk of diabetes in high risk children PMCID: PMC1173447 *BMJ.* 2000 October 28; 321(7268):1040.

302  Cantani A, Micera M. Neonatal cow milk sensitisation in 143 case-reports: role of early exposure to cow's milk formula. (PMID:16128043) *Eur Rev Med Pharmacol Sci* 2005; 9(4):227–30.

303  Katz Y, Rajuan N, Goldberg MR, Eisenberg E, et al. Early exposure to cow's milk protein is protective against IgE-mediated cow's milk protein allergy. (PMID:20541249) *J All Clinical Immunology* 2010, 126(1):77-82.e1. DOI: 10.1016/j.jaci.2010.04.020

immediately after birth and occasionally in the next few days (the usual pattern in Australian hospitals in the 1970s, and still occurring) is much more harmful than giving repeated doses constantly, beginning after some days of mother-feeding to protect the gut.[304] (Industry-funded studies often recruit children only after a couple of weeks of breastfeeding.) An early study by Coombs showed that neonatal exposure of guinea pigs to cows' milk on the second day after birth resulted in nine of the thirty-eight developing persistent antibodies to cows' milk, while the remaining twenty-nine became negative, or tolerant, over time. So the outcome of the same intervention can be quite different, depending on factors in the animals themselves, and other factors that have shaped their response. What makes the difference?

## Comp feeding and family history of allergy

Does the outcome of comp feeding depend on the family's allergy history? And does that history depend on their infant feeding? What might make sense of some apparent contradictions in both study results and practical experience is knowing a great deal more about the mothers who are feeding, and their tolerance of the antigens being fed. A little bit of formula given to the baby of a mother *herself made allergic by milk as a child* may have a different outcome from the same dose given to the child of a *non-allergic* mother. We have known since the 1980s that the same dose of allergenic food fed to lactating women results in very different levels of antigens in their milk[305]: to some had had none, others much more.

Samples of breast milk and serum were taken from 29 women at various stages of lactation before and after they had eaten 1 raw egg and half a pint of milk. Researchers found:

Beta-Lactoglobulin, 10 out of 19    Ovalbumin, 13 out of 22    Ovomucoid, 7 out of 9
Concentrations: ranging from 110 pg/ml to 6.4 ng/ml.
Maximum levels in breast milk were attained 4 or 6 hours after ingestion.
Antigen was detected in blood: 1–2 hours earlier than in milk

Figure 2-5-2 Antigens in milk

What determines the difference in milk levels? What effect do they have? Another Finnish study, which considered the effects of 'atopic heredity' (allergy such as asthma, rhinoconjunctivitis, and eczema in previous generations)[306] concluded that "The long-term effect of breastfeeding was dual: in children with atopic heredity, breastfeeding protected against atopy, whereas in children without atopic heredity, it increased the risk of atopy." They looked at four groups of four-year-olds.

---

304  El-Merhibi A, Lymn K, Kanter I, Penttila IA. Early oral ovalbumin exposure during maternal milk feeding prevents spontaneous allergic sensitisation in allergy-prone rat pups. (PMCID:PMC3235444) *Clin Dev Immunol* 2012, 2012:396232 DOI: 10.1155/2012/396232

305  Kilshaw PJ, Cant AJ. The passage of maternal dietary proteins into human breast milk. (PMID:6746107) *Int Arch Allergy Appl Immunol* 1984; 75(1):8–15

306  Siltanen M, Kajosaari M, Poussa T, Saarinen KM, Savilahti E. A dual long-term effect of breastfeeding on atopy in relation to heredity in children at 4 years of age. *(PMID:12757455) Allergy 2003; 58(6):524–30.*

- Group A had a positive atopic history and was 'breastfed exclusively' and then solely breastfed for at least 3 months (quaintly described as 'long'!) with solids at a mean of 4.4 months (range 4–6) and mean duration of partial breastfeeding around 10 months

- Group B had a negative atopic history and 'long exclusive breastfeeding' with solids at a mean of 4.4 months (range 4–6.5) and mean duration of partial breastfeeding around 10 months

- Group C had positive atopic history and 'early cows' milk-based feeding plus breastfeeding till around 5.4 months, solids at a mean of 3.6 months (range 2–5)

- Group D a negative atopic history and 'early cows' milk-based feeding plus breastfeeding till around 5 months; solids at a mean of 3.4 months (range 2.5–5)

The study found that '... in children with atopic heredity [A and C], 'exclusive breastfeeding' protected against atopy. So not feeding cows' milk formula neonatally reduced the rates of allergy in high-risk children. How explain a higher rate in the lower risk group? The study definitions were interesting. 'Breastfed exclusively' included supplements of pasteurised breastmilk (an unknown quantity) or whey hydrolysate (known to be capable of causing reactions, though fewer than regular formula). Cows' milk fed (Groups C and D) meant children had consumed at least 450 ml of cows' milk in the first two weeks of life – followed by three months of some breastfeeding (with what solids beginning in the middle of that?). Comparing groups B and D it can be seen that this study's definition of exclusive breastfeeding, and the earlier introduction of other solids, increased the risk of allergy being reported in those with no atopic history.

There are a huge number of possibilities here. Maternal diet would have been an important variable. We need to know more about those mothers. It seems possible that the allergic mothers in group A didn't drink cows milk in pregnancy or lactation, while the non-allergic in group B did, which could have affected tolerance of those proteins. And how can we rule out intra-uterine sensitisation in any of the groups? Is the dose important? Over 450 ml is a substantial amount.in the first four days. Some animal studies have found timing and dose critical to results: tiny doses sensitising, large doses suppressing normal immune reactions. Some find adjuvants fed with food important to creating sensitisation. Should mothers without known allergy keep eating such foods themselves during partial breastfeeding in the hope of creating tolerance? Were those non-atopic mothers, or their babies, the ones through whom allergy has now entered that family tree for the first time, so that the next generation is at higher risk of immune disorder if this study were to be repeated?

We don't really know, of course, and this study does not suggest for one moment that babies might be better off not breastfed exclusively, whether from an allergic family or not. A breastfed baby's immune system might simply be more active, if misguided, than an immune system distorted by artificial feeding which leaves a baby vulnerable to infectious and metabolic disease. Studying allergy in isolation from other health and developmental issues can sometimes lead to the wrong conclusions! As when I read recently that

> There is no global support for any significant impact [on allergy] of breast-feeding in industrialized countries. Swedish infants are breast-fed, and this is still the case in 70% of the babies at 3 months... These figures are not mirrored by any lower prevalence of allergies as compared with other industrialized countries with a much lower rate of breast-feeding ... It is also noteworthy that the rapid increase in the rate of breast-feeding in Sweden in the 1970s was not accompanied by any slowing of the increasing incidence of allergies.[307]

All true, regrettably. But so one-dimensional and unaware of the past and its likely impacts, and ignoring infant formula changes. Breastfeeding rates in Sweden were very low before that resurgence, which happened to coincide with newer, hyperallergenic whey-dominant formulas being fed in hospitals from the 1960s and 1970s. And babies 'breastfed' in Sweden have rarely been solely breastfed: we have no idea what allergy rates may have been without the reality of mixed feeding, and that other reality of breastfeeding mothers having been bottle fed in the previous generation. Nor can we be sure that exclusive breastfeeding is practised even now: it remains the exception, resisted as unnecessarily restrictive by many – those who don't think of gut colonisation as important. I view these studies through the lens of the experience of families I have worked with, and have attempted to depict this in the sketch below.

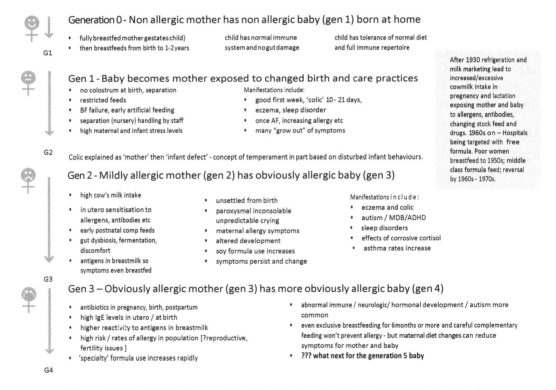

Figure 2-5-3 A sketch of some infant feeding trends Diagram by Catherine Horsfall

I see both the Swedish experience and the Siltanen et al study as supporting the milk hypothesis: the idea that much Western allergy was produced by the compounding effect of

307  Björkstén B. Pediatric Allergy Research – are we on the right track? *Pediatr Allergy Immunol* 2014; 25(1): 4–6. DOI: 10.1111/pai.12184

formula feeding in communities where women who were then non-allergic (let's call them Generation 1, gestated by non-allergic mothers) – attempted to breastfeed, in different decades in particular places. They were often unsuccessful (thanks in part to perinatal stresses and practices limiting breastfeeding. Many of their Gen-2 children, perhaps fed sugar water in hospital, and no longer breastfed to 9-12 months but early switched to home-made cows' milk mixtures, became allergic. A huge increase in eczema was noted around the 1920-30s, and accurately attributed to such cows' milk bottle-feeding.

These largely bottle-fed Gen-2 children then went on to gestate the Gen-3 babies in the 1950-60s, the educated following bad advice in parent manuals which ensured they weaned early. Many affluent Gen-3 children were artificially fed from birth after a bit of colostrum feeding, and very few were exclusively breastfed for any length of time, wherever bottle-feeding had been adopted by the middle classes. It was disadvantaged/poor Gen-3 children who breastfed for financial reasons, although where subsidised formula-feeding was available, soon only about 20 per cent of the total population breastfed at all, mostly the disadvantaged without access to free formula.

Sensitised and/or reacting, by the 1970s and 1980s Gen-3 women (many reacting against past practices and wanting to get back to nature) gestated Gen-4 babies, birthing them in hospitals where industry marketing had ensured that comp-feeding had become universal, and breastfeeding difficulties usual. Educated women had often not been breastfed, much less exclusively breastfed for six months. Their almost universally comp-fed Gen-4 babies of the 1970s and 1980s were unsettled from birth if sensitised in utero; others began to scream with colic (as their mothers had done) ten to twenty-one days after birth, as it takes time for dysbiosis or antibody reactions to increase to the point of creating symptoms. These 1980s Gen-4 babies are now adults[308] and after a lifetime of greater chemical exposure and antibiotics (rarely used before 1960–70, and even less so in animal feeds) are now birthing.

Nowadays advantaged Gen-4 women, many sensitised or allergic, are actively attempting to breastfeed *exclusively*, some because they are aware of allergy problems, others because they know it's better for their baby and all babies. Few succeed in protecting the child's microbiome from insult. They are still being subjected to antibiotics before or during or after birth, while comp feeding practices continue in many places. Additionally, vaccination practices now extend back into the immediate postpartum period, another new development with potential immune significance. Allergic Gen-4 mothers produce allergic Gen-5 babies unless they address the problems before pregnancy. These mothers almost always in time that dietary changes help them as much as their crying babies. A vocal minority of these mothers have found that extensively hydrolysed formulas improve serious allergic problems in their older children, and have even become active advocates for formula-feeding from birth, since breastfeeding clearly did not produce problem-free

308  Colen's controversial comparative study of differently fed siblings used this population: her subjects were drawn from children born 1957–65 (when poorer women breastfed) together with a sample from the next generation of children birthed by the girls in that earlier sample. See Colen CG, Ramey DM. Is Breast Truly Best? Estimating the Effects of Breastfeeding on Long-term Child Health and Wellbeing in the United States Using Sibling Comparisons, *Soc Sci Med* (2014), DOI: 10.1016/j.socscimed.2014.01.027. There are many potential confounders of inter-sibling and inter-generational studies not considered in the analysis.

children for them. (Though it can, as with my two recently-born grandchildren, when physiological care of both mother and baby is possible: and mothers can worry because their young fully-breastfed babies are too plump and placid! What I see as the norm for solely breastfed babies is unusual in our society.)

All these changes in breastfeeding demographics and experience and related care – different in every society, every generation, every social class – need to be considered as part of the issue of biodiversity and microbiomic changes, as they have certainly had impacts on gene expression, immune development, hormones, and mother-infant interactions through generations. Alison Fleming outlined this intergenerational health and behaviour connection some years ago. The article from which this next figure is taken is well worth reading.

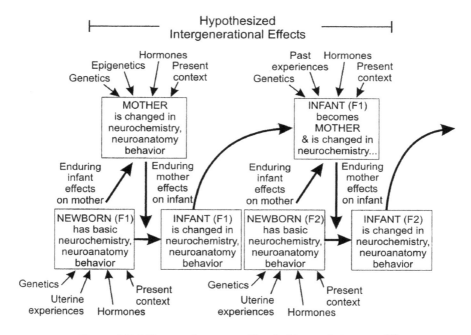

Figure 2-5-4 How mothers may affect babies and vice versa[309]

Epigenetic changes accumulate. These might be the origins of gene variants that are linked to different outcomes of US research into the impact of breastfeeding on sensitisation to foods. For example, in multi-ethnic, but largely African-American families,[310] the presence of particular gene variants (polymorphisms) was strongly associated with sensitisation to common foods measured by certain tests. And in this US population, with those gene variants, ever-breastfed children had a higher risk of developing food sensitisation than the never-breastfed.[311]

---

309  Republished with permission of Elsevier Ltd, from Fleming AS, O'Day DH, Kraemer GW. Neurobiology of mother-infant interactions: experience and CNS plasticity across development and generations. *Neurosci Biobehav Rev* 1999; 23(5):673–85. DOI: 10.1016/S0149-7634(99)00011-1; permission conveyed through Science Direct.

310  Hong X, Wang G, Liu X, Kumar R et al. Gene Polymorphisms, Breastfeeding and Development of Food Sensitisation in Early Childhood *J Allergy Clin Immunol.* 2011; 128(2): 374–381.e2. DOI:10.1016/j.jaci.2011.05.007.

311  Studies of ever-breastfed versus never-breastfed children are almost impossible to interpret, and only studies that include truly breastfed children and fully artificially fed children *and their families* will provide answers.

Should those genetic variants linked to sensitisation have been looked for in the mothers and even grandmothers as well? Did bottle-feeding in the previous generation account for the presence of the gene variant? At what point in the family line can such variants first be documented? American women now breastfeeding – perhaps especially African-American women – may well have been damaged genetically and nutritionally by generations of artificial feeding. After all the risk of death from asthma is four times higher[312] in that community, and even allowing for other variables, that is a huge difference. After generations of low breastfeeding rates, inter-generational genetic damage done to the mothers *as children by infant formula* might manifest as breastfeeding-associated damage in their children. Or indeed, the medications used by mothers suffering from infant-allergy-induced symptoms may need to be controlled for: is a higher rate of wheeze in children of allergy sufferers the result of reaction-suppressing medications used by mothers during pregnancy? Or used during months of lactation? The fact that Canadian children who are breastfed have less asthma[313] may relate to differences in their parents' and grandparents' feeding history and medication use.

After all, remember that earlier study (page 93) showing the effects of formula exposure in hospital and exclusive breastfeeding thereafter: heightening IgG responses, which persisted to two years, with the effect greatest *in those breastfed for less than two months*, as though longer breastfeeding reduced an undesirable effect. The same factors may or may not be at work here: it is not possible to know from the design of this later study whether these mostly African-American children were formula-exposed in hospital in the twenty-four to seventy-two hours before study enrolment. That would depend on how strictly the hospital followed Baby-Friendly Hospital Initiative (BFHI) guidelines. It would also be interesting to check early formula exposure (noting the brands and batches involved) against the presence of gene polymorphisms in both cord blood and the infant blood samples collected six to twelve months later. There is evidence of genetic changes over time in infants, and it might well be linked to early feeding and antibiotic exposure. Or it might simply be a result of stress, which suggests that birth and neonatal events should be added as potential confounders to study.

However, reading this study raised some questions. For the group, a rate of 21 per cent for those 'exclusively' breastfed to four months or more (27 per cent of those who began breastfeeding) is quite an achievement, especially given a 35 per cent Caesarean section rate, which almost certainly meant antibiotic exposure and probably formula-feeding.[314] But then, the infant feeding data were self-reported no earlier than six to twelve months postpartum, at a follow-

312  US Department of Health and Human Services: *HHS Action Plan to Reduce Racial and Ethnic Health Disparities* http://www.minorityhealth.hhs.gov/npa/files/Plans/HHS/HHS_Plan_complete.pdf

313  Ye M, Mandhane PJ, Senthilselvan A. Association of breastfeeding with asthma in young Aboriginal children in Canada. (PMID:23248799) *Canad Respirat J* 2012, 19(6):361–66

314  Where mother and baby are separated, C-sections often lead to artificial feeding. This is because of the effects of the medication and stress on both mother and baby. C-sections can slightly delay the normal onset of breastmilk production – but in themselves are not a reason for breastfeeding failure. The culprit in most cases is medical anxiety, resulting in unnecessary interventions and separation of mother and child, or worse, false perceptions of convenience, A senior industry scientist has suggested that there should be 'recommendations for allergic reasons against the usage of cesarean sections for convenience … We know that in industrial countries they are made for the convenience of the surgeon or the mother rather than for good obstetrical considerations.' Guesry P, quoted in Isolauri E, Walker WA, op. cit., p. 174.

up visit, with no evidence that researchers sought to validate early exclusive breastfeeding in hospital or in the days before study enrolment. Mothers simply stated that they had given no formula or other solids for more than, or less than, four months.

(The authors noted that recall bias was possible, but thought it would affect both groups equally. That to me is very unlikely. When mothers know that healthworkers think that breastfeeding is a good thing, they are more likely – consciously or unconsciously – to exaggerate the duration or the exclusivity of breastfeeding,[315] and less likely to admit that they chose to formula-feed from birth or give the odd bottle while breastfeeding. In mothers' groups it is not uncommon to hear women sharing the little white lies they tell healthworkers 'to keep them happy'. And mothers would have to be questioned closely[316] and in detail soon after the birth to establish the likelihood of their baby having been given formula in the first days after birth. As mentioned earlier, this is not always noted in records, and is sometimes flatly and untruthfully denied by healthworkers. Like mothers, some doctors and nurses have a tendency to say what they think will please, rather than tell a truth that might upset.

So we can't be sure about those 'exclusively breastfeeding' rates. It's so difficult to establish who's really been fed what, that all these studies can only be inconclusive. However, it is regrettably possible that in the African-American generation referred to above, breastfeeding, designed by nature to stimulate the infant immune system, may be doing so inappropriately and causing more reactivity to harmless foods – while still also protecting against pathogens, cancer,[317] dysnutrition and other forms of ill-health, of course. But then, what does proof of sensitisation mean? As the study authors said,

> Finally, it should be noted that food sensitisation as measured in this study is often part of a biological response to an allergen, but that alone does not necessarily mean a clinical reaction to a food, therefore, caution is needed when extending our findings to food allergy.' [That 'when' should have been 'before'.]

It might prove to be the case that adverse food reactions are now more common in some populations of breastfed children, especially African-American ones with certain gene variants. This certainly wasn't true historically, if contemporary observers can be trusted. But even if it were to be proved so, being protected against allergic disease while being more likely to die of other diseases would not be a good trade.

The one certain take-home message of this study is that breastfeeding makes a difference, interacting with our genome. Just what that difference means for the non-allergic and the

---

315  Gillespie B, d'Arcy H, Schwartz K, Bobo J, Foxman B. Recall of age of weaning and other breastfeeding variables. *International Breastfeeding Journal* 2006, 1:4 (9 March 2006).

316  A1984 UK study showed that when this is done, at least a third of 'solely breastfed' babies had been comp fed: see Cant A, Marsden RA, Kilshaw PJ. Egg and cows' milk hypersensitivity in exclusively breast fed infants with eczema, and detection of egg protein in breast milk.(PMCID:PMC1417254) *Br Med J (Clin Res Ed)* 1985; 291(6500):932–35.

317  Another new discovery: the presence of cancer-killing factors in breastmilk. See Davanzo R, Zauli G, Monasta L, Vecchi Brumatti L et al. Human colostrum and breast milk contain high levels of TNF-related apoptosis-inducing ligand (TRAIL). (PMID:22529245) *J Hum Lact* 2013; 29(1):23–25.

already-allergic family is not yet clear. But the fact of difference says that infant formula is not the same as breastfeeding, and that it therefore needs to be proven that the difference it makes to the expression of our genome is not harmful to the individual and the population. As the researchers say,

> ... this study suggests that significant gene–breast-feeding interactions are involved in the development of FS [food sensitization]. Given the undoubted health benefits of breast-feeding, our findings should not lead to a change in the general recommendations for breast-feeding. Rather our findings should lead to further studies that would allow for a better understanding of the effect of breast-feeding on allergic diseases in the context of individual genetic variation. The type of information yielded by such studies might enable physicians to provide more personalized medical care and advice to mothers in the future, with the potential to decrease the risk of allergic disease in their children.

It may be that using only expensive extensively-hydrolysed formula (E-HF) is less harmful than using the so-called hypo-allergenic (=less allergenic, labelled HA) or usual (= more allergenic) varieties. It may be that for some atopic children, some early postnatal exposure to antigens like cows' milk could moderate reactions engendered by prenatal exposure to those allergens. We don't know. If we don't know, we stay with Mother Nature's brew, not industry's.

Whether or not comp-feeding could ever be justified for any sub-group, it still changes normal microbiome development and gut function and every other aspect of normal development investigated to date. And it was and remains a disaster for the breastfeeding dyad, usually decreasing both maternal confidence and milk production. Even if the amounts given are small, the willingness of doctors to give formula to breastfed babies proclaims medical confidence in the complete safety of the product. What's more, the infant formula is not the only factor: many can linings and plastic bottles and teats used by babies can also contribute BPA and similar chemicals, linked with asthma and allergies in a huge recent study.[318] Breasts are a safer delivery system – the biodiversity they offer is preferable!

Research will have to identify ways to manage these problems without sacrificing breastfeeding. All that might be needed is managing individual maternal diet, ending neonatal comp-feeding, and reducing or eliminating antibiotic exposure and any other neonatal gut-altering challenges, while enabling good lactation. We won't know until it has been rigorously tried. Instead, the number of neonatal challenges an infant is put through seems to be increasing: vitamin K injections (perhaps using peanut or soy[319] or castor bean oils), Hep B vaccination ... Sometimes these are necessary and important, but we need to consider very carefully any trade-offs here. And when there clearly are risks to all available options, *as there are,* parents' informed decisions must be respected.

---

318  Hsu NY, Wu PC, Bornehag CG, Sundell J, Su HJ Feeding bottles usage and the prevalence of childhood allergy and asthma. (PMID:22291844) *Clin Dev Immunol* 2012, 2012:158248. DOI: 10.1155/2012/158248

319  Fraser H. *The peanut allergy epidemic* (Skyhorse Publishing, 2011) p. 53. Lecithin E322 is soy-derived. Castor bean is another legume, and a gut irritant.

## Studies and media silence or clamour

A large Finnish study[320] published in 1999 supports the idea that feeding infant formula to breastfed infants in hospital increases the likelihood of proven cows' milk allergy. Formula, pasteurised donor milk, and whey hydrolysates were the comp feeds given to 87 per cent of 6209 infants (and note that sad fact: only 824 out of over 6000 mothers birthing in these hospitals were enabled to feed their own babies without any comp feeds!) Formula resulted in a higher rate of allergy than either of the other feeds. Parental history of atopy also affected the results, and even some exclusively breastfed infants developed allergy in this Finnish population (which had a high usage of dairy products and a history of artificial feeding prior to a 1970s revival of breastfeeding from a very low base, see Figure 3-11-3 on page 441).

But other studies, more widely quoted by the world's press and formula advocates, came to different conclusions. One study[321] (by the group that earlier identified higher IgG levels in comp-fed babies) is still being cited as 'proving' that brief neonatal exposure to infant formula based on cows' milk is harmless. In fact it proves no such thing. It simply shows that one cows' milk formula is not much worse than the alternative that the same formula company supplied. (Nearly 10 per cent of all the children developed clinical disease under 12 months. There was no exclusively breastfed control group. How was this study justified to the ethics committee?)

Exactly what did the study assess? Whether early exposure to a company-supplied lower-protein cows' milk formula, or to a cows'-milk-free 'placebo formula', resulted in more diagnoses of the classic allergic disorders, eczema or asthma, in the first two years of life. According to the researchers, the 'placebo product designed for this study was based on a maltodextrin, glucose, and mineral solution emulsified with vegetable fats, visibly indistinguishable from infant formula.' Maltodextrin made from wheat, or corn, or potato?[322] What vegetable fats, and how highly purified? Who decided what to include? All children reported on (not all those in the study) received one or other comp feed at least three times under three days old.

The published report did not disclose the exact contents of the placebo formula (also made and supplied by the formula company), so that the likely effects of its ingredients on the gut, and thus on antigen uptake, could be assessed. The theory that early exposure while still breastfeeding induces tolerance (see page 168) suggests that there could be more or different reactions to the foods consumed by the lower-protein 'placebo' group in their second year of life or later.

A placebo is generally intended to be a harmless alternative. But substances other than intact proteins can also cause immune responses and gut damage and microbiomic change.

320  Saarinen KM, Juntunen-Backman K, Järvenpää AL, Kuitunen P, Lope L, Renlund M, Siivola M, Savilahti E. Supplementary feeding in maternity hospitals and the risk of cow's milk allergy: A prospective study of 6209 infants. (PMID:10452771) *J All Clin Immunol* 1999; 104(2 Pt 1):457–61.

321  de Jong MH, Scharp-van der Linden VTM, Aalberse RC. Randomised controlled trial of brief neonatal exposure to cows' milk on the development of atopy. *Arch Dis Child* 1998;79:126–30.

322  Packets of many foodstuffs (but not infant formula) tell the purchaser that the maltodextrin used is (from corn) or (from wheat) or (from potato) or whatever starchy food is available.. Why doesn't infant formula?

Many fats and carbohydrates are in fact antigenic either because of included protein traces (membrane proteins in oils, for example) or by hapten[323] formation, where complexes formed during digestion cause symptoms. The detection limit for protein in the so-called placebo was low, but the human body is more sensitive than any laboratory test. And was that test – for all of the hundreds of cows' milk proteins or just a few? – also done by the same company supplying both formulas?

This possibly-protein-free placebo formula study looked at a narrow band of IgE-related symptoms indicating atopic sensitivity. It did include recurrent gastrointestinal symptoms clearly related to food, as recorded by parents , but not behavioural symptoms. Only medically diagnosed eczema, asthma and rhinitis were included: how many breastfed children were not taken to doctors for diagnosis because symptoms were mild or episodic, or were considered 'normal'? In my experience, quite a few. However, the clinical examination and questionnaires recorded should have given reasonably accurate and consistent results in diagnosis of the allergy symptoms chosen.

All foodstuffs – placebo or bovine – will affect the gut microbiome. That's just a fact. (Another fact: that differences in gut microbiota relate to allergy.)[324] Such effects were not recorded, as no detailed study of infant gut flora was undertaken (and the small exclusively breastfed group were not used in the analysis – more on this later.) In fact, for the first three days after enrolment, which seems to have been immediately after birth, healthy breastfed babies were randomised to be given three feeds of either formula each day, to me an astonishing amount of non-breastmilk going into the neonatal gut, displacing the physiologically small amounts of colostrum and early milk. Each sachet was made up with 60 ml of water, and sometimes 'replaced' breastfeeds. How can such studies get past ethical committees, given what we know about colostrum and neonatal gut development? What does this experiment say about the (unjustified) assumptions of both doctors and parents about the total safety of infant formula? What might future lawyers say about such experiments on babies, when so many go on to develop allergy, even those with no apparent inherited risk?

Interestingly, and not unexpectedly, there was a high rate – around 10 per cent in the first year of life – of IgE mediated allergic disease in both of these highly comp-fed groups, regardless of the family risk of allergy. There was a trend towards cows' milk formula producing a higher rate of allergic disease than the placebo, although the trend did not reach statistical significance. Even more worrying, by the age of five, 25 per cent of both formula-exposed groups proved positive for atopic disease; and the study did not record other disease often associated with allergy, such as ear infections. Far from growing out of allergy, these comp-fed Dutch children seemed to be growing into it, suggesting that their immune systems were ill-equipped to deal with ongoing environmental and dietary challenges; and more of their parents also tested positive. These rates were higher than those reported from other studies, suggesting that while both comps produced much the same rate of allergy, it was a higher rate than previously recorded. And there was no exclusively breastfed control

---

323  Haptens are small molecules combined with a larger carrier such as a protein, and can cause immune reactions.
324  Penders J, Thijs C, van den Brandt P, Kummeling I et al. Gut microbiota composition and development of atopic manifestations in infancy. *Gut* 2007; 56: 661-7. DOI: 10.1136/gut2006.100164

group. Atopic families were confidently said to be over-represented in the study sample, but that statement was based on a national estimate of allergy prevalence, and most of such estimates are very conservative, if community experience is any guide.

What reduced my confidence in the results of this group's first study were its final words:

> ... A second study is underway, focusing on respiratory symptoms at the age of five years, *as a next step in dispelling the fears* related to the concept of 'the dangerous bottle'. [The italics are mine.]

Perhaps that ensured both the company's willing participation and the study's global reporting. We can't have parents believing that bottles could be dangerous! And what does it say that this slipped past pre-publication editing: that those critiquing the study shared those assumptions, and so missed this evidence of bias?

For shouldn't the aim of that second study have been an impartial 'to assess relative risk of respiratory allergy'? Science aims to describe reality, fearful or otherwise as the facts suggest, and it seems like advocacy, not good science, to announce such motivations or prejudge findings of future work in this manner. Studies like this (carefully avoiding the inclusion of exclusively breastfed children and children solely formula-fed from birth) are important in creating reasonable doubt about the possibility that formula is seriously harmful. While there is doubt, continued use, and continued marketing by endorsement, is legally permissible. Morally? I have my doubts.

As noted above, the second study[325] of these same children at age five showed similar high rates of allergy in both comp-fed groups of children then solely breastfed for at least six weeks, of around 25 per cent. And sure enough, the researchers concluded that 'Early and brief exposure to cows' milk in *(briefly)* breastfed children is not associated with atopic disease or allergic symptoms up to age five.' That is, no more than the rates to be found in other briefly-breastfed children exposed early to the second formula supplied by the same funding company. I concluded from this second paper only that the Dutch low-protein cows' milk formula supplied was no worse than the mystery placebo formula, and that very short periods of exclusive breastfeeding *after being comp-fed* don't undo whatever harm was done by *both* formulas. (If even that subsequent breastfeeding was truly exclusive: the brief mention of 'glucose solution and fennel seed water' in the first study raised a query for me about other possible comp feeds used in Holland. Fennel seed water reminded me that I would never have considered lemon a likely substance for newborns to be exposed to if I had not seen a dish of cut lemons beside every mother in a Swedish hospital, asked what for, to be told it was nipple prophylaxis.)[326]

---

325 de Jong MH, Scharp-van der Linden VTM, Aalberse R, Heymans HAS et al. The effect of brief neonatal exposure to cows' milk on atopic symptoms up to age 5. *Arch Dis Child* 2002;86:365–69.

326 One small triumph: a Swedish midwife later told me at an ILCA conference that my response had ended the practice. I asked straight-faced whether an abraded or damaged penis was always daily treated with lemon juice to prevent infection.

In short, the study showed me that early and brief exposure to *anything other than breastmilk* is associated with atopic disease or allergic symptoms up to age five. But remember that the analysis excluded two groups: those said to be exclusively breastfed from birth, and those never to have received breastmilk. Without those missing groups of children fully and exclusively breastfed from birth, or never breastfed from birth, we won't know what might have been possible in the allergy-prone Dutch population created by artificial feeding, where only 54% of mothers reported breastfeeding solely (after 3 days of three comp feeds) until 6 weeks of age. Others and I have asked for a comparison of allergy rates in the excluded group that was fully breastfed from birth, and that solely formula-fed from birth. I asked specifically for this data in 2012 and again in 2014, and could not obtain it. The information must be on record, but money to analyse that data was not available.

I wonder was this because the company did not approve of the release of this information? I have been told that such things can happen, when results emerge that the sponsor company does not like. A 1990s trial in bottle-fed infants with diarrhoea found that a newer low lactose-free formula, for example, was worse than an older formula; the researchers discovered that the contract's fine print meant the formula company's legal department had to vet publications, and the work was never published. The researcher who told me was furious, but could do nothing. Publication bias may well be preceded by reporting bias where infant formula is concerned. Or perhaps the Dutch researchers fear that parents of breastfed children given formula might not like to find out that the risk of allergy for their children could have been less, or the disease less severe, had those children been breastfed fully from birth to 6 months as WHO advises. And Dutch parents who solely bottle-fed from birth might be angry that no one advised them not to do so, but to give some colostrum at least to help the newborn gut. I can only speculate about why this information is not made public. To summarise the study:

1422 comp-fed infants , were given up to three 60ml feeds for 3 days after birth

824 of 1422 then "breastfed exclusively to 6 weeks" (54%).

Of those, data for 777 infants analysed; results are tabled

| 365 of the 707 fed cows' milk formula | | | 412 of the 715 fed low-protein formula | |
|---|---|---|---|---|
| Age | Allergic disease or symptoms | Immune markers | Allergic disease or symptoms | Immune markers |
| 1 year | 10% | RAST+ 9.4% ↑IgE 5.8% | 9.3% | RAST+ 7.9% ↑IgE 4.1% |
| 2 years | 9.6% | | 10.2% | |
| 5 years | 26.3% | ↑IgE 5.3% | 25% | ↑IgE 3% |

Figure 2-5-5 Allergy in Dutch comp-fed children

There are some important issues to notice about this study:

NO results for truly exclusively-breastfed-from-birth children; low breastfeeding in population

NO data reported separately for the children fully formula fed from birth

**Published conclusions, widely believed and cited:**

'no difference in sensitisation' between 2 groups of comp-fed, briefly breastfed, children: TRUE. Why would one be expected?

'Early brief exposure to CMP in BF children is not associated with atopic disease or allergic symptoms to age 5': UNPROVEN

**What this study says to me:**

Both formulas provided by the company are associated with high rates of allergic symptoms.

Elevated immune markers persist in virtually all cows' milk-exposed infants, but in only half of the children fed the alternative formula. Which suggests more protein results in greater reactivity five years later.

Early cows' milk protein exposure in children then breastfed for short periods results in high levels of allergic symptoms and atopic disease at the age of five years. So does exposure to other alien foodstuffs in this population.

Holland has a huge problem with allergy, it would seem from these studies. I added the reported figures in the Obvious Allergic Disease and the Possible Allergic Disease categories found in Table 14 of this second study: almost half of these children might possibly be allergic, and a quarter obviously is at age five!

Does this reflect the Dutch use of milk over the centuries? Have there been genomic effects? Major industries in any country do not take kindly to suggestions that their product has caused or may cause harm. Is this why researchers feel the need to reassure and dispel fears?

And once again, we have a widely publicised study with no control group of children exclusively breastfed from birth, and breastfeeding encouraged to 'at least six weeks'. A very short-term goal, twenty weeks less than WHO's suggested six months, so that formula use was endorsed for 46 weeks of the year by professionals! Research funding for such studies as these is certainly worthwhile for industry.

I would like to see an independent re-analysis including the excluded infants, those either solely formula-fed from birth, or breastfed exclusively from birth. Their data were irrelevant to a study which only wanted to compare two specific formulas. But that study was then used to justify far broader claims, that early and brief exposure to cows' milk formula made no difference to outcomes in any group of children, not just those fed two same-company-made formulas. To me, that makes the omission of these two groups from analysis highly problematic. Strictly relevant or not, results of analysis might be very interesting all the same, even the numbers mean results can only be suggestive. Will analysis show that those babies without 'early and brief exposure' *to any formula,* and who really were exclusively breastfed to 6 months[327] do much better in regard to allergy than those solely formula fed from birth, *with no drop of breastmilk*? These are the two groups we need to know about, because parents are being told it is safe to feed formula from birth.

## Proper independent consumer research

I am reminded of my 1990s visit to a prominent US allergy researcher who had tested the allergenicity of a casein hydrolysate formula. The tins of product had been supplied direct from the company funding the research. After many adverse reactions the researchers had stopped the trial, themselves checked the powder supplied, and found it contained considerable amounts of intact protein. The company subsequently provided another batch, which produced better results, and those results were then published.[328] Surely products used in research should be sourced independently off the shelf at retail, so they are identical to those parents will purchase? This is standard practice when consumer organisations assess products. But researchers' uncritical trust in the infant formula industry seems to be absolute. Does history suggest that such trust is justified?

To my knowledge nothing was ever published about the adverse reactions that stopped the trial. Ben Goldacre is particularly scathing about the effects of such selective data: read his highly entertaining book.[329]

And so we do not know the most important thing parents want to know: if both formulas produced more problems than complete breastfeeding, as could be expected, since both would distort the normal development of the gut microbiome. Exclusively breastfed control groups (not exposed to other foods or antibiotics) define the current normal for any population. Though, as I keep on saying, this *present normal* reflects past experience with foods and other allergens, and so even this may be a deviation from any possible human *optimum*.

Nor was this one study relevant to the products parents buy to feed their children. The experimental formula in this study contained just 11.1 g/L of protein. This was a very low figure for a formula made in the 1990s, when protein content in leading brands was usually around 15–18 g/L. Formula in 2013 still contains 13–18 g/L. It would be interesting to follow up on these children fed lower-protein formula, as it is concern about obesity that is driving the reduction in protein content of formula. (See page 289)

So between Denmark in 1985, Holland in 1992–94, Finland since 1980, and Australia in the 1990s, there are significant differences to explain. Yet even if study methodology were to

---

327  If any children *were* breastfed to six months despite the implicit endorsement by trusted health professionals of infant formula as safe.

328  Trial director (personal communication). I promised to preserve his anonymity.

329  Goldacre B. *Bad Pharma. How drug companies mislead doctors and harm patients.* (Fourth Estate Press 2012)

be standardised, this variability is exactly what the milk hypothesis would predict: results will all depend on past population history as well as present experience, on maternal diet as well as direct infant exposure, on genes as well as the environment, on the composition of the specific batch of formula as well as the theoretical recipe which the factory was trying to match.

However, even despite the great variability of contexts, amounts, definitions, and exposures, a recent survey of all known studies investigating the effect of early supplementary feeds of formula to breastfed children has concluded that it almost doubles the risk of cows' milk allergy.[330] The author concluded:

> The first weeks of a baby's life is a critical period for the immune system in its determination of what is harmful and what is harmless. Many of the studies that showed a link between breastfed infants being given irregular CMF [cows' milk formula] and the development of CMA [cows' milk allergy] had strong prospective designs, were able to show causality and did not depend on participants to remember events. Mothers who wish to breastfeed and are offered or advised to supplement their newborn baby with CMF should be made aware of the risks of doing so, as they are currently made aware of the risks of not supplementing.

So the better-designed studies do show causal links between early cows' milk exposure and allergy. I wonder why so many, so much worse, studies are still funded?

Soothill said decades ago, 'Early artificial feeding, including supplements, should never be done unnecessarily.'[331] His perspective certainly fits with my experience in Australian families: protect babies from comp feeds and they are easier and happier babies than those exposed to cows' milk, and their mothers are not distressed and depressed by inexplicable infant misery. While of course I cannot prove it, I usually suspect comp feeds have done the damage (rather than say, in utero sensitisation) when a previously placid breastfed baby starts to fuss while at the breast and cry inconsolably between day ten and twenty-one. (For more about this see Book 3, Chapter 4, the practical help sections.)

If the effects are heritable and interactive, why would we be surprised that some of the outcomes may seem paradoxical, leading to fewer reports of infant allergy in one generation, or one region, and more reports in the next generation or a different region, when infant gestators had been differently fed?

Above all, why should such reports of problems in now-breastfed children undermine confidence in breastfeeding? Even if breastfeeding in any one time or place were to be associated with *more* infant allergy where mothers are themselves badly affected – and I hasten to say that *hasn't* been shown – there is still no way that infant formula could ever

---

330   Smith HA. Formula supplementation and the risk of cow's milk allergy. *British Journal of Midwifery*, 2012; 20 (5) 345–50.

331   Soothill JF, Hayward AR, Wood CBS. *Paediatric Immunology*. (Blackwell 1983) p. 116.

be a better choice for infant motor development[332] or cognitive development[333] or language development[334] or overall immune and cardiovascular function lifelong.

All major allergy and paediatric groups recommend exclusive breastfeeding for at least 4 months, most supporting the WHO policy of around 6 months. How can comps continue when they are not necessary? And how can we tolerate obstetric practice which makes them necessary? We know that they affect the likelihood of successful lactation. Many studies have found that , as one said, 'the practice of giving pre-lacteal feeds is a key determinant of early cessation of full breastfeeding.'[335]

## Comp feeds support breastfeeding?
## Another widely reported study

Of course that is so. But a tiny study of just forty mothers[336] may have persuaded some (who didn't read it carefully) that infant formula is harmless, even beneficial, because it supports maternal breastfeeding. Like that Dutch study, the media coverage of this forces me to discuss it. The study authors' conclusion: giving restricted small quantities of infant formula up until the time of mature milk production means more breastfeeding for longer, as more mothers were solely breastfeeding at three months.

This widely publicised study looked at the effects of giving 10 ml of expensive extensively hydrolysed infant (E-HF) formula by syringe after every breastfeed, within twenty-four to forty-eight hours after birth, to infants who had lost 5 per cent or more from birth weight under thirty-six hours old. The comps were to be continued 'until the onset of mature milk production', likely to be day 4 at latest. A control group of mothers were instructed in 'soothing techniques', and *advised to* breastfeed exclusively for the duration of their hospital stay. Follow-up at one week and three months showed that the deliberately comp-fed babies were much more likely to be fully breastfed than those assigned to no comps, and free to feed their babies as they chose.

Those given the study's 10 ml feeds drank much less infant formula in their first week of life (an average of 116 ml, at most 226 ml) than the other mothers. The group advised to breastfeed exclusively in fact fed an average of 262 ml (at most 673 ml) of various formulas

332  Chiu WC, Liao HF, Chang PJ, Chen PC, Chen YC. Duration of breast feeding and risk of developmental delay in Taiwanese children: a nationwide birth cohort study. *Paediatr Perinat Epidemiol.* 2011 Nov;25(6):519–27. DOI: 10.1111/j.1365-3016.2011.01236.x. Epub 2011 Sep 15.

333  Mortensen EL, Michaelsen KF, Sanders SA, Reinisch JM. The association between duration of breastfeeding and adult intelligence. *JAMA.* 2002 May 8;287(18):2365–71; Sacker A, Quigley MA, Kelly YJ. Breastfeeding and developmental delay: findings from the millennium cohort study. *Pediatrics.* 2006 Sep;118(3):e682–9.

334  Whitehouse AJ, Robinson M, Li J, Oddy WH. *Duration of breast feeding and language ability in middle childhood.* Paediatric and perinatal epidemiology 2011, 25(1):44–52.(MED:21133968) DOI: 10.1111/j.1365-3016.2010.01161.x

335  Lakati AS, Makokha OA, Binns CW, Kombe Y. The effect of pre-lacteal feeding on full breastfeeding in Nairobi, Kenya. (PMID:21516965) *East African Journal of Public Health* 2010, 7(3):258–62.

336  Flaherman VJ, Aby J, Burgos AE, Lee KA, Cabana MD, Newman TB. Effect of Early Limited Formula on Duration and Exclusivity of Breastfeeding in At-Risk Infants: An RCT. *Pediatrics;* originally published online May 13, 2013; DOI: 10.1542/peds.2012-2809.

to their babies in the first week. It was not stated whether the no comps/supposed to be 'exclusively breastfeeding' control group of mothers gave this formula in hospital, or only in the days after discharge; nor was the day of discharge given for either group.

Not surprisingly, the group of babies fed the greater volume of infant formula in the first week of life were much less likely to be breastfeeding at three months of age. Exclusive breastfeeding, according to the global definitions, involves nothing but human milk from birth. So when the figures are examined, it seems that of the forty mothers who entered the study, at most eight babies of mothers[337] in the control group could have been genuinely exclusively breastfed at three months (overall 20 per cent, compared with the stated national figure of 30 per cent). Should the researchers be happy about that?

The conclusions that I draw from this study are:

- using only tiny amounts of an extensively-hydrolysed brand for only 2–3 days does less harm than allowing mothers free use of both bottles and normal allergenic infant formula for the first week;
- the more infant formula in total given by mothers in the first week, the lower the chance of continuing to breastfeed;
- maternal anxiety about their initial milk supply needs to be addressed with effective education and support after hospital discharge and if need be small quantities of donated breastmilk (not gut-altering infant formula);
- health professionals are unaware of the power of their modelling the use of infant formula, and are ignoring the WHO-preferred option of using donated human milk where necessary.

None of those conclusions is surprising or new. There were other aspects of this study that deserved comment:

- The study was of infants who had lost 5 per cent or more from birth weight under thirty-six hours. There was no discussion of the difficulty of establishing true infant birth weight when IV fluids have been given in labour, so that 'weight losses' may have been real in some infants, but simply a reduction of fluid overload in others. Unless we know this, we can't judge whether the intervention was either needed or useful in preventing further weight loss, though we can know that it altered the infant microbiome.
- The higher parity of mothers in the intervention group, and the lower gestational age of infants in the control group, recorded in the study, may well have influenced outcomes, making continued breastfeeding more likely in the restricted comps group;
- The apparently high stated rate (eleven of forty mothers) of delayed onset of lactation across both groups strongly suggests sub-optimal obstetric and postnatal practices, which undermine breastfeeding initiation.

---

337 Maybe not even that: the 8 women who were classified as exclusively breastfeeding (EBF) when asked at one month may not be the same women classified as EBF at 2 or 3 months.

Allaying mothers' fears about the adequacy of their milk supply (by giving babies very small doses of formula by syringe) did indeed result in less formula use overall in the first week. And so greater breastfeeding success at three months. But was giving formula the best way to achieve that? Would, for example, 'kangaroo care' – keeping babies skin to skin and allowing frequent feeding – have achieved the same ends without the potential for altering infant gut development? And what about using donor human milk, and thus proclaiming by actions, not words, the second-rate nature of infant formula?[338] It is sad that any infant formula was even considered for these seemingly quite healthy babies without any research into the consequences for their gut development.

Yes – surprisingly in a study done so recently, there was no documentation of the unavoidable effects on gut microbiota, and the possibility that the effects of derangement of the microbiome might be subtle and very long-term. The authors were aware of the possibility that giving formula so soon after birth could have adverse health results for some babies, but wondered if this might be balanced by greater breastfeeding duration. Is it ethical to experiment without at least attempting to document results other than duration of breastfeeding? (It was pleasing that apparently many mothers had the sense to refuse to participate in the trial – maybe because they had been clearly advised that this might not be safe.) For example, given the research interest in the microbiota, could not the researchers have arranged for studies of the evolution of gut flora in both groups?

Nor was there any apparent awareness of the powerful psychological impact of official medical approval of formula complementation, which may have influenced the rate of breastfeeding in both groups. Did it also influence formula or brand choice post discharge? Did anyone look? Physicians who recommend such practices should take care to think of the likely results of their actions.

Nor was there discussion of strategies (besides giving formula) to create greater maternal confidence that unsettled infant behaviour was not simply hunger; or if it was, strategies for meeting that infant need for suckling and sustenance. Feed frequencies of eight to twelve times a day are mentioned in the article, when in the first days of life babies are at the breast much more often if access is unrestricted. Gastric emptying times of ninety minutes make three-hour intervals absurd.

This study fits neatly into the Western mindset, evidenced in so many actions and books written by health professionals until recently: 'When breastfeeding is a problem, formula is the answer.' But is it? There may well be serious consequences for health professionals who cause babies to be exposed to artificial feeding unnecessarily. And necessity has been

---

338  Informed mothers are increasingly making their own arrangements in this regard: one mother recently helped by her neighbour to provide enough high-calorie milk for her preterm infant in the stressful early days following major blood loss has just told me proudly that she has now passed on that gift by giving a desperate mother of twins five litres of her own excess milk. Good on them both! This is why pregnant women need to be connected to breastfeeding networks before birth, just in case …

clearly outlined in the Baby-Friendly Hospital Initiative's Global Criteria;[339] it is no longer a matter of one staff person's opinion, however high in the hierarchy.

## Comp feeding: legal implications and duty of care

How many mothers would be willing to test the possibilities of comp feeds or formula-feeding if fully informed in writing of the real nature of formula? That it is non-sterile, contains fats made by genetically altered marine algae and soil fungi, and may come with industrially produced bacteria as well as foods for those bacteria to grow on; that these substances will affect gut development in ways that cannot be predicted and have not been monitored.

And that safer alternatives[340] exist: breastfeeding, or if that is difficult or impossible (and it rarely is with the right support) assistance with expressing milk, or the use of donor human milk?

Not to give this information could quite fairly be seen as a failure of the doctor's legal duty to warn of material risk.[341] And if mothers are not given that information, how can any consent they give be informed?[342] And if mothers do not give informed consent to the use of such products – as most mothers in the twentieth century certainly did not! – legal opinion is that giving the product to their child may constitute the offence of battery.[343] I think it might also be argued nowadays to be a 'lack of reasonable skill and care', the basis of many negligence lawsuits; or 'the loss of a chance for a better outcome', which surely the unnecessary distortion of the infant microbiome causes.

An interesting question that arises is the possible reporting obligation of those who are aware that unnecessary fluids have been given, with their attendant risks. According to one expert group, insured medical practitioners have a duty to report all incidents that they might reasonably know could lead to a claim at a later date, or they will not be covered by their medical insurance. Adverse events that must be notified are those where:

- a patient suffers a major complication

---

339 Acceptable medical reasons for supplementation are outlined in a variety of national documents and at http://www.who.int/nutrition/publications/infantfeeding/WHO_NMH_NHD_09.01/en/

340 While all options carry risks, I think the greater safety of these alternatives (assuming due care in preparation) is conclusively proven.

341 'A risk is material if in the circumstances of a particular case a reasonable person in the plaintiff's position, if warned of the risk, would be likely to attach significance to it, **or** if the doctor is or should be reasonably aware that the patient if warned of the risk would be likely to attach significance to it.' (FJ Purnell SC. Negligence and Birth Injuries. Transcript of talk at PSANZ (Perinatal Society of Australia and New Zealand) Conference Canberra March 2001.)

342 What informed consent means for legal defence cases in Australia is discussed at length in the manual of the Medical Defence Association of Victoria, *Medicine and the Law: A practical guide for Doctors.* (MDAV 2006). For the medical duty to disclose risks , and the loss of a chance for a better outcome, see Ch. 17.

343 This has already been argued in one Washington DC court. I predict that with a few decades such a case will be successful. Awareness of this risk is driving the use of 'informed consent' forms which are frequently quite inadequate in content and process of administration, but which may enable hospitals to say the mother consented.

- there is an error in providing health care

- an adverse outcome results in serious anger in the patient or his family

- the doctor concerned is aware that something has happened (including a complaint, investigation, or enquiry) which is thought may lead to a claim.

How soon will it be before there are plaintiff lawyers considering cases of NEC or sepsis or meningitis or juvenile diabetes or even eczema where infant formula has been given to a neonate? When the importance of exclusive breastfeeding is becoming ever more obvious, and parents are often angry that their wishes are disregarded, only the current confusion of scientific studies protects those responsible.

It could be argued in court that

- world and national health authorities already consider it an error to subject infants to unnecessary artificial feeds (or to put it another way, unjustified dietary assaults), particularly where parents are not warned of risks and so do not give informed consent; or there is no proof that they gave such consent;

- not supporting and enabling women to provide their breastmilk for sick infants, or not maintaining a breastmilk bank, results in the loss of a chance of a better outcome;

- hospitals that do not encourage reporting of incidents of needless exposure to formula, or that fail to take seriously the reports of concerned staff about routine practices, are failing in their duty of care;

- staff who do not consider such practices reportable incidents, and so fail to notify their insurers, will not be covered if claims are made. And given what we are learning about the lifelong effects of early artificial feeding, those claims might arise decades later.

To some this may seem far-fetched. In the 1970s pregnant women, with medical blessing, smoked in hospital wards, making me vomit as I recovered from primary and secondary postpartum haemorrhages. It seemed far-fetched then to imagine smoking in public places would end, but public health awareness increased and the public demanded protection. Infant formula is not poison, not tobacco, and is currently necessary for the survival of many babies. But formula is still a risk, and a needless one wherever breastmilk is available, which is wherever women are lactating and society values breastmilk. (In Leipzig in 1989, just 95 paid donors supplied 10,000 litres of breastmilk over and above the needs of their own infants, and breastfed longer in order to do so.[344]) Imagine the consequences if infant formula were to be seen as a risk, 'the tobacco of the twenty-first century,'[345] in as short a space of time. Such a recognition is possible, even likely, despite the powerful forces arrayed against it.

When and how will the message about the potential and real harms of inappropriate formulas reach health professionals? Possibly when industry begins to market their solutions to

---

344 I visited this milkbank then and was given this information. See ALCA News 1990;
345 Professor Peter Hartmann made this statement at a conference some years ago.

the problem they have caused: formulas with synbiotics, mixtures of both probiotics and prebiotics, which result in a gut microbiome and infant faeces more like that of [**but not the same as**] the breastfed infant. If the usual marketing patterns are followed, marketing of synbiotics will be done through inferences and exaggerated claims believed by uncritical health professionals and vested interests, and popularised via the social media and websites. It may not be far away now![346] There must surely be some intelligent commentators who will ask questions about the practice of feeding industrially produced bacteria to infants as we learn more about how bacteria can share genes and morph into different strains of greater virulence.

But of course it's possible that this recognition will be delayed by the fact of formula faeces and breastmilk faeces becoming more alike in some ways. It seems possible that once enough of the industry-produced bugs are being consumed in yoghurts by mothers, fed to babies, and spread everywhere in the postnatal environment, breastfeeding mothers will pick up the bugs of industry's choice. Hospital comp feeds are the perfect vehicle for changing maternal microbiomes via their breastfeeding infants. Feed the bugs to the newborn baby, bugs colonise baby, mother handles baby, changes nappies, kisses and fondles baby, is herself colonised, and so mother's milk may come to contain the patented commercial products industry has chosen as suitable for inclusion in infant feeds.[347] Those pathways designed to sample the biodiverse natural environment and react appropriately could ensure that breastfeeding mother's microbiota includes formula-derived organisms! So, ironically, breastmilk could become more like formula, and industry can then claim that formula is more like breastmilk ... If I were a marketing manager, I'd see the provision to hospitals of ready-to-feed formula in neat single doses as an investment likely to repay its cost. Then if a food company, I'd sell yoghurt containing the infant formula bacteria and market it as organisms found in mother's milk ... If they're not there already, they soon may be!

## Healthy gut healthy life

We understand now that 'humans are mostly a scaffold for the bacteria that live in and on us,' as Wassenaar says. Microbes outnumber human cells ten times over. Only about one percent of the bacteria we share our lives with have even been characterised. There is a standard set of approximately 23,000 genes in each human cell, and over a million different bacterial genes in our microbiome. And all these cells and their genes may interact,[348] affecting every aspect of our human lives. Which makes the establishment of the infant microbiome a process fundamental to health.

---

346 Closa-Monasterolo R, Gispert-Llaurado M, Luque V, Ferre N et al. Safety and efficacy of inulin and oligofructose supplementation in infant formula: Results from a randomised clinical trial. *Clinical Nutrition* 2013. Doi: 10.1016/j.clnu.2013.02.009). Recruitment was in the first month, not from birth.

347 Perhaps as with GM corn in Canada, mothers will have to pay for the privilege of being contaminated with patented products. Will mothers need a licence to make milk containing patented probiotics? Mad, I know, but who would have guessed that an organic crop contaminated by pollen from a neighbour's GM crop would result in confiscation of the organic crop, not damages awarded against the polluters?

348 Wassenaar TM. *Bacteria: the benign, the bad and the beautiful* (Wiley-Blackwell, 2011) pp. 141–42.

There is nothing controversial about the importance of early gut colonisation for lifelong health – it has been researched for decades.[349] Nor should there be any controversy about the adverse effects of formula on gut colonisation. Infant formula manufacturers have been trying for a century to improve how formula affects the infant gut microbiome. Yet scientists say that

> This collection of resident commensal microbes performs many important physiological functions and plays a central role in the development of the immune system. We hypothesize that alterations in the microbiome interfere with immune system maturation, resulting in impairment of IgA production, reduced abundance of regulatory T cells, and Th2-skewing of baseline immune responses which drive aberrant responses to innocuous (food) antigens.[350]

It is understood by almost all health professionals that babies really should not be exposed to strange foods soon after birth. Yet the astounding exception to that is infant formula. Formula is not seen for what it is: a variable broth of different heavily processed industrially concocted foodstuffs. Even by those who should know better, formula is seen as a breastmilk analogue, 'artificial breast milk' – which, emphatically, it is not, as its history demonstrates.

This ignorance can reach ludicrous heights. One midwife warned a mother against a faint smear of ultra-purified anhydrous lanolin (wool fat) on a baby's lip: it could alter gut flora, which would be dangerous. She issued this warning soon after giving a comp feed to a newborn! Infant formula is still being given to hundreds of thousands of newborn babies needlessly by such midwives and doctors, who have heard about the importance of gut flora, yet behave as though infant formula is magically safe, incapable of having harmful biological effects. Some do not even realise that they are feeding babies cows' milk. More than one mother has heard the cry, 'We'd never do that, we only use infant formula.' Yes – infant formula which contains whey and/or casein proteins and lactose from cows' milk, and a lot more besides, including industrially produced bacteria ... and a midwife who gives formula worried about a smear of lanolin! If, unknown to her, that mother were to be HIV-positive, that midwife would have dramatically increased the risk of infant HIV infection[351] by her single bottle of formula – not the mother by an external trace of lanolin.

Even pasteurised (which means heat-damaged) breastmilk would be preferable as a short-term supplement were any needed. This was once normal in the UK and Australia. In a country hospital in 1979 the staff boiled some of my bountiful day-four-since-birth breastmilk for a big baby whose birth had been traumatic and whose mother was shattered: he settled down beautifully, having screamed every time infant formula was offered. However, heating breastmilk not only alters nutrients, it destroys the normal microflora

---

349 Balmer SE, Wharton BA Diet and faecal flora in the newborn: breast milk and infant formula. (PMID:2696432) *Arch Dis Child* 1989, 64(12):1672–77; Perkkiö M, Savilahti E. Time of appearance of immunoglobulin-containing cells in the mucosa of the neonatal intestine. (PMID:7191555) *Pediatric Research* 1980, 14(8):953–55.

350 Feehley T, Stefka AT, Cao S, Nagler CR. Microbial regulation of allergic responses to food. (PMID:22941410) *Semin Immunopathol* 2012, 34(5):671–88

351 Henrick BM, Nag K, Yao XD, Drannik AGet al. Milk matters: soluble Toll-like receptor 2 (sTLR2) in breast milk significantly inhibits HIV-1 infection and inflammation. (PMID:22792230) *PLoS One* 2012, 7(7):e40138.

present in it, increasing the risk of the infant being colonised by less beneficial bacteria from the hospital environment unless the mother still provides much skin contact. This is something to remember when assessing trials that use pasteurised donor breastmilk as a placebo or for purposes of comparison. Cooking transforms foods.[352] We need to know a lot more about how it transforms breastmilk. Is breastmilk becoming more like formula, rather than formula becoming more like breastmilk?

Meanwhile, my advice to every pregnant mother is simple – express some colostrum antenatally or access donor milk, take in a frozen supply when you go to hospital, and refuse to allow any non-human food to be given to your new baby. If baby needs extra calories, provide them from your own milk: look up lacto-engineering in the index of this book. You may not need to do anything but breastfeed if you and your partner or a trusted helper can keep your baby skin to skin and you feed often, effectively and for as long as baby wants to stay at breast. (Often means as often as baby is interested, but at least every two hours in the first days after birth.) But it is reassuring to know a safe alternative is there for your baby, when staff members really don't believe exclusive breastfeeding is important. As well, keep your baby skin to skin: 'kangaroo care' means baby has lower energy needs, because your body helps regulate her temperature and breathing, and dramatically lowers levels of stress hormones.[353] That means lower levels of stress hormones, faster growth and a happier baby. Well-treated like this, preterm babies can even grow at in utero rates: a grandchild of mine just did in 2014. Go prepared with simple cloth slings or even just large stretchy wraps.

By reducing your own stress levels, that frozen milk supply increases the likelihood that you will be giving it away to some other mother, because you didn't need it yourself. (That's 'nutritional insurance'.) And if you do use it, or if you are separated from your baby for any reason, remember that like any other liquid, every drop you give that does not come from you needs to be made by you in future, so work on expressing and building up your supply as soon as possible. Always remember that the baby is yours, not the hospital's. Of course small or sick babies may need special care, but skin contact and breastmilk are still optimal and even lifesaving.[354]

By contrast, complementary feeds are creating dysbiosis in your baby's gut, as well as undermining your confidence in lactation and as a mother. Make it clear they are never to be given without your fully informed consent. Especially if your baby is preterm, as a diet containing cows' milk protein products increases the risk of both serious sickness and death.[355]

---

352  Here I must urge everyone interested in this topic to read Michael Pollan's *Cooked: a natural history of transformation.* (Allen Lane 2013) and his other books, such as *In Defence of Food*.
353  Bergman J, Bergman N. *Hold Your Prem*. Available from www.kangaroomothercare.com
354  Wight NE, Morton JA, Kim JH. *Best Medicine: human milk in the NICU*. (Hale Publishing 2008.)
355  Abrams, SA, Schanler RJ, Lee ML et al. Greater morbidity and mortality in ELBW infants fed a diet containing cow milk protein products. *Breastfeeding Medicine* 2014; 9 (56): 281-285. DOI: 10.1089/bfm2014.0024

# 2.6 Other potentially damaging factors

Early postnatal feeds are only one of many influences on immune development, highlighted here because they are *too often totally avoidable*. Other negative influences can be harder to avoid, and some may provide benefits that make them necessary despite any negative side effects.

## Antibiotic use

Babies are great survivors. Most babies seem to tolerate or deal effectively with alien proteins, pathogens, and the gut effects of the broad-spectrum antibiotics given to mother or baby. Obviously even today many children and mothers die for want of those same antibiotics, the twentieth century's magical silver bullet. But now we know that antibiotics affect normal gut development and function. Which means that they should never be used unnecessarily – as at present, they often are.[356] Scientists unaware of usual hospital practices may not realise that in some birthing centres it is a rare baby who is not exposed to antibiotics, either directly, or via the placenta, or via the mother's milk. If mothers test positive for Strep B, a course of antibiotics can be routine, despite the controversy around this practice.[357] Wherever there are high intervention or surgical delivery rates, antibiotics are routinely prescribed to prevent infection. If a mother runs a fever after birth – sometimes simply a marker of immune activation – some are quick to give antibiotics 'as a precaution'. And situations causing antibiotic prescription can also be associated with lower breastfeeding rates, multiplying the damage, and confounding research into the effects of both artificial feeding and antibiotics on the microbiome.

Of course antibiotic exposure can come via many other routes. This has been discussed earlier in the section on the Biodiversity hypothesis and also in relation to stock feed (see page 387 and page 389). Does this almost ubiquitous antibiotic exposure matter later in life? Unsurprisingly, the answer appears to be yes:

> Colonisation of the gut immediately after birth has been shown to be different in allergic and non-allergic infants, and colonisation is now recognised to play a key role in 'allergy' development. Colonisation is likely to be affected by the use of broad-spectrum antibiotics in the neonatal period. While most of the studies on food 'allergy' relate to children, it is clear that these effects track into adult life.[358]

---

356  The routine use of ampicillin antenatally to prevent group-B strep sepsis has resulted in 'a massive increase in coliform sepsis which additionally is resistant to ampicillin' Bedford-Russell AB, quoted in Isolauri E, Walker WA (eds), op. cit., p. 174. And, I would add, microbiomic distortion in all exposed mothers and children.

357  Wickham S (2010). Antibiotics for Group B Strep: are they effective? *Essentially MIDIRS* 1(1): 27 – 30; http://www.sarawickham.com/research-updates/whether-and-how-to-treat-group-b-strep-the-continuing-gulf-between-evidence-and-practice/

358   Blair M, Stewart-Brown S, Waterston T, Crowther R., *Child Public Health* (OUP 2010) p. 197

## Other perinatal stressors and gut closure

Decades ago, Professor John Gerrard noted that:

> ... the later development of allergy seems often to be triggered by infections ... measles and even ordinary inoculations may trigger the development of an allergy to cows' milk. Viral infections in infancy are often associated with a rise in IgE levels. We would speculate that such infections may act as adjuvants in initiating the development of new allergies.[359]

Developing tolerance to foods depends on how the gut handles antigens, and stress is critical to whether tolerance or reactivity result. The consumption of antigens by laboratory animals has long been known to result in tolerance – provided that the animals were not already sensitised before they ate the food, and that the animals were not exposed to adjuvants like pertussis at the time of food exposure. Adjuvants are substances that trigger immune reactions, and so increase the likelihood that the body will not ignore the other presenting antigens. In the 1980s, Professor RC Coombes from Cambridge told me that pertussis inoculation reliably created food allergy in guinea pigs, and this is backed up by recent studies.[360] Human babies too seem less likely to develop tolerance to foods fed to them while they are also subject to immune stressors and gut-altering substances, or lacking vital hormones and enzymes and anti-oxidants supplied by fresh breastmilk.

Separation from the mother's body with its regulatory support, traumatic procedures like circumcision or surgery, viruses or other microbes damaging the gut: these are conditions likely to affect the development of tolerance of strange foods. All have been associated with a higher risk of allergy in children (but, I hasten to add, don't necessarily cause such problems for every baby!) The gut is designed to be permeable ('leaky') after birth, to allow uptake of useful cells from maternal colostrum and later milk. Maternal immune cells have been found in infant urinary tracts, for example. Permeability decreases over the first month, faster in breastfed children than in those not exclusively breastfed. A recent poster presentation by a Russian paediatrician showed that in a group of 51 babies, greater gut permeability for longer after birth was associated with higher rates of allergy.[361] Did the inflammation of allergy cause the greater permeability or vice versa? Do stress hormones have this effect on the gut? Or is this simply a gene-linked variation of the normal closure process, which was of no importance when alien foods were not given? Could delayed gut closure even be protective for solely breastfed infants? How much does permeability alter throughout life, and what causes it to? These are all ongoing research questions.

---

359   Gerrard J. op. cit., p. 438.

360   'There was a positive association between pertussis infection and atopic disorders in the pertussis-vaccinated group only. From the present study, it cannot be concluded whether this association is causal or due to reverse causation.' Bernsen RM, Nagelkerke NJ, Thijs C, van der Wouden JC. Reported pertussis infection and risk of atopy in 8- to 12-yr-old vaccinated and non-vaccinated children. *Ped Allergy Immunol* 2008, 19(1):46 – 52.

361   Makarova S, Borovik T, Skvortsova V, Yatsyk G et al.. Increased gut permeability in newborns with food allergy. *Clinical and Translational Allergy* 2013; Suppl 3 (3) p. 94. http://www.ctajournal.com/content/3/S3/P94 DOI:10.1186/2045-7022-3-S3-P94

# Pollution and chemical contamination

Industrialisation brought many changes to communities. None would prove more dramatic than the change in infant feeding. In the early twentieth century, in the first generations of formula-feeding, it was very clear to some doctors that bottle-fed babies had hugely different rates of gut distress and visible allergic disease such as eczema.[362] But babies survived and grew fat, and that was the litmus test for infant formulas of the time, not whether children suffered more distress and disease.

Industrialisation has brought with it a toxic load of chemicals that can affect the baby in utero and contaminate both formula and the mother's milk – and through it the breastfed child, especially the firstborn of an older woman who smokes, for example. There have been some deeply disturbing analyses of this issue of chemical risks and environmental degradation, none better than the stunning scientific writing of Sandra Steingraber, which every parent and scientist alike should read.[363]

Artificial feeding is one (unnecessary) way in which many of these chemicals reach the vulnerable child, via the product, the water needed to make it up, and the feeding equipment used. Until relatively recently, all three were sources of lead contamination, for example, and children have died from such exposures. But – to a lesser degree now than ever before in affluent communities – breastmilk is also contaminated, even though a woman's body filters and sometimes alters environmental substances before feeding them to her baby. This is probably one reason why the effects of postnatal exposure are so much less than the harms of prenatal exposure: exposure to PCBs via breastfeeding was unrelated to cognitive performance, whereas prenatal exposure was damaging.[364]

 Mothers can exercise more control over their milk than they can over the formula they buy, so fear of contamination is simply not a reason for a mother to avoid breastfeeding. Neither is smoking; not only is ingesting formula going to add to the infant's problems, but breastmilk can reduce the harms of passive smoking to the child.[365] Chemically exposed mothers need to breastfeed to help their child deal with the toxins. Smokers need to breastfeed. (And cut down or quit!) And lead-lighting is definitely not an occupation for anyone of childbearing age, unless extreme care is taken to avoid contamination!

A group of concerned Dutch doctors have spelt out what they see as the environmental risks (such as Maillard compounds in formula, smoking, household chemicals, air pollution, lead, methyl mercury, etc.) to infants, related to the most common childhood problems:

---

362 One classic study found seven times the rate of eczema in artificially fed children compared with breastfed ones. Grulee GG, Sanford HN, Herron PH. Breast and Artificial Feeding. *JAMA* 1934; 103: 735.

363 See the bibliography for more, but begin with the eminently readable *Raising Elijah: protecting our children in an age of environmental crisis*. (Da Capo Press, 2011)

364 Jacobson JL, Jacobson SW, Humphrey HE. Effects of in utero exposure to polychlorinated biphenyls and related contaminants on cognitive functioning in young children. (PMID:2104928) *J Pediatr* 1990, 116(1):38–45

365 Yilmaz G, Hizli S, Karacan C, Yurdakök K et al. Effect of passive smoking on growth and infection rates of breast-fed and non-breast-fed infants. (PMID:19400822) *Pediatrics International* 2009, 51(3):352–58. DOI: 10.1111/j.1442-200X.2008.02757.x

Prematurity. Intra-uterine growth restriction. Testicular dysgenesis syndrome. Type I and Type II diabetes. Asthma, atopy and hay fever. Autism. Attention deficit hyperactivity disorder (ADHD). Learning disabilities. Cancer. Obesity. Hearing problems.[366]

The doctors recommended promoting breastfeeding amongst other things. For more on this, read the very recent Policy Statement and Technical Report released by the American Academy of Pediatrics.[367] Let's hope that paediatricians will take the lead in every country.

Meanwhile women can lower their own and their children's pesticide intake by buying only organic foods in pregnancy and lactation, and by avoiding lot-fed beef, battery chicken, regular dairy products[368] and so on – as well as avoiding tobacco (a toxin-laden product), and pesticide-resistant GM cereal crops. In the nature of things, such crops ought to have more pesticide than organic cereals. Even a week on an organic diet has been shown to lower pesticide intake markedly.[369] Organic foods are said by some to taste better, and their purchase supports farmers who've cleaned up their land, restoring a normal biodiverse microbial ecosystem and healthy soil structure. A better microbial balance on the land, and in farm animals, can mean parents are more likely to be exposed to beneficial bacteria. Antibiotic-resistant bacteria are commonplace in industrial agriculture,[370] and industrial agriculture has to be involved in the production of the vast quantity of raw materials needed to make infant formula on an industrial scale and schedule.

## The uterine environment and stress

Anyone considering childbearing might find an account of Pottenger's cats thought-provoking. In controlled studies, cats fed cooked, not fresh, food degenerated over two or three generations, suffering a range of health problems, infertility, skeletal malformation, and so on. In animal studies, poor reproductive function can result from their diet and from stress. There is ample evidence that stress in pregnancy affects allergy outcomes.[371] In the human animal, diet and/or stress could perhaps help explain the need for in vitro fertility treatments, declining sperm counts and the epidemic of polycystic ovary syndrome (PCOS), although of course other environmental factors are implicated, such as smoking, ubiquitous oestrogen-like chemicals, mould toxins, diesel particulate in the

366  van den Hazel P, Zuurbier M, Babisch W, Bartonova A et al. Today's epidemics in children: possible relations to environmental pollution and suggested preventive measures. (PMID:17000565) *Acta Paediatrica* Supplement 2006, 95(453):18–25.
367  Roberts JR, Karr CJ, Health CoE. Pesticide exposure in children. *Pediatrics* 2012; 130 (6) e1757 -e1763. DOI: 10.1542/peds.2012-1757
368  Dagnelie PC, van Staveren WA, Roos AH et al. Nutrients and contaminants in milk from mothers on macrobiotic and omnivorous diets. *Eur J Clin Nutr* 1992; 46: 355–66.
369  Oates L, Cohen M, Braun L, Schembri A et al. Reduction in urinary organophosphate pesticide metabolites in adults after a week-long organic diet. *Environmental Research* 2014; 132:105–11. DOI: 10.1016/j. envres.2014.03.021 Online report: http://theconversation.com/eating-organic-food-significantly-lowers-pesticide-exposure-study-26055
370  Pollan M. *Cooked: a natural history of transformation.* (Allen Lane 2013)
371  de Marco R, Pesce G, Girardi P, Marchetti P et al. Foetal exposure to maternal stressful events increases the risk of having asthma and atopic diseases in childhood. *Pediatr Allergy Immunol* 2012: 00

air,[372] antibiotics,[373] caffeine, as well as food processing, feeding equipment and ingredients, and even something as simple as a lack of Vitamin D due to reduced sun exposure. Some of these will be discussed in Book 2.

Pregnancy is the period of greatest vulnerability to large harms from small exposures as well as genetic influences. No one doubts the importance of a healthy pregnancy in the creation of a healthy child, although again, it is surprising how resilient human infants can be, and some apparently perfectly healthy children emerge despite worryingly bad maternal diets and stresses. But remember that the egg that is to become a fertilised embryo was created a generation before, inside the womb of the grandmother, where we all begin. So stressors during more than one pregnancy may influence the development of any child. Grandparents contribute the genes that make the mother and her eggs (and influence which of those genes are expressed); mother's egg contributes half the baby's genes and father's sperm the other half. All those genes have the potential to be expressed in different ways, with very different outcomes. .

There is some evidence that the childhood nutrition of grandparents affects outcomes like diabetes and coronary artery disease in their offspring.[374] Both fathers[375] and mothers influence health outcomes, genetically and epigenetically. So do grandparents, with some of the effects being gender specific. For example, one study showed that the paternal grandfather's poor nutrition in middle childhood was linked to a greater risk of early death in grandsons, but not granddaughters, while the paternal grandmother's poor nutrition was reflected in a higher mortality risk for granddaughters. This effect is obviously mediated through the father in some way. As Whitelaw said, and as a mother I noted with some relief, 'these findings go some way towards shifting the balance of responsibility for the unborn away from the mother.'[376]

But of course the growing baby's uterine environment is influenced by many factors affecting the mother, among them her diet and health, stress levels and medications, toxic exposures and lifestyle habits. As noted earlier, the antibodies she supplies after the eighteenth week will last around three months postpartum, allowing the infant time to start making its own antibodies while being protected to some degree both by maternal immune cells (including IgG and IgA) secreted generously in her breastmilk. But intra-uterine sensitisation to allergens is possible, and elevated infant IgE blood levels at birth (as measured in cord

372 Morgenstern V, Zutavern A, Cyrys J, Brockow I et al. GINI/LISA Study Groups. Atopic diseases, allergic sensitisation, and exposure to traffic-related air pollution in children. (PMID:18337595) *Am J Respir Crit Care Med* 2008, 177(12):1331–37.

373 Flöistrup H, Swartz J, Bergström A, Alm JS et al. Parsifal Study Group. Allergic disease and sensitisation in Steiner school children. (PMID:16387585) *J Allergy Clin Immunol* 2006, 117(1):59–66

374 Kaati G, Bygren LO, Edvinsson S. Cardiovascular and diabetes mortality determined by nutrition during parents' and grandparents' slow growth period.(PMID:12404098) *Eur J Hum Genet* 2002, 10(11):682–88; Kaati G, Bygren LO, Pembrey M, Sjöström M. Transgenerational response to nutrition, early life circumstances and longevity. (PMID:17457370) *Eur J Hum Genet* 2007; 15(7):784–90

375 Bygren LO, Kaati G, Edvinsson S. Longevity determined by paternal ancestors' nutrition during their slow growth period. (PMID:11368478)*Acta Biotheor* 2001, 49(1):53–59.; Pembrey ME, Bygren LO, Kaati G, Edvinsson S et al.. Sex-specific, male-line transgenerational responses in humans.(PMID:16391557) *Eur J Hum Genet* 2006;14(2):159–66.

376 Whitelaw E. Sins of the fathers and their fathers. *Eur J Hum Genet* 2006; 14: 131–2.

blood), together with family history, can predict postpartum allergy.[377] Whatever the allergen exposures, the ways in which women's bodies deal with them affects how the baby will react, with either tolerance or hypersensitivity. But it is not all down to this mother in this pregnancy: she herself is the product of her environment and heredity. And the father's health also influences allergy outcomes, though to a lesser extent than the mother's. Most mothers find it helpful to know that others share responsibility for the health of her child: the child's father and both their parents and grandparents are all involved.

## Vaccination: a plea for rationality on all sides

I support vaccination. It has saved millions of lives. Yet there is still much we do not know about it. The perception is that vaccine effects are targeted and specific, but it is emerging that vaccines can have many non-specific effects as well. Much of what is now being discovered is very positive, such as the preliminary evidence that the measles vaccine reduces deaths from infections other than measles, and the BCG vaccine – designed to protect against tuberculosis (TB) – stimulates an immune reaction against bladder cancer. Vaccines, like all treatments, have side effects, for good or ill; they can alter individual immunity in more ways than specifically intended.[378] But in general they do vastly more good than harm, and early childhood vaccinations are among the most effective.

That said, in any discussion of factors that affect the development of the infant immune system, it is impossible to ignore the role of vaccination. It is implicit in what has been said already about viruses acting as adjuvants: some early infant vaccines are live or killed viruses. Vaccines themselves contain many ingredients, some of which, like peanut oil (see page 325) may not be listed in the extensive US CDC database available online.[379] Some of these are known allergens, present in tiny quantities but capable of causing reactions in a minority of infants. Despite all that, most parents, even those with known allergies, sensibly choose to protect their children by vaccinating them.

There is evidence that breastfeeding reduces the severity and in some cases even prevents infection by some of the most feared childhood diseases, such as whooping cough[380] and measles,[381] among others. To be clear, just as with vaccines, the protection given by breastfeeding is by no means total protection: some breastfed infants (and some vaccinated

377  Hansen LG, Host A, Halken S, Holmskov A, Husby S et al. Cord blood IgE. III. Prediction of IgE high-response and allergy. A follow-up at the age of 18 months. *Allergy* 1992; 47 (4 pt 2): 404–10.

378  An accessible discussion of this is found in Brooks M. Small shot, big impact. *New Scientist* 2013; 2930: 39–41. See also http://www.newscientist.com/article/dn24027-booster-shots-the-accidental-advantages-of-vaccines.html, where this story is updated.

379  http://www.cdc.gov/vaccines/pubs/pinkbook/downloads/appendices/b/excipient-table-2.pdf.

380  Quinello C, Quintilio W, Carneiro-Sampaio M, Palmeira P. Passive acquisition of protective antibodies reactive with Bordetella pertussis in newborns via placental transfer and breast-feeding. (PMID:20591078) *Scand J Immunol.* 2010; 72(1):66–73. DOI: 10.1111/j.1365-3083.2010.02410.x 'Our data demonstrated the effectiveness of anti-pertussis antibodies in bacterial pathogenesis neutralisation, emphasising the importance of placental transfer and breast-feeding in protecting infants against respiratory infections caused by Bordetella pertussis'.

381  Silfverdal SA, Ehlin A, Montgomery SM. Breast-feeding and a subsequent diagnosis of measles. (PMID:19133867) *Acta Paediatrica* 2009, 98(4):715–19. DOI: 10.1111/j.1651-2227.2008.01180.x ; Nikitiuk NF. The antimeasles immunity in infants in the 1st year of life. (PMID:10876898) *Zhurnal Mikrobiologii, Epidemiologii, i Immunobiologii* 2000(1):63–65.

ones) will contract these diseases. Continued breastfeeding assists recovery from any disease contracted. Recovering from the natural disease usually means lifelong immunity, with protective antibody passed on in breastmilk to one's children.

Even so, some breastfed children will die from these diseases, and the odds seem to be that not as many would, if they had been vaccinated. But would breastfed babies (solely breastfed from birth) benefit from being spared unnecessary microbiome disturbance for just a few months, with vaccine schedules for the breastfed infant beginning – as they used to – only at three to four months, not straight after birth? Development in body size and immune function suggests infants might cope better at that age, as they once seemed to, if maternal observation is any guide. Why should vaccination policies and schedules for artificially fed and exclusively breastfed babies be identical when the exclusively breastfed child is naturally less at risk of any severe infection? Are young breastfed babies being put at needless risk in an attempt to protect the mixed-fed and artificially fed?

Some parents have a lot of questions about vaccinations, but they are urged to simply follow orders blindly. In Australia they are even paid to do as they are told, and their questions go unanswered. Yet there are risks, and industry knows it. And while those risks are in general much lower than the disease risks the vaccine is preventing, and serious damage is very rare, that is no consolation if it is your child who is badly affected.

Here are some of the questions discussed among concerned parents.

- How many new immune challenges – microbes and vaccines – can safely go into one small rapidly developing newborn at the same time?

- Are immune reactions synergistic, so that offering new foods and vaccines at the same time, or vaccinating when a child's immune system is already challenged, is partly responsible for adverse immune reactions?

- Are the food and antibiotic traces in vaccines more of a problem now than in the past?[382]

- Could vaccination doses relate to body weight, not days since birth?

- What about the effects of adjuvants and trace residues?[383]

- Are repeat vaccinations really necessary and safe if the child has reacted obviously to the first or second dose?

- Do we vaccinate artificially fed infants against so many viruses because children under three are in childcare centres, known to cause high cortisol levels and be major vectors of disease transmission?

- Would it be safer or better to vaccinate mothers in late pregnancy or during lactation? (Obviously not in early pregnancy with live viruses!!)

---

382  It seems that antibodies against egg proteins are linked to a greater risk of allergy: but were vaccine traces responsible for sensitisation? Kukkonen AK, Savilahti EM, Haahtela T, Savilahti E, et al. Ovalbumin-specific immunoglobulins A and G levels at age 2 years are associated with the occurrence of atopic disorders. (PMID:21771118) *Clin Exper Allergy* 2011, 41(10):1414–21. What about bovine protein traces? Peanut oil?

383  Dórea JG, Marques RC. Infants' exposure to aluminum from vaccines and breast milk during the first 6 months. (PMID:20010978) *J Exposure Sci Envir Epidem* 2010; 20(7):598–601. DOI: 10.1038/jes.2009.64

It would make economic sense to pay breastfeeding women to care for their own children, for twelve to thirty-six months, within their own ecological environments, with a *guaranteed right to return to work* after that. Childcare places babies at greater risk of infection[384], as well as psychological distress.[385] The increased medical costs that even quality public-funded childcare would create for taxpayers were said to be the reason the Finnish government chose generous support for parents to care for their own children for the first three years of life over taxpayer-funded empires of commercial infant day-care.[386] Systems that force women to return to work by giving money only to support commercial daycare, or in the form of rebates on money paid, or taxes, may be costing us a great deal more. How many women would care for their own children if paid to do so, and how would that transform suburbs, allowing mothers to find local support?

Let me repeat – I support vaccination, just as I support the use of antibiotics, when safe, effective, and necessary. Major diseases like polio, smallpox, diphtheria, whooping cough, tetanus and measles have been dramatically reduced by vaccination. Vaccination is a fundamentally important health strategy world wide, and anti-vaccination lobbyists should not claim any one study as proof of harm, or urge a total boycott of all vaccination; to do so is irresponsible.

However, the success of those first childhood vaccines like diphtheria, tetanus and whooping cough does not mean that we can go on pushing more and more vaccines into ever younger, smaller, more allergic babies with impunity. Six vaccines at once, and a young child developed paralysis in the leg that had been injected with five of them: was that coincidence or unnecessary risk?[387] A till-then-placid solely breastfed six-week-old baby screaming in pain within hours of a live rotavirus dose, with bloody diarrhoea and reactions to foods in maternal diet thereafter, is no coincidence. I have seen it happen, and that child was at almost zero risk of rotavirus infection: never in child care and fully breastfed. Basic science says that a live virus can cause gut damage, and that damage can cause pain and further problems.

Wherever this is possible (and I acknowledge that it is often impossible in mass vaccination programmes) there needs to be serious discussion about every individual vaccine, and

---

384 Najnin N, Forbes A, Sinclair M, Leder K. Risk factors for community-based reports of gastrointestinal, respiratory, and dermal symptoms: findings from a cohort study in Australia. (PMID:24240632) Free full text article *J Epidemiol* 2014, 24(1):39-46 DOI: 10.2188/jea.JE20130082; Sacri AS, De Serres G, Quach C, Boulianne N et al. Transmission of acute gastroenteritis and respiratory illness from children to parents. (PMID:24476955) *Pediatr Infect Dis J* 2014, 33(6):583-588 DOI: 10.1097/INF.0000000000000220

385 James O. *How not to F*** them up* ( Vermilion Press 2010)

386 Mikko Vienonen (personal communication). Australia, like many other countries, chose to develop profit-making taxpayer-funded empires of commercial infant daycare by providing tax rebates only to parents who put their child into group care by strangers. Our first woman Prime Minister got paid parental leave enshrined in law, an egalitarian scheme which guaranteed all women only 18 weeks' leave paid at the basic wage. The new government's proposed scheme (matching women's wages, up to $150,000, for six months) clearly meant that those who least need help would receive most of the financial assistance with child-rearing. Such unfairness angered many, and the scheme has not proceeded . But six months should be the minimum leave period, and would pay for itself if women breastfed longer.

387 Edwards EA, Grant CC, Huang QS, Powell KF et al. A case of vaccine-associated paralytic poliomyelitis. (PMID:10940185) *J Paediatr Child Health* 2000; 36(4):408–11.DOI: 10.1046/j.1440-1754.2000.00514.x

every individual brand, for each child – not the all-or-none, do-as-you're-told polarised stances of today. Besides being unjustified, that's counterproductive and plain dumb. It seems to me that the lack of honest discussion and individualised advice undermines trust in the system. And so an obviously bad reaction to an unnecessary rotavirus vaccine at 6 weeks may reduce the chance of a baby getting a pertussis or diphtheria vaccine at three months. When rotavirus in exclusively breastfed children is both much less likely, and a milder disease, than pertussis or diphtheria, that is not a good outcome. It can take a great deal of explanation to persuade a mother to put her baby at risk of a second reaction. Her instinct is to protect by avoidance, not to take any unnecessary risk.

In my personal experience, such individualised and respectful discussion was once possible in 1970s Victoria, Australia, when community-based maternal and child health nurses still had time to see mothers other than by appointment, and went through a lengthy checklist and discussion of potential risk factors in that individual child. The 1975 National Health and Medical Research Council (NHMRC) Guidelines[388] in fact stressed the needs for 'hygiene, valid consent and thorough pre-immunisation assessment', which included checking previous reactions, and whether the baby was unwell on the day. It seemed to be routine back then to advise a parent to wait if a child was ill, and not complete the full course in the event of evident seroconversion, i.e., a strong reaction to a previous dose. Experienced nurses who daily saw healthy children (not just sick ones) vetted babies, who then presented for mass immunisation by sessional visiting doctors in community centres. Waiting another month or two for the next dose was not seen as a problem in the age before commercial childcare facilities. Is such discussion, time and care possible when seeing a private doctor whose standard consultation lasts ten minutes, and whose practice means she has much less knowledge of normal children than those experienced community-based nurses did? Is the imperative drive for vaccination even of very young fully breastfed babies the direct result of mass commercial childcare? (And are mothers of infants going back to work aware that increased illness for the family is a likely cost of commercial daycare, and that, as Oliver James argues in *How not to f\*\*\* them up*, this is the worst form of care for very young children?)

Reporting of adverse reactions was encouraged in the 1970s. Nowadays parents are often reassured so dogmatically that the vaccine had nothing to do with the reaction that official reporting seems unlikely to happen. Certainly no one wanted to know about the baby I mentioned earlier: having rung the hospital where the child was seen in distress, and the official immunisation answering machines, saying that I wanted to report an adverse event, I received no call back. The mother, dealing with a now very unhappy baby reacting to her dietary intake, was in no position to follow this up any further. Nor was I. Denying parental perceptions of such clearly-linked outcomes undermines trust in the system. Yet vaccines are grown on milk, others on egg, or bovine products, or monkey kidney cells, any of which may have contributed inadvertently to gut damage and sensitisation in this baby. Why would that mother trust dogmatic vaccination advocates again?

 Dogmatic insistence on all three doses of the triple antigen vaccine is contrary to what I was told in the 1970s was accepted practice, when experienced maternal and child health

---

388   NHMRC Immunisation Procedures. (NHMRC 1975) copy on file.

nurses would point out that a child who had reacted strongly to a first or second dose of this vaccine had clearly seroconverted, which was the aim of the multiple doses, and so obviously did not need the third early dose, but should return for boosters in due course. In reading horror stories of vaccine-damaged children, it was remarkable how often the damaged children had been given a subsequent dose (often of a vaccine grown on bovine products like milk or calf serum) after earlier reactions were deemed unimportant – despite parental misgivings. Why insist on three doses, supposedly to be sure of seroconversion, when there is clear evidence of an immune reaction having taken place after two? Why, when there is a UK study of vaccination and hospital records which 'found an increased relative risk for convulsions 0–3 days after the DPT vaccination. *The effect was limited to the third dose of vaccine.*'[389] (They didn't say whether parents reported that these children had reacted to the second.) How much damage was done?

If any parent of an allergic child asks me what to do about a third dose after strong reactions to previous doses, I tell them about that UK study. Consent to vaccination is not informed if such information is withheld. Vaccination is powerful enough to deserve respect. Infants are different enough to deserve respect too.

Parents certainly do need to vaccinate against major known killer diseases like diphtheria, whooping cough, tetanus, measles and polio, while evaluating the risks of any vaccines that could be seen as experimental, or even optional in their circumstances. For instance, some parents of a healthy term baby might reasonably decide that vaccination against Hep B immediately after birth, or rotavirus before twelve weeks, is unnecessary if the mother has herself been vaccinated and is exclusively breastfeeding a thriving baby. Others, aware that their baby is to go into early childcare thanks to a lack of maternity leave, or unable to breastfeed fully for other reasons, might think Hep B at birth and rotavirus vaccines at six weeks a very good idea. That's for parents to decide. (And parents of infants in childcare need to be sure any childcare workers are vaccinated and will be scrupulous about handwashing.)

The technicalities of vaccine timing and dose aside, let's come back to allergy. Allergy researchers trying to make sense of their national data may need to know in detail *what has been in their nation's vaccines,* as well as what foods and antibiotics went into babies in maternity hospitals. A PubMed search revealed that this is a subject of intense interest already, as allergists are aware that immune stimulation – whether by live viruses or foods or vaccines or aluminium or other vaccine adjuvants[390] – does indeed have an effect on atopy (immune reactions narrowly defined) as well as the infant microbiome. And the presence of peanut oil and wild viruses in early vaccines – freely admitted now by scientists in charge of those programmes[391] – was not without consequences. There are now more (still rare) cases of paralytic polio due to vaccine strains than due to the wild virus, which

---

389  Farrington P, Pugh S, Colville A, Flower A et al. A new method for active surveillance of adverse events from diphtheria/tetanus/pertussis and measles/mumps/rubella vaccines.(PMID:7619183) *Lancet* 1995; 345(8949):567–69.

390  Terhune TD, Deth RC. How aluminum adjuvants could promote and enhance non-target IgE synthesis in a genetically-vulnerable sub-population. (PMID:22967010) *J Immunotoxicology* 2013; 10(2):210–22.

391  Butel JS. Simian Virus 40, poliovirus vaccines, and human cancer: research progress versus media and public interests *Bulletin WHO,* 2000, 78 (2) 195–97. http://www.who.int/bulletin/archives/78(2)195.pdf

has been eradicated in some developed countries.[392] There have been no cases in Sweden where the killed vaccine was standard, and this seems a safer bet – but is this option always available for parents who ask?

Vaccination is important, and parents need to be able to trust those responsible for such programmes. It seems natural to be suspicious about potential risks, especially in a system where multinational companies agree to manufacture highly profitable goods *only on condition that they do not bear the burden of compensating anyone harmed by their products*. No fault compensation schemes have been created in many countries, protecting vaccine manufacturers from injury claims, after large payouts in civil courts. Vaccination protects many children, but does injure a tiny minority.

It seems natural that governments never want to admit fault in the product they insist that parents use, even pay them to use. It would help build parental trust if

- vaccines were developed and produced only by not-for-profit ethical global entities,
- reporting of adverse events was actively encouraged,
- independent tribunals (including consumer advocates) existed to hear claims of damage and
- needed compensation or assistance was funded by vaccine profits, so that those who make the profits pay for any damage they cause.

I have been extremely reluctant to raise the subject of vaccination, but in any discussion of immune disorder, so powerful a positive immunological event as vaccination cannot be omitted just because I suspect that some readers will misrepresent what I'm saying. Allergy complicates vaccination decisions. I have seen allergic children affected by vaccination on the standard schedules, with the standard doses. I have talked to healthworkers whose own babies were given only single carefully chosen vaccines not multivalent vaccines, only when baby was well, not after obvious seroconversion has happened, not after adverse reactions to an earlier shot, and so on. I have talked with too many intelligent parents who have sought to discuss the best process and products for their individual allergic child – only to be dismissed as cranks for taking their responsibility as parents seriously. Educated women will not just obey doctors' orders and take the government payment for being obedient,[393] and it is such vocal parents with access to modern media who lead the current backlash against vaccination in western communities. If health workers will not listen, parents will speak out, and others will listen to them.

I recall startlingly similar reactions to parents who fought to have food allergy recognised as real and serious against the prevailing medical wisdom of the 1970s and 1980s. Those parents have since been thoroughly vindicated: most healthworkers finally recognise the problems parents had seen decades before. Respect for parental perspectives is needed, to

---

392  Soto NE, Lutwick LI. Poliovirus immunisations. What goes around, comes around. PMID:10198803) *Infect Dis Clin North Am* 1999; 13(1):265–78, ix.

393  The Australian government has made an annual payment of $726 contingent on proof of full vaccination or approved exemption. Yet there is controversy about paying women to breastfeed or to supply breastmilk?

avoid another whooping cough debacle, and to head off virulent anti-vaccination claims by affected parents. In the UK Dr Richard Halvorsen has tried to address these parental concerns.[394] A pro-vaccination US paediatrician, Dr Robert Sears, has also tried to address such concerns[395] (and for his pains, been publicly misrepresented by a vaccine patent-holder, in the pages of *Pediatrics*[396]). The ensuing correspondence outlined a wide variety of opinions, and makes it clear (to me at least) that polarisation of this debate into pro- and anti-vaccination camps is not helping babies, or society. Parents need to be told all the truths, not simply some, by both camps, and their choices respected. At present those who refuse vaccination are being scapegoated, blamed for much that is not their doing. It may be that every nation in fact needs a minority of unvaccinated children: eliminating the disease altogether may prove impossible in such an interconnected world.

For perhaps it should be noted that having a breastfeeding mother who survived a disease might even be more effective than vaccination, in creating long-lasting ongoing human immunity, if a small Russian study (for which I confess to having read only the abstract) is accurate:

> The serological survey of 138 infants aged 8 months and 138 mothers having had protective titres of specific antibodies to measles during pregnancy was made. The study revealed that passively transferred antibodies to measles circulated in infants for a longer time and were detected more frequently under the conditions of breastfeeding by mothers having had measles (up to 93.7% of infants). In artificially fed infants, born of mothers having had no measles, but previously vaccinated against this infection, antibodies to measles were detected in rather rare cases (only in 7.3%). In infants, artificially fed, but born of mothers having had measles, the level of antibodies to measles was practically unchanged (81.6%).[397]

This is only a small study, and I have not researched this topic in depth, but the accepted orthodox vaccination literature makes it clear that vaccination does not generally create such lifelong maternal immunity, and the creation of protective antibodies by vaccination is limited. Maternal exposure to the virus itself may mean that passively transferred maternal antibodies will protect against infection in the vulnerable first months of life, no matter whether the child was breastfed or not. So there is a silver lining for mothers who have experienced infective diseases: their infants may be born better protected, and their breastfeeding adds another layer of protection. That fact raises an even bigger question: was the nineteenth to mid twentieth century rise in the severity and frequency of childhood infectious diseases in any western country even partly due to the decline of breastfeeding exclusivity and duration?

Since mothers can and do transfer immune protections both during pregnancy and via their milk, vaccination research could also consider what maternal exposures would be of benefit to the baby without risking the mother's health. When it comes to common

---

394 Halvorsen R. *Vaccines: a parents' guide* (Gibson Square, London 3rd ed. 2013)
395 Sears RW. *The Vaccine Book: Making the Right Decision for Your Child.* (Little Brown & Co. 2011)
396 As I have no doubt I will be misrepresented! Offit PA, Moser CA. The Problem With Dr Bob's Alternative Vaccine Schedule. *Pediatrics* 2009; 123 (1) e164 -e169. DOI: 10.1542/peds.2008-2189. http://pediatrics.aappublications.org/content/123/1/e164
397 Nikitiuk NF. op. cit.

diseases that we want to protect babies from, should we vaccinate women before they get pregnant, when pregnant, or while they are lactating? Or not at all? What genetic changes might this involve? Would women recently immunised against rotavirus, for example, transfer protection to an extent that means we do not need to challenge the tiny baby's gut with doses of live virus, endangering its fragile microbiome, and in some cases generating disease in parents as well as infant? Or is adult rotavirus vaccination problematic? That's worth thinking about rationally, assuming rational debate is possible in such a polarised and profitable field as vaccination!

This is not my area of expertise, and I can only raise questions. But whenever humans intervene in nature there can be unintended consequences. Cases of viral disease can be traced to the vaccine used,[398] and it was recently discovered that a trial vaccine actually increased the virulence of the malaria parasite.[399] There is evidence that vaccinating chickens with attenuated viruses has created a lethal combination virus,[400] which some have speculated may increase the risk of a bird-flu pandemic. As I write, this is of concern again in China, and cases are being found which have had no obvious connection with poultry. Surely this means that agencies should be vaccinating only when truly necessary, and staying alert for signs of pathogen adaptation that could involve an increase in virulence? Just as with antibiotics, too much of a Good Thing might be dangerous.

Surely too, this means that all natural protections, like breastfeeding, should be valued and protected and promoted by all those devoting billions to vaccination programmes? In 2007 the American Academy of Pediatrics even created a poster stating 'Breastfeeding. Baby's First Immunization.'[401] Breastmilk is the baby's first and most powerful multivalent and ongoing vaccination. Why is that not strongly highlighted in all vaccination literature? Because no one makes money from it? Because formula-feeding parents don't want to hear it? I reckon so, myself. But even vaccination itself cannot do as much for an infant's immune system as breastfeeding does.

## An aside: vitamin K injections immediately after birth

Parental decisions about vitamin K injections need to be informed. While not a vaccination, Vitamin K injections immediately after birth also need to be investigated in relation to gut and immune development, and a thorough risk-benefit analysis done. Both the brief pain of the injection and the abnormally high vitamin K blood levels achieved need to be justified, as it is counter-intuitive to think that breastmilk's vitamin K content is not all the normal human baby needs. Does such high Vitamin K affect the microbiome? But of course infant starvation can

---

398 Troy SB, Ferreyra-Reyes L, Huang C, Mahmud N et al. Use of a novel real-time PCR assay to detect oral polio vaccine shedding and reversion in stool and sewage samples after a Mexican national immunisation day. (PMID:21411577). *J Clin Microbiol* 2011; 49(5):1777–83.

399 Pro-vaccination lobbyists must read Barclay VC, Sim D, Chan BHK, Nell LA, Rabaa MA et al. (2012) The Evolutionary Consequences of Blood-Stage Vaccination on the Rodent Malaria Plasmodium chabaudi. *PLoS Biol* 10(7): e1001368. DOI:10.1371/journal.pbio.1001368.

400 http://news.sciencemag.org/sciencenow/2012/07/chicken-vaccines-combine-to-prod.html Lee S-W, Markham PF, Coppo MJ, Legione AR et al. Attenuated Vaccines Can Recombine to Form Virulent Field Viruses. *Science* 2012; 337 (6091):188 DOI: 10.1126/science.1217134

401 https://www2.aap.org/breastfeeding/curriculum/documents/pdf/BFIZPoster.pdf

result in low Vitamin K levels: newborns need to be thriving on breastmilk. In one reported case of catastrophic brain bleeding the course of lactation was said to have been 'uneventful', but the child was barely back to birth weight at three weeks. That is not uneventful, but inadequate lactation. In another, signs of deficiency reported to health professionals were ignored as their significance was not realised. The problem in both cases was inadequate milk intake. That is, not too little vitamin K in the milk, just too little milk in the baby.

However, poor maternal diet can also result in low vitamin K breastmilk levels. Pregnant women and breastfeeding mothers should be advised to get plenty of vitamin K themselves, from plant foods like spinach, asparagus, broccoli, beans, soy beans, and strawberries, along with eggs and meat. Classic Vitamin K deficiency bleeding was once seasonal and related to the winter lack of fresh foods, in the days before refrigeration; it presented soon after birth. Whether late onset VKBD is more likely to have been caused by too little milk in the baby or too little vitamin K in the milk should be carefully explored in every case that presents. Unless it is completely safe – and I don't think we know that – universal prophylaxis is hard to justify when so many breastfed babies never have symptoms, and so many are given artificial feeds with added vitamin K from birth. The discovery that too much iron can be harmful should have taught us not to presume the safety of anything fed to all infants.

Any parents who refuse the injection must be educated about the need for vigilance, especially if the baby is not gaining weight well. They must seek urgent medical care if any of the above signs emerge. Detection of these early symptoms and administration of vitamin K can prevent late-onset catastrophic brain bleeds.

> Parents should be made aware of signs of possible low newborn vitamin K levels:
>
> * poor weight gain ( which suggests low breastmilk fat - and vit K - intake)
>
> * bruising easily
>
> * continued bleeding from an injection or cut (circumcision, e.g.)
>
> * oozing from the umbilical stump
>
> * blood in stools or urine

Figure 2-6-1 Signs of low  infant Vitamin K levels

Where preterm infants are concerned, parents need to realise that the issue of what to do about any post-birth injections is affected by their lower body stores of nutrients, greater vulnerability, possible medications, and greater risk of infection during a longer hospital stay. The safety of these post-birth injections in the short term seems proven, so following current protocols is advisable. There are more important issues that may require parental challenges to current practice, such as ensuring virtually constant skin to skin contact and exclusive human milk use. However, continuous evaluation of the possible longer-term effects of these neonatal stresses remains important: many past practices have been found to have unexpected side effects.

# 2.7. Outcomes: bodies built on formula or/and breastmilk

## From community belief to scientific acceptance

The knowledge that early diet and environment influence lifelong health, and the health of children to come, has a long history both in Western medicine and popular culture. Read any late-nineteenth or early twentieth-century medical text on infant feeding and this would be taken for granted, long before research proved it to be true.[402] The health of the infant was of enormous concern to society because of the observed fact that unhealthy survivors of childhood faced lifelong debility and produced unhealthy offspring.

There is a long and continuous thread of this belief in the lifelong importance of infant feeding right through the early part of the twentieth century, and yet today, the idea that early infant nutrition, in and out of the womb, can alter health outcomes in later life and also over generations is somehow startling – when applied to humans. Animal breeders everywhere have known this for a very long time, and it is no longer controversial to researchers in the field.

Yet many parents remain unaware that it is now completely accepted that nutrition, like many other things, affects gene expression and influences health lifelong.[403] For example, at eighteen, adolescents breastfed in infancy are more likely to have antibodies to proteins linked with arthritis and atherosclerosis.[404] This implies that they will better resist these conditions. Arthritis has a well-established food link.[405]

Regrettably but inevitably, science does not always underpin medical practice – and as incentives, and therefore incentive bias, rest more and more with commercial entities than with patients and the public as a whole, it seems likely that this will only get worse. A major online report summarises some of what is now known about nutrition and disease in adult life. The UK Department of Health had asked its Scientific Advisory Committee on Nutrition (SACN) to:

> Review the influence of maternal, fetal and child nutrition, including growth and development in utero and up to the age of 5 years, on the development of chronic disease in later life in the offspring.

---

402  See also Smith GD, Kuh D. Does early nutrition affect later health? Views from the 1930s and 1940s. In Smith DF (ed) *Nutrition in Britain: Science, Scientists and Politics in the Twentieth Century.* (Routledge, London 1997).

403  Phillips CM. Nutrigenetics and metabolic disease: current status and implications for personalised nutrition. *Nutrients* 2013; 5(1):32–57. (PMCID:PMC3571637) Free full text article.

404  Victora GD, Bilate AM, Socorro-Silva A, Caldas C et al. Mother-child immunological interactions in early life affect long-term humoral autoreactivity to heat shock protein 60 at age 18 years. *J Autoimmun* 2007; 29(1):38–43. DOI: 10.1016/j.jaut.2007.02.018.

405  Hvatum M, Kanerud L, Hällgren R, Brandtzaeg P. The gut-joint axis: cross reactive food antibodies in rheumatoid arthritis. (PMID:16484508) *Gut* 2006; 55(9):1240–47.

Identify opportunities for nutritional intervention that could influence the risk of chronic disease in later life in the offspring.[406]

Their June 2011 Report begins:

- Cardiovascular disease, type 2 diabetes and cancer, are leading causes of death in the UK and present a major contemporary public health challenge. The causes are complex. Many environmental exposures modify risk, but diet and lifestyle play a significant part. This report examines the contribution of nutritional exposures in early life.

- Fetal life and early childhood are periods of rapid growth and development (see Chapter 3). Imbalanced nutrient supply* at this stage [in utero and postpartum] may alter body structure and function in a way that increases risk of chronic disease and, in girls, may modify the ability to meet the nutritional and other stresses of reproduction. The nutritional status of the population therefore has implications for the health of both current and future generations.

- Human observational evidence demonstrates associations between growth in early life** and adult chronic disease risk (see Chapter 4). Experimental evidence suggests that at least some of these associations may be causal and offers insight into mechanisms (see Chapter 5).[407]

Note: * *Infant formula is imbalanced nutrition, compared to breastmilk. **Formula distorts growth compared to normal breastfeeding.*

In short, this official considered report is saying that infant nutrition matters for life, and not just to the generation nourished, as effects can be inherited. And there is further evidence of this fact.

The UK Millennium Cohort consists of over 18,000 children born in 2000, an ongoing massive research project.[408] As part of the project, early nutrition and patterns of breastfeeding are being documented, and the effects on child health and development recorded. Analysis of the data has resulted in a number of studies showing that even in a country where artificial feeding became almost universal, and many of those now breastfeeding would have been formula-exposed during infancy, breastfeeding a child still protects health and facilitates better development – or more accurately, allows the child to experience biologically normal health and development, which artificial feeding compromises.

In the 1970s German researchers published important studies indicating that early nutrition played a major part in determining lifelong development, including gender orientation, diabetes, and heart disease. The controversial Professor Gunter Dorner used the term 'qualitative dysnutrition' to describe bottle-feeding; and argued that

---

406  www.sacn.gov.uk/.../sacn_early_nutrition_final_report_20_6_11.pdf
407  ibid.
408  Dex S, Joshi H (eds). *Children of the 21st Century. From birth to nine months.* (2005); Hansen K, Joshi H, Dex S. *Children of the 21st Century, The first five years.* (both from Policy Press, University of Bristol, 2010).

qualitative as well as quantitative dysnutrition during the first trimenon of postnatal life was found to lead to long-lasting mental, psychological and/or physical ill-effects in the human. Females who were completely bottlefed during neonatal life showed significantly decreased school achievements as well as significantly decreased learning capacity and social adaptability at sixteen years of age as compared to females who were purely breastfed or breast- plus bottlefed in neonatal life. Males who were artificially overfed during neonatal life also showed significantly decreased school achievements and significantly decreased learning capacity in adolescence as compared to males with normal weight development in neonatal life.[409]

There's now enough accumulated evidence to support such claims, radical as they seemed at the time. Dysnutrition describes what has been standard practice – artificial feeding. Whenever the outcomes of this dysnutrition are common, that there is a risk of their being mistaken for normal. Western communities have lost sight of what is physiologically normal – the only real human normal – and re-adjusted expectations of maternal and child health and behaviour to the defective standards now considered usual for formula-fed people.

Dorner's work was largely ignored, possibly because his studies on homosexuality were controversial,[410] and almost certainly because his emphasis on infant feeding (as well as foetal nutrition) was deeply unwelcome at a time when few women breastfed in the Western world. Subsequent research focused more on the pre-birth or foetal origins of adult disease after the seminal studies of David Barker and his colleagues,[411] which had led to the 1991 Ciba Symposium.

This interest has evolved into a worldwide movement exploring the developmental origins of health and disease (DOHaD). Given the extreme vulnerability of the foetus, it is not surprising that the research focus until recently has been more on foetal development than

---

409  Dörner G, Grychtolik H. Long-lasting ill-effects of neonatal qualitative and/or quantitative dysnutrition in the human. *Endokrinologie* 1978, 71(1):81–88.; *Issue dedicated to Professor Günter Dörner on the occasion of his 60th birthday.* (PMID:2689188) *Exp Clin Endocrinol* 1989; 94(1–2):1–225.

410  Dorner claimed that animal studies showed clear gender effects of qualitative dysnutrition; that manipulating animal diet could create homosexuality. He was condemned for trying to manipulate nutrition to prevent homosexuality. Where his framing of homosexuality as a disorder legitimised appalling treatment of homosexual people, those objections absolutely stand. But while his writing about his findings reflected the prevailing homophobia, the questions he raised about the biological mechanisms that contribute to the development of gender identity and sexuality are important ones which are still to be adequately explored. Understanding how biology contributes to and interacts with gender identity is valuable to everyone. Now that we know more about the reproductive impacts of oestrogen analogues and other developmental agents and toxins, his ideas seem much less implausible. Sigusch V, Schorsch E, Dannecker M, Schmidt G. Official statement by the German Society for Sex Research (Deutsche Gesellschaft für Sexualforschung e.V.) on the research of Prof. Dr. Günter Dörner on the subject of homosexuality. (PMID:7181651) *Arch Sex Behav* 1982, 11(5):445–49. For instance, one group found evidence that there are effects on gender-role play in 42-month-old children. See Adgent MA, Daniels JL, Edwards LJ, Siega-Riz AM et al. Early-life Soy exposure and gender role play behavior in Children. *Environ Health Perspect.* 2011; 119(12):1811–16.

411  Barker proposed and chaired the important 1990 Ciba Symposium 156, published as *The Childhood Environment and Adult Disease* (Wiley 1991). See also Barker DJ, Osmond C. Infant mortality, childhood nutrition, and ischaemic heart disease in England and Wales. *Lancet.* 1986;1(8489):1077–1081; Barker DJ, Winter PD, Osmond C, Margetts B et al. Weight in infancy and death from ischaemic heart disease. *Lancet.* 1989;2(8663):577–580; Barker DJ, Gluckman PD, Godfrey KM et al. Fetal nutrition and cardiovascular disease in adult life. *Lancet* 1993; 341(8850): 938–941.

postnatal nutrition and development. However, it is possible that the postnatal period is at least as important.[412] It may even be more so, because postnatal intervention has fewer risks than prenatal, and is more possible. I suspect that optimal postpartum infant nutrition can even repair some intra-uterine damage or defect. Why? Because I have seen some astonishing improvements in damaged children lucky enough to have been exclusively fed breastmilk (usually despite negativity about the value of doing so). And some clever research on red and white mice has now shown that milk stem cells reach the young and make normal tissues in many locations.[413] Only the milk could have provided the cells, as the young were cross fostered, as in the wallaby experiments that showed such dramatic effects of milk in controlling infant development. Less than optimal in utero development may be remedied by such mechanisms, helping to explain better outcomes in children born with congenital disorders such as Down's syndrome, or phenylketonuria, for example.

One fascinating piece of practical human research decades ago illustrated one way that early infant feeding alters immune responses for life. Where organ transplantation was concerned, a number of studies showed that 'Breast-fed patients showed dramatic improvements in graft function rates compared to non-breast-fed counterparts at all intervals studied (P less than or equal to 0.001)'.[414] Transplant specialists have shown that if, as an adult, you need an organ transplant, your best chance of success is to have an organ donated by someone related to your mother, but only if your mother breastfed you. If she didn't, maternal kinship adds no greater chance of success.[415]

So we are more like Mum immunologically if we were breastfed. This is because there is greater transfer of maternal cells or antigens during breastfeeding than anyone has realised until recently, so that a child not breastfed is indeed less like Mother, and more likely to react badly to transplanted antigens.

A recent abstract stated:

> Recent experimental and clinical studies suggest that exposure of the fetus to non-inherited maternal antigens (NIMAs) during pregnancy has an impact on allogeneic transplantations performed later in life. We have reported that NIMA exposure by breastfeeding further potentiates the tolerogenic NIMA effect mediated by in utero NIMA exposure during pregnancy in mice of allogeneic hematopoietic stem cell transplantation (HSCT). Breastfeeding generates Foxp3(+) regulatory T cells that suppress anti-maternal immunity and persist until adulthood. These results reveal a previously unknown impact of breastfeeding on the outcome of allogeneic HSCT [hematopoietic stem cell transplantation, the transplantation of bone marrow or other blood-forming cells].[416]

---

412  Cf. Geddes D, op. cit.

413  Wilson C. Breast milk stem cells build baby. *New Scientist*, 2014; 2994: Online at http://www.newscientist.com/article/dn26492-breast-milk-stem-cells-may-be-incorporated-into-baby.html

414  Kois WE, Campbell DA Jr, Lorber MI, Sweeton JC, Dafoe DC Influence of breast feeding on subsequent reactivity to a related renal allograft. (PMID:6379295) *J Surg Res* 1984, 37(2):89–93. DOI: 10.1016/0022-4804(84)90166–5

415  ibid.

416  Aoyama K, Matsuoka KI, Teshima T. Breast milk and transplantation tolerance.(PMID:21327152) Free resource *Chimerism* 2010, 1(1):19–20.

The point is that breastfeeding may suppress anti-maternal immune reactions. Our children tolerate our donated cells better if they were breastfed. Does that affect transfusions as well as transplants?

But again, to talk of the outcome as better with breastfeeding subtly implies that the norm is what happens with artificial feeding. Is the difference in outcomes due to breastfeeding, or to its alternative? It might also be that there is an unrecognised uptake of bovine cellular materials, which make the formula-fed child biologically less like its human mother, and more likely to reject her cells: I have seen no studies investigating this possibility. Milk is powerful whether it comes from a cow or a woman, and bovine milk evolved to build calves, not humans. If we consider it normal for humans to have this greater tolerance of maternal cells, and breastfeeding to be the means to achieve it, then we are looking again at negative effects of bovine milk. Remarkable as the idea may seem, the question needs to be asked and answered.

Some babies are known to be at greater risk of harm than others because of the ticket they drew in the genetic lottery of life. Their genome may mean that they are more likely to be harmed by unnatural feeding or other adverse environmental factors. Earlier I referred to this in African-Americans. Another study reports that a genetic variant in fatty acid metabolism influences the degree to which not being breastfed reduced childhood IQ.[417] As usual, the study definitions of 'breastfed' were poor and retrospectively reported, relying on maternal report in a written questionnaire when children were two or three years old, and one group was drawn from a birth register sample of twins. (Modern multiples,[418] like preterm infants, are more likely to have been exposed to infant formula in hospital or soon after.) However, the study results suggest a clear interaction between the presence of a particular gene and the effect of artificial feeding on cognitive development.

Children can carry gene variants that affect their sensitivity to their environment, predisposing some to damage. Genes that make a child vulnerable to damage in one environment or when exposed to particular stresses may also allow them to excel if nurtured differently. It is to be hoped that this is not used by the formula industry to suggest that the harms of artificial feeding derive from the child's parents, not their product! After all, only one of those two contributors – parental genes or infant formula – is unnecessary.

In fact, the results simply confirm that breastfeeding is more important to some children than to others in preventing some conditions, in ways we have not yet uncovered and

---

417 Caspi A, Williams B, Kim-Cohen J, Craig IW et al. Moderation of breastfeeding effects on the IQ by genetic variation in fatty acid metabolism. (PMID:17984066) *Proceedings of the National Academy of Sciences* USA 2007, 104(47):18860–65 Note that again, even in a study which takes it for granted that breastfeeding is overall relatively beneficial compared to formula. The assumption is that breastfeeding 'affects' the IQ, rather than being the default which enables the natural development of the child's brain.

418 Early in the twentieth century, strenuous efforts were made to ensure that at least initially, multiples and prems were breastmilk-fed, as survival was at risk in the pre-antibiotic, low-tech era . See authors such as Mary Crosse and Julius Hess in the Bibliography. A recent cluster of severe gastrointestinal problems affecting fifteen children in a Melbourne Australia NICU says the dangers are still real. Damage can be done by infectious agents, by alien proteins, or by the products of digestion of formula fats and proteins: it does not require the presence of a specific pathogen for infant formula to damage babies' sensitive guts.

probably never will. It is a safe bet that there will be many more discoveries in this field now we have some tools to research it. No doubt there are many more such gene–environment interactions, potentiating greater or lesser susceptibility to harm from the lack of breastfeeding or the realities of formula feeding. Family histories could probably indicate how that susceptibility would show up in life, as vulnerabilities can 'run in the family'.

It has long been known that gender can affect susceptibility to certain disorders, and traditional practices of longer breastfeeding for boys[419] may reflect community awareness of the male sex's greater vulnerability.[420] Sadly, boys are now more likely to be weaned earlier than girls in some Western communities where breastfeeding is linked with overt sexuality.[421] Yet the process of making breastmilk almost certainly recognises differences in infant gender: studies in both cows and monkeys have shown differences in quantity and composition of milk for male and female young, reflecting (and possibly contributing to) normal sex-related differences in growth patterns. As the research biologist reporting this at a meeting of the American Academy of Sciences said, 'We think it's important – and it's not – to make different deodorants for men and women, and yet we kind of approach formula as though boys and girls have the same developmental priorities.'[422] And they don't. Will we see pink and blue infant formula anytime soon, I wonder? How much of the discordant development of artificially fed infants may be due to sex-related unsuitability of the cows' milk mixes? Another question not yet asked by regulatory agencies allowing formula to be sold without independent investigation of outcomes.

So far I have discussed the immune impact of early formula feeds as if symptoms of these effects will always manifest in infancy. Not so. If a child is sensitised and then breastfed, there may be no sign of immune distortion for decades. It may take a different and unrelated trigger to precipitate symptoms. As Murch said, 'It is quite a common pattern that an adult may manifest sensitisation for the first time later on.'[423]

A viral infection – or perhaps a vaccination – may unmask the sensitivity created by early exposure in a child with a particular genetic predisposition. And in later life autoimmune disease may develop: in Murch's study sample, 25 per cent of the mothers of allergic children have developed autoimmunity,[424] compared with only 10 per cent in the (obviously older) grandparents. Common autoimmune problems usually emerge later in life, so that one would expect the grandparents to have higher rates than their daughters. However, the younger women's problems may also be a sign of the increasing prevalence and severity of immune disorder once it has penetrated populations.

---

419  Nath DC, Goswami G. Determinants of breast-feeding patterns in an urban society of India. (PMID:9198314) *Human Biology* 1997; 69(4):557–73.

420  Hill CM, Ball HL. Parental manipulation of postnatal survival and wellbeing: are parental sex preferences adaptive? In Pollard TM, Hyatt SB. *Sex, Gender and Health*. (Cambridge University Press 1999).

421  Scott JA, Aitkin I, Binns CW, Aroni RA. Factors associated with the duration of breastfeeding amongst women in Perth, Australia.(PMID:10342541) *Acta Paediatrica* 1999; 88(4):416–21. DOI: 10.1080/08035259950169800

422  Neergaard L. Animal mothers' milk differs by infant sex. *Seattle Times*, 14 Feb 2014. http://seattletimes.com/html/nationworld/2022917697_apxmedmothersmilk.html

423  Murch S. Oral tolerance and gut maturation. In Isolauri E, Walker WA, op. cit, p. 147.

424  ibid., p. 149.

So the harms done to us – or indeed to our parents – by poor infant feeding practices in the past may account for much of our own immune problems, and those of our children. And the harms we do now to our children by not fully breastfeeding them may compound that inherited harm, and be reflected in the generations to come. Diabetologists and cardiovascular physicians take note: an experienced British paediatrician who had worked in Indonesia for decades told me in the 1980s that he had seen only one case of childhood diabetes in all that time: an artificially fed child of an expatriate family. On his return to the UK he was shocked by the rate of juvenile diabetes he met.

As we struggle to understand why our miserable unwell children have such problems, we need to consider our family history. Parents with distressed breastfed babies were once dogmatically told that nothing they ate would affect their baby, and nothing they did could affect their genes. We now know that neither claim is true. Gene function depends on gene expression, and both what we ourselves eat, and what we give our babies to eat, influences gene expression. Women's milk is the only food for which newborns are evolutionarily adapted.

What milk does for infants and their immune system is incredibly complicated. It isn't just a matter of the right microbes and resistance to disease; it's also a matter of how the immune system is structured and functions. Consider this review, available online, which

> presents milk as a materno-neonatal relay system functioning by transfer of preferential amino acids, which increase plasma levels of glucose-dependent insulinotropic polypeptide (GIP), glucagon-like peptide-1 (GLP-1), insulin, growth hormone (GH) and insulin-like growth factor-1 (IGF-1) for mTORC1 activation. Importantly, milk exosomes, which regularly contain microRNA-21, most likely represent a genetic transfection system enhancing mTORC1-driven metabolic processes.[425]

In short, milk is a 'genetic transfection system'; in relatively plain English a functionally active nutrient system promoting neonatal growth of mammals. As Melnik says elsewhere,

> Milk is not 'just food' but represents a most sophisticated signalling system of mammalian evolution promoting a regulatory network for species-specific controlled m-TORC1 driven postnatal growth and metabolic programming. Milk signalling is mediated by milk-derived BCAAs, which stimulate the secretion of insulin and IGF-1. Exaggerated m-TORC-1 signalling induced by formula feeding appears to represent the underlying mechanism explaining exaggerated postnatal growth, aberrant adipogenic, hypothalamic and allergenic programming, laying the foundation for the development of the chronic diseases of civilisation, i.e., obesity, type 2 diabetes, dyslipoproteinaemia, arterial hypertension, allergic and autoimmune diseases.[426]

Milk influences much more than weight gain, that sole criterion used to assess infant formula adequacy for too long. Cows' milk makes normal calves, human milk normal humans.

---

425 Melnik BC, John SM, Schmitz G. Milk is not just food but most likely a genetic transfection system activating mTORC1 signaling for postnatal growth. *Nutr J* 2013;12:103. (PMID:23883112) Free full text article.

426 Melnik BC. *Formula feeding promotes adipogenic, diabetogenic, hypertonic and allergic mTORC-1 programming.* In Preedy V, Watson RR, Zibardi S (eds), op. cit. (Wageningen Academic Publishers 2014) p. 545.

# Early diet and intergenerational effects

Until at least the 1970s, Cow & Gate, manufacturers of formula and infant foods, used the slogan, 'What you feed them now matters forever', a perhaps unwitting acknowledgement of the intergenerational impacts of infant nutrition. That is a true statement, even if also a piece of advertising puffery. Why say it? The eugenics movement was big at the time of formula development, making heredity in health a key issue of public policy, and advertisers have always researched and tapped into community beliefs. And the community has always believed that what babies eat affects their character as well as their body.

Everything in the body is inter-related, just as everything in the environment is. There is a discipline called psycho-neuro-immuno-endocrinology, because minds, nervous systems, brains, immune systems and hormones all interact. Just as the ankle bone's connected to the shin bone, so how our brain functions will affect how our immune system works, and our gut affects our brain, and so on and vice versa. If by four months we are seeing differences in bodily development in one area, it seems reasonable to think that there will be deviations in others, and consequences from those deviations. The fact that breastmilk contains hormones and nerve growth factors and multiple active immune cells all adds up to differences in development of every infant bodily organ, as well as the immune system. A more efficient or less-stressed kidney or liver may more rapidly clear toxins, for example. A more acid stomach acts as a better barrier to food microorganisms reaching the gut.[427] Normal gut transit times remove allergens and pathogens from the bowel faster than in the artificially fed child, in whom their slower passage allows more time for multiplication, colonisation and harm.

Much more research is needed into the way artificial feeding alters normal immunological, genetic and other outcomes. The immune disorder epidemic must have its roots in such deviations of development. Many people in every generation inherit genes that code for allergic and autoimmune disease. Not all those with the genes develop the disease. Even in the same family, one child will develop 'allergy' and another won't. Many factors can be at work, such as: interbirth intervals and related maternal depletion; other stressors leading to high cortisol levels; innate immune differences and chemical exposures. By affecting how genes are expressed, these factors can trigger damaging disease.

The Report from the UK Department of Health's Scientific Advisory Committee on Nutrition (SACN) notes:

> Molecular mechanisms can explain how fetal nutrient supply alters phenotype at the cellular and tissue level (section 5.2). For example, animal studies show that imbalanced supply of those nutrients involved in the methylation cycle may induce changes in observable characteristics through epigenetic regulation. The role of epigenetics in human disease is becoming more widely appreciated. Altered methylation of DNA has been

---

427 Usowicz AG, Dab SB, Emery JR, McCann EM et al. Does gastric acid protect the preterm infant from bacteria in unheated human milk? (PMID:3345705) *Early Hum Dev* 1988, 16(1):27–33.

associated with some cancers and atherosclerosis. Epigenetic effects can also account for inter-generational effects observed in animal models.[428]

Epigenetics[429] is the study of how environmental factors influence the expression of inherited genes without altering DNA, and how gene expression affects health and development. Epigenetics hunts for the precise mechanisms that explain which genes are expressed and which suppressed, and which are transmitted to offspring.[430] Subtle mechanisms (including DNA methylation, histone modifications, RNA silencing, and so on) can explain the intractable differences from what might have been. Some, possibly many, genes will be expressed differently because of qualitatively different nutrition immediately after birth.

And even if genes aren't altered, simply the way they are expressed, the effects of such damage can continue through generations. For example, a recent mouse study of folic acid deficiency showed that two subsequent generations were affected, not because the deficiency changed the actual genes they inherited – it couldn't – but because epigenetic modifiers to those genes were inherited along with the genes themselves,[431] until recently thought impossible. In another study recently reported, maternal food deprivation in the period before birth resulted in more diabetes in two generations, *both offspring and their offspring,* fed normally after birth.[432] Transgenerational epigenetic changes exist, and infant formula effects on genes are prime candidates for such transgenerational impacts. These too could be cumulative, each generation adding further issues to those inherited. The concept of intergenerational amplification (or amelioration) of immune problems, or progressive degeneration (or rehabilitation) of immune systems, seems to me to be a priority for research.

What was once a debate about whether nature or nurture is most responsible for developmental differences has been recast. It is now clear that nurture (before and after birth) affects what nature (genes) bestows, activating some genes while suppressing others, and modifying the genome transmitted to the next generation. Therefore, early nutrition and maternal care has not only lifelong, but intergenerational effects. Nature and nurture are linked scientifically, and interact. We inherit a unique genome, and our unique environment, from conception onwards, will help to sculpt that genome, adapting the child to the environment, and making it more like its family as well. This is a basic tenet of the rapidly expanding field of evolutionary medicine, which makes use of the principles of evolution to understand disease and develop treatments.[433]

---

428  *The influence of maternal, fetal and child nutrition on the development of chronic disease in later life.* Downloadable at http://www.sacn.gov.uk/reports_position_statements/index.html

429  As always, *New Scientist* provides a readable summary for the novice: see Bird A. Epigenetics. *New Scientist* 5 January 2013 pp. i–viii.

430  Texts are emerging: Gilber SF, Epel D. *Ecological Developmental Biology: integrating epigenetics, medicine and evolution* (Sinauer Associates 2009), is one useful overview.

431  Geddes L. Lack of folic acid in pregnancy hits generations. *New Scientist* 5 October 2013 p. 14

432  Saini A. Epigenetics: genes, environment and the generation game. *The Observer,* 7 Sept 2014. Comments provide interesting further reading re possible mechanisms.

433  Trevathan W, McKenna J, Smith EO. (eds) *Evolutionary Medicine.* (OUP 1999); Trevathan W. *Ancient Bodies, Modern Lives,.* (OUP 2010); *Evolutionary Medicine and Health* (OUP 2009).

Every child's environment is different: birth order and intra-uterine influences are never the same for any two children in the same family, even for identical twins. What is more, it seems that the transfer of cells (both ways) between mother and baby in utero may be more extensive than previously imagined.[434] And so may the transfer of cells, including pluripotent stem cells, through breastfeeding (see page 174). We don't need aborted foetuses or invasive procedures to have a rich source of stem cells for stem-cell therapy; breastmilk provides them for every baby. Those stem cells in breastmilk, only recently discovered,[435] may also have some repair capacity, as well as helping the infant adapt to the post-birth environment. Breastfeeding may well come to be recognised as universally available stem-cell therapy for infants: no one can provide that so cheaply! And the neurotransmitters, growth factors, immune cells, hormones, enzymes, and all the thousands of other astonishingly complex bioactive factors in human milk[436] may be far more relevant to the origins of adult behaviour and disease than has ever been suspected, preventing immune distortion or even repairing damaged chromosomes.

At a clinical level, it can be simple to correlate allergic severity with feeding history: in fact the client often does it for you. 'My mum breastfed my sister and she's healthy as can be, but she couldn't feed me for more than a week and I've had coeliac disease since I was little ...'[437] 'I was born in America and Mum took the bottles they gave her and fed me, but my brother was born here in Australia and she insisted on breastfeeding, and he has no problems ...' Or the reverse: 'There's always been allergy in our family, and Mum breastfed me to try to prevent it, but it hasn't worked.' Such comments are important, although inconclusive, clues.

Most research studies don't give all the details of feeding, and average together very different experiences, as do meta-analyses and reviews. In the real world it can sometimes take hours of conversation for some relevant factor to emerge, triggered by some remark. Ongoing studies may be failing to ask some key questions about intergenerational issues and neonatal exposures in specific nations or cultures.

A classic example of this is the recent sibling study[438] widely reported as showing that the benefits of breastfeeding were 'overstated'. This will be discussed in more detail later. (See page 163) The authors say, 'When we get more advantaged moms selecting

---

434  A really interesting review of what is called microchimerism can be found online: see Gammill HS, Nelson JL *Naturally acquired microchimerism.* (PMID:19924635) *Internat J Dev Biol* 2010; 54(2–3):531–43 and other articles by these authors.

435  Indumathi S, Dhanasekaran M, Rajkumar JS, Sudarsanam D Exploring the stem cell and non-stem cell constituents of human breast milk. (PMID:22940915) *Cytotechnology* 2012.; Hassiotou, F, Beltran, A, Chetwynd, E. Stuebe, AM et al. (2012), Breastmilk Is a Novel Source of Stem Cells with Multilineage Differentiation Potential. *Stem Cells*, 30: 2164–2174. DOI: 10.1002/stem.1188; Twigger AJ, Hodgetts S, Filgueira L, Hartmann PE et al. From breast milk to brains: the potential of stem cells in human milk. (PMID:23515086) *J Hum Lact* 2013; 29(2):136–39.

436  Hamosh M, op. cit. for an excellent online summary, now out of date as so much new research has happened, but giving a good clear overview in plain language.

437  Yes, associated with artificial feeding; see Palma GD, Capilla A, Nova E, Castillejo G et al. Influence of milk-feeding type and genetic risk of developing coeliac disease on intestinal microbiota of infants: the PROFICEL study. (PMID:22319588) Free full text article *PLoS One* 2012; 7(2):e30791DOI: 10.1371/journal.pone.0030791

438  Colen et al, op. cit.

into breast-feeding and we know those traits also will affect the health outcomes, it's not clear what's affecting an outcome like obesity – is it breast-feeding itself or those other background characteristics?' A valid question, which makes it all the more remarkable that the study authors would make any conclusions about breastfeeding or bottle-feeding from retrospectively self-reported feeding methods in a mixture of two very different generations:

- children born between 1957 and 1965 (when poor women breastfed) plus
- children (born in the period 1985–96) of the girls in the earlier cohort. (By 1985 poor US women were getting free formula from WIC, and it was advantaged women who breastfed.)

So the breastfeeding mothers could have been a curious mix of both poor and advantaged women! We need to know a lot more about those involved in this study.

But science is finally providing some answers as to whether it is the demographics or the breastmilk. **Absolutely it is both,** but bodies are **constructed** from food, not maternal diplomas. **And it is also a *third* factor**: not only the presence or absence of breastfeeding, but also the presence of particular infant formulas. They not only lack things in breastmilk, they provide things NOT in breastmilk. And that has effects, as the history in Book 2 will make clear.

# Research into the effects of formula

New scientific technologies make it possible to identify and explain some genetic differences and their contribution to disease. Yet comparative studies of the effects of artificial feeding on gene expression or chromosomal damage have not seemed an urgent priority, even after the realisation that the microbiome affects gene expression in heritable ways.

Strangely, this is despite the fact that preliminary studies a decade ago revealed more chromosomal and DNA damage in artificially fed infants.[439]

Specifically, there needs to be independent research into whether, as might be expected on first principles, all infant formulas damage DNA, or only some; and how each infant formula affects gene expression in children. Proof of low levels of DNA damage might even become a requirement for approval of the product by national authorities. It is quite possible that there could be significant differences between brands, as there are significant differences in the ingredients, the formulations, and the complex processing of each formula product.

---

439 Dündaröz R, Aydin H, Ulucan H, Baltaci V et al. Rates of chromosomal damage are significantly higher in children as young as 9–12 months. Preliminary study on DNA damage in non breast-fed infants. *Pediatrics International* (2002) 44, 127–130.; Shoji H, Shimizu T, Shinohara K, Oguchi S, et al. Suppressive effects of breast milk on oxidative DNA damage in very low birthweight infants. (2004). *Arch Dis Child Fetal and Neonatal Edition* 89:F13

And standardising the processing does not standardise the effects on humans,[440] each being so individual.

These differences may well become more marked as different varieties of patented bacteria ('probiotics') are added to formulas, mostly without specific labelling of the species, so parents can never know what bacteria their child ate. If significant differences between formulas are discovered, parents should have access to the results, so they know which formulas do most damage to infant DNA and gene expression. This would certainly result in the worst products being de-marketed, and less harmful products gaining market share.

Understandably perhaps, despite the huge biological plausibility of the idea, many people who have used the product will refuse to believe that any infant formula could be harmful until the precise mechanisms and pathways are proven beyond doubt. Again, proof of innocence is assumed for formula, despite the vast accumulation of animal and human evidence of its distortion of normal development, and industry's own attempts to improve it. But who will fund long-term studies to determine what genetic damage is done by any particular infant formula, or by all of them? None of the major long term studies currently available and being used to create meta-analyses and reviews has seen the importance of either exclusive breastfeeding in current and maternal generations or of the substantial differences between formulas within and between those generations. Yet maternal obesity and maternal intelligence will obviously have an impact on child development. Follow-up studies could outline what that damage does in the next generation who inherit that altered genetic material and are gestated in those altered bodies. Could the bottle-fed fare better? 'Pigs might fly,' said one expert reader. It is more rational to assume that alterations to normal infant development are not benefits. Thus, while starting independent research that will take decades, we should be working to make breastfeeding possible and breastmilk available now, even if being fed breastmilk by bottle is not the same as being breastfed.[441]

## Testing and labelling formula

When testing the safety of new additives to infant formula, researchers set up trials that compare certain outcomes in babies fed standard formula with babies fed the formula with the new additive. As we have seen, they may, and often do, include babies breastfed for days or even weeks before they are randomly assigned to using a test formula or the standard brand, as their supplement to or total replacement for breastmilk. Mothers who actively choose to formula feed from birth are becoming a minority in some locations, which makes true comparisons of formulas difficult. Their babies' outcomes are usually averaged with outcomes from babies initially breastfed and then moved on to formula by the mother: as noted earlier and in other trials, there can be reluctance to disclose the results of the fully and only artificially fed. When families are pressed for money, the availability of an ongoing

440 Meulenbroek LA, Oliveira S, den Hartog Jager CF et al. The degree of whey hydrolysis does not uniformly affect in vitro basophil and T cell responses of cow's milk allergic patients.(PMID:24330309) *Clin Exp Allergy* 2013. DOI: 10.1111/cea.12254

441 Krogh C, Biggar RJ, Fischer TK, Lindholm M et al. Bottle-feeding and the Risk of Pyloric Stenosis. (PMID:22945411) *Pediatrics* 2012; 130(4):e943–9; Noel-Weiss j, Boersma S, Kujawa-Myles S. Questioning current definitions for breastfeeding research. *Internat Breastfeed Jl* 2012, 7:9 DOI:10.1186/1746-4358-7–9

supply of free formula might be a powerful inducement to join a trial – if a mother doubts her ability to feed her baby, as many do, and trusts infant formula. Logically, this mixing of groups has the potential to influence the prevalence and severity rates of problems in both groups in the short time of the study. Any breastmilk given to the bottle-fed is likely to reduce the apparent harms of formula, while any formula given to the breastfed is likely to increase problems for them. Symptoms created by formula in both groups can then be seen as 'normal' in countries where bottle feeding has been endemic for generations, especially when babies are gestated in maternal bodies affected by it.

It seems obvious to me that if we want to be able to assure parents (as formula labels do) that any one formula is 'suitable to use from birth', we should have access to reliable data about the outcomes in those children who have used that particular formula from birth: their growth while reliant on that formula alone, their later health and cognitive development, or at the very least, the development of their brains.[442] Instead, we label formula as 'suitable' on the basis of studies done where children may have been fed breastmilk for days or even weeks before starting on some past formula. And we allow images of any healthy babies, perhaps breastfed, to be used to advertise infant formula, rather than requiring companies to depict on their websites and in advertising only infants fed their particular formula for at least four months. The European Parliament has just banned 'pictures of infants, or other pictures or text which may idealise the use of such formula' (although graphic representations intended for easy identification of the formula re permitted, as are illustrations of advised preparation.) Will the rest of the world follow? Will the companies voluntarily change labels world-wide?[443] Again, watch out for flying pigs.

If such individual testing of each formula from birth cannot be done for practical or ethical reasons, then perhaps the warnings once used on US puppy formulas should be on infant formula labels. In 1981, Borden's Esbilac labels urged dog owners not to wean pups prematurely: 'Feeding newborn mammals a milk formula always entails some risk ... From birth through the second week all puppies should receive their mother's milk ...'[444] The human equivalent of two weeks for dogs is three to four months for babies: pups start to initiate semi-solid feeding at twenty-one days, although dog milk alone supports growth until at least twenty-eight days.[445] Since puppy formulas fed too early could kill or sicken more pups, sales will be greater when pups get mothers' milk initially, develop a healthy gut and then go on to replacement feeds. It is rare for pedigree dogs or cats to be taken from their mothers under four weeks of age, as breeders know that formulas can be responsible for digestive troubles. We are less careful of the human young. It does seem odd that major US companies have been more careful about feeding dogs than babies! And it seems even

442  Deoni S, DC, Piryatinksy I, O'Muircheartaigh J, et al. Breastfeeding and early white matter development: A cross-sectional study. *NeuroImage*, 2013; DOI: 10.1016/j.neuroimage.2013.05.090

443  Scattergood G. Infant pictures ban on baby formulas backed by MEPs. Food Manufacture.co.uk June 11, 2013 http://foodmanufacture.co.uk/content/view/print 782594.

444  Domestic use of infant formula: Hearing before the Subcommittee on Oversight and Investigations of the Committee on Energy and Commerce, House of Representatives, Ninety-seventh Congress, first session, June 17, 1981. p. 24. Can be accessed from http://nla.gov.au/nla.cat-vn3853323

445  Oftedal O. Lactation in the dog: milk composition and intake by puppies. *J Nutr* 1984, 114(5):803–12. See http://jn.nutrition.org/content/114/5/803.full.pdf

odder that there is such resistance to warning parents about food for babies, as has been proposed in Australia in 2013.[446]

Obviously I see newborn artificial feeding as an important factor in the emergence of widespread allergy and intolerances in the twentieth century. But why was this not immediately obvious as a consequence of infant feeding before 1930? Because those babies were gestated by healthy females themselves breastfed as babies and not overdosed with cows milk? Does this explain some inter-country differences today, such as the different results obtained between the Americanised Philippines and China? Why did it take some generations for formula-using developed nations to experience not just isolated cases, but epidemics of anaphylaxis, autoimmune disease, and sudden unexpected infant deaths? In my view, because harms accumulate through generations. Some foods that are now common allergens had been eaten for centuries without causing epidemics of allergic disease (but they were not being fed to infants as trace amounts in formulas). Indeed, many have been staple foods for whole populations, and some still are. For example, while developed nations struggle with a serious peanut allergy problem, groundnuts – another term for peanuts – are an essential protein source in countries where this allergy is currently virtually unknown. Allergic reactions are on record past and present, but not on the same scale until the second half of the twentieth century.[447] Immune disorders now afflict between 23 and 50 million Americans, depending on how the statistics are collated.[448]

A greater prevalence of distress and disease among artificially fed infants is not always obvious to parents. Many people can tell of a 'breastfed' baby with visible allergy problems. Assertive bottle feeders often claim that their children have no such problems. Whether breastfeeding (variously defined) is protective against infant allergy or not is now questioned. However, most studies that carefully chart feeding histories accurately and prospectively show that babies completely and exclusively breastfed from birth have much lower rates of 'allergy', as those Finnish and Australian studies testify (see page 106 and page 96). These are often swamped in meta-analyses by larger industry-supported studies with poorer definitions.

But as previously shown, children who truly have been exclusively breastfed are very rare. They are often children fortunate enough to have determined and educated mothers who get the support they need to persevere through difficulties. Even rarer are exclusively breastfed children who were gestated by completely breastfed mothers, and so on back through at least three generations. Yet these are the children who in theory should form the control population for any study of the harms or otherwise of infant formula through the generations. Does any data – reliable data, that includes comp feeds given without parents' knowledge or consent – exist to identify such children?

---

446  A FSANZ proposal to include such warnings is unlikely to succeed under the Abbott industry-friendly government. http://www.examiner.com.au/story/1776896/bid-to-get-formula-warnings/

447  And these epidemics are recent. As a young woman in the 1960s I remember laughing about how American friends all seemed to have an allergist as well as a psychologist, while I knew very few people who saw either variety of health professional. As a new mother in the 1970s, I heard child health nurses saying the same thing.

448  Schmidt CW. Questions persist: environmental factors in auto-immune disease. *Envir Health Perspect* 2011; 119: a248–53. DOI: 1289/ehp.119-a248

As noted earlier, in many existing studies there is a lamentable muddying of feeding categories, so that, for example, infants are classified as 'breastfed' when they drink one bottle or less of formula per day, and 'formula-fed' when they drink more than that regardless of earlier breastfeeding. These methodologically flawed studies can be expected to show few differences between such groups at twelve months of age.[449] I have to say, I find it hard to think of a comparably contained area of research in which such sloppy and inconsistent definitions of a major variable (infant feeding method) are so commonly used when the stakes are so drastic an intervention as total dietary substitution. Until rigorous and well-designed studies are done, there will be little 'scientific evidence', and some people assume that means there is proof of safety and equivalence. Never believe the results of studies until you have checked the definitions!

We've seen all this with tobacco and smoking. It took fifty years to get smoke-free air in many places; in some countries it hasn't happened yet as industry power is greater than the will, or the ability, of politicians to protect public health. Yet common sense, basic science, and human experience have indicated since the sixteenth century that smoking was likely to be bad for humans and should be proved safe before being promoted or being put on unrestricted sale ... Whose was the burden of proof? Those who objected to such a profitable enterprise had to prove it unsafe. The tobacco industry spent hundreds of millions on obfuscating the facts and producing poor science, publishing ill-defined studies that attempted to pin the blame on everything except the real culprit, and employing amoral (immoral?) scientists to manipulate and even outright falsify the evidence to undermine the proof of tobacco's harms.[450]

They did this because it was 'fiscally responsible', a way to discharge the company's overly narrow responsibility to maximise shareholder returns. Telling the truth and co-operating with what was clearly in the public interest both medically and financially could perhaps not be permitted if it might reduce shareholders' profits. Never mind that that same public of course included those same shareholders, many of whom might have lost more in medical bills – and more importantly, years of life – than they gained from the companies' profits! The same skewed legal obligations and pressures (and massive personal financial incentives) exist for those in charge of the large corporations that produce formula.

Some of the harm done by artificial feeding is likely to be due to both the damaging effects on infant genomes and microbiomes of not being breastfed, and also of being formula-fed. What was missing and what replaced it quite likely both have and have had separate negative effects. We are not talking solely about loss of benefits, but also of presenting harms, when comparing the outcomes of infant diets.

Thus recording the precise details of, and controlling for, variants of both breastfeeding and artificial feeding should be routine in all studies looking at child health and development. As a relatively benign example, where a particular immigrant group has found a particular

---

449  Auerbach KG, Renfrew MJ, Minchin MK. Infant Feeding Comparisons: a hazard to infant health? *J Hum Lact* 1991; 7:63. DOI: 10.1177/089033449100700226.

450  Michaels D. *Doubt is their Product: How Industry's Assault on Science Threatens Your Health.* (OUP 2008).

formula to produce more rapid growth than others, the brand may become associated with that ethnicity (and indirectly with other infant nutrition or child-rearing practices of that community), as one product did in an Australian Vietnamese community at one time.[451] This can confuse researchers who do not understand the mechanisms driving brand choice, or who fail to establish all confounding variables. It was not being Vietnamese, or being a migrant, or being socially disadvantaged, that made for overfed babies, it was using that brand, which the community reasonably saw as better because it made bigger babies.

More importantly, taking care in the design of research makes it easier to pinpoint other problems that result in damage to children. Consider, for example, the powder structure that made one 1980s formula more likely to settle and compact in the tin, and thus be over-concentrated by parents who were unwittingly serving a greater density of powder when measuring out the correct volume.[452] This had to result in more rapid growth, along with greater stress to cardiovascular systems, kidneys and brains. This cannot easily be identified as a problem unless all details of each formula given to each child are recorded in studies, and any better or worse outcomes associated with a given brand noted.

Or consider the still-excessively high levels of aluminium, ten to forty times higher than in breastmilk, which can still cause neurodevelopmental problems. In 2010 a study warned:

> Every effort should be made by manufacturers to reduce the aluminium content to an achievable practical minimum while at the same time manufacturers should be compelled to indicate the level of contamination by aluminium on the packaged product ... There is evidence of both immediate and delayed toxicity in infants, and especially preterm infants.[453]

Problems like compacting powder or aluminium contamination, a serious concern,[454] are widely talked about only after they have been identified and a remedy found: too late to prevent damage to some children. In other words, they get attention only when they can be used as the basis of marketing strategies by industry people: our brand has less sugar, contains more or less x or y or z or some brand-new ingredient essential to your child ... now. Of course, that means our brand didn't have whatever desirable feature is now being touted before, but nobody draws attention to unpalatable facts. (There is much more about such problems, including both intentional and unintentional additives, in Chapter 3.)

There has to date been little awareness of the role of nutrient-induced genetic damage in disease or 'allergy' reviews. This is because it has been usual since the second half of the twentieth century to dismiss any advantage of breastfed babies as being due to socioeconomic status, maternal education or both. Over-controlling for the wrong social

---

451  Dr Martha Morrow (personal communication).

452  It's worth noting that this wasn't parental incompetence: highly trained scientists have experienced difficulty in mixing formula to correct concentrations according to the preparation instructions.

453  Burrell SA, Exley C. There is (still) too much aluminium in infant formulas. (PMID:20807425) Free resource *BMC Pediatr* 2010, 10:63.

454  Krewski D, Yokel RA, Nieboer E, Borchelt D et al. Human health risk assessment for aluminium, aluminium oxide, and aluminium hydroxide. *J Toxicol Environ Health B Crit Rev* 2007; 10 Suppl 1:1–269. (PMCID:PMC2782734) Free full text article.

confounders and omitting other more biologically important ones will always minimise the perceived damage of artificial feeding. The end result is that major reviews, even the 2013 one supported by the World Health Organization,[455] are being cited by formula advocates as proof that there are no adverse long-term consequences of infant feeding – though that was not what the report concluded, and the report did not touch upon many of the concerns I raise in this book.

## Early diet, intelligence and health across generations

One inconvenient fact is rarely noted by those who believe that any advantages a breastfed baby might have are due to its parents' class or education. The socioeconomic groups linked with breastfeeding have switched over the last hundred years, while the link with better health and better outcomes remained constant.

In the second half of the twentieth century it was advantaged women who breastfed, and their babies are healthier and smarter than those of lower socioeconomic groups, as we have been conditioned to expect. But in the nineteenth century and up to the middle of the twentieth century the reverse was true: it was poorer women who breastfed. It is on record that their breastfed babies were less likely to die than the not-breastfed babies of affluent families. Smart children have a chance to escape the poverty trap via education, academic scholarships or by excelling in their work. Even in the twentieth century of universal education, breastfeeding has meant a greater likelihood of social mobility, with adults who had been breastfed as children more likely to have risen in the UK social class structure when all other confounders were controlled for.[456]

In a review of studies done from the 1920s to the late 1980s, I found that not one study suggested that artificially fed children were smarter: it was always breastfed children, regardless of their parents' socio-economic status.[457] With one exception. One school-based study in the 1920s[458] showed that breastfed children did better, as expected, but infants *exclusively breastfed for longer than twelve months* did almost as badly in school as those fed contemporary infant formulas. Breastmilk alone will rarely provide sufficient protein for all aspects of growth after twelve months. In that timeframe and demographic, to be exclusively breastfed for more than twelve months was due to poverty, the lack of other food in the household, in the days before food stamps and income support. This result shows that inadequate food intake, not breastmilk per se, harms childhood development. It also tends to validate the positive cognitive advantage of exclusive breastfeeding for six and nine months (also shown in that same study), and supports the current emphasis on

455 Horta BL, Victora C. Long term consequences of breastfeeding: a systematic review. (WHO 2013) Available for download at www.who.int/maternal_child.../breastfeeding_long_term_effects/en/
456 Sacker A, Kelly Y, Iacovou M, et al. Breast feeding and intergenerational social mobility: what are the mechanisms? *Arch Dis Child* 98(9):666-671. DOI:10.1136/archdischild-2012-303199; see also Quigley MA. Breast feeding, causal effects and inequalities. *Arch. Dis. Child.* 2013; 98:654–55.
457 I spent months researching this for my July 21, 1991 presentation at the ILCA conference in Miami Florida USA. A tape may still be available from First Tape Inc or from ILCA itself.
458 Terman LM. *Genetic studies of genius* (Stanford University Press 1926) vol 1: Mental and physical traits of a thousand gifted children.

the need for good quality complementary foods *as well as breastmilk* after nine months at the very latest.

The advantage of breastfeeding for cognitive development remained constant in all social classes over the century, despite the shifts in the association of breastfeeding from poorer groups between the 1920s and 1950s, to the advantaged after 1970.[459] And there are multiple contributory factors to this effect:[460] as Wyeth advertised, 'There's more to IQ than being born with it.'[461]

Maternal intelligence is seen by many as contributory to infant cognitive development, as doubtless it is. However, for some, it is a sufficient explanation, with the biological mechanisms needing no elucidation.

> In a meta-analysis of observational studies in 2006, Der and colleagues showed that when maternal intelligence is accounted for, the differences in children's performance are no longer evident, suggesting that apparent benefits of breastfeeding could be due to effects of residual confounding*[37].[462]

Could be, of course. Anything is possible. And vested interests will cite this speculation as proof: 'could be' or 'might be' rapidly becomes 'was proved to be' in the popular press when infant formula is in question. But how do we explain the increasing number of cognitively impaired children in communities where maternal education has increased? What are the actual mechanisms by which greater maternal intelligence is inherited? (It is not true that greater intelligence always means better or more responsive caregiving.) And how do we explain away the fact that for prems at least, it is the milk that matters: an intelligent and informed mother's choice to breastfeed is not predictive of any IQ advantage. In the famous study of preterms randomised to get banked breastmilk or infant formula, mothers who wanted to, but did not provide any breastmilk, had infants whose IQ at seven to eight years was the same as that of children whose mothers chose to bottle feed from birth (i.e., more than twelve points less than those being breastfed at hospital discharge.)[463] There is no evidence that being more intelligent meant greater success at breastmilk expression!

459  Breastfeeding, social class, and change-over time. *Am J Publ Health* 1959; 49: 365. http://www.ncbi.nlm.nih. gov/pmc/articles/PMC1372695/ See also, Meyer *Infant Foods and Feeding Practices.* (CCThomas Ill 1960) pp. 46–8.

460  Committee on Nutrition of the British Paediatric Association. Is breast feeding beneficial in the UK? *Arch Dis Child.* 1994; 71(4): 376–380. PMCID: PMC1030026.

461  In handouts (collected in the year 2000) suggesting that new ingredients in their formulas 'IMPROVED INFANT IQ' and caused 'BETTER VISUAL ACUITY'.

462  Robinson S, Fall C. Infant Nutrition and Later Health: A Review of Current Evidence. *Nutrients* 2012, *4*, 859–74; DOI:10.3390/nu4080859; citing Der G, Batty GD, Deary IJ. Effect of breast feeding on intelligence in children: Prospective study, sibling pairs analysis, and meta-analysis. *BMJ* 2006, *333*, 945. *The presence of a confounding variable affects the variables being studied so that results do not reflect the actual relationship between those variables. For example, in a study on a possible link between drowning and beer consumption, a confounding variable would be the season, summer. Residual confounding is the confounding that remains after unsuccessful attempts to adjust for it.

463   Lucas A, Morley R, Cole TJ, Lister G et al. Breastmilk and subsequent intelligence quotient in children born preterm. *Lancet* 1992; 339(8788):26-4.  DOI: 10.1016/0140-6736(92)91329-7

Even if we were to accept that maternal intelligence is a sufficient explanation for any child's better cognitive development, why do we assume that maternal intelligence is itself innate? What influenced the mother's cognitive development? How was the mother herself fed as an infant? Was the 'unintelligent' mother who reduces her child's potential herself a victim of artificial feeding? And did her failure to breastfeed arise from her lack of education and self-confidence and social support? Did this reduce the mutuality and responsiveness that lactation hormones and more physical connectedness and skin contact might have created? In short, was both the less intelligent mother's cognitive development, *and her mothering*, compromised by a bottle-fed start to life? Does her lack of education (not the same as intelligence though sometimes used as a proxy measure) reflect socio-economic limitations in times and places where education is expensive?

When researchers (and parents) dismiss the possibility of a direct effect of infant feeding on intelligence, how do they explain away the measurable physical differences in infant brains that are increasingly becoming apparent, like the differences in myelination and greater amount of white matter in breastfed children's brains mentioned earlier? Did the studies used to come to the conclusion that maternal intelligence explained infant intelligence include any/many children breastfed exclusively for months? Drane and Logemann have commented on some of the factors that need to be considered, which all increase the measurable differences.[464]

It is all too convenient for Western researchers and industry to adjust the data and so reduce the raw cognitive differences between groups of children. The assumptions underlying those adjustments and confounders need critical scrutiny, once cognitive and physical development is seen as affected inter-generationally. So too, do the assumptions made plain by talking about 'apparent benefits of breastfeeding', rather than 'apparent harms of artificial feeding' (i.e., not breastfeeding). To say that breastfeeding halves a risk is less striking than saying that formula feeding doubles a risk. The biggest residual confounder never controlled for might be artificial feeding damage in previous generations.

If there are specific groups today stuck in poverty traps, infant feeding can be an important contributing factor. There is a growing realisation that early adversity or stress – which for an infant can include lack of frequent skin contact and the physicality of breastfeeding – affects lifelong development. Dysnutrition – poor quality food, which formula is by comparison with breastmilk – affects lifelong development. Illness is more likely in households where babies are not breastfed. So too may be absenteeism from employment due to childhood illness and adult illness by contagion;[465] and the financial costs of artificial feeding are greater than those of breastfeeding. These factors can all increase household stress. Chronic as well as episodic or dramatic stress causes biological changes that can affect both brain and immune functioning, putting some children 'on a lifelong trajectory

---

464  Drane DL, Logemann JA. A critical evaluation of the evidence on the association between type of infant feeding and cognitive development.(PMID:11101022) *Paediatr Perinat Epidemiol* 2000; 14(4):349–56.

465  Cohen R, Mrtek MB, Mrtek RG. Comparison of maternal absenteeism and infant illness rates among breast-feeding and formula-feeding women in two corporations. (PMID:10160049) *Am J Health Promot* 1995; 10(2):148–53.

of increasing risk.'[466] And that trajectory puts them at risk of 'psychiatric disorders that involve enhanced anxiety and/or social dysfunction', which can be both inherited and transmitted.[467] Such disorders

> may be dependent not only on the specific alleles of genes that are inherited from one's parents and on one's own experiences, but also on the experiences of one's parents when they were young.[468]

Infant and adult diet can contribute in many ways to the development and severity of psychiatric disorders. To me, this all suggests that there are many ways in which artificial feeding contributes to increased household stress, yet it has not been investigated as a potential stressor; rather, it has been assumed to have no particular effect on stress levels in poor households, or even to be a benefit by allowing babies to be cared for while their mothers work. Socio-economic status is controlled for, without investigating fully what aspects of socioeconomic status are powerful. For this reason the harm done to poor families both by the presence of artificial feeding, and the lack of breastfeeding, may be underestimated. Would those households be so stressed if the mother had been assisted to enjoy breastfeeding, and made financially secure while doing so? Hardly likely.

To formula advocates suggesting that breastfeeding *per se* has little effect, and that socioeconomic rank or maternal education is more important, I cheerfully acknowledge that the potential for confounding variables is enormous in this area. But this cuts both ways. As just one example, the quality of interactive and responsive care given to any child is *not* solely determined by socioeconomic rank, however much money makes it easier to cope with daily life. Otherwise the modern megarich would be the best-parented people in history, and our ancestors would be lucky to have survived long enough to produce us! Less facetiously, corporate mum may go to work and leave baby in the care of the newly imported *au pair* or another uneducated low-paid carer, for example (although truth to tell some babies may be better served by an affectionate and responsive, if uneducated, mother substitute, than by frustrated blood kin.)[469] Affluent families in Australia with a room to spare find that there are not enough au pairs available in 2014; nannies are increasingly sought and may have no broader education than a basic diploma.[470] Living in Singapore in the 1970s, we were told that it was common for the infants of educated working women to be left in the care of less-educated Malay families until around two years of age, when they were considered old enough to be brought back to the home for the (often Filipina) servant or amah to care for them (along with doing the housework and cooking). Simply classifying

466  Sokolowski M, Boyce WT, McEwen BS. Scarred for Life? *New Scientist* 2013; 2901: 28–30.

467  Saavedra-Rodríguez L, Feig LA. Chronic social instability induces anxiety and defective social interactions across generations. (PMID:22906514) *Biol Psychiatr* 2013; 73(1):44–53.

468  ibid. Oliver James's reflections on childhood impacts on parental behaviour are riveting reading. See Bibliography.

469  Though for any child, subsequently losing a carer to whom they have become attached is a major trauma with lifelong consequences. Sarah Blaffer-Hrdy's *Mother Nature* (Pantheon Press 1999) describes how she resolved these tensions through the recruitment of an allo-mother, a woman to share the mothering task. See also James O. *They F*** You Up: How to Survive Family Life*. (Bloomsbury Publishing 2006).

470  http://www.news.com.au/lifestyle/parenting/childcare-agencies-struggling-to-find-staff-in-australia-looking-offshore/story-fnet085v-1226718780613

outcomes in children by the mother's ethnicity or employment or education level would be misleading; knowledge of the care the infant received would be important. I rarely see any mention of this in studies that focus on maternal education.

For there are attentive and neglectful mothers in all strata of society. Neurobiology suggests that an affectionate, responsive, tactile and breastfeeding – but perhaps poor – mother will almost certainly help her young baby's cognitive and immune development far more than a self-absorbed, contact-avoidant, bottle-feeding (but wealthy) mother or partner, as the case may be. Of course poverty makes life harder, while wealth can make possible some remediation of developmental problems. But regardless of parental education, or environment, or income, not breastfeeding any child increases the microbial and contamination risks inherent in both poor living conditions and commercial childcare. As Professor Lawrence Gartner, chair of the American Academy of Pediatrics (AAP) Section on Breastfeeding, said in *Newsweek* years ago: 'It's hard to come out and say "your baby's going to be stupider or sicker if you don't breastfeed." But that's what the literature says.'[471] Indeed it does.

In summary, if intelligence is heritable, and it is to some degree, then how you were fed, how your brain developed, and how your genes were expressed, will matter not only to you, but also to your children, and maybe to their children as well, if your children cannot heal the damage.

Many of the differences in structure and content of formulas will affect brains, as will be discussed in many chapters of the history. Where new disorders limiting intellectual development are emerging, suspicion about infant feeding and its intergenerational effects seems justified from basic science and first principles. As far back as 1988 researchers noted the link between formula and what was then termed 'pervasive developmental disorders.'[472] The link was not widely publicised. A US paediatrician noted for his breastfeeding advocacy over many years argues that such disorders can largely be prevented.[473] Perhaps his experience matches mine: that autism is emerging in the third or fourth generations affected by formula-feeding, the children of the 1980s and 1990s, at far greater rates than in previous generations. Does it take a multi-generational load (with what genomic distortions?) before sporadic cases turn into an epidemic?

---

471 Gartner L. in *Your Child from Birth to Three. Newsweek* special edition, April 1997, p. 32.
472 Burd L, Fisher W, Kerbeshian J, Vesely B, Durgin B, Reep P. A comparison of breastfeeding rates among children with pervasive developmental disorder, and controls. (PMID:3225319). *J Dev Behav Pediatr* 1988, 9(5):247–51.
473 Gordon J. *Preventing Autism: what you can do to protect your children.* (John Wiley 2013.) This could just as easily be titled, 'How to have a healthy child.'

# Autism, mental health, immune disorder, and artificial feeding

Is infant feeding a causal factor in autism? And if so, what might be the links? There are studies[474] showing an association with artificial feeding, not surprisingly. But if the link was a simple causal one it ought to have been identified by now. It is likely that there are a number of interacting factors affecting a perhaps genetically vulnerable child, so no parent should feel that this is a problem they have caused, however they fed their child. But there are a number of impacts of artificial feeding that might pre-dispose, trigger, or even directly cause autism, such as:

- the different balance of amino acids in the blood of infants fed artificial formulas, some of which act as neurotransmitters in the brain (see Protein quality issues on page 270 onwards);
- the defective myelination of the artificially fed brain (see footnote on page 147);
- other damaging effects on the programming of brain development;
- excessive levels of minerals or heavy metals in infant formula;
- the lack of powerful hormones and growth factors found in breastmilk;
- more frequent infections necessitating antibiotics;
- higher levels of pro-inflammatory fats and their impact (see page 315);
- and of course the gut effects of artificial feeding and the unnatural microbiome it creates (which can include bacteria that produce toxins affecting the brain).

(Many of these factors are discussed in Chapter 3, as they relate to infant formula composition and its changes. To avoid repetition, I suggest reading the whole before making a judgement about this issue.)

Is it 'just' that some nasty, more virulent bugs, of the Clostridial family for instance, have mutated – as some certainly have in animals – and bottle-feeding facilitates their entrenchment in the gut where they produce toxins absorbed into blood and affecting the brain? Autism is definitely associated both with food hypersensitivities and with gut dysbiosis (microbial imbalance – the wrong mix of some nasty microbes)[475]. A truly remarkable Canadian mother, Ellen Bolte, has shown this beyond all reasonable doubt in her son's case, and convinced many sceptics.[476] Following her instincts, and her conviction that her autistic son had regressed after antibiotics altered his gut flora, she prevailed upon researchers to dose him with powerful antibiotics that kill Clostridia: and saw dramatic improvements in his functioning. It would be interesting if trials involving faecal transplants

---

474 Tanoue Y, Oda S. Weaning time of children with infantile autism.(PMID:2793787) *J Autism Dev Disord* 1989, 19(3):425–34.; Schultz ST, Klonoff-Cohen HS, Wingard DL, Akshoomoff NA et al. Breastfeeding, infant formula supplementation, and Autistic Disorder: the results of a parent survey. (PMID:16978397) *Int Breastfeed J* 2006, 1:16.

475 Finegold SM, Downes J, Summanen PH Microbiology of regressive autism.(PMID:22202440) *Anaerobe* 2012, 18(2):260–62.

476 A documentary about this family, *The Autism Enigma*, can be seen on ABC iview, and the story can be read at http://atguelph.uoguelph.ca/2012/07/gut-bacteria-may-hold-key-to-autism/

for patients with severe colitis[477] were to be extended to autistic children, preferably before too much learning time has been lost. Since then we have had research showing that the gut-brain connection is a two-way street, with the gut influencing the brain as well as the brain influencing the gut.[478] The concurrence of gut problems and mental disorders in autism and other forms of cerebral dysfunction seems to me unlikely to be coincidence.

Then there is the relative oxytocin deficit of artificially fed infants not given the repeated skin to skin contact of breastfeeding, and lacking oxytocin in the milk they drink. Researchers studying oxytocin know that lactation hormones have powerful effects on shaping both infant and maternal brains.[479] There is evidence that the brains of those with autism are different from as young as six months,[480] which suggests early influences at work. Autism researchers have even identified areas of the brain affected by a lack of oxytocin, and seen some improvement with its administration.[481] In a recent presentation Dr Touraj Shafai argued that 'there is extensive and credible evidence [which he reviewed] that Autism Spectrum Disorders are associated with oxytocin deficit and dysfunction.'[482] It is notable in this connection that contact aversion is one of the diagnostic markers of autism spectrum disorder.

How about the undoubted effects of oxytocin[483] and infant feeding on brain development? Is that important in autism? We know now that when the brains of healthy children of matched socio-economic status are examined using MRI scanning techniques, there are significant differences between those exclusively breastfed for just three months, and those mixed fed or those formula-fed. By the age of two, there were substantial differences in brain growth in exactly the areas of the brain associated with language, emotional function, and cognition.[484] It might take only a small but significant digression soon after birth to create those differences by the age of two. Which is why it is really important that investigators using MRI or any other techniques to document normal brain development over time ensure that they are looking at brains developed by breastmilk: some studies

477 Youngster I, Russell GH, Pindar C, Ziv-Baran T et al. Oral, Capsulized, Frozen Fecal Microbiota Transplantation for Relapsing Clostridium difficile Infection. *JAMA*. Published online October 11, 2014. DOI:10.1001/jama.2014.13875.

478 Tillisch K, Labus J, Kilpatrick L, Jiang Z, et al Consumption of fermented milk product with probiotic modulates brain activity. (PMID:23474283) *Gastroenterology* 2013;144(7):1394-401, 1401.e1–4.

479 Uvnas Moberg K. *The Oxytocin Factor. Tapping the hormone of calm, love, and healing.* (da Capo Press 2003).

480 Wolff JJ, Gu H, Gerig G, Elison JT et al. IBIS Network. Differences in white matter fiber tract development present from 6 to 24 months in infants with autism. (PMID:22362397) *Am J Psychiatry* 2012, 169(6):589–600.

481 Tachibana M, Kagitani-Shimono K, Mohri I, Yamamoto T et al. Long-term administration of intranasal oxytocin is a safe and promising therapy for early adolescent boys with autism spectrum disorders. *J Child Adolesc Psychopharm* 2013; 23(2):123–27. (PMID:23480321); Anagnostou E, Soorya L, Chaplin W, Bartz J et al. Intranasal oxytocin versus placebo in the treatment of adults with autism spectrum disorders: a randomised controlled trial. *Molecular Autism* 2012; 3(1):16. (PMID:23216716).

482 Shafai T. Presentation, *The Impact of infant feeding methods; breastfeeding, breast-milk or formula-feeding on the prevalence of autism spectrum disorders* at the Global Online Lactation (GOLD) conference, May 2012.

483 Feldman R, Gordon I, Influs M, Gutbir T, Ebstein RP. Parental Oxytocin and Early Caregiving Jointly Shape Children's Oxytocin Response and Social Reciprocity. *Neuropsychopharmacology*. (PMID:23325323); Groppe SE, Gossen A, Rademacher L, Hahn A et al. Oxytocin Influences Processing of Socially Relevant Cues in the Ventral Tegmental Area of the Human Brain. *Biol Psychiatry* 2013. (PMID:23419544).

484 Deoni S, DC, Piryatinksy I, O'Muircheartaigh J, et al. Breastfeeding and early white matter development: A cross-sectional study. *NeuroImage*, 2013; DOI: 10.1016/j.neuroimage.2013.05.090.

make no mention of infant feeding, yet offer their findings as reference norms.[485] The 'usual is normal' assumption allowed obesity to become an epidemic before it was recognised as distortion of normal development!

A 2012 case study of 102 children with autism spectrum disorders (ASDs) and matched controls evaluated the association between suboptimal breastfeeding practices and autism spectrum disorders. ASDs were associated with late initiation of breastfeeding (which may mean formula being given even before colostrum), lack of colostrum, prelacteal feeding, and bottle-feeding generally. The risk decreased in a dose-response fashion over increasing periods of both exclusive breastfeeding, and continued breastfeeding. The authors concluded that 'increased ASD risk is generally associated with suboptimal breast-feeding practices'.[486] Has anyone seen that splashed across the media?

If, as some formula advocates want to argue, autism is a purely inherited defect, which is not in any way affected by postnatal influences or even prenatal gestational ones, how do we explain such consistent associations? What is the evidence for it being purely inherited when changes to gut bacteria can bring about improvement? However multi-faceted autism's causes, the association of damage with too little or no breastfeeding across generations is there, albeit unpredictably. (A little formula may damage one child's genome while a larger exposure may not visibly harm another child: disease will arise from the interaction, not necessarily the dose.) No review I have seen has even dared ask if autism is a long-term consequence of formula feeding.

And a word of warning here: widespread trends to bottle-feed breastmilk – as a way of facilitating mothers returning to work – are removing the benefits of physical closeness and skin contact, of freshly expressed hormones, of infant control of intake and relative cream levels. In addition, bottle-feeding even fresh breastmilk increases the risks of chemical exposure and contamination, infection, and decreased infant ability to recognise satiety. It is not just the milk but also the feeding method that matters,[487] although clearly, even bottled fresh breastmilk is preferable to formula. But how much of the damage commonly attributed to prematurity, or the problems of multiple-birth children, is in fact the result of the common avoidable practice of depriving preterm or small babies or multiples of skin-to-skin contact and breastmilk?

Neurobiology is explaining more about brain development and behaviour, and those explanations are revealing the impact of early nutrition and care on that development and later behaviour. The hypothesis that early life events explain much later disease, both physical and psychological, via metabolic programming is becoming more widely accepted in scientific circles – more widely than it is publicised to the parents who have to make

---

485 Blüml S, Wisnowski JL, Nelson MD Jr, Paquette L et al. Metabolic maturation of the human brain from birth through adolescence: insights from in vivo magnetic resonance spectroscopy. *Cerebral Cortex* 2013, 23(12):2944–55 DOI: 10.1093/cercor/bhs283.

486 Al-Farsi YM, Al-Sharbati MM, Waly MI, Al-Farsi OA, Al-Shafaee MA, Al-Khaduri MM, Trivedi MS, Deth RC Effect of suboptimal breast-feeding on occurrence of autism: a case-control study. (PMID:22541054) *Nutrition* 2012, 28(7-8):e27-32.. DOI: 10.1016/j.nut.2012.01.007

487 Noel-Weiss op. cit.

and live with the consequences of infant feeding decisions, or to the health professionals advising them. Many professional conferences, even of midwives or paediatricians, include few updates on infant feeding research other than those sponsored by companies.

And if the act of breastfeeding affects maternal behaviour – as both human and animal research evidence suggests – than not only nutrition, but also care, is different, which in itself can clearly have intergenerational effects. Fleming's diagram (see Figure 2-5-4 on page 102) of the effects of mothers on their offspring and vice versa[488] summarises the feedback loops which clearly exist and account for a great deal of human social disadvantage. Anyone doubting this should search Pubmed for articles authored by Fleming AS. Yes, much of the work is in mammals other than humans but mammalian biology is powerful and much of it shared. How else could we accept formulas based on the development of rats and pigs?

Of course it should also be noted that diet beyond infancy is also important to cognitive function. 'Eat your way to dementia' is the title of a recent New Scientist review[489] of the cognitive impacts of Western diet. But infancy is also the time when basic metabolic processes are set in train that can influence later responses to diet. The issue of diet beyond infancy is more widely accepted as being critical – but how adult diet affects us is itself influenced by our diet in infancy. What we ate then affects how we process what we eat now … and to some extent what we prefer to eat now, as taste preferences are also established in childhood.[490]

Interestingly, many cultures have long believed that babies' personalities were influenced by what they ate; that those fed cows' milk were more bovine than those fed human milk, for example. While these crude generalisations were once rightly ridiculed, science is now providing explanations for some of the observations communities have passed down. Infants fed diluted cows' milk and bread sops in traditional cultures would indeed be substantially less intelligent (more bovine) than those breastfed, if they survived. And if they reproduced, their children could start life disadvantaged. This need not have any direct epigenetic effect, but it may. And the substantial differences in protein quantity and quality over the last century in milk-based formulas to date have still not eliminated IQ differences between solely breastfed and artificially fed children – differences that in some studies can match the effects of low-level lead exposure.[491] Why do we worry about one and not the other?

Ongoing research into cerebral effects, with their known and unknown consequences for transmission both genetically and socially, is not all that is needed. The possibility

---

488 Fleming AS, O'Day DH, Kraemer GW. Neurobiology of mother-infant interactions: experience and central nervous system plasticity across development and generations. (PMID:10392659) *Neurosci Biobehav Rev* 1999, 23(5):673–85. DOI: 10.1016/S0149-7634(99)00011-1.

489 Trivedi B. Eat your way to dementia. *New Scientist* 1 Sept 2012, pp. 32–37.

490 Trabulsi JC, Mennella JA. Diet, sensitive periods in flavour learning, and growth. (PMID:22724643) *Int Rev Psychiatry* 2012; 24(3):219–30.

491 Mortenson EL, Michaelsen KF, Sanders SA, Reinisch JM. The association between duration of breastfeeding and adult intelligence, *JAMA* 2002;287:2365-2371. 'The adjusted difference between test scores of individuals breastfed for <1 months and those breastfed for 7–9 months was 6.6 points for the Full Scale WAIS and 2.1 points for the BPP, representing one half and one fifth of a standard deviation, respectively.'

of intergenerational amplification of immune problems, or progressive degeneration of immune systems, needs to be explored in depth through more than one generation. Allergists and immunologists have long documented a greater likelihood of immune dysfunction in children whose parents or siblings are allergic. When both parents are allergic, the risk is exponentially higher. Despite this, neither neurologists nor even allergists enquire about previous generations and their feeding history.

Yet Frances Pottenger's remarkable experiments with diet in some 900 cats through several generations[492] (referred to on page 124) indicated that drastic effects of constant poor feeding from birth show up by the third and fourth generation (which is about where affluent Western nations are in relation to mass artificial feeding) and include a wide range of problems including reproductive defects and infertility. (It's harder to test intelligence in a cat.) Encouragingly, his studies also indicate that in cats, deficits could be reversed by generations of good nutrition. If so, perhaps parents can make a positive difference to what their child has inherited – and it is clearly worth trying. Beginning of course, with the mother, and with the child's nutrition before and after birth.

I have earlier mentioned the Finnish Allergy Group and its national strategy for the prevention and treatment of allergy. This can be accessed online.[493] But a broader national strategy is needed, devoted to optimal infant feeding. For the preventive approach that has never been tried in any country is the one I have used with considerable success in many families: maximising the power of breastfeeding to heal and induce food tolerance in children once the mother's own food allergy problems have been identified and dealt with. Instead of relying on ersatz industrial remedies, it harnesses the power of mammalian milk. For more on this, see Book 3.

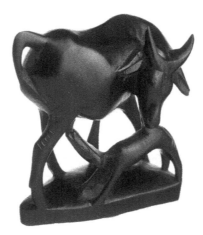

Figure 2-7-1 The enteromammary system illustrated by Indonesian craftsmen. Photo © James W Maher

492 Pottenger FM. *Pottenger's Cats: a study in nutrition.* (Pottenger-Price Nutrition Foundation 1983).
493 Haahtela T, Von Hertzen L, Mäkelä M, Hannuksela M and the Allergy Programme Working Group Finnish Allergy Programme 2008–2018 – time to act and change the course. *Allergy* 2008; 63 (6): 634–645. DOI: 10.1111/j.1398-9995.2008.01712.x.

# 2.8 Testing the milk hypothesis

Designing experiments to test the milk hypothesis relies on a clear understanding of the complexities of the issues and the definitions[494], and why past studies into differences between breastfed and artificially fed infants have produced limited results. It also requires detailed knowledge of both human milk feeding and the substitutes that have adulterated or replaced it over time, in the relevant local culture and time. This does not mean that such experiments are impossible, just difficult.

## Problems with researching the idea

It is not ethical or possible to randomise babies to being breastfed or artificially fed. In every society in every age there can be differences between mothers who breastfeed and those who do not. Lucas et al's classic study of preterms showed that the choice to breastfeed made no difference to the infants' cognitive outcomes, but the milk received certainly did[495]. (Children of mothers who chose to breastfeed but were unable to carry through their choice had outcomes as poor as those who chose to formula feed.) Are researchers giving the appropriate weight to maternal intent and maternal milk?

It is easily forgotten that breastfeeding itself influences mothers and mothering styles at least as much as the converse. This is a feedback loop, as Fleming illustrates: (see Figure 2-5-4). And cultural contexts of breastfeeding change. In the first half of the twentieth century, poor women breastfed while advantaged women used infant formula. The well off also usually had access to medical care, good quality food and water, and relatively safe environments (no open community cess-pits, e.g.) In some past studies, when the women breastfeeding were poor, failing to control adequately for socio-economic status and maternal education reduced differences in outcome. Better research techniques were not available until after a major demographic shift had occurred, and it was advantaged women who breastfed. The new association of breastfeeding with advantage, and the ability of researchers to control for socio-economic status and maternal education, meant that better recorded outcomes were often assumed to be due to that advantage, not to the milk. But is it reasonable to assume that the nutrition that creates the child is less important to health than a mother's education? When education was accounted for in the study previously mentioned, it was the amount of mother's milk that mattered.

Of the existing studies, as we have seen, many have not been well designed or carefully executed:

- almost no research uses as the basis for comparison the human biological norm: around six months of nothing but breastmilk, gradually tapering off over a couple

---

494  WHO. *Indicators for assessing infant and young child feeding practices* : conclusions of a consensus meeting held 6–8 November 2007 in Washington D.C., USA. (WHO 2008) online at http://www.who.int/maternal_child_adolescent/documents/9789241596664/en/

495 Lucas A, Morley R, Cole TJ, Lister G et al. Breast milk and subsequent intelligence quotient in children born preterm. (PMID:1346280) Lancet 1992, 339(8788):261-264. DOI: 10.1016/0140-6736(92)91329-7

of years minimum, in conjunction with an increase in family foods of suitable quality and quantity

- very little research uses globally accepted definitions of breastfeeding – for example, the study which classified all children breastfed for less than six months as bottle fed, and those having any breastfeeds at 6 months or more as breastfed![496]

- almost no research compares infants fully formula-fed from birth, without any colostrum or breastmilk, and those fully breastfed from birth with no additives. In fact, infant formula companies encourage limited early breastfeeding so strongly nowadays (pushing supplementation) that I suspect that they are fully aware that differences would be marked if groups of solely artificially fed from birth children were used in studies. Mixed feeding is the panacea that will save the companies' bottom line, and gullible formula advocates are helping them push it as the best solution for western women.

- all failure to distinguish accurately between breastfed infants and artificially fed infants (and degrees of mixed feeding) increases the likelihood of null (no difference) results, and reduces the likelihood of results that show the damage done by artificial feeding

- data about feeding methods are gathered in unreliable ways: asking parents, sometimes months or years later, who tend to over-report their breastfeeding rates,[497] and who may in any case not be aware of their child's exposure to artificial feeding in the early days of hospital. Nine of thirty-nine Danish mothers of allergic fully-breastfed babies had no idea they had been exposed to cows' milk in hospital.

- qualitative aspects of research have been flawed:

- exactly which formula or formulas were fed, at which stages of the child's development? Which batches? Formulas are all very different and affect babies differently,[498] yet there is almost no published – let alone publicised – research available that systematically compares brand and batch. Some other details to consider:

  - was the formula batch supplied by the company (and perhaps subject to special quality control, as has happened) or bought on the retail market?

  - how close were the actual contents of the formula tin to the ingredients listed on the outside, given the wide latitude needed for industrial products with a long shelf-life?

  - was the now formula-fed child breastfed in hospital or given antibiotics?

  - If a placebo was used, what was it, who supplied it, was it tested for reactivity?

---

496  Wigg NR, Tong S, McMichael AJ, Baghurst P et al. Does breastfeeding at 6 months predict cognitive development? *ANZ J Pub Hlth* 1998; 22:232–36.

497  Gillespie B et al. op. cit. Knowing that breastfeeding is considered 'better' ensures this over-reporting. It is my experience that, like healthworkers, many mothers say what they know others hope to hear, or approve of.

498  Check out sites like http://www.productreview.com.au/c/baby-formulas.html

The Colen et al sibling study (see p. 144-5) argued that breastfeeding benefits are overstated. This had some of the flaws listed above such as using retrospective 'ever' versus 'never' breastfed records. As well, "all the scenarios we can call to mind in which siblings are fed differently favour the breastfed sibling." Not so in my experience: the small, sick, difficult, or allergic baby is often breastfed longer. Reasons for using breast or bottle can relate to perceived child or family health issues, as well as birth order dynamics, and both affect and are affected by interbirth intervals (not mentioned). An earlier sibling comparison study[499] had cogently discussed some other problems of comparisons within families.

But one defect that stands out to me is an apparent lack of awareness of the significant population shift from predominantly disadvantaged women breastfeeding in the 1950s–60s (from which period the 1979 cohort was drawn) to the 1986–2010 cohorts (when advantaged women had taken up breastfeeding again, but were birthing in hospitals where children were routinely exposed to bovine milk and antibiotics). To me, this study doesn't just compare apples and oranges, but a whole fruit salad of possibilities, in a representative (?) sample, 94% of whom had medical insurance. Let's make that concrete. Women self-reporting breastfeeding duration years after weaning could have included, for example:

- malnourished women living in poor conditions who breastfed in the 1950s (producing children who typically may have bottle-fed in the 1980s);
- advantaged bottle-feeding mothers of the 1950–60s;
- their evaporated-milk-fed allergic daughters feeding infants by the 1970–90s;
- among the latter group, those whose infants were exposed to free formula in hospital from the 1960s (almost all in some hospitals) and those who were not;
- allergic mothers (themselves either formula or breastfed) of the 1980–90s who breastfed – some while consuming a litre of cow's milk daily – because they were aware of research suggesting breastfeeding could reduce allergies;
- disadvantaged mothers in any decade who were persuaded to give a few breastfeeds in hospital but gave up within a week or two and used infant formula.
- women with immune disorders as a result of their artificial feeding in infancy

The bottle feeding women could have included

- women healthy because gestated and breastfed in the 1950s by disadvantaged mothers who (like their own mothers in the 1930s) had no alternative before free WIC formula was arranged by industry and the USDA
- advantaged women in any decade whose advantaged mothers had tried and found breastfeeding too difficult, giving up after a few days, weeks or months
- allergic women who gave their babies colostrum, but who always intended to bottle feed and didn't count a few hospital feeds as important;
- women (themselves breastfed) whose first experience of breastfeeding was so painful and difficult that they chose to formula feed solely from birth.

499 Evenhouse E, Reilly S. Improved Estimates of the Benefits of Breastfeeding Using Sibling Comparisons to Reduce Selection Bias. *Health Serv Res.* 2005; 40(6 Pt 1): 1781–1802. PMCID: PMC1361236 DOI: 10.1111/j.1475-6773.2004.00453.x. Free online, this showed significant benefit to the breastfed. Worth reading.

The combination of all these possibilities increases the likelihood that differences between the ever-breastfed and the never-breastfed will be blurred. To get any significant difference in studies using self-reported 'ever versus never' categories is to me astonishing. And what about the impact of family birth order in sibling studies? It would be interesting to know how many first-borns were breastfed in each decade. Unsupported first-time mothers often give up breastfeeding relatively quickly in a culture where bottle feeding is considered safe and is in fact normal practice, as it was by 1950 in America. How many of the breastfed in each era were subsequent siblings, breastfed because of the firstborn's problems; equally, how many siblings in each era were bottle-fed from birth after failed breastfeeding of the firstborn? How does birth order affect outcomes being measured?

For me, the bottom line is that without detailed questioning, and even with it sometimes, retrospective self reporting may not give reliable details of early bovine milk exposure in hospital and exclusive breastfeeding. Few studies that I have seen to date get reliable data about prior generations' actual feeding history in the first week of life. Yet knowing such details, or at least being able to assess probabilities by knowing the local context and actual hospital practices, is critical to clinical practice as a lactation consultant advising distressed mothers about their distressed infants. Parents will tell me that their babies have never been given formula, but if they reveal that the baby was in a nursery for more than a very short time, the odds are that the baby was comp-fed. That history was almost always true of the Australian mothers themselves, even if some of their babies had been more fortunate since the Baby-Friendly Hospital Initiative has affected hospital practices. And those comp-fed previous generation mothers mostly gestated babies while consuming large amounts of milk.

I am looking at this issue from my local Australian context of women who have succeeded in establishing full breastfeeding despite many obstacles and early setbacks and who then go on to experience breastfeeding as so rewarding that they continue for what in many overseas studies would be seen as "extended" periods, at least twelve months and often longer. That length of time is normal breastfeeding for me. I have helped many such women go on to have another child who is not exposed to bovine protein, and to breastfeed even longer, especially if the baby is thought to be the last child. The same mother, but the difference is qualitative: a normal microbiome makes for a peaceful baby. It would not surprise me to find that there are significant differences in gut bacteria (as well as immune factors) between colicky and peaceful babies. (See the section on Colic in Book 3.)

What matters now is the outcome in the present generation. But if there are powerful intergenerational impacts that have reduced the effectiveness of breastmilk's ability to help a child adapt to the environment, we need to know. Incremental damage through generations cannot be instantly removed, but the evidence strongly suggests it can be gradually reversed by better nutrition and care. Industry may well have a role to play in assisting adults to overcome problems partly created by their early nutrition. The plethora of bacteria now on sale may include some strains or mixes that do help restore better gut function to adults. But the most helpful thing industry could do would be to stress the need for early exclusive breastmilk feeding of all infants in the first weeks of life, stop providing convenient supplies of infant formula to hospitals, and stop pushing formula for supplementation of breastfed infants.

## 2.9  The infant feeding issue in the broader context

In Western nations, processed industrially produced foods are now normalised for all stages of the life cycle, from birth to death. In many countries the same major global food companies dominate markets. Countries that still have affordable fresh food can still choose whether to value and protect it, including the freshest of all, women's milk, delivered by breast to baby. Increasingly the choice appears to be between wellness and illness, and adults are making that choice for the next generation. The replacement of breastfeeding in every country where industrially manufactured artificial milks have become normal has a great deal to do with the epidemic of 'allergy' that follows, or so it seems from the reality of all the families I've seen over thirty-five years.

Babies truly are what they eat. They build their bodies from the food they consume, and those bodies have then to deal with the chemical and toxic and microbiological assaults their environment presents. Without an efficiently functioning gut, immune system, and brain, babies will deal less well with those challenges and much discomfort and dis-ease will result. Artificial feeding was and is harmful, and its effects are intergenerational. All artificially fed babies are not the babies they would have been if breastfed. Each child is a non-repeatable, unique experiment.

As I see it, no single industrial-era change is as fundamental or powerful a challenge to normal human development as:

1. the replacement of women's milk by synthetic industrial mixes falsely promoted as 'so good as to make no real difference'
2. the quasi-force feeding of those industrial milks to virtually all hospitalised newborns in the period after 1960
3. the continued expansion of the use of industrial milks to at least twelve months of life or even longer.

For me, decades of clinical and personal experience suggest that intergenerational harms of artificial feeding accumulate. Animal studies support that idea: from Pottenger's cats to rat and mouse and pig and deer and rabbit studies. They're all in PubMed if you want to search and read. Human studies are harder to do, but are emerging. Daily I see that the harms done to past generations by poor infant feeding live on in the descendants of the artificially fed, in unpredictable ways related to their genomic uniqueness.

We are what we eat, and what our forebears have eaten. In this perspective, for example, the coeliac epidemic, the obesity epidemic and the autism epidemic may all be outcomes of two or three generations of harm – even though either condition could also arise de novo in any child exposed to a toxic overload in any one generation. For one bottle-fed child, autism may arise from the gut dysbiosis inherited at birth from an obese mother herself artificially fed as a child, together with a protein overload from artificial feeding. For another child, of a breastfed mother, gut dysbiosis may result later, from exposure to a virulent pathogen acquired via NICU staff or infant food or day-care or contact with health professionals. In both cases, the observed onset of symptomatic gut disease or regressive autism could be triggered by infection, or vaccination,[500] or multiple antibiotic doses that facilitate clostridial overgrowth. A child fully breastfed for six months by a mother herself fully breastfed for six months might be exposed to identical risk factors, even at higher doses, and come to no harm. We could postulate as many different hypothetical pathways as there are lives and genomes, for each life is unique, just as each mother's milk is.

The research to prove this beyond dispute will take time: intergenerational studies in humans have been rare and seen by some as impractical, and the number of potential confounding variables is mind-blowing. For even simple issues it can take decades to establish relative certainty in science: for decades, self-interested parties disputed the blindingly obvious fact that sucking thousands of toxic, even radioactive, chemicals into human lungs would undoubtedly cause cancer. (And then there's climate change!) Someone had to prove it did, and the first to try were invariably rubbished by someone who didn't like them saying it.

However, few people are aware of just how many indicators there are that the presence of artificial feeding, or the absence of breastfeeding, or both those two separate impacts synergistically, have a significant impact on human health and disease. Without wanting to distract from the main focus of this book, immune disorder, it seemed wrong not to include at least an outline summary of what research currently indicates overall about both natural and artificial feeding, and to reference a few detailed treatments of this topic for any possible Doubting Thomases. There is much more about many of these aspects in the following chapters: what follows is just a partial overview.

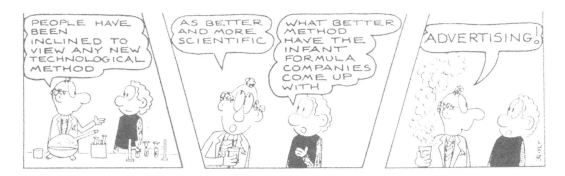

Figure 2-9-1 A better method? Image from *Protecting Infant Health: a healthworker's guide to the International Code of Marketing of Breastmilk Substitutes.* (ICDC 1993 edition)

---

500  While I know of others, Valerie Foley's son Billy is clearly one such case. She writes intelligently and passionately on this topic and its controversies at jumpontherollercoaster.blogspot.com.au and has published *The Autism Experience* ( Jane Curry Publishing, Sydney 2012).

# 2.10 A selective summary: breastfeeding

We all benefit from breastfeeding, though only a minority of women breastfeed. Scandinavian countries, often leaders in societal change, not only encourage breastfeeding, they have created social structures which make it possible. Norway literally values it, including breastmilk production in its annual GDP,[501] as every country should: there is no more 'domestic' product, after all, even if it prevents illness and reduces public health expenditures in a myriad of ways.

Breastfeeding:

- provides for normal infant development, including development of a protective microbiome
- prevents countless infant deaths and even more episodes of illness
- uses fewer resources and creates less waste
- reduces demand on health services throughout the life of the breastfed individual
- increases the health of the breastfed baby's family by reducing the severity of diseases brought into the home from childcare or kindergarten, and so increases workplace productivity
- creates individuals who are healthier, smarter, happier and better adjusted (than those same individuals would be if not breastfed), thus reducing demands on social services, policing and other government services
- benefits infants in areas with endemic HIV, resulting in reduced risk of acquiring HIV infection compared to infants on a mixed diet of human milk and other foods and/or commercial infant formula
- would save $13 billion[502] per year in the US alone, if 90 per cent of US mothers would breastfeed exclusively for six months; similarly, UK calculations show massive health budget savings. [503]

## The milk of humankind: a short summary

Like blood, breastmilk is a complex living tissue that profoundly influences infants' biochemistry, metabolism, body composition, and microbiome (the complex interacting population of micro-organisms in the gut that are essential for normal functioning, aiding digestion, food tolerance, growth and development). In fact, breastmilk has recently been shown to contain at least 700 different species of beneficial bacteria ('probiotics') as well as nutrition – 200 or more prebiotic oligosaccharides for instance – tailored to help the bacteria grow.[504] What formula matches that? A baby's first small doses of colostrum

501  Smith J, Ingham L. Mothers' milk and measures of economic output. *Feminist Economics* 2005; 11(1):41–62.

502  Bartick M, Reinhold A. The burden of suboptimal breastfeeding in the United States: a pediatric cost analysis. *Pediatrics* 2010;125(5):e1048–56. See also Smith JP. 'Lost Milk?' Counting the economic value of breast milk in gross domestic product. *J Hum Lact* 2013; 29 (4): 537–46.

503  S Pokhrel, M A Quigley, J Fox-Rushbyet al. Potential economic impacts from improving breastfeeding rates. (PMID:25477310) *Arch Dis Child* 2014; DOI: 10.1136/archdischild-2014-306701

504  Cabrera-Rubio R, Collado MC, Laitinen K, Salminen S, et al. op. cit.

begin to establish the normal, protective gut microbiome. Breastmilk provides the perfect mix, adapted to suit the environment in which the baby will live and the food that will be available.

Breastmilk in fact samples the total environment and provides it to the baby in a buffered form, which the infant body is biologically able to handle, and which is likely to induce tolerance rather than reactivity.

> Breastmilk mediated transfer of innocuous environmental and self-antigens can help in the education of the infant immune system towards tolerance induction. Tolerogenic potential of breast milk will be different between mothers and will depend on her antigen exposure, her immune responses to transferred antigen, her mammary gland permeability, her milk levels of growth factors, microbiota influencing factors and tolerogenic molecules.'[505]

And, of course, the mother's own infant feeding, and her mother's before her, can influence all those factors: the intergenerational hypothesis helps explain all that variability between mothers.

Breastmilk is a 'bioactive fluid', dynamic and interactive, changing with the needs of babies. Every mother's breastmilk is unique, adapted to the sex of her child, adapted to its developmental needs, and responsive to the child's suckling behaviour, which itself adapts to the milk provided. Babies drink less by volume of a high fat milk, and the fat in milk can range from 2–13 per cent between samples (time of day, interval between feeds, degree of breast emptying, and method of collection can influence these figures.) Persistent lengthy feeders willing to suckle on the breast long after the initial let-downs will get more fat than the baby who chooses to stop feeding once the easy rushes of milk stop. Some babies feed little and often, others long and slow. Some babies like gulping down large volumes as the letdown occurs, others pull off and wait till the flow slows. Infant oral structures influence how effectively and long they feed before tiring, and that can influence the interval to the next feed ... every baby, every breast, every mother, is unique. The art of breastfeeding is learning to adapt to one another so that both thrive: breastfeeding can teach responsiveness.

The biochemistry of breastmilk is complex, and changes during the weeks and months of breastfeeding as a baby grows and develops: amounts and types of protein and fatty acids and other ingredients change as infant developmental needs change. Breastmilk composition also changes through the day, and even during each feed. As a baby feeds, and the first breast drains, the fat content of the milk steadily increases, doubling on average from the beginning of the feed to the end. The second breast has benefitted from milk let-downs while the first is being fed from, so that it begins as a richer milk than the first breast did. Often the baby will stop feeding after one side, or only a few minutes on the second side, as the fat-rich milk leads to the baby feeling satisfied and knowing when to stop, an essential ability in avoiding obesity in adulthood. There is evidence that breastfed babies are less likely to grow into overweight or obese children, at risk of the chronic diseases

---

505  Macchiaverni P, Tulic MK, Verhasselt V. Antigens in breast milk. In Zibadi et al 2013 p. 455.

associated with excessive weight; the longer they are breastfed, the greater the protective effect, which could last into adulthood.

Some of this is due to the many hormones and other bioactive factors found in breastmilk, the significance of which is finally being explored. Surprising findings are emerging. It may be that the levels of a variety of hormones in breastmilk programme infant development in unforeseen ways. For instance, only recently has it been realised that receptors in the infant gut take up cortisol, which may affect personality development later in childhood.[506] Women's milk – with all those hormones – is the only food for which newborns are evolutionarily adapted. It is the perfect start to good nutrition from birth, providing all the food babies need for around the first six months or so of life.

Breastmilk protects children against serious illness and death. The longer they are breastfed (and after about 6 months, given suitable complementary foods alongside breastfeeding), the greater the protection against disease. Some specifics are listed under artificial feeding, which both increases the risk and severity of infection, and the consequences of early antibiotic exposure due to illness.[507] (32 per cent of children who received antibiotics before their first birthday were overweight at age twelve, compared to just 18 per cent of those who didn't.[508])

Preterm infants especially benefit from breastmilk, not only in NICU (neonatal intensive care unit), but also well into the first year, with fewer hospital readmissions. Breastfeeding – or even just breastmilk feeding – has positive effects on the long-term neurodevelopment of these tiny babies, and is associated with higher intelligence scores and teacher's ratings.

Fortunate babies still being breastfed when they start eating solids and drinking water have two immune systems to help deal with any threats: mother's via her milk, and their own new, healthy and effective immune system, constructed by breastfeeding.

Early infant nutrition, in and out of the womb, affects health outcomes both in later life[509] and over generations. Animal breeders have known it for centuries, and it is no longer controversial to serious researchers in the field, even if formula advocates choose to live in denial.

## Breastmilk and smarter babies

Breastfeeding fuels and shapes any child's neurodevelopment; this has been discussed earlier. Is this due to maternal intelligence or biology? Surely both. Breastfed babies have greater amounts of white matter in their brains, and are less likely to develop autism. Breastmilk's complex essential fatty acids are needed for normal neurological and eye development, and infants have a limited capacity to synthesise these. The changing balance of the 184

---

506  Hinde K. op. cit.
507  Azad MB, Bridgman SL, Becker AB, Kozyrskyj AL. Infant antibiotic exposure and the development of childhood overweight and central adiposity. *Int J Obes.* 2014 Jul 11. DOI: 10.1038/ijo.2014.119.
508  Cox LM, Yamanishi S, Sohn J, Alekseyenko AV et al. Altering the Intestinal Microbiota during a Critical Developmental Window Has Lasting Metabolic Consequences. *Cell* 2014. http://dx.doi.org/10.1016/j.cell.2014.05.052
509  Fewtrell M. The long-term benefits of having been breastfed. *Current Pediatrics* 2004; 14: 97–103.

fatty acids found in breastmilk coincides with different stages of infant brain development that utilise more of the different varieties. The fats found in formula are not a perfect match for breastmilk fats and do not change with the child's growth. Choline, a water soluble B vitamin, is important in neurotransmission and cell membranes, important for both memory and muscle function. The breastmilk forms of choline result in enhanced uptake by brain and other tissues.[510] The amounts and the types of both free choline and choline metabolites differ between breastmilk and formula; neither cow and soy formula has a choline metabolite profile that matches human milk, as the figure below[511] shows clearly. So even if advertising proclaimed that infant formula 'contains Choline, important to neurotransmission' it would not be telling the whole truth. These differences do make a difference!

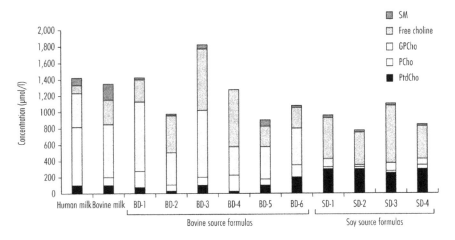

Figure 2-10-1 Differences between choline in milk and in artificial substitutes. (© Wageningen Academic Publishers 2013)

I can cover only a few of the nutrient differences between the foods that the baby grows on. Many more have been outlined previously, and others will be discussed in Book 2. Consider the many factors related to infant feeding that we know influence intelligence, summarised earlier.

There are many types and levels of evidence now available, none of which suggests that formula-fed infants are smarter, regardless of the groups studied, whether in Belorussia[512] or Boston.[513] Even massive over-controlling cannot talk away this difference.

---

510   Davenport C, Caudill MA. Choline and milk. In Zibadi, Watson and Preedy, op. cit., p. 345.

511   ibid p. 334. Image © Wageningen Academic Publishers 2013.

512   Kramer MS, Aboud F, Mironova E, Vanilovich I et al. Breastfeeding and Child Cognitive Development. New Evidence From a Large Randomized Trial. *Arch Gen Psychiatry*. 2008; 65(5):578–84. DOI: 10.1001/archpsyc.65.5.578.

513   Chapman DJ. Does breastfeeding result in smarter children? A closer look. *J Hum Lact* 2013; 29 (4): 444–5. Commenting on Belfort MB, Rifas-Shiman SL, Kleinman KP, Guthrie LB et al. Infant feeding and childhood cognition at ages 3 and 7 years: Effects of breastfeeding duration and exclusivity. (PMID:23896931) *JAMA Pediatr* 2013, 167(9):836–44.

# Breastfeeding and happy families

Pleasant sensory stimulation is as essential as good food for normal child growth and development. Mammals have evolved over millions of years to suckle their young, with mothers and babies in close skin-to-skin contact, facilitating the sharing of their microbiomes, and mutually influencing moods and behaviours. Human infants are the only primates to feed and sleep apart from their mothers (and then only in some societies). The cost of this in terms of maternal and child emotional, physical and intellectual wellbeing is still being determined.

Breastfeeding is a powerful intimate psychosocial interaction and relationship, which has long-lasting hormone-mediated biological effects on both breastfeeder and breastfed. A breastfeeding baby is necessarily held against the mother's body, skin to skin, with the physical intimacy of skin and eye contact strengthening attachment, and reducing energy needs and stress levels in them both. Lactation hormones such as oxytocin and prolactin have powerful and beneficial effects on both the infant's and mother's brains and the mother's body, reducing stress and helping emotional bonding. Anyone unaware of how profoundly this is true can read more in Kerstin Uvnas-Moberg's work on oxytocin.[514]

Breastfeeding fully as WHO suggests (exclusively for 6 months and then into the second year and beyond) may also protect children from developing ADHD (attention deficit hyperactivity disorder) and autism. Breastfeeding has also been linked to better mental health in childhood and adolescence. An association exists between breastfeeding for six months or longer and a reduction in mental health problems throughout childhood and adolescence.[515] All of these reductions in behavioural and cognitive problems remove pressures for everyone in the family, making everyone – not just the child in question – happier and healthier. As eminent researcher into the social origins of violence, James W Prescott, recently said, 'Bottle-feeding may be the single worst invention of the twentieth century'.[516]

# Breastfeeding and mothers

The health risks to women of not breastfeeding babies they have gestated are substantial.[517] Breastfeeding is a biological norm; all deviations are to greater or lesser degree abnormal by definition. All have consequences. Mothers' short- and long-term health is protected by successful breastfeeding, which:

---

514  Uvnas Moberg K. op. cit.

515  Oddy WH, Kendall GE, Li J, Jacoby P et al. The Long-Term Effects of Breastfeeding on Child and Adolescent Mental Health: A Pregnancy Cohort Study Followed for 14 Years. *J Pediatrics* 2010, 156(4):568–74; press release at http://www.childhealthresearch.org.au/news-events/media-releases/2010/january/new-study-shows-long-term-mental-health-benefits-from-extended-breastfeeding.aspx

516  Prescott. JW. Nurturant versus non-nurturant environments and the failure of the environment of evolutionary adaptedness, in Narvaez D, Panksepp J, Schore AN, Gleason T (eds) *Evolution, Early Experience and Human Development.* (Oxford Uni Press 2012) p. 427.

517  Groer M, Kendall-Tackett KA. *How breastfeeding protects women's health: the psychoneuroimmunology of human lactation.* (Thomas Hale Publishing 2008); Labbok M; Bobrow KL, Quigley MA, Green J et al. Persistent effects of women's parity and breastfeeding patterns on their body mass index: results from the Million Women Study. *Int J Obesity* (2013) 37, 712–717; DOI:10.1038/ijo.2012.76

- stimulates oxytocin release, which in turn helps the uterus contract, reducing the risk of haemorrhage and anaemia
- helps adjustment to the new role of motherhood, with lactation hormones buffering stress[518] and providing affectional rewards
- improves maternal mood and mental functioning[519]
- improves the quality of maternal sleep[520]
- delays menstruation and fertility, allowing mothers to space children more effectively and recover fully after the birth
- helps weight loss and a return to the woman's usual weight
- improves mineral metabolism, increasing lumbar spine density by 1.5 per cent per breastfed child,[521] thus reducing the risk of osteoporosis[522] and hip fracture[523] in later life
- lowers the risk of pre-menopausal breast cancer,[524] and possibly protects against post-menopausal breast cancer[525]
- reduces the domestic work and expense that are part of formula-feeding.

Breastfeeding women are at lower lifetime risk of

- ovarian,[526] cervical[527] and endometrial cancers

518  Kinsley CH, Meyer E. Maternal mentality. *Scientific American Mind* 2011; 22 (3): 25–30. (PMID:16468436); Hillerer KM, Jacobs VR, Fischer T, Aigner L. The maternal brain: an organ with peripartal plasticity. (PMID:24883213) Free full text article *Neural Plast* 2014, 2014:574159 DOI: 10.1155/2014/574159

519  Kinsley CH, Bardi M, Karelina K, Rima B et al. Motherhood induces and maintains behavioral and neural plasticity across the lifespan in the rat.(PMID:18074214) *Arch Sex Behav* 2008; 37 (1): 43–56. DOI: 10.1007/s10508-007-9277-x; Mezzacappa ES, Katkin ES. Breastfeeding is associated with reduced perceived stress and negative moods. *Health Psychology* 2002; 21: 187–93; Heinrichs M, Neumann I, Ehlert U. Lactation and stress; protective effects of breastfeeding in humans. *Stress* 2002; 5: 195–203.

520  Blyton DM, Sullivan CE, Edwards N. Lactation is associated with an increase in slow wave sleep. *J Sleep Res* 2002; 11: 297–303. See also Middlemiss W, Kendall-Tackett K (eds) *The Science of Mother Infant Sleep* (Praeclarus Press 2013)

521  Hreschyshyn MM, Hopkins A, Zylstra S et al. Associations of parity, breastfeeding, and birth control pills with lumbar spine and femoral neck bone densities. *Am J Obstet Gynecol* 1988; 159: 318–22; Koetting CA; Wardlaw GM. Wrist, spine, and hip bone density in women with variable histories of lactation. *Am J Clin Nutr* 1988; 48: 1479–81.

522  Paton LM. Pregnancy and lactation have no long-term deleterious effect on measures of bone mineral in healthy women: a twin study. *Am J Clin Nutr.* 2003; 77:707–14.

523  Bjørnerem A, Ahmed LA, Jørgensen L, Størmer J et al. Breastfeeding protects against hip fracture in postmenopausal women: the Tromsø study. (PMID:21898594) *J Bone Miner Res* 2011, 26(12):2843–50. DOI: 10.1002/jbmr.496

524  McTiernan A, Thomas DB. Evidence for a protective effect of lactation on risk of breast cancer in young women. *Am J Epidemiol* 1986; 124: 353–8.

525  Collaborative Group on Hormonal Factors in Breast Cancer. Breast cancer and breastfeeding: collaborative reanalysis of individual data from 47 epidemiological studies in 30 countries, including 50302 women with breast cancer and 96973 women without the disease. (PMID:12133652) *Lancet* 2002; 360(9328):187–95.

526  Cancer and Steroid Hormone Study, CDC/NICHHD. The reduction in risk of ovarian cancer associated with oral contraceptive use. *N Engl J Med 1987;* 316: 650–5; 1987; 317: 508–9; Li DP, Du C, Zhang ZM, Li GX et al. Breastfeeding and ovarian cancer risk: a systematic review and meta-analysis of 40 epidemiological studies. (PMID:24998548) *Asian Pac J Cancer Prev* 2014; 15(12):4829–37 DOI: 10.1177/0890334413475838.

527  Brock KE, Berry G, Brinton LA et al. Sexual, reproductive and contraceptive risk factors for carcinoma-in-situ for the uterine cervix in Sydney. *Med J Austr* 1989; 150: 125–30.

- cardiovascular disease[528]
- cancer in later life for survivors of childhood cancer[529]
- rheumatoid arthritis,[530] type 2 diabetes, metabolic syndrome[531]
- gall bladder[532] problems.

Duration of breastfeeding is important to some of these outcomes, as those studies from Iran, and those looking at cancer and arthritis make clear. The effects are significant: for rheumatoid arthritis, for example, the authors state that

> The risk was lower with increasing duration of breastfeeding [adjusted odds ratio (OR) 0.54 (95% CI 0.29, 1.01) for breastfeeding at least 36 months; P for trend = 0.04]. Compared with those who had never breastfed, breastfeeding was associated with half the risk of RA.

When breastfeeding is the physiological norm, that should be said as 'Not breastfeeding doubled the risk of rheumatoid arthritis', a painful, even crippling, condition.

For normal breastfeeding (till around the age of two or longer) to be possible, breastfeeding needs to be supported as a cultural norm. Here Islam and the Vatican[533] agree. The Holy Quran suggests that new mothers should breastfeed for two years – as a result, many Iranian mothers lactate for as long as WHO recommends, into the second year and beyond. And reduced risk of metabolic syndrome is clear.

Some of the increased risks of disease in mothers who have not breastfed their babies also apply to women who choose, or are forced by circumstances, to remain childless. Breast cancer was once considered 'the nuns' disease', as high rates were recorded among women living in religious communities, as well as other nulliparous women, proverbial 'old maids'. Lactation is part of women's biological reproductive cycle, and the absence of normal breastfeeding from a female life confers increased risks. (So too does the absence of pregnancy. There the cost-benefit analysis is more complicated, as the risks of birth itself are avoided, and in many places those risks are heavy. ) Advice to all young childless

---

528  Schwarz EB. Infant feeding in America: enough to break a mother's heart? (PMID:24112066) *Breastfeed Med* 2013; 8:454–57.

529  Both being breastfed and breastfeeding their children reduces the risk for women who survive childhood cancer. Ogg SW, Hudson MM, Randolph ME, Klosky JL. Protective effects of breastfeeding for mothers surviving childhood cancer. *Journal of Cancer Survivorship*, 2011; DOI 10.1007/s11764-010-0169-z

530  Adab P, Jiang CQ, Rankin E, Tsang YW, et al. Breastfeeding practice, oral contraceptive use and risk of rheumatoid arthritis among Chinese women: the Guangzhou Biobank Cohort Study.(PMID:24395920) *Rheumatology* 2014; 53(5):860–66. DOI: 10.1093/rheumatology/ket456; Pikwer W, Bergstrom U, Nilsson JA et al. Breastfeeding but not use of oral contraceptives is associated with a reduced risk of RA. *Ann Rheum Dis* 2009; 68:526–30.

531  Ramezani Tehrani F, Momenan AA, Khomami MB & Azizi F. Does lactation protect mothers against metabolic syndrome? Findings from the Tehran Lipid and Glucose Study. *J Obstet Gynaecol Res* 2014; 40(3):736–42; Tørris C1, Thune I, Emaus A, Finstad SE et al. Duration of lactation, maternal metabolic profile, and body composition in the Norwegian EBBA I-study. *Breastfeed Med* 2013; 8(1):8–15. DOI: 10.1089/bfm.2012.0048. Epub 2012 Oct 11

532  Liu B, Beral V, Balkwill A, et al., Childbearing, breastfeeding, other reproductive factors and the subsequent risk of hospitalization for gallbladder disease. *Int J Epidemiol*, 2009; 38(1):312–18.

533  Glatz C. Pope to moms: it's OK to breastfeed, even in the Sistine Chapel. *Catholic News Service*. http://www.catholicnews.com/data/stories/cns/1400120.htm

women could include a rational use of hormonal contraception when young, with an eye to reducing breast cancer risk, not merely to avoiding pregnancy[534] in heterosexual females. Whether childless by choice or circumstance, women should not face a greater risk of serious illness due to ignorance of a real risk. It remains to be seen what impact women delaying childbirth until their thirties or forties will have on reproductive cancer rates a few decades from now; the choice of contraceptive method may be critical.

I am continually astonished by formula fantasists who ignore the impact on *women's* health when trying to persuade other mothers in affluent countries that infant feeding makes no real difference to their children.

## Breastmilk as medicine for adults

Twentieth century doctors seemed unaware that for centuries breastmilk had been used as medicine for the sick and elderly, as well as the best start for babies. Given how essential breastmilk is for healthy human development, it's surprising how little research there has been into its makeup until recently. Science is now beginning to discover why it is so effective.

As noted earlier, breastmilk contains 'pluripotent' stem cells, which can be 'reprogrammed' by the body to form different types of human tissues. Experiments that have involved injecting stem cells into humans suggest that it is entirely possible that such reprograming occurs within any human body where there is damage recognised by the immune system. And mouse experiments described earlier make it clear that stem cells are transferred via milk. Perhaps the stem cells repair some intra-uterine or perinatal damage: birth is itself a stressful process. Breastmilk is an obvious ethical source of stem cells for adult stem cell therapy.

That's just one example; the neurotransmitters, growth factors, immune cells, hormones, enzymes and all the thousands of other astonishingly complex bioactive factors in human milk may be far more relevant to adult health and disease than has ever been suspected, preventing immune distortion or even repairing damaged chromosomes. Infant formula cannot provide these, now or ever.

Breastmilk may also help address the increasing global problem of multiply resistant pathogens. As mentioned earlier, recent research has found that the breastmilk-derived complex called HAMLET – human α-lactalbumin made lethal to tumour cells – kills cancer cells while stimulating an innate immune response in surrounding healthy tissue. HAMLET can also cause bacteria like Multiply Resistant Staphylococcus aureus (golden staph, MRSA) to become once again sensitive to antibiotics.[535] Doses of breastmilk could be prescribed to such MRSA patients, to see if such a simple therapy could be effective. Of course the pharmaceutical industry can be expected to see it as more profitable to patent[536]

534  Britt K, Short R. The plight of nuns: hazards of nulliparity.(PMID:22153781) *Lancet* 2012; 379(9834): 2322–23.
535  Marks LR, Clementi EA, Hakansson AP. Sensitization of Staphylococcus aureus to Methicillin and other antibiotics In vitro and In vivo in the presence of HAMLET. (PMID:23650551). *PloS one* 2013, 8(5):e63158. DOI: 10.1371/journal.pone.0063158
536  A search at http://www.freepatentsonline.com is very revealing.

breastmilk ingredients and market them at greater cost than breastmilk donated (or even sold) by compassionate women. Norwegian experience (see box below) is that breastmilk works even on multiply resistant strains in already sick infants!

Recent studies are discovering the effects of breastfeeding on the generation of T-cells to suppress anti-maternal immunity.[537] It is becoming increasingly clear just how powerful breastmilk is. And I suspect that if the world could access all the research locked away in the files of infant formula companies, we would know a great deal more about it, and see infant formula as simply unacceptable.

There is much more detail about many aspects of this throughout Book 2. The US Surgeon General concluded that 'infant feeding should not be considered as a lifestyle choice but rather as a basic health issue'.[538] It is also a basic equity issue. Taxpayers should see the support of breastfeeding as an investment that saves them money, and consider compensating the women who provide such a social benefit, which may entail unfair financial disadvantage.

## Breastmilk and superbugs

Breastmilk can be the difference between life and death for infants, even in highly developed nations such as Norway. Breastmilk's immune memory cells can rapidly attack multiply resistant bugs, as Norwegian doctors well know. Dr Gro Nylander tells the story of an outbreak in a paediatric ward of a diarrhoeal disease rare in Norway, but common overseas. There had been two deaths, and several children were gravely ill. Modern antibiotics failed. So a search was made for breastfeeding women who had migrated from countries where the disease was common. Such women were found; they donated breastmilk with disease-specific antibodies; the milk was fed to the sick children: all recovered. And the outbreak ended.[539]

How many babies have died and will die in American, Canadian, British and Australian hospitals because doctors do not think of fresh breastmilk as both safe and potentially lifesaving? How much suffering could be averted by using breastmilk as a potent resource?

Communities that for centuries used breastmilk as medicine for the sick and elderly are vindicated!

---

537   Aoyama K, Matsuoka KI, Teshima T. Breast milk and transplantation tolerance.(PMID:21327152) Free resource *Chimerism* 2010, 1(1):19–20.

538   www.surgeongeneral.gov/topics/breastfeeding/Accessed March 28, 2011

539   Nylander G. op. cit., p. 126.

# 2.11 A selective summary: infant formulas

*Formula.* The word conjures images of scientists in white coats. As it is meant to. It conjures images of constant precision and exactness in ingredients. (Even though the breastmilk it replaces is in fact a unique bespoke product tailored for and by each individual child, as described earlier.) It implies predictable outcomes. (Even though the uniqueness of every child means the extent of any harm cannot be predicted.)

But what is formula? Artificial breastmilk, it is emphatically not, even if this is claimed in the *Irish Examiner* as true as recently as 2012, and by the Operations Manager for Danone, who should know better.[540] Artificial substitutes for breastmilk are now, and always have been, grossly inadequate on many levels, even the simplest – but utterly impossible – one of matching the nutritional content of breastmilk. Book 2 will detail formula's ever-changing nature and problems. This is the merest outline of some overall concerns.

In 1861 von Liebig called his mixture 'a soup for babies'. He was right. Infant formula is in fact a non-sterile, variable soup[541] (or dehydrated soup powder) of different heavily processed industrially concocted foodstuffs drawn from a variety of animal, plant, fungal, algal and other sources brought together from many sources, even many different countries.

Formula has been based on animal milk proteins (whey or casein), animal meat (beef and sheep hearts, chicken meat), and soy beans, with additives such as DHA and ARA (essential fatty acids) sourced from egg yolks, fish, or genetically engineered fungi and algae, oils from known allergens like peanuts, cottonseed, corn and sesame, and carbohydrates sourced from common western allergens like wheat and corn. Lately ingredients sourced from apples to peas are being used. Infant formula is really much more like an ever-changing soup – a variety of different soups, in fact – than a single food like milk. Infant formulas are not milks – no mammal ever produced them, though herds of mammals may have contributed one or more of the major raw ingredients, while fields and industrial plants contribute others.

Even less are they 'babymilks': no baby ever made them, and given a choice of breastmilk, no baby would ever want them; and they are not what babies need for normal development.

These unpredictable industrial soups lack the complex, species-specific bioactive properties of breastmilk, and to the extent that they contain milks from other species, may provide bioactive factors appropriate for those species, and quite inappropriate for humans.

A hundred years after these mixes began to be fed to whole populations of children (unwitting guinea pigs) in industrialised nations, scientists are still trying to remedy newly identified deficiencies and excesses. Only recently, for example, has it been shown

---

540 Ketch C. Danone expanding in Cork to capitalise on 2015 quota cessation. *Irish Examiner,* 25 October 2012. See http://www.irishexaminer.com/farming/general/danone-expanding-in-cork-to-capitalise-on-2015-quota-cessation-211924.html

541 Wikipedia says a soup is a primarily liquid food, generally served warm (but may be cool or cold), that is made by combining ingredients such as meat and vegetables with stock, juice, water, or another liquid.

that digested formula (but not digested breastmilk) is toxic to human intestinal cells.[542] Scientists have only just realised that they need to know not just what goes into babies, but what by-products are created while it's being digested inside them.

Labelling on infant formulas is often inadequate or misleading, making it difficult or impossible for parents to make informed choices. To complicate matters further, formulas are all different, even from batch to batch, let alone brand to brand. Those produced by the same company with the same name may contain different ingredients in different countries, making it difficult for parents travelling with infants.

It doesn't take a genius or a biochemist to recognise that feeding babies new and often untested soups by bottles was bound to cause problems, most of them unforeseen.

# Known hazards of artificial feeding

First and foremost, it alters babies' bodies, in small ways and large, in preterm and term infants, from what those bodies would have been if breastfed. Their brains, their bones,[543] their biomes. For example, by four months of age, the formula fed infant's thymus is half the size of the exclusively breastfed infant's, 'possibly because breastmilk provides the important growth factor IL-7 to the infant's immune system, thereby enhancing thymic output of T cells.'[544]

And it exposes babies to needless risk. The risk of SIDS is increased by at least 50 per cent.[545] Most parents believe formula is sterile. It isn't,[546] despite 100 years of advertising it as pure and uncontaminated. Industrially produced powdered formula *cannot be* sterilised without risking damage to heat-sensitive vitamins. Liquid ready-to-feed formula can be sterilised, but liquid formula is more heat damaged than powder (see page 251) Once any container of infant formula is opened, it will inevitably become contaminated with ambient microbes, and deteriorate rapidly if it is not stored correctly. Even if formula does not itself introduce pathogens to the infant, it creates the wrong environment in the infant gut for friendly bacteria, and favours instead the growth of pathogens omnipresent in hospital and home environments, for many of which the mother's immune system cannot have prepared the baby during pregnancy.

Mixing formula correctly introduces more potential problems: getting accurate measurements of formula and water, using sterilised bottles that don't retain traces of chlorine or other harmful chemicals; ensuring water is not contaminated with harmful chemicals or bacteria, checking the temperature to avoid burns, ensuring the teat or bottle isn't leaching harmful plasticisers into the formula, and so on.

---

542  Penn AH et al, op. cit.
543  Bishop NJ, Dahlenburg SL, Fewtrell MS, Morley R et al. Early diet of preterm infants and bone mineralisation at age five years. *Acta Paediatr* 1996: 85:230–6.
544  Brandtzaeg P. *Immune aspects of milk: an overview,* in Zibadi S, Watson RR, Preedy VR (eds), op. cit.. (Wageningen Academic Press 2013) p. 70.
545  ibid., p. 73.
546  Jason J. Prevention of invasive Cronobacter infections in young infants fed powdered infant formulas. *Pediatrics* 2012; 130(5):e1076–84. (PMID:23045556)

The processing and packaging of any industrial product, infant formula included, leaves traces of substances such as aluminium, cadmium, cobalt and nickel and so on.[547] For many years lead solder was used in making infant formula cans, and the US discovered particularly high lead levels in liquid infant formula (5–50 mcg per 100 ml).[548] In 1979, shortly before I fed my third child cans of liquid US-made soy formula, over 90 per cent of all US-produced cans used lead solder, according to the National Food Processors' Association.[549] In the 1980s disturbing levels of lead, cadmium, aluminium, and other heavy metals were found in some formulas. (See 3.9 Unavoidable contaminants on page 367 ) The problem has not gone away, as you will read.

Infant formulas, like all other mass-produced foodstuffs, are also occasionally contaminated with insects, broken glass, metal fragments, plastic, machine oil,[550] and so forth. Formulas have also had to be modified over the years after certain ingredients proved harmful to babies. This list is a small sample of much more to be found in the next chapter of this book.

- Vitamin K was added after acute bleeding episodes in antibiotic-exposed infants fed early casein hydrolysates like Nutramigen (a hydrolysate is a compound in which proteins have been broken down into amino acids);
- fat blends were changed after skin lesions developed in infants;
- megaloblastic anaemia resulted from low folic acid and Vitamin C levels;
- cases of goitre from early soy formulas led to iodine being added;
- overheating led to B6-deficient formula brain-damaging babies, so that heat-stable pyridoxine was added in 1953;
- excess Vitamin D caused hypercalcaemia in more than 200 children.

In the 1980s, when some of today's parents were babies:

- different formulas were found to be deficient in vitamin B-6, vitamin A, copper, thiamine, linoleic acid, zinc, folacin and vitamin D
- various formulas were unfit for food because they could not pass through a bottle nipple, they were curdled, smelt 'off', were discoloured, lumpy, brown
- some were contaminated with a variety of bacteria, moulds and toxins
- some were contaminated with lead and other heavy metals

In the 1990s problems with various formula included:

- contamination with Klebsiella pneumoniae, Pseudomonas aeruginosa and Salmonella bacteria

547 Dabeka RW. Survey of lead, cadmium, cobalt and nickel in infant formulas and evaporated milks and estimation of dietary intakes of the elements by infants 0–12 months old. *Sci Total Environ.* 1989;89:279–289. PubMed.

548 Walker B. Lead content of milk and infant formula. *J Food Prot* 1980; 43 (30 178–79; see also the September 1980 issue of *Food Chemical News*.

549 Reported in *Food Chemical News* July 2, 1990, p. 52.

550 Judge D. Switching to food-grade lubricants provides safety solution. *Machinery Lubrication* July 2005. Customer discovery in Danish milk product reported in *Straits Times* 12 July 2002. Earlier UK incident reported in *The Sentinel* 1 September 2000. Not reported in medical literature.

- sour taste, curdling or lumpiness
- incorrect labelling and preparation instructions
- contamination with lead, cadmium, arsenic or excessive magnesium and ...
- substitution of adult food for formula, capable of causing dehydration or severe medical problems in infants
- failure to list ingredients fully

The next table lists some known recalls[551] in the 2000s.

| 2005 | Enfamil LactoFree with Lipil | Mead Johnson | Off odor, clumping Parent identified. |
|---|---|---|---|
| | Humana soy | Israel: imported | thiamine deficient |
| | Similac Advance with Iron | Ross/Abbott | Rigid PVC inclusion |
| 2006 | Enfamil AR Gentlease | Mead Johnson | 'aluminium dust'/metal shavings Parent identified. |
| 2007 | Alimentum Advance | Abbott | Vitamin C omission. Parent identified. |
| | Similac Special care | Abbott/Ross | Iron deficient |
| 2008 | Calcilo | Ross/Abbott | |
| 2009 | Neocate | Nutricia | Protein-deficient |
| 2010 | Similac: many varieties | Abbott/Ross | Beetle debris Parent identified. |
| 2011 | Aptamil, Milumil | Milupa | |
| | AR Digest | Novalac | Salmonella traces |
| 2012 | Meiji Japan | Meiji | Radioactivity |
| 2012 | Good Start | Gerber/Nestle | Foul odour |
| 2012 | Damil | Fasska | Salmonella |
| 2013 | Karicare stage 1 and Gold Stage 2 NZ, | Nutricia/ Danone | *Clostridia sporogenes*, mistaken for *C. botulinum.* |
| | Baby's Only Organic | Nature's One USA | arsenic (from brown rice syrup used) |
| 2014 | Nan Pro 2 (Philippines) | Nestlé | lacked fatty acids; factory noted error |
| 2014 | S26 original progress | Aspen Australia | dead lizard in powder made in Singapore |

Figure 2-11-1 Some known recalls in the 2000s.

Although rare given the volume of formula produced, and the massive costs to the company, recalls do happen; some are discussed in Book 2. It is worth noting that if both company

551 See also http://www.naba-breastfeeding.org/images/Formula%20Recalls-W.pdf

quality control and government inspection was *as thorough as parents assume it to be*, problems would be identified by the company before the product was marketed. Yet I keep noticing in press coverage that recalls happen because some consumer (the child) gets sick, or some purchaser/carer notices an off smell or odd texture or colour or debris (usually heat-damaged ingredients, often metal fragments, allegedly a whole gecko in July 2014 in formula manufactured in a modern Singapore plant[552]). Consumer complaints triggered factory inspections and created the well-documented Abbott beetle-in-formula recall, for example. (Seepage 492).

As well,

> In February 2006, China's quarantine authority ordered a ban on faulty milk powder Mead Johnson had produced. This order came on the heels of the company's recall of this Gentlease-branded product sold in the United States. Also identified as defective was Enfamil Lipil, a product sold in South Korea. Mead Johnson recalled both products due to unidentified metal particles contained in the milk powder.[553]

In addition, as the product becomes ever more expensive, economically motivated criminal fraud involving infant formula has increased, with dangerous substitutions, re-labelling, and counterfeiting of formula recorded in America and many other countries. Melamine in Chinese milk products was not the only case of wicked deliberate substitutions not identified by infant formula manufacturers before children were damaged. In 2014 a German formula company had to defend its products as safe amid allegations that an importer had added milk powder to extend the volume and then re-packaged the product.[554] One representative of a major formula maker has privately expressed to me deep concern about some mixtures being shipped as infant formula to Asia. Even terrorists have made money out of infant formula![555] No wonder a Chinese firm is now offering an insurance policy to recompense (rich) parents in the event of infant formula recalls.[556]

The infant food industry is actively trying to reduce known – but not publicised – risks of artificial feeding, such as the high levels of particular milk antigens, the adverse effects on gut flora (microbiome), the lack or excess of many ingredients in modern infant formula, the presence of known pathogens in powdered formula, and more. Formula-feeding parents need to be careful in their selection of infant formula, to reduce the known risks as best they can. (More about that in Book 3.)

A breastfeeding woman needn't worry, provided that her lifestyle is not bizarre: she has perfectly constituted and far safer and fresher milk instantly available, at the right

---

552  Visentin L. Mother finds lizard in baby formula. *Sydney Morning Herald* 13 July 2014. http://www.smh.com.au/national/mother-finds-lizard-in-baby-formula-20140713-zt5v6.html

553  http://www.fda.gov/NewsEvents/Newsroom/PressAnnouncements/2006/ucm108604.htm

554  http://www.dairyreporter.com/Regulation-Safety/No-evidence-that-Nutradefense-infant-formula-unsafe-in-China-Hero

555  Olson DT, Financing Terror. *Law Enforcement Bulletin* 2007; 76 (2); 1–5. Carter T. The Terror-Mob Crimes Link: Organized crime leaders and terrorists cross paths in cyberspace. *ABA Journal* 2014. Online at http://www.abajournal.com/magazine/article/organized_crime_leaders_and_terrorists_cross_paths_in_cyberspace/

556  http://www.dairyreporter.com/Markets/Chinese-retailer-introduces-infant-formula-recall-insurance

temperature, without the need for cash outlays. She can know what constitutes a risk to her milk and her child and to a far greater extent, those risks are within her control. And, as P!nk said, she is a walking antibiotic for her baby. What formula can match that?

# Formulas and disease

The epidemic of immune dysfunction described in this book has its roots deep in the period when artificial feeding began, when, for example, Grulee found eczema seven times more common in artificially fed infants.[557] That ratio changed over the century as the milk hypothesis would predict. As those made allergic by infant feeding gestated the next generation, the rates in breastfed infants rose.

Immune disorder grew steadily with the growth of artificial feeding in Western countries, and I confidently predict that it will continue to expand worldwide, especially in countries like China and Vietnam and India, now uncritically adopting Western infant feeding practices: formula sales in Asia are increasing 23 per cent annually. Allergy and autoimmune disease will increase and intensify in a few decades, affecting whole populations, unless we address the root causes over the next generations. I am convinced that those root causes include infant feeding, and that its importance is seriously underestimated.

Formula-feeding needs to be suspected and well-researched as a potential contributory or causal factor in *every one* of the many serious immunological and degenerative diseases that are more common in societies where artificial feeding is normative. Wherever the question is well-researched, whether the problem is childhood cancer[558] or constipation,[559] depression or diabetes, leukaemia, or liver disease,[560] the problem is more common in those not solely breastfed for the first half year of life. And those born with an inherited condition such as alpha-1 anti-trypsin deficiency are at risk of severe disease or even death if not breastfed.[561] What I will list here is only the tip of an iceberg. Other diseases such as leukodystrophy and any demyelinating disorder seem to me prime candidates for research into the effects of early nutritional damage. An excellent online source[562] for those who want to read more about this has been compiled for Evergreen Perinatal Education by Gina

557  Grulee CG, Hanford HN. The influence of breast and artificial feeding on infantile eczema. *J Pediatr* 1936; 8: 223–5.

558  Davis MK, Savitz DA, Graubard DI. Infant feeding and childhood cancer. *Lancet* 1988; 8607, ii: 365–8; Bener A, Denic S, Galadri S. longer breastfeeding and protection against childhood leukemia and lymphomas. *Eur J Cancer* 2001; 37: 234–38.

559  Andiran F, Dayl S, Mete E. Cows milk consumption and anal fissure in infants and young children. *J Pediatr Child Health* 2003; 39: 329–31.

560  Nobili V, Bedogni G, Alisi A, Pietrobattista A et al. A protective effect of breastfeeding on the progression of non-alcoholic fatty liver disease. *Arch Dis Child* [2009, 94(10):801–05. (PMID:19556219); Nobili V, Day C. Childhood NAFLD: a ticking time-bomb? *Gut* 2009; 58(11):1442. (PMID:19834114. Is the liver yet another target organ damaged by food allergy? See Brown C, Haringman N, Davies C, Gore C et al. High prevalence of food sensitisation in young children with liver disease: a clue to food allergy pathogenesis? (PMID:23050587) *Pediatr Allergy Immunol* 2012; 23(8):771–78.

561  Udall JN Jr, Dixon M, Newman AP, Wright JA et al. Liver disease in alpha 1-antitrypsin deficiency. A retrospective analysis of the influence of early breast- vs bottle-feeding. *JAMA.* 1985; 253(18):2679–82; McGilligan KM, Thomas DW, Eckhert CD. Alpha-1-antitrypsin concentration in human milk. *Pediatr Res* 1987; 22(3):268–70. (PMID:3498927)

562  http://www.evergreenperinataleducation.com/upload/OutcomesofBreastfeeding_Nov2013.pdf

Wall IBCLC, and the Bibliography points to other resources. Obstetrician Alison Steube's online article is a good conservative summary.[563] Any doubting Thomas (or Thomasina) simply should make a point of reading much more. New information is being generated all the time, *none of it reassuring,* such as the increased awareness of the effects of processing and industry's attempts to deal with these (See Measureing formula realities and processing effects on page 534). This table makes that clear.

| Short-term risks | Long-term risks |
| --- | --- |
| Feeding intolerance | Metabolic programming (nutritional imprinting) |
| Infantile colic | Hypertension |
| Necrotizing enterocolitis | Obesity |
| Increased osmolarity and renal solute load | Hyperlipidemia |
|     Increased sodium intake | Type I and II diabetes |
|     Dehydration | Allergy |
| Allergy |     Wheezing |
|     Cow's milk protein allergy |     Asthma |
| Infectious risks |     Atopic dermatitis |
|     Otitis media | Attention Deficit and Hyperactivity Disorder (due to |
|     Bacterial contamination |     soy proteins?)? |
|         Gastroenteritis | Economic burden |
|         Sepsis | |
|     Probiotics: sepsis? | |
| Chemical exposure due to economically motivated | |
|     adulteration | |
|         Acrylamide | |
|         Glutamate | |
|         Melamine | |
|         Manganese | |
| Neurotoxicity? | |
| Reproductive toxicity | |
|     Phytoestrogens: endocrine disruptors? | |

Figure 2-11-2 Reported risks and complications of infant formulas.[564]
Image © Wageningen Academic Publishers 2013.

The damage done by known environmental toxins is almost certainly compounded in child bodies constructed from infant formulas. Such foods, and the feeding technology, inevitably expose children to such chemicals and contaminants at the most vulnerable stages of development after birth. What we know suggests that formula damage and toxic chemical

563  Steube A. The risks of not breastfeeding. *Rev Obstet Gynecol* 2009; 2(4): 222–31. PMCID: PMC2812877.
564  Korkmaz A, Surmeli-Onay O. Powdered and liquid formulas: clinical and nutritional aspects. In Preedy, Watson Zibadi, op. cit., p. 166

damage will be synergistic. Take cigarette smoke, for example: formula use and smoking independently and synergistically increase hospitalisation for respiratory disease.[565]

The role of infant formula and its feeding in promoting lifelong ill health and obesity[566] is becoming increasingly obvious, and some recent studies explore its effects on genetic materials, as well as brain and reproductive development. Poor research continues to confuse the issue, creating doubt, which allows profits to grow. (It is hard not to see this as an intentional effect, especially after reading a little about corporate practices such as those outlined by David Michaels in *Doubt Is Their Product*).

The extent of the harm done has yet to be catalogued, and there is genuine uncertainty about the degree of the problem, and how contributory factors interact. But there is no doubt that there is a problem. What is beyond dispute is that – among other things – a formula-fed baby is at greater risk of:

- childhood leukaemia and other cancer
- sudden unexplained infant death (SUDI)
- obesity, and the later 'non-communicable diseases' that develop from obesity
- hospitalisation for gastrointestinal illnesses such as diarrhoea, NEC (necrotising enterocolitis: dying intestinal tissue, or basically gut gangrene)
- hospitalisation for respiratory tract infections such as bronchiolitis, other vial diseases, and pneumonia
- poorer cognitive development
- meningitis and other serious viral and bacterial infections
- snoring, sleep apnoea, dental malocclusion (bad bite) and other orthodontic problems, with their effects on faces, speech, and self-confidence
- otitis media, or middle-ear infections, which can lead to deafness and are associated with language and literacy problems at school
- asthma and allergies such as atopic dermatitis
- urinary tract infections
- metabolic disorders
- bacteraemia (bacteria in the blood)
- inflammatory bowel disease, coeliac disease, Crohn's disease
- type 1 diabetes
- worse outcomes if born with PKU[567] or other enzyme deficiency
- maternal abuse and neglect

565 Chen Y. Synergistic effect of passive smoking and artificial feeding on hospitalisation for respiratory illness in early childhood. (PMID:2785023) *Chest* 1989, 95(5):1004–07.
566 See Oddy WH. Infant feeding and obesity risk in the child. *Breastfeed Rev* 2012; 20 (2): 7–12.
567 Riva E, Agostini C, Biasucci G et al. Early breastfeeding is linked to higher intelligence quotient scores in dietary-treated phenylketonuric children. *Acta Paediatr* 1996; 85: 56–8

Formula-feeding also increases risks to the mother's health. It

- delays the mother's recovery from childbirth
- fails to postpone menstruation and fertility, making it more difficult for her to space her children effectively and recover fully after the birth
- increases the risk of pre-menopausal breast cancer, and possibly fails to protect against post-menopausal breast cancer
- delays the uterus returning to the size it was before pregnancy, making haemorrhage and anaemia more likely
- increases the risk of ovarian and endometrial cancers
- encourages weight retention and delays the return to the woman's usual weight
- worsens bone mineralisation, thus increasing the risk of osteoporosis and hip fracture in later life
- promotes inflammation that increases risks of auto-immune disease such as rheumatoid arthritis or both juvenile and adult-onset diabetes
- may make post-natal depression more likely or longer lasting, while abrupt weaning to formula may trigger psychosis
- increases the domestic work and expense that are part of formula-feeding (important in all households other than those wealthy enough for infant care to be delegated to lower-paid carers)
- makes adjustment to the maternal role more difficult by not automatically supplying hormones that reduce maternal stress and improve maternal sleep. (Bottle-feeding mothers who ensure frequent skin-to-skin contact with their baby can induce limited releases of prolactin and oxytocin by so doing. But they remain in a hormonally-abnormal state compared with breastfeeding mothers, with fertility returning well ahead of the evolutionary norm.)

## Infant formula's collateral damage

So artificial feeding and its equipment exposes mothers to risks as well as their babies. Infant risks include distorted growth patterns, microbiomic distortion, chemical contamination, facial deformity and subsequent problems with dentition, speech and hearing, not to mention unknown psychological risks through contact deprivation in the first years of life. I know that bottle-feeding parents can provide skin contact and closeness, and many make a point of doing so. But there is clear proof in the marketplace that others do not – specially designed bottles for small hands, handles for bottles, bottle props or even indwelling tubes in bottles for the child who can't hold the bottle (see 'murder bottles' on page 216). And breastfeeding is impossible without sensations of physical closeness: there are no takeaway breasts.

The collateral damage and costs to society and the planet of artificial feeding are enormous, though as yet not widely recognised. Just think of the milk produced and its environmental costs, the packaging materials needlessly used, the plastics produced and discarded in landfill, the water wasted, the transport resources and costs, the pollution and litter created – all needless if women breastfeed. And stop to think about the health problems being generated by all that waste, once again problems experienced most often by those already disadvantaged. Commercial incinerators and rubbish dumps are never located in affluent suburbs! The dioxins created by waste incineration can be recycled through milk packaging[568] and so reach even breastfeeding mothers and babies. A table listing just some of infant formula's collateral damage is below.

## Some of infant formula's collateral damage

- Population growth and higher reproductive cancer rates due to loss of natural contraception, greater need for artificial alternatives that have human and environmental side effects.

- Environmental damage (e.g., from increased herds, palm oil plantations, energy used in production and distribution, plus increased population and consumption).

- Wasted natural resources (e.g., energy, containers, labelling, advertising, marketing, global transport, waste disposal)

- Increased health costs (more frequent or more serious illness or both, from cancer to CVD, in women and children; higher rates of metabolic syndrome, osteoporosis, associated fractures, and thus dependent elders with poorer quality of life)

- More post-partum maternal haemorrhage and anaemia, shorter interbirth intervals and so greater rates of maternal depletion and death.

- Altered human microbiome and decreased human immune repertoire, thus poorer responsiveness to existing and newly emergent microbial threats.

- Societal costs of lower IQ (at both ends of the distribution curve particularly).

- Increased early-life exposure to compounds shown to have effects on reproductive tissue: possible effects on fertility and gender behaviour

- Increased antibiotic use and resistance (due to both bovine herd effects and higher illness rates in children).

- SIDS epidemic facilitated by prone sleeping in response to greater infant distress.

- NEC epidemic among premature infants fed bovine protein

- Damage and death from higher rates of maternal child abuse, neglect, and non-accidental injury

- Cultural loss and family dislocation especially among oppressed minorities

- Societal costs of increased rates of mental disorders: depression, autism, schizophrenia, attachment difficulties.

- Increased social inequity as the disadvantaged are further disadvantaged by artificial feeding, reducing chances of social mobility.

Figure 2-11-3 Some of infant formula's collateral damage

---

568 *Food Chemical News* 14 August 1989, pp. 18–19.

All these harms have their greatest impact on disadvantaged peoples, communities, and individuals, contributing to social and global inequality. Indigenous peoples in particular have suffered more than dominant elites as a result of the loss of traditional normal infant feeding practices such as sustained breastfeeding beyond twelve months of life. Chronic otitis media, for example, virtually unknown among the Inuit before bottle feeding,[569] is a greater danger where antibiotics are not easily obtained. Adult onset diabetes, strongly associated with infant formula feeding among the Pima Indians of North America,[570] is harder to manage in conditions of disadvantage or poverty. So too is asthma, much more common in children not exclusively breastfed.[571] Formula-fed babies are already fatter at twelve months[572] and are more likely to become obese wherever fresh food is hard to access. Poverty's disadvantages are deepened by bottle-feeding artificial formulas. And vice versa.

## Formula and allergies

Allergy and autoimmune disorders have increased in parallel with significant changes in infant formula ingredients and manufacture, which led to infants being exposed very young to known toxins as well as some of Western society's most common allergens. Some of the most common allergens are: milk, soy, eggs, wheat, peanuts, corn.

These have all been fed to infants in artificial substitutes for breastmilk, and some still are. It is reasonable to ask whether these are common allergens *because* they were used in formula in the nineteenth and early twentieth century. Independent research is needed into precisely when and where they were first given to neonates, in relation to allergy prevalence. That exposure to alien proteins via infant formula has sensitised babies is part of the milk hypothesis.

Not surprisingly, formula manufacturers have taken advantage of the rise in allergies to produce extensively hydrolysed and hypoallergenic varieties of formula that can be tolerated by the increasing numbers of babies allergic to the proteins they or their parents were exposed to in 'ordinary' formula. By the next generation we can expect to see infants reacting to those formulas, and new ones created. There is much more about these issues in Books 2 and 3.

569 Schaefer O. Otitis media and bottle-feeding. An epidemiological study of infant feeding habits and incidence of recurrent and chronic middle ear disease in Canadian Eskimos. (PMID:5133823) *Can J Public Health* 1971; 62(6):478–89.

570 Pettit DJ, Forman MR, Hanson RL, Knowles WC et al Breastfeeding and incidence of NIDDM in Pima Indians. *Lancet* 1997; 350: 166–68. I asked Dr. Pettit to review infant feeding in relation to diabetes for a 1995 conference I organised under the auspices of ALCA Vic Branch and the Mercy Hospital, Melbourne. This study was the result. Unlike me, he had not expected to find such a correlation, but had data that could be used to ask and answer the question. The results were clear-cut.

571 Ye M, Mandhane PJ, Senthilselvan A. Association of breastfeeding with asthma in young Aboriginal children in Canada. (PMID:23248799) Free full text article *Can Respir J* 2012; 19(6):361–66.

572 Gale C, Logan KM, Santhakumaran S, Parkinson JR et al. Effect of breastfeeding versus formula feeding on infant body composition: systematic review and meta-analysis. *Am J Clin Nutr* 2012 95; 656–69.

# 2.12 Conclusions, or beginnings?

Despite all that, it has to be said that few of the specific associations between infant formula and western ill health mentioned throughout this book has been, or can ever be, proven beyond all shadow of doubt. Only because in science, *nothing* is ever proved *beyond doubt*: we rely on a working consensus based on evaluation of available evidence. Just as with climate issues, scientific consensus about the link between artificial feeding and ill-health *has* been reached, despite continuing debate about many details, and many successful efforts to create doubt in the minds of those without access to the scientific literature. Bloggers oversimplify and distort selective findings and makes sweeping claims of safety that industry would not dare to do. (That these are usually well-intentioned, motivated to make other women feel better about their use of infant formula, is sad, because women and children may die as a result of their misplaced advocacy.) Doubt weakens any popular or national will to change that might inconvenience those profiting from the status quo. Breastfeeding advocates have shoestring budgets, while the merchants of doubt[573] are often well-paid.

However, the infant formula industry actually agrees with the basic facts underpinning my milk hypothesis, and can be relied upon to spread the word, though with their own very different spin on it. Consider this statement by Danone/Nutricia researchers:

> Accumulating evidence suggests that nutrition during pregnancy and early postnatal life is one of the most important environmental cues that programs microbiological, metabolic, and immunologic development. The neonatal period is crucial for the early microbial colonisation of the almost sterile gastrointestinal tract of the newborn infant. These first colonisers play an important role in host health because they are involved in nutritional, immunologic, and physiologic functions. Evidence from animal and human studies indicates that the composition of the gut microbiota has an effect on body composition, digestion, and metabolic homeostasis. Furthermore, the functionality of the metabolism develops after birth when the newborn is first exposed to nutrition via the gastrointestinal tract. Exposure to environmental microbial components is also suggested to have a key role in the maturation process of the immune system, and in turn the immune system shapes the composition of the microbiota.[574]

Well, of course I agree with all that. It's what this book is arguing is fact, not supposition. And in the real world, those concerned with existing health problems are rapidly developing microbial therapies to address disorders related to gut dysbiosis. For the infant formula industry, the logical consequences of those facts are also clear:

> Therefore, the use of nutritional strategies to program the microbiota composition to favor a more beneficial bacterial population and to support the development of the metabolic

573  Michaels D. *Merchants of Doubt:* op. cit.

574  Nauta AJ, Kaouther BA, Knol J, Garssen J et al. Relevance of pre- and postnatal nutrition to development and interplay between the microbiota and metabolic and immune systems. *Am J Clin Nutr* 2013; 98 (2): 586S-593S. DOI: 10.3945/ ajcn.112.039644

and immune systems may provide a good opportunity to prevent later health problems such as obesity, diabetes, and allergy.[575]

True, true. And it is very important for those already affected that such strategies are developed. But it simply does not seem to dawn on industry or some health care professionals – or if it does, they certainly do not publicise the idea – that the perfect 'nutritional strategy' already exists. *It is human lactation and breastfeeding.* I believe that women's milk matters so much that society needs to be actively enabling breastfeeding, not pressuring mothers for whom breastfeeding is often impossible, and financially penalising those who take time out of the workforce to make breastfeeding their children a priority.

There are libraries of powerful scientific research about lactation and epigenetics and child development. Recent discoveries showing substantial differences in brain development in very young children should persuade any sane person that it is critical to recognise the importance of breastfeeding. No one has to prove that this is harmful: industry has to prove it is safe to distort brain growth, preferably obtaining fully informed consent from the parents of its human guinea pigs. Similarly, animal research that shows profound impacts on maternal behaviour, cascading inter-generationally, does not really have to prove its relevance to humans. We are mammals, and while we have perhaps more complex skills and language, evolution has not set us that far apart biologically from the rest of our kind. Lactation is still a fundamental biological process that affects women's health and happiness. A very recent short film on YouTube tries to express how deeply.[576]

But what convinced me so profoundly that I have spent a lifetime in this crusade was not just the science. It was my own lived experience, described in Appendix 3. It was the lived experience and emotions of the hundreds of families I have dealt with since 1976. And it was also the reality of infant formula development in the twentieth century. Book 2 relates that history; Book 3 summarises the experience, and offers a strategy that has helped some people.

The same old lie about formula being 'just like breastmilk' has been told for decades – since the days of evaporated milk formulas (which nobody now claims are anything like breastmilk), and even right in the middle of scandals that brought down one major formula brand. 'Only Osterfeed gets it right' preceded the seven million-pound recall and eventual disappearance of the brand. After hearing the same old lie for decades about products that have been remixed, redesigned and reformulated many times over, there is no particular reason to believe that a 2014 formulation is any closer to breastmilk in composition or effect than earlier efforts. The same claim was made about its predecessor and undoubtedly will be made again about its replacement. Neptune is (usually) closer to the Sun than Pluto is, but it's still not close!

Like other educated western parents, even the best formula advocates and bloggers, I once thought I knew enough about infant formula development to be sure of its safety

---

575  ibid.
576  Clare Boyle, Love Breastfeeding https://www.youtube.com/watch?v=k4i7gj8BsB8

and efficacy in a developed country. I used it during weaning or when convenient, as most women of my generation did. That was before I began reading *industry's scientific* literature. I now understand that what little most educated western parents 'know' is a pastiche promoted by industry marketing, and written by industry collaborators who, naturally, do not emphasise any problems before they have come up with something they can sell as solutions.

As I view the history of artificial feeding, it is not a triumphal progress from perfection to perfection, as advertising has always, illogically, claimed. What Ben Goldacre has said about drug development is very pertinent to infant formula development (much of it by those same drug companies[577]):

> Drugs are tested by the people who manufacture them, in poorly designed trials, on hopelessly small numbers of weird, unrepresentative patients, and analysed using techniques which are flawed by design, in such a way that they exaggerate the benefits of treatments. Unsurprisingly, these trials tend to produce results that favour the manufacturer. When trials throw up results that companies don't like, they are perfectly entitled to hide them from doctors and patients, so we only ever see a distorted picture of any drug's true effects. Regulators see most of the trial data, but only from early on in a drug's life, and even then they don't give this data to doctors or patients, or even to other parts of government. This distorted evidence is then communicated and applied in a distorted fashion. In their forty years of practice after leaving medical school, doctors hear about what works through ad hoc oral traditions, from sales reps, colleagues or journals. But those colleagues can be in the pay of drug companies – often undisclosed – and the journals are too. And so are the patient groups. And finally, academic papers, which everyone thinks of as objective, are often covertly planned and written by people who work directly for the companies, without disclosure.[578]

Every last word of Goldacre's summary is as true for infant formula as for other manufactured medical interventions. Formula corporations employ nearly all the world's experts in this area directly or indirectly, and these are the people consulted when proposals for regulation are made. With nutrients and additives, the infant formula corporations have created problems that harm children, then gradually minimised the harms as they became known, lowering protein levels, changing fat blends, reducing unsuspected contaminants, adding missing ingredients discovered through deficiency disease in children or the latest scientific revelation about breastmilk[579] ... the history tells the story.

But even after sufficient proof is in to convince most of the open-minded and informed, it takes decades to change public policy and practice. It does not help either that there are small armies of skilled and highly paid practitioners deliberately, and with extraordinary

---

577   Big Pharma players grew out of the profits from infant formula sales, among them Glaxo and Mead Johnson.

578   Goldacre B. *Bad Pharma. How drug companies mislead doctors and harm patients.* (Fourth Estate Press 2012) Another must-read book for anyone concerned with health.

579   Missing ingredients not mentioned elsewhere in this book are the polyamines, functional compounds thought to be important in gut, liver and pancreas maturation, and the prevention of allergy. First discovered in breastmilk only in 1974, infant formula contains 10 times less, and industry is looking for ways to add them. They can be toxic in excess, however. See Gomez-Gallego C, Periago MJ, Ros G. Infant formula and polyamines in Preedy et al, op. cit., Ch. 16.

cunning, actively spreading lies and concealing inconvenient truths[580] that threaten profits: anyone who doubts that statement should read more widely and be less trustful, especially where billions of dollars, not to mention high-powered careers and the egos that go with them, are at stake.

But the evidence about the harms of artificial feeding is accumulating, and awareness is growing in the scientific community. This book has taken so long to write partly because there is so much more evidence now than there was when I first started talking about the, to me, obvious intergenerational harms of artificial feeding, to course attendees in the 1980s.[581] (People who pay attention to mothers and history and use their common sense could learn a great deal that science might investigate subsequently, to reveal mechanisms of causation. We mothers might get the connections wrong, but our observations are usually accurate. )

By tinkering with infant diet, and undermining breastfeeding, I believe the formula corporations have largely created the global epidemics of obesity and autoimmune disease. What new epidemics will be created as it experiments on babies to find the right blend of microbes and their foods? How dare industry imagine that it can predict the ongoing interaction and evolution of live organisms (some genetically modified and patented) fed to babies? Can parents give informed consent, when so much is locked away as commercial-in-confidence? What regulations can ensure that harms are prevented or identified, when foods for infants are not subject even to the critical scrutiny involved in drug regulation, which many see as inadequate?

It could reasonably be argued that, being a newborn's whole diet for up to six months, infant formula is far more powerful than any drug prescribed for a limited period of time, and so should be regulated much more tightly than any drug. Once industry alters the microbiome of a generation of children, there can be no way of knowing the consequences, and perhaps no way of reining in the effects, for adults and their descendants. Microbes can and do make their own history faster than we make ours. Naturally industry resists any suggestion that tighter global regulation is needed. But the scientists think that it is. As some said,

> It is vital that the increasingly globalised food supply is better regulated, that safety breaches are minimised, and that researchers develop more accurate methods of detecting possible contamination in foods ... Enzyme linked immunosorbent assays, enzymatic amino acid analysis, and colorimetric methods are being used with greater frequency by standards auditors and regulatory agencies world-wide, *although they are still considered too costly and too time-consuming for routine use.*[582]

So even though we are developing the tools that make it possible to detect gross adulteration, these are too expensive? The history of infant formula outlined in Book 2 is proof that clever men simply cannot make 'artificial breast milk' that is as good as the

---

580  See Michaels D. op. cit.

581  A former student then working in research later forwarded me one of the earliest papers on epigenetics with a note saying something like 'This looks like being the explanation for the intergenerational effects you talk about.' She was right. I rejoiced to read it, in those ancient times before open access to PubMed online.

582  Gadoth A, Somers NL. Melamine: adulteration of infant formula, health impacts, and regulatory response.. In Preedy, Watson, Zibadi op. cit., p. 453

milk of ordinary women, though some have always believed this to be a possibility – and a gormless few still do and probably always will. That history consists of brilliant but blinkered research, resulting in accidents and discoveries from adverse outcomes in the unsuspecting experimental subjects provided by loving but deceived parents.

Those parents, and their babies, have paid the price for any improvements made over time; and yes, there have been many such improvements, or errors rectified, as I record. It is true that fewer babies die now as a direct result of formula feeding, at least in the tiny affluent fractions of mankind. But babies still die, even in the USA, which has a truly shameful infant mortality rate for so rich a nation. And in America as around the world, the dead babies are still disproportionately from ethnic minorities and First Nations and other vulnerable groups more often exposed to alien foods too young. And the sales of formula in Asia undoubtedly mean more deaths and damage than ever before in history.

## So to summarise Book 1, my milk hypothesis and its basis:

I believe that feeding babies infant formula and not breastmilk – along with other factors such as abnormal birthing, the needless use of antibiotics, and chemical pollution in all its forms – are key causative factors not only of the 'allergy' epidemic, but also of many other 'diseases of affluence', some of which might perhaps be better labelled 'diseases of artificial feeding'. Researchers need to consider whether NCDs (called Non-Communicable Diseases because not being transmitted horizontally within populations) are in fact being communicated vertically, that is, inter-generationally, in many cases. They are indeed communicable, and communicated in many cases, from parent to child.

I think there is ample evidence to support the idea that women's milk today is far more important to human health in present and future generations than the public and the health professions generally realise. I know that my milk hypothesis is not yet proven beyond reasonable doubt by rigorous science – just like more widely accepted hypotheses, which in fact blend seamlessly with this milk hypothesis. I feel as though these scientists are all focussing on small parts of the whole, while just not seeing the largest elephant in the room of global maternal and child health!

Because parents do affect their children in so many ways, the population-scale experiment of artificial feeding has made definitive scientific proof difficult to obtain: each human child is an experiment of one, and the result of a unique history, as is each community.

By now, however, there is available both accumulating biological evidence that supports the milk hypothesis, and newer technology to investigate its mechanisms of action. The differences in reproductive tissue development seen at four months, or the increase in DNA damage, may be straws in the wind. But the gale may not be far off, once enough scientists and media break both the mental shackles of formula safety propaganda, and the cultural shackles of fearing to make vocal affluent women anxious or angry.

But there are many forms of evidence other than the scientific, with its inherent limitation of working towards relative certainty by a process of proving error.

The cumulative experience of those who work with breastfed babies, and the documented reality of infant formula harms from its beginnings till now, are also forms of evidence I consider important, though they too have their limitations.

The normal physiology and evolutionary history of human infants and their mothers are also forms of evidence: complex interactive systems that are derailed with negative consequences.

And whenever definitive proof of causation is difficult, the default position guiding medical science should always be to work from first principles: First Do No Harm, or in other words, 'avoid unnecessary interventions'. Mother Nature has done better work than Big Pharma over a longer time frame to ensure the health and survival of humankind.

I am convinced that infant feeding is a critical and unpredictable variable in child development, not because of scientific proof about one disease, or even all of them – and the list keeps growing. I am convinced because of basic human immunobiology and the science of lactation. The highly specialised nature of human milk, evolving as both protection and food, tells anyone with a grain of common sense that there must be negative consequences from not feeding babies the thousands of interactive live components in that living milk. That is my belief. I think it more rational than a global blind faith that any serious negative consequences to artificial feeding would be immediately obvious in very limited studies funded mostly by vested interests. The history of capitalism says otherwise; so does the concept of programming.

'Programming' refers to the fact that infants, especially human infants, are born 'immature' – or more flexible and responsive than adults – in many ways. This allows them to adapt to more aspects of the environment that will shape their development. Some can even adapt to weird methods of infant feeding and survive without extreme obvious damage. If this were not so, the artificial feeding experiment could never have succeeded. Programming of development is far from a new belief, but is starting to receive new acknowledgment in scientific circles. This new/old scientific perspective highlights the absolute importance of the milk of human kind being fed to the infants of human kind.

Human infants are also born more dependent on their mothers than virtually every other animal, including the vast majority of mammals (many of which can at least start moving under their own power much earlier than human infants). The growth of our brain makes a large head that creates problems in birthing, unless the infant is born early. Which means that a suitable food must be immediately and reliably available to continue development that otherwise might have happened in utero. Bowlby was so right to see the human infant as an 'obligate extra-utero gestate.' That is, in plain English, as little creatures whose healthy development requires a prolonged after-birth period of maternal care almost as complete as gestation, with food, warmth, and contact security all essential. Breastfeeding, and the breastfeeder's exposure to the infant's environment, can both reasonably be seen as necessities for the healthiest possible development of children; indeed human milk, with its transfer of nutrients and immune assistance, can be seen as a replacement for the umbilicus. The assistance of an adult immune system mediated by milk and skin contact is a fundamental part of the child's interaction with its environment. Milk is a powerful pathway into the environment the child must grow to deal with as an independent being. Milk matters.

My passion on this topic has developed from my decades of learning, from evidence as scientists define it and as historians understand it, and from the evidence of parental experience, mine and countless others. I am appalled that in my lifetime artificial feeding has grown from an enterprise worth only two billion dollars in 1979 to one worth thirty to fifty billion dollars.[583] This modern plague is distorting health worldwide. My hope is that readers will find the following history of formula both interesting and shocking – and perhaps life changing. Read Book 2, and see whether you agree with this summary by a researcher:

> The vigorous change from the evolutionarily highly conserved system of breastfeeding to artificial infant feeding during a most sensitive and vulnerable window of metabolic, hypothalamic and immunological programming apparently represents the most serious error of modern medicine, laying the foundation for the worldwide epidemic of diseases of civilisation. [584]

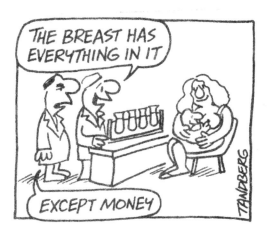

Figure 2-12-1 Tandberg says it all. Image © Ron Tandberg 1996. Used with permission.

---

583 Renfrew R. 7% growth for 50billion global infant nutrition market.
Zenith International, April 2014. http://www.zenithinternational.com/articles/1355?7%25+growth+for+%2450+Billion+global+infant+nutrition+market. See also The Statistics Portal, baby food market sales value, 2010 and 2015. http://www.statista.com/statistics/249469/global-baby-food-market-size-2015/ It can be difficult to obtain a breakdown by product and by company, although these were once available in Australia. The industry has become shy since about 2004.

584 Melnik BC in Preedy, Watson & Zibadi, op. cit., p. 548

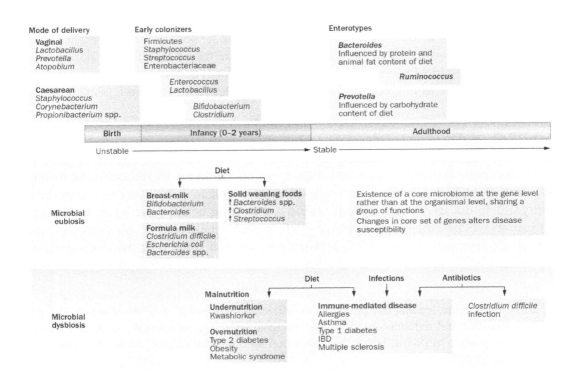

Figure 2-12-2 Diet, gut microbiota and dysbiosis. Image from Jain N, Walker WA.  Diet and host–microbial crosstalk in postnatal intestinal immune homeostasis. *Nat Rev Gastroenterol Hepatol* 2015; 12, 14–25; doi:10.1038/nrgastro.2014.153 Reprinted by permission from Macmillan Publishers Ltd: *Nature Reviews Gastroenterology & Hepatology* 2015;12, 14–25 , © 2015

On page 88, I referred to a serious inconsistency in this diagram. Its existence illustrates beautifully the power and pervasiveness of the myth of infant formula equivalence. Can you spot it? Yes, it's the fact that 'formula milk' and breastmilk are listed together in the section titled 'microbial eubiosis',  even though the diagram clearly shows that formula results in a microbiome different from the  human norm, breastmilk. That to me, by definition, is dysbiosis. So 'formula milk' belongs in the section titled 'microbial dysbiosis'. Formula is in fact the infancy diet that introduces or entrenches potential and actual pathogens in the infant gut. Why else are manufacturers spending vast sums to change what it does, to try to achieve the outcome of a microbiome ever more like that of the breastfed infant? Yet all the research, as well as clinical experience, tells us that they have not achieved that outcome, and probably never will. What infant formula produces is dysbiosis, at the most critical point in a child's life, when the gut directs so much other development. Let's start telling the truth about this to parents, not just the scientific community.

# BOOK 2

# Creating a 'perfect' breastmilk substitute: reality and myths

# Foreword

In 1985, I had just completed graduate work in anthropology, after spending two years immersed in the Bambara culture of Mali, West Africa, where formula was essentially unheard of. Among the many interesting things I learned from Bambara women was that the transfer of breast milk from mother to child was what linked them together. Breast milk was made from a woman's blood, and breastfeeding created bonds of kinship between a mother and any child she breastfed. I was then nursing my first child, and I went on to nurse two more, to do further research on breastfeeding and weaning, and to be an outspoken advocate for mothers and their children.

In 1985, a number of scholarly books concerned with breastfeeding were published, including Maureen Minchin's *Breastfeeding Matters*. I vividly remember reading her book for the first time and thinking, "Finally, someone who gets it. Someone who understands the value of breast milk and breastfeeding for normal human development." Now, some thirty years later, I am delighted and profoundly grateful that Maureen Minchin has, yet again, put her heart and soul into another book on the importance of infant feeding. This three-part book is an exhaustive survey of how much more we now know about both why and how breastfeeding matters – to our children, to us as mothers, and to all of us as members of the human community. So much that is written about infant formula begins from the assumption that formula is both necessary and safe, a close second-best to breastmilk. The reality is that infant formula is not now, and indeed can never be, anywhere close to breast milk in terms of its health-promoting and nutritional qualities. The reality is that the widespread acceptance of infant formula as a replacement for breast milk and breastfeeding continues to cause enormous amounts of misery and suffering for children and parents alike.

Book Two explores the fascinating and disturbing history of the attempts to create a substitute for mother's milk that wouldn't automatically kill infants, but would allow many of them to survive with only apparently mild to moderate impairments in their immunological systems, cognitive resources and metabolic processes. Minchin has brought together a wide-ranging and extensive set of resources that will give readers a deeper understanding of how imperfect and problematic infant formula still is today. And she reminds us, once again, that breastfeeding truly matters. To borrow her own words . . . "breastfeeding my children taught me how to be a mother . . . the bonds breastfeeding creates are unbreakable." Indeed, breastfeeding does matter, for so many reasons.

Katherine A. Dettwyler, Ph.D.
Anthropology professor at the University of Delaware;
author, *Breastfeeding: biocultural perspectives*, and
*Dancing Skeletons: life and death in West Africa*.

# CHAPTER 3

# Infant formula, past, present and future

"A century ago, babies who couldn't be breast-fed usually didn't survive. Today, although breast-feeding is still the best nourishment for infants, infant formula is a close enough second that babies not only survive but thrive." So said a 1996 article in the official organ of the US Food and Drug Administration, *FDA Consumer*.[585] One heading summed up what many twentieth-century parents believed: 'Infant Formula (Artificial Breast Milk)'.

That single quotation contains two powerful myths: most babies died on early formulas, and (all) babies thrive on modern formulas.

The fact is that firstly, despite not being breastfed, many babies have always survived, and always will, especially when clean water and antibiotics are available. Infant mortality rates of 400 per 1000 are horrendous, but even then the majority survive: many impaired, and only the well-breastfed able to reach their full potential. Not all survivors will have children, but many of the damaged will, as Western history demonstrates. And secondly, most early-formula-fed babies did indeed 'thrive' (in the limited sense of grow or increase), many quite excessively: obesity has become a global problem, and even industry scientists acknowledge the contribution of the distorted growth parameters produced by infant formula.

Infant survival rates and growth improved as cows' milk formulas replaced older and even worse options, but early 20th century parents knew that breastfeeding was important to child health. Not until the second half of the twentieth century did western parents and professionals alike believe that industrial mixes were virtually equivalent to breastmilk. Millions more, even from child-centred cultures, are buying into this dominant western myth, that babies truly *thrive* on breastmilk substitutes. "Thrive" conveys a sense of healthy

---

585 Stehlin I. 'Infant formula, second best but good enough'. *FDA Consumer*, June 1996. This is no longer found on the USFDA website, but is still on the web, with FDA attribution, at athttp://pregnancy.about.com/od/formula/Infant_Formula_Artificial_Breast_Milk.htm http://pregnancy.about.com/cs/breastfeedinginfo/l/blbreastorbottl.htm

flourishing, maximising potential, optimal development, not just increasing in size. How did we get to this point, and is that assumption of almost equivalence justified? Is our current formula a 'close-enough second' as the USFDA trumpeted to the world in 1996? Is 'near enough good enough' for babies' brains and bodies?

That belief in equivalence, in 'artificial breastmilk', is perhaps the single most powerful myth ever created, allowing humans to abandon a fundamental survival mechanism, lactation and breastfeeding. Companies have consistently marketed their current formulas as almost equivalent breastmilk substitutes, so close as to make no real difference, even as perfect foods for infants, "richer" in nutrients than breastmilk. They have consistently played on parents' fears, knowing that protecting their young is a basic animal instinct. They still do. Politicians and professionals and parents have believed them, and many still do. Who or what does infant formula protect? Just how perfect was, and is, infant formula? Are today's formulas, as industry claims, 'a perfect mix of science and love'?

The following overview, a partial interpretative history, should put paid to any such foolish notions. Within a loose chronology, it outlines some selected aspects of how infant formula has developed over time. This exposes some of its many defects and their impacts that – considered collectively[586] – are to me the strongest evidence to date for my Milk Hypothesis.

I hope that this book will give rise to much more specifically targeted and detailed histories, work that describes in greater depth just when, and how, and which infant formulas have invaded and affected different populations and sub-cultures world-wide. And describes it from a perspective more akin to mine, that such substitution for the real thing can only be a fundamental mistake. To date, even those who have written well about infant feeding have usually done so from *within* the dominant assumptions of safety and near-equivalence the infant formula industry has cultivated. I believe that both infant formula itself, and the loss of breastfeeding, are keys to far more substantial change in nations, in cultures, and in human bodies, than has yet been realised. I hope this history helps explain why so many have missed seeing the wood of subtle and fundamental damage for the trees of survival and immediate growth.

# 3.1 Background to a nutrition revolution

Babies are born to be breastfed. A wealth of evidence supports the World Health Organization's (WHO) global recommendation of breastfeeding solely for six months, and partially for at least the first couple of years. This evolutionarily normal pattern of infant feeding often results in inter-birth intervals of between three and four years.[587] This has obvious benefits for the health and wellbeing of women, who benefit from lactation hormones and can replenish their body stores before the next pregnancy. Historically, any

---

586  New information about details that I may have got wrong is highly unlikely to change the overall weight of the argument from the evidence of formulas' constant need for improvement and modification. Every month brings new discoveries about formulas' problems and mammalian milks' 'incredible sophistication."

587  Potts M, Short RV *Ever since Adam and Eve: the evolution of human sexuality* (Cambridge University Press, 1998) pp. 152–4.

artificial feeding meant many more frequent births, in times of high infant and maternal mortality. Women's key role was producing children. Patrilineal families accepted as usual the toll this took. A woman was readily replaced if too-frequent childbearing exhausted or killed her, as it still does today in cultures where access to fertility control is difficult.

In our own family history, for example, a clergy wife, Mary Ann Wright, died at the age of forty-seven after producing nineteen children between 1816 and 1839. Almost every year (after her marriage at the age of twenty-one) brought a baby; the longest interbirth interval was two years, after a set of twins. The widower re-married, naturally, and went on to a ripe old age. Where a woman died after producing a mere six or seven children, her successor would often produce as many: such large families were the foundation of the unprecedented population explosion that has resulted in huge environmental pressures on the planet. It was widely understood across social classes that breastfeeding reduced fertility: unacceptable to many men, as the high infectious disease rates meant some children would die young. Mary Ann could not have breastfed her children even for six months, or fewer babies would have been born. Most of her children survived infancy (which says that they were at least initially wet-nursed), and went on to populate the far-flung British Empire, with sons in the civil service or armed forces in Australia, New Zealand, Ceylon, India, South Africa, and England, and daughters marrying well. The family prospered. That was what children were for, in the aspiring middle class.

For more affluent families, children could be of value as pawns in the marriage mart (though we know from Jane Austen, daughters could be a burden as well as the source of family enrichment.) There was a longstanding tradition of Western upper-class mothers not themselves breastfeeding, to increase family size. Wealthier families chose wet nurses to feed their infants, despite many concerns – moral and practical – about the consequences; and also despite the grief and pain this undoubtedly caused some birth mothers, who had little choice but to be brood stock, producing and giving up their children to the care of others after a brief breastfeeding interlude or none.

For poorer families, children were of value as potential caregivers for the very old and very young, and as workers, contributing pitiful wages that could mean the difference between survival and utter destitution. While breastfeeding could result in lower infant mortality in slum conditions, poorer women often breastfed for lack of any alternative, although breastfeeding could also restrict their earning capacity. Loss of a woman's income could mean starvation. However, not fully breastfeeding also increased the likelihood of another pregnancy and birth, with its attendant risks. Repeated childbearing and breastfeeding by women on desperately poor diets resulted in maternal depletion syndromes that shortened women's lives (now as then). Poverty and poor complementary feeding diet resulted in high infant death rates during weaning, as they do today in poor communities. Farming out young children to be hand-reared or dry-nursed was frequently fatal.

So: *where many babies were wanted,* breastfeeding duration was often limited to hasten the return of fertility: early weaning was encouraged, and wet nurses used to increase survival chances of mother-weaned babies. This association of breastfeeding with lower-class status persisted over time in Anglophone society, and not until the Western breastfeeding revival of the 1970s would this be reversed. Using wet nurses was widespread wherever it could be afforded; it was even nationally organised in France.[588] Some mothers mourned the loss of breastfeeding, others who had experienced nipple pain and mastitis regarded the whole process of lactation with distaste and fear: infection could be fatal in the days before antibiotics. Breastfeeding then as now was a cause of immense emotional concern,[589] and a pressure on women who wanted their babies to live and thrive. To have enough milk to feed their babies often meant reliance on other women's milk at times, then as now.

Where *many babies were not especially wanted, but were seen as valuable* if they arrived, breastfeeding was encouraged both to decrease fertility and increase survival chances. By the late nineteenth century it was realised that for a nation to have labourers and armies, poor babies needed to survive. By the early twentieth century those in power would support moves to improve the feeding practices of the poor.

Where *babies were not wanted and could not be reared* by poor families or single mothers, abandonment, or artificial feeding, or both, was often the tacitly approved means to an early death, though charities tried to keep 'foundlings' (literally found babies) alive. Selective infanticide, pre- or postpartum, deliberate or unintentional, is almost inevitable wherever fertility control is impossible. All this has been well documented by Valerie Fildes,[590] Sarah Blaffer Hrdy,[591] and many others.[592]

Equally well documented is the rise of dairying, and the growth in some communities of the use of animal milks, whether the mares' milk favoured by the Mongols or the cow, goat, and asses' milks used in parts of the Western world. Holland's astonishing seventeenth-century achievements in yield per cow allowed milk to become both a dietary staple and valued export, along with the cheeses and other milk products preserved using salt. Other European farmers took note of what had been achieved, and cheese became a dietary staple in England, now reflected in the modern English pub's invention of the 'ploughman's lunch' of bread, cheese and pickles. Deborah Valenze has documented how 'milk products that were part of customary diets among rural people became thought of as fashionable and desirable for everyone, including urban elites.' Her fascinating book, *Milk: a local and*

---

588  Sussman D. *Selling mothers' milk: the wet nursing business in France 1715–1914* (University of Illinois Press, 1982); Budin P. *The Nursling* (Caxton Publishing House, London 1907; online at http://www.neonatology.org/classics/nursling/figures/title.gif ) Wet nurses were employed to feed premature infants in some American hospitals well into the twentieth century: see Hess JH, Lunden E. *The care and nursing of the premature infant* (Lippincott 1949).

589  For some glimpse of the complex realities, see the essays in Sullivan D, Connolly M (ed) *Unbuttoned. Women open up about the pleasures, pains and politics of breastfeeding.* (Harvard Common Press 2009).

590  Fildes V. *Breasts bottles and babies* (Edinburgh University Press, 1986); *Wet nursing: a history from antiquity to the present* (Blackwell, 1988)

591  Blaffer Hrdy S. *Mother nature: natural selection and the female of the species* (Chatto & Windus, London, 1999); Hausfater G, Blaffer Hrdy S (eds) *Infanticide: comparative and evolutionary perspectives* (Aldine de Gruyter, 1984)

592  Ransel DL. *Mothers of misery: child abandonment in Russia* (Princeton University Press, 1988); Golden J. *A social history of wet nursing in America* (Cambridge University Press, 1996); Sussman D. op. cit.; Potts M, Short RV, op. cit.

*global history*,[593] also describes how milk has been seen and used in Western countries until modern times, but does not go into much detail about changing infant formulas and the decline of breastfeeding, even though so much of the world's milk – in 2011, 1.8 million metric tons a year,[594] 23 per cent of all whey powder produced globally, 12 per cent of all skim milk powder,[595] and rising – now goes into infant formula.

Throughout the nineteenth century, urbanisation, industrialisation and increasing population mobility resulted in the loosening of social constraints that helped keep partners together. Many more women had to fend for themselves and their children as men died in unsafe workplaces, or moved to find work and often with that, new de facto partners. Life was short by modern standards. Maternal malnutrition among the poor was endemic. Infant mortality rates were high, and linked to infant feeding methods: communities that breastfed had lower infant mortality and hospitalisation rates – the Irish poor in England being remarkable for this – so that 'the comparative fewness of Irish in a town could raise the infant death rate, as in Preston.'[596] Preston was the factory town with the second worst diarrhoeal death rate in England, but Mr Pilkington, the Medical Officer of Health, stated that babies of poorly-paid Irish labourers were comparatively exempt 'due to the fact that the latter are almost always fed at the breast.' How sad that modern Irish breastfeeding rates fell to be among the worst in the developed world!

But then as now, maternal ignorance was often blamed for child deaths, rather than unsuitable feeding and poverty. 'Untaught, the human mother is inferior to the cat, inferior even to many insects, which know by instinct how to rear their young rightly.'[597] Such attitudes towards women shaped much of what was to come by way of mothercraft.

The fact that wealthy women did not nurse their own babies required justification. Over the eighteenth and nineteenth centuries there emerged a widespread medical belief that cultured, educated, 'refined' women were incapable of adequate lactation. Some even prophesied that lactation would become extinct in 'the higher orders of society'. Then as now, mothers' milk was talked of as better for babies and more convenient, but also as highly variable, unreliable, and a drain on the mother. (Despite metabolic adaptation, it can indeed be depleting where the mother is seriously malnourished or has other drains on her health. The sane solution is to feed the mother and avoid damaging regimes on her body, not to wean the baby.) Then as now, babies were damaged or killed by makeshift substitutes for breastmilk – paps, gruels, watery porridges, and so on. Some porridges and paps were made with flour and water, or breadcrumbs and small beer. As noted earlier, wet-nursing in western society had many uncomfortable social and ethical dimensions.

---

593 Valenze D. *Milk, a global and local history* (Yale University Press, 2011)
594 Lidefelt J-O. Infant Nutrition. 2011 Investor Seminar for AAK (Danish supplier of vegetable oils to the formula industry) http://www.aak.com/Global/Investor/Infant%20Nutrition%20presentation%20201111115.pdf
595 Lafougere C. Global developments in the infant formula sector. Eucolait General Assembly Helsinki May 2013. http://www.eucolait.be/all-files/general-assembly/2013-helsinki/14397-christophe-lafougere-infant-milk-formula-final/download.
596 Smith FB. *The people's health 1830–1910* (ANU Press Canberra, 1979) p. 91.
597 Dwork D. *War is good for babies and other young children: a history of the infant and child welfare movement in England 1898–1918* (Tavistock Publications London, 1987) p. 16

A better alternative to wet-nursing seemed an urgent necessity, when maternal lactation seemed to be so unreliable, or else was impractical in both industrial settings where poor women were employed, and in polite society.

Thus by the nineteenth century a growing market existed for a substitutes for breastmilk. Scientists, then as now, addressed the issue, often because of the death of their own children. They did not investigate the causes of poor lactation and lactation-related difficulties; they sought to supplement or replace both maternal lactation and wet-nursing. Their stated goal was to replicate human milk; they had complete confidence that this could be done, and that it needed to be done. Then as now, these chemists were not modest in their claims about their products, or far-sighted about questions other than the immediately urgent one of infant survival and growth. They did not understand the physiology of human lactation, and would have dismissed any surviving oral traditions of folk medicine relating to lactation as 'old wives' tales'. It did not occur to them that lactation failure might be avoidable and treatable, or that maternal depletion might be the result of the many artificial demands placed on women's bodies, not least the too-frequent pregnancies (a consequence of lactation failure). Their wives could not successfully breastfeed, so perhaps lactation was becoming extinct in the whole species: Lactation 'is being atrophied in the modern woman; the higher their civilisation, the less able they are to suckle their infants.'[598] But science and industry would ride to the rescue of hungry babies and replace problematic wet-nursing (which they actively campaigned against). The development of nineteenth-century technologies that made animal milks safer, and canned foods possible, was to revolutionise infant feeding.

There are some first-rate histories of infant feeding which deserve explicit recognition here. Valerie Fildes produced two superb books: *Breasts, bottles and babies,*[599] covering the period 1500–1800 in Europe; and *Wet nursing: a history from antiquity to the present.*[600] Rima Apple's *Mothers and medicine*[601] and Jacqueline Wolf's *Don't kill your baby*[602] offer a far more detailed examination of the decline of breastfeeding and development of the early infant formulas in America in the first half of the twentieth century. An excellent recent Canadian history provides a useful comparison.[603] And I must mention Christina Hardyment's scholarly yet delightfully ironic *Dream babies: child care from Locke to Spock,*[604] which covers aspects of child care from 1750 to the present. The broad-brush historical picture I have painted needs to be complemented by the finer detail these scholars and others provide: I am well aware that a more nuanced and complex picture can be drawn in different societies, but that is not within the scope of this outline history of infant formula. The Bibliography lists these and

598 Spargo J. *The common sense of the milk question* (Macmillan NY 1910) p. 17.
599 Fildes V. *Breasts, bottles and babies* (Edinburgh University Press, 1986).
600 *Wet nursing: a history from antiquity to the present (Basil Blackwell Press, 1988)*
601 Apple RD. *Mothers and medicine: a social history of infant feeding 1890–1950* (University of Wisconsin Press, 1987).
602 Wolf JH. *Don't kill your baby: public health and the decline of breastfeeding in the nineteenth and twentieth centuries* (Ohio State University, 2001).
603 Nathoo T, Ostry A. *The one best way? Breastfeeding history, policy and politics in Canada* (Wilfrid Laurier University Press, 2009).
604 Hardyment C. *Dream babies: childcare advice from Locke to Spock* ( Jonathan Cape Ltd London, 1983); updated *Locke to Gina Ford* in the 2007 edition published by Frances Lincoln, London.

many other notable works, all of which have contributed to my understanding of the issue as well as my enjoyment of reading.

But none of these books focuses on the larger whole of twentieth-century infant formula development after 1950 and its impacts, while some seem to me subtly permeated by the pervasive industry myth that current infant formulas are good enough and quite safe, so long as parents are careful. After reading how infant formula has changed, and why, the reader (and many authors) may reconsider industry's constant claim to have come as close as possible to breastmilk and breastfeeding. No doubt when escaping a predator, a turtle comes as close as possible to a cheetah in traversing ground: does the comparison tell you anything meaningful about either animal?

## The 'infant formula' story begins

The story of the product now referred to as 'infant formula' begins with the availability of condensed and dried skim milk, and crude initial chemical analysis methods soon applied to milk components. William Prout's analysis of foods as consisting of 'three great classes, the saccharine, the oily, and the albuminous', was validated by chemists such as Justus von Liebig, who worked tirelessly to create portable and non-perishable foodstuffs such as the beef tea and beef extract that became staples in Victorian times.

Pioneer chemists such as Edward Frankland and von Liebig soon began creating recipes or formulas for alternative 'infant foods', based on cows' milk and cereals, with varying amounts of carbohydrate, fats and protein. Despite damaging deficiencies, these foods were then claimed to be virtually identical to mother's milk, a claim that would be repeated with every new discovery. In 1867 *Home and Hearth* advertised Liebig's 'perfect baby food', a cereal powder to be dissolved in warm milk. (This was more accurately called a soup – bouillie or zuppe – in Europe.) In the same year chemist Henri Nestlé produced the first 'complete' infant food, Farine Lactée, one to which only water was added: it was a powder of malt, milk, sugar, and wheat flour. His son survived this, and so a food empire began. Other patent foods advertised in the mid nineteenth century were mixtures of wheat flour, malt flour and cows' milk, cooked with a little bicarbonate; a powder containing less milk and some pea flour, to be added to fresh cows' milk; others which added malted starches and grape sugar to cereal flours. Of course, in these days before microbiology, herd testing and heat treatment of milk, even unsterile dried milk powders could be bacterially safer than raw milk.

Basically, with these first formulas, cereal-based and gluten-containing infant soups were being fed – as they had been in the porridges and paps – to very young infants, and as always, some of these infants survived. *This was a generation of gluten-exposed infants, and probably the beginnings of the epidemic of gluten intolerance to come in Western nations, as we now know that exposure to gluten under three months of age increases the likelihood of sensitivity.*

However, in the era before antibiotics, only the healthiest of these nineteenth- and early twentieth-century children would survive the potent interactions between germs, gut disturbances and dietary deficiencies, and live to breed the next generation. Any upper respiratory or ear infection could be fatal, and artificial feeding has always been associated with higher rates of such infections, though rarely remarked on before 1980 except in the case of Inuit families.[605] In an age where every family expected to lose some children to infectious diseases, the adverse health impacts of these early baby foods would have been accepted as unavoidable in the overall high toll of infant and young child mortality. But it is also not surprising that, as these artificial substitutes for mothers' milk grew in popularity in the last quarter of the nineteenth century in England, the mortality rate actually rose despite some public health improvements. [606]

These nineteenth-century foods for babies were patented, right from the start, as infant formulas still are. They were described as perfect infant foods, as infant formulas still are: in 2012 Wyeth even claimed to provide 'the perfect mix of science and love.' Such modesty! Initially many were advertised as suitable both for infants and for under-nourished mothers or invalids. They were a key part of an era of tonic foods and drinks, usually cereal-based, and were advertised widely in journals aimed at the increasing numbers of now literate women with the money to buy them.

The increase in female education that characterised the nineteenth century – and was deplored by many men – meant that popular print resources reached more women then ever.[607] Young Mrs Beeton's famous book, a triumph of marketing, was just one omnibus of home management and infant care; she obviously did not enjoy breastfeeding, seeing it as 'a period of privation and penance' for the mother, which required the use of malt liquor 'to support her strength during the exhausting process'.[608] A pioneer bottle-feeder of considerable influence, Isabella Beeton died of puerperal fever at the age of twenty-eight, a week after giving birth to her fourth child; two of her children had died before her, her first at three months old, after six days of diarrhoeal disease. Her own death may have been related to the custom of wealthy women to wait until the child was three days old before putting it to the breast.[609] Mastitis was often involved in cases of puerperal fever, and damaged nipples could also be a portal of fatal infection in the pre-antibiotic era. Strangely, the role of infant feeding was not considered in the otherwise excellent recent account of Beeton's life and times,[610] despite her statement that lactation was more likely to be successful in 'the nerveless cow' than in women! Isabella's fate was deeply ironic. She was one of the first in what has become a veritable library of unsuccessful breastfeeders advising other women badly about

605 Schaefer O. Otitis media and bottle-feeding: an epidemiological study of infant feeding habits and incidence of recurrent and chronic middle ear disease in Canadian Eskimos. (PMID:5133823) *Can J Public Health* 1971; 62(6):478–89.

606 Dwork, op. cit.

607 The growth of popular publications and their content is well described in Hughes, K. *The short life and long times of Mrs Beeton.* (Harper Perennial, 2006).

608 *Mrs Beeton's book of household management* (Chancellor Press London, 1982; Facsimile edition of the original published in 1861) p. 1035.

609 Smith FB, op. cit. p. 83.

610 Hughes, K. op. cit. Syphilis may well have been involved, as Hughes posits, but to omit consideration of Isabella's failed breastfeeding as a factor in the health of both mother and child is unwarranted, given Beeton's writing on the subject.

breastfeeding[611], with many remaining ignorant of the causes of their own problems. And that ignorance may have been fatal for her, as well as for some of her readers.

Figure 3-1-1 Frightening mothers into formula feeding

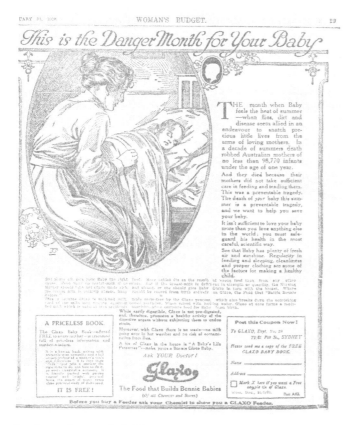

Other home compendia were similarly depressing about breastfeeding: the Ward Lock Home Book stressing that 'should a mother give her milk to her child when she has been suffering from agitation caused by sorrow or fright, she will likely kill it', so that 'even mild worry should be avoided strenuously.'[612] Doubtless then as now many women worried about being worried – or 'stressed' in twentieth-century parlance – or else worried about what to feed their babies instead of their toxic milk. Hardly helpful advice!

Articles in ladies' journals undermined the confidence of women readers, suggesting that their milk might not be good enough in quantity or quality, and that supplements would benefit both mother and child. Then as now, there were many messages that breastfeeding was just too difficult or painful for any woman to succeed, or that the stress of modern life was incompatible with breastfeeding, while artificial feeding was convenient and safe.[613] Advertisements for patent foods also vilified wet nurses, playing on the complex emotions that can be generated by giving one's child to other women to breastfeed. Marketing also made unjustified claims about patent foods' safety and convenience, as formula advertisements ever since have done. Read the fine print in the foregoing Glaxo advertisement from 1920, and you will see the recurrent themes of industry advertising.

---

611  Check out what Beeton has to say about alcohol intake for both mothers and wet-nurses, for example! Though she was aware of diet affecting maternal milk long before some doctors. She includes many old wives' tales that were still current a hundred years after her book was published.

612  *Home book, a domestic cyclopaedia forming a companion volume to Mrs Beeton's book of household management* (Ward Lock & Co, nd) p. 419.

613  It has always surprised me that the advice of those who have not succeeded at breastfeeding is considered authoritative, while the failed athlete or morbidly obese dietician would generally not be accepted as a reliable guide in their own field, however interesting their personal story might be.

That lactation faltered or failed in the real world of women then was understandable. But when mothers do not understand the reasons for their breastfeeding failure, they can become unconsciously invested in seeing other women fail. Other mothers' success can feel like a reproach, or a proof of their own inadequacy, even of their unfitness as mothers. This is never helped by insensitive pressure to breastfeed. When articulate mothers react against and rationalise their own inability to breastfeed successfully, the advice they give helps bring about breastfeeding failure for other women (then as now). Mothers can heavily influence their daughters' breastfeeding outcomes. Literate women,[614] society's opinion leaders, in America[615] and Australia and Britain alike, led the way to formula feeding.[616] Some even became active formula advocates, distributing the products free to poor families in seriously mistaken gestures of benevolence that were in fact excellent marketing strategies for commercial products. Modelling the elite's use of any product is classic marketing strategy, which is why industry is happy to give free supplies to wealthy women of note, such as assorted royals. Royal babies were worth more than their weight in gold to firms lucky enough to supply such households.

Figure 3-1-2 Formula as the choice of the social elite

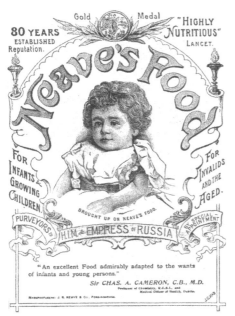

Many 'hand-fed' babies survived, as the innate adaptability of human babies is phenomenal: some survive the strangest diets, though not without damage. And some babies grew enormous by comparison with breastfed children, since their nutrient intake vastly exceeded what was needed for normal growth. Thus began the advertising cult of hugely fat babies, promoted as success stories by companies such as Mellin's and Mead Johnson and Nestlé, in their free handout literature, and via baby shows. Western mothers today might be appalled by the morbidly-obese Michelin-man blobs in industry publications (see the advertising images of babies below). Pritchard's trenchant criticism is memorable:

These patent foods were, and I regret to say, still are the delight of mothers ... the infant grows visibly and ponderably fatter, and to the parents' inexpressible delight presents the appearance of an infant Hercules. Who cannot recognise at sight a patent-food baby veiling under his outward serenity the germs of latent and inevitable trouble? Large, square-headed,

614  The influence of literacy on women's self-awareness and decision-making about infant care is well described in Mein Smith P. *Mothers and king baby: infant survival and welfare in an imperial world: Australia 1880–1950* (Macmillan Press, 1997). Anyone discussing the influence of welfare services in Australia should read this excellent detailed account.

615  Levenstein H. Best for babies or preventable infanticide? The controversy over artificial feeding of infants in America 1880-1920. *J Am Hist* 1983; 70 (1): 75–94.

616  My third book, *Breastfeeding matters* (1985) first made the point that affluent women led the way into and out of bottle-feeding following the advice of health professionals, and that industry followed almost as much as it led the trend. As I see it, this is still the case.

fatuously complacent, pot-bellied, spade handed and dumpy-footed, for all the world presenting the appearance of animated jelly.[617]

But to mothers then, even these fat-encased stupefied pupae were wonderfully reassuring, a proof that babies 'thrived' on the patent food. And after all, weight gain was the measure industry has always used to judge the success of infant formula! To call a baby 'fat as a little pig' was to compliment the mother in early twentieth-century England.[618] At 28 pounds in weight, aged eleven months, Master Buck was fat as a little pig indeed! Miss Dodson, 25 pounds at 9 months, seemed less happy with her lot.[619]

Figure 3-1-3 Patent food babies

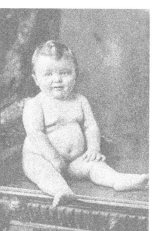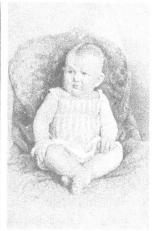

It should perhaps be said here that mothers' love of the fat baby is global, and very understandable. Many healthy breastfed babies kept in arms (to keep them safe in unsafe environments) do rapidly grow plump, stacking on up to 500 grams a week for a time, while being incredibly healthy and at no risk of later obesity. The condition such babies put on in the first months helps them survive epidemics and the malnutrition that threatens during the danger times of weaning and being off the breast altogether. For parents to value weight gain in young babies is sensible –when it is the right sort of weight gain. Seeing wealthier women with chubby babies attracts mimicry of their presumed methods of feeding. The mother who publicly feeds even breastmilk from a bottle can be inadvertently discouraging breastfeeding and promoting artificial formula feeding from a bottle.

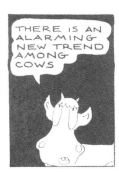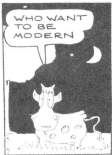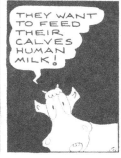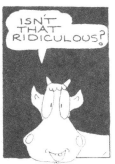

Figure 3-1-4 A modern trend in cows. Image from *Protecting Infant Health: a healthworker's guide to the Internaitonal Code of Marketing of Breastmilk Substitutes.* (ICDC 1993 edition)

617  Cited in Mepham TB. 'Humanizing milk': the formulation of artificial feeds for infants 1850–1910. *Medical history,* 1993; 37:225–49
618  Ross E. *Love and toil: motherhood in outcast London 1870–1918* (Oxford University Press, 1993) p. 141.
619  Images from Mellin G. *How to feed babies and invalids.* (Cassell &Co, 1893).

# 3.2 Making cows' milk safe enough to use industrially

Milk will always carry bacteria to the offspring, and help create a favourable microbiome. Hand-expressed cows' milk is a fragile product, inevitably contaminated (which is good for calves) due to the location of udders near anuses, and so spoiling within hours at room temperatures. Thus societies with domesticated lactating animals usually fermented or heated or otherwise sanitised or preserved milk, while many developed tolerance of its usual pathogens, from living in the same environment, even under the same roof in winter, as their animals. But in the early twentieth century milk was still seen as a dangerous product, with good reason, as the recent death of a child underlines.[620]

Decades before, the first steps towards making raw cows' milk a safer food for an urban public had been taken. In 1863, French chemist and biologist Louis Pasteur invented a method of killing harmful bacteria in food that could be heat-treated; in 1886 Franz Ritter von Soxhlet developed a better method. 'Pasteurisation' was born. It was very experimental and varied, and was not universally approved for infants' milk: some doctors expressed concerns about the effects of heat treatment on milk components. Raw cows' milk freshly produced and fed is indeed a different product from heat-treated or stale milk: 'new' milk had been used in the past as therapy for adults with digestive disorders, with some reported success. Raw milk[621] of varying quality, often then boiled, was the mainstay of very early artificial feeding: diluted and supplemented with sugars and starches and even oils. Sugars used included lactose, sucrose, and cereal-derived malt; after 1912 'dextri-maltose' produced from potato starch was an alternative to lactose in some US formulas, and even cheaper corn by-products would take over once the agricultural boom in corn developed.

There were many problems with fresh milk which technology would gradually address. Cream had long been skimmed off for making butter, leaving variable amounts in fresh milk. In 1871 the development of a mechanised cream separator allowed cream to be treated as a separate industrial material and product. Some of the early homemade 'formulas' used skim milk to which a percentage of cream, or 'top milk', was added back, in varying amounts depending on infant caloric needs and tolerance. This continued well into the twentieth century, and early child health manuals gave details of how to identify infant fat excess or

---

620 In December 2014 raw milk bought from a healthfood store has been implicated in the death of a child and illness in others.

621 According to one review, 'there is a growing body of epidemiological evidence suggesting that consumption of unprocessed cow's milk does not increase but rather decreases the risk of asthma, hay fever and atopic sensitisation.' See Braun-Fahrländer C, von Mutius E. 'Can farm milk consumption prevent allergic diseases?' *Clinical and Experimental Allergy*, 2011, 41(1):29–35. DOI: 10.1111/j.1365-2222.2010.03665.x. This may be the result of intact immune factors such as TGF-β. Oddy WH. Transforming growth factor β in milk. In Zibadi et al, op. cit., Ch. 23. Raw milk remains contentious in the United States and other countries, for medical and economic reasons. 'Raw' milk is the term now used for what was once called 'fresh' milk. Yet heat-treated milk is not called 'cooked' or 'processed', but 'pasteurised' – though there are other processes involved as well. See Schmid R. *The Untold Story of Milk*. (New Trends Publishing, 2009.)

intolerances from infant faeces,[622] something most health professionals today would rarely diagnose.

# Concentrating and preserving milk

Fresh milk had obvious limitations. It was easily recognised as sour or curdled, and was bulky and difficult to transport. From 1856 Gail Borden had experimented with condensing milk by boiling off some of its 87 per cent water content. The American Civil War dramatically boosted the fledgling condensed-milk industry, as cans were included in army rations, and soldiers developed a taste for tinned milk. Condensed (skimmed or whole) milk had sugar added as a preservative, along with some stabilising salt. To differentiate his own product from that of other plants he licensed, Borden changed the name of his condensed milk to Eagle Brand.

In 1866, two American brothers, Charles A and George H Page, founded the Anglo-Swiss Condensed Milk Company in Switzerland. One of their employees, John Baptist Meyenberg, suggested that the company use a similar process but eliminate the addition of sugar to produce an evaporated milk. Meyenberg's idea was rejected. Convinced that his idea held merit, Meyenberg quit the company and emigrated to the United States. By 1885, Meyenberg was producing the first commercial brand of evaporated milk at his Highland Park, Illinois, plant, the Helvetica Milk Condensing Company. Back in Switzerland, after fierce competition with Nestlé's Farine Lactée, or cereal milk mix, Anglo-Swiss were to merge with Nestlé in 1905. Industry consolidation has always been a feature of the baby food business.

The use of sweetened condensed (skimmed or whole) milk for infant feeding had increased during the 1870s in America. This was to lead to epidemics of scurvy, rickets, wasting and death everywhere, but especially in the tropics where it was widely used till the mid twentieth century. In 1907, the Nestlé Company began full-scale manufacturing in Australia, its second-largest export market. Warehouses were built in Singapore, Hong Kong, and Bombay to supply the rapidly growing Asian markets for canned milk products,[623] much of it condensed milks, still widely used in coffee and other drinks, even fruit juices like green mango.

Condensed-milk plants were soon established all over America as well as in Europe. Evaporated milk plants followed. Meyenberg moved from Illinois to Kent in Washington State, where the Pacific Coast Condensed Milk Company, on 6 September 1899, produced the first fifty-five cases of evaporated milk, called Carnation Sterilised Cream. Nicknamed 'Cheese John', Meyenberg had to educate local dairymen to produce clean, high-quality milk, as hygiene standards could be appalling. By 1902, thanks to adept marketing, Carnation milk was a favourite brand among grocers, and soon the image of Carnation's

---

622  This proved useful clinically when dealing with a fully breastfed baby with white stools but no signs of illness; it emerged that this busy mother of three had been living on chocolate; the problem disappeared when she changed her diet!

623  It was in Singapore in 1939 that Dr Cicely Williams would publicly condemn the murderous results of using condensed milks for infant feeding, and then go on to experience the power of breastfeeding to protect the lives of all the children born (and their mothers) in the Japanese camp where they were imprisoned.

'contented cows' (Holsteins, almost certainly making A1 milk[624]) was familiar in the US. Ironically, Nestlé would buy Carnation in 1985 in its attempt to penetrate the lucrative US formula market.

Evaporated and condensed milks are both concentrated milk from which the water has been removed, and the terms were used interchangeably at times. Evaporated milk is milk concentrated to half or less of its original bulk by evaporation under high pressures and temperatures, without the addition of sugar. Condensed milk is essentially evaporated milk with sugar[625] added. In the late 1880s, a Texas grocer, Eldridge Amos Stuart, had developed a method of processing canned, sterilised, evaporated milk, an improvement in microbiological terms. In 1899, Stuart partnered with Meyenberg to supply Klondike gold miners with evaporated milk in 16-ounce cans. All such mass movements of men into areas lacking infrastructure, or off to wars, created opportunities for lucrative and large-scale contracts for canned goods manufacturers, which they were quick to exploit. By 1910, a single machine could produce 35,000 cans per day.[626]

Homogenisation was soon added to the processing of concentrated milk, after an article in an issue of *Scientific American* on 16 April 1904.[627] This could be done before or after pasteurisation, as the milk needed to be heated to 60°C (140°F) to liquidise the fat before it was forced through fine filters and broken into smaller particles more evenly dispersed through the milk. This increased the stability of the condensed product, and the inactivation of milk lipases (enzymes that break down fats) lengthened its shelf life. But homogenisation was not widely used for milk sold fresh for drinking until at least the 1950s, according to dairy texts. The milk tasted different to those used to fresh whole milk. There is still debate about the effects of the process on absorption and digestion. The combination of turbulence, pressure and heat destroys the natural milk fat globule membrane, which contains components thought to be beneficial. These are lost even in a much gentler process such as making cream into butter. But homogenisation was useful because it allowed valuable milk fat to be removed without this being so obvious to consumers, leading to the setting of a standard for whole milk of not less than 4 per cent (later 3.5 per cent or even 3.2 per cent) fat.

Because early evaporated milk lacked sugar, a stabilising salt and carrageenan were added, beginning American infants' exposure to this product, forbidden by EU infant formula regulations because of suspected links with gut inflammation.[628] (See page 397.) But awareness of the inadequacy of condensed milk for infant feeding was growing by the end of

---

624 The reference here is to differing casein proteins in milk from different breeds of cow, thought to have different immunological impacts. cf. Woodford K. *Devil in the milk: illness health and politics. A1 and A2 milk* (Craig Potton Publishing Nelson New Zealand, 2007). See also the health professional resources on the website http://www.a2milk.com.au. This is discussed further in chapter 3.5 "Basic Ingredients Protein".

625 Slavery in the Caribbean and America had made sugar more available and cheaper than it once had been.

626 Levenstein H. *Revolution at the table* (University of California Press, 2001) p. 37

627 *How products are made: evaporated and condensed milk* – Background, History, Raw Materials, The manufacturing process – Evaporated milk, Condensed milk – Quality control. http://www.madehow.com/Volume-6/Evaporated-and-Condensed-Milk.html#b#ixzz1oIC4KtMZ

628 Carrageenan health hazards were discussed in *Food Chemical News,* 17 June 1985. See also http://www.cornucopia.org/wp-content/uploads/2013/02/Carrageenan-Report1.pdf

the nineteenth century, as characteristic nutritional deficiency diseases became common: failure to thrive, rickets, bottle caries, and so on. These would be exported to tropical climates along with the condensed milk that kept so much better in the heat. Condensed milk would allow rubber plantations to employ women as tappers, with their infants kept in a central location and fed sweetened condensed milk from large communal vessels. These were the abuses that led to Cicely Williams' famous speech, *Milk and murder.*[629]

## Drying and powdering milk

Powdered milks provided the solution. Milk drying into powder had first been done by a slow vacuum process of little commercial value. Glaxo developed high temperature roller drying in the early twentieth century.[630] This allowed the production of full-cream milk powders, products with a relatively short shelf life, as the fats rapidly went rancid with exposure to air. Cow & Gate and Nestlé were among the first to use this unsterile dried milk for infant formulas. (Powdered infant formulas are necessarily still unsterile – see page 390). Waste skim milk from butter factories was also turned into dried skim-milk powder, which kept longer. While the companies instituted quality control mechanisms to reduce the level of contamination in milks they processed, these early powders were undoubtedly both contaminated and heat-damaged. (And over time, some bacteria adapted to living in the most carefully managed processing facilities, becoming resistant to drying and even to heat.)[631]

Once roller drying made supplies of tinned dried milk available, municipal officers in UK and US cities bought dried milk patent foods for distribution to overworked malnourished women struggling to cope with large families. Ironically, in so doing, these health authorities increased the likelihood of yet another conception – and maternal death in childbirth or after – by undermining lactational amenorrhea. But in the days before widespread access to refrigeration, dried powdered milks could be cleaner than milk available to urban populations.

## 'Clean' milk and official support for ersatz substitutes

New industrial processes were part of a growing awareness of the need for cleaner fresh milk. Rural families might have access to fresh cows' milk. The urban poor could not afford 'clean' milk. Several decades after Robert Milham Harvey's 1830s articles about the need for pure milk from well-fed cows, 'clean milk' movements spread in the UK, the US and Australia. These early twentieth-century initiatives provided better quality fresh milk from regulated city depots, facilitating elite take up of artificial feeding. This milk was mostly sold below cost, but the price was greater than really poor families could afford, making it an aspirational product. And if they did purchase, families still had to adapt the milk to

---

629 Dr. Cicely Williams, Singapore 1939. http://wphna.org/wp-content/uploads/2014/03/1939_Cicely_Williams_Milk_and_murder.pdf.

630 Infant feeding products generated the profits that created massive pharmaceutical giants like Glaxo. See Jones E. *The business of medicine.* (Profile Books London 2001) and Davenport-Hines RPT, Slinn J. *Glaxo: a history to 1962* (Cambridge University Press 1992)

631 Yan Q, Power KA, Cooney S, Fox E, et al. Complete genome sequence and phenotype microarray analysis of Cronobacter sakazakii SP291: a persistent isolate...(PMID:24032028) *Frontiers in Microbiology* 2013; 4:256.

make it suitable for infant feeding, introducing further risks of contamination, especially in the ill ventilated and unsewered homes of many working people.

Again, one of the unanticipated results of the clean milk movements was to undermine breastfeeding – by validating artificial feeding as adequate and safe. Whatever authorities said about breastfeeding being better, they were not making it possible, but were actually spending money on making artificial feeding available instead. Actions always speak louder than words. Had authorities paid women to breastfeed, or even fed hungry breastfeeding women, women might have believed breastfeeding was valuable. By investing instead in artificial feeding, authorities were endorsing that as important and safe, and making it normal. One UK medical officer of health, Dr John Sykes, found that 'Mothers were sedulously weaning their babies in order to follow the detailed advice of the medical officer of health in the method of hand feeding'[632] – the exact opposite of what he had hoped for when he had fliers distributed encouraging breastfeeding but also giving advice about artificial feeding.

Then as now, mothers got the message that artificial feeding was endorsed by health professionals, and infant feeding products were made to seem desirable by the modelling of more advantaged mothers.

The poverty that was usual for the Western underclass[633] is almost unimaginable, though still usual in many parts of the world, including within affluent societies. Women were worn threadbare with work and childbearing while eating only the food left over by the men of the household (who always ate best of all, and often ingested calories from alcohol as well) and their children. It is not surprising that grossly malnourished women thought lactation a drain on their scarce physical resources, and welcomed the idea of a safe method of hand-rearing the latest, not-necessarily-wanted, arrival.

Only a few far-sighted reformers realised that feeding pregnant and lactating women was the practical solution. In 1904 in Paris, under the banner of L'Oeuvre du Lait Maternel, there were five restaurants that provided free meals for such women. When this was tried in England, the meals cost more and the system was far more bureaucratic. While the French were even willing to pay mothers who breastfed, the British seemed unable to comprehend the idea of direct assistance to the women who needed it most. That was, until there were agricultural surpluses to be managed, as with milk in the 1930s, or peanuts in 1968 USA. Somehow it seems that in countries like the UK and America and Australia, farmers and businesses have always been more worthy of taxpayer support than the undeserving urban poor.[634]

---

632 Lewis J. *The politics of motherhood* (Croom Helm London, 1980) p. 96

633 The good old days were not so good for women. See Ross E. *Love and toil: motherhood in outcast London 1870–1918* (Oxford University Press, 1993); Hewitt M. *Wives and mothers in Victorian industry* (Rockliff, London, 1958); McCalman J. *Struggletown: public and private life in Richmond 1900–1965* (MUP, 1985); Valenze D. *The first industrial woman* (Oxford University Press, 1995)

634 *Food Politics blog, currently browsing posts about: Farm-bill.* http://www.foodpolitics.com/tag/farm-bill/

# Changes in infant feeding equipment and technology

Feeding technology and equipment also developed in the nineteenth and twentieth centuries, and in so doing, would eventually reduce some of the risks of artificial feeding.

Latex teats had been first invented in 1842, as foul tasting objects that became hard and black. Lead could be added to make them appear white, or they could be varnished. They were not widely used until the late nineteenth or early twentieth century, according to one source.[635] As a replacement for tanned animal teats (ugh!) or leather sucking cloths, they were an obvious short-term improvement. However, many were tied to the bottle (or hollowed-out animal horn) with twine, and Mrs Beeton in 1861 advised against removing the teat when washing the bottle in warm water. Beside its obvious microbiological hazard, the legacy of such neonatal exposure to latex in teats may also have been a significant factor in the twentieth-century problem of latex anaphylaxis. It is interesting however, that not until 2004 was an article published documenting infant latex allergic reactions caused by teats, dummies and other routinely–used latex objects.[636]

Latex teats evolved over time to be brown or yellow and more flexible, though still strong smelling and tasting. Accepted as the normal way of enabling self-feeding by quite young infants, they were not superseded until the development of clear and less strong-tasting silicone teats in 1970. In the 1980s in Australia, rival marketers publicised the hazards of the chemical plasticisers used to make latex durable: parents had to balance the risks of exposure to a potential carcinogen (nitrosamines) with the risk of choking, as the silicone teats tended to split, and some broke off in the baby's mouth.[637] Many different chemicals, some now known to be biologically active, have been used as plasticisers. In 1990, a British Standard was created covering the 'Specification for babies' elastomeric feeding bottle teats' (BS 7368:1990). I know of no public discussion of the chemicals in silicone teats as yet.

Teats remain problematic in two areas: hygiene, and impact on infant oral development.[638] Until the 1980s there had been little discussion and analysis of how babies breastfeed, although teat manufacturers claimed to mimic this. As I discussed in the 1985 and all subsequent editions of *Breastfeeding matters,*[639] NUK's claims seem unsubstantiated by any literature they supplied in response to my 1980s request (some of the literature was circular, i.e., it cited two French theses as proof, documents which, when obtained from France, were found to cite NUK claims as fact). NUK literature amusingly said the design was based on plaster casts of the breast after feeding, though most breasts I have seen rapidly resume their usual shape ... Which does not resemble a NUK teat!

---

635 In Australia a 1986 *Choice* article was the catalyst for a major change to silicone. Although Choice has since advised parents that the risks of nitrosamines are now considered negligible, most parents prefer to avoid even negligible but unnecessary risks.

636 Kimata H. Latex allergy in infants younger than 1 year. (PMID:15663567) *Clin Exp Allergy* 2004; 34(12):1910–15.

637 A number of instances were reported by INFACT Canada, and there were recalls in the UK and Australia of teats and pacifiers. See *ALCA News*, 1991; 2(3):35–6

638 Montaldo L. Montaldo P. Bottle feeding and dentition. In Preedy, op. cit., ch.32

639 Minchin MK. *Breastfeeding Matters: what we need to know about infant feeding.* (Alma Publications 1998)

I have seen no evidence to date to refute the idea that the long-term use of so-called orthodontic teats can result in more facial malocclusion than simpler long cylindrical teats. In Australia in the early 1990s, NUK withdrew such advertisements under threat of prosecution for breaches of the Trades Practices Act, which forbids false and misleading advertising.[640] Such marketing claims have since re-emerged. If there is any new research to prove the old claims, I should be delighted to read it and publicly amend this critique.

Lack of strict regulation of bottles and teats in Australia meant that anything can be claimed without a solid research basis. And the cost of taking companies to court for false and misleading advertising seems to have discouraged later prosecutions for obvious untruths in advertising. Meanwhile, some parents go on assuming that 'They wouldn't be allowed to say it if it wasn't true'. Wherever governments fall over themselves to support industry, alas, industry is allowed to say whatever they believe will sell the product. In the case of teats, many marketers beside NUK make the ludicrous claim that they resemble, or behave like, a woman's breast in the infant's mouth. To my knowledge there is none that does, except *perhaps* a very new one, in one limited way. To date only small studies have been published. Ongoing research will reveal whether the new Medela teat results in fewer problems of adjustment to breastfeeding for initially bottle-fed infants.[641] Advertising claims that they consider exceed what the research proves have caused some breastfeeding groups to refuse Medela sponsorship on the grounds that Medela is violating the International Code by advertising bottles with teats.

Glass (and steel) feeding bottles also developed from the mid-nineteenth century, with many different styles and designs. *The Lancet* commended one in 1858, because it was easier to clean than the narrow-necked type previously used.[642] These replaced both 'pap boats', which were easier to keep clean, and a variety of other utensils, like hollowed out cows' horns, which were not. And what about the feeding bottles themselves? Many mothers still rely on the markings on bottles to measure the amount of water needed to make up the powder. Yet sometimes bottles are so badly constructed that on the same bottle, the written levels do not correspond[643] with the embossed levels! Baby bottles need to be either a very precise glass tool, or else a plain object with no markings, with mothers educated to make up formula in a glass jug that has exact, easily read, markings, then transfer the liquid to the feeding bottle. Baby bottles cannot be trusted to be exact: mothers should monitor this possibility.

Glass bottles are too heavy for young infant self-feeding. This is a practical advantage as it means babies are not left alone to self-feed. But it is a problem if the major purpose of artificial feeding is 'convenience', i.e., to allow the baby to get on with feeding with no contact with, or assistance from, another human. Hence an obliging nineteenth century industry created flat-based glass bottles containing a glass tube connected to a long piece of rubber tubing

---

640 Denise Drane and I collaborated on a literature review informing that threat of prosecution. I have this on file.
641 Geddes DT, Kent JC, Mitsoulas LR, and Hartmann PE. Tongue movement and intra-oral vacuum in breastfeeding infants. *Early human development* 2008. 84(7):471–7. See also the Medela site: http://www. medela.com/AU/en/breastfeeding/products/breastmilk-feeding/calma-feeding-device.html
642 *Lancet* 1858; April 24, p. 415.
643 Dr Karleeen Gribble, personal communication 2014.

with a teat on the end (see below). Not surprisingly, these were impossible to keep clean. Soon known as 'murder bottles', they were banned only by France in 1912.[644] Variants still exist in countries that, like Australia, do not create or enforce legal standards for basic infant feeding equipment. The Swedish cow horn with leather teat is no longer seen, but there is little to choose between the other two feeding modes in the following photograph.

The 'Podee feeding bottle', bought on the Internet in 2012, is a modern example of the feeding-tube-in-bottle designed to ensure babies can feed themselves in any position, even lying down, as the tube end always sits in the pool of milk that gravity creates.[645] In 2013 I watched videos on YouTube showing how a two-week-old sleeping baby can be prompted to feed himself in car or crib, without mother having to do more than pinch his cheeks and stimulate sucking. She doesn't have to pick him up or wake him up, he doesn't have to manage to hold the bottle either: it's hands-free feeding.[646] And the Podee website showed three-week-old twins (one swaddled) feeding themselves lying propped on their backs in their crib, while the commentary says that these bottles are works of genius, and 'this is how America will stay one step ahead of China. One simple step for feeding. One giant step for USA. The Podee.'[647] Good grief!

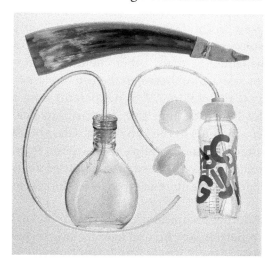

Figure 3-2-1 Murder bottles past, present and future? Photo © James W Maher.

Lighter plastic bottles began to replace glass only in the second half of the twentieth century, although to many it seems they have always been there. In fact, the growth of the plastic industry from its beginnings in the 1920s almost exactly mirrors the growth of the infant formula industry, which it facilitated. And the benefits and problems has plastic has brought with it, and industry's appalling management of the problems, provide eerie parallels, as a fascinating recent book made clear to me.[648]

Plastic bottles have been produced in various compositions and designs, some very odd, and many explicitly encouraging the dangerous practice of infant self-feeding, possible earlier in life when bottles are lighter. Plastic bottles have become almost universal in Australia since 1970, and few parents see leaving a child to self-feed as neglectful or dangerous, despite

644  See *Breastfeeding matters* pp. 104–5
645  http://www.podeeaustralia.com is the website I checked it in December 2014 and an image of two tots propped in chairs looking into space as they fed greeted me.. Watch the videos and look at the expressions on babies' faces.
646  http://www.youtube.com/watch?v=xXHoZKBOgY8, watched 29 March 2013.
647  http://www.youtube.com/watch?feature=player_embedded&v=2bwFZpE01_M
648  Freinkel L. *Plastic: a toxic love story.* (Text Publishing, 2011) Highly recommended reading!

weak injunctions not to do so from health authorities. (Who will be brave enough to create a public health education campaign about reducing the risks of bottle-feeding itself?)

Parental awareness of the risks to normal development of chemicals used in plastic bottles grew in the 1990s, and Bisphenol A in polycarbonate bottles was declared a hazardous substance by Canada in 2008. Whether it is or not, it is still found in some baby bottles, as would be many other chemicals less well known or researched. A recent study found an association between the use of plastic feeding bottles and asthma and allergy in seven-year-old children.[649] Some parents now actively search out glass bottles as a safer option for infant feeding. They are easier to clean thoroughly, and do not contribute oestrogenic compounds to the baby's diet. Glass bottles can also be sterilised without warping (and so altering dilution ratios of powdered formula). One Australian hospital was alerted to this issue after autoclaved plastic bottles would no longer stand upright. The shrinkage made a significant difference to water volumes, inadvertently concentrating the formula.[650]

Another technical problem in making up infant formula is simply getting the ratio of water to nutrients right, and here feeding technology still fails carers. Whether liquid or powder base is used, making up infant formula is notoriously imprecise, not because mothers are careless, but because the technology is both variable and unreliable. As the authoritative report *Infant milks in the UK* (June 2013) stated clearly:

> The potential for harm to infants from making up powdered formula milk feeds incorrectly is serious. Over-concentration of feeds may lead to hypernatraemic dehydration or obesity, while under-concentration may lead to growth faltering (Department of Health and Social Security, 1974; Chambers and Steel, 1975). A systematic review of formula feed preparation (Renfrew et al, 2008) reported that errors in reconstituting feeds were commonly reported and that there was considerable inconsistency in the size of scoops between milk brands. In addition there appears to be little information provided to parents antenatally on how to make up bottles appropriately. A study in which mothers at clinics were asked to measure powdered milk with the same scoop found wide variations in the amount of powder used, ranging from 2.75g to 5.2g per levelled scoop (Jeffs, 1989). Pre-weighed sachets of milk powder have been suggested as a way to reduce volume errors, although where part packets are required to make up smaller or larger feeds, it is likely that errors will still occur. Renfrew et al (2008) recommended that there should be a consistent approach in terms of uniform instructions in the making up of feeds and in scoop sizes to avoid confusion, led by the Food Standards Agency and the Department of Health, but these recommendations do not appear to have been taken forward. When preparing this report we made up powdered formula for the main first milk brands following the manufacturers' instructions, and 900 g of dried powder made between 6,625 ml and 7,520 ml of milk, suggesting some varieties in the energy density of milks per scoop if the final products meet similar compositional standards.

It is surely not impossible for the few major multinational infant formula manufacturers to take responsibility for standardising scoop to water ratios, and then clearly identifying

---

649  Hsu NY, Wu PC, Bornehag CG, Sundell J, Su HJ. *Feeding bottles usage and the prevalence of childhood allergy and asthma.* (PMID:22291844). *Clin Dev Immunol*, 2012, 2012:158248.

650  Sue Cox, International Board Certified Lactation Consultant (IBCLC). Personal communication.

their scoops as solely for a particular named formula. Leading paediatric nutritionist Dorothy Francis called for this in the 1990s, saying that this had then been achieved in the UK.[651] Because powder density of different products varies, a standardised ratio would not eliminate the problems created by using the wrong scoop for any formula. But at least mothers could become accustomed to the same ratio of water to powder! Embossed brand names would further reduce the possibility for error, as would advising mothers to destroy every used scoop: a change in processing like that which made the powder 'fluffier due to the process of agglomeration'[652] might mean no scoop should be kept for re-use, even with a later can of the same brand-name formula.

However, it's laughable to think that carers can ever use a scoop precisely enough to ensure consistency in formula content. Industry scientists know full well, and acknowledge to other scientists, that there can be no absolute consistency about what is in the can to begin with. As well, powders settle and compact in the can over time, especially when subject to vibration (from nearby traffic, say) so that scoops hold more as the use-by date approaches. Processing errors can also occur, for example during the process of agglomeration. Even acknowledging the inevitable, intended or unavoidable degree of variability, formula can vary significantly from what is intended or expected. Formula composition needs to be closely monitored; there is no evidence that regulatory agencies or consumer interests do this frequently or with any regularity.

There are a myriad of influences on actual formula content, so that if ever a doctor really needs to know precisely what a child is drinking, it would be necessary to analyse every bottle made up during the period of diagnosis, or at a minimum, to analyse the formula batch and the caregiver's methods of preparation. No doctor should assume that the nutrient intake of a child can be calculated from the can label, when the content of the bottle may be at a 150 per cent concentration or 75 per cent dilution! (See page 248.)

New technologies have been developed through the century, many adapted to make bottle-feeding more convenient for carers. Microwaving is another example of a new technology used for infant feeding without real knowledge of what it might do to the nutrients in infant formula or their bioavailability. Parents are warned that heat spots may form: this has led to some parents shaking bottles which then exploded, burning parent and child, once so severely that the baby's hand was partially amputated.[653] Babies have suffered serious full palatal thickness burns and scalds from localised hot spots unnoticed before the baby was fed.[654]

---

651  Full Assessment report: Subject Proposal P93: Revision of Standard R7 Infant Formula. Online http://www.foodstandards.gov.au/code/proposals/documents/P93%20Full%20Assesment%20Report.pdf

652  One Australian Wyeth product compacted too readily, which led to consistent over-feeding, so this change was necessary. I still have the advertising flier about its new fluffiness on file. Who drinks fluff? But it's meant to sound soft and cuddly. Curious about agglomeration? Go read http://www.niro.com/niro/cmsdoc.nsf/webdoc/webb7nrh3r; http://www.engineersjournal.ie/agglomerate-breakage-during-pneumatic-conveying/

653  Dixon JJ, Burd DA, Roberts DG. Severe burns resulting from an exploding teat on a bottle of infant formula milk heated in a microwave oven. (PMID: 9232290) *Burns*, 1997; 23(3):268–9

654  Hibbard RA, Blevins R. Palatal burn due to bottlewarming in a microwave oven. *Pediatrics*, 1988;82:382–4

But those dangers are immediate and painful, and readily noted. Damage done to nutrients would be less obvious and perhaps seriously damaging. Microwave ovens do profoundly alter protein structure: do they affect nutrient bioavailability for infants? Do they affect different formulas differently?[655] Only those unaware of the complexity of interactions between formula ingredients would think these are idle questions. One 1992 study[656] boldly stated that under the specific conditions they used of heating casein-dominant formula for short periods, no loss of vitamin C or riboflavin was reported. Well, fine (though contested by a questioner who found huge losses), but that tells us nothing much about other types of formulas and other formula ingredients and their interactions. To think the dilemma resolved because the most heat-labile components survived is a little premature, methinks. And the unevenness of heating in microwaves means that bacteria or spores might well survive. No authority, either health professional or industry body, recommends using microwave ovens for heating infant formula. But some parents do it all the time because it is convenient. Research into consequences other than burns is overdue.

Changes to feeding equipment, and above all, the availability of disinfectants and clean water, do make artificial feeding less hazardous in affluent households. Today, in less affluent areas, contaminated water combined with unsterile formula still kills millions of children. In such places the local equivalent of an open pap boat, or a cup, is still recommended by WHO as safer than feeding bottles. But wherever it happens, artificial feeding per se still carries the risk of death, and not just for preterm or sick infants. And parents everywhere can be too casual about important hygiene measures like hand-washing.

Many of the pioneers of the infant formula industry were health professionals, and their lack of concern about replacing breastmilk seems inexcusable. However, they did not have the luxury of hindsight to see the consequences of obsessing about substitutes, rather than focussing on protecting and promoting maternal breastfeeding. Negative unintended consequences – perhaps I should call it 'collateral damage'? – litter the past. But finding a name to camouflage the extent of horrific harms does not end either the harms, or the moral responsibility for them.

655 Hettiarachchi CA, Melton LD, Gerrard JA, Loveday SM. Formation of β-lactoglobulin nanofibrils by microwave heating gives a peptide composition different from conventional heating.(PMID: 22877308) *Biomacromolecules*, 2012; 13(9). pp. 2868–80. DOI: 10.1021/bm300896r
656 Sigman-Grant M, Bush G, Anantheswaran R. Microwave heating of infant formula: a dilemma resolved. *Pediatrics* 1992; 90:3 412–15

# 3.3 Scaling up production and propaganda for the 'perfect' substitute

The expansion and mechanisation of the dairy industry continued despite adverse economic conditions after the First World War. Fresh milk sales plummeted in the 1930s Depression, as people simply could not afford dairy products. Farmers were at risk of going under, as the price paid for their milk was often less than the cost of production. Milk for processing brought very poor returns. UK and US governments stepped in with price setting, farm subsidies, price supports, and schemes to encourage consumption of agricultural surpluses. In the UK, the Milk Marketing Board[657] was created in 1933 as a centralised buying agency with a guaranteed floor price for fresh milk; its remit extended to education and reform in dairy practice, and improvement of herd quality.[658] In fact, the Milk Marketing Board's commitment to buy all milk offered to it led to a massive increase in UK milk production and the number of dairy farms. The Milk Board then built creameries around the UK to process the surplus milk into butter and cheese. Novel schemes for increasing fresh-milk consumption were then developed as a means of providing national food security, subsidising agriculture as well as improving the nutrition of the underfed working classes. Governments continued to look at new schemes to improve child health among the poor, as well as to dispose of any gluts from agricultural production. The UK Milk Marketing Board in 1934 had supported a study of 8000 hungry malnourished children. The study had shown that 200ml of free milk daily accelerated their growth, as well as improved their ability to learn – which of course almost any regular supplemental protein and calories probably would have done. However, the growth was seen to be due not simply to healthy food supplementation, but to certain unique properties of milk, by this time being marketed as a uniquely necessary food for children.

This Milk in Schools Scheme started in 1934; the Industrial Milk Scheme supplied workers on a similar basis, and Welfare Schemes made cheap milk available to 'nursing and expectant mothers and children.[659] The UK's National Dried Milk scheme in July 1940 was to reflect both the lessons learned in the First World War, and build on the work of the Milk Marketing Board, making powdered milk available cheaply to feed infants (and incidentally increasing the cost of milk to other consumers). Again, war had ramped up government procurement of foods for feeding troops, and so increased the likelihood of over-production once armies were disbanded and civilians had to find the money to pay for such foods.

In the United States, control over milk distribution had been consolidated in the 1920s into the hands of giant holding companies such as National Dairy Products and Borden. They developed a marketing organisation that inundated schools with posters advising all children to consume a daily quart of milk (nearly a litre!). Supplying the US Army overseas had created a demand for increased milk production, and when the war was over, new markets had to be found. Over time, school milk, school lunches, export incentives and

---

657 Pepperall RA. *The Milk Marketing Board* (Clare, Son & Co Ltd, Somerset, 1948).
658 The Accredited Scheme improved hygiene standards, while in 1935 the Attested Scheme certified that herds were free of bovine tuberculosis. Milk produced by herds in both schemes was worth a significant premium.
659 Pepperall discusses these under the heading of 'Developing the market for milk'. op. cit., Ch. 7.

assistance all developed to use up milk gluts and to address widespread malnutrition alike. Milk lakes and butter mountains are costly to dispose of: governments usually step in to prop up the agricultural sector, as they may face justifiable social unrest if people are going hungry while a glut of food decays. In the US the Department of Agriculture (USDA) was to become the world's largest purchaser of infant formula, to be distributed free to poor families via food stamp schemes (from 1939), and from 1972 via the WIC (Women, Infants and Children) scheme. Infant formula has even been exported at taxpayer expense as part of foreign aid packages.[660] With the best of intentions, but very little intelligent forethought about damage limitation in this crucial area, governments became principal agents in the twentieth-century decline of breastfeeding. Some remain so, wherever social policies are developed without thought for the likely effects on women's ability to breastfeed optimally.

After 1900 death rates were dropping: after 1910, ice boxes and later refrigerators had reduced bacterial growth in milk, and clean water and sanitation in cities reduced infant morbidity and mortality. It would still take, in the period 1900–30, a wide-ranging coalition of diverse forces, well described by Valenze,[661] to bring about much needed hygiene reforms in national milk supplies.

From the 1920s onwards consumers everywhere witnessed a snowfall of propaganda documenting the miracles worked by milk, especially for women and children. Organisations of dairy interests, staffed in part by home economists, medical experts and nutritionists, generated campaign posters, pamphlets and recipe books. Buoyed by their own funded research, the British National Milk Publicity Council, established in 1920, united producers, distributors and representatives of the medical professions. This early co-option of health professionals into groups funded by the large milk interests continued throughout the twentieth century.

## How did artificial feeding come to be accepted?

Apart from the risk to life, there are many disorders that beset the hand-fed child more often than the baby at the breast: the sleepless child who screams with flatulence and colic is nearly always the hand-fed infant; the infant who fails to gain weight and drives

---

660 In fact the US Federal Trade Commission (FTC) investigated possible price-fixing by the formula industry, and while no formal charges were laid, in January 1992 Mead Johnson agreed not to engage in pre-bid communications, to stop advertising infant formula, and to donate 3.1 million pounds of formula to the USDA for charitable distribution at home and abroad. Some of this the US government then exported at its own cost into the newly emergent Eastern European market as humanitarian and trade aid. The aid was clearly to the US formula industry! And the cost of transport may well have exceeded the cost of the formula. I learned of an unconscionable US export exercise when a WHO Europe official rang me to ask where to locate an alternative sources of a low-phenylalanine formula needed to prevent brain damage in PKU children (those lacking the enzyme to metabolise the amino acid phenylalanine). I was told that the US company supplying Poland was refusing supply until the Polish government took out a US dollar loan to build a plant that could service Eastern Europe with their product. Poland has a high rate of PKU, a genetic disorder. I was sickened to hear that the elder President Bush had taken a small supply with him as a present on a visit to Poland, while this blackmail by an American company was underway. I advised WHO Europe about exclusive breastfeeding and alternate sources of low-phenylalanine formula, but never heard the outcome. These are the scandals that never make press headlines, as it is in no one's interest (except babies) to publish them. All I can do is bear witness.

661 Valenze D. *Milk, a global and local history* (Yale University Press, 2011).

doctors and parents to their wits' end in the effort to find one that will suit is the hand-fed infant; rickets is almost entirely a disease of the hand-fed infant; convulsions are also much commoner in these infants. Let us beware then, how we counsel a mother not to suckle her child; it is a heavy responsibility, and one which I venture to think is often taken too lightly.[662]

Like Dr Still, some doctors did see the problems as they arose. As 'human infants tend[ed] more and more to become a parasite of the milch cow',[663] epidemics of diarrhoeal disease, scurvy and rickets continued, with a rise in eczema and skin problems being noted in medical literature by the 1930s. Even so, only a passionate minority of doctors in any country spoke out strongly against the encroaching tide of artificial feeding. Then, as now, many doctors simply followed where industry led. And industry reached and persuaded both doctors and parents, with talk of improving breastmilk, perfect 'uncontaminated germ-free'[664] mixes, protecting infants from disease 'like the breastfed baby'[665], helping women cope ... themes that played on powerful emotions (as they still do). Parents and doctors alike could see some children growing fat on artificial foods; they believed this to be a proof of safety. How could they realise it was a precursor to Western epidemics of diseases like obesity, diabetes, cardiovascular and autoimmune diseases, which were not then known to have their origins in childhood? Most doctors were genuinely trying to save the lives of infants when they endorsed products that ironically lead to a greater loss of infant life than many wars. And wars would help promote artificial feeding!

## How war helped artificial feeding

This is well discussed by Dwork in her thought-provoking history of the emergence of the infant welfare movement in the UK, entitled *War is good for babies and other young children*.[666] Medical men of the early twentieth century thought preventing infant mortality a national patriotic duty, both to strengthen the nation's workers and in order to ensure a steady supply of soldiers:

> 'Men with long-lost teeth [needed to deal with hard tack rations], or suffering from the consequences of rickets, were of no use' in the Boer War. 'We cannot get soldiers or men ready-made. We must go back to infancy and motherhood.'[667]

---

662  Still GF. *Common Disorders and Diseases of Childhood* (Oxford Medical Publications London 1910).

663  Holt, WL. Medical milk commissions and the importance of a pure milk supply. *Cal State J Med.*, 1909 April; 7(4):136–42. Holt was quoting one Dr McCleary, but went on to say that 'most children fed on pure cows' milk in accordance with carefully worked out principles of our modern specialists like himself thrive very well.' How would he know unless they were studied lifelong?

664  Glaxo advertisement in *Woman's Budget*, April 10, 1920, p. 29.

665  ibid.

666  Dwork D, op. cit.

667  Saleeby CW. The problem of the future. In *Mothercraft: a selection from courses of lectures on infant care delivered under the auspices of the National Society for the Prevention of Infant Mortality*. Published by the National League for Physical Education and Improvement, London. Part 1, 2nd edition, 1916.

Army recruiters during the second Boer War (1899–1902) had rejected many volunteers because of poor health, poor physique, and rotten teeth.[668] In the UK after 1904 there was widespread concern about the future of the Empire in the face of a declining birth rate and the rising infant mortality rate in the last quarter of the nineteenth century, well documented after the passage of the registration of births was made mandatory in 1874.[669] The *British Medical Journal* pontificated that the lack of a clean milk supply was at the root of the problem, and failed to see that for health authorities to provide milk for infant feeding might perhaps undermine breastfeeding.

Scarcity of milk in the later stages of the First World War (due to destruction of European herds and scarcity of shipping) created coalitions of concerned middle-class women and health professionals urging governments to ensure that sufficient fresh milk was available for children, along with reliable supplies of infant foods. Powdered milks provided the solution.

Living in conflict zones has always made infant survival precarious. Only breastfed babies survived the Siege of Paris in 1871, despite numerous efforts to create breastmilk substitutes that would keep other babies alive.[670] In wartime, breastfeeding rates are usually higher than in peacetime, because families know that supplies of any food cannot be guaranteed. But while this is true, war also encourages milk production and places new burdens on lactating women. Wartime requisitions of milk for making canned food to feed troops interferes with regular supplies, at the same time as war damage in conflict zones reduces herd sizes. This increases prices and profits, which in turn encourages milk production and canning in safer areas. As noted earlier, the American Civil War had made the novel condensed and evaporated milks familiar and popular with hungry men, and survivors looked for these foods after demobilisation.[671]

Similarly, the twentieth century's major mechanised wars have promoted both artificial feeding and government control of, and subsidies for, milk supplies of all kinds. Nestlé's worldwide production of dried milks doubled during the First World War, largely through government contracts. Glaxo too prospered from the war. Women were needed in factories for war work, but babies had to be fed. The First World War accelerated the trend towards free distribution of artificial feeding products, as the UK Ministry of Food bought bulk supplies of the newly developed tinned powdered milks, making them available cheaply and with official blessing. America's Food Administration was conceived amid the food crisis of 1916–17.[672] Protection of the national food supply was seen as a government responsibility in this era, and this would entail managing both scarcity and glut. The responsibility for feeding troops created scarcities. Once armies are demobilised, surpluses will develop, as they did in both the US and the UK by the 1930s.

---

668 There had been fewer such complaints from the first Boer War of 1880–81, perhaps because the men enlisting then had been breastfed and survived infancy in the 1860s, before patent foods took off among the poor.
669 Dwork D, op. cit. p. 6
670 Newman G. *Infant mortality: a social problem* (Methuen, 1906).
671 Fisher JC. *Food in the American military* (McFarland and Co., Jefferson, 2010).
672 Levenstein p. 137.

Later in the century, the Second World War (1939–45) also influenced the availability of ingredients and diverted attention from oversight of ongoing feeding problems. It boosted all milk product sales, including formula, as governments bought in stocks of powdered milk in case of shortages, supplied rations to armies, and created schemes so that poor families could access free or cheap formula – because God forbid that mothers should stay home to feed and care for their babies when the arms factories needed workers! And, of course, the provision of government-subsidised formula was seen as an endorsement that artificial feeding was safe – 'they wouldn't do it otherwise, would they'.

## Mathematics and paediatrics

In America from the 1890s onwards, complicated methods of infant feeding had been developed. Precise and frequently changing formulations were promoted and prescribed by a bevy of doctors involved in infant feeding, that 'portal to a profitable practice'[673] for the emerging specialty of child doctors. Some of the early milk manufacturers actively courted doctors, and some were doctors themselves. The American profession of paediatrics grew as artificial feeding required individualised care involving stool examination, growth monitoring, and adjusting the strength of the formula, sometimes weekly, perhaps changing the amounts of added fat). Thomas Morgan Rotch was one of the leading lights in American 'percentage methods' of milk manipulation. Only the newly emerging breed of paediatricians felt confident to advise mothers about how much of the product to use with how much water and what other additives. Obviously closely supervised medical care was the preserve of the affluent, society's opinion leaders. Percentage feeding was seen as the epitome of skill, and reached heights of absurdity hard to credit now. The first edition of the official *Victorian Government Guidelines on Infant Feeding*[674] contained dozens of tables showing how to vary the percentages of fats, carbohydrates and so on, all 'for the use of members of the medical and nursing professions'. Dr Vera Scantlebury was appointed Director of Infant Welfare in the Public Health Department of Victoria in 1926, and created these Guidelines. Rotch would have approved. In 1893 he had said: 'It would hardly seem necessary to suggest that the proper authority for establishing rules for substitute feeding should emanate from the medical profession, and not from non-medical capitalists. Yet when we study the history of substitute feeding as it is represented all over the world, the part which the family physician plays, in comparison with the numberless patent and proprietary foods administered by nurses, is a humiliating one, which should no longer be tolerated.'[675] He has a point, mind you.

Scantlebury's second edition in 1933 contains just five pages of information about breastfeeding, and the rest of the 113 pages were about artificial feeding, with some thirty-six tables showing how to vary concentrations. But by the 1930s such complicated and time-consuming methods for adapting fresh milk (using sugars, cream, barley water, lime

---

673  Apple RD. 'To be used only under the direction of a physician': commercial infant feeding and medical practice, 1870–1940. (PMID:6998527) *Bull Hist Med* 1980, 54(3):402–17.

674  *A Guide to infant feeding for the use of members of the medical and nursing professions* (Public Health Department Victoria, 1929.) Noted in *The Argus*, 4 October 1929, p. 10.

675  Apple RD. *Mothers and medicine*, op. cit., p. 24.

water and more besides) were going out of fashion in America. Individualised supervision of the bottle-fed infant was – then as now – a luxury society could not afford to provide for any but the wealthy who could afford private doctors. Doctors then recommended either simple homemade formulas using the now-accepted evaporated milks, or patented industrial brands, some of which they had helped create: Drs Gerstenberger and Ruh created SMA (Synthetic Milk Adapted) in 1915, and fed it to babies in Cleveland in 1918.[676]

The nexus (to this day still a close one, though increasingly challenged) between infant formula manufacturers and American paediatrics originated in businessmen wooing doctors who had invented likely products, then scaling up production to commercial and hugely profitable levels. Their vision was international from the early days: SMA was invented in 1918, and exported to England and the Philippines by 1925![677]

As the artificial feeding industry burgeoned, so did the disciplines dependent on it, not only for financial support, but also for an endless supply of clients with feeding problems. Not natural feeding problems: paediatricians were simply not trained to deal with mastitis, for instance, or fissured nipples. The breasts that fed the baby were simply not their province. In fact, for many doctors, the solution to any infant's breastfeeding problem was to find a suitable formula, and stop messing about with a process that could only be unsatisfactory and possibly embarrassing. In America the specialty of paediatrics grew along with the infant formula industry. Rima Apple's work documents this so brilliantly that I am skipping the early genesis of the important nexus between healthworkers and industry: read her books!

From 1900 to 1950 there were of course many important advances in paediatrics, as doctors worked out ever more ingenious ways to identify and deal with child ailments of every kind. Great progress was made, especially compared with what had gone before the era of antibiotics. By the 1940s paediatricians were excited about many things other than feeding babies; neonatology was developing with its focus on the medical care of small and sick children. This can all be read in the official histories of paediatrics, which celebrate the successes of the growing discipline, which evolved differently in the UK from the USA. I too salute those achievements, from which their spectacular failure with infant feeding does not detract. Yet I note that, as with infant feeding, some of those successes were also bought at considerable cost to the infants on whom new treatments were trialled.[678]

I also salute the courage of that minority of paediatricians, obstetricians and physicians, some of them pioneering women, who resolutely held the line that breastfeeding was always better than formula feeding, and that every effort must be made to protect, promote and support it. For their efforts they were usually regarded as old-fashioned or slightly odd,

---

676  http://www.wyethnutrition.com.hk/tn.aspx?id=abu4&l=en. Accessed 14 March 2013.
677  Wyeth website, in 2013 http://www.pfizernutrition.com.hk/tn.aspx?id=abu4&l=en. Accessed 20/5/2013. Previously found on Wyeth US website, prior to sale and break-up of Wyeth formula markets. Only Wyeth Hong Kong (now owned by Nestle) retains some of this history.
678  Look up Retrolental fibroplasia and Pinks Disease if you think that overstated. Or check out the series Robertson AF. Reflections on errors in neonatology: I. The 'Hands-Off' years, 1920 to 1950. (PMID:12556927) *J Perinatol* 2003, 23(1):48–55.

if not positively barmy or fanatical. (Those using that term fanatic should be aware that one definition is 'someone who is right before you are'.) Harold Waller, Cicely Williams, Mavis Gunther, Niles Newton, Alan Cunningham, Derek and Patrice Jelliffe, Michael Latham, were all fanatics in that sense, now heroes to those who study human lactation.

Early patent formulas had been advertised everywhere that might reach mothers. Doctors didn't approve of this, or of the cans providing detailed instructions about how to make up the formula: both could mean that mothers chose and used formula without ever seeing doctors. Rima Apple has documented how the American Medical Association solved the problem: by giving its Gold Seal of approval only to brands which removed all instructions from the cans,[679] so that mothers were *obliged* to consult doctors about making up the product – or just guess what to do if they couldn't afford doctors. Industry agreed to this as the cost of getting the AMA Gold Seal, despite the obvious negative consequences for infants whose mothers could not afford medical fees. Industry marketing focussed on the medical profession. Marketing of patent products to doctors focussed on the physician's control and convenience and economic benefit, ironically echoing Cadogan's famous dictum that it was 'time for the business of feeding to be controlled by Men of Sense.'[680] What a business it has become!

Many of the doctors involved in formula development (then as now?) were idealists who truly believed their products were better than milk made by malnourished or dirty women, so little did they know about human milk at the time. In 1929 Marriott's study had purported to show that evaporated milk was 'superior' to mother's milk as newborns fed on it regained their birth weight faster than those exclusively breastfed or given supplemental bottles of cows' milk mixes.[681] It was especially good for preterm babies, he thought, little knowing that he was endorsing a change that would see up to seven per cent of all preterm US children struck down by necrotising enterocolitis (NEC) or sepsis, and twenty to twenty-five per cent of affected infants –about one percent of all premature babies – die, with many more left nutritional cripples with short bowel syndrome and liver problems. (See page 436).

Studies like Marriott's were widely publicised, which helped to silence the critics of artificial feeding. Journals were openly or subtly co-opted by industry, which of course supported their existence through advertising. Industry had always claimed identity with breastmilk, along with a subtle or blatant suggestion of superiority and greater reliability. The intractable and persistent problem of excess protein, for instance, could be made a virtue: Lactogen, created in 1921, was 'nearly identical to mother's milk, but richer in the protein needed for building bone and muscle'. (No suggestion of excess leading to kidney damage and obesity there!) Good, because like breastmilk, and even better because different, richer, stronger, more reliable ... Surely that is having one's cake and eating it too! This sort of advertising went largely unchallenged.

---

679  Apple R op. cit.

680  Colon AR, Colon PA. *A history of pediatrics* (Greenwood Press, 1999) citing Cadogan W. *An essay on nursing and the management of children from their birth to three years of age* (36 pp essay, written 1748, published 1768).

681  Marriott WM, Schoenthal L. An experimental study of the use of unsweetened evaporated milk for the preparation of infant feeding. *Arch Ped.* 1929; 46:135–48.

Thus began the absurd and still-current trend in medical literature for proponents of breastfeeding to feel obliged to prove breastmilk superior to infant formula before making any claims about its benefits, while infant formula advocates were never publicly challenged to prove what they asserted or inferred or implied – that their product was safe, or equivalent to, or as close to breastmilk as possible,[682] and perhaps even better in modern environments.

Journals were openly or subtly co-opted by industry, which of course supported their existence through advertising.[683] In 1948 the journal *Pediatrics* began publication, the voice of the American Academy of Pediatrics. The advertising content of early issues makes it clear that infant gut distress was then common, and many panaceas are proposed, including soy and goat formulas, early so-called 'hypoallergenics' (later significantly altered), including a meat-based[684] formula made from beef hearts. Two or three generations into mass artificial feeding already by the 1950s, America led the world in complications and complicated formulas. New formulas were constantly being devised to deal with the problems the old ones created. Some of the many formulas that are now never heard of include Allergilac, Bremil, Formil, Frailac, Vi-Lactogen, Golden Ostermilk, Lactropon, Milumil (became Aptamil), Modilac, Nektarmil, Nido, Osterfeed, Pelargon, Trufood, Utilac, Varamel ... and many more. Clearly these were as good as possible at the time – but not good enough to continue in use once science revealed their defects, or they were publicly associated with some problem. No one trumpeted either their defects or their demise.

Developmental paediatrics also was born in the period before 1960. So the 'normal' Western baby that paediatric textbooks described was based on the usual bottle-fed infant. Doctors work with sick people: they saw a lot more artificially fed babies, and saw more of them, because the breastfed ones were healthier, and in this period many families saw a doctor only as a last resort.

New brain and conduct disorders were emerging in this period, again most notably in the US. Parents were usually considered responsible. Parents could become unwilling to admit problems in children as their nurture was blamed: autism, for example, described first in 1943, was blamed on 'cold' mothers.[685] By the 1950s the US stereotype of normal child behaviour was expanding to include what seem in retrospect very like ADHD children. Dennis the Menace – hyperactive, uncontrollable, hard to discipline – was seen by many older non-American parents as a badly brought-up brat. Such impulsive out-of-control

---

682  'Next to breast milk, it's the best milk.'

683  In the interest of shelf space, libraries have stripped journals of advertising sections before binding annual volumes. This can give a false impression of the extent to which marketing was conducted through professional journals. Only where unbound issues survive can industry advertising be evaluated. I am grateful for those who mislaid the odd issue long ago so that the year's journals, being an incomplete set, were not bound.

684  Gerber discontinued this product in 1985, after a recall due to excess vitamin A levels. However, in 1990 a single batch was again made for a 'severely mentally and physically retarded' asthmatic allergic fifteeen-year-old, Raymond Dunn Jr, who could not tolerate other food. See http://articles.latimes.com/1990-04-06/news/mn-667_1_gerber-make-formula. He died, painfully, in 1995. http://community.seattletimes.nwsource.com/archive/?date=19950126&slug=2101545

685  Jacobsen K. Diagnostic politics: the curious case of Kanner's syndrome. (PMID: 21877421) *History of Psychiatry*, 2010, 21(84 Pt 4):436–54.

children were totally outside the older generation's wide experience of children. Brain-disordered and learning-disabled children would become more common in Australia by the 1980s, although again parents were met with patronising denial and what felt like blame from doctors.

> A classic example of this: a mother whose overactive four year old was diagnosed as simply defiant, and an attention-seeking behavioural problem, because of his habit of soiling his pants, then going to his mother for clean up. We were watching him play happily outside, when suddenly he stopped and looked distressed, and his mother said angrily, "He's done it again, and he'll be in here asking me to clean him up." I urged her to consider what we had just witnessed, a child happily engaged with water play, suddenly interrupted by a bodily action which surprised him: clearly something other than volition had triggered a bowel movement. After reviewing the history, I suggested diet changes. Not only the encopresis but also episodic otitis media and temper tantrums disappeared. The result: different child, different mother, different relationship. Tell me that makes no difference to a life, and I'll know you've never had children!

No one researched infant feeding methods in these children, but from what we now suspect about the impact on brain development of the wrong amino acid balance at critical times, it would have been a good idea. As Dorner said, the

> ... tryptophan to neutral amino acids ratio in the blood is thought to control the synthesis of serotonin in the brain. Serotonin deficiency in the developing brain based on a decreased plasma tryptophan to neutral amino acids ratio may contribute to developmental obesity and/or permanent changes of mental capacity and social adaptability as observed in human subjects who had been formula-fed as compared to those who had been breast-fed in neonatal life.[686]

It may also be significant that US formula makers were using high levels of what are now known to be pro-inflammatory fats, while British societies were still pushing cod liver oil (omega 3 fats included) into children. Such impulsive out-of-control children[687] were totally outside the older generation's wide experience of children. Brain-disordered and learning-disabled children would become more common in Australia by the 1980s, although again parents were met with patronising denial and what felt like blame from doctors. See further on these issues in chapters on protein and fats in formula.

## 'Experts' undermine breastfeeding

Powdered patent formulas were still relatively expensive before 1950, however, except in the UK where National Dried Milk was supplied – and that was largely just what its name

---

686 Bewer G, Lubs H. Changes of the plasma tryptophan to neutral amino acids ratio in formula-fed infants: possible effects on brain development. (PMID:6686152) *Exper Clin Endocrinol* 1983; 82(3):368–7.

687 The best parent guide to such problems is found in Dr Doris Rapp's book, *Is This Your Child? Discovering and treating unrecognised allergies in children and adults.* (Quill NY 1991).

said. Evaporated milk, readily available in smaller quantities and by then trusted as safe, began to be widely used from the 1930s, although formulas for adapting fresh milk remained popular up until the 1950s in countries like Australia where urban homes had a milkman calling or a local suburban dairy, and farms kept a 'house cow' for milking, often a Jersey (providing probably A2 milk, lower in the beta-casein linked with health problems,[688] as well as more cream for butter-making). In Australia the dried milk powders continued to be used as well, thanks to the network of maternal and child health centres established in the first half of the century, which oversaw infant feeding for a significant part of the population. The Victorian Department of Public Health official guide gave detailed tables of recipes for formula to be made from dried, fresh or evaporated milk right up until the (last) 1978 edition; it also included full details of the just four patent brands then on the Victorian market.[689]

No matter how well the products were advertised, there would have been a smaller market for them had women been breastfeeding easily and successfully. But responsive breastfeeding had been undermined, even countermanded. The early twentieth century had seen the emergence of widely read, popular, moralistic and dogmatic writings about infant care by 'men of sense' such as Frederick Truby King and William Holt. Such men wished to support and actively promote breastfeeding, but apparently knew almost nothing about it. Their schedules and rules and timed feeds caused dwindling supplies and breastfeeding failure for many literate middle class women.

However, the direct influence of such authors was probably less than that of the many free infant care booklets provided by formula makers, advertised widely, and available to nurses and mothers alike. Of course the booklets echoed what those prominent doctors said: the infant formula industry has been unfairly blamed for inventing much bad advice about infant feeding that was in fact copied from the writings or practice of ill-informed doctors.[690]

The underlying theme of these writings, almost all by men whose at-home wives and servants would care for their children, was regulating and controlling infant behaviour in inflexible patterns to suit the convenience of the household's adults. This is easier said than done, when dealing with inborn needs and instinctive behaviours that reflect millennia of evolutionary development, and which mandate physical closeness and flexible feeding patterns. Perhaps men's success in controlling women's behaviour up until the 1970s contributed to their joint expectation that infants could be similarly controlled.

---

688  Woodford K, op. cit. This was still common in 1950s rural Australia, where I lived on a dairy farm, and as a child milked cows and made butter.

689  Campbell K, Wilmot E. *A guide to the care of the young child. A textbook for workers in the field of maternal and child health* (Dept of Health, Victoria, 1978). Subsequent guidelines have been far less informative about practical matters of artificial feeding.

690  Successful marketing strategies of companies like Mead Johnson co-opted health professionals so effectively that it is hard to sort out the chicken from the egg: did these doctors think what they did because industry had suborned them or their predecessors? Did industry truly respect what doctors thought or was it conscious of having recruited them? Some 1980s industry reps spoke to me of how cheaply other health professionals could be got 'on side' to promote their products – with obvious contempt.

Control of baby was certainly more possible with arbitrary large feedings of sedating bovine protein, which alters infant sleep patterns and brain behaviour.[691] Those doctors were unaware that bovine opioids can sedate a child, and were working from the assumption that the 'good baby' does not cry, and 'naughty' babies must be trained not to. Few understood that the techniques they advised could lead to learned helplessness and emotional scarring: like Dr Spock, they themselves were often the damaged products of such techniques.

Infant nurture was widely believed to determine adult physical and moral outcomes.[692] Responsive parenting was not an idea that fitted an authoritarian time when both women and children were taught to know their place, and to fit in with the household. Infant attachment was seen as needing to be transformed into independence as soon as possible; attachment was not a goal of parenting. Similarly, the clothing of the time made breastfeeding a chore, and frequent breastfeeding an absurdity for some women; while public breastfeeding in some circles would have been a scandal. 'Respectability' was a societal norm. The respectable woman's place was in the home, and breastfeeding helped keep her there. Which is precisely why some early twentieth-century women saw artificial feeding as liberation, unlike their sisters in the 1970s.

All writers on the subject of infant feeding in those days extolled breastmilk as perfect – but in theory, and only from some women (see the list on page 479). Breastfeeding was really seen as unreliable, uncontrollable, and incomplete, weak and fallible. This mirrored attitudes to women themselves, then seen as intellectual inferiors, needing to be subject to male control. Uncritical faith in science, combined with what can now be recognised as monumental ignorance and hubris, engendered certainty that a product as good as or superior to women's milk could be produced by clever scientists. The model of nutrition these men were working from saw the child as a depository for nutrients: get the amounts of each component right, as they were sure they could, or even had, and the results would be an improvement on nature. (The whole nature vs. nurture debate was a constant influence on infant care and feeding.)

Assisted by astute marketing, the popular perception of cows' milk changed from dubious (because contaminated and infected) to essential. Social historians have found that in just one generation there was a shift away from valuing meat-bone-based vegetable-rich soups. When asked about the best food for growing a healthy child, grandmothers responded 'soup'. Their daughters replied 'milk'.[693] By which they did not mean their own.

That was just one example of the abrupt disjunction between generations of women that came about with the increasing intrusion into family life of well-meaning health professionals. In Australia, historian Janet McCalman has said that the 1930s 'saw the beginning of the end of easy breastfeeding'.[694] McCalman documented the split between the

---

691  Which, like any unnecessary sedative, reduces infant arousal and increases the risk of death; and of course, if that failed, other more powerful sedatives, from opium to alcohol, were still available.
692  Hardyment and Apple both describe this well. See Bibliography.
693  Murcott A. *Sociology of food and eating: essays on the sociological significance of food* (Gower International Library of Research & Practice, 1983)
694  *Struggletown*, op. cit. p. 209.

generations brought about by involvement with the developing maternal and child health care system in an inner urban Australian neighbourhood. Instead of looking to mothers and aunts and cousins for advice, women now looked to the new breed of health professional, often childless, full of the new 'scientific' knowledge created by male 'experts'. And so they struggled with breastfeeding and soon weaned their babies.

Poor families in the UK were drawn into artificial feeding by free or low-cost supplies of 'National Dried Milk' and vitamins provided by child health clinics. They were emulating women in higher-status groups – many recruited unwillingly to artificial feeding by following poor lactation management advice from Truby King and his ilk.

Similar schemes of giving free or low-cost substitutes for breastmilk had multiplied around the world after 1940: in Chile, clinics providing free milk to address malnutrition issues caused the breastfeeding rates to plummet disastrously.[695] In areas with clean water, most artificially fed infants survived and grew, and often grew fat;[696] but there was little research into other outcomes. To generations used to high infant mortality and morbidity rates, as long as most babies survived and grew, artificial feeding must be reasonably safe. And in comparison to some other forms of artificial feeding, post Second World War infant formula probably did offer much better survival chances when used in the context of available antibiotics and clean water. Any apparent increase in paediatric disorders was initially explained, as it often still is, as better recognition of longstanding problems, despite the contrary evidence of experienced mothers and grandmothers.

## Women's changing roles

Traditionally, it had been unusual for educated women to seek paid employment after marriage. In some professions, such as nursing and teaching in Australia, employment of married women was actively forbidden, and less formal but still powerfully oppressive barriers of social opprobrium were in place elsewhere. But ever since the 1920s, many women have needed paid work, as so many were left widowed or single after the Great War of 1914–18. The Great Depression and increasing industrialisation of Western society had meant that people had to find new occupations. Servants became less affordable for the middle classes, and housing became an issue for a group that traditionally had lived in, with bed and board provided. Agriculture became more mechanised, and farm labourers (and their families) became redundant. As the 1930s progressed and the armed forces began to soak up male labour, women would be needed once again in the war factories and on the land.

All these changes in women's roles contributed to the reality of formula being necessary, or just more convenient, in a world where breastfeeding was simply not expected or accommodated – because mothers had previously been excluded from that working world. And rather than society changing to accommodate mothers entering or re-entering the workforce in greater numbers, such women were expected to avoid 'discomforting' or 'provoking' men. As women

---

695  Jelliffe DB, Jelliffe EFP. *Human milk in the modern world* (Oxford University Press, 1978) p. 234.
696  By 1964, the height of the bottle-feeding era, the average weight of a six-month-old baby was a kilo heavier than in earlier decades.

began to enter 'male' occupations, anxieties arose about men seeing women breastfeeding – a sight once routinely depicted in public and even sacred art, and normal in many non-Western societies, even those with strict ideas about female modesty. But Western cultural attitudes to sexuality and breasts were changing, along with movies and marketing. All this made public breastfeeding a more heavily charged topic. With women having so many battles to fight, breastfeeding became less possible and less acceptable socially.

## Not so perfect?

No talk of risk reached parents who had chosen artificial feeding, and who quite reasonably thought the product totally safe. The only publicised problems and warnings related to carer negligence, that is to the misuse of the product. Parents had no idea that infant formula was not, and could rarely be, a sterile product, much less that the powder itself may allow omnipresent mould spores or bacteria to grow, if left at room temperature.

Even now, almost a century later, parents are still shocked to read the WHO website statement that powdered infant formula is not a sterile product.[697] Some governments have not yet adopted the WHO advice about water temperature for formula preparation to reduce the risk of meningitis, sepsis and death.

Industry has largely ignored it, if formula cans are evidence. All those I checked in March 2012 in Australia advise making up formula in the tepid or lukewarm water in which microbes thrive.[698] Most labels did not tell parents that formula powder is not sterile. None advised storing opened tins at temperatures that would retard mould or bacterial growth. While the development of antibiotics would come to mean that fewer artificially fed infants of the wealthy die as a result of infectious disease, some of it transmitted by infant formula, such diseases are still often fatal in poor communities. And every summer many formula-fed infants are still admitted to hospital with diarrhoea, and every winter with respiratory disease. But the infant formula tins only warn parents that the misuse – not the use – of their product is risky. The truth is that both use and misuse are risky, to differing degrees depending on the family context.

No mention of such microbial hazards marred the twentieth century assumption that industrial milks were safe. 'Closeness to breastmilk' remained the reassuring marketing theme, together with further subtle and overt undermining of perceptions of breastmilk quality and reliability. A theme that lasted in advertising for decades was something like 'When breastfeeding fails or is insufficient ...' Not 'if ever', or 'in the rare event that', but 'when', because we all know it surely will fail or be insufficient before baby can eat family foods. Great for maternal confidence. So is the current claim that one formula is 'the perfect blend of science and love': clearly mothers' milk can't compete, as mothers know they are not perfect, or scientific. And despite the evidence of thriving babies of mothers on even poor diets, every formula tin advises women that good diet is necessary for breastfeeding mothers ...

---

697  Available at http://www.who.int/foodsafety/publications/micro/pif2007/en/
698  Contrary to the clear advice in the WHO/FAO document above.

## Built-in obstacles to breastfeeding: healthworkers as formula advocates

The medicalisation of birth and breastfeeding advanced at different rates in different nations. Britain in the 1950s was still in an era of stringency and recovery from the Second World War, and the creation of its National Health Service was reshaping the medical landscape. America was generally in the lead in the rush to medicalise women's birthing and breastfeeding, helped along by architectural hospital plans supplied by obliging infant formula makers.[699] Buildings made to these plans were designed to separate babies from their unclean mothers – the product of an era that obsessed about hygiene, especially in the 'lower classes', yet failed to recognise that hospital staff are much more likely to be disease carriers. Dates and extent may vary, but the process of institutional interference with and suppression of breastfeeding followed a similar trajectory around the English-speaking world, shaped by increasingly international commercial forces, and the dominance of American paediatric publications and obstetric literature – a dominance created and underpinned by advertising and grant income from industry.[700]

At the beginning of the 1920s, artificial feeding had been seen as experimental, and mostly a supplement to initial breastfeeding. But by the 1940s, infant formula had become an accepted part of life. Enough babies had been bottle-fed for some of its damage to be obvious to formula makers, who continued to revise formulas in response. But still most babies began life with a little breastfeeding, as the pundits all advised. Formulas were thus being introduced only after some days or weeks of breastfeeding, which undoubtedly increased the likelihood of gut tolerance.

It was usual from the 1940s right up until the 1980s in Australia for hospital staff to insist that a baby must be 'settled' on a feeding regime, whether breast or bottle, before leaving hospital. If a mother was struggling with breastfeeding, this meant swapping to the bottle before going home. As mothers gave up breastfeeding increasingly early, the colostrum myth emerged: the idea that colostrum, the first milk secreted, contains special protective qualities that breastmilk doesn't. In animal rearing, intense efforts to obtain colostrum will be made if any valuable young animal cannot be mother-fed, as farmers are aware that the infant animal gut allows cells to pass into the blood and is easily damaged, with devastating diarrhoea the consequence of artificial feeding. Colostrum was known to provide some protection against large molecules passing through the gut wall into the bloodstream. The process of the gut becoming less permeable to large molecules is referred to as 'gut closure', and it took days or weeks in some animals. However, gut closure was (wrongly) believed to have happened before birth in human babies or very soon after, and so it was assumed that alien proteins could be safely fed, preferably with the baby's gut primed with a little

---

699  Domestic use of infant formula: hearing before the Subcommittee on Oversight and Investigations of the Committee on Energy and Commerce, House of Representatives, Ninety-seventh Congress, first session, June 17, 1981. pp. 32–3. Can be accessed from http://nla.gov.au/nla.cat-vn3853323.

700  In his San Francisco home, Dr Bill Silverman in 1984 showed me correspondence with the AAP estimating that every US paediatrician would need to pay an additional US$70 annually, without industry advertising in the AAP's flagship journal, *Pediatrics*.

colostrum with its unknown protective properties, not then categorised or understood. We now know that colostrum actively 'paints' the gut with protective immune cells. And it is thought that infant gut closure can take weeks, and that oxidative stress of any kind increases permeability, while the anti-oxidative power of breastmilk and the presence in milk of EPO (erythropoetin) modulate this process.[701]

Perhaps the colostrum myth was an instinctive attempt to rationalise the increasing number of mothers sent home from hospital bottle-feeding, as interventionist hospital births and restrictive hospital practices interfered with normal physiological lactation. As early as 1952 Illingworth et al suggested more flexible feeding practices; they were largely ignored.[702]

Medical ignorance also contributed. In England and Australia, where governments subsidised medical care for citizens, general practitioners acted in conjunction with community health midwives or nurses, as first-line consultants for all child care. General practitioners referred to private paediatricians only in cases of unusual child disease or abnormality. Paediatricians outside the United States initially had little to do with well babies, and many left breastfeeding management to nurses and midwives in both the hospital or the community. Their role has since expanded as allergy and developmental disorders have become more common, but even in those cases there are other avenues of referral, such as to allergists or psychologists. Until recently, many paediatricians have not been educated about human lactation and, not knowing how to solve breastfeeding problems, tended to advise the use of infant formulas, about which they had been assiduously 'educated' by industry. Similarly, neonatologists working in special care units have been willing to accept industry products a little too uncritically, as the story of fortifiers illustrates (see 3.11 The 1980s: bettering breastmilk on page 427). And until the 1980s and the publication of *Successful Breastfeeding: a guide for midwives* by the UK's Royal College of Midwives, many midwifery staff were as ignorant as the doctors whose orders they deferred to in matters of feeding. Scientific research into human lactation was just beginning to take off with the creation of the International Society for Research into Human Milk and Lactation (ISRHML) in 1984, and lactation was not well understood by most frontline healthworkers. Dr Mavis Gunther had been one of the pioneers of such research from the 1940s onwards, when her observation of a woman in labour, whose breasts ejected milk with each contraction, led her to hypothesize that oxytocin was responsible for milk ejection. She was frustrated[703] by her inability to get doctors to take lactation seriously. It was animal physiologists who first took up her challenge to research human lactation in the late 1960s,[704] and progress was slow.

---

701 Westerbeek E, Stahl B, van Elburg RM. Human milk and intestinal permeability. In Zibadi et al, op. cit., p. 105.

702 Illingworth RS, Stone DG, Jowett GH. Self-demand feeding in a maternity unit. *Lancet* 1952; i: 683–87.

703 Gunther's book *Infant Feeding* (Methuen 1972) had been important in solving my breastfeeding problems in mid 1976. So I visited her in 1983 and 1987 to tell her how she had contributed to *Breastfeeding Matters*.

704 Peaker M. in Crowther SM, Reynolds LA, Tansey EM (eds). *The resurgence of breastfeeding, 1975–2000*, electronic resource: http://www2.history.qmul.ac.uk/research/modbiomed/Publications/wit_vols/44865.pdf. The transcript of a Witness Seminar held by the Wellcome Trust Centre for the History of Medicine at UCL, London, on 24 April 2007. Also available as a book, p. 40.

# 3.4 Going global: perfecting formula feeding 1950s–1980s

The postwar world changed dramatically. America was buoyant and expanding, and goodwill from her allies was at an all-time high, especially countries like the UK and Australia. By the 1960s, Australia had become a rapidly expanding market as the decade of postwar immigration and the baby boom had increased the population from under seven million to over ten million. Modernity was whatever was American, baby feeding included. Dr Benjamin Spock[705] soon outsold Truby King: his influence was global in the Anglophone world by 1960, despite his tragic experience as both parent and partner.

One unexpected outcome was that the 'American position'[706] for sleeping babies – putting babies down to sleep on their stomachs, or prone – became fashionable by the 1960s and 1970s, after Spock recommended it in his 1956 edition.[707] That happened despite decades of warnings that babies sleeping on their tummies were more likely to die. As they did, in the SIDS epidemic that accompanied the rise in prone sleeping. Warnings about any link between sleeping face down and 'suffocation' were opposed on the grounds that they would make parents of dead babies feel guilty, after one study showed that babies could breathe under blankets.[708] Spock's endorsement of the face-down posture was in line with prominent US paediatricians like Joseph Garland whose Harvard University Press book in 1932 had stated that colic was less likely to occur in babies 'accustomed to sleeping for a part of their time on their stomachs, for in this position gas is more readily expelled from the bowel.'[709] Prone sleeping was never traditional in Western society, and was actively denounced in others, but accompanied the rise in distress from artificial feeding. It was all about settling the distressed baby, like those described in the many *Pediatrics* advertisements for infant formulas. Garland, a Harvard lecturer in 1932, went on to become editor of the prestigious New England Journal of Medicine; the 'American position' went on to facilitate the twentieth century epidemic of cot death, part of formula's collateral damage.

---

705 Maier T, *Dr Spock. an American life* reveals much about the man and incidentally, perhaps the consequences of artificial feeding. As the baby of a neurotic upper-class mother Ben had suffered from the 'summer complaint' so common in bottle-fed babies, diarrhoea; later his success at Yale was due not to academic ability but to rowing. His first wife, who helped write the famous book, had a tragic life: a premature baby who died, repeated miscarriages, problems with alcohol and prescription drugs for mental illness, spells in institutions. Of their two sons, the first was reared on strict four-hourly bottle feeds, was dyslexic and struggled at school; the second, more than a decade younger, had been diagnosed with coeliac disease by the age of two. Spock's grandson was schizophrenic and suicided. http://www.nytimes.com/books/98/05/17/reviews/980517.17bolotit.html

706 Called that by two older maternal and child health nurses when I was a 1970s new mother.

707 Spock recommended it as 'the usual starting position for infant sleep.' and though back-sleeping increased the risk of choking on vomit.

708 Gilbert R, Salanti G, Harden M, and See S. Infant sleeping position and the sudden infant death syndrome: systematic review of observational studies and historical review of recommendations from 1940 to 2002 *Int. J. Epidemiol.* First published online April 20, 2005 DOI:10.1093/ije/dyi088. A must-read article on this topic.

709 Garland J. *The youngest in the family* (Harvard University Press, 1932) pp. 144–5. He also suggested that 'bandaging the mouth tightly shut will often serve to break the habit' of ruminating infants spitting back their food (p. 142). I guess it would. Pity about the risk of choking though.

Endorsed by health professionals and hospitals, bottle-feeding was by now as American as Uncle Sam. It was a symbol of modernity, an agent of freedom for those women who could afford to employ poorly paid women to care for their children, or who had relatives with whom babies could be left for care. And, as movie-goers revelled in the Hollywood-led obsession with breasts as sex symbols, bottle-feeding meant freedom from messiness[710] and embarrassment as well.[711] In addition, men could reclaim women's breasts as their private property, not compete with the baby. It was an irresistible package for an increasingly self-centred and sexualised culture. And it was immensely profitable for the companies: in America Ross Laboratories, a division of Abbott Laboratories, made the market-leading formula, Similac; Mead Johnson, a subsidiary of Bristol Myers, sold Enfamil; and between them these two controlled most US sales, with Wyeth, owned by American Home Products (making SMA) trailing in third place. Despite huge marketing budgets, the profit margins on infant formula were enormous by comparison with other products: 15–25 per cent in 1979, in a global market of just $2000 million, or two billion, of which a quarter was the US home market.[712]

American 'formula' feeding was soon being exported. Wyeth brought its new nitrogen-packed formula, SMA, to Britain in 1956, and sales increased rapidly, 'an advance to which TV advertising has contributed', according to the UK Competition Commission.[713] No need for companies to keep producing printed advice for mothers on the scale they once had: women could be reached by more powerfully persuasive means. Wyeth had introduced liquid concentrate cans, and in 1961 developed a 'humanised' powder formula, SMA Gold Cap-S-26.[714] More on this in on page 310.

## What type of formula where?

British and Australian and New Zealand infant feeding still revolved around dried mik products made up at home. The 1950s market leader in the UK was of course Glaxo's product, the free National Dried Milk; in Australia it was Nestlé's Lactogen, which had supplanted Glaxo (both minimally altered dried milk powders) and would be joined by the 'humanised' product Nan in 1959. Condensed milks were by then used only in illness and on the advice of the network of child health nurses (although as late as the 1970s an 'emergency' recipe using condensed milk was written into my solely breastfed son's child health record).

---

710 Not only from oxytocin-triggered milk ejection during sexual play, but an end to leaky breasts staining clothes, and mortification when this occurred in public.

711 Some of the ramifications are well-explored in Rodriguez-Garcia R, Frazier L. Cultural paradoxes relating to sexuality and breastfeeding, *J Hum Lact*, 1995; 11(2):111–15.

712 Borgholtz P. Economic and business aspects of infant formula promotion: implications for health professionals. In Jelliffe DB, Jelliffe EFP (eds) *Advances in International Maternal and Child Health* volume 2. (OUP 1982) pp. 158–203. This deserves a wider reading.

713 http://webarchive.nationalarchives.gov.uk/+/http://www.competition commission.org.uk/rep_pub/reports/1960_1969/fulltext/038c02.pdf

714 Wharton B. Food and child health in Britain. In Bond JT, Filer LJ, Leveille GA, Thomson AT, Weil WB (eds) *Infant and child feeding*. (Academic Press, San Diego 1981) p. 160.

North America was different. There, infant feeding had not been predominantly based on dried milk powder; evaporated milk was the staple. In 1960, 80 per cent of US infants were drinking homemade evaporated liquid milk mixtures, used with fresh orange juice and cod-liver oil or vitamin drops for the first few months, with other solids introduced ever earlier. The other 20 per cent were fed some of the more expensive patent formulas in handy cans, or were breastfed for ever shorter periods. By nine to twelve months, children were supposed to be eating family foods, including regular full cream milk. Evaporated milk continued to be part of the whole family's diet as it was cheap and kept well. It was still used in the 1990s by poor families, and its deficiencies were revealed in an article in 1999, which followed up eighteen-month-old children fed such formulas. The abstract speaks for itself.

In parts of Canada including Newfoundland and Labrador and among Aboriginal peoples, infants still consume evaporated milk (EM) formulas for cultural and economic reasons. At 3 and 6 months, full-term infants fed EM (n = 30) received low intakes of iron, thiamine, selenium and had higher weight velocity than breastfed (BF, n = 29) infants. EM infants had greater anemia, lowered transketolase activity (thiamine) and lowered glutathione peroxidase (selenium) activity (p < 0.05). To determine the later effect of early feeding deficit on nutritional status, we examined these same infants at 18 months of age. At that time, there were no differences in dietary intakes of energy, protein, zinc, copper, selenium and iron, nor in plasma levels of zinc, copper, vitamin C, nor in red blood cell activity levels of glutathione reductase (riboflavin), transketolase, glutathione peroxidase, nor in superoxide dismutase. However, EM infants weighed more and were more likely to visit a physician, have anemia, and have iron depletion than were BF infants. We conclude that infants consuming evaporated milk formulas should receive iron supplements throughout infancy.[715]

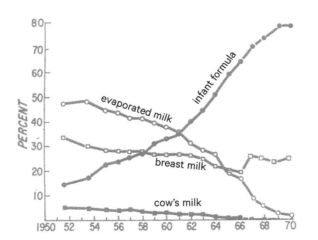

Figure 3-4-1 Infant feeding at hospital discharge 1950-1970 USA[716] © NY Academy of Medicine

More expensive US patent formulas gained ground in the 1940s, and with the 1951 introduction of liquid concentrates to which only water was added, their popularity increased. By 1970 fewer than 10 per cent of families were using evaporated milk mixes; by 1972 the figure often cited was less than 5 per cent, with 70 per cent or more now using the patent brands[717] at hospital discharge, and more within a week or two as breastfeeding was abandoned. The shift to 'humanised' patent foods happened in

715 Friel JK, Andrews WL, Edgecombe C, McCloy UR, et al. Eighteen-month follow-up of infants fed evaporated milk formula. (PMID: 10489720) *Can J Public Hlth*, 1999; 90(4):240–3. Personally, I concluded that Canada needs to educate parents not to use evaporated milk!

716 Fomon SJ. A pediatrician looks at early nutrition. *Bull NY Acad Med* 1971; 47(6): 569-578. PMCID: PMC175004. Free online. © NY Academy of Medicine. Image modified: feed labels added.

717 Cone, in Bond et al., op. cit., p. 27.

two decades, and this was what America exported to the world. 'Infant formulas' they were now called, and in the era of naïve science worship, that misleading[718] wording worked well, inspiring confidence.

# The decline of breastfeeding, and the growth of popular marketing

The period after the Second World War was one in which women were reassessing their roles and seeking greater freedom. Reassured that modern formula was safe, and would not harm their precious children, more and more women felt free to escape the real tyranny of (needlessly and unfairly) closeted breastfeeding, with its restrictions on their lives. With increasing prosperity, and government-subsidised formula, poor families saw infant formula as an investment that permitted women to continue paid work. So in countries like the UK and Australia, breastfeeding rates plummeted as disadvantaged groups (the women who had still been breastfeeding in the 1940s) followed their middle-class sisters into artificial feeding. Not until activist educated mothers took the lead would this tide turn, and then only slowly and partially, as the mother to mother support volunteers lacked the millions necessary to match industry's universal reach.

The worldwide decline in breastfeeding was phenomenal. By the 1970s in many countries only 25 per cent of babies ever breastfed (and of course, many mothers gave up breastfeeding soon after beginning, then as now). In Chile, for example, breastfeeding rates dropped from 95 per cent in 1960 to 10 per cent in 1968. Many who worked with poor families around the world could not avoid seeing the damage infant formula was doing.[719] Kenyans created a new word, 'chupa-itis' or bottle disease, for diarrhoea.[720] The National Council of Churches' Inter-Faith Center on Corporate Responsibility (ICCR) took up the cudgels for child victims.[721] Catholic nuns and doctors alike had accused companies of being irresponsible for marketing their wares so slickly around the world. (Perhaps the Catholic Church could mobilise its global power to protect infants from commercial exploitation of all sorts nowadays!)

Companies naturally responded by vilifying their critics. Bristol Myers/Mead Johnson gave $10,000 to right-wing Ernest Lefever's Ethics and Public Policy Center, who contracted with *Fortune Magazine* editor Herman Nickel to study the infant formula controversy. This resulted in critics being described as 'Marxists marching under the banner of Christ',[722] and

---

718  Few scientific formulas would work reliably or predictably if they allowed as much leeway with ingredients as any infant formula does!

719  Notable early publicists of the problem were Dr Derrick Jelliffe, Director of the Caribbean Food and Nutrition Institute in Jamaica, and Dr Caterine Wennen, along with Dr Bo Vahlqvist. See Richeter J. *Holding corporations accountable* (Zed Books, London, 2001) p. 50

720  The Kiswahili word for bottle is chupa.

721  ibid., p. 53 et seq.

722  Nickel H, in *Fortune,* 16 June 1980. For more on this see Nestle M. *Food politics: how the food industry influences nutrition and health* (University of California Press, 2007), p. 150 (no relation to the company!). There is an excellent account of aspects of the controversy in this book, but I would like to see the author look more closely at the major American players, who have largely escaped scrutiny, although she notes that they were enjoying profits of 15–20 per cent on sales, unheard of for foodstuffs with such huge marketing budgets.

corporation haters. Nestlé was also soon exposed as having given Lefever's Center some $25,000, a fact often cited while Mead Johnson's funding role is not mentioned.

Industry portrayed itself (and still does) as supporting breastfeeding while simply trying to replace dangerous high-solute cows' milk in the infant diet. Companies tried hard to avoid being seen as undermining breastfeeding. They asserted that they were not competing for the share of the market held by breastfeeding: they encouraged breastfeeding 'if possible'. No, they were trying to capture the market share of full-cream whole cows' milk, which should not be given to infants.[723] This latter claim was technically true, but for it rang a little hollow, because most mothers never used full-cream cows' milk: they took whole cows' milk in liquid or powdered form, diluted it by adding carbohydrate and water, and fed it along with supplements of vitamins and iron. Some early formulas were not much different from that, yet all would claim, as one put it, to contain 'All the things that are in mother's milk'.[724] Widespread marketing (TV, magazines, detailing to doctors) of formula presented the newer formula versions as modern, safe and very close to breastmilk (just as the older ones had). All paid lip service to breastfeeding as the ideal, with a persistent sub-text that of course not all women can breastfeed.

The irony of marketing formula by promoting breastfeeding was not lost on marketing experts. As one said in 1980,

> There can't be many manufacturers whose main advertising platform is to advise customers to use a competitive product. What's more, the competitive product is free and no one makes any profit at all. But the paradox doesn't end there: advertising the competitor is likely the shrewdest and best way of promoting the product in question. That product is baby milk.[725]

And that is still true. The more wonderful breastfeeding was, the better the formula seemed, when 'so close nowadays as not to make any real difference'. The 'next best milk', in fact. Which is another sly statement which can be read both as 'a successor to,' or a supplanter of, breastmilk, not just as an admission of breastmilk's superiority. If companies want to tell women breastfeeding is best, they would inform them of the risks of not breastfeeding, and they would be believed where 'fanatics' are not.

While the initial strategy was supposedly to oust older formulas based on evaporated or powdered cows' milk, the dual message about closeness to breastmilk and women's inability to breastfeed obviously facilitated early weaning.[726] Affluent mothers then went on with formula feeding, as is now happening in China and India and the Middle East.[727] (See Growing the world market on  page 493)

---

723  American Academy of Pediatrics (AAP) Committee on Nutrition. The use of whole cow's milk in infancy. *Pediatrics* 1983; 72:2 253–55
724  Richter op. cit. p. 50.
725  Anon. Baby's milk: soft sell success . *Marketing* 1980; May 14.
726  An excellent chapter outlining promotional strategies of these transnational corporations is Borgoltz, PA. op. cit.
727  http://www.ubic-consulting.com/template/fs/documents/Nutraceuticals/Ingredients-in-the-world-infant-formula-market.pdf. Downloaded 30 March 2013.

As always, where elites lead, the less advantaged follow. Many postwar American marketing images showed bottle-feeding women as elite women– sophisticated, coiffed, wearing smart clothes and jewellery – and breastfeeding mothers as dishevelled or blowsily exposed in night attire, without even a wedding ring on display, much less jewellery. The bottle-feeding mothers were smiling and gazing into their child's eyes, the breastfeeding mothers often shadowed or unsmiling, headless torsos or huge bare breasts, with flat shoes and frumpy clothes.

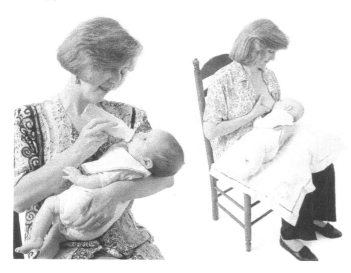

Figure 3-4-2 Images of mothers: which is more attractive?

Yet when a breastfeeding mother was used to advertise a formula's claim of closeness to breastmilk, as they were at times, her image would be one of intense closeness and intimacy. Bottle feeding at night was imaged only by those selling heating devices for bottles, or suggesting fathers would do night feeds: the industry subtly promoted the idea that only by competing for feeding rights could fathers have equal access to their child, while suggesting to mothers that this would relieve their workload. No doubt there are some families where this was the case, but they were not breastfeeding families. Having to express milk so a partner can do token feeds adds to a woman's workload; using formula in the bottle may give her mastitis and an unsettled baby to deal with.

In British countries, healthworkers tried to persuade mothers to feed for at least the first few days in hospital. This was in some ways counterproductive, as the subliminal message became 'valuable antibodies are in colostrum, milk is not all that important'. That healthworker emphasis on the value of colostrum and even a few days of breastfeeding was in some ways the best of both worlds for companies, as initial breastfeeding made little difference to profit, but could improve infant tolerance of formula once it was introduced.

## Emerging allergy

For formula companies did know that their products caused problems for some babies: they had never stopped trying to create less allergenic formulas, from Cow & Gate's Allergilac to Ross Labs Isomil or Mead Johnson's Nutramigen, repeatedly reformulated.

Eczema was widely understood to be much more common in formula-fed babies: and so was gut distress. Yet there was little or no long-term research about 'allergy' in first or later generation bottle-fed children, some of whom were becoming breastfeeding mothers, and having problems with their own children. As late as the 1980s, intelligent educated mothers who tried to get help for their food-allergic child were often dismissed by hospital-based doctors as manifesting the 'muesli-belt syndrome'. Patronising dismissal of mothers' concerns was all too often the hallmark of the medical profession in this postwar era of mother-blaming, as I know all too well. I believe that attitude delayed recognition of the emerging epidemics, such as autoimmune and developmental disorders. These are discussed in subsequent chapters.

## Humanising the industrial product: the power of language

The term 'humanised' formula was once again used as healthworkers sought to discriminate between older homemade formulas and new 'complete' ones. 'Humanised' is an imprecise and changing term, which really just implies the equivalence of artificial formulas to breastmilk, the human product.

Biochemist Dr. Ben Mepham's account of the specifics of early foods claiming to be 'humanised' is unrivalled for explanatory detail.[728] In the early part of the twentieth century 'humanised' was applied at times to homemade formulas made by breaking down cows' milk with water and sugar. In 1915 Gerstenberger's SMA[729] (Synthetic Milk Adapted) was the first single formula in which the total fat content was adapted to approximate human milk: it was humanised, because it contained roughly 4.6 per cent fat. Then 'humanised' referred to the so-called 'complete' American formulas of the 1940s onwards. Later, in the 1970s, it was claimed by companies making brands with fat blends only of vegetable oils, without butterfat or lard. (That was a bit odd, when cows, as mammals, are closer to humans than plants!) Next it would refer to changes in protein balance, one of the battlegrounds of the 1980s marketing campaigns. In fact, it was a ragbag term, never defined, but emotionally persuasive.

Ironically, by the 1960s and 1970s, some companies openly criticised past formulas as unsuitable. In some cases they were distancing themselves from their own products, which had made identical claims of closeness to breastmilk. Yet the old formulas, now criticised as unsuitable and unsatisfactory, are paradoxically still cited as reassurance that the new improved ones of the same name, or by the same company, can be trusted to be an infant's sole food for months! Companies appeal to the past as proof of current trustworthiness and authority. 'Trusted by generations' say the cans. 'We've been in the business of making formula for 100 years', 'Your mother trusted us, and now you should' is a common marketing theme. Full-page advertisements in every influential medical and nursing journal were the norm, and those journals and associations turned a blind eye to the idea that this could undermine breastfeeding.

The 1960s claim that a product was 'humanised' distanced infant formula from cows' milk, so successfully that even hospital nurses were sometimes unaware that the product was

---

728　Mepham TB. Humanizing milk: the formulation of artificial feeds for infants, 1850–1910. *Medical History* 1993; 37: 225–49.

729　Parents of children afflicted with and dying of Spinal Muscular Atrophy (SMA) dislike seeing the formula's slogan 'Every baby deserves SMA'. Now that Wyeth is owned by Nestlé, the brand name (and its objectionable advertising and imagery) might finally be targeted for change.

based on milk.[730] The term 'humanised' alters the linguistic and emotional associations around formula, which in fact has been becoming ever more industrialised and highly processed throughout the twentieth century. Health professionals should have been deriding and denouncing this manipulative, if not outright deceptive, language. Medical authorities and journals allowing it to go unchallenged, suggest that they were gullible, ignorant, or complicit. As an industry spokesman rightly said in 1975,[731]

> For over 25 years industry has praised breast-milk as the ideal feeding and that which provides a model for humanized milk. This message has been transmitted to physicians and mothers through promotional literature. Humanized milk formulas owe their success to having been promoted as close equivalents to breastmilk and providing comparable clinical benefits.

As close as possible: what does that mean? When hearing that formulas are 'as close to breastmilk as possible', parents should realise that those possibilities are limited not only by cost, but also by insuperable scientific, financial, manufacturing and engineering constraints. It is still not possible to produce anything like breastmilk, any more than we can produce artificial blood. The differences between living tissues and industrially produced stopgap substitutes are intractable. If the previous 'perfect' products need to be replaced, why should we believe that the latest ones won't be similarly defective? If the new ones are sensitive and gentle, why are rough and insensitive ones still sold? Or is there really no difference: surely if there were, there would be no second-class product for sale? Do the companies even believe that the differences matter? If they do, it would be deeply unethical for them to continue to make second-rate products. If they don't, how can they justify charging so much more for the 'gold' than their previous formula? Where are the long-term comparative studies to tell us what formula is better overall? A grandmother will say with no sense of irony that her grandchild will do well on brand X because her daughter did, not knowing that the new formula is not the same as the old (even if the name remains the same), and not seeing any connection to her daughter's – or her own – lifelong health issues. I have had some fascinating dialogues with such women, who usually end up enraged, not with me, but about what they did not know about products they trusted so implicitly.

Personally, I agree with Dr Sykes, who in 1903 stated that 'The only way to humanise cows' milk is to pass it through a mother.'[732] The term should be banned from advertising worldwide, as nothing will ever make a collection of inert ingredients from around the world 'human'. Human milk is the unique milk a woman's body makes for her unique child (or others), influenced by that child's sex[733] and feeding patterns. Infant formula should be named in the French style, industrial milks – milk made by industry, or ersatz, or artificial substitutes for breastmilk. Formulas are not baby milk – babies do not lactate – and the

---

730 'We'd never give them cows' milk, we only use infant formula,' was heard by many parents, myself included!

731 Sehring DA,. Infant feeding trends in an industrialised culture. *Mod Prob Pediatr.*, 1975; 15:231. Cited in Jelliffe, *Human milk in the modern world,* op. cit., p. 340.

732 Lewis J. op. cit., p. 96.

733 Hinde K. http://www.abc.net.au/radionational/programs/healthreport/the-effect-of-breastfeeding-on-infants/5587144#transcript Downloaded August 16, 2014.

product is not particularly good for babies either, wherever there is the better alternative of women's milk.

Stop for a moment, and think some more about language and how industry uses it to persuade. In marketing, formula is described as close to breastmilk or even more insidiously, nearly identical to 'mother's milk', capturing something of the maternal care factor by the reference. Talk of 'human milk' somehow disembodies it, making it generic and objective and standardised when in fact it is individualised. A recent major work even uses 'human breast milk' in its title, as though animals other than humans have breasts, and milk is made by all humans, male and female.

By contrast, we rarely refer to cows' milk as udder milk, or even bovine milk, because it is the females, cows, that lactate. Why do we never talk of or read about women's milk? Women's milk is simply milk made by women, a more generic but striking term than mothers' milk. Certainly, rare cases of male lactation have been recorded,[734] but even more rarely would those breasts feed a child. When enough men have functional breasts, induce lactation and breastfeed, we could accurately be gender-neutral and describe breastmilk as human milk or breastmilk. Until then women's milk is the more accurate collective term, and mother's milk the specific individual term. Indeed, for humans, women's milk could be the definition of 'milk', not the udder product! Think about the potential emotional significance of women claiming their own unique resource, being aware of its importance to human survival, and being proud of what they alone can do for their child – and for other children, quite often.

It's worth noting in passing that some scientists were not fooled into thinking formulas 'humanised'. In 1973 Crawford termed contemporary formula 'a collection of proteins, minerals, vitamins and some vegetable oil foisted on an uninformed public as being as nutritious as human milk.'[735]

And in 1977 Leif Hambraeus wrote that formula feeding represents 'the largest in vivo experiment without a control series'.[736]

Which is precisely why Professor Zef Ebrahim pointed out that:

> ... artificial feeding carries risks. Infants who are fed artificially are biologically different from those who are breastfed. Their blood carries a different pattern of amino acids, some of which may be high enough to cause anxiety. The composition of their body fat is different. They are fed a variety of carbohydrates to which no other mammalian species is exposed in neonatal life. They have higher plasma osmolality, urea, and electrolyte levels. Their guts are colonised by a potentially invasive type of micro-flora, at the same time as they

734 Ploss HH, Bartels M, Bartels P. *Woman: an historical, gynaecological and anthropological compendium* (WM Heinemann Medical Books 1935) vol 3, pp. 213–16.

735 Crawford MA, Msuya PM, Munhambo MA. Structural lipids and their polyoenic constituents in human milk. In Calli G, Jacini J, Pecle A (eds). *Dietary lipids and postnatal development* (Raven Press NY, 1973) p. 41. Cited in Jelliffe. *Human milk in the modern world* op. cit., p. 207.

736 Hambraeus L. Proprietary milks versus human breastmilk: a critical approach from the nutritional point of view. *Pediatr Clin N Am*, 1977; 24:17.

are exposed to large amounts of foreign protein resulting in an immunologic response. In addition, they are deprived of the various immune factors present in human milk. All these factors need to be taken into consideration every time a decision is made not to breastfeed an infant, for inherent in such a decision are known and unknown risks to the infant.[737]

All that is still true, no matter how formula has changed since then. How could health professionals be ignorant of this? How could they know this yet advise formula feeding? How could parents take such things into consideration when health professionals told them none of that? And why didn't they?

## Co-option, co-operation, corruption and copping out: capturing healthcar

In the brilliant light of hindsight, so many health professionals were so gullible. But they have to be seen in the context of the times. Their education had not covered infant feeding; they were trained to respect authority and accept authoritative statements; rote learning rather than critical thinking dominated the curriculum in the days before evidence-based medicine; there was little pressure for ongoing education, much of which was supplied by industry anyway. Most health professionals were well-intentioned ethical people who could not envisage that babies' interests might be sacrificed to company profits. They trusted company reps to know that what they were saying was true. Company reps trusted the company to be telling them the whole truth about the product, and were drilled about how to sell it. But this was not 'truth, the whole truth, and nothing but the truth.' Partial truths can be misleading. I have since met some very disillusioned formula industry reps!

Besides, health professionals probably wanted and needed to believe that formula was safe and 'close to breastmilk nowadays'. By the 1970s and 80s, breastfeeding women were presenting with problems they could not solve. Largely trained in the era of bottle-feeding, very few had much clinical experience or even abstract knowledge of lactation or of breastfeeding. The books of the era were little help. Almost every mother came home from hospital with breastfeeding problems after a 4–5 day stay.[738] Many hospital staff didn't even know how lactation and breastfeeding worked. Suffering was expected as nipples fissured and mastitis flared. Early warning signs like nipple compression stripes were seen as normal, and breastfeeding was expected to be painful. Hospital schedules and rules and supplements could have been designed deliberately to interfere with normal lactation, in the name of hygiene, staff convenience, and cost saving. Mothers and babies had to fit in with absurd routines.

So much easier, then, if babies could be sated and sedated with bottles of formula, and mothers could be despatched home with a sample can considerately left behind for the purpose by a charming rep who even remembered the nurse or doctor's name (with the help

---

737  Ebrahim GJ. *Breastfeeding, the biological option* (Macmillan, 1978) p. 59.
738  Reiger K. *Our bodies, our babies: the forgotten women's movement* (Melbourne University Press, 2001) gives an excellent outline of typical birthing experiences in Australia at this time.

of very detailed confidential files kept by companies and passed on between reps[739]) and who brought little tokens of appreciation to brighten their day. After all, 'humanised' formula was so much better nowadays, and they wouldn't say that if it wasn't true ... would they?

Healthworkers of the 1970s had often artificially fed their own children, and many (if not most hospital staff) had never seen a lactating breast working well. Many positively resisted the rising tide of scientific information suggesting that artificial feeding damaged children: just as for any other parent, it is not easy to stand back and acknowledge that something you have done in good faith may have harmed those you care about. If anything, it might well have been much harder for health professionals to do so. Healthcare is a vocation as much as a career. Doing what was best for babies was part of their professional and personal identity. How much more difficult would it be to accept such evidence? Much easier emotionally to ignore what hasn't been definitively proven, and condemn as fanatics those who took it seriously. And who did they think they were, these uppity mothers' groups telling women how to succeed at breastfeeding? In the hierarchical world of the health professional trained in the postwar era, mothers were to take advice, not give it.[740] Assertive women who wanted to birth or breastfeed in ways that conflicted with established practice were not appreciated, much less encouraged, by many such healthworkers. Change would come as women mobilised around childbirth education and breastfeeding, but it came slowly and piecemeal.

The 1960s US transition to patent brand names had been facilitated by US hospital contracts that ensured all parents saw the health–care system modelling the use of a particular infant formula as safe and effective. Mead Johnson was possibly the first company to provide free supplies of ready-to-feed formula to US hospitals in 1959. Wyeth supplied four-ounce bottles of SMA, distilled water, and 5 per cent glucose in 1963, along with sterilised teat units.[741] Abbott/Ross Laboratories, makers of Similac, pioneered convenient single ready-to-feed (RTF) units in 1963. Their Ross Hospital Feeding System was designed, as the Sales Training Manual put it, 'to provide an easy and convenient means of getting infants started on Similac ... and ultimately sent home with instructions that the mother continues to use Similac.'[742] Industrial/patent formula makers had long targeted both health professionals and hospitals as important marketing tools. Their stated goal was 'to make the physician a low-pressure salesman for our products.'[743] Not until 1969 were such freebies given to UK hospitals, when Ross exported SMA, 'the first ready-to-feed milk to UK maternity units',

---

739  One former salesperson confessed to being shocked by some of the private detail that was passed on in company card files which breached accepted standards of confidentiality, and was sure that health professionals had no idea the company kept such records of their lives and prescribing behaviours.

740  Some mothers' groups agreed, and – in the interests of gaining medical approval – insisted that their well-trained volunteers should never give advice: just make suggestions. Of course many mothers think that suggestions from a better informed woman are advice! It's a fine distinction.

741  *Wyeth infant formulas: a distinguished history of nutritional research and development.* Company literature collected in USA, 1984. On file.

742  Confronting the infant formula giants. *The Corporate Examiner*, 1982; vol. II, issue 7–8, p. 2. Interfaith Centre on Corporate Responsibility (ICCR)

743  ibid.

and with it the practice of locking in 'contracts for the milk kitchens in each of the major maternity units' using financial and other inducements.[744]

Free supplies of formula to hospitals developed first in the US, where Ross's Similac was the brand favoured by physicians. Parents exposed to brands in hospitals assumed those fed to their babies to be the best choice: an internal Abbott Ross training manual for sales staff claimed that brand loyalty was as high as 93 per cent, i.e., that 93 per cent of parents would buy that brand after going home.[745] A Canadian study documented this powerful influence.[746] (see image below). A more recent study showed that such parents were less likely to switch formula brands[747] as well, although there are few good reasons not to do so.

Figure 3-4-3 Hospital samples and maternal choice of formula brand.

The fight to get hospitals to accept product was intense, and various incentives were offered. In the US this could be a million-dollar payment to the hospital for exclusive rights to give parents take-home gifts of formula and even bottles, all – of course – company branded. Mead Johnson even bought the US rights to use Beatrix Potter's iconic Peter Rabbit in

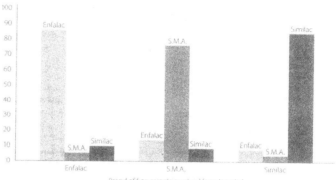

its US marketing giveaways, on lovely tote bags: ironic when baby rabbits would die if fed cows' milk, being seriously lactose-intolerant. The condition of any such gifts (and all the companies provided similar things) was that the maternity hospital would enter a contract to use only its brand of formula for all term infants, and to see that 'every new mother will leave a municipal hospital with a free one-day supply of Similac.'[748] No one told the mothers that was why they were getting a particular brand: it smelt uneasily like corruption. In Italy it is now being investigated as just that.[749]

In Australia, I considered the most despicable incentive of which I had direct knowledge was the American company waiving payment for its so-called 'human milk fortifiers', then in vogue for adulterating breastmilk given to preterm infants (see 3.11 The 1980s: bettering

---

744  Prof. Forrester Cockburn, in Crowther et al, op. cit. p. 53.

745  ibid.; also Borgoltz, op. cit., p. 186. Ross Abbott's Similac was sold in Australia. The product was a little-used casein-dominant mix, available as a liquid concentrate only in chemists by the 1970s. It remained the dominant formula in America through the 1980s, while in Australia in March 1990 its market share was just 5 per cent according to data supplied by industry at the time.

746  Image from 1985 Breastfeeding Promotion KiT. Nathoo T, Ostry A. Op. cit., p. 136. ©All Rights Reserved. Canadian Infant Feeding Patterns: Results of a National Survey". Health Canada, 1982. Reproduced with permission from the Minister of Health, 2015.

747  Huang Y, Labiner-Wolfe J, Huang H, Choiniere CJ, Fein SB. Association of health profession and direct-to-consumer marketing with infant formula choice and switching. *Birth*, 2013; 40(1):24–31. DOI: 10.1111/birt.12025.

748  *New York Times,* 27 September 1981.

749  http://www.reuters.com/article/2014/11/21/us-italy-breastmilk-arrests-idUSKCN0J51TZ20141121

breastmilk on page 427). The company priced these tiny sachets of cows' milk and minerals at a ridiculous cost, and then claimed that cost as part of the value of their 'gift' to any hospital which would sign an exclusivity contract to use only its formula. (Some would see this as a bribe, others leverage, or even extortion.) Copies of such contracts were hard to get, but I was given one by an outraged midwife. Which Australian hospital was naïve or base enough to sign one? By contrast with the $1.50 for each tiny allergenic sachet (to be added to 25 ml breastmilk), their hospital-invoiced price of 100 ml glass bottles of ready-to-feed formula shipped into Australia was a nominal 25 cents,[750] and to my knowledge never rose above 50 cents in later years.

Convenient ready-to-feed (RTF) formula saved Australian and UK staff time making up powdered formula (a task many hated); in the US, where formula preparation had often been outsourced, they saved hospitals big bills from commercial milk laboratories.[751] In addition, they saved staff time in other ways: a fractious baby could be dosed, and there would be no need to waste time on trying to get a breastfeed into him or her. Hold the baby at an angle with its head back, apply the bottle and milk will flow: baby will swallow. (The alternative is choking.) Staff insisted that mothers 'get baby settled on breast or bottle' before discharge 4–5 days postpartum. If the mother was having problems breastfeeding, obviously that meant she 'chose' formula. What choices did she have?

## Expanding choices and consequences: liquid or powder, when, where?

As the industry consolidated and expanded globally after 1950, many types of infant formula emerged. As noted earlier, Anglophone countries have varied widely in the physical form of the infant formula products used, and this is significant for many reasons. In Australia and New Zealand, use of industrial formulas has always been predominantly in the form of cans of dry milk-based powder, an economical way of packaging and transporting infant food over long distances in small markets. In the UK, charity and then government supplies of baby milks were also of tinned powdered milk, the cheapest option. But in North America most formula sold by the 1970s and 1980s was liquid. Following on from liquid evaporated milks, formula concentrates had been produced by US companies from 1951, first in 390 ml (lead-soldered) cans. There were increased risks of microbial growth if any liquid product was inadequately sealed, or not kept at 4 degrees Celsius or less, and heavy metals like lead transferred more readily from can solder into liquid formula than into powder. As well, new chemicals had to be added as stabilisers, or the liquid formulas would separate or curdle, while iron could cause the fats to oxidise and so the liquid formula could develop an obnoxious taste.

Liquid concentrates had come first. Parents were to add an equal amount of water, and failure to do so, presumably by the illiterate or careless or distracted, resulted in infant deaths. Equally, once the ready-to-feed liquid formulas were produced, some parents diluted these as they had the earlier concentrates.

750  Noted in *ALCA News*, 1990; 1 (2):25; see also *ALCA News*, 1992; 3(1); 6–7.
751  Fomon SJ. *Infant nutrition* (1974 2nd ed.) p. 13.

From 1964, quart (950 ml) cans of liquid ready-to-feed (RTF) infant formula were made available, and Fomon sees this as the principal reason for consumers moving away from the cheaper home-prepared formula: convenience won out over price.[752] Ready-to-feed infant formula varieties were to be poured straight from the can into the bottle, and minimised preparation error as far as dilution and water quality were concerned.[753] They were soon the most popular type of formula in America, and possibly made bottle feeding by the poor less likely to result in illness. By 1970 fewer than 10 per cent of American parents used the older homemade evaporated milk formulas; by 1973 the figure was just 5 per cent.[754]

This weighty liquid alternative to infant formula powder was affordable in part thanks to US government subsidies to industry and agriculture. In the late 1960s, the US government had focussed on feeding low-income Americans. The 1967 US National Nutrition Survey had shown that many lower-income children suffered from anaemia and poor growth, adversely affecting brains and so cognitive ability, and that many poor mothers did not get adequate food in pregnancy. In 1972, Congress created the Special Supplemental Nutrition Program for Women, Infants, and Children, to be known as WIC. Congress funded the program for two years with the US Department of Agriculture (USDA) in charge of it. Thus the main US purchaser of all infant formula from the mid 1960s onwards was the USDA, which paid full retail prices for infant formula purchased in bulk, then handed it out free to poor families via food stamp and relief programs, then WIC.

This massive government purchase at full cost (by all but a couple of US states)[755] must surely be what allowed US companies to provide free supplies to hospitals, and cross-subsidised retail sales so that liquid formula was cheaper in America in the 1970s than powdered formula was in Australia, despite the extra weight, manufacturing, and transport costs. When visiting supermarkets in the United States in 1983 I was astonished at the low price of ready-to-feed quart/950 ml cans, which took up masses of shelf space in supermarkets.

Being able to pour formula from the can into a baby bottle was what made formula-feeding convenient, and to some degree safer for disadvantaged families. Preparing powder carefully never was, and never will be, convenient. Even midwives used to hate being on duty in hospital 'milk rooms': in the courses I taught for two decades, this was a common rueful admission. Errors could be fatal, as when six of eleven infants died after salt was accidentally added instead of sugar.[756] In 1980 only around 5 per cent of commercial US formula sales were of powder. Then came the first Oil Shock and the inflation of the 1980s, and powder sales rose. When industry profits from USDA/WIC purchases went down in the 1990s, formula prices rose and so did formula powder sales. In 1994, the figure was

752  Fomon SJ. Infant feeding in the 20th century: formula and beikost. J Nutr 2001; 131: 409S-420S Infant feeding in the 20th century: formula and beikost. *J Nutr* 2001; 131: 409S-420S

753  Lucas A, Lockton S, Davies PS. Randomised trial of a ready-to-feed compared with powdered formula. (PMID: 1519960) *Arch Dis Child,* 1992; 67(7):935–9. Free full text article. DOI: 10.1136/adc.67.7.935.

754  Fomon SJ (1974), op. cit., pp. 14–15; see also Cone TE. In Bond J., et al. *History of infant and child feeding* (Academic Press, 1981) p. 30, citing Fomon's data: no independent national statistics exist, but these figures were sourced from industry, with whom Fomon worked closely.

755  Kent G. WIC's promotion of infant formula in the United States. *International Breastfeeding Journal* 2006, 1:8 DOI:10.1186/1746-4358-1-8

756  Finberg L, Kiley L, Luttrell CN. Mass accidental salt poisoning in infancy. *JAMA,* 1963; 184:121

44 per cent; by 2008, 83 per cent of US infant formula sales would be of powder.[757] The boom years of RTF infant formula in affluent America were over. The following image from Fomon's useful overview article[758] illustrates these dramatic shifts.

To my knowledge, no other country has ever recorded such a high use of ready to feed liquid patent formula. Probably no other country could have afforded to. No other country had such generous government subsidies to formula manufacturers and agriculture in general. US taxpayers have funded artificial feeding and dairy producers on a massive scale: corporate socialism on an unparalleled scale, which makes a mockery of talk of free trade.

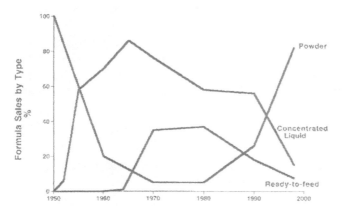

Figure 3-4-4 US sales of different types of infant formula 1950-1998 © American Society of Nutrition

Using liquid ready-to-feed or concentrated formulas has its own potential hazards of contamination and microbial growth, as well as dilution, over-concentration, and heat damage to contents. Serious problems are on record, where parents made mistakes in dilution or failed to notice off odours or can swelling. Formula company water sources used to make up the liquid formula have been contaminated; the wells involved were closed due to groundwater contamination with known carcinogens.[759] It is reasonable to think that the practice of fracking for coal seam gas will increase this risk to liquid infant formulas, and add costs to retail prices as formula companies try to guard against such eventualities without knowing what chemicals may have been used, and therefore should be tested for, in groundwater. There are already reports of contaminated water supplies as storage units leak. (And a Texas jury has just awarded damages to a family harmed by their neighbour's wells.[760])

But in general, the use of liquid formulas also avoids or reduces many basic problems[761] relating to water quality, preparation hygiene and scoop contents. Machines ought to be more accurate in measuring powder than scoop-users.[762] All studies show wide variation in the composition of made-up powdered formulas, even when Australian scientists attempted

757 Oliveira V, Prell M, Smallwood D, and Frazao E. *WIC and the retail price of infant formula.* Food Assistance and Nutrition Research Report 39–1. Available online.

758 Fomon SJ (2001) op. cit.. 1950-1998 © Republished with permission of American Society of Nutrition, from *Journal of Nutrition* 2001 131 (Supplement); permission conveyed through Copyright Clearance Center, Inc.

759 *Food Chemical News,* November 28,1983; p. 29.

760 Morris J. Texas family plagued with ailments gets $3M in 1st-of-its-kind fracking judgment. CNN April 26, 2014 – http://edition.cnn.com/2014/04/25/justice/texas-family-wins-fracking-lawsuit/

761 An excellent review is Renfrew MJ, Ansell P, Macleod KL, op. cit.

762 As far back as 1973 researchers found that 'the variations 93–111 per cent when following the instructions carefully raises the question of whether the scoop is a satisfactory measure at all.' Shaw JC, Jones A, Gunther M. Mineral content of brands of milk for infant feeding. (PMID: 4739637) *Br Med J,* 1973, 2(5857):12–5

to accurately reconstitute the product. Scientists consciously trying to get it right did better than parents: their range was 80–120 per cent of the recommended strength, while parents made up bottles with strengths ranging from 66–150 per cent of that recommended.[763]

Interestingly, in that study the formula that showed the highest mean concentration was the same one that Vietnamese mothers believed made bigger babies ( a belief that induces them to give infant formula soon after birth, in Melbourne or in Sydney.)[764] They were right! That was the brand later reformulated to be 'fluffier' (see page 216).

In Leeds in 2001, I did a presentation to the local Infant Feeding Consortium on making artificial feeding safer. As always, the realisation dawned that the risks of the process are inherent and utterly unavoidable.[765] Professor Mary Renfrew then set in train what became two excellent reviews of the processes of artificial feeding: these are essential reading for health professionals.

The first, on making up feeds, stated:

> ... it is important to minimise the risks associated with breast milk substitutes. Specifically, parents need to know which ways of giving their babies formula feeds are the simplest, most accurate, and cost effective. It is important to identify the outcomes as well as the sources of error in making up feeds – what contribution do they make to infant mortality and morbidity?[766]

The authors recommended that

> The range of ways in which manufacturers package and sell breast milk substitutes needs to be examined; they themselves recognise that risks are introduced in the reconstitution of their products. Some consistency in approach would be a step forward, perhaps moving towards uniform instructions and scoop sizes for the reconstitution of all products and brands. This would avoid confusion for parents when changing from one product to another, and help health professionals teach parents how to make up feeds more accurately. A source of unbiased information is needed to inform parents and health professionals about the differences between the available formulae, including the different forms in which they are sold. In the UK there is an important role in this regard for both the Food Standards Agency and the Department of Health.[767]

And of course, similar agencies in other countries need to take this on.

---

763 Bennett J, Gibson RA. Accuracy of infant formula preparation by Adelaide caregivers. *Breastfeeding Review*, 1988 (November issue) pp. 59–61. See also Lilburne AM, Oates RK, Thompson S, Tong L. Infant feeding in Sydney: a survey of mothers who bottle feed. (PMID: 3355446) *Aust Paediatr J,* 1988, 24(1):49–54. Renfrew MJ, McLoughlin M, McFadden A., op. cit.

764 Nguyen ND, Allen JR, Peat JK, Schofield WN et al.. Growth and feeding practices of Vietnamese infants in Australia. (PMID:14749758) *Eur J Clin Nutr* 2004 Feb;58(2):356–62.

765 What I was saying was so obvious if only the process was thought about step by step. I have often heard from experienced health professionals after such presentations, 'I knew all that, but I'd never put it all together and thought about it.' Such is the power of custom and massive advertising budgets to suppress critical thought.

766 Renfrew MJ, Ansell P, Macleod KL. op. cit.

767 ibid.

The later publication from the York Mother and Child Health unit was a systematic review of cleaning and sterilising feeding equipment, which concluded that:

> There is a lack of good-quality evidence on effective ways of cleaning and sterilising infant feeding equipment in the home. The evidence base does not answer the question about which of the methods in common use is most effective or most likely to be used by parents. Hand-washing before handling feeding equipment remains important. Further research on the range of methods used in the home environment, including assessment of the views of parents and carers, is required.[768]

Indeed – in every country where artificial feeding is carried out.

The UK and WHO materials about safer bottle-feeding alluded to elsewhere are key outcomes of this long-overdue concern. But industry is well aware of the problems. To jump ahead in time to the present era, the ultimate high-end formula-making product is a logical extension of food preparation trends: the Nestlé automated formula-preparation machine, Babynes. This controls the formula dose, eliminates bacteria, and is done in a flash: and those with deep pockets are almost certainly buying it and becoming totally dependent on a gizmo to feed their baby. That has serious downsides when one thinks of all that can go wrong with being dependent on machinery in modern life – including the potential for further avenues of microbial contamination. However, it's likely that this again makes formula feeding safer microbiologically for the rich, though it does nothing about the inherent defects of the artificial formula itself and is clearly not going to help those most likely to need it, poor families everywhere. Competitors will emerge, and a formula maker will become yet another expensive outlay parents can be persuaded to consider buying to prove that they love their babies. Governments and health authorities should instead market those natural devices that control the dose in response to consumer demand, eliminate multiple risks, require no special cleaning, and always work even in power outages, fire, flood and famine – women's breasts.

A 1999 study showed that failure to comply with recommendations for making up formula was high for several practices with clear health implications: 33 per cent of mothers mixed formula with warm tap water (microbes, lead, copper), and up to 48 per cent heated bottles in a microwave oven (burns, nutrient damage, formation of toxic agents). Mothers of two-month-old infants who received instruction from a health care professional and who breastfed showed increased compliance, but few demographic characteristics, such as education, were related. The longer made-up formula was left unrefrigerated, the higher the rates of diarrhoea.[769]

Unlike the rest of the world, at this time US health authorities did not mandate boiling water for making up formula from either powder or liquid concentrates, perhaps because they were aware that this was impossible for some of those who bottle-feed and live in impermanent and sub-standard accommodation, perhaps because of misplaced confidence

---

768   Renfrew MJ, McLoughlin M, McFadden A. op. cit.

769   Fein SB, Falci CD. Infant formula preparation, handling, and related practices in the United States. (PMID: 10524388) *J Am Diet Assoc*, 1999, 99(10):1234–40. DOI: 10.1016/S0002-8223(99)00304-

in the safety of urban tap water, and failure to consider the hazards of groundwater.[770] But perhaps also because of an implicit bureaucratic recognition that to raise public awareness of the need for extreme care with artificial feeding might lead to irresistible public demand for the affordable services that make this possible: reliable and cheap power, very clean water, decent living conditions and the income that makes them possible.[771]

Illness and deaths across all social classes were – and still are – blamed not on faulty or contaminated formula, but on careless mothers reconstituting it in unsafe conditions. Carers are always to blame. Hygiene in the home was the solution. As though poor families anywhere, including in affluent nations, can provide safe conditions for such a potentially hazardous task with an intrinsically hazardous product: it requires access to clean water, soap and utensils, affordable fuel, and safe preparation spaces! As poverty, urban decay, homelessness and drug use increases in wealthy nations, how many babies are fed in conditions no mother is responsible for? How many are non-Anglo, Indigenous or poor or immigrant or otherwise disadvantaged? And babies can still die even when affluent mothers take the greatest care to follow instructions on the label.[772] As this study just cited makes clear, formula-borne bacteria can infect healthy, term (not just hospitalised preterm) young infants. Invasive infection is extremely unusual in infants not fed powdered milk products.[773] Thus the study author encouraged breastfeeding and/or the use of ready-to-feed liquid formula for infants under two months, the latter an option for the wealthy bottle feeder. 'There are very few studies comparing the clinical and nutritional effects of powdered and liquid formulas ... liquid formulas have been easily accepted worldwide because of their advantages of sterility and ease of use in routine neonatal care.'[774]

However, sterilisation of liquid formula creates higher levels of heat-damaged protein by-products, so first we need to know more about the so-called glycation products produced.[775] Half a century after the appearance of liquid formulas, these advanced glycation end products (AGEs) are now of concern, as they have been linked to higher rates of regurgitation and delayed growth in infants.[776] And, while saying no direct human evidence of harm as yet exists, researchers flag a wide variety of possible concerns – insulin sensitivity, kidney damage, bone health among them – so that they advise no or limited re-heating of reconstituted infant formula, and avoidance (except where absolutely necessary) of the most heat-damaged products, the hydrolysed formulas.[777] And there are many other differences between powdered formula and liquid formula, even within the same brand.[778]

---

770 Rogan WJ, Brady MT, Committee on Environmental Health, Committee on Infectious Diseases. Drinking water from private wells and risks to children. (PMID:19482745) *Pediatrics* 2009, 123(6):e1123–37.

771 Barbara Ehrenreich's attempt to live as a minimum wage worker should be read by those who assume that all Americans live in suitable housing with access to affordable, reliable water and power. See Ehrenreich B. *Nickel and dimed* (Metropolitan Books, 2001).

772 Jason J. Prevention of invasive cronbacter infections in young infants fed powdered infant formulas. (PMID: 23045556) *Pediatrics*, 2012, 130(5):e1076–84.

773 Ibid.

774 Ibid p. 167.

775 Sebekova K, Klenovics S, Brouder Sebekova K. In Preedy V, Watson RR, Zibardi S (eds) op. cit, Ch. 26

776 Korkmaz A, Surmeli-Onay O. Powdered and liquid infant formulas: clinical and nutritional aspects. Ibid., ch. 10.

777 Sebekova K et al., op. cit.

778 Korkmaz A, Surmeli-Onay O. op. cit.

# Invisible risk

Whether powder or liquid, all infant formulas carry risks. It is certain that with such a low index of suspicion around infant formula, and such defective – or non-existent – education of families and carers, many cases of formula-induced illness in previously healthy babies have been overlooked, or wrongly attributed to parental carelessness or ignorance. Parental ignorance is hardly culpable or surprising in a society where knowledge is not universally available, but it is always punished, often quite unfairly, if it results in harm to a baby. But there is little real risk of punishment for others who feed a baby formula. The financial consequences of proven formula-linked illness could be huge, so health professionals will sometimes help the company to cover up the fact of contaminated or defective formula, as it might well put their institution or themselves at legal risk for endorsing or supplying or feeding the product. Silence is of course rationalised as a matter of not upsetting other parents. I have known staff to be threatened with job loss after urging senior staff to report a batch of clearly defective ready to feed formula, quietly replaced by the company.

Despite this cone-of-silence protection afforded formula, some instances of such formula problems have been publicly recorded in Western nations in every decade (see Figure 2-11-1 on page 179). One classic example occurred in the UK.

> Just before Christmas 1985, considerable public concern was aroused when Ostermilk baby foods and some other milk products were withdrawn following an outbreak of Salmonella Ealing food poisoning. The manufacturer was the Plymouth-based Farley Health Products although the factory where the problem occurred was in Kendal, Cumbria.[779]

This £8 million recall led to Glaxo Smith Kline putting Farley's into liquidation, and its two manufacturing plants were sold to Boots in 1986 for £18 million. But the brand had never recovered from the reputational damage done by the recall, although Boots ploughed millions into promoting it. Boots sold the Ostermilk brands to Heinz for £94 million in 1994, and Heinz Nurture replaced Farley's Ostermilk. Both Milupa, initially a German-based manufacturer, and Wyeth UK had gained market share meanwhile. Then in 1996–7 it was Milupa formula that was the source of Salmonella anatum infections in infants.[780]

There have been other outbreaks of infection due to Salmonella in infant formula, and an open access article[781] outlines those proved to have occurred in the twenty years from 1985. It pointed out the inevitability of under-reporting and the extreme difficulty of identifying formula as the source. It provided a useful table of the many countries involved: USA, Canada, France, UK, Korea, and in the latest cases discussed, many countries from a single

779 Goldie FJ. Farley health products: a case history, *British Food Journal,* 1988; 90(1):20–1

780 www.independent.co.uk/news/milupa-offers-milk-refund-1285144.html Like Wyeth, Milupa has changed over time. A German bakery firm which first produced infant cereals, Milupa sold an infant formula, Milumil, from 1964. A rival Dutch firm, Nutricia, bought the UK's Cow and Gate in 1981 and then Milupa in 1995 as well as New Zealand's Karicare brands and Douglas Pharmaceuticals' SHS International (1996); a name change in 1998 to Royal Numico followed, and later, in 2007, Numico was bought by French rival Danone, still buying up milk production facilities in NZ in 2014. See http://www.fundinguniverse.com/company-histories/royal-numico-n-v-history/ and http://www.dairyreporter.com/Manufacturers/Danone-Nutricia-set-to-acquire-NZ-infant-formula-operations

781 Cahill SM, Wachsmuth IK, Costarrica Mde L, Ben Embarek PK. op. cit.

source, due to the international trade in infant formula. Cases continue to be reported. In 2012 Salmonella-infected Belgian infant formula caused disease in Russia.[782] Such disease is not confined to mild cases of diarrhoea: babies have died, and been brain damaged by meningitis.

A similar problem had been discovered in Australia in the mid-1970s. After a couple of expensive and fruitless searches for the source of microbial contamination of its infant formula, the company went back into making milk products, and exported the infant formula into Asia.[783] The same factory made milk foods for the elderly, and a cluster of deaths in a geriatric facility revealed these as the source of infection. The resulting investigation unearthed the formula problem[784] and its unethical 'solution'. No company worker had acted as a whistleblower, though many would have known of the problem; no one knows how many babies – who typically live singly, not in clusters – were affected.

Nowadays such actions by major infant formula companies seem inconceivable (just as they did then), not least because better international accountability has been created by greater consumer awareness. But then it is inconceivable to normal people that, simply to make money, anyone would add melamine to milk for infant formula,[785] or that anyone would deliberately counterfeit formula by putting fake labels of expensive hydrolysed brands on to cheaper tins, or add detergent powder, or sell those or outdated products over the internet. Yet such vile actions have harmed and killed babies.[786] Wicked things still happen in the twenty-first century! So much so that a new database is being established to record fraudulent and counterfeited food ingredients from 1980 onwards.[787] It expects to have many thousands of entries, and infant formula products will be among them. And not only in China do such things occur. The USFDA has prosecuted dairy farmers and milk transporters for adulterating milk with water and salt, a firm selling milk loaded with antibiotic residues, and an individual rebranding infant formula.[788]

It is of course not always greed or malice which puts babies at risk. Accidental or careless mistakes can be just as deadly.

> Another major recall occurred in 2001 when preparation instructions were translated incorrectly into Spanish and printed on the labels of some 3.7 million cans of powder Nutramigen [Mead Johnson] formula and 930,000 32-ounce cans of the ready-to-use version. In 2004, a blunder in translating preparation instructions from English to Spanish again resulted in a product recall when the FDA reported that following instructions on

---

782  Astley M. 24 January 2012. http://www.foodqualitynews.com/Food-Alerts/Belgian-baby-formula-linked-Salmonella-outbreak-sickens-16-in-Russia

783  Craven JA. Salmonella contamination of dried milk products. *Vic Vet Proc.*, 1978; 36:56

784  Forsyth JR, Bennett NM, Hogben S, Hutchinson EM, Rouch G, Tan A, Taplin J. The year of the Salmonella seekers – 1977. (PMID: 14705299) *Aust N Z J Public Health*, 2003, 27(4):385–9.

785  Moore JC, Spink J, Lipp M. Development and application of a database of food ingredient fraud and economically motivated adulteration from 1980 to 2010. *J Food Sci*, 2012; 77(4):R118–26.

786  Kent G. *Regulating Infant Formula* (Hale Publishing 2011) ch. 5 deals with this.

787  Moore JC, Spink J, Lipp M. Development and application of a database of food ingredient fraud and economically motivated adulteration from1980 to 2010. *J Food Sci*, 2012; 77(4): R118–126.

788  Check out http://www.fda.gov/ICECI/EnforcementActions/EnforcementStory/EnforcementStoryArchive/ucm109460.htm

both the 16-ounce powder infant formula and the 32-ounce ready-to-use infant formula could cause serious health problems.'

And not just the labels, but the product can be entirely wrong, as when a milk-based adult supplement was substituted for soy formula, much of which is consumed by infants allergic to milk protein. Only a mother smelling her child's formula identified Vanilla Sustacal instead of Prosobee.[789] Another failure of presumed-fail-safe in-house quality control?

The needless death toll of infants due to defective feeding had not ended anywhere by the 1980s, or even in 2014. It has merely been reduced (a century late) in those affluent communities where governments subsidise costs and mothers are educated and have access to clean water. As the global market expands and more communities adopt artificial feeding, the absolute number of infant deaths per year will be constantly rising from the one million that James Grant, Director of UNICEF, estimated in 1981, when he began the Child Survival and Development Revolution, with breastfeeding as a core strategy.[790]

At the international public health level, awareness of the risks of formula feeding has never been greater. Yet among elite Western women, complacency about the safety of our current infant formula continues, epitomised in the comments made in an ABC radio interview by one former obstetrician and an equally ignorant respondent.[791] It will be interesting to know whether such complacency survives in anyone reading the following chapters about infant formula's most basic ingredients and its additives over time. In every decade, every company has claimed to be producing the best possible infant formula, referencing it to breastmilk.

The next few chapters focus on the basic ingredients of infant formula and how these have changed over time. The ingredients of course have to be sourced and assembled. Few people seem to realise the complexity of that assembly and production process, so a copyright diagram illustrating that process is added below, courtesy of GEA Liquids Technology. To me it is astonishing that so much formula is produced with so few recorded problems, when a pinhole in any part of the assembly could allow microbes in: industry works hard to contain, but cannot eliminate, that risk. Few people also seem to realise just how much change there has been even in formula's fundamental major components, protein, fat and carbohydrates, and how much of that change is still ongoing. Few people seem to understand how much latitude there is in infant formula regulations, allowing very different infant formulas all to comply. In fact, I think it safe to say that no one in the world knows which infant formula is 'best'. Possibly those involved in designing formulas all believe that theirs is best, but they have funded very little publicly-scrutinised comparative research to support such beliefs. There are significant differences between formulas, but what difference they make to children remains unknown without lifetime comparative

789  Lodato, Patti. Mead Johnson & Company. *International Directory of Company Histories*. 2007. Encyclopedia. com. (May 31, 2014). http://www.encyclopedia.com/doc/1G2-3480000067.html

790  UNICEF *State of the world's children* Report, 1981. See also Jolly R (ed) *Jim Grant: UNICEF Visionary*. Available online at http://www.unicef.org/publications/files/Jim-Grant-LR.pdf

791  Paying for breastmilk? *Life Matters*, Radio National 18 December 2013. http://www.abc.net.au/radionational/programs/lifematters/paying-for-breastmilk/5159118

studies. So as for any infant formula being 'the perfect mix of science and love' ... judge for yourself.

The historical thread from the 1980s will be picked up again in Chapter 3.11. Before going on to consider the ingredients, consider the process involved in producing infant formula.

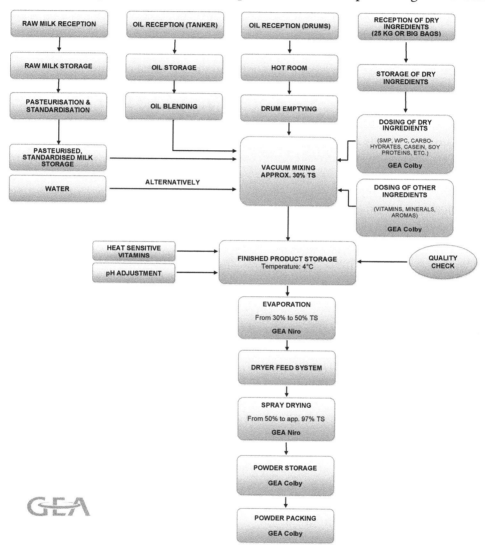

Figure 3-4-5 Compiling an infant formula. © GEA Liquid Technologies

# 3.5 Basic ingredients: Protein

## Problems and potential

For over a hundred years the basis of most artificial feeding has been cows' milk. To a farmer, cows' milk was just that – milk from a cow, nothing added, nothing subtracted (except maybe a little cream skimmed off). But cows' milk varies in composition, and throughout its history has been diluted and adulterated to increase profits on a product sold by volume. Standards have been set to define the minimal requirements for nutrients in cows' milk.[792] These standards are themselves variable: in Australia whole milk should contain 30 g/L (g/L (grams per litre) protein (3 per cent) and 32 g/L fat; it varies slightly in other countries, up to 35 g/L fat, for example. Any excess fat and protein above required legal standards for whole milk may be removed for use in other products like cheese – or it may not. People used to supermarket milk can be surprised by the richness and flavours of fresh farm milk!

Broadly speaking, cows' milk is a complex mixture of proteins and fats made by the bovine mammary gland, and soluble proteins, carbohydrates, minerals, and immune components contributed from blood. It is solidly white because its proteins, predominantly caseins, reflect light.[793] When exposed to acid or to calf stomach enzymes like rennet, this white mix curdles, leaving solids and a clear liquid: curds and whey (or junket if you are old enough to remember that). Paediatric literature from 1900 onwards had talked of making cows' milk easier to digest by modifying the curd to break down, or denature, the casein proteins it contains. Acids, enzymes, and heat can all break down proteins. But no process can stop an alien milk from harming some of those exposed to it. Mechanisms whereby harm is done are all lumped together as hypersensitivity to, or intolerance of cows' milk, as though the problem is the child, not the food it is being given. Whether IgE immune-mediated allergy or other non-IgE-mediated disease like FPIES,[794] the numbers are growing with each generation. And so is the complexity of the protein mixes infants are exposed to.

Breastmilk protein shares broad similarities with cows' milk, but is markedly different. From among the four major groups of proteins (mucins or milk fat globule membrane proteins, wheys, caseins, and peptones (low molecular weight proteins), some 761 distinct proteins have been identified. Research is focussed on identifying what each does and its potential for commercial exploitation.

## Curds and whey

Casein, one whole class of proteins in milk, is the basis of cheese, and also has a wide variety of industrial uses such as paint, glue and plastics. Casein solids can readily be extracted

---

792  Codex Alimentarius (FAO/WHO, 2006)

793  When any unhomogenised milk is allowed to stand, cream separates out and rises to the top. So when breastmilk is allowed to stand, milk beneath the cream layer is translucent because its proteins are predominantly non-reflecting whey.

794  Kemp AS, Hill DJ, Allen KJ, Anderson K. Guidelines for the use of infant formula to treat cows milk protein allergy: an Australian consensus panel opinion. *Med J Aust* 2008; 188(2):109–12.

from milk. The leftover translucent liquid is whey, sweet because it contains lactose (milk sugar), and made up of many different whey proteins along with minerals and more. Lactose can be extracted from whey, and once was sold in tins as milk sugar, to be added to homemade formulas. Nowadays, the protein, carbohydrate and mineral-rich whey can be refined to varying degrees until only a watery residue remains, and governments have allowed this 'permeate' to be disposed of by adding it back into the supposedly 'whole' milk to 'standardise' it.[795] Standardised milk and fresh whole milk taste quite different to anyone brought up on a dairy farm, and have some different properties.

The ratio of casein proteins to whey proteins in cows' milk is roughly 80:20; there are hundreds of different proteins in total, just as there are in any mammalian milk. Back in the 1970s and 1980s, companies taught sales reps (who taught healthworkers) that the ratio of casein to whey in breastmilk was 40:60, and announced they had achieved this ratio in their new so-called humanised infant formulas. In fact, breastmilk protein ratios alter over lactation, but start at about 10:90 in colostrum, averages about 30:70, and later is around 50:50. Some formulas began to mimic the notional 40:60 ratio of casein proteins to whey by the 1970s: any clinic nurses in practice then were deluged with literature about the importance of the whey:casein ratio.

A formula is called whey-dominant if there is more whey-derived protein than casein-derived protein in the mix, and casein-dominant if the reverse applies. So any percentage above 50 can determine 'dominance' of the source protein. Nowadays most artificially fed babies on cows' milk formulas are getting more whey than casein as a protein source; some formulas are now 100 per cent whey-based; and casein dominant formulas are still on the market.

Before 1950 the major formula feeding products in Australia, as in the UK, had been the standard roller-dried full- and half-cream dried milk powder products, and in second place, homemade formulas using dried and evaporated milks. Brand name powdered infant formulas – Lactogen, Ostermilk, Cow & Gate, and National Dried Milk (1940–77) – were little more than modified dried cows' milk plus lactose/sucrose plus vitamins A, D, and C and iron. Each brand gave varying instructions for home manufacture of the formula for baby to drink. In the USA, homemade formulas made with liquid evaporated milk dominated. Thus most pre-1960 formulas were casein-dominant, with proteins in the 80:20 casein:whey ratio. Formula protein levels at this time were from 21 g/L up to 36 g/L.

# From pig-swill to infant formula!

A 2013 presentation to the Eurolait[796] General Assembly in Helsinki contains that phrase. As Christophe Lafougere said in support of it,

> in less than one generation dairy proteins will have gone from feeding pigs to feeding kids, and in so doing created one of the highest added-value, high-volume dairy products

---

795  http://www.nutritionaustralia.org/national/resource/permeate---everything-you-need-know-about-milk-standardisation

796  Eucolait is the European dairy producers organisation.

ever seen, one which is playing a major role in keeping the world milk price and all dairy commodity process high and trending ever higher.[797]

As noted above, whey is a complex mixture of sugars, proteins, and minerals. Before the 1960s whey was a waste product that had few uses – some factories handed it back to the farmer to dispose of! Other factories simply poured the waste into local creeks, or down mineshafts, leading to the pollution of groundwater and wells many miles away. Two notable cases causing major economic loss were the pollution of a bore supplying a poultry processing plant and a well supplying a brewery.[798] Environmental protection laws – regulation backed by policing – caused industry to act more responsibly, to its own benefit as well as that of the community – though there are still exceptions! (see page 524). The prospect of steep fines for environmental vandalism is always unwelcome and usually resented, but does force change on those responsible for making profits for shareholders. As a dairy text put it,

> Traditionally whey was regarded by the dairy industry as an undesirable waste product, of low commercial value, which presented the industry with problems of disposal. However, the imposition of strict controls on the disposal of waste necessitated the construction and operation of effluent treatment plants, which proved costly for the industry. This, together with the recognition that whey was a potentially valuable source of nutrients, stimulated interest in the development of commercially viable processes to convert liquid whey into valuable products, suitable for human and animal foods.[799]

From 1950 onwards was a time of rapid technological change for the dairy industry, partly as a result of such regulatory pressures, and in order to retrieve valuable nutrients being wasted. Electrodialysis in the 1950s, and ion exchange and then ultrafiltration in the 1960s, allowed whey residues to be used as a formula protein source, by lowering the excessive mineral content. The new technologies meant that tonnes of whey protein became available relatively cheaply. Buttermilk (the residues from cream that had been separated from whole milk for butter making) was another Cinderella waste product that was soon reclaimed for sale and later fractionation (breaking up into useful parts). Soon there were huge advances in dairy technology that allowed production of specific milk components and protein fractions (via gel filtration and other processes).[800]

The page opposite illustrates the process of breaking down whole milk to obtain whey powder concentrates; the next image shows what happens to that concentrate.

---

797  Lafougere C. Global developments in the infant formula sector. Eucolait General Assembly Helsinki May 2013. http://www.eucolait.be/all-files/general-assembly/2013-helsinki/14397-christophe-lafougere-infant-milk-formula-final/download.

798  Varnam AH and Sutherland JP *Milk and milk products: technology, chemistry and microbiology* (Chapman & Hall, London, 1994) p. 160. As children walking to school in South Gippsland in the 1950s, we saw the pipe running from our local butter factory to one enterprising pig farmer's property.

799  Mulvihill DM. Functional Milk protein products chapter in Andrews AT, Varley J.(eds) *Biochemistry of Milk Products*. (Royal Society of Chemistry, Cambridge, 1994) p. 99.

800  Packard V. *Human milk and infant formula*. See also Andrews AT, Varley J.(eds) *Biochemistry of Milk Products*. (Royal Society of Chemistry, Cambridge, 1994) p. 99.

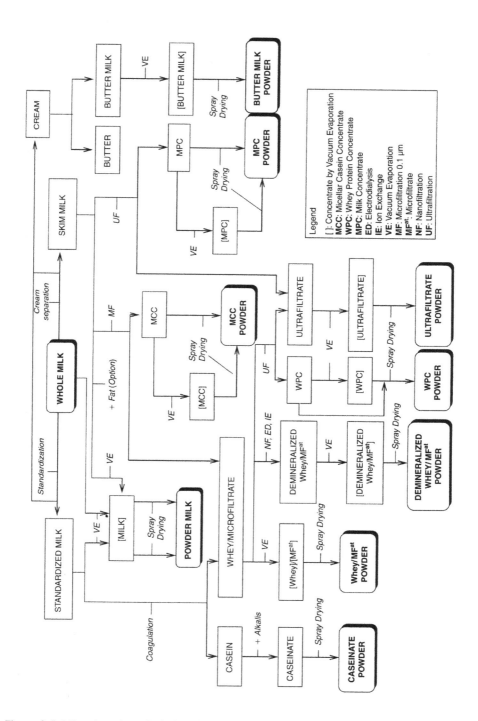

Figure 3-5-1 Fractionation of whole milk to obtain Whey powder concentrates[801] © Elsevier

801 Republished with permission of Elsevier Ltd. Copyright image from Thompson A, Boland M, Singh H. (eds) *Milk Proteins from Expression to Food* (Academic Press 2009) p. 285. Permission conveyed through Copyright Clearance Center.

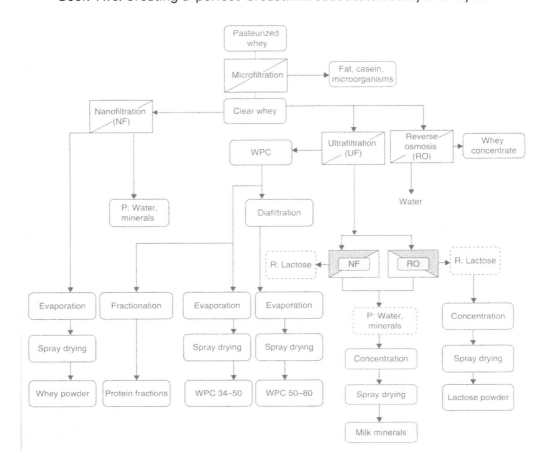

Figure 3-5-2 Whey powder manufacturing flow chart[802] © John Wiley & Sons Ltd.

These processes involve the use of acids, alcohol, alkalis, bacteria, catalysts and enzymes, all potential sources of trace residues, contaminants, and consequences. This diagram above indicates the complexity of these processes just looking at the whey fractions. Caseins and fats head off down other tracks, as can be seen in the next diagram.

## Whey to go: how it is processed

Once enough demineralised whey was available, in the 1970s and 1980s, companies conducted a strong global marketing campaign for whey-dominant formulas as the choice for first formulas, for at least the first few months of life. Wyeth claimed to have made the first 'humanised' whey-dominant formula, SMA (Synthetic Milk Adapted) Gold Cap in the UK, SMA in the US, or in Australia, S-26, in 1961: after 25 previous formulations had been deemed unsatisfactory.[803] Unlike iPhones, where a higher number promises innovation and is desirable, an ever-changing number for infant formula might raise questions about the suitability of the old product for its purpose. And a key marketing strategy for any baby product is to claim a long history of safe usage, and the credibility of past figures such as

802  Park and Haenlein, *Milk and Milk Products in Human Nutrition*, op. cit., p. 482. © John Wiley &Sons Ltd.
803  https://www.meandmychild.com.au/S-26/How_S26_got_its_name/ Downloaded 8 March 2011.

Sir Frederick Truby King[804] (who might well turn in his grave to be associated with some current marketing practices.)

Yet despite touting its 'humanised' product as so much better, Wyeth continued to market its casein-dominant formula SMA as well. SMA, established in the UK after 1956, had become available in Australia in 1959, through Wyeth's pharmacy distribution systems. Both S26 and SMA were more expensive than their competitors, and only available through chemists, both factors which made S26 seem a better and more desirable product, perhaps even more of a medicine than a food. And it harnessed the active good will of pharmacists,[805] respected healthworkers who recommended it as preferable to competitors sold through grocery systems. Wyeth would rapidly increase market share in Australia by its dual strategy of detailing to health professionals and supplying hospitals with giveaways, while confining its retail sales to pharmacies, giving that profession an incentive to believe, and to tell mothers, that the Wyeth product was an improvement over others. In fact by the end of the 1980s Wyeth's S-26 had become the market-leading formula in Australia.[806]

Until this time in Australia Nestlé formula has been the market leader, and would remain a less expensive option, as Nestle distributed formula along with coffee and other foods to grocery outlets, and spent less on advertising. Nan would be the 'humanised' and cheaper competitor to S26, and replaced casein-dominant Lactogen over time. (Lactogen was re-positioned as the second stage formula for older infants.) But Nestle would lose market share, as being more expensive actually works to sell infant formula: even the poorest families want to give their children the best, and many assume a more expensive pharmacy-only product is better.

American marketing practices pushed the whey-dominants to health professionals and hospitals, and so to more affluent opinion leaders. Simple but misleading graphics, sometimes superimposed on curvaceous female bodies, showed how unlike cows' milk was to breastmilk, and how close formulas supposedly were.[807] When the first whey-dominant formulas were being advertised, one such Wyeth image, (later adapted by Nutricia as shown here) put types of ingredients in coloured strips. The colour blocks seemed almost the same size, just a tiny extra bar for immune proteins. In this later Nutricia (Danone) materials, 'enzymes and antibodies' were the only difference –except that cows milk had no minerals, unless these had been combined into the salts section! This seems to

---

804  A basic biography can be found online. A useful outline of his impact on infant feeding in NZ can be found in Apple RD. The medicalisation of infant feeding in the United States and New Zealand. *J Hum Lact* 1994; 10: 31–37. See also Beasley A, Trlin A (eds). *Breastfeeding in New Zealand: practice, problems and policy.* (Dunmore Press, 1998).

805  Pharmacists in the 1980s told me that Wyeth formula made them little profit, as their margins were slight, but it acted as a loss leader, bringing parents in, and they might also purchase other items once there.

806  American-made formerly-Wyeth-S26-formula is currently on sale in Australia as the Advanced Kare product imported and sold by a discount chemist chain. Wyeth chose in the mid 1990s to sell its US factories (but not brand name SMA or S26) to PBM Nutritionals after a period of making formula in America only for export.

807  I have files of such materials, which have also been catalogued in publications of the International Code Documentation Centre (ICDC), IBFAN's office in Penang, Malaysia. Go see what you think, and purchase their materials for healthworkers, such as Protecting Infant Health. http://www.ibfan-icdc.org/index.php/about-us

me quite inaccurate and misleading as a representation of what is in both breastmilk and formula. See what you think.

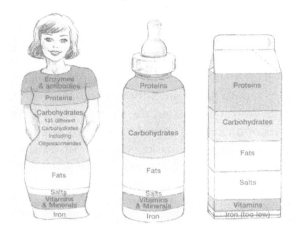

Figure 3-5-3 Comparisons of formula to women's milk (marketing materials)

This same style of (what I see as misleading) diagram appears in an open access 2003 article[808] by a Wyeth scientist writing about the newest formulas with increased concentrations of lactalbumin. In that article the usual whey-dominant formulas were, as you can see, now very different from human milk, while the new experimental one was of course much closer, if one uses the categories chosen. The fact that there are literally hundreds of different proteins spread across those four categories, that they are different between bovine and human milk, and that each, and the quantity of each, may be important to human health, is not conveyed by such pictographs.

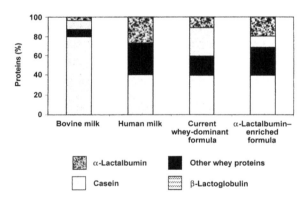

Figure 3-5-4 Comparing formulas in blocks again © American Society of Nutrition

Being a small but concentrated market where in-hospital use and sampling heavily influenced parental uptake of brands, Australia seems to have been a significant launch nation for whey-dominant formula: by the mid 1980s there were few advocates for casein-dominant first formulas, although they were still available, and in fact remained the market leaders in the USA. Mead Johnson had reformulated its US Enfamil[809] to 60:40 whey dominant in the 1980s, and their entry into the Australian market with Enfalac and later the low-lactose Olac,[810] increased marketing activity (and it seems to me, almost single-handedly persuaded parents and health professionals that crying babies were 'lactose–intolerant'. Many doctors would soon suggest lower-lactose formulas even to breastfeeding mothers).

808   Lien EL. Infant formulas with increased concentrations of alpha-lactalbumin. *Am J Clin Nutr* 2003;
     77(6):1555s–8s. (PMID: 12812154). © American Society of Nutrition.

809   Enfamil was created in 1959 as a typical casein-dominant formula with 9 per cent of its calories as protein.It was
     re-formulated in the USA as a 60:40 whey dominant, following Enfalac in Australia.

810   Olac was created in the 1930s as the first high-protein infant formula to include only vegetable oils and no
     lactose. It (or a version of it) was introduced to Australia in the 1980 by Mead Johnson, who pushed the idea of
     lactose intolerance as the cause of crying.

Marketing about whey-casein ratios has varied by country: top US and UK brands were all casein-dominant initially, but marketing shifted this to whey-dominant products over the 1980s – with the exception of Similac (Abbott/Ross), never a huge seller in Australia, but the market leader in America at this time. Even in 2012 Australian SMA still has a casein:whey ratio of 80:20, although in 1997 UK SMA (also Wyeth) had changed from 82:18 to 48:52 casein:whey ratio. While in the USA, the leading brand, Ross/Abbott's Similac, was casein-dominant until the 1990s, when it changed to 48:52. Meanwhile, their organic formula, and the leading organic formula, Nature's One, remains an 80:20 casein-dominant. And some of the newer hypo-allergenic/sensitive formulas can be 100 per cent hydrolysed whey. Which is or was better? What difference does it make lifelong? No one knows.

Using whey for formula-making made sense for the companies, as it was both available and cheap protein. It was marketed as ending the longstanding issue of casein being harder to digest, and constipating. The principal marketing claims from all brands related to easier digestibility, stool characteristics and gut transit times. It was claimed that the old ratio of 80:20 casein:whey unduly increased infant gastric emptying times, and was associated with constipation. (Excess mineral intake of the casein-dominant older formulas was certainly associated with lactobezoars in preterm infants, gut 'stones' or concretions that required surgical removal.[811]) By the 1970s and 1980s there was plenty of advertising making such claims, though there was not a lot of independent research to support them. It is surprising that regulatory agencies permit such claims when there is some evidence that in fact gastric emptying times for whey- and casein-based first formulas are similar.[812] And in 1995 formula-fed babies still had harder stools than breastfed babies.[813] And longer gastric emptying times.

## How much protein is too much?

The total protein load in infant formulas had varied over the century, but on the whole the first formulas had aimed for around 20–25 g/L (grams per litre) of protein, based on the (mistaken) belief that breastmilk supplied around 15 g/L. (The extra in formula was to compensate for lower bioavailability). The new humanised formulas of the 1960s and 1970s would lower this amount considerably, with first formulas around 15–18 g/L in formulas of between 60–70 kcal/100mL. For by the 1970s there were concerns about the effects of high levels of protein on infant bodies, principally kidneys and brains.[814] This level was still excessive. Said a 1981 standard gastroenterology text:

---

811  Robertson AF. Reflections on errors in neonatology III. The 'experienced' years, 1970 to 2000. *J Perinatol* 2003; 23:240–9. DOI:10.1038/sj.jp.7210873

812  Thorkelsson T, Mimouni F, Namgung R, Fernández-Ulloa M, Krug-Wispé S, Tsang RC. Similar gastric emptying rates for casein- and whey-predominant formulas in preterm infants (MED:7808829) *Pediatric Research*, 1994, 36(3):329–33. DOI: 10.1203/00006450-199409000-00010

813  Quinlan PT, Lockton S, Irwin J, Lucas AL. The relationship between stool hardness and stool composition in breast- and formula-fed infants. (PMID: 7884622) *J Pediatr Gastroenterol Nutr*, 1995; 20(1):81–90.

814  Janas LM, Picciano MF, Hatch TF. Indices of protein metabolism in term infants fed either human milk or formulas with reduced protein concentration and various whey/casein ratios. (PMID: 3495653) *The Journal of Pediatrics*, 1987, 110(6):838–48.

> The infant formula industry has formulated its products with significantly greater protein levels than the minimum required ... levels are about 40 per cent greater than the level of protein found to be adequate in feeding trials ...
>
> [Formula with too much protein] will not have any advantages as far as growth [sic], but will stress the metabolic and excretory systems of the infant. Excessive protein intakes during critical periods of development may have negative long-term effects on the infant.[815]

'Stressing the metabolic and excretory systems' translates into, among other effects, high rates of dehydration leading to convulsions and brain damage: bottle-fed infants were known to be at greater risk each summer, and deaths resulted. Scientific research on the metabolic effects of amino acids began to investigate possible connections with diminished kidney health and brain function. Parents heard nothing of such concerns being related to formula composition, later expanded to look at links with diabetes and obesity.[816] They were simply told to offer water to bottle-fed infants in warm weather. This often became offer water to all infants in hot weather, undermining breastfeeding. Yet if, for instance, the larger kidneys that develop in bottle fed babies (see page 535) also have fewer nephrons, kidney function could be affected lifelong. And kidney disorders have risen in countries like Australia.

This research into protein quantity led to a call for industry to reduce the total protein intake in artificially fed infants. But knowing how much to aim for is not simple. Before moving on with this issue of total protein intake, there are two important caveats.

Firstly, it takes more of the less-well-utilised cow protein (and even more of the soy protein) to support adequate growth. Because breastmilk protein is very bioavailable, very little in total is needed for good growth. And as research looked more closely, it became evident that all the protein in breastmilk was not being used for growth: up to 10 per cent was excreted intact in faeces.[817] Its function was protection in the gut. What is more, during months of lactation, the protein content of breastmilk changes.

The accepted average figure now for breastmilk protein is just nine grams per litre (9g/L). So breastfed babies' bodies break down around a gram of protein per 100 ml or just 10 grams per day if they drink a litre of breastmilk (many don't). If from one to four months, they drank the average 750 ml per 24 hours, that falls by 25 per cent to about seven grams per day.

By contrast, Figure 3-5-5 on page 268 shows formula-fed babies' bodies must still digest much more protein, even though the amount has steadily dropped all century. Gunther documented a 1970s protein range in UK and American formulas of 15–29 g/L.[818] Take the average today of 14–16 grams of protein per litre per day and do the sums. The infant body is *metabolising and excreting the wastes from more than twice, sometimes more than three times,* the protein that

815  Benton D. Protein in the diet of neonates. In Lebenthal E (ed). *Textbook of gastroenterology and nutrition* vol. 1 (Raven Press NY, 1981) p. 388

816  Gibbs BG, Forste R. Socioeconomic status, infant feeding practices and early childhood obesity. (PMID: 23554385) *Pediatric Obesity*, 2013. DOI: 10.1111/j.2047-6310.2013.00155.x

817  Davidson LA, Lönnerdal B. Persistence of human milk proteins in the breast-fed infant. (PMID: 3661174) *Acta Paediatrica Scandinavica*, 1987; 76(5):733–40. DOI: 10.1111/j.1651-2227.1987.tb10557.x

818  Gunther M. *Infant feeding* (Penguin Books, 1973) Fig. 11.

the breastfed baby's body copes with. Some formula labels advise mothers to feed over a litre per day; I have seen total doses of up to 1200 ml suggested. So add another 20 per cent to the average of around 15 grams a litre and those babies drinking 1200mL were processing 18 grams of protein per day. That is a serious difference that kidney researchers and obesity researchers should be considering: more anon. Then remember that 15–17 grams is in fact a lot less than the 23–29 g/L a previous bottle-fed generation might have been exposed to!

Secondly, what any formula label says is in the tin is just an approximation of what is aimed at, written around any relevant regulations. As Wharton asked,

> Recommendations, guidelines, regulations and directives are all very well, but can the food industry meet them? What are the tolerance limits around a stated concentration on the label? ... If the regulation is say, 1.8–3g per 100kcal *[that's roughly 12–21 g/L]* and the label claim for a particular product is 2.2g *[15.4 g/L]* what are the limits of variability around this in individual batches of the product? A variation of say 15 per cent would give a range of 1.9 to 2.5 [13–17.5 g/L] values still within the regulatory limits, but somewhat different from those the pediatrician thinks he has prescribed.

> Pediatricians are fond of discussing and studying quite small changes in the protein intake of infants. This is relevant in nutritional terms, but whether it is relevant in the real world, where variations around stated label concentrations could be greater than the fine tuning suggested by physiological experiments, remains to be shown.[819]

And greater it will always be, for practical reasons. The figure on the label is the minimum a company must guarantee will be there for the whole product shelf life. It is not an exact scientific measure of what is there when the formula is fed to the baby. It simply cannot be. Amounts can vary considerably. As an eminent Nestlé scientist, Pierre Guesry, says,

> What is in the can should be more than or equal to what is on the label *[for the entire life of the product]*. This is why, to be on the safe side, we tend to add a little more. The second point is that we work with an unstable raw material. Cows' milk is not constant. In spring there is more fat; during the winter, when the animals receive other types of food, there is less fat. Because of this, the protein/energy ratio is quite variable. We try to measure what is in the raw material and to adapt it, but this is not very easy to do on a day-to-day basis. This explains one type of variability.[820]

And that variability adds to the total protein load of any infant in ways that can only be guessed at. Protein levels in formula have been dropping steadily since this realisation. But what are the safe limits? Too little protein compromises physical growth and cause stunting, but too much has the reverse effect, promoting obesity[821] in the populations so

---

819  Wharton BA, International recommendations on protein intakes in infancy: some points for discussion in Raiha N (ed). *Protein metabolism during infancy* (Nestec/Raven Press NY, 1993) p. 80. Online at http://www. nestlenutrition-institute.org/Resources/Library/Free/workshop/Publication00033/Pages/publication00033. aspx

820  ibid., p. 83. Dr Guesry was responding to the presentation by Dr Brian Wharton.

821  Weber M, Grote V, Closa-Monasterolo R, Escribano J et al. Lower protein content in infant formula reduces BMI and obesity risk at school age: follow-up of a randomized trial. (PMID:24622805) *Am J Clin Nutr* 2014, 99(5):1041-1051. DOI: 10.3945/ajcn.113.064071

overfed. One of the relatively simple issues industry has had to deal with is deciding the quantity of protein allowed in infant formula.

Working out just how to establish the upper and lower level of protein in infant formula was not easy. A Ross Laboratories scientist, JD Benson, discussed this at an AOAC (Association of Official Analytical Chemists) Conference on Production, Regulation and Analysis of Infant Formula May 1985. The Proceedings record him as saying:

> Protein is one of the nine nutrients that have both a minimum and maximum prescribed. The minimal level is based on both the protein content of human milk – 1.6g/100kcal [11 g/L] – and experiments where formulas with protein levels at 1.8g/100kcal [12 g/L] have been fed and have produced growth equivalent to the breast-fed infant. The current minimal regulation is the same as that proposed in 1971. [15g/L] The 1980 recommendation differs from previous recommendations in that a maximum is now included. Establishing a maximal level for protein recognizes that excessive protein not only offers no advantage but because of renal solute load may be deleterious. Milk-based infant formulas contain approximately 2.3g protein per 100kcal [15.4 g/L].

There are some problems with this. As noted earlier, human milk protein at 9g/L is in fact significantly less than even the 12 g/L cited here, substantially different in quality,[822] and the amino acid balances change as the baby grows.

Benson went on to say:

> The standard also states that the protein must have a protein efficiency ratio (PER) at least 70 per cent that of casein. Interestingly, PER reflects the protein quality for a growing rat. In PER-type studies with human milk, rats did not grow optimally, providing some doubts about the utility of PER studies for evaluation of protein for human infants. [823]

Again, it is not often realised that the animal models used to assess the quality of the protein used in infant formula are variable and all have problems. If a rat won't grow on human milk, what can we conclude from its growth on formulas? Pigs are also used, as they are said to be physiologically similar to humans, and 'Because piglets grow at a faster rate than human infants they have more stringent dietary requirements. Therefore a diet which supports healthy growth in the piglet will probably be more than adequate for the human infant.'[824] Spot the problem with that logic? Outside Hollywood no one ever met a talking pig, and no pig made it through university. It is just possible, methinks, that some important parameters of development will not be adequately evaluated using pig growth, while it is increasingly certain that a 'more than adequate diet' for humans is harmful.

---

822  A figure of 7–9/L is now accepted as the amount of protein breastfed infants ingest, compared with the 15–29 g/L usual for formulas through the twentieth century. (The 12 g/L formula mentioned above was experimental in 1985; most first formulas in the 1980s contained a minimum of at least 15 g/L, as the 1971 Codex Alimentarius standard required.)

823  Benson JD. Nutrient guidelines for infant formula. In AOAC. 1985. Production, regulation and analysis of infant formula. *Proceedings* of the Topical Conference, Association of Official Analytical Chemists, Arlington, Va.

824  Ibid.

## Calculating how much of what proteins in infant formula

Most people assume that if a formula can says it has 1.8grams of protein per 100 kilocalories, that is an exact figure derived from analysis of the batch of formula. No, it's an approximation of what should be there if the cows' milk base didn't vary too greatly from the reference values for standard cows milk. (In general that's near enough when milk from many cows is pooled, but there are sufficient differences that some companies made infant formula only at certain times of year when cows' milk approximated the theory.) But even without that possible variance, formula protein content varies. Why?

- Regulations for allowable amounts of protein vary within a wide range. The Codex and EU upper limit for first stage infant formula protein is 3g/100kcal (the USFDA 4.5g/100kcal); the lower limit set by all three regulators is 1.8g/100kcal, but this is likely to be lowered.

- The upper limit for second stage or follow on formula is considerably higher, so that a child who swaps early from Stage 1 to Stage 2 will have quite a different cows milk protein intake than a child who drinks only Stage 1 formula for the first year of life (along with other foods).

- What the limits mean as protein per litre of formula depends on the actual caloric value of the formula. The regulations are stated as amounts per 100kilocalories. Under all global regulations, formula can contain 60-70 kcal per 100mL, or 600-700kcal per litre. Thus a declared (1.8 grams per 100kcal) formula contains just 1.2 grams of protein per 100mL (12grams of protein per litre) only when the total caloric value per 100mL is 66.6kcal. If the caloric value were to be 70kcal/100mL, the protein content would be 12.6g/L; if only 60kcal/100ml there would be 10.8g/L protein in 100mL made up formula. Details of aimed-for kcal/100mL are found on the label. Once they were usually around 67-68 kcal/100mL. Now some are 65kcal/100ML and some companies are changing to 60kcal. [The equation: kcals x protein ÷ 100 = protein per 100m; multiply by 10 for a litre.]

- What that change can mean for whey and casein intakes varies again, with the whey:casein ratio of the recipe used in the formula. [The equation: protein per 100mL x ratios = amount of either whey proteins or caseins. ]

- And what really is in the can vary again, with the variability involved in complex manufacturing processes. A variability of plus or minus 15% has been suggested as a minimum. [The equation: multiply preceding figures by 115%. Extra is more likely than deficiency because of overages..]

Over a year of infant formula consumption, there are big differences in infants' total intakes of casein and whey proteins, depending on all the above factors, as well as on infant appetite. And the total daily volume of formula varies of course, with four month old formula-fed infants drinking on average some 200mL more than breastfed infants' average 750mL per day. But for a conservative estimate of 150 litres of formula in the first six months of life, the figures below indicate how differently infants are fed an ingredient essential for growth, which in excess can be harmful.

| g/L, whey: casein ratio | Total protein, no 'overage' or variation | Total Whey for 150L FIF | Total Caseins 150L FIF | Where found or seen on labels – samples only |
|---|---|---|---|---|
| Womens' milk: 7-9g/L | 1350gms/150L | Varies with baby's age, 90:10 to 50:50 | | Human milk – total protein less, and intake volume less. |
| 11g/L 100:1 | 1650gms | Not stated | | BOKAAL research formula |
| 12g/L 100:1 | 1800gms | 1800gms | 0 | UK, EU, Codex, US minimum |
| 12g/L 60:40 | | 1080 gms | 720gms | W:C ratio not specified |
| 13g/L 70:30 | 1950gms | 1365gms | 585gms | Nan 2012 |
| 13g/L 65:35 | | 1268gms | 682gms | S26 Gold 2012 |
| 14g/L 60:40 | 2000gms | 1200gms | 800gms | Karicare/Aptamil 2012; Novalac Gold 2012 |
| 15g/L 60:40 | 2250gms | 1350gms | 900gms | 1980s S26, Nan, Enfalac* |
| 15g/L 18:82 | | 450gms | 1800gms | SMA Aust 2012, UK 1996 |
| 15g/L 52:48 | | 1170gms | 1080gms | SMA UK from 1997 |
| 1970-1980s formulas mostly 15-18g/L , specialty formulas higher than FIFs | | | | |
| 16g/L 20:80 | 2400gms | 480gms | 1920gms | AR formulas |
| 17g/L 30:70 | 2550gms | 765gms | 1785gms | Lactogen 1980s |
| 17g/L 18:82 | | 459gms | 2091gms | Similac 1984 |
| 18g/L 60:40 | 2700gms | 1800gms | 1200gms | Aptamil 1984, Mamia 2012, Baby's Own Organic 2104 |
| 19g/L 20:80 | 2850 gms | 570gms | 2280gms | Aptamil AR 2012 |
| 20g/L 20:80 | 3000gms | 600gms | 2400gms | UK, EU, Codex maximum |
| 20g/L 70:30 | | 2100gms | 900gms | Alprem 1980s |
| 22.5g/L 60:40 | 3375gms | 2025gms | 1350gms | Codex 72/1976 |
| 22g/L | 3300gms | varied | varied | Nutramigen, Pregestimil, Lofenalac |
| 24g/L 60:40 | 3600gms | 2160gms | 1440gms | Enfalac Prem, Ostermilk |
| 27g/L | 4050 gms | 1950-1960s formulas were 22-27g/L (Fomon 1993 p. 19) | | |
| 30g/L60:40 | 4500gms | 2700gms | 1800gms | US maximum 4.5g/L |
| 36g/L 60:40 | 5400gms | 3240gms | 2160gms | Similac Advance 1970s; France max |

Figure 3-5-5 Protein intakes for 150L of different infant formulas

Most health professionals wrongly state that there is no real difference between brands, even though parents commonly report that changing formulas can make a difference to the baby's behaviour. Multiply the above figures by at least 115% to reflect natural variability and 'overages." *Yet the range of casein intake is from zero to 2760grams, whey proteins from 450 to 3726grams.* Are these intake differences important to brain development in the first six months of life? I can't say, but given what parents of autistic children report about improvements on casein-free and gluten-free diets I would like to know. Perhaps those parents are wrong. Perhaps this means nothing. After all, breastmilk varies too, though not like this. But I couldn't find anything researching possible longterm outcomes of such differences in protein quantity and quality. And this huge casein/whey intake variability has all happened over the timeframe in which the incidence of brain disorders in children has dramatically increased. Independent studies comparing health outcomes of named formula brands with different compositions are scarce. Meanwhile, estimates of infants' per kilogram daily need for protein have dropped (but were only around 1.2g/kg/day in the 1990s, for infants from around four months of age.) My gut feeling is that industry is changing over to increased amounts of whey protein and lower total protein because they know more about this than I do!

Working out the upper and lower limits of total protein for infant formula is an ongoing process. This is a political as well as a scientific issue, with participants in the meetings of the Codex Committee on Nutrition and Foods for Special Dietary Uses, which met in Bonn in November 2005, Germany to revise the Codex standard for infant formula, recording that

> the US delegation requested that both maximum values and guidance values should not be lower than values used for formulas already on the market, even if such levels have not been subjected to systematic evaluation of their biological effects and safety.[825]

US industry was saying that current levels shouldn't be lowered when we don't know for sure that current levels are too high – even if scientists think they should be lowered, and industry is trying to reduce them. Consensus within Europe seems to have been reached with the 2006 EU Directive on Infant Formulae and Follow On Formulae. The minimum set was 1.8g/100kcal; the maximum to 3g/100kcal. That's twelve to 20 grams per litre, for formula with a caloric value of 67kcal/100ml. This was adopted as the global limit by the Codex Committee. But the caloric value of the formula can range from 60 to 70kcals/100mL. So the extremes could in fact be a minimum of just under 11g/L to over 21g/L, without breaching any regulations. That should accommodate all first infant formula still on the market!

But perhaps 11–21g/L is not a wide enough range. The US Infant Formula Regulations still allow the 1971 protein content range of 1.8 to 4.5g/100kcal, an upper limit of 50 per

825 Koletzko B. Standards for infant formula milk. Commercial interests may be strongest driver of what goes into formula milk. *BMJ*. 2006; 332: 621–622. PMCID:1403284 DOI: 10.1136/bmj.332.7542.621

cent more than the EU regulations, which would mean even old first formulas with almost 30grams of protein per litre could be legally sold. Whether such pragmatic demands shaped the outcome of US or Codex or deliberations is unknown to those outside the process. It is absolutely usual for government regulators, advised by industry consultants, to set wide limits to accommodate existing formulas and give industry time to modify their products without financial penalty. (The issue of lead in infant formula makes that very clear – see page 368).

As noted earlier, the protein content of newborn formulas made by major companies had dropped by the 1980s to a range of 1.5 to 1.7 g/100 ml (15–17 g/L). Meanwhile, major manufacturers now aim for the midpoint-to-lower end of the allowed range if current Australian labels represent reality: a quick check of brands in 2014 indicated protein content of 12–16g/L for first infant formulas. Higher protein concentrations are found in stage two and three formulas for normal infants, and in pre- and post-discharge formulas for preterm or growth-retarded infants.

If the total daily protein intake over months is significant for the development of obesity, or the casein intake significant for brain function, some children would seem to be more at risk than others. Consider the summary table below (or skip it if you don't need proof of that statement.)

The trend in protein content of normal formulas is clearly downwards, as concerns about the link with childhood obesity gain some media attention. Industry acknowledges this as fact: the Business Development Manager of Arla Food Ingredients, a Danish firm, says formula fed babies typically ingest 50–80 per cent more protein than breastfed babies, that this results in more rapid growth, and that there is 'strong scientific evidence that this can lead to obesity and other health concerns in later life.'[826] But all the indications are that the current levels of protein in formula are indeed too high. In fact, in 2014 an article asks 'Infant formula lower in protein and better for brains: are we there yet?' No, is the correct answer.

## Protein quality issues

So much for protein *quantity*. But protein *quality* was also an issue by the 1980s. Protein is broken down (mostly by our helpful gut bacteria) into its constituent amino acids, in different ratios depending on the food source. The balance of these amino acids determines how much can be used by the body, and how much must be excreted via the kidneys. Those amino acids circulate in the blood; they influence many aspects of development, so the ratios and types are important to much more than physical growth. It was thought that using whey protein would make formula more like human milk. But the amino acid structure of human whey proteins is different from that of cows' whey. In fact, not until the 1990s was human milk composition

---

826  Mullaney L. Get the breast of infant formulation. Food Manufacture.co newsletter. July 2, 2013. Online at: http://www.foodmanufacture.co.uk/NPD/Get-the-breast-of-infant-formulation; http://www.foodmanufacture.co.uk/NPD/The-quest-for-breast-milk

revealed in great detail, and it differed substantially from the theoretical construct companies had been trying to match all century.

Researchers at the time had concluded not only that protein levels were excessive, but also that 'feeding bovine whey to the full term infant is not more desirable than feeding bovine casein'.[827] Plasma amino acid levels differed between those fed whey- and casein-dominant formulas,[828] with some infants fed whey-dominant formulas having levels of tyrosine 'high enough to cause anxiety about brain damage, impairment of intelligence, and later learning disabilities.'[829] So the second concern about protein is not the total amount, but the amino acid composition of the protein in infant formula.

A wide variety of products remain on the market. Both whey-dominant and casein-dominant infant formulas are sold for use from birth; in some cases the casein-dominant is advised only from three months. This suggests that any research has shown confusing results, or else that it makes little difference. Despite that, from the 1970s, whey-dominant formula took over as the recommended choice for a first formula, though at different rates in different markets. Whey-dominant is now recommended for young babies by most health authorities. Comparative long-term studies by brand of brain and kidney function (as well as growth and childhood obesity) might help us know if there are any important differences in outcome. There may be. The fact that industry is still changing the balance of the amino acids and dairy companies are specialising in providing different blends suggests that these early whey-dominants were far from perfect matches for breastmilk! But again, a major change was adopted because of beliefs rather than rock-solid evidence.

## What caseins?

What complicates matters further is the fact that there are many different whey and casein proteins. Not all bovine caseins are the same, and the differences result in different balances of amino acids in infant blood. Cows' milk varies in the amount of the four major groups of casein proteins. In large-scale dairying large volumes of milk are wanted, so black and white breeds (Holsteins, Friesians) have been popular. These almost always produce A1 milk, which contains more of some casein proteins largely absent from the milk of A2 cows. Jerseys are more often A2 types, but produce lower volumes of milk, usually with more fat. Professor Keith Woodford, a New Zealand agricultural scientist, has shown, I think definitively, that the genetic profile of the cow determines the by-products of casein digestion, and that there are potentially very significant differences in those by-products between A1 and A2 cows. In New Zealand and Australia this has resulted in herds being bred and certified as free of the A1 casein variant, and the marketing of A2 milk, which some families report tastes better and has fewer adverse effects than regular supermarket

---

827 Janas LM, Picciano MF, Hatch TF. Indices of protein metabolism in term infants fed either human milk or formulas with reduced protein concentration and various whey/casein ratios. (PMID: 3495653) *The Journal of Pediatrics*, 1987, 110(6):838–48.

828 Janas LM, Picciano MF, Hatch TF. Indices of protein metabolism in term infants fed human milk, whey-predominant formula, or cows' milk formula. (PMID: 3872443) *J Pediatr*, 1985, 75(4):775–84.

829 Jelliffe DB Jelliffe EFP. *Adverse effects of foods*, (Plenum Press, 1982) p. 544

milk. The product has become so successful in Australia that competitors are attempting to discredit it.[830]

The digestion by-products of the caseins in A1 milk include several biologically-active beta-casomorphins, or BCMs, one of which, BCM7, acts on the brain in some of the ways other opioids do, including sedation.[831] Breastmilk casein too is digested and produces some beta-casomorphin, even some BCM7, but only one hundredth the amount, and 'it is also less biologically active, so that when it comes to relative opioid effect, human milk has less than one-thousandth the potential potency of A1 cows' milk.'[832]

Over months of a daily intake of up to a litre or more, there will be a substantially different protein intake, both in quantity and quality, between breast and artificially fed infants, perhaps especially if the milk used in formula-making is from A1 (rather than A2) type cows. It is quite possible that formulas, with different amino acid patterns, do alter normal brain patterns, doing more than sedating the baby in this sensitive period of brain development. We won't know until it has been researched, and the A2 industry has fewer resources just now than the established dairy industry.[833] However, having launched an infant formula aimed at the burgeoning Chinese market in 2013,[834] A2 producers are probably looking forward to higher returns on their investment. After all, the A2 formula in Australia and online has been positioned as the Platinum option, which tops Gold! I'm waiting for the Diamond range ...

## Potential consequences of excess caseins

Parents accustomed to taking pills to sleep may think opioid sedation of little consequence, perhaps even a blessing. But altering normal infant sleep rhythms and arousal patterns is a risk: ready arousal is seen as protective against SIDS, and is a characteristic of normal (i.e., exclusively breastfed) babies.[835] Sleep researchers need to emphasise to parents that all very young babies are at risk when sedated, whether by alcohol, opium, barbiturates, anti-histamines (historically, all used to sedate babies) illegal or prescription drugs, or cows' milk. Research could be done to see if the recorded deviations from normal infant sleep cycles are greater with casein-dominant formulas made from A1 variant herds. That means researchers would need to know more about where the milk in the formula came from, or else analyse its casomorphin content. Labelling could declare the likely range of BCM7 content. Parents could then decide whether any possibly greater relative risk of infant death is less important than the theoretical possibility, often never realised, of just a little more sleep.

---

830 http://www.smh.com.au/national/rival-seeks-to-water-down-a2-milk-claims-20140523-38uef.html

831 This is discussed in Woodford K. *The Devil in the Milk* ( Craig Potton Publishing 2007)

832 ibid.p.

833 It would not surprise me to discover that a large dairy co-ops will be gradually changing herd intake from A1 to A2 over the many years it takes to replace a full herd of valuable cows. If they do, it is likely that much infant formula marketing material will then focus on the risks of BCM7 and advantages of A2 milk.

834 http://www.news.com.au/lifestyle/food/formula-scare-source-of-new-business-for-australian-company-specialising-in-8216a28217-digestionfriendly-milk/story-fneuz92c-1226691601421

835 Horne RS, Parslow PM, Ferens D, Watts AM, Adamson TM. Comparison of evoked arousability in breast and formula fed infants. *Arch Dis Child*, 2004, 89(1):22–5. (PMID: 14709496).

In fact, if more sleep is important to prospective parents, formula should be avoided altogether – several recent studies have shown a significant gain in sleep time[836] for breastfeeding parents, and one has urged educators to inform parents that choosing formula feeding does not result in more sleep in the first twelve weeks.[837] Such myths persist in the face of scientific evidence because there is simply so much misinformation available globally, some of it on websites that claim to be helping bottle-feeding parents (see below).

Given the amino acid/neurotransmitter differences between formulas, comparative studies of infant brain function, sleep, and perhaps even population studies of SUDI rates, might be very interesting. Is the recorded late-twentieth-century drop in cot death rates partly due to infant formula amino acid changes as well as the change in sleep position, just as the twentieth-century epidemic paralleled the move to high-protein artificial feeding with its gastric discontents and so tummy sleeping? For more on cot death, once known as SIDS, now Sudden Unexpected Death in Infancy (SUDI), see page 234. An Australian SIDS group agreed, then rejected, and now has agreed, that artificial feeding is a risk factor for sudden unexpected death of infants. The article[838] explaining this reversion to an earlier status quo is worth reading, along with the responses to it.

Neurotransmitter levels are only one aspect of the SIDS puzzle. It is also worth reading Dr Mavis Gunther's 1970s thoughts, and pondering how many babies might have lived had she been taken seriously in 1975 [839] when she stated that 'Statistically speaking a baby sleeping on his side or back is safer than one put to sleep on his belly.'[840]

And autism researchers too might take note of quantitative and qualitative infant formula changes, including total protein and casein intakes in the first year of life. It was parents who identified diet as a problem for their autistic children, and the diet that both researchers and parents now recommend suggests lowering casein (and gluten) intake. Coincidence? Does amino acid balance/neurotransmitter levels affect other late-emerging developmental disorders as well?

I noted earlier that companies marketing whey-dominant formulas as more easily digested and not causing constipation, still made and sold casein-dominant formulas, touting them for 'hungry babies' and as 'keeping tummies full for longer'[841] and as more satisfying. As far back as 1985 a small double-blind crossover study found no difference in crying time or volume of formula consumed.[842] No one listened. I can still find no evidence that higher

836  Doan T, Gardiner A, Gay CL, Lee KA. Breast-feeding increases sleep duration of new parents. (PMID: 17700096) *J Perinat Neonat Nurs* 2007, 21(3):200–6.

837  Montgomery-Downs HE, Clawges HM, Santy EE. Infant feeding methods and maternal sleep and daytime functioning. (PMID: 21059713) *Pediatrics*, 2010, 126(6):e1562–8.

838  Young J, Watson K, Ellis L, Raven L. *Responding to evidence: breastfeed baby if you can – the sixth public health recommendation to reduce the risk of sudden and unexpected death in infancy.* (PMID: 22724308) *Breastfeed Rev*, 2012, 20(1):7–15.

839  Gunther M. The neonate's immunity gap, breast feeding and cot death. (PMID: 48624) *Lancet*, 1975, 1(7904):441–2

840  Gunther M. *Infant feeding* (Penguin, 1973) p. 71.

841  In 2012 Australia, SMA made this claim.

842  Brooke OG, Wood C. Investigation of the 'satisfying' quality of infant formula milks. *Arch Dis Child* 1985; 60(6): 577–79.

casein intake results in longer inter-feed intervals or more settled infant behaviour. And frankly, I would be very worried if higher casein intakes mean that babies slept abnormally long or deeply. But what is the popular understanding of all this? Websites are full of it:

> I have a 6 wk old baby who is a very big and hungry baby. She is taking 120 ml every 2–3 hours. A UK friend of mine's baby was feeding lots and she put her on a stronger hungry baby formula. The ones in the UK are whey based and then casein based is the hungrier baby formula. Here the casein based is step 2. So would she be ok to have the stage 2 if she does not seem to be settling for long after feeds? If this is the difference and the UK milks do this hungrier baby milk I should be ok to put her on a stage 2 for a more full milk?[843]

No, you wouldn't be okay, gailbaby. Definitely not. Casein-based FIFs are not FOFs. And switching to either is probably pointless as a way to make babies go longer between feeds.[844]

How clearly are companies telling mothers what to do about the products? Not very clearly, it would seem. One mother had a baby who by ten weeks was taking 250 ml every three hours, or 1.5–2 litres a day. On another website mums shared ideas about adding extra scoops of powder or heaped scoops of thickeners because babies fell asleep after bottles of 180 ml and didn't last three or four hours between feeds. Companies and individuals that offer mothers forums to chat on should employ some competent staff to monitor posts, so that they do not spread harmful advice unnoticed – as is only reasonable to anticipate that they will (unintentionally or otherwise).

## FIF or FOF? Whey, casein, follow-on formulas and complicated choices

Maternal confusion about the nature and use of stage one and stage two and follow-on formulas is widespread if that website is any guide. And not surprisingly. In 2011, UK formula label information was as follows.[845]

Whey-dominant first infant formula (FIF-W) products are recommended by authorities, and marketed as suitable from birth. These are labelled with a prominent figure '1'.

Casein-dominant first infant formulas (FIF-C) were labelled either 1 or 2, depending on the manufacturer. Labels state they can be used from birth for hungry babies.

So UK parents could choose either whey or casein-dominant first infant formula for use from birth. Infant formulas by definition are claimed to be complete foods, whether whey or casein-dominant.

---

843   Search 'hungry baby formula' at The Bub Hub or any similar parenting site, and see how confused and confusing this all is. This was gailbaby on 29.09.2008.

844   Thorkelsson et al. Similar gastric emptying rates for casein- and whey-predominant formulas in preterm infants. (1994) http://onlinelibrary.wiley.com/o/cochrane/clcentral/articles/691/CN-00108691/frame.html

845   Australian brands are just as confusing – that is to say, brands on sale in Australia, as most major brands are imported, and there is very little formula on sale in Australia that is made and/or owned by Australians. As technology developed, newer plants were built in the growth markets of Asia – Singapore, Vietnam, China. Australian plants mostly make formula for export.

In Australia and New Zealand as in the UK, FIF use tended to be two-stage. The casein-dominant FIF was mostly used from three months of age, first as a sole food, then with other foods after four months. In fact the FIF-C was usually a surviving familiar older formula that had been superseded by the newer, more expensive, premium whey-dominant product or FIF-W. So for Nestlé in Australia, for example, Nan was the new whey-dominant and Lactogen survived as a cheaper alternative; Wyeth retained SMA while selling S-26 as the preferable first whey-dominant formula; in the UK SMA Goldcap was the whey-dominant and SMA Original the casein-dominant.

Figure 3-5-6 Stage three formula with prominent numeral two

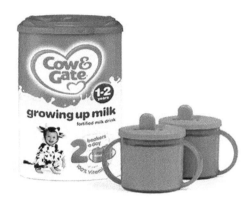

Confusion has perhaps been greatest in any country like the UK or New Zealand where some companies have labelled their whey-dominant first infant formula with the numeral 1 (let's call it FIF-W1), and advise swapping at three months to their casein-dominant (FIFC-1 but labelled 2, though it is NOT a follow-on formula, or FOF). These casein-dominants are increasingly called 'hungry baby formula'. In fact, it was in New Zealand that I first saw older casein-dominant FIFs advertised as being for 'hungry babies' from three months. (Obviously some babies are never hungry?) Perhaps soon only genuine follow-on formulas for babies over 6 months will be labelled 2? It has not helped that the Cow and Gate website currently shows has a huge figure 2 on the front of its Toddler formula (Stage 3 for most global companies), part of a claim about a daily intake of two 150mL beakers.[846] So a label with a prominent figure 2 on it might be a formula for newborns, for children over 6 months, or for children over a year old: why blame illiterate parents for feeding the wrong stuff to young infants?

## What does all this mean for protein intakes from FIFs?

The reality was that an 'extra hungry first formula' contains a theoretical total of 16 g/L of protein, of which 13 g is casein and just 3 g whey: a casein:whey ratio of 81:19. This contrasts with the same company's whey-dominant first formula, also labelled 1, which has a total of 13 g/L protein, of which just 3 g is casein and 10 g/L whey: a casein:whey ratio of 23:77. Overall, there is only 3 g difference in total protein intake, for every litre of formula. But there is a more than four-fold difference in casein intake, and thus a very different amino acid profile. Are both equally suitable for a baby under six months? Will the extra 10 g of casein per litre over time affect brain development differently? A baby can drink more than 150 litres in six months, after all, and many children are now predominantly formula-fed till twelve months. Does this matter? And does it matter that the artificially fed child's body has to deal with roughly twice the amount of total protein that the breastfed child's body will? If you're getting confused by the numbers, go back to the previous Figure 3-5-3 on page 262.

846  See http://www.cowandgate.co.uk/article/growing-up-milk-1-to-2-years

Now for the follow-on formulas, or FOFs. These were explicitly defined as incomplete products, to be part of a weaning diet, not suitable as whole foods. In most countries these are now described as second stage, post six months, not to be used under six months, and usually with a large number 2 visible on the can. But in one case, the FOF was labelled 3, as that company's whey-dominant was labelled 1, its casein-dominant 2. In other countries, 3 is the number placed on the newest addition to the formula range, so-called Toddler formula or Fortified Milk for children older than twelve months. Anything labelled 3 is nutritionally even less suitable for infants under six months than FOFs (not FIFs) labelled 2.

FIFs 1 and 2 may be suitable for babies under six months, but all FOFs and toddler formulas are absolutely not suitable for young babies. Because the FIFs labelled 2 (the casein-dominants) were always introduced around 3–4 months, and because FOFs are called names that suggest it is an advance, or progress, for babies to move on to them, some babies are fed FOFs earlier than six months. To their detriment, presumably.

## Why higher protein for Follow On Formulas anyway?

The global problem of protein-calorie malnutrition in weanling chidren was one rationalisation for allowing higher protein levels in FOFs. As the AOAC report[847] stated, in the majority of countries, 'Once weaning has started, the trend is to reduce the amount of breastmilk/formula fed per day (500ml). In such a situation it is imperative that the formula contains a protein level above that of human milk or the original infant formula.' But expensive processed foods cannot be the solution. For protein-calorie malnutrition is most common in poor communities where usual family foods are low in protein and fat, the most expensive food items in any society. In these communities any infant formula is unaffordable, where not subsidised by governments, and represents a bad return on any money available to buy food.

In Anglophone countries industry encouraged the continued drinking of large amounts of formula, up to a litre or more according to can labels. Because of cost, many families moved on to ordinary cows' milk and other foods after 6 months of formula feeding. So the stated rationale there for creating a second stage follow-on formula was different: the need for lower caloric intake[848] in a population where obesity was becoming a concern by the 1970s. In 1971, Ross had

> pioneered by introducing our product Advance ... designed to be used in the transition from infant formula or breast feeding to cows' milk ... Advance can be used to help control total calories consumed as solid foods are introduced.[849]

By 1978 Ross had Advance in the WIC program. The manager of government sales for Ross Abbott stated that 'Advance was approved by USDA primarily because of an increasing

---

847  *Production regulation and analysis of infant formula.* (AOAC Conference Proceedings 1985) p. 48.
848  Ross Cassette Information Program HR457, 3rd period, 1978; Advance Public Health Promotion. Transcript recording of Ron Bernard, Advance product manager, with Jerry Martin, manager of government sales (copy on file).
849  Smart WD. Pediatric Nutritionals, transcript of Abbott Laboratories Investor Seminar, June 4, 1981 (file copy).

concern by WIC programs about the need for a lower-calorie feeding.' Lower than what? And for how many years was it lower-calorie? The strategy in fact was to replace full cream cows' milk with an iron-fortified alternative – unnecessary if complementary iron-rich foods were given – and extend the total period of formula feeding with this then 'considerably cheaper' product. Increased duration of formula feeding had been the principal source of market growth for Ross in recent years according to Smart, a Ross vice president.[850]

Advance was to provide more protein than breastmilk, but less than cows' milk, and 20 per cent fewer calories than standard infant formula. The range of protein allowed in the FOFs was made wider partly because it was assumed that daily volume of intake would drop as infants eat other foods after four to six months.

However, does infant volume of formula intake drop when a child 'advances' from FIF to FOF? Who would know without research? Label-suggested daily intake for FOFs range from 300–630–1200 ml, while protein levels in FOFs on the Australian market in 2012 ranged from 15 to 25 g/L. That means a protein intake range daily of 10–25 g/day from this food alone. This goes against the trend of lowering infant formula protein as a safety measure, to reduce stress on brain and kidneys and decrease the likelihood of obesity. The stage one formulas on sale ranged from 13–18 g/L, recommended daily intakes ranged from 920–1150 ml, and daily protein intake would therefore range from 13–18 g – theoretically of course, if the formula protein content was precisely what the label said, the product did not include overages, and was made up with inhuman precision. None of which would be true in the real world. Compare the two types

| Daily intake | 15g/L protein | 25g/L protein |
|---|---|---|
| 300mL | 4.5g | 7.5g |
| 600mL | 9g | 15g |
| 1200mL | 18g | 30g |

Figure 3-5-7 Protein intake from 15-25g/L FoFs

The protein needs of infants from 6-12 months have been estimated as being roughly 1.4grams per kilogram bodyweight per day. The child getting a varied weaning diet can easily get the amount they need from foods including dairy products other than infant formulas. And in animal foods iron will be present along with other important minerals and trace elements.

In 2013 FOFs have again come under fire as unnecessary, as the World Health Assembly declared them to be in 1986.[851] They should also be condemned as confusing and unsafe. The global infant formula industry should ensure that labels warn of the dangers of confusing a FOF with a FIF, and advise parents that it is not 'progress' to move from a self-styled complete infant formula to one that both increases protein, and omits ingredients presumed to be in complementary foods. Yet in my experience of mothers, formula is seen

---

850  ibid.
851  WHA 39.28.

as the main part of the child's diet for the whole first year, and complementary feeding is hit and miss, with unreliable coverage of essential intakes.

And how much of what protein? What do we know about comparative amino acid profiles *by brand* of FIF and FOF? By the 1980s scientific research on the metabolic effects of amino acids was suggesting connections between artificial feeding and childhood and adult onset diabetes (an emerging epidemic) and obesity,[852] as well as kidney health and brain function. Parents heard little or nothing of such concerns, as all along infant formula has been presumed innocent/safe until conclusive proof of causation becomes available. There have even been misleading diagrams plotting amino acid content of formula against breastmilk, suggesting that the closeness of the lines mean that the protein quantity and quality did not differ significantly. Was this true? A leading researcher would state in 1994:

> simply by changing the quantity of protein or the whey/casein ratio ... it is not possible to reach an amino acid profile in term infants equal to that found in breastfed infants. Plasma amino acid concentrations under critical periods of development will affect amino acid transport to the central nervous system and by this, possibly the long-term outcome.[853]

Quality changes to the balance of proteins in formula are ongoing, as technology makes it possible to manipulate milk proteins.[854] This is because of the growing realisation of the complexity of milk proteins, their multiple bioactive components, the importance of non-protein nitrogen (NPN), and their multiple complicated interactions with other ingredients and one another. Proteins are polymers of twenty different amino acids, and there are hundreds of proteins in any mammalian milk. Proteins are involved in virtually all body functions. They are needed for all tissue growth and for hormone and immune responses: antibody production, for example. Some proteins have quite specific functions in mineral transport. Blood concentrations of some amino acids directly affect serotonin and dopamine levels and with them brain development.[855] Blood amino acid levels of infants on current whey-dominant formulas – compared with breastfed infants – have elevated threonine while those on current casein-dominant formulas have elevated phenylalanine and tyrosine.[856] This is interesting science, but tells us nothing about any individual baby. Except perhaps that regularly checking blood amino acid levels of any preterm, unwell or poorly developing artificially fed baby should be routine, provided the laboratory uses a reference standard based on breastfed children. Abnormal plasma amino acid levels in infants might be rapidly reversed by a diet of human milk, a perfectly feasible option in any society aware of its value. And as mentioned elsewhere, dairy companies now fractionate whey and create multiple new mixes of amino acids, touting them as –of course – 'closer to breastmilk' – indeed, one online page was headed 'Trial praises Arla breast milk.' By which

852  Gibbs BG, Forste R. Socioeconomic status, infant feeding practices and early childhood obesity. (PMID: 23554385) *Pediatric Obesity*, 2013. DOI: 10.1111/j.2047-6310.2013.00155.x.

853  Raiha NCR. Milk protein quantity and quality in human milk and infant formulae. *Acta Pediatr Scand*.1994; S402:57–8.

854  Thompson A, Boland M, Singh H (eds). *Milk Proteins: From Expression to Food*. (Academic Press 2009).

855  Wurtman RJ. Synapse formation and cognitive brain development: effect of docosahexaenoic acid and other dietary constituents. (PMID: 18803968) *Metabolism: Clinical and Experimental*, 2008, 57 Suppl 2:S6–10.

856  Darling PB, Dunn M, Gilani GS, Ball RO, Pencharz PB. Phenylalanine kinetics differ between formula-fed and human milk-fed preterm infants. (PMID: 15465744) *J Nutr*, 2004; 134(10):2540–54.

they meant infant formula with added Lacprodan OPN-10, or osteopontin. Danish Arla Foods is scaling up production; it will be marketed in Asia[857] where naïve consumers expect any new additive to make one formula superior to the others.

But even without these latest added fractions, casein to whey ratios remained confusing. I noted earlier that in 1997 the Wyeth UK formula called SMA changed from 82:18 to 48:52 casein:whey ratio. Yet in 2012 in Australia an ex-Wyeth US formula called SMA (made in Singapore) still has a casein:whey ratio of 80:20. An Australian-SMA baby taken to the UK and fed SMA (or vice versa) would be having a major dietary change without the parents being aware, unless they were careful label readers. Some companies no longer disclose whey:casein ratios on the label, though it can sometimes be calculated from nutrition information tables which give amounts for whey and casein. (Some don't provide even that information.)

## Specific protein changes: cysteine, taurine, carnitine ...

Proteins in infant formula have been a subject of considerable research effort. From the 1960s onwards, the development of specialised milk-based products and protein fractions allowed an explosion of 'specialty formulas', as described on page 286. Specific amino acids were researched and changes made to formulations, to deal with rare metabolic problems, and also to correct deficiencies in formulas for term infants. Cysteine was added, having been found to be essential for infants, partly as a source of taurine. Such changes were widely touted as vital: taurine for example, was added in 1984 after its importance to cats, and later, retinal and central nervous system (CNS) development in preterm infants was established.[858] Most health professionals had never known about taurine's possible effect on eyes before they were inundated with company literature arguing that it was essential, and soon every formula included added taurine. This was despite the scepticism expressed by some scientists even a decade later, who in 1994 thought it 'difficult to prove that it has any useful function', adding about its inclusion in formula, 'We could probably spend a couple of hours debating whether this is only window dressing ...'[859] Another said 'As David Rassin stated, there are no data proving that taurine should be incorporated in formulas for full-term infants. So there is some other reason for its presence overriding the factual data.'[860] (Increased sales figures, perhaps? Or just keeping up with the Joneses?)

It *was* clear that retinal development was affected in infants subjected to long-term tube feeding that lacked taurine. (Did anyone tell their parents?) Researchers have since argued that taurine could provide protection against DNA damage[861] and also long-term

---

857 http://www.dairyreporter.com/Ingredients/Protein-could-boost-nutritional-profile-of-infant-formula

858 Chesney RW. Taurine: its biological role and clinical implications. PMID: 3909770 *Advances in Pediatrics*, 1985, 32:1–42; Heird, WC Taurine in neonatal nutrition – revisited. *Arch Dis Child Fetal Neonatal Ed*, 2004; 89: 473–474.

859 Rassin DK. Essential and non-essential amino acids in neonatal nutrition, in Raiha N (ed). *Protein metabolism during infancy* op. cit., Nestlé Nutrition Workshop no. 33, 1993 p. 118.

860 Uauy-Dagach R, Quan R. Significance of nucleic acids, nucleotides, and related compounds in infant nutrition in ibid., p. 209

861 Ergun MA, Soysal Y, Kismet E, Akay C, Dundaroz R, Ilhan Ml, Imirzalioglu N. Investigating the in vitro effect of taurine on the infant lymphocytes by sister chromatid exchange. *Pediatrics International* (2006) 48, 284–6. DOI: 10.1111/j.1442-200X.2006.02205.x

neurodevelopment.[862] Which implies that its lack had been allowing DNA and cognitive damage to occur ... perhaps this was responsible for the higher rate of chromosomal damage noted in infants not breastfed? Or those researchers might be quite wrong ... in science there is little that is proven beyond doubt.

By the end of the 1980s a new race seems to have begun, to add some new ingredient to formula that competitors did not yet have. Just as I did in the 1970s, educated mothers scrutinise formula labels, looking to see what one might have that another doesn't, assuming that any extra additive had been proved to be better for babies, not just for sales. Carnitine was added to some formulas, so it was assumed to be a necessary additive. Was it? A very senior Nestlé scientist was scathing:

> Cows' milk whey is full of carnitine and all infant formulas based on cows' milk contain a level of carnitine equal to or higher than breast milk. It is only in soy formulas that you need to add carnitine. To add it to cow's-milk-based formula is nonsense.[863]

Yet again, the experts say, as with taurine,

> The same thing is happening with carnitine. We found that normal full term infants fed with soya milk, which is devoid of carnitine, can synthesize carnitine very well. The problem of carnitine deficiency is probably limited to preterm babies.[864]

Does this mean excesses of carnitine are being included in formulas for term babies? Does it matter? The problem would be less if companies were not restricted to declaring on labels only what they intentionally add to infant formula. The overall composition of the product should be declared when composite ingredients like bovine milk are included. Seeing carnitine declared on a label might mean the company added more just so they could advertise its presence, even though all bovine-based formulas contain plenty.

Breastfed babies benefit from many other minor proteins, including the immunoglobulins, hormones such as oxytocin and prolactin, and proteins involved in vitamin and mineral transport such as transferrin and lactoferrin. Industry in the 1980s also experimented with adding bovine lactoferrin, which might improve iron bioavailability as human lactoferrin does in the breastfed infant. (It didn't; see more on page 521.) This and other potential formula additives are dealt with in 3.15 Infant forumla in the twenty-first century on page 533.

## Processing effects on proteins

From about 1990, it was realised that even different manufacturing processes within and between companies affected protein quality. It took until the 1990s before it was realised that methods for processing whey can have different effects on human blood lipid levels. Ultrafiltration (the cheaper method) results in 'significantly higher values of total

---

862  Wharton BA, Marley R, Isaacs EB, et al. Low plasma taurine and infant development. *Arch Dis Child Fetal Neonatal Ed* 2004;89.

863  Guesry P. commenting on p. 119 of Raiha N (ed) Nestlé Workshop no 33; http://www.nestlenutrition-institute. org/resources/library/Secured/workshop/Documents/Publication00033/npe_33_105.pdf

864  Marini A, in discussion Raiha N (ed) Nestlé Workshop no 33, ibid. p. 118.

cholesterol and low-density lipoprotein (LDL) cholesterol in infants' when compared with levels in infants fed electrodialysed whey. The researchers concluded 'Plasma lipid profile in infancy is influenced by dietary protein, not only by the casein-to-whey ratio, but also by the method of whey deionization.'[865]

So the composition of ultrafiltered whey protein varied from that of electrodialysed whey protein, and that affects babies' blood and body. There were also different effects from varying heat treatments of formula. Companies do not advise parents about how the whey used in any formula has been filtered or heat-treated!

Researchers into cardiovascular disease should be aware of such variations in milk content and bioactivity, as they may be relevant to studies of comparative outcomes of infant feeding. Some formula may be more damaging than others, in short. Industry endorsed this idea in marketing, claiming in advertisements that 'prevention should start as soon as possible' by avoiding the 'unnecessary risks' of the competitors' fat blends.[866] Compared with breastfeeding, cardiovascular outcomes in adulthood are worse in those fed artificially as infants, but the results may be more marked in groups or countries or time periods – or in those fed brands using whey protein concentrate produced by ultrafiltration. A global database with details of the production techniques used in each manufacturing plant, and the countries where those products are fed to infants, could be useful. Who would want to set it up?

## Individual whey proteins

Both bovine whey and casein can be broken down into ever more individual proteins (there are hundreds in any mammalian milk). Whey is made up of alpha lactalbumin (around 13 per cent) and beta lactoglobulin (58 per cent) plus other proteins. Beta lactoglobulin is a known major allergen, and the amino acid structure of alpha-lactalbumin is seen as better. The now greater commercial availability of alpha-lactalbumin is helping industry to create lower protein reformulations of old formulas.[867] Lien, a Wyeth scientist, explained that

> ... lactalbumin is rich in tryptophan, which is typically the limiting[868] amino acid in formula, and as a result *[of being able to use alpha-lactalbumin]* formulas have been developed with lower *[total]* protein but higher tryptophan concentrations. This type of formula may offer a number of advantages to the neonate, which include producing plasma tryptophan concentrations equal to those found in breastfed infants, and obviating the need for the body to dispose of excess nitrogen loads.[869]

865 Weizman Z, Ursacha C, Leader D, Zegerman C. Whey deionization method of infant formula affects plasma lipids. *J Pediatr Gastroenterol Nutr.* 1997; 25:529–32.
866 S-26 advertising: 'Cardiovascular problems: prevention is better than cure' below a cartoon of a smiling mother bottle feeding her clinically obese baby with a basket of S-26 beside her ... See Figure 3-6-1 on page 311.
867 Lien EL. Infant formulas with increased concentrations of alpha-lactalbumin. (PMID: 12812154) *Am J Clin NUtr,* 2003, 77(6):1555S–8S.
868 Protein synthesis requires a balance of amino acids, a shortfall of any one can be a limiting factor, requiring the body to excrete other amino acids that can't be used for lack of tryptophan. More tryptophan from alpha-lactalbumin means the total amount of protein can be lowered a little.
869 ibid.

So, possibly good for kidneys, though it will only reduce the extra load on bottle-fed infant kidneys. Still, will it make a difference to the Western world's already high rate of renal disease? And if it does, will anyone acknowledge that infant formula helped create that expensive public health problem? We learned in 2004 that there is a difference in kidney growth and size at three months in the formula-fed infant, although by eighteen months the difference was no longer apparent. Said the researchers, 'The consequences of such increased kidney growth on kidney functions later in life are unknown.'[870] In that last sentence, for 'increased' substitute 'early unnaturally rapid' and think about programming effects, and ponder why the effects still remain unknown to date. Again, language either disguises the possibility of risk or suggests it – and industry marketing has controlled the language, and with it, the public perception of infant feeding.

Adding alpha-lactalbumin and so reducing total protein seems to be a laudable attempt to do a number of things:

- to redress known amino acid imbalances that affect brain function;
- to reduce the burden on young kidneys which have to excrete protein breakdown products;
- to allow the lowering of total protein content to around 11–13g/L, perhaps reducing the risk of obesity;[871] and
- to perhaps reduce allergenicity by decreasing relative infant intakes of beta-lactoglobulin (the dominant whey protein and allergen).

That would all be good, and such formulas now typically state that they contain 13 g/L. However, milk will still cause allergic reactions. No single major allergen is apparent in cows' milk, according to either the challenge tests or laboratory procedures. Casein (now decreased), alpha-lactalbumin (now increased), and beta-lactoglobulin (reduced) all show a high proportion of positive reactions.[872] And the extraction processes that produce commercial quantities of alpha-lactalbumin may prove to alter its properties or leave residues ... And any protein fed at a vulnerable time may become more of a problem allergen in the next generation ... Any unexpected negative side effects of adding this particular highly-processed whey protein will emerge in time.

## Protein degradation products: another concern?

Producing alpha lactalbumin in bulk requires specialised breakdown of large quantities of heat treated milk whey. Figure 3-5-8[873] outlines this process, which involves a variety of filtrations and finally spray drying.

870  Macé K, Steenhout P, Klassen P et al. Protein quality and quantity in cows' milk based formula for healthy term infants: past, present and future. In. Rigo J, Zeigler E. *Protein and energy requirements in infancy and childhood* (Karger AG/Nestec Ltd, 2006) p. 196 Nestle Nutrition workshop no 58

871  Haschke F. discussion in Clemens RA, Hernell O and Michaelsen KF *Milk and milk products in human nutrition* (Nestlé Pediatric Series,v.67, Karger, 2011) p. 26.

872  Savilahti E, Kuitunen M. Allergenicity of cows' milk proteins. (PMID: 1447629) *J Pediatrics*, 1992, 121(5 Pt 2):S12–20

873  From Parke & Haenlein op. cit., p. 483. ©John Wiley &Sons Ltd.

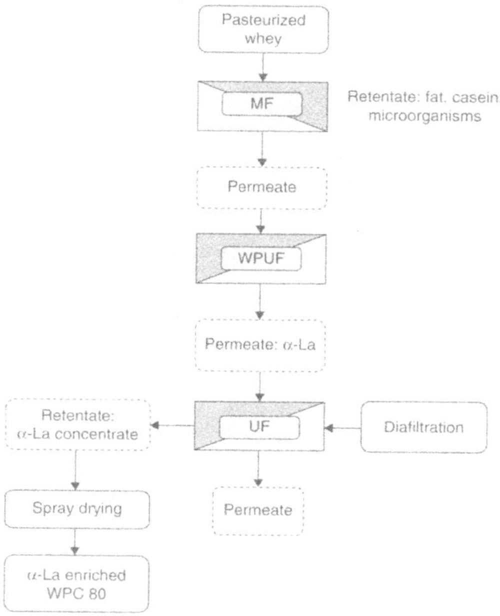

Figure 3-5-8 Making alpha lactalbumin powder for use in infant formula © John Wiley & Sons Ltd

The spray drying process (next page) is itself a complicated two or three stage drying system, since the 1980s producing instantised powders. Looking even at simple diagrams of what is involved in this one step, I appreciate the French term for infant formula, 'industrial milks.'

Milk is complex, and every process it is subjected to changes it, sometimes quite unpredictably. This is true of other ingredients as well: the damage that heat-produced trans-fats can do (see page 314) was not predicted, or even recognised for decades. Yet nowadays we know that

> Most studies confirm a higher degree of damage in infant formulas compared to regular milk products. Differences between various types of infant formulas, such as liquid, powdered or hypoallergenic formulas depend on the analyzed markers and brands ...[874]

None of which is information published where parents can access it easily. Reassuringly perhaps, the authors hasten to add that

> 'A considerable portion of protein degradation products in infant formulas can be avoided when process parameters and the quality of the ingredients are carefully controlled.'[875]

As of course infant formula manufacturing always would be. Wouldn't it? We know how infallibly large-scale manufacturing processes go on, with never a human error or computer malfunction or machine failure or inadvertent contamination or ingredient defect ... Hmmm. Less reassuringly, the authors of that study add: 'The nutritional consequences of thermal degradation products in infant formulas are largely unknown.'[876]

So there's another set of potential outcomes to investigate in the children fed products containing degraded protein ... when science has identified the metabolites. Those heat-damaged ingredients and the new compounds produced will be the subject of a lot of study. After all, it has just been discovered that some other formula metabolites are toxic to the infant gut (see page 321).

---

874  Pischetsrieder M, Henle T. Glycation products in infant formulas: chemical, analytical and physiological aspects. (PMID: 20953645) *Amino acids*, 2012, 42(4):1111–18. DOI: 10.1007/s00726-010-0775-0
875  ibid.
876  ibid.

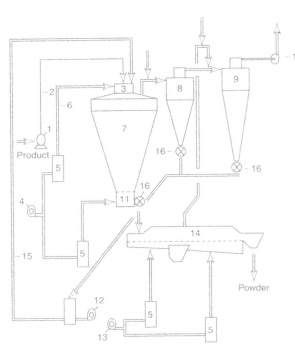

1 – Feed pump
2 – Feed flow
3 – Sprayer/Air disperser
4 – Inlet air fan
5 – Air heater
6 – Drying air
7 – Drying chamber
8 – Primary cyclone

9 – Secondary cyclone
10 – Outlet air fan
11 – Integrated fluid bed
12 – Pressure conveying system
13 – Vibro-fluidizer air fan
14 – Vibro-fluidizer
15 – Fines reincorporating
16 – Rotary valve

Figure 3-5-9 A multiple effect spray drier[877]

Which brings me to the controversial subject of allergy and infant feeding, where common sense says formula feeding has been a disaster, but enough doubt has been created to obscure common sense.

# Bad reactions: protein and allergy

Protein in infant formula is obviously relevant to allergy and food hypersensitivity issues (hereafter referred to as allergy, in its original meaning of an adverse reaction to a substance others find harmless). All changes to infant formula have complex consequences. The change from casein-dominant to whey-dominant formulas is no exception.

To recap: the 1970s increase of bovine whey in formula would reduce infant intakes of some important casein antigens, but also greatly increase infant intakes of beta-lactoglobulin, a known major bovine antigen, soon to be implicated in colic in breastfed babies.[878] Yet by the twenty-first century industry is reducing beta-lactoglobulin in the hope of reducing allergy. No regulatory authority asked for comparative 'allergy' outcome trials before the change to whey-dominants occurred, so they were not produced so far as I could discover. (Even today some companies assume that a footnote stating 'data on record at the company' should be sufficient proof of any marketing claims.) Thus the timing of this change from casein-dominant to whey-dominant formulas, and then to 100 per cent whey formulas, could be worth noting, if looking for factors associated with the newly emerging global allergy epidemic. Comparative sales data by brand and type may well be available from pharmacy and grocery wholesalers, if industry does not supply them.

Secondly, it should be noted that simply changing the vehicle that allergens are delivered in (from diluted whole milk or evaporated milk – with milk fats – of the pre-1960 mixes

---

877  Published with permission of Elsevier Ltd. Copyright image from Thompson A, Boland M, Singh H. (eds)*Milk Proteins from Expression to Food* (Academic Press 2009) p. 289. Permission conveyed through Copyright Clearance Center Inc.

878  Jakobsson I, Lindberg T, Benediktsson B, Hansson BG. Dietary bovine beta-lactoglobulin is transferred to human milk. (PMID: 4003058) *Acta Paediatr Scand,* 1985, 74(3):342–5.

to the modern whey-dominant mixes with vegetable oils) has the potential to change the allergenicity of what is presented to the baby. Those who wonder about rising allergy rates in Western communities need to know that a study found that

> The fat content of a challenge vehicle has a profound effect on the reaction experienced after allergen ingestion. This is another factor to be considered in assessing the risk of certain foods to food-allergic consumers and adds another dimension to clinical, research and regulatory practice.[879]

Quite possibly the changes of fats as well as the changes of proteins that increasingly occurred over the twentieth century make a difference to the effect of formula on infants. For more on this see Chapter 3.7, Basic ingredients: Formula fats and fictions.

Companies knew perfectly well by the 1970s that the problem of infant allergy was exploding. Industry has to stay ahead of popular knowledge of problems to be able to mould the discussion to sell its products. They had all been busy for decades trying to create less allergenic formulas, after all! The solution for these babies could also be found, at a cost. 'Allergy' research had been funded by companies well aware that not all children tolerated cows' milk products. (This did not stop bovine formulas being advertised as suitable for all children from birth!) A variety of soy proteins, beef hearts, goats' milk and so on had all saved the lives of babies intolerant of regular formula – and had caused symptoms themselves. Enzymatic or acid hydrolysis of cows' milk protein allowed older casein hydrolysate formulas to be reformulated, causing fewer problems for some (not all) allergic children. These formulas still tasted revolting: one company scientist talking about hydrolysates said '... it tasted – well I mean you would never drink it. But you would probably have a hard time when the formula bottle was open to be in the same room with it.'[880] Like mud, said another. A taste test at one Baby Friendly Hospital Initiative (BFHI) National Advisory Council meeting in Melbourne Australia found some adults unwilling to sip a teaspoon of the new formula a baby was being asked to swallow every feed, every day. Some of the formulas with these new fats smelt revolting – some still do – as did the baby's stools.

Attempts to improve taste and smell used fungal enzymes (peptidases) to 'de-bitter' the casein hydrolysates. The belief was of course that no trace of these fungal enzymes would remain in the product, a belief later questioned as unproven and, from first principles, unlikely. Whey hydrolysates were developed as well, using different products (acids, alkalis or enzymes) to break down the milk proteins, with different results, and different trace residues.

The 1980s saw another major development in the protein used in first infant formulas, when Nestlé broke into the well-protected US market via the purchase of Carnation. This was to be a game-changer in more ways than market share. The formula they launched used only partially hydrolysed bovine whey protein, which they claimed would be 'gentler' for sensitive stomachs, and might help prevent allergy. It was labelled hypoallergenic (HA),

---

879 Grimshaw KE, King RM, Nordlee JA, Hefle SL, et al. Presentation of allergen in different food preparations affects the nature of the allergic reaction – a case series. (PMID: 14616872) *Clin Exp Allergy*, 2003; 33(11):1581–5.
880 November 2002 FDA Food Advisory Committee Meeting on Infant Formulas p. 69.

meaning less allergy-producing than the previous types, whether casein- or whey-based. It was also labelled as unsuitable for infants with established allergy. The product, Carnation Good Start, was the equivalent of Nan HA in Australia and Europe, and soon the other major companies were marketing similar HA products as first formulas. Whey-protein-only formulas, many partially hydrolysed, were now in the mix for parents making choices about infant formula.

## Partially or extensively hydrolysed protein in formula?

These whey-based, so-called 'gentle' or 'sensitive' or 'comfort' formulas are still allergenic. The US Food and Drug Administration (FDA) considered an application from companies to allow companies to make the claim in advertising that such whey-protein partially hydrolysed infant formula (W-PHF) reduced the risk of eczema, or atopic dermatitis (AD). Not surprisingly,

> The FDA concluded there is little to very little evidence, respectively, to support a qualified health claim concerning the relationship between intake of W-PHF and a reduced risk of AD in partially breastfed and exclusively formula-fed infants throughout the first year after birth and up to 3 years of age. [In fact,] the FDA required a warning statement ... that partially hydrolyzed infant formulas are not hypoallergenic and should not be fed to infants who are allergic to milk or to infants with existing milk allergy symptoms.[881]

Does the existence of these self-styled 'gentler' and 'sensitive' formulas mean that other formulas are rough and insensitive? Bullies all? If the partially hydrolysed less-allergenic gentler, sensitive varieties are so much better, why are the older formulas still produced? Much of the expense of infant formula relates to economies of scale, after all. If these hypo-allergenics are better for babies, then they should become the default routine formula everywhere, and companies could then reduce the price!

Perhaps it is in the companies' best interests, when introducing these new formulas, to keep other types of formula on the market? After all, some children's blood even reacts to extensively hydrolysed infant formulas.[882] That is not surprising when there is little real knowledge of just what the massive technological changes have done to the formula's ingredients besides break them down into smaller parts. Novel formulas such as these might have adverse developmental or growth outcomes when used long term, and no one can know that until thousands of babies have been reared on them and studied. Not until 2009 did we have a study claiming that ten-year-old children who had been fed three different named hydrolysate formulas during infancy had growth similar to children exclusively breastfed during infancy.[883] That's possibly important when obesity is such an issue, but does that apply across different cultures? In discussion of this paper, the lack of relevant

881  Chung CS, Yamini S, Trumbo PR FDA's Health Claim Review: Whey-protein Partially Hydrolyzed Infant Formula and Atopic Dermatitis. (PMID:22778306) *Pediatrics* 2012, 130(2):e408–14.

882  Dean TP, Adler BR, Ruge F, Warner JO. In vitro allergenicity of cows' milk substitutes. (PMID:8472190). *Clinical and Experimental Allergo*logy 1993, 23(3):205–10. DOI: 10.1111/j.1365-2222.1993.tb00883.

883  Rzehak P, Sausenthaler S, Koletzko S, Reinhardt D, et al. Long-term effects of hydrolyzed protein infant formulas on growth – extended follow-up to 10 y of age: results from the German Infant Nutritional Intervention (GINI) study. (PMID:21849601) *Am J Clin Nutr* 2011, 94(6 suppl):1803s–1807s

research was highlighted, and the point made that 'one cannot conclude that long-term growth of children who were fed *other* hydrolysates would be similar.'[884] And the roll call of superseded infant formulas no longer made includes several so-called hypo-allergenics, presumably discarded by their makers for some good reason. So once again, where are the by-brand comparative studies of infant formula?

Although industry must be getting better at doing so, it is impossible to predict exactly how things will turn out when the target population is changing, and so is the processing. Note what this recent review says on processing and allergenicity:

> Hypoallergenic formulas can be prepared by hydrolysis and further processing, such as heat treatment, ultrafiltration, and application of high pressure. Attempts have been made to classify formulas into partial and extensively hydrolyzed products according to the degree of protein fragmentation, but *there is no agreement on the criteria on which to base this classification* ... Nevertheless, hydrolyzed formulas have until now proved a useful and widely used protein source for infants suffering from CMA [cows' milk allergy]. Because undigested protein can still be present as residue at the end of proteolysis [protein splitting],[43] further processing is necessary in combination with enzymatic treatment. Another attempt to eliminate antigenicity involves the use of proteolysis combined with high pressure. Different authors have shown increased fragmentation of BLG [betalactoglobulin] if proteolysis occurs after or during the application of high pressure.[44] The partial ineffectiveness of proteolysis under ordinary atmospheric conditions may be because of the inability of enzymes to reach epitopes that are less exposed. Heat treatment is also often combined with proteolysis to unfold the protein and modify the 3-dimensional structure of conformational epitopes. However, thermal denaturation can also cause the formation of aggregates with greater resistance to hydrolytic attack, as is the case with BLG [beta lactoglobulin].[885]

So new compounds get formed for the baby's gut to handle, and we won't really know the outcomes until it's been tried on enough children over time, and then only if we set up research now. Yet hydrolysates of various kinds have been in use in Western countries for over seventy years. And if they do result in less obesity (i.e., more normal growth, akin to the breastfed), perhaps they *should* become normative for those who have to be artificially fed. Such formulas may be more or less acceptable to babies, and if their higher cost is not an issue, parents may buy them. But parents should not be misled into buying them in the hope of completely preventing allergy. And most children do not have to be part of this ongoing experiment with their growth and their lives.

Commercial confidentiality cloak many details parents might like to know, in order to be able to make an informed choice of feeding product. Advertising has never reflected the reality that some children would and will have intractable problems with artificial feeding. Industry knows that, but in its marketing there was always another product to try, and an assumed happy ending. No one knew in the 1970s that the end result of multiple formula

884  Clemens RA, Hernell O, Michaelsen KF. *Milk and Milk Products in Human Nutrition* op. cit., p. 158.
885  World Allergy Organization (WAO) Diagnosis and Rationale for Action against Cow's Milk Allergy (DRACMA) Guidelines. *World Allergy Organ J.* 2010 ; 3(4): 57–161. PMCID: PMC3488907. DOI: 10.1097/WOX.0b013e3181defeb9 Published online 2010 April 23.

changes might be a child of five still reliant for its survival on an expensive tinned powder. There seem to be more of such children than ever before. The myth of all children 'growing out of allergy' is still powerful.

From the 1980s onwards, the experience of formula feeding for many children was a miserable pilgrim's progress from cows' milk formula to low-lactose milk formula (wrongly labelled lactose-free or LF) to lower-allergen or hypoallergenic milk formula: all at increasing cost and symptom severity. Some babies even did an extra detour via soy formula before or after low lactose formula: usually finding that in the first couple of weeks things seemed to improve (as one allergen, cows' milk, was removed) only to get worse after that (as allergic sensitisation to soy developed). In the 1990s some babies sidestepped via the anti-reflux (AR) formula products with added thickening starches and gums, and usually a high casein:whey ratio. Then they could progress to those vile-tasting hydrolysates or if even that failed, the amino acid-based formulas, if their child was damaged enough to convince a doctor to prescribe these. Parents had to keep paying out for yet another experiment, and hope that their baby would tolerate the next option better than the last. Thanks to clever media management, at no stage was this obvious increase in allergy seen as due to infant formula itself, or to the twentieth century's experiment of artificial feeding. And at no stage in this miserable progress was re-lactation considered, or human milk feeding, other than by a few empowered women with social support.

Another major drug manufacturer, Bayer, saw opportunity in some common ailments of children: colic, reflux, constipation and diarrhoea. Bayer bought into the multi-billion dollar infant formula market with products overtly marketed for such problems, and with another one titled Sweet Dreams (for hungry babies). Infant formula can cause colic, insomnia, reflux, constipation and diarrhoea in some children, but no formula has yet been proved to prevent or end these conditions in all children. However, these Bayer formulas include some novel food sources such as apple, banana, cornstarch and 'cream of rice'. I suspect that these foods are likely to rise up the popular 'allergy' rankings (although slowly, as these products were not huge sellers.)[886]

I have seen no published scientific evidence to support Bayer's emotive marketing claims, nor – more importantly – comparative allergy studies on these formulas. Independent proof that any new ingredients in formulas for infants under six months of age – such as pomegranate![887] – do not cause sensitivity or allergy reactions should be mandatory prior to mass marketing. Parents assume that such research takes place before any regulatory approval, not realising that even studies of a few hundred healthy babies may not reveal side effects that could appear when many thousands of children –including theirs – are fed

---

886 A trade journal, *Retail pharmacy*, published from 1991–2008 an annual *State of the industry* report giving market share details for pharmacy sales, and a brief analysis of trends. Other data gathering organisations exist, though some charge large amounts for any information. It would have cost almost $20,000 to get up-to-date data on infant formula world and national market value.

887 Mead Johnson has a patent on 'Nutritional compositions containing punicalagins' – search 'infant formula' at the US patent office at http://patft.uspto.gov/netahtml/PTO/search-bool.html for other fascinating details of what companies have done and possibly plan to do.

the formula as sole diet for months. 'Post-market survelliance' needs to be comprehensive, organised, and independent for subtle problems to be noticed. It presently is none of those.

Of course the cows' milk-exposed children of the 1960s and 1970s have had children, some of whom are now having their own children. Allergy is even more common and more unpredictable in each subsequent generation. So the medical profession has finally recognised the now endemic problem. More about this later.

## Growing babies or Michelin men?

Whey-dominant formulas, from 1962 on, changed infant diet in yet another potentially very significant way. 'Fat absorption from a whey predominant formula is greater than from a casein predominant, so the metabolisable energy available to the baby is greater.'[888] They increased infant caloric intake. So did the much more saturated fats like palm and coconut oil, very readily absorbed. Both had potential implications for the development of childhood obesity, the other epidemic in the making. There were and are still many unanswered questions about how much infant formula protein is enough or too much. And in the twenty-first century we have even more reason to be concerned about our lack of knowledge. Consider these excerpts from the abstracts in an important industry-funded symposium, available in print and online:

> Milk seems to have a specific stimulating effect on linear growth ... it is not known which components in milk stimulate growth. Possible components are proteins, minerals, vitamins or combinations of these. Cows' milk proteins have a high protein quality, and whey has a slightly higher quality than casein, according to some indices based on amino acid composition. Studies ... suggest that whey protein has the potential to increase muscle mass. Whether whey improves body composition to a larger extent than other milk proteins is not clear ... *[And I would add here, the implication that more lean muscle mass is always an improvement is an assumption based on a cultural prejudice – MM].* The mechanism behind a possible growth-stimulating effect of milk is likely to be through a stimulation of insulin-like growth factor-I (IGF-I) synthesis and maybe insulin secretion ... The effects of milk on linear growth and adult height may have both positive and negative implications.[889]

Indeed. It gets more complicated.

> There is increasing awareness that childhood circumstances influence disease risk in adulthood. As well as being strongly influenced by genes/genetic factors, stature acts as a marker for early-life exposures, such as diet, and is associated with risk of several chronic diseases in adulthood. Height is also a marker for levels of insulin-like growth factor one (IGF-1) in childhood. Levels of IGF-1 are nutritionally regulated and are therefore

---

888 Wharton BA. International recommendations on protein intake in infancy: some points for discussion. In Raiha N (ed). *Protein metabolism during infancy* op. cit., (Nestec/Raven Press NY, 1993) p.77–78. http://www.nestlenutrition-institute.org/Resources/Library/Free/workshop/Publication00033/Pages/publication00033.aspx

889 Mølgaard C, Larnkjær A, Arnberg K, Michaelsen KF. Milk and growth in children: the effects of whey and casein. in Clemens RA, Hernell O, Michaelsen KF (eds). *Milk and milk products in human nutrition* op. cit., p. 67. Online: http://www.nestlenutrition-institute.org/Resources/Library/Free/workshop/BookNNIW67/Pages/booknniw67.aspx

modifiable. Milk intake in childhood and in adulthood is positively associated with higher levels of circulating IGF-1 and, in children, higher circulating IGF-1 promotes linear growth. Studies conducted by our team and others, however, indicate that the effect of milk is complicated because consumption in childhood appears to have long-term programming effects which are opposite to the immediate effects of consuming milk. Specifically, studies suggest that the long-term effect of higher levels of milk intake in early childhood is opposite to the expected short-term effect, because milk intake in early-life is inversely associated with IgF-1 levels throughout adult life. We hypothesise that this long-term programming effect is via a resetting of pituitary control in response to raised levels of IgF-1 in childhood. Such a programming effect of milk intake in early life could potentially have implications for cancer and ischaemic heart disease risk many years later.[890]

What does this suggest? *That infant formula distorts normal growth patterns (as the WHO-funded Multicentre Growth Reference Study – MGRS – makes clear) in a variety of ways, and the effect is lifelong, and may be linked to rates of heart disease (and obesity and diabetes[891] and cancer).[892]* This is not an eccentric opinion. Read the summary table opposite, from a chapter on formula feeding and neurodevelopment.

Distorted growth can take many forms and have outcomes that are unpredictable with our current level of knowledge. But again, research should start from the assumption that what happens to healthy breastfed children is the human norm and that deviations must be proved safe, not that the human norm needs to be justified. After all, *we have just learned that both being breastfed, and breastfeeding their children, reduces the risk of cancer for women who survived childhood cancer.*[893] That is important to know, and I suspect cancer researchers ought to be looking at the potential for breastmilk to inhibit cancer proliferation in adults.

Studies were beginning to ask these questions, consistently finding a higher risk of obesity for artificially fed infants.[894] The early-protein-exposure hypothesis was generated. A 2012 open access online article[895] reviews this topic extremely well, with the author identifying one mechanism which probably explains the link between the excess protein intake of the artificially fed infant and subsequent obesity: its multiple effects on a central cell regulator, named mTORC-1. As the author sees it, a

---

890  Martin RM, Holly JMP, Gunnell D. Milk and linear growth: programming of the IGF-1 axis and implication for health in adulthood. ibid., p. 79.

891  Sadauskaite-Kuehne V, Ludvigsson J, Padaiga Z, Jasinskiene E, et al. Longer breastfeeding is an independent protective factor against development of type 1 diabetes mellitus in childhood. *Diabetes Metab. Res. Rev.* 2004; 20 (2): 150–7. DOI:10.1002/dmrr.425. PMID 15037991.

892  Both being breastfed and breastfeeding their children reduces the risk for women who survive childhood cancer. Ogg SW, Hudson MM, Randolph ME, Klosky JL. Protective effects of breastfeeding for mothers surviving childhood cancer. *Journal of Cancer Survivorship*, 2011; DOI 10.1007/s11764-010-0169-z.

893  It has certainly prolonged life in the historical past. See Ploss and Bartels, op cit., vol 3, chapter XII, titled Woman's milk as a medicine and magical agency.

894  Kramer MS. Do breast-feeding and delayed introduction of solid foods protect against subsequent obesity? *The Journal of Pediatrics.* 1981; 98(6):883–7; Von Kries R, Koletzko B, Sauerwald T, et al. Breast feeding and obesity: cross sectional study. *British Medical Journal,* 1999; 318(7203):147–50.

895  Melnik. B C Excessive Leucine-mTORC1-signalling of cows' milk-based infant formula: the missing link to understand early childhood obesity. *J Obes*, 2012; 2012:197653. Published online 19 March 2012. DOI: 10.1155/2012/197653.

Infant formula feeding in comparison to breastfeeding results in excessive serum levels of leucine, insulin, and IGF-1, explaining exaggerated mTORC1-dependent early adipogenic [fat-generating] programming, the promoting mechanism for early onset of childhood obesity ... Exaggerated formula-induced mTORC1 signalling appears to be the most critical factor for the early development of childhood obesity and other mTORC1-driven chronic diseases of civilization, especially T2D [type 2 diabetes] and cancer.[896]

Maybe he's right, and maybe there are other biological explanations relating both to protein and fat in formulas. Experimental infant formulas with higher nutrient content have indeed resulted in increased fat mass in childhood, something no twenty-first century parent would be happy to learn.[897]

| | |
|---|---|
| Brain development | • A suboptimal early nutrition could cause cognitive impairments in childhood. |
| | • Human milk has a high concentration of n-3 and n-6 long chain polyunsaturated fatty acids (LCPUFA), which are crucial for normal development of CNS, and which deposit in the brain and in other nervous tissues during the perinatal period. |
| | • Docosahexaenoic acid, the most abundant n-3 LCPUFA in the brain, has been positively related to an optimal neurological development and a major visual acuity. |
| | • Studies on preterm infants fed a formula enriched with LCPUFAs have shown beneficial effects on retinal and cognitive development (a greater sensitivity to light and a more mature visual acuity) and short-term neurological outcomes. |
| | • Even if studies on term infants have demonstrated weaker effects, there are sufficient data to support the usage of term formulas enriched with LCPUFAs. |
| Bone health | • Formula feeding has been related to an increased bone cells turnover, with subsequent higher risk of late degenerative bone disease, compared to human milk feeding. |
| Risk of cardiovascular disease | • Two main factors might influence the risk of cardiovascular disease: breast milk (BM) and post-natal growth. |
| | • BM feeding has been related to lower risk of cardiovascular diseases, hypercholesterolemia, obesity (as leptine resistance), type II diabetes, high blood pressure. |
| | • A rapid post-natal growth increases the risk of the metabolic syndrome and has been related to endothelial dysfunction (lower flow-mediated dilatation of the brachial artery), which could be the cause of a premature atherosclerosis in adolescence. |
| Obesity | • The acceleration in weight gain, in the first 24 months, is a negative predictor of overweight in childhood. |
| | • Formula milk has been related to an increased risk of obesity, which seems to be linked to protein content (55-80% higher in formula milk than in breast milk). |
| | • An excessive protein intake stimulates a higher secretion of insulin and insulin-like growth factor 1, which enhance the adipogenic activity and lead to an accelerated growth during the first two years, with a documented higher body mass index in childhood. |
| Immune system | • LCPUFAs have been related to the prevention of allergic diseases, due to their anti-inflammatory and immunomodulating properties. They may have some slight beneficial effect in established allergic diseases, such as asthma and atopic dermatitis, particularly if they are introduced in the diet during pregnancy or in the early postnatal period. |

Figure 3-5-10 Long-term consequences of nutritional programming.[898]

---

896 Melnik BC. *Formula feeding promotes adipogenic, diabetogenic, hypertonic and allergenic m-TORC1 programming.* In Preedy et al (2014) op cit., p. 545

897 Singhal A, Kennedy K, Lanigan J, Fewtrell M, et al. Nutrition in infancy and long-term risk of obesity: evidence from 2 randomized controlled trials. (PMID: 20881062) *Am J Clin Nutr*, 2010; 92(5):1133–44. DOI: 10.3945/ajcn.2010.29302.

898 Monari C, Aceti A, Faldella G. *Formula feeding and neurodevelopment.* In Preedy et al op. cit., p. 621. © Wageningen Academic Publishers

Maybe he's right, and maybe there are other biological explanations relating both to protein and fat in formulas. Experimental infant formulas with higher nutrient content have indeed resulted in increased fat mass in childhood, something no twenty-first century parent would be happy to learn.[899]

## Overall dietary protein intake per day

One point that should be made is this: not only do quantity and quality of protein in infant formula matter, but also the total overall dietary intake of protein by the child on a daily, monthly, and yearly basis. So the amounts of formula recommended by industry to be fed to babies of different ages every day and over their early childhood is important. Again, this varies widely, though the formulas are all said to be made to the same energy density, between 65 and 75 kcal/100 ml, most usually 67 or 70 kcal if can labels are accurate.[900] Figure 3.5.5 illustrates what this could mean to protein intakes for 150 litres of infant formula Authorities might like to give parents a little guidance as to how much is too much, even of a good thing.

## Protein in the twenty-first century

Where are we now in relation to protein? Changes in formula quantity and quality have been a recurring theme in this history. There is no doubt that infant formula these days is a far cry from the old evaporated milk mixes. If a mother has to formula-feed for whatever reason, that is a positive to focus on, while accepting that even the best of the current substitutes for breastmilk must fall far short of the ideal (and we still don't know which formula is 'best' or worst, of course). The most technologically competent infant formula companies have long realised that they cannot match breastmilk, but increasingly see the potential for minor proteins to improve their mixes – nutritionally and commercially (see on page 533).

Where has the protein story got to in the twenty-first century? Still plenty of unanswered questions, as the experts outline.

> The development of infant formula with optimized protein quality and quantity has been, and still is, the subject of intense investigation. A better understanding of the protein composition of breast milk and infant needs, in association with technological breakthroughs in cow's milk fractionation, has led to the development of infant formulas with a protein content that is closer to that of human milk [but still light years away – MM] Today, infant formulas with a protein/energy ratio of 1.8 g/100 kcal [12 g/L] are

899  Singhal A, Kennedy K, Lanigan J, Fewtrell M, et al. Nutrition in infancy and long-term risk of obesity: evidence from 2 randomized controlled trials. (PMID: 20881062) *Am J Clin Nutr*, 2010; 92(5):1133–44. DOI: 10.3945/ajcn.2010.29302.

900  To work out the grams of protein per litre (g/L) from the labelled amount of protein in grams per 100kilocalories (g/100kcal), multiply the stated energy density of the formula (legally ranging from 60 to 70kcal per 100mL) by the stated grams of protein per 100kcal (say 2.2g) and divide by 100. Any reduction in energy density will mean a reduction in total protein intake. A 70kcal formula x 2.2 ÷ 100 = 15.4 g/L of protein; a 60kcal formula x 2.2 =13.2g/L. I used 66.6 kcals in my calculations, as 67-68kcal/100mL was common on labels, and it made for easier conversion: 2/3rds of the 100mL amount. It underestimated some brands. To translate kcal to kJ, multiply by 4.18.

commercially available. These formulas have been shown to be safe and nutritionally adequate for term infants. However, the short-term and potentially long-term metabolic benefits of formulas with reduced protein content have still to be elucidated and are currently under investigation *[i.e., children survive and grow on them but we don't know their other effects, and they are currently for sale in some markets – perhaps obesity will decline?].* In addition to providing amino acids as building blocks for growth, milk is the source of numerous bioactive factors/hormones which are involved in multiple physiological processes. Continuous efforts are being made to identify new bioactive compounds in human milk. However, a better understanding of their biological functions in suckling infants as well as a comparison with their bovine counterparts is needed. *[This generation of infants are the guinea pigs we will learn from.]* Technological processes, which preserve some bioactive factors in cow's milk, already exist. These processes could be applied to infant formulas.[901] *[More experiments envisaged.]*

In short, the protein story is still ongoing. The perfect mix is proving elusive. The quantity of protein in first formulas (FIFs) has been more than halved over the century, which is almost certainly a good thing, and may be resulting in a decline in early childhood obesity rates. (But rhose already obese have affected their children in utero.)

The quality of protein, its amino acid makeup, has been changed, which is also probably a good thing; only time will tell. The next step, into adding yet more bioactive proteins (See Chapter 3.14 on page 517 and Chapter 3.15 on page 533) will also be problematic.[902] Formulas are still different from one another in protein makeup, and we still have almost no independent comparative studies to guide parents in their choice of brand.

In short, it's still a lottery. I advise parents to

- avoid the highest protein formulas,
- look for the lowest calorie content per 100mL,
- read about the source and outcomes of any new protein additives, and
- monitor their child's growth on WHO growth charts,
- trust their instincts, and consult if concerned about anything

After all, in the period of these changes to infant formula protein content, the incidence of severe gut inflammatory diseases in infants has risen. Is that intergenerational damage compounding harms, or is it just the result of those changes in the foods infants are still exposed to far too often in western hospitals? Do FPIES researchers understand the importance of knowing exactly and in detail what a child has been exposed to before and after birth, before thinking that this problem typically 'occurs at the first introduction of

---

901 Macé K, Steenhout P, Klassen P, Donnet A. Protein quality and quantity in cows' milk-based formula for healthy term infants: past, present and future. (PMID: 16902335) *Nestlé Nutr Workshop Ser Pediatr Program,* 2006, 58:189–203; discussion 203–5.

902 Lönnerdal B. Infant formula and infant nutrition: bioactive proteins of human milk and implications for composition of infant formulas. (PMID:24452231) *Am J Clin Nutr* 2014; 99(3):712S-7S DOI: 10.3945/ajcn.113.071993.

cows' milk to the diet'? The fact that FPIES 'has not been reported in exclusively breastfed infants'[903] seems significant.

## Milking mothers for human protein

So why not invest in human production of human milk protein? Breastmilk is not a scarce resource, just an under-utilised one. Many women produce more than they need, and almost all could. The formula companies are well enough informed to know the time is coming when only human milk or products made from human milk will be considered safe for use in neonatal intensive care units (NICUs) around the world. Safe for the NICUs, and the infant formula companies, that is. Lawsuits will soon start if parents realise that the child who died of sepsis or NEC might well be alive if the NICU had provided only human milk or products. Any infant death is a fact to be investigated and causation noted. As Raiha said, in some countries anything other than exclusive human milk feeding of preterm infants is considered unethical.[904] It is not surprising that Ross, Abbott's formula arm, has created a co-promotional arrangement with Prolacta Bioscience Inc, 'the pioneer in standardised human milk-based nutritional products for premature infants'. Which is to say, the first commercial operation selling products made from women's donated milk.[905] This privately owned company should recoup its investment fairly swiftly, now that one American state, Kentucky, has virtually mandated that only human milk be used in neonatal intensive care nurseries (NICUs).[906] Ross/Abbott has a representative on Prolacta's Board.

But of course paying mothers for their milk raises numerous ethical issues, and could simply prove to be another way to exploit poor women and harm their babies. It need not be so, as the East German and Scandinavian experience has shown. It could result in poor women breastfeeding longer and valuing their milk both for their child and for its contribution to household income and their own well-being. It is absolutely worth exploring. At present women can make money from their milk only via the porn industry, where exploitation of women is rife, and they may be forced to perform other sexual acts not of their own choosing.[907]

Mothers' own milk is always preferable to any other breastmilk. Industrial processing of human milk will alter it and reduce its benefits, making it more like infant formula. Even so, human-milk-derived additives are likely to be superior to bovine additives, even after industrial processing. But only a tiny proportion of eligible infants will ever have access to them unless they too are heavily taxpayer-subsidised. And sadly, their availability and use could even undermine the likelihood of many more babies being mother-fed, unless and until all obstetricians and paediatricians learn about normal infant feeding and actively support and enable it in healthcare facilities. Heat-treated breastmilk is no substitute for

903  Kemp AS, Hill DJ et al, op. cit.
904  Raiha, N (ed) *Protein metabolism during infancy,* op. cit.
905  http://www.prolacta.com. Note that everyone but the women doing the work of producing milk will be making money from women's bodies.
906  http://www.marketwatch.com/story/prolacta-praises-landmark-legislation-in-kentucky-mandating-human-milk-diet-for-preemies-in-jeopardy-of-intestinal-disease-2013-05-07
907  Porter T. International Business Times. 29/12/2014. http://www.ibtimes.co.uk/chinese-police-break-adult-breastfeeding-prostitution-ring-1481180

the real thing: fresh mother's own milk. Quite simple technologies can increase the caloric density of that milk. Well-documented, evidence-based changes to NICUs[908] can increase the chances of mothers producing enough of their own milk, and also reduce the infant stress that causes them to burn more calories needlessly.[909] It takes education, effort, and constant support, but motivated mothers can bring home an exclusively human-milk-fed preterm baby and have that baby fully mother-fed within a week and watch her gain weight at an average 50 grams per day: in 2014 one of my grandchildren did just that, and a more peaceful baby it would be hard to find. For more on this see Concentrating and preserving milk on page 209.

## Soy protein based infant formulas and their problems

The previous discussion of protein in formula focussed on the difficulties of cows' milk based formulas. What about the other common protein source, soy? It too has been used for a century, and undergone major changes in that time. The first report[910] of the use of soy in infant feeding was in 1909. Starting out as mixes of soy flour and other ingredients, soy formulas were clearly unsatisfactory, even in the 1950s and 1960s causing intense windiness and loose malodorous stools, worse-smelling than cows' milk formula stools. (Only those who have experience of fully-breastfed babies realise that baby poo is not always revolting and stomach-churning. This is one of the side effects of the different microbiomes created by different feedings.) Excess flatus and stinky stools were predictable as soybeans contain indigestible carbohydrates that even the adult body cannot readily metabolise, and also an inhibitor of the enzyme trypsin, needed for digestion. (Different processing inactivated this inhibitor, improving the quality of soy protein.)[911]

Early soy formulas had multiple problems – and so did the infants fed them! The addition of iodine ended the problem of goitre seen by several investigators, although there are still questions about soy exposure and auto-immune thyroid disease, and infants with congenital hypothyroidism are more difficult to treat if being fed soy rather than bovine formula.[912] Various vitamin deficiencies were addressed after being identified in infants fed early soy formulas: fat-soluble vitamins A and K had to be added back as they had been removed from soybeans by organic solvents; B vitamins destroyed in processing had to be added after reports of infants with thiamin deficiency.

Processing soybeans to create soy protein isolate improved available protein quality. Mead Johnson created the first soy isolate formula in the 1960s, and by the 1970s soy protein isolate formulas had almost completely replaced the older soy flour formulas. Eminent formula researcher Samuel J. Fomon catalogued the mishaps above and others relating to soy formulas. In 1974 he would write that 'It is apparent that nutritional adequacy may vary

908  Nyqvist KH, Anderson GC, Bergman N, Cattaneo A et al. Towards universal Kangaroo Mother Care: recommendations and report from the First European conference and Seventh International Workshop on Kangaroo Mother Care. (PMID:20219044) *Acta Paediatr* 2010, 99(6):820–26.

909  Arnold LD. *Human Milk in the NICU: policy into practice*. (Jones & Bartlett 2009) For a fuller appreciation of what this entails, see Dr. Uwe Ewald, Uppsala University Hospital Sweden, talking about the merits of their Family-Centered Care approach, in a 35 minute video, which –along with other useful resources, can be accessed from http://www.babyfirst.com/en/neonatal-care/nicu-designs.php.

910  Ruhrah J. The soy bean in infant feeding: preliminary report. *Arch Pediatr* 1909; 26: 494–501.

911  Fomon (1974), op. cit., p. 387.

912  Vandenplas Y, Turck D. *Soy protein infant formula in infant nutrition*, in Preedy op. cit, p. 214.

considerably from one product to another. Extensive clinical testing of new products is desirable before they are marketed.'[913] This would be proved by the Syntex Neo-Mull-Soy disaster that would lead to the 1980 Infant Formula Act (see The Syntex disaster and the Infant Formula Act of 1980 on page 407). It is a call still being made, because it is still not happening.

Nowadays soy formulas consist of soy protein isolate combined with pro-inflammatory vegetable oils, sugars (either sucrose or corn syrup solids, the dried form of corn syrup known as glucose syrup in the USA), and needed vitamins and minerals. Some ingredients (like protein) are present at higher levels than in bovine formula because they are less bioavailable in soy formulas. Soy protein contains too little of some amino acids, and is therefore fortified with methionine, an amino acid in plentiful supply in cows' milk. Homemade soy formulas are unable to address this issue, or the others still to be investigated.

Modern soy formulas do not contain any lactose. But the use of soy formula for infants with galactosaemia remains controversial as they contain stachyose and raffinose, carbohydrates which 'may produce alpha-1,4-galactose that may cause flatulence and diarrhoea in sensitive individuals and contribute to elevated galactose1-P values' in the blood of galactosaemics.[914]

Soy formulas are often used for infants who react badly to cows' milk formulas, even though the UK's Chief Medical Officer has advised that they should not be used for this purpose for infants under six months old.[915] Yet parents of children with bovine protein allergy, and others with lactose intolerance, often find that soy formulas reduce symptoms of gut distress, at least for a couple of weeks before the baby starts reacting to soy protein – which is not uncommon.[916] Most authorities do not suggest using soy, but instead advise extensively-hydrolysed formulas to treat bovine protein allergy. However, the use of pig-pancreas-derived enzymes in the process of hydrolysis may make hydrolysates unacceptable for religious reasons.[917] As well, perhaps 17.5 per cent of infants allergic to cows' milk will also react to even extensive-hydrolysates;[918] and some parents will not be able to afford such expensive alternatives: soy formula is no dearer than bovine products.

Why was soy chosen as an alternate protein source, when in some countries (New Zealand especially) goats' milk formula developed as an alternative to cows' milk? Because soy was a cheap product growing on America's vast acres, offering limitless availability. Soy formula has spread from America with the US companies' expansion, though it always remained unpopular in the Francophone world. Goats were likely to be just as expensive as cows,

---

913  ibid., p. 390.

914  Vandenplas Y, Turck D. op. cit., In Preedy, Watson, Zibadi (eds) op. cit., p. 212.

915  First Steps Nutrition Trust has an excellent monograph free online about the British versions of these milks: Crawley H, Westland S. *Infant milks in the UK: a practical guide for health professionals*. June 2013, p. 54 http://www.firststepsnutrition.org/pdfs/Infant_milks_June13.pdf

916  Rozenfeld F, Docena GH, Anon Mc, Fossati CA. Detection and identification of a soy protein component that cross-reacts with caseins from cows milk. *Clin Exp Immunol* 2002; 130: 49–58.

917  ibid., p. 215.

918  Rancé F, Brondeau V, Abbal M. Utilite des prick-tests dans le 'screening' de l'allergie immédiate aux proteines: 156 cas. *Allergie et Immunologie* 2002; 34 (3): 71–3. 202 reactions were described in Cantani A, Micera M. Immunogenicity of hydrolysate formulas in children. *JACI* 2000; 10(5) 261–76.

or perhaps even more so. Yield per goat is lower after all, and goats may not be as docile as cows. But in the 21st century the use of goats' milk for infant formula is increasing,[919], and the search for other commercially-viable mammalian milks continues. Soy formula use may decrease, even though babies grew and apparently thrived on soy, as that overdue research reveals some subtle problems.

Soy formulas (SF) have been used widely in America and quite commonly in Australia since 1970, and children raised on them do not stand out as visibly different from those raised on cows' milk formulas (CMF). However, in 2013 those Arkansas researchers (see Soy formulas and infant development on page 38) report that in the first year of life

> Infants fed CMF and SF had significantly different fat and bone accretion trajectories, and all infants fed formula were significantly different from infants fed BM [breastmilk]. Infants fed SF had a leaner body phenotype throughout the first year of life, lower bone mineralization by age 3 months, and greater bone mineral accretion during the first year of life compared with infants fed BM or CMF. Although the body composition profiles are strikingly different in these 3 diet groups, the implications for long-term health outcomes and bone health remain unclear.' [920]

Again, babies fed soy develop differently from those fed breastmilk, and from those fed cows' milk formula. Which divergence from the normal (breastmilk-fed) is less desirable? Only the absolute need for an alternative to cows' milk in a bottle-feeding culture ensured that soy formulas were well established before such concerns about their effects on infant development were raised. Over the twentieth century, the growth of infants fed soy formula had been assessed using solely the old criterion of growth in largely bottle fed term infants. Now there are other concerns.

The first is soy formula's often-high levels of metals such as aluminium, manganese, and silicon. Soybeans naturally pick up minerals from soil and concentrate them. For more on aluminium and manganese, see Chapter 3.9 on page 367. Amounts of silicone range from 746 to 13,811 ng/mL [nanogram/millilitre].[921] Media hype surrounds the problem of silicone breast implants and women's milk, yet the milk of breastfeeding women with silicon implants contains approximately 56 ng/ml, a little more than normal.[922]

> Silicon levels were analyzed in breast milk, whole blood, cow's milk, and 26 brands of infant formulas. Comparing implanted women to controls, mean silicon levels were not significantly different in breast milk (55.45 +/- 35 and 51.05 +/- 31 ng/ml, respectively) or in blood (79.29 +/- 87 and 103.76 +/- 112 ng/ml, respectively). Mean silicon level measured in store-bought cow's milk was 708.94 ng/ml, and that for 26 brands of commercially available infant formula was 4402.5 ng/ml (ng/ml = parts per billion). We

---

919  http://www.dairyreporter.com/Manufacturers/FDA-wants-more-goat-s-milk-formula-on-US-market-Hyproca-Nutrition/

920  Andres A, Casey PH, Cleves MA, Badger TM. Body fat and bone mineral content of infants fed breast milk, cow's milk formula, or soy formula during the first year of life. (PMID:23375908) *J Pediatr* 2013; 163(1):49–54.

921  Semple JL, Lugowski SJ, Baines CJ, Smith DC, McHugh A. Breast milk contamination and silicone implants: preliminary results using silicon as a proxy measurement for silicone. (PMID: 9703094) *Plast Reconstr Surg,* 1998; 102(2):528–33.

922  ibid.

concluded that lactating women with silicone implants are similar to control women with respect to levels of silicon in their breast milk and blood. Silicon levels are 10 times higher in cow's milk and even higher in infant formulas.[923]

Can those levels possibly be harmless? Why are they not publicised whenever concerns about breast implants and breastfeeding emerge?

Secondly, the safety of trans-fatty acids made from soybeans is questionable. When this was first raised, commercial interests replied that definite scientific proof was lacking, and to restrict their use would be to 'destroy the biggest cash crop in the US'.[924] The issue of trans-fats is discussed on page 313. As these are created by heat, they will not easily disappear from fat-containing heat-processed foods. While doing all it can to decrease the levels of trans-fats, industry is resisting pressure to provide label information about levels of trans-fats. So again, parents cannot make any informed choice to lower the level of these pro-inflammatory ingredients.

Thirdly, concern has grown about the immune effects of oestrogen-like plant compounds (referred to as phyto-oestrogens or isoflavones) in soy. Phyto-oestrogens in soy and cows' milk are endocrine disrupters, inhibiting a thyroid enzyme, thyroid peroxidase. Children with autoimmune thyroid disease are more likely to have been fed soy formula as infants.[925] And questions have been raised about the impact of a soy formula diet on infant response to vaccinations.[926]

Fourthly, not only immune effects are of concern. The potential impact of high doses of such oestrogen analogues on reproductive organs and related sexual characteristics of developing infants is worrying. As noted earlier, Arkansas studies show *small but measurable differences in reproductive tissue growth* between breast-, cow- and soy-fed infants *at just four months of age* (see page 38). And a recent abstract talks of 'reduced breastfeeding [i.e., increased artificial feeding – MM] and soy formula feeding as potential risk factors for acquired cryptorchidism'[927] [undescended testicles, or 'balls' in common slang]. It says

> Although additional studies are needed, hormonally active components of breast milk and soy formula could influence the establishment of normal testis position in the first months of life, leading to apparent ascent of testes in childhood.[928]

923  ibid.

924  Food Chemical News 25 February 1985, pp. 28–30.

925  Fort P, Moses N, Fasano M, Goldberg T et al. Breast and soy-formula feedings in early infancy and the prevalence of autoimmune thyroid disease in children. *(PMID: 2338464) J Am Coll Nutr*, 1990; 9(2):164–7.

926  Zoppi G, Mantovanelli F, Pittschieler K, Delem A et al. Response to RIT 4237 oral rotavirus vaccine in human milk, adapted-and **soy-formula** fed infants. (PMID:2556883) Acta Paediatr Scand 1989; 78(5):759–62; Businco L, Bruno G, Grandolfo ME, Novello F et al. Soy formula feeding and immunological response in babies of atopic families. (PMID:2570322) Lancet 1989; 2(8663):625–26.

927  Barthold JS, Hossain J, Olivant-Fisher A, Reilly A et al. Altered infant feeding patterns in boys with acquired nonsyndromic cryptorchidism. (PMID: 23081935) *Birth Defects Research. Part A, Clinical and Molecular Teratology*, 2012; 94(11):900–7.

928  ibid.

As written, that makes breastfeeding sound like a risk factor along with soy. In fact the study shows that it is the lack of breastfeeding and the presence of soy, which creates risk. So let's re-write that more plainly: 'Formula feeding, especially soy formula, may increase the risk of babies' testicles remaining inside the body after birth, instead of moving down.' Similarly, the title might be not 'altered feeding patterns in boys with acquired nonsyndromic cryptorchidism' but 'increased risk of acquired nonsyndromic cryptorchidism in boys not exclusively breastfed'. Or just 'association of infant formula feeding with undescended testicles', if the proof is still lacking. Although we know that exposure to endocrine disrupters affects reproductive characteristics of every species studied, from alligators[929] to polar bears![930]

This concern has finally resulted in, and the media fuss ended with, high-level medical advice to use cows' milk based formulas and avoid soy-based formulas for infants less than six months of age. The UK Committee on Toxicity of Chemicals in Food, Consumer Products and the Environment (COT) concluded in 2003 that phyto-oestrogens or isoflavones posed a potential risk to the future reproductive health of infants, and the European Society for Paediatric Gastroenterology Hepatology and Nutrition (ESPGHAN) recommends that extensively hydrolysed cows' milk formulas are used instead of soy formulas, which should be avoided for infants under six months.[931] In 2012 Australia's NHMRC noted that soy formula was a suitable substitute for cows' milk formula only when used under medical supervision, though how supervision affects soy's underlying nutritional characteristics, or just *what* supervision *what doctors* should provide, is not spelt out. It is not a usual medical responsibility to scientifically measure changes in infant reproductive development, much less to follow up minor deviations in infancy through to middle age ...

Is soy protein so dangerous that it should be eliminated as a source of food for infants, or is it not? Where is the sense in any medical authorities saying avoid soy for six months, while allowing the unrestricted sale of soy formula labelled as suitable to use from birth? A significant number of children are reared on soy, despite the allergy authorities' misgivings. What then is the point of the warnings? To make sure that parents are the ones held responsible for any ill effects, since they chose to use the formula against authoritative advice? At least some parents believe 'The government wouldn't let them sell it if it was dangerous.'[932]

Yet it may be, for that and other reasons. An infant's exposure to cadmium is six times greater from soy formula than cows' milk formula,[933] and toxic metals and other mineral imbalances

---

929 Finger JW Jr, Gogal RM Jr. Endocrine-disrupting chemical exposure and the American alligator: a review of the potential role of environmental estrogens on the immune system of a top trophic carnivore. (PMID:24051988) *Arch Environ Contam Toxicol* 2013, 65(4):704–14

930 Sonne C, Letcher RJ, Bechshøft TØ, Rigét FF et al. Two decades of biomonitoring polar bear health in Greenland: a review. (PMCID:PMC3305763) *Acta Vet Scand* 2012, 54(suppl 1):s15–s15.

931 ESPGHAN Committee on Nutrition, Agostoni C, Axelsson I, Goulet O, Koletzko B, et al. Soy protein infant formulae and follow-on formulae: a commentary by the ESPGHAN Committee on Nutrition. (PMID: 16641572) *J Pediatr Gastroenterol Nutr*, 2006; 42(4):352–61.

932 That has been said to me times without number.

933 Eklund, G., Oskarsson, A. Exposure of cadmium from infant formulas and weaning foods. *Food Addit. Contam.*, 1999; 16:509–19.

are of increasing concern in relation to the development of autism. A recent study claims that 'for the 1,967 autistic children aged 0–15-year-old, we were able to demonstrate not only the critical epigenetic factor (zinc- and magnesium-deficiency and/or high burdens of aluminium, cadmium and lead) but also the presence of another critical factor, an 'infantile window' in neurodevelopment and for therapy probably.'[934] What the study did not do was examine in detail the feeding histories of these children and their mothers, which might explain both the differences in body burden and neurological development. There are many concerns about both types of formula, not just soy.

Is it only because of the high rates of cows' milk allergy in Western infants that medical authorities continue to tolerate the open sale of soy formula? It is, after all, the cheap alternative for poorer families who cannot obtain very expensive hydrolysates or elemental formulas at taxpayer expense, or under a health or insurance plan. In practice, assertive and lucky mothers win through the system to reach an allergy specialist and are prescribed expensive formulas – for much less than the cost of soy or cows' milk formulas. In the UK formula is accessible to all children by prescription according to need. In theory this is true in Australia as well, but only after a trial of soy formula has failed, resulting in allergy to soy *as well as* bovine protein. In Australia, the government agency insists on proven intolerance of soy formula before authorising subsidised supplies[935] of hydrolysates on scripts from specialists.[936] (Making sure a child has two major allergens rather than one seems hardly cost-effective!)

Where is the justice in less assertive/educated/affluent parents paying much more for over-the-counter soy formula to reduce their child's symptoms of cows' milk allergy, then watching as their child progresses to being allergic to both milk and soy? And while it is accepted that 20–40 per cent of those allergic to bovine protein go on to develop soy allergy, how much of that is because they were first exposed to soy products, like soy oil, in the cows' milk based formula? Should soy oil and any other soy product be allowed in cows' milk formulas now it has become such a common allergen? Where authorities recommend that soy formula should not be used under six months, as in the UK, have they tested the soy oil in bovine formula? Did researchers in Europe test soy oil when deciding to ban sesame and cottonseed oils in infant formula?

Soy formulas given from birth do not prevent allergy.[937] Many children allergic to cows' milk protein will also become allergic to soy protein, and hidden dietary soy protein can be as at least as difficult to deal with as hidden milk protein. ESPGHAN says that 'There is no evidence supporting the use of soy protein formulae for the prevention or management of infantile colic, regurgitation, or prolonged crying.' All true.

---

934  Yasuda H, Yasuda Y, Tsutsui T. Estimation of autistic children by metallomics analysis. *Scientific Reports* 2013, 3, DOI:10.1038/srep02254.

935  The equivalent price of 4 large cans – or up to 10 cans in some cases – of regular formula for the price of a script, around $35 if without a health care card; $6 otherwise. A regular can of cows' milk formula costs $20–$25. See NPS Medicine Wise. Changes to PBS listings of synthetic infant formulas. Online at http://www.nps.org.au/publications/health-professional/nps-radar/2012/july-2012/brief-item-infant-formula

936  http://www.nps.org.au/publications/health-professional/nps-radar/2012/july-2012/brief-item-infant-formula

937  Osborne DA, Sinn J. Formulas containing hydrolysed protein for prevention of allergy and food intolerance in infants. *Cochrane Database Systematic Review* (2006 Oct 18;(4):CD003664).

But in the real world there are babies who cry less, and are healthier, on soy formula than they were on cows' milk formula, and many of their parents will not be able to afford more expensive alternatives, or perhaps even be aware that such alternatives exist and are subsidised. Parents will go with what reduces or stops distress in their individual child. That is quite often a change to soy formula, although the improvement may not last. Good quality complementary feeding after four to six months, widening the diet as soon as possible with unprocessed foods, and getting the child eating healthy family meals by twelve months, will reduce the plant oestrogen load in the child's total diet, whether soy of cows' milk formula fed. Will that be enough to avoid harm from oestrogen analogues? No one knows, but it's sensible to do it anyway.

Meanwhile, where is the long-term follow-up for all infants fed soy formulas from 1970? Where is the detailed research into past infant feeding practices and their relationship to present problems such as premature puberty, endometriosis, polycystic ovarian syndrome, early development of large fibroids, male and female infertility, age and experience of menopause, and any hormone mediated disorder? IVF clinics might be an interesting place to start such research, although of course the demographics for such clinics cannot be fully representative of national populations. (It takes money to access IVF.) The worst effects of any infant formula are likely to be compounded by poverty and poor diet during later infancy and childhood, so that overall the disadvantaged in countries like the US and Australia can always expect to be more greatly disadvantaged by infant formula than the more affluent. Soy formula may prove to have been no worse than the cows' milk formula it replaced for families dealing with the under-publicised problems of artificial feeding. And the limitations of the group definitions in the Arkansas studies need to be borne in mind when considering their conclusions: outcomes might be worse for those fully formula-fed from birth, with zero breastmilk intake.

## Soy protein formula and other oestrogen mimics

The issue of the reproductive effects of soy also has to be seen in conjunction with concerns about other oestrogen-mimicking chemicals. If there was reason for concern about the effects of oestrogen mimics in soy, were health authorities aware that cows' milk contains more bioactive oestrogen analogues? That these can be at high levels depending on the cows' diet? That such chemicals can be found in cows' milk formula and baby food can linings and baby bottles? Since these compounds (including a whole family of phthalates and Bisphenol A) do seem to affect the reproductive organs and sexual behaviour of virtually every animal studied, why has so little been done about those other sources of exposure for the babies? Too expensive, no alternative?

The use of some plasticisers in infant feeding bottles was finally ended in Anglophone countries after 2000, once alternatives that were free of Bisphenol A (BPA-free) were on the market.[938] When in 2013 the US decided to ban BPA in formula packaging materials, it

---

938 Environment Working Group (EWG) has an excellent timeline/history of the use of BPA and its demise: see Timeline: BPA from Invention to Phase-out. http://www.ewg.org/reports/bpatimeline [http://www.ewg.org/research/timeline-bpa-invention-phase-out[?]. Retrieved 26 April 2012.

was careful to stress that it did so not because any harms were proven, but solely because the product was no longer used by US industry: on 'abandonment grounds'. Of course, once a product is no longer used, there is no risk of offending industry in banning it,[939] but also not much point in doing so, and little public health gain!

All of these concerns had been around for twenty years or more before they were acted on. Parents had been quick to ask for BPA-free bottles, and industry to advertise their availability. But what plasticisers are used instead? All plastic leaches chemicals into fats that it contacts. Are the chemicals now leaching into fatty foods any better or worse than BPA? And few people tell parents that their own greatest intake of phthalates is likely to be ingested as coatings on delayed-release medications such as theophylline and omeprazole.

Again, Western health authorities differ in their concern about these issues. Some see no real risk in BPA, as levels in formula remain below the official threshold of risk (a level always set in consultation with industry about what is technically feasible or measurable). Perhaps they are right, and that exposure alone will do no real harm. (So don't panic!) But authorities seem to ignore the fact that this is only one of multiple chemical exposures, that our babies swim in a sea of novel chemical contamination, which comes at them through every aspect of their environment. Every exposure that can readily be avoided is one small lightening of a body burden that may well have effects beyond those we currently see.

A US government-funded research team at the University of Illinois has a five-year $8 million grant to examine how substances used in food packaging affect the health and development of children.[940] Note that it is the taxpayer funding the study decades after industry began using the products, with assurances of safety but little proof. All the research on these issues needs to take the solely-fully-exclusively-from birth breastfed child as the norm for development, not the child fed on cows' milk formula or exposed to it neonatally.

## Other proteins and infant formula: make your own?

There is nothing magical about cows' milk or soy or any other ingredient commonly used to make infant formula. They are protein sources that are dependent on intensive agriculture to be 'reasonably-priced and commercially available'. Infant formulas can be made from many foods. Beef hearts were used in Gerber's Meat Base Formula until 1985.[941] Lamb is being tried in America,[942] donkey milk or almonds in Italy,[943] and rice in Spain.[944] Chicken and rice have routinely been used in recipes for allergic children, and some have done well

939 There can also be economic advantage to local industry, as imports may still contain the banned product. Similarly, large manufacturing concerns can usually afford to make changes more reasdily than smaller firms.

940 http://news.illinois.edu/news/10/1021bpa_schantz_flaws.html

941 http://articles.latimes.com/1990-04-06/news/mn-667_1_gerber-make-formula

942 Weisselberg B, Dayal Y, Thompson JF, Doyle MS, et al. A lamb-meat-based formula for infants allergic to casein hydrolysate formulas. (PMID: 8902326) *Clin Pediatr* (Phila) 1996, 35(10):491–5.

943 Salpietro CD, Gangemi S, Briuglia S, Meo A, et al. The almond milk: a new approach to the management of cow-milk allergy/intolerance in infants. (PMID: 16172596) *Minerva Pediatr* 2005; 57(4):173–80.

944 *Reche M, Pascual C, Fiandor A, Polanco I, et al. The effect of a partially hydrolysed formula based on rice protein in the treatment of infants with cows' milk protein allergy. (PMID: 20337976) Pediatr Allergy Immunol 2010; 21(4 pt 1):577–85.*

on these. Allergy texts have recipes for dieticians to construct such formulas, though these are rarely seen as intended for sole use for many months, and may not have been evaluated against international standards for an infant formula.

That said, because cows' milk and soy have been commercially available, and so many babies have been fed them, these are the proteins about which we know most in relation to infant feeding. Many deficiencies and hazards have emerged and been compensated for by the reduction of this, the addition of that, a change of processing temperature, as the companies learned from their mistakes.

I want to emphasize that this book is not an attempt to persuade parents to shun modern industrial infant formula when they need to use it. Infant formula is a highly complex food mixture. History tells us that above all, babies need food, and also that suitable mixtures are very hard to get right before babies are of an age to eat family foods, around six months or so. History also tells us that carefully prepared recent industrial formulas are something most young babies can and do survive and grow on. Formula may be to breastmilk what dehydrated industrial fast food is to gourmet fresh organic food, but it does enable babies to grow, and almost all survive, mostly without catastrophic harm, in affluent parts of modern societies. No one can hope to mimic these complex foods by making homemade formulas. Yes, children will survive pretty much anything – but with consequences. This is a field in which a little knowledge misapplied could be a very dangerous thing. Some of the YouTube videos on making your own infant formula horrify those with knowledge of infant nutrition and food safety.

But, and it is a big but, that doesn't make industrial formula a good choice when breastmilk could be available, or a mere matter of personal preference. Industrial formula is just the least bad alternative for most babies who can't be fed breastmilk, for whatever reason. Survival and growth are a lottery in which genes, nutrition and environment all play a part. As I've pointed out, some babies always have survived and grown 'normally' on deficient diets (including animal milks and infant formulas that now would be totally unacceptable, as well as 'modern' ones). But experimenting with homemade formulas or other foods as the sole diet for a very young baby could be disastrous.[945] Some websites do offer recipes for homemade mixtures in preference to industrial formulas for babies under six months old. These may well be fine for short periods, or as a small supplement to breastmilk, thanks to babies' innate survival capacities: they would not be supported if they were obviously and quickly lethal! Children do grow on formulas such as those promulgated by the Weston A Price Foundation (WAP), which – with the support of credible nutritionists – has publicised homemade formulas with multiple protein sources for decades. Is this because most babies who progress to using such formulas were breastfed initially, or still are, and the WAP formulas simply serve as a rich complementary diet? How good or bad are such formulas nutritionally as sole foods from birth? Shouldn't orthodox paediatric dietitians give parents some detailed analysis of these, rather than dismissing or ignoring them? Parents should be

---

945 Unless starvation is the other option, of course! Fourreau D, Peretti N, Hengy B, Gillet Y, et al. [Pediatric nutrition: Severe deficiency complications by using vegetable beverages, four cases report]. (PMID: 23021957) *Presse Medicale* 2013; 42(2):e37–43. DOI: 10.1016/j.lpm.2012.05.029.

free to make decisions about their child's nutrition, and the basic principle of using fresh food is sound enough, but what are the outcomes for the infants? Is there more or less Type 1 diabetes, for instance, in infants reared on commercial or homemade formulas? What impact is there on kidneys and circulation? Surely paediatric and nutrition authorities could address this issue?

Scientologists may still use the very 1950s Hubbard formula of cows' milk plus barley water plus corn syrup, which almost certainly fails to meet any accepted infant formula regulations, yet surprisingly seems not to have been publicly denounced by US or other paediatric authorities. Has anyone sought to study the outcomes of such a diet in children born into Scientologist families? It's clear that it can cause scurvy, for starters.[946] Its use was recorded in Australia in August 1991[947] and the recipe and how to make it is online at official Scientology sites.[948] Why is the US government so keen to stop the use of fresh/raw cows milk by adults, but doing nothing about such recipes?

Creating or adopting a DIY (do-it-yourself) infant formula (such as the one created by an ancient Roman, according to L Ron Hubbard) means that parents – and maybe the websites and books – would be responsible for the consequences. If the effects are less than ideal, that can be hard to bear, and parental anxiety levels would be high. And if old-fashioned DIY formula given to very young infants resulted in obvious illness, parents certainly would be considered culpable by health professionals and perhaps even legal authorities.[949] (When parents have ignored standard medical advice and inadvertently harmed their child, it sometimes seems as though they are to be punished for not respecting the social hierarchy. No punishment could be as painful as the death of a loved child. Well-intentioned and caring parents deserve compassion and education, not condemnation, however daft or disastrous their feeding decisions.)

So I'd suggest strongly that it's better for parents of young infants to stick with scrupulous use of current industrial infant formulas, assuming breastfeeding is impossible and safe sources of human milk unavailable. Industry and its paediatric endorsers are legally responsible for any problems that may emerge from their use, and it's vanishingly unlikely that any individual could create a superior product single-handed. After all, even formula companies with multiple laboratories and massive budgets find that getting a substitute feed even mostly right enough is very hard to do. Unexpected side effects can emerge with every change of ingredient, however minor it may seem.

If such homemade formulas prove anything, it is the incredible adaptability of the omnivore human infant, who develops best on mothers' milk, but can cope with a comminuted

946 Burk C, Molodow R, Infantile scurvy: an old diagnosis revisited with a modern dietary twist. *Am J Clin Dermatol*. 2007;8(2):103–6.

947 *ALCA News* 1991; 2(2):18. Copies of record in National Library of Australia.

948 http://www.scientologycourses.org/courses-view/children/step/read-healthy-babies.html The level of nutritional knowledge can be judged from a statement that 'mixed milk powder, glucose and water' adds up to 'total carbohydrate.' Downloaded 12.05.2013.

949 Parents have been jailed: see http://www.nytimes.com/2003/04/05/nyregion/couple-guilty-of-assault-in-vegan-case.html

chicken diet,[950] and does not look noticeably different even when fed an evaporated milk mixture or sometimes appalling alternatives. Proteins, fats and carbohydrates come in many forms, and the harms done by deviating from nature's blueprint for these, in breastmilk, do not always reveal themselves externally. Children – mostly poor or Indigenous children – in Newfoundland and other parts of Canada were still being fed on evaporated milk mixtures in the 1990s and apparently 'thriving', even if iron supplementation is recommended as needed to lower rates of anaemia.[951] And evidently even those fed the 2200-year-old Roman formula grew within the wide range of apparently normal enough, or surely their Scientologist parents might have been concerned. No sane person expects every artificially fed child to develop horns, or show immediate obvious differences from the normal breastfed child – the range of human normal is very wide, and genetics plays a large part in external appearances; protein source is just one influence among many.

## But wait, there's more: milk protein in mothers' diets before and after birth

Another major change in Western diet after 1930 was the huge increase in bovine milk protein intake by women during pregnancy and lactation. Some believed it impossible for bovine protein to find its way from mothers' gut into breastmilk and cause reactions, but nevertheless, it did. This is discussed at greater length elsewhere, but is included here as a reminder that the content of human milk could be affected adversely by the same proteins that would cause problems when fed in formula. And as I have emphasized in Book One, it may be the concurrence of excess maternal milk intake during pregnancy together with neonatal exposure via comp feeds and then continuing exposure to those proteins via breastmilk which creates the greatest levels of infant sensitisation.

Company marketing of milk-based products had always urged consumption by pregnant and lactating women and invalids, as well as infants. Many of the tonic foods (usually based on cereals and milk) of the early twentieth century were aimed at the widest of markets, and indeed, malnourished women may have benefitted – if they could afford to consume such foods, and if they came from that minority of humans tolerant of lactose after infancy.[952] Ubiquitous marketing by dairy interests created a perception that milk was somehow special for those at nutritional risk: they did not just need more quality food; they needed processed or fresh milk foods.

Not until the boom after the Second World War and full employment were the poor able to consume large amounts of fresh milk. By the 1960s and 1970s pregnant women were being

---

950 Paediatric dietitians' texts such as Shaw V, Lawson M. *Clinical paediatric dietetics*, (John Wiley & Sons, 2008) contain information about comminuted, or ground, chicken diet

951 Friel JK, Andrews WL, Edgecombe C, McCloy UR, et al. Eighteen-month follow-up of infants fed evaporated milk formula. (PMID: 10489720)*Can J Public Hlth*, 1999; 90(4):240–3.

952 When milk foods provided by relief agencies were given to malnourished displaced persons in refugee camps after the Second World War, many became seriously ill as a result of lactose intolerance; some thought the camp organisers were poisoning them.

urged to drink up to a litre of milk, and some drank a great deal more, up to 2 litres.[953] It was once routine in some hospitals for postpartum women to have a large jug of a dried milk drink such as Bonlac put beside the bed to be drunk that day, on the spurious grounds that this would help them make breastmilk!

Some research in the late 1980s suggested that high milk intakes during pregnancy greatly amplify the antigen exposure of the infant (see Figure 2-2-3 on page 25). This was perhaps especially likely if the mother herself had been sensitised by formula exposure as a child, and was milk-reactive. And this may be a very important factor in the intergenerational amplification of immune problems, or progressive degeneration of inherited immune systems, which I posit as part of the milk hypothesis. Many women realise their long-standing sensitivity only when breastfeeding a 'fussy' baby, and changing their diet ends symptoms in both mother and baby.

However, despite further publication in 1991,[954] I could find no follow up studies or even much discussion of this obviously important possibility. What happened to this research? There is plenty of evidence that maternal pregnancy diet affects infants,[955] but what about the environmental antigens in bovine milk consumed in pregnancy? Children have been born with severe milk protein allergy problems such as rectal bleeding[956].

> Following up intra-uterine sensitisation with exposure to bovine protein in infant formula is a recipe for misery. I've dealt with many families over allergy issues in a young breastfed firstborn. Most are extremely anxious when having a later child, only to be astonished at the difference avoiding hospital infant formula and antibiotics can make: they can hardly believe that they have a placid contented baby. Only then do they really believe what I told them about the cause of the firstborn's problems!

What was not discussed in this chapter on infant formula protein is the rationale for, and use of, genetic engineering techniques to produce new 'human' proteins for inclusion in infant formula. This can be found in Chapter 3.14 on page 517, in which various aspects of gene technology and their potential use in infant formula making are discussed.

---

953   One mother was drinking five pints (2.8 L) of milk and the cream of another three pints (1.7 L) a day in order to make good milk. Illingworth RS. *The Normal Child* (Churchill Livingstone 7th edition 1979) p. 23.

954   Collins AM, Roberton DM, Hosking CS, Flannery GR. Bovine milk, including pasteurised milk, contains antibodies directed against allergens of clinical importance to man. (PMID: 1809694) *Internat arch allergy appl immunol*, 1991;96(4):362–7. I tracked down this researcher but got no reply to emails. See *La Trobe University Bulletin* February 1992 for an outline of this research. [http://catalogue.nla.gov.au/Record/1778852]

955   Polte T, Hansen G. Maternal tolerance achieved during pregnancy is transferred to the offspring via breast milk and persistently protects the offspring from allergic asthma. (PMID: 18778271) *Clin Exp Allergy*, 2008, 38(12):1950–8.

956   Alabsi HS, Reschak GL, Fustino NJ, Beltroy EP, et al. Neonatal eosinophilic gastroenteritis: possible in utero sensitization to cows' milk protein. (PMID: 23985469) *Neonatal Netw*, 2013; 32(5):316–22.

# 3.6 Basic Ingredients: Formula fats and fictions

If the quality of protein is important to infant formula, so too is the quality of fats. Fats are the single largest energy source for babies, essential for healthy growth, and much more besides. They provide much of the flavour and odour of any product, and are involved in immune function, as a recent review pointed out:

> Recent work has emphasized the fundamental contribution of adipose tissue to the immune system. Immune function is metabolically expensive, involving a variety of costs, including the defense and repair of specific tissues, the metabolic cost of fever, and the production and maintenance of lymphocytes and other immune agents (Romanyukha et al., 2006). Ironically, these costs also include the growth and metabolism of the pathogens themselves. Again, adipose tissue not only provides energy for immune function, but also anatomically specific molecular precursors for immune agents (Mattacks et al., 2004; Pond, 2003) and a range of pro- and anti-inflammatory cytokines that play numerous roles in both immune defense and the repair of damaged tissues (Atanassova et al., 2007; Badman and Flier, 2007; Permana and Reardon, 2007).[957]

Fats occur in both human and cows' milk in a wide variety of forms, which are broken down during digestion by acids or enzymes, into their constituent fatty acids. Other free fatty acids can also be present in milk. There are short-chain and long-chain fatty acids, saturated and unsaturated and polyunsaturated … a chemistry textbook of differences, creating different fat profiles for every mammalian milk.[958] Only the complicated fatty acid profile of human milk fats is ideal for human babies. Some fats derive from blood and body fats, others are made by the mammary gland. Milk fat is secreted into milk as droplets surrounded by a complex protein-containing membrane (the milk-fat globule membrane), about which more anon. All animal milks are very different in the mix of fats they contain, and human milk fats are quite different from bovine milk fats. Since formula began, industry has been trying without success to match breastmilk fats. A world expert, Professor Peter Hartmann, subjected recent infant formula to gas chromatograph analysis and found multiple divergences from breastmilk composition, with fatty acid spikes that show little relationship to breastmilk fatty acid spikes, and some unknown spikes that are simply absent from breastmilk. Infant formula fatty acid profiles are all quite different, and will change with every change of fats (and their processing) in the formula.

Whatever the fats used in various infant formulas, none can match the unique blends found in breastmilk, and all have been subject to change, both during processing and after, in the can. Women have always given their babies fresh, newly made fats, including the long-chain polyunsaturates that industry is touting now as necessary to visual and brain development. Any woman's breastmilk fat reflects her diet and her body composition, but is not completely constrained by these.[959] De novo synthesis of fats is universal and uniquely

957    Wells JC. The evolution of human adiposity and obesity: where did it all go wrong? *Dis Model Mech*, 2012; 5(5):595–607 (PMCID:PMC3424456); Hurley WL, Theil PK. Perspectives on immunoglobulins in colostrum and milk. *Nutrients*, 2011; 3(4):442–74. (PMCID:PMC3257684).

958    Jensen RG (ed). *Handbook of milk composition.* (Academic Press London 1995).

959    Lawrence RA. *Breastfeeding: a guide for the medical profession* (CV Mosby, 2005 6th edn) pp. 118–25.

flexible, and some comes from maternal body stores. Some mothers produce higher fat milk than others, but mothers quite specifically and automatically make more of the different types of fats that their babies need at different stages of growth. So in the early days after birth, human milk contains more of the long chain fats needed for brain cell growth. Then later, when myelination of the brain and central nervous system is the major growth process, human milk contains more of the phospholipids used in myelination.[960] Mothers' bodies are so attuned to their infants' that even the ratios of specific fats in breastmilk vary in harmony with the baby's stages of brain development.[961] And babies get more fat as the feed progresses, as fat levels in milk rise as the breast empties.[962] The hungry baby who persists longer gets more cream; the already replete baby stops as the milk gets richer. This may help explain why babies fed at the breast develop better satiety feedback mechanisms: even when older, they will stop drinking before a cup or bottle is empty, whereas bottle-fed babies tend to consume the lot, with its uniform taste, regardless of quantity.[963] That way obesity lies, as industry now acknowledges[964] in yet another 'blame the parents' exercise. No one knew in the 1970s that what was fed to an infant under six months of age could program development lifelong. In the US, obesity concerns by then had led to an increasing use of skim milk for infants between four and six months. Fomon's research team showed that while this led to loss of skin-fold thickness, it also led to big increases in overall food intake, potentially more dangerous.[965] (Although obesity obviously relates to total energy intake, and both quantity and quality of fats, it is also related to protein and carbohydrate intake and is discussed further in those chapters.)

Technically referred to as lipids, fats are broken down by acids and enzymes, lipases, in a process referred to as lipolysis. Animal milks contain such enzymes and the process of lipolysis begins immediately milk is expressed, although heat both changes the fats and inactivates the milk enzymes, extending the shelf life of animal milks. In the body, digestive processes are complex and dependent both on the nature of the fats provided and the host gut microbiome. The specific chemical formula of the fatty acid can destroy viruses and promote or hinder gut absorption. Fats also influence gut transit: constipation is still more common in artificially fed infants.[966] And they influence brain development and function.

## Animal or vegetable fats for formula?

Initially, bovine milk fat (cream) was the usual source of fat in infant foods, with frequent adjustments of cream content usual in the early percentage formulas (see Mathematics and

960  Harbord MG, Finn JP, Hall-Craggs. Myelination patterns on magnetic resonance of children with developmental delay. *Dev Med Child Neurol* 1990; 32: 295–03. As do children with autism.

961  Daly SEJ, Kent JC, Atwood CS, Warner BJ, et al. Breastmilk fat content increases with the degree of breast emptying (AGR:FNI93002536) *Proceedings Nutrition Society of Australia.* 1991; 16:126.

962  Lawrence op. cit., p. 120.

963  Brown A, Lee M. Breastfeeding during the first year promotes satiety responsiveness in children aged 18–24 mths. *Pediatr Obes.* 2012;7(5):382–90.

964  Gray N. 'Overeating' infant formula linked to higher risk of obesity. *Dairy Reporter* 4 September 2013. Implicit in that is 'It's not our product that's the problem, it's how parents use it'. Sorry, but it's both, and perfect use is an impossible dream.

965  Fomon SJ. Infant feeding in the 20th century: formula and beikost. *J Nutr*, 2001; 131(2):409–20s.

966  Straarup, 2006 Hale TW, Hartmann PE, op. cit., p. 52.

paediatrics on page 223). Older formulas using butterfat recorded levels of around 22 g/L, but there has been a relatively small variation in the total amount of fat in formula since then, with ranges on labels claiming to include around 33–37 g/L, based on breastmilk's theoretical average 40 g/L.[967] A mixture of lard (pork fat) and cod-liver oil was tried briefly, and linseed and cottonseed oils were also used. Beef tallow (old-fashioned 'dripping' in British parlance) was sometimes also part of those mixtures, though its processing allowed it to be labelled 'oleo' or oleo oil, which once was used as a cheap lamp oil.

Cottonseed oil was in fact the cause of a small and largely forgotten American allergy epidemic that started in the late 1930s, peaked in the late 1940s, and sharply declined during the 1950s; cottonseed allergy now is little heard of. Cottonseed oil was 'a useless by product of cottonseed pressing (which produced the stuffing for mattresses and upholstery, and cottonseed meal used for animal feed).'[968] Margarine and shortening changed quickly from being based on pig fat, and cottonseed oil was marketed extensively as a replacement for both lard and tallow. A well-researched book on peanut allergy states an FDA investigation found that cottonseed-crushing protocols had led to the contamination of many other oils also used in food. 'While this discovery explained how many people were unwittingly exposed to the oil, it did not explain how so many had suddenly become sensitised to it ... Doctors responded to the outbreak with a flurry of analyses and opinions, none of which managed to unearth the functional cause of this mass sensitisation.'[969] No investigation of the formulas fed to those people in infancy was undertaken. And I have never seen any report of the contemporary pesticide content of food oils derived from a chemical-intensive crop like cotton, which few then thought would become part of the human food chain. (Such chemical toxicants/contaminants could act as adjuvants to create allergy that would not have occurred if the crop had been organically grown, perhaps.)

By the 1950s cottonseed oil was no longer being used in infant formula; soy oil had largely replaced it (and soy proteins are similar to those of that other legume, peanuts, about to develop as a problem allergen – see page 325). Soy oil was to become ubiquitous, found in everything from vaccinations to cosmetics, as well as manufactured foodstuffs like infant formula. In the days before mandatory labelling, few people were even aware that cottonseed oil had been used in foods. The cottonseed epidemic declined as the use of cottonseed declined. Coincidence? Fraser points out that cottonseed oil was also used as part of the delivery system in many drugs and early vaccines, and where the excipient fats were emulsified with casein or egg lecithin as early as 1913.[970] Again, the combinations may have been the sensitising mix. The cottonseed epidemic was an important but overlooked early warning about the dangers of fats, which carry more than calories into infant formulas and skin creams.

In the next era of formula-making, from the 1950s on, these first fats would be reduced or replaced by tropical and seed oils (and in the US, legume oils like peanut and soy) as world

---

967    Jensen, 1995, Hale TW, Hartmann PE, op. cit., p. 50.
968    Gillespie D. *Toxic oil* (Viking Penguin, 2012) p. 30..
969    Fraser H. op. cit., p. 12.
970    ibid., p. 90.

markets opened up, and palm and coconut oils became plentiful and above all, cheap. Patents were filed, as they had been all century, to protect new infant formula developments from being used by other manufacturers (a practice not necessarily in the best interests of bottle-fed infants!). What follows is an excerpt from a 1972 Wyeth patent application. Note two things as you read: the immense potential variability of the fat mixtures in formula, and the reasons given for rejecting or choosing certain fat sources.

## Humanised fat compositions and infant formulas thereof

The object of this invention is to provide a 'humanised' fat mixture suitable for use in infant formulas … using commercially available, reasonably priced fats and oils.

More particularly, this invention concerns new and novel edible, highly assimilable, fat compositions with a fatty acid composition resembling that of human milk fat consisting of, by weight, from about 15 percent to about 45 percent of oleic oil; from about 10 percent to about 45 percent of oleo oil; from 0 percent to about 25 percent of a seed oil selected from the group consisting of soybean oil, corn oil, peanut oil, sunflower seed oil and cottonseed oil; from about 10 percent to about 35 percent of a member selected from the group consisting of coconut oil and babassu oil;[971] and from 0 percent to about 2 percent of soy lecithin: and infant formulas incorporating said edible oil composition. Among the palmitic acid oils and lauric acid oils, the ones listed above include all members of these classes. The other commercial animal fats (butter, lard, mutton tallow) are not used* because of economic considerations (butter), religious prejudice (lard) and relative unavailability (mutton tallow). The other available seed oils are not considered suitable for various reasons: linseed [previously included] because it contains over 50 percent linolenic acid; olive oil because of uneconomical price, safflower because it contains over 70 percent linoleic acid; sesame seed oil because of the presence of phenolic compounds and sunflower oil because of unavailability. [my italics]

Excerpts from US Patent no 3649295 (A) lodged by American Home Products (then owners of Wyeth) in 1972. Online at the official US Patents Office website (http://patft.uspto.gov/), where you can search by patent number.

Note that in the above patent application, butter was considered uneconomic, and only 'reasonably-priced' fat sources were listed. Butter, or milk fat, was usual in British dominions and Europe where it was cheap. Wyeth in 1961 had developed its 'humanised' powder formula, known in the UK as SMA Gold Cap-S-26.[972] This was a lower-mineral whey-base formula with vegetable oils, beef fat, and carrageenan, which would be manufactured and marketed as S-26 in Australia by the 1960s. By the 1980s Mead Johnson had gone one step further and launched an only-vegetable-oil Olac in Australia, while Enfamil was re-formulated in the USA. These mixes of 'all vegetable oils' were claimed to be more digestible, and to result in less offensive vomit and stools, as they lack certain free volatile fatty acids. Advertising also suggested that they might reduce the risk of cardiovascular disease, as in this rather apt next figure, showing an obese infant being bottle fed by an inattentive mother.

---

971   Babassu oil comes from an Amazonian palm.
972   Wharton B. Food and Child Health in Britain. In Bond JT et al., op. cit., p. 160.

Thus the 1980s saw a major change in countries where milk fat had been used until then, such as Australia and Europe. 'Animal fats' were openly condemned by those selling only 'all-vegetable blends'.[973] As indicated above, this change had occurred earlier in American infant formulas, which had long used cheap corn and soy oil rather than more expensive cream or butterfat, and then had added in the saturated tropical oils as well. Later, these saturated tree oils like palm and coconut would temporarily fall from favour, and corn oil was also questioned, with one industry advertisement suggesting a link to corn allergy. (Animal studies would show that using corn/coconut oil mixes decreased brain accretion of gamma-linoleic acid(GLA) and increased linolenic acid (LA), and queried the impact on membrane function and learning behaviour.)[974]

Figure 3-6-1 Preventing cardiovascular disease?

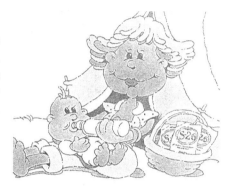

CARDIOVASCULAR PROBLEMS:
PREVENTION IS BETTER
THAN CURE

Further changes were possible once seed oils became cheaper, when new varieties of rapeseed (renamed canola[975]) came onto the market. Further genetic modification to other oilseed plants (some by traditional selective breeding, and some using genetic engineering techniques) followed, making the oils more predictable for use in formula, margarines, and other fatty foods: high oleic safflower oil, for example.

This move to vegetable oils was despite Fomon's 1974 statement that 'serum concentrations of cholesterol in infants receiving formulas containing butterfat are more similar to those of breastfed infants than is true of infants receiving formulas containing mixtures of vegetable oils.'[976] Somehow 'vegetable oils' sounded, well, nicer than 'animal fat'. Just as the term 'humanised' sounds better than 'industrial' or 'artificial', and so was used long after its prohibition by the 1981 International Code of Marketing of Breastmilk Substitutes – Article 9.2. Marketers know their business.

Oddly enough, some disguised animal fat did survive this push for 'all vegetable' oils. Oleo, which few parents would have recognised as destearinated beef tallow or lard, remained in some formulas for decades. I hope observant Jews and Muslims and Hindus and vegetarians understood what it was. Printed material supplied by a Wyeth rep lecturing students in a 1990s Australian maternal and child health course stated: 'the amount of beef oil [oleo] in Wyeth formulas is minute (1.3 per cent weight per volume). The formulas are not strictly kosher but many Jewish mothers do use Wyeth formulas since the amount of beef in the

973  None are vegetable oils; they're seed oils, legume oils, fruit oils, or algal or fungal oils. They are vegetable in the broadest sense, that is, only in being neither animal nor mineral oils.
974  Hrboticky N, MacKinnon MJ, Innis SM. Effect of a vegetable oil formula rich in linoleic acid on tissue fatty acid accretion in the brain, liver, plasma, and erythrocytes of infant piglets. (PMID:2305703) *Am J Clin Nutr* 1990; 51(2):173–82.
975  Canadian oil, low acid = canola, formerly known as rapeseed. The selectively bred strain contained less erucic acid, a known toxin.
976  Fomon (1974) op. cit., p. 380.

formulas is so minute.'[977] Asked about this, she was reported to have replied, 'Ours is only a little bit not kosher.' Like being a little bit not pregnant?

And milk fat continued to be used in countries where it was readily available, in Nestle's product in Australia, and some European formulas, for example. So for a time some infant formulas contained cholesterol, while others contained none. Another confounder for studies of cardiovascular outcomes comparing breastfed and artificially fed infants? After 'Whether formula-fed', researchers need to ask '*Which* formula fed', then consult a global database about what that formula contained at the time in question. Of course industry claimed the changes would help heart health.

## Swallowing cholesterol

Cholesterol was becoming a bogey by the 1970s and 1980s. Thanks to Ancel Keys's selective manipulation of demographic data, and the association between the presence of cholesterol in arteries and heart disease, a simplistic belief spread that cholesterol was the cause of heart disease. The US 1980 Dietary Guidelines were accepted uncritically by dietitians and health authorities alike, despite the fact that the US Department of Agriculture helped draft them! Fat was Bad. Cholesterol was Bad.[978] The food industry in general, infant formula companies included, helped spread this myth, despite the ubiquity of cholesterol in human cells. This later developed into only Some Cholesterol was Bad, the LDL or low density lipoprotein variety. Saturated fats contained cholesterol, and whole populations, beginning with the US, were advised to switch to unsaturated fats, usually cheap, heat-treated, chemically-extracted, vegetable oils. Formula companies emphasised that cholesterol and/or high levels of saturated fats were not present in their formulas.

Conflicting schools of thought soon developed about whether infants need to be exposed to cholesterol early in life to develop appropriate metabolic processes for life. Breastmilk contains substantial amounts of (human) cholesterol, after all, and it is needed in brains. There is still uncertainty about the impact of early exposure to (bovine) cholesterol on infant or adult cholesterol metabolism.[979] Primate studies seem to suggest that early (species-specific) exposure to cholesterol is protective rather than damaging, programming the body to manage cholesterol better.[980] As Innis and Hamilton said,

---

977 Notes on infant feeding.Wyeth Pharmaceuticals. File JC:ajl:02/91. Archived material provided by MCH student present at course.

978 A recent *Time* magazine article reviewed the history of America's dietary guidelines re fat intake: see Walsh B. Don't Blame Fat. *Time*. June 23, 2014; 183 (24): 1723.

979 Wang J, Wu Z, Li D, Li N et al. Nutrition, epigenetics, and metabolic syndrome. (PMCID:PMC3353821) *Antioxid Redox Signal* 2012; 17(2):282–301

980 McGill HC Jr, Mott GE, Lewis DS, McMahan CA, Jackson EM. Early determinants of adult metabolic regulation: effects of infant nutrition on adult lipid and lipoprotein metabolism. (PMID: 8710234) *Nutr Rev* 1996; 54(2 pt 2):s31–40.

> Studies in the developing young of other species suggest that up-regulation of cholesterol synthesis or turnover and excretion, at stages when these pathways are acquiring functional maturity, may have lasting effects on cholesterol metabolism.[981]

Since then, we have come to realise that most of the cholesterol in our bodies (if we don't live on junk food) is not only essential, but made there for a purpose. The natural presumption would be that when cholesterol is in breastmilk, it's important to normal development, or the breast itself, or both. So some companies are now putting cholesterol back into formulas.

But bovine cholesterol is not human cholesterol. Homogenisation and heating alter the composition of fats, and exposure to oxygen during these processes also increases the risk of rancidity unless other chemicals (natural or synthetic anti-oxidants) inhibit this. Oxidation, as well as hydrogenation, can create dangerous trans-fatty acids from seed oils. The Australian discovery of high levels of oxidised cholesterol created by formula production involving twice heating milk (starting with powdered milk which is reconstituted, mixed with other ingredients, then dried again, sometimes more than once) may have influenced one company's decision to sell an infant formula factory[982] and relocate to new plant, using different processes. Some plants use three heat treatments; each has effects.

## Impacts of processing fats

Hydrogenation of fats (used to solidify vegetable oils to form margarine, for example) was shown to increase industrial *trans* fats, and these were shown to be harmful, although enshrined on the GRAS (generally recognised as safe) list created by the USFDA in 1958 (see page 397). British scientist JC Annand argued that such processing increased the atherogenicity (formation of deposits in arteries) of milk fats and allergenicity of milk proteins,[983] and the rise of US heart disease rates fits rather well with the rise in artificial infant feeding from the late nineteenth century. Even homogenisation of milk could be harmful: the combination of turbulence, pressure and heat destroys the natural milk fat globule membrane, and a new membrane is formed which includes a much greater proportion of casein and whey proteins. Different structure often results in differences in function and metabolism. The original milk fat globule membrane (MFGM) contains components thought to be beneficial, which are lost even in a much gentler process such as simply making cream into butter. The health impact of these changes on milk fat used in formula and elsewhere is still under-researched, although there is some evidence that raw cows' milk, while risky because contaminated, is beneficial because it contains active immune factors![984] But as noted earlier, homogenisation also allowed valuable milk fat to be

981 Innis SM, Hamilton JJ. Effects of developmental changes and early nutrition on cholesterol metabolism in infancy: a review. *J Am Coll Nutr* 1992; 11 (Suppl 1): 63S68S.

982 An ex-industry employee asserted this was the case, but I was unable to document it, so I am not citing the company involved. However, it probably was cheaper to relocate production to another country offering huge tax concessions and build new plant there, than to attempt to update old equipment in a country where taxpayers were not overtly subsidising production.

983 Annand JC. Denatured bovine immunoglobulin pathogenic in atherosclerosis. (PMID: 3964356) *Atherosclerosis,* 1986; 59(3):347–51.

984 Astley M. Raw milk consumption cuts infant respiratory infection. *Dairy Reporter* 23 October 2014.

removed, and a standard of not less than 3.5 per cent fat for whole milk had to be set. (The natural range of fat in milk can be from just under 4 per cent to over 6 per cent in Jerseys).[985] The standard for whole milk varies over time and between countries, as do the protocols for heat treatment.

Increasingly in 2013 formula companies use whey protein concentrates and skimmed milk in their mixtures: products that have undergone processing to remove those valuable milk fats, along with heat treatments for pasteurisation and drying to powder. 'Commercially available reasonably priced oils' are used instead of cream. Has this been an improvement? Multiple studies have since suggested that for a much wider variety of reasons, both the child who is not breastfed[986] and the mother who does not breastfeed[987] are at greater risk of coronary artery disease and poorer cardiovascular health, with differences in offspring emerging as early as adolescence.[988] These findings too are still debated, and the lack of feeding detail in studies makes clarity impossible.

So some believed in the 1980s– a belief since questioned – that heat-treated vegetable oils were less likely to damage arteries. This was hard to prove without long-term studies that were not set in train in the 1970s. Vietnam War autopsies had revealed significant plaque in young adult coronary arteries: the arteries of young men brought up on American formulas and polyunsaturated margarine, not having been breastfed as babies or brought up with cream and butter.[989] But what proportion of these was fed the all-vegetable-oil formula and how many were instead fed on the homemade evaporated milk mixes? No one will ever know. The marketing departments of formula and margarine companies were free to create popular myths which can be hard to expose as unfounded, wherever little evidence exists.

Yet how to reduce artery-damaging *trans* fatty acid levels in all processed foods (including formula) is now a big issue for the processed food industry. But of course some industry sponsored studies soon emerged showing trans-fats in the breastmilk of women eating processed foods containing high levels of such fats.[990] Such papers often ignored the otherwise very different profile of breastmilk, and the strong likelihood of little damage to infants from the quantities of trans-fats actually present in breastmilk.[991] Yet breastfeeding women are able to lower the trans-fats in their milk simply by avoiding foods containing highly processed and hydrogenated fats, while formula fats must always be heat-treated.

985   Park and Haenlein op. cit., p. 71.
986   Matturri L, Ottaviani G, Corti G, Lavezzi AM. Pathogenesis of early atherosclerotic lesions in infants. (PMID: 15239349) *Pathology, Research and Practice*, 2004,200(5):403–10.
987   Schwarz EB, McClure CK, Tepper PG, Thurston R, Janssen I, Matthews KA, Sutton-Tyrrell K. Lactation and maternal measures of subclinical cardiovascular disease. (PMID: 20027032) *Obstetrics and Gynecology*, 2010, 115(1):41–8.
988   Labayen I, Ruiz JR, Ortega FB, Loit HM, Harro J, Villa I, Veidebaum T, Sjostrom M. Exclusive breastfeeding duration and cardiorespiratory fitness in children and adolescents. (PMID: 22237059) *Am J Clin Nutr*, 2012 95(2):498–505.
989   Osborn GR. Aetiology of coronary artery disease. (PMID: 5131544) *Med J Aust*, 1971, 2(20):1039–40. Research cited in Jelliffe DB, Jelliffe EFP. *Human milk in the modern world* op. cit., p. 255.
990   Chen ZY, Pelletier G, Hollywood R, Ratnayake WM. Trans fatty acid isomers in Canadian human milk. (PMID:7760684) *Lipids* 1995, 30(1):1521.
991   Chappell JE, Clandinin MT, Kearney-Volpe C. Trans fatty acids in human milk lipids: influence of maternal diet and weight loss. *Am J Clin Nutr*, 1985; 42(1):49–56. (PMID: 4040321).

Chapter 3: Infant formula, past, present and future
3.6 Basic Ingredients: Formula fats and fictions
| 315

And breastmilk has many other mitigating anti-oxidant and anti-inflammatory compounds not found in industrially processed milks. There is increasing concern about the pro-inflammatory effects of many plant oils.

Concerns about the exclusive use of vegetable oils in infant formula have included possible links not only with cardiovascular disease, but also with allergic sensitisation and poor bone mineralisation.[992] Later concerns would emerge about possible negative effects of vegetable oil blends on bone density.[993] So will we start to see more osteoporosis 50–60 years after 'all vegetable' formulas dominated the market, in 2020–30? Some harms of artificial feeding emerge only decades later, by which time they can be explained in many different ways – or more likely ignored, as we currently ignore the harms done by formulas of fifty years ago in people still living today. All long-term studies of population health always need to factor in changing infant formulas over the time.

## A fishy tale of fungi and algae and eggs

The patent application quoted earlier makes it clear that fat blends will change as markets dictate and research suggests something cheaper or new and of high marketing value. The 1980s all-vegetable fat blends were soon found wanting, with their very high omega-6 (linoleic acid) content and lack of omega-3 long-chain polyunsaturated fatty acids (LCPUFAs, like arachidonic acid and docosahexaenoic acid, AA and DHA). Too much linolenic acid was proved to be pro-inflammatory, when not balanced by adequate amounts of anti-inflammatory factors such as the omega-3 fatty acids. It also became clear that infants could not synthesise enough of these essential omega-3 polyunsaturated fats, though it had been assumed that they could.

Industry will never be able to match the changing balance of the 184 fatty acids found in breastmilk.[994] But industry became aware of the need to provide at least some of those neglected fats, always found in breastmilk, though in varying amounts. So industry moved to find a 'commercially available, reasonably-priced' source of omega-3 fats, which their own products had in fact ousted from Western childhood diets.

Longstanding practices of giving babies and children fish-oil supplements, and egg yolk[995] at six months, had disappeared with the move to 'complete' infant formulas from the 1960s in America, and 1970s elsewhere. (Do many of my readers remember Hypol or cod-

992  Clandinin MT, Larsen B, Van Aerde J. Reduced bone mineralization in infants fed palm olein-containing formula: a randomized, double-blinded, prospective trial. *Pediatrics*, September 2004; 114(3):899–900; author reply 899–900. PubMed PMID: 15342879. http://pediatrics.aappublications.org/content/114/3/899.long

993  Litmanovitz I, Davidson K, Eliakim A, Regev RH, et al. High Beta-palmitate formula and bone strength in term infants: a randomized, double-blind, controlled trial (PMCID:PMC3528957). *Calcif Tissue Int*, 2013; 92(1):35–41.

994  Jensen RG (1995) op. cit., p. 536. In the early days after birth, breastmilk contains more of the fats needed for brain cell growth; later it contains more of the fats needed for myelination of the central nervous system.

995  Egg yolks contain these fats and were once routinely added to infant diet at around six months of age, enriching mashed vegetables, for example. Only the introduction of egg white was delayed. Allergy researchers need to know in detail what was suggested in each country.

liver oil doses as children?[996]) 'Old wives' had always said that eating fish (which contains those omega-3 LCPUFAs) is good for the brain. And they were right. By the 1990s, two or three decades after the abandonment of cod-liver oil for babies, the omega-3 LCPUFAs in breastmilk were being linked to better vision and cognition, and industry was looking for sources to use as formula additives. Recent research suggests the absence of such fats in pregnancy and infant diet may also have been part of the reason for higher allergy rates.[997]

Why did fish oil for babies fall out of favour? Because when the so-called 'humanised' formulas came along, companies adding vitamin A and D to formula were concerned that an excess intake of fat-soluble vitamins, especially vitamin D, was toxic. After some inadvertent overdoses, and a British epidemic of hypercalcaemia,[998] paediatric authorities emphasised that industrial formulas were complete, and must not be supplemented with any fat-soluble vitamin drops. Initially cod liver oil had been part of such supplements; the oil base used would have varied over time.

Thus by perhaps the late 1970s on, certainly the 1980s, LCPUFAs were entirely absent from American and Australian infant diet (other than breastfed babies). The UK was the possible exception: a 1980 recommendation was that vitamin drops (which might have contained cod liver oil as the source of vitamins A and D) be given up to five years of age. What were the consequences of this absence of omega-3 fats from the diet of artificially fed children? Was it linked to the emergence of so many brain disorders in that period? Another unmonitored experiment ... As is the simple fact of breaching basic dietary rules of variety and moderation of intake by depending on one processed food.

One early attempt to add LCPUFAs to infant formula may have increased the prevalence of egg 'allergy', and perhaps also increased infant reactions to vaccines grown on egg cultures. Egg phospholipids[999] were used in experimental formulas, and indeed might still be in use somewhere in the world. Publications about the allergic outcomes of such exposures seem impossible to locate. But then, judging from the public record, allergy seems not to have been an outcome studied when formula changes were made. Comparative studies between brands, or with reformulations, may be on record in the company archives, but they are rare in scientific literature. And we cannot conclude anything from the fact that the research did not result in egg phospholipids being added to all formula: it may have proved impossible to standardise egg lipid composition, as it varies with the hen's age![1000] Or to locate a large

996   And Saunders Malt Extract for extra nutrition, as if we needed it!

997   D'Vaz N, Meldrum SJ, Dunstan JA, Martino D, et al. Postnatal fish oil supplementation in high-risk infants to prevent allergy: randomized controlled trial. (PMID: 22945403) *Pediatrics*, 2012; 130(4):674–82.

998   Wharton BA, Darke SJ. Infantile hypercalcaemia. In Jelliffe DB, Jelliffe EFP. *Adverse effects of foods*, op. cit., Ch. 33.

999   Sala-Vila A, Campoy C, Castellote AI, Garrido FJ, Rivero M, Rodríguez-Palmero M, López-Sabater MC. Influence of dietary source of docosahexaenoic and arachidonic acids on their incorporation into membrane phospholipids of red blood cells in term infants. (PMID: 16326086) *Prostaglandins, Leukotrienes, and Essential Fatty Acids*, 2006, 74(2):143–8; Chávez-Servín JL, Castellote AI, Martín M, Chifré R et al. Stability during storage of LC-PUFA-supplemented infant formula containing single cell oil or egg yolk. *Food Chem*, 2009, 113(2):484–92. DOI: 10.1016/j.foodchem.2008.07.082.

1000   Nielsen H. Hen age and fatty acid composition of egg yolk lipid. (PMID: 95682990 *British Poultry Science*, 1998; 39(1):53–6. DOI: 10.1080/00071669889394.

enough supply at an affordable price. As Professor Berthold Koletzko was later to say, 'commercial interests may be the strongest driver of what goes into formula milk'.[1001] And 'commercially available, reasonably priced' is the economic mantra.

Fish oils made a big comeback to child diet. Tuna canneries were able to offer fish heads as a source for oil extraction, and the technology was developed to process these quickly to minimise oxidation (and the development of strong odours and tastes.) By the early 1990s fish oils were packaged in capsules, with drops to be added separately to infant formula. Milkarra in Australia was one such experiment. This was said to have proved ineffective because the oil adhered to the (plastic) baby bottles. This would not only make bottles very hard to clean, but would also very obviously lead to them developing a strong smell from any film or residue clinging to the surface, while a biofilm of microbes could also form. Plastic facilitates such biofilms, and infant formula is an excellent growth medium for bacterial formation of biofilms.[1002] I suspect that the awkwardness of adding one or two drops from small blister packs to each bottle as it was being made up, one at a time, ensured that this method of supplementation, however logical, would never take off. It was a useful stopgap though, as anything known to be jeopardising infant brain and visual development ran the risk of undermining the entire infant formula market and having families return to breastfeeding in droves. Again, the reticence of breastfeeding advocates (and their concern about how other mothers might feel about talk of risks) ensured that this game-changing awareness that formula lacked ingredients needed for optimal brain growth was not widely publicised, although in the 1980s I included this fact in a video made by a South Australian hospital with funding from Nestlé! I have been unable to locate follow-up studies looking at rates of 'allergy' to fish or seafood in exposed infants and of course, the children they will produce in the next decades. I would hope that might be part of the USFDA's 'extensive post-marketing surveillance' that I keep hearing about, but cannot locate.

Adding fish oil to the infant formula in cans was initially impossible: it oxidised rapidly, creating problems of taste and shelf life. Fish oil was also expensive, and to get enough for the world's vast formula industry would empty the oceans of fish. (Some companies are using tuna oil as of 2012, but most are using synthetic mixes.) Large-scale long-term reliable availability of omega-3 fats was needed, together with a way of protecting these fats from oxygen. Industrial-scale synthetic production was the solution, along with new technology to micro-encapsulate the oils. And so a new industry was born.

## Gold from oil: Martek's miracle

Founded in 1985 as a spin-off from the aerospace industry, new American biotech company Martek Biosciences had by 1994 put into a formula (for sale in Europe, not America) patented omega-3-rich oils, DHASCO and ARASCO, made by genetically modified soil fungi and marine algae. These organisms were cultured on a large scale, described in industry literature as follows:

---

1001  Koletzko B. Standards for infant formula milk. *BMJ*, 2006; 332:621–2.
1002  Oh S-W, Chen P-C, Kang D-H. Biofilm formation by *Enterobacter sakazakii* grown in artificial broth and infant milk formula on plastic surface (Agr:Ind43982644) *J Rapid Method Autom Microbiol*. 2007; 15(4):311–19.

Brewed in 130-gallon vats of water surrounded by fluorescent bulbs and injected with a mix of nitrates, potassium, phosphates, carbon dioxide, and other elements, Martek's algae typically doubled its weight within five to 24 hours and was ready to harvest within a week.[1003]

Martek described what followed as:

The oil is then separated from the dried biomass by hexane extraction and centrifugation and/or filtration, followed by winterization.[1004] The hexane phase undergoes additional centrifugation/filtration to remove solids then the winterized oil is heated and treated with acid. Subsequently, the oil is treated with caustic, centrifuged, bleached and deodorized.

That's a lot of heavy-duty processing! But a single 130-gallon container yielded as much as $25 million worth of algae a year.[1005] Extracted with chemicals including hexane, and tasting of their fungal and algal origins, these oils were truly unpalatable, even after bleaching and deodorising. It is to be hoped that they have been so thoroughly purified that no traces of algal or fungal protein could be transferred with the oil the brew produced.

Other proteins have been, and caused reactions. A new technique, micro-encapsulation,[1006] had made it possible to use these oils to add omega-3 to powdered infant formula, with a reasonable length of shelf life. Micro-encapsulation coated the volatile oils with edible proteins, protecting them from oxidation. How much thought was given to the proteins used, initially milk and soy, which caused reactions in allergic children? And what proteins are now used, and has anyone checked to see if they are sensitising? After long years of unprofitable research and development, Martek became a multi-million dollar success once more infant formula companies relied on its patented products. It would be sold for over US$1 billion in 2010.[1007] That billion dollars will be recouped from customers, of course: which helps to explain price rises in infant formula.

As was usual, the US-designed products were first trialled in infant formula outside the United States. Not until the following decade, in 2001, were these fungal and algal oils added to US infant formula, and even then, the regulatory authority, the FDA, did not formally approve them.[1008] As is now routine (see page 409), the USFDA has merely noted that they are present in US products, and asked for 'extensive post-marketing surveillance' – but has no power to compel industry to provide such reports. The FDA replied to a Freedom of Information Act request by Cornucopia Institute that up to 2009 none of the companies marketing these oils had reported adverse reactions to the FDA, despite some 98 self-

---

1003 http://www.fundinguniverse.com/company-histories/martek-biosciences-corporation-history/ Accessed 7 August 2013

1004 The process of removing components with high melting point (e.g. waxes) from some vegetable oils, by cooling, filtering and centrifugal forces.

1005 http://www.fundinguniverse.com/company-histories/martek-biosciences-corporation-history/ Accessed 7 August 2013

1006 US Patent no EP 2166874 A1 (text from WO2008157629A1) describes this in detail.

1007 This is claimed as a triumph brought about with the help of publicly funded tertiary institutions: see http://www.mtech.umd.edu/news/news_story.php?id=5408

1008 Kent G. Regulating fatty acids in infant formula: critical assessment of U.S. policies and practices. *Intl Breastf J* 2014, 9:2 DOI:10.1186/1746-4358-9-2.

reported adverse reactions by 2008.[1009] But once the oils had been added to US formula, political lobbying ensured US government programs promoted them (see page 324).

Some other companies are now patenting and producing versions of these essential fats, made by different organisms, extracted using different chemical processes, and coated with different ingredients. A German manufacturer uses 'specially prepared egg-yolk lipids.'[1010] Others are using carbohydrates. The globally advertised link with possible cognitive benefits has enabled infant formula prices to be raised far beyond the additional cost of the ingredient added. (One report stated that in the period 1983–96, formula prices had increased 200 per cent while the cost of milk had risen 30 per cent.) That topic is another book in itself, which I hope someone with access to global market data will write. But as always, there were some unexpected side effects: when outcomes were assessed, it was found that some microbial oil supplements were associated with growth retardation in children fed formulas containing them, and this had to be explained by research.[1011] No matter what fats are used, the end-products of oxidation are very different to those found in breastmilk whether fresh or stored, as Michalski has shown. See Figure 3-6-2 on page 324.

Many people are concerned about these products, among them the Cornucopia Institute, a US non-profit group that supports 'the ecological principles and economic wisdom underlying sustainable and organic agriculture'.[1012] Infant formula is one of their ongoing concerns, and I recommend their website, the report they produced: *Replacing mother — imitating human breast milk in the laboratory*,[1013] and their submission to the National Organics Standards Board in relation to the use of these microbial oils.[1014]

These latest altered-fat infant formula products were labelled as 'Gold' formulas, talked about as premium formulas, and sold at a much higher price. Yet so far the jury is still out on how much difference, if any, these make when added to formula for term infants. A number of reviews and meta-analyses – the latest in 2012[1015] – keep concluding that

> LCPUFA supplementation of infant formulas failed to show any significant effect on improving early infant cognition. Further research is needed to determine if LCPUFA supplementation of infant formula has benefits for later cognitive development or other measures of neurodevelopment.[1016]

What did marketing tell parents about the effects on intelligence? The marketing of the omega-3s in formula used every visual and verbal trick in the book to suggest that the addition of these fats would improve brain development, long before the research was

1009 Spinning suspect ingredients in baby formula http://cornucopiaorg/2012/02/ spinning-suspect-ingredients-in-baby-formula/
1010 Sawatzki G, Georgi G, Kohn G. Pitfalls in the design and manufacture of infant formulae. (PMID: 7841620) *Acta Paediatr Suppl,* 1994; 402:40–5. Do allergy researchers know and have they tested this?
1011 ibid.
1012 www.cornucopia.org/home
1013 Online at http://www.cornucopia.org/2008/01/replacing-mother-infant-formula-report/
1014 http://www.cornucopia.org/NOSB_DHAletter.pdf
1015 Qawasmi A, Landeros-Weisenberger A, Leckman JF, Bloch MH. Meta-analysis of Long-Chain Polyunsaturated Fatty Acid supplementation of formula and infant cognition. (PMID: 22641753) *Pediatrics,* 2012; 129(6):1141–9.
1016 ibid.

available to say whether it did or not. Babies with mortarboards, reading Einstein's theory of relativity; A+ signs on labels and blackboards (Mead Johnson), misleading text like 'There's more to IQ than being born with it' (Wyeth). True, of course. Breastmilk and nurture is needed to optimise genetic inheritance. But what conclusion is suggested when that slogan is on an advertisement for any food product? As the new formulations went on sale, parents were bombarded with sly and subtle marketing claims of improved IQ. Misleading syllogisms abounded, as always:

- Omega-3 fats in breastmilk help brain development (true)
- Omega-3 fats are important for eyesight (true)
- Omega-3 fats are now in our formulas (true, but not the same as in breastmilk)

Therefore ... what? What is the logical conclusion? Not what most parents are being nudged to assume. Some companies clearly breached advertising and even legal (not to mention ethical) standards in their efforts to promote the considerably more expensive formula products. Mead Johnson has been found guilty in three US lawsuits filed by PBM, the makers of store-brand formula, for claiming that only Mead Johnson products contained the nutrients needed for good visual development. Mead Johnson advertisements showing blurry images resolving into sharp focus (implicitly because of formula fatty acid composition) were judged misleading, but the company kept on airing them.[1017] But where penalties for misleading advertising are less than the profits from increased market share, would we expect any billion-dollar industry to stop advertising? Why not just offset any fines against the profits? (And are legal expenses tax-deductible, so indirectly taxpayers foot the bill?)

The universal presence of these LCPUFAs in breastmilk, whatever the mother's diet, suggests that they are important nutrients. But the presence of these (human) fats in human milk doesn't prove that different, synthetic, algal and fungal mixes will be as important, effective,[1018] or even safe, in formula! It may be better for formula to include them, perhaps especially pre-term formulas. But once again, a change has been made to infant diet that requires careful long-term scrutiny to see what all the results are. It is a new experiment, and should be monitored long-term and in depth, to see what difference changed brains make through the lifespan.

For almost immediately after these fungal and algal oils were put into formula, there were clinical reports of intractable diarrhoea and allergic reactions to formulas that included these novel fats. The following letter is typical of reports from lactation consultants.

---

1017  See http://www.cbsnews.com/8301-505123_162-42744908/strike-five-why-mead-johnson-keeps-airing-misleading-baby-formula-ads/ Accessed 8 August 2013.
1018  Gould JF, Smithers LG, Makrides M. The effect of maternal omega-3 (n-3) LCPUFA supplementation during pregnancy on early childhood cognitive and visual development: a systematic review and meta-analysis of randomized controlled trials. (PMID: 23364006) *Am J Clin Nutr*, 2013; 97(3):531–44. DOI: 10.3945/ajcn.112.045781.

I have received telephone calls from 2 mothers in the past year in relation to their babies having severe reactions to infant formula.

Both mothers were breastfeeding their babies; but intended to gradually wean their babies onto formula.

Mother 1 explained that her baby had a small amount of formula at about 4 weeks of age, and vomited some of it afterwards. At 4 months the infant was given a bottle of formula. The reaction included severe vomiting and collapse, requiring ambulance transfer to hospital.

Mother 2 attempted to give her 4 month old infant a bottle of formula; but the baby refused to take it, possibly swallowing about one mouthful of milk. The infant was put into bed; but was unusually restless and crying intermittently for about 20 minutes. When he was checked he was found to have a rash and to be 'swollen all over', so was taken to hospital immediately. (The only other time this infant had 'formula' was 24 hours after birth for low blood sugar whilst in Special Care Nursery).

The mothers and infants were linked with an allergy clinic and recommended to continue to breastfeed. Both mothers contacted me as they wanted some further information about maintaining a good milk supply. Have you had any other reports of reactions to artificial baby milks becoming more severe and/or more common?

Some reactions, in young infants, and in children allergic to cows' milk and soy and living on so-called hypoallergenic formulas, were severe. The allergic children may have been affected by the proteins used for micro-encapsulation: milk and soy![1019] The babies may have been reacting to other antigens, including fungal and algal protein traces, or traces of the chemicals used to break up the algal biomass and extract the oils, or the products of digestion of these strange fats in their guts. (Research has recently shown that fatty acids from formula fats can be cytotoxic, killing intestinal cells.)[1020] After adverse outcome reports, Martek changed the encapsulating proteins for use in hypoallergenic formula products. It is not clear what proteins they now use, but no doubt time (and enough allergic reactions) will tell.

Where a community trusts infant formula implicitly, that evidence is likely to be slower to emerge, because other causes for symptoms are more likely to be assumed and formula analysis not carried out. But what does it say about the tunnel vision of an industry that it would put Western society's most common allergens in formulas for allergic children? What does it say about the depth of thought of the industry buyers of fungal and algal oils that they did not investigate what proteins coated the encapsulated oils they were buying?

---

1019 This was reported on Martek's own website, in a press release splashing the news of the new hypoallergenic blend for hypoallergenic formulas. However, while I downloaded it at the time, and reported it widely, I can no longer find that information on the Martek website.

1020 Penn AH, Altshuler AE, Small JW, Taylor SF et al. Digested formula but not digested fresh human milk causes death of intestinal cells *in vitro*: implications for necrotising enterocolitis. *Pediatric Research* 2012; 72: 560–7 DOI:10.1038/pr.2012.125

Everyone assumes safety, and no regulator ensures it. Only parents can protect their children, but they should not have to! This is a social responsibility.

# Structured oils as sources of LCPUFAs

Already however, another new fat contender is emerging: a novel 'designer fat' created from hazelnut oil, that contains DHA and ARA at the same positions found on fats in human milk.[1021] We are told that Novozym 435 lipase was used to produce palmitic acid-enriched hazelnut oil. (Novozym 435 is in fact 'Lipase acrylic resin from Candida antarctica' a genetically engineered enzyme from a fungus.) Extra virgin olive oil is being treated in a similar fashion.[1022]

The scientists involved have extensively analysed their human milk fat mimics and concluded that 'the new DHA and ARA source is suitable for the supplementation of infant formulas.'[1023] In their paper, there was no discussion of allergenicity, yet allergens found in hazelnut oil cross-react with birch and other plant pollens; hazelnut allergy is common in European countries that use hazelnuts extensively. And one of those hazelnut allergens belongs to the group of lipid-transfer proteins that were recently identified as plant pan-allergens. What is more, those allergenic proteins were demonstrated to be stable against heat treatment.[1024]

Plant pan-allergens are related to proteins found widely in plants, proteins that are responsible for many cross-reactions to different foods that contain them.[1025] And being heat-stable, such allergens may persist unaltered into infant formula. Yet hazelnut oils may still prove nutritionally better than fungal and algal oils, about which *Science Daily* writes:

> Currently, DHA and ARA ... from algae are added to many formulas, but concerns exist about the digestibility of these algae-derived fatty acids, which are not exactly identical to those in human milk.[1026]

Hundreds of thousands of babies have now been fed these 'oils from a single-cell source'. (That is how these oils are identified on formula cans. It does sound better than 'fungal' or 'algal' oils.) What to make of all that? Wait and see. A recent study has shown for the first time that a neurotoxic amino acid called β-methylamino-L-alanine, or BMAA, produced by blue-green algae, is linked with motor neurone disease.[1027] These are *not* the algae used

1021  Turan D, Yeşilçubuk NS, Akoh CC. Production of human milk fat analogue containing docosahexaenoic and arachidonic acids, *J. Agric. Food Chem.*, 2012; 60 (17) pp. 4402–7. DOI: 10.1021/jf3012272.

1022  Pande G, Sabir JSM, Baeshen NA, Akoh CC. Enzymatic Synthesis of Extra Virgin Olive Oil Based Infant Formula Fat Analogues Containing ARA and DHA: One-Stage and Two-Stage Syntheses. *J Agric Food Chem* 2013; 61 (44):10590–10598.

1023  ibid.

1024  http://www.food-allergens.de/symposium-3-1/hazelnut/hazelnut-allergens.htm

1025  Hauser M, Roulias A, Ferreira F, Egger M. Panallergens and their impact on the allergic patient. *Allergy Asthma Clin Immunol.*, 2010; 6(1):1. DOI: 10.1186/1710-1492-6-1. PMCID: PMC2830198.

1026  *Science Daily*, May 2012 www.sciencedaily.com/releases/2012/05/120523115053.htm citing Turan D, Yeşilçubuk NS, Akoh CC. Production of human milk fat analogue containing docosahexaenoic and arachidonic acids. *J Agric Food Chem*, 2012; 60 (17):4402. DOI: 10.1021/jf3012272.

1027  Dunlop RA, Cox PA, Banack SA, Rodgers KJ (2013) The non-protein amino acid BMAA is misincorporated into human proteins in place of l-Serine causing protein misfolding and aggregation. PLOS ONE 8(9): e75376. DOI:10.1371/journal.pone.0075376

by Martek or other makers for the formula industry. The point I'm making is that we didn't know until now that such a nasty disease could be linked to *any* algae. Can we be sure that no such nasty surprises will emerge from fungi and algae genetically modified by enzymes from such a huge variety of novel sources, all being sought by an industry keen to grab a slice of an enormous emerging market? There are some unavoidable risks in any infant feeding, but who decides about relative risk and benefit?

Of course it is possible that something which is helpful, or at least harmless, for some children, in communities where mothers' diets are abnormally low in that ingredient, may also be hazardous in other contexts. Although these fats have been added to infant formula for almost twenty years now, a follow-up study of 311 Danish preterm babies suggests that too much might have some detrimental effects, in girls anyway.

> The results from the study indicate that DHA status at 9 months may not have a pronounced beneficial effect on psychomotor development in early childhood, and that communicative skills at 3 years of age *may even be inversely associated* with early red-blood-cell DHA levels in girls.[1028]

Some older children might receive too much of a probably Good Thing for newborns. If confirmed, this study, the first to look at red blood cell DHA levels for weanlings, surely has implications for the widespread addition of these oils to foods at later stages of childhood.

Is there any current science which might help explain detrimental effects of LCPUFAs in infant formula, and their benefit in breastmilk? PUFAs in breastmilk and formula behave very differently. All unsaturated fats are highly susceptible to oxidation, which is affected by many factors such as temperature, storage time, exposure to light or to metal ions, and so on. Human milk can be stored more safely than formula: even after a week, breastmilk is remarkably stable against oxidation, thanks to its low iron and many anti-oxidants, which decrease in concentration over lactation but increase in activity.[1029] By contrast, the polyunsaturated fatty acids in infant formula oxidise very rapidly once exposed to air, particularly when LCPUFAs have been added and large amounts of iron are present (as in premium/Gold formulas). The end products formed by oxidation are highly reactive and their potential impact on infant health is currently debated.

> It is thus important to quantify and prevent the presence of such components in infant food. Despite high PUFA in breastmilk, peroxidation products are in fact present only in trace amounts. This is presumably due to breastmilk containing anti-oxidants such as vitamin E and to the protective structure of the MFGM (milk-fat-globule membranes), since they have been shown to protect PUFA against oxidation. (Song et al 1997) In contrast, *even a*

---

1028 Engel S, Tronhjem KM, Hellgren LI, Michaelsen KF et al. Docosahexaenoic acid status at 9 months is inversely associated with communicative skills in 3-year-old girls. (PMID:22642227) *Matern Child Nutr* 2013; 9(4):499–510.

1029 Westerbeek EAM, Stahl B, van Elburg RM Human milk and intestinal permeability. In Zibadi, Watson and Preedy, op. cit., p. 105.

*few minutes after milk preparation,* infant formula contains substantial amounts of MDA, 4-HHE, and 4-HNE.[1030] (see table below)

| | 4-HHE/n-3 PUFA ratio (ng/g) | 4-HNE/n-6 PUFA ratio (ng/g) | MDA/PUFA ratio (ng/g) |
|---|---|---|---|
| Breast milk | | | |
| Freshly expressed | 190±10 | 4±0 | 640±190 |
| Stored 1 day at 18 °C | 160±70 | 25±10 | 720±160 |
| Stored 1 week at 4 °C | 180±30 | 25±13 | 1,280±830 |
| Infant formula | | | |
| Powder (diss. at 37 °C)[1] | 3,600±310 | 1,100±1000 | 13,800±4,900 |
| Liquid at opening | | | |
| Regular | 695±205 | 25±7 | 2,800±300 |
| Added PUFA | 5,600 | 620 | 8,200 |
| Liquid stored 1 day at 4 °C | | | |
| Regular | 800±200 | 20±10 | 7,300±2,900 |
| Added PUFA | | | 23,700 |

[1] 2 regular, 1 PUFA-enriched.

Figure 3-6-2 Some end-products of oxidation, breastmilk and formula[1031] © Wageningen Academic Publishers

These substances can accumulate in the gut and contribute to chronic intestinal disorders and cancer; they can affect enzyme functioning and alter insulin signalling. Thus the author went on to 'wonder whether low but chronic exposure to both HHE-4 and HNE-4 via oxidised lipids in infant formula would produce some deleterious effects on infant metabolism,' and to call for research as to safe threshold levels.

Meanwhile, to me this is yet another reason why parents should be advised – as WHO says – not to make batches of formula hours before feeding, and to feed made-up formula immediately. Chilling reduces the rate of oxidation, but does not prevent it.

## The USA goes for Gold (fats in formula)

Public acceptance of these new oils was not inevitable, especially if issues like their potential for rapid oxidation had been discussed. The higher cost involved was also a major disincentive in America. But President Bush came to the aid of American industry yet again. When Congress re-authorised the US Women Infants and Children (WIC) program in 2004, industry was permitted to dictate to WIC what formulas they will supply to parents via the tender system.[1032] Not surprisingly, knowing how dramatically WIC use affects retail

---

1030 Michalski MC. Lipids and milk fat globule properties in human milk. p. 329. Ch. 16 In Zibadi, Watson and Preedy, op. cit.

1031 ibid, p. 330. © Wageningen Academic Publishers

1032 See WIC Policy Memorandum #4-2004, Implementation of the Infant Formula Cost Containment Provisions of P.L. 108–265, 30 July 2004. Online at http://www.fns.usda.gov/sites/default/files/2004-4-InfantFormulaCostContainment.pdf

sales, US manufacturers offered their Gold (expensive) brands, not those without these microbial oils. This has forced many US States' WIC programs to provide and so promote the expensive new brands. The consequences:

> After adjusting for inflation, net wholesale prices increased by an average 73 percent for 26 fluid ounces of reconstituted formula between States' contracts in effect in December 2008 and the States' previous contracts. As a result of the increase in real net wholesale prices, WIC paid about $127 million more for infant formula over the course of a year. This was equivalent to the cost of supporting 134,200 persons in WIC for a year or about 2 percent of all women, infants, and children participating in WIC in fiscal year 2008. Seventy-two percent of the increase in real net wholesale price was due to an increase in the real wholesale price of infant formula. All rebate contracts in effect in December 2008 were based on formulas supplemented with the fatty acids docosahexaenoic acid (DHA) and arachidonic acid.[1033]

As noted earlier, WIC is not an open access programme, something all poor citizens are entitled to access. The help it can offer hungry families lucky enough to get on its books is limited to what its budget will support. So the trade–off for possible (as yet unproven) benefits to term infants is that other families go hungry. (For more on this see page 491) And increasingly, perhaps live in cars, or on the street, or beg – or turn to crime to feed their children.

## Peanut oil and allergy

As a result of clinical experience, not intelligent foresight, many manufacturers have quietly shunned at least one previous fat source. From around 1940 peanut oil had replaced cottonseed oil in American food, drugs and vaccines. By the 1990s the peanut allergy epidemic had emerged, and was causing deaths in every Western nation (though fewer than milk protein was causing, by a long shot.[1034])

The Australian Infant Formula Standard was under review through the 1990s. I remember well an apparently unanimous[1035] ANZFA (the-then Australian and New Zealand Food Authority, now FSANZ) teleconference agreeing that the proposed new Infant Formula Standard must insist on the exclusion of peanut oil. This did not make it into the final published Australian Standard. When I later called to ask ANZFA staff about the omission, I was told that the formula industry had assured the regulatory agency[1036] that a specific exclusion was unnecessary as they did not use peanut oil, and singling out peanut oil as forbidden might

---

1033 Oliveira V, Frazão E, and Smallwood D. *Rising infant formula costs to the WIC Program: recent trends in rebates and wholesale prices*, ERR-93, US Department of Agriculture, Economic Research Service, February 2010. p. III.

1034 Macdougall CF, Cant AJ, Colver AF. How dangerous is food allergy in childhood? The incidence of severe and fatal allergic reactions across the UK and Ireland. (PMID: 11919093) *Arch Dis Child*, 2002; 86(4):236–9. DOI: 10.1136/adc.86.4.236.

1035 joint Australia/New Zealand telephone conference call in which I participated; noted from memory, though no doubt the notes are somewhere in my filing system!

1036 From the NFA, National Food Authority, to ANZFA, and now FSANZ, Food Safety Australia and New Zealand. I have been told that cutbacks caused significant losses of experienced personnel over that time, and increased dependency on contractors, rather than in-house independent expertise.

alarm parents. I translated that mentally into, 'might alert parents and allergy researchers to the fact that peanut oil was being used in the past'. Some Sydney allergy specialists were openly incredulous when I told them that peanut oil had ever been used in some infant feeding products. And as late as 1991 Moneret-Vautrin recorded peanut oil in eleven of forty-five infant formulas analysed.[1037] No one other than Heather Fraser[1038] has openly publicised the fact that peanut oil was also in many vaccines and medications like vitamin K injections.

The EU has since prohibited the use of sesame and cottonseed oils in formula,[1039] but not banned peanut oil. That strikes me as odd, suggesting that it might still be in use by some companies.[1040] Some allergists are still pondering how a protein so harmless for whole populations (notably in mostly-breastfeeding Africa) has become such a problem for others. Those same specialists were well aware that peanut oil had been in eczema and nipple creams,[1041] and had suggested both as potential causes of allergy. They were also happy to implicate maternal diet, reluctant to implicate formula feeding. Yet if breastfeeding were to be the cause, peanut allergy would be highest in those breastfeeding populations that rely on groundnuts/peanuts in pregnancy and lactation: some African populations, where until recently peanut allergy has been virtually unknown. And a recent UK study found that peanut allergy in children was associated with skin care products used on oozing rashes, but 'not at all associated with maternal ingestion of peanut products during lactation.'[1042] In fact, a recent study in mice suggests that exposure via breastmilk might be protective, that peanut traces in milk 'may prevent rather than priming allergic sensitisation'[1043] which is what I'd expect in animals not already allergic.

In Australia the last brand label that I saw peanut oil listed on was a specialty formula that used medium chain triglycerides (MCTs) as well; a neonatologist told me that the oil has also been part of a widely used vitamin supplement given to preterms (who are at increased risk of immune disorder). This could be an especially damaging mix, as MCTs have recently been shown to 'promote allergic sensitisation and anaphylaxis by affecting antigen absorption and

1037  Moneret-Vautrin DA, Hatahet R, Kanny G, Ait-Djafer Z. Allergenic peanut oil in milk formulas.
      (PMID:1682569) *Lancet* 1991; 338(8775):1149; Moneret-Vautrin DA, Hatahet R, Kanny G. Risks of milk
      formulas containing peanut oil contaminated with peanut allergens in infants with atopic dermatitis.
      (PMID:7951761) *Pediatr Allergy Immunol* 1994; 5(3):184–188.
1038  Fraser H. op. cit.
1039  EU Commission Directive 2006/141/EC on infant formulae and follow-on formulae. Online see http://
      ec.europa.eu/food/food/labellingnutrition/children/formulae_en.htm
1040  Infant formula regulations are always carefully written around industry realities. Anyone who doubts that is
      out of touch with reality!
1041  Vadas P, Wai Y, Burks W, Perelman B. Detection of peanut allergens in breast milk of lactating women.
      (PMID:11277829) *JAMA* 2001: 285(13):1746–1748. Immediately rehashed as Stock S. Peanut allergy can
      be carried in breastmilk. *Weekend Australian* April 21, 2001, p. 7. The *Daily Telegraph* (July 21, 1996) had
      screamed 'Breast oil linked to allergies in babies' after the discovery of peanut oil in widely used creams.
1042  Friedman NJ, Zeiger RS. The role of breast-feeding in the development of allergies and asthma.
      (PMID:15940141) *J Allergy Clin Immunol* 2005; 115(6):1238–1248 DOI: 10.1016/j.jaci.2005.01.069
1043  Bernard H, Ah-Leung S, Drumare MF, Feraudet-Tarisse C et al. Peanut allergens are rapidly transferred in
      human breast milk and can prevent sensitization in mice. (PMID:24773443) *Allergy* 2014, 69(7):888–897]DOI:
      10.1111/all.12411

Chapter 3: Infant formula, past, present and future
3.6 Basic Ingredients: Formula fats and fictions
| 327

availability and by stimulating T(H)2=Th2 responses.'[1044] These fats stimulated absorption of antigens into Peyer patches in the gut, from whence they could reach the bloodstream. 'A single gavage of peanut protein with MCT, as well as prolonged feeding in MCT-based diets, caused spontaneous allergic sensitisation.'[1045] Neocate contained peanut oil (together with beef fat, pork fat and coconut oil) until 1991, according to David.[1046] Peanut oil was also still in use elsewhere in the 1990s: an Indian group discussed adding it to cows' milk based formulae,[1047] and French paediatricians reported cases of atopic dermatitis (eczema) where infant formula was the only source of exposure to peanut oil; they stated that 'Owing to the growing incidence of peanut hypersensitivity, the elimination of peanut oil from all milk formulas, food for babies, and ointments, seems to be highly advisable.[1048]

Yet in 1997 those Indian researchers reported that 'the present study suggests that a vegetable oil such as peanut oil could be used in milk fat to improve the essential fatty acid (EFA) status of infants.'[1049] And it was also being fed to preterm infants via intravenous fat emulsions.[1050] Nowadays, peanut oil is not only still in use where explicit labelling is not required, as in the USA, but is seen as one way of lowering levels of trans-fats, since everyone has become aware that trans-fats are so damaging to cardiovascular systems.

It must be said that one study of 10 adults showed that when ultra-refined peanut oil is blind-tested against unrefined oils, there might be no immediate obvious reaction from *adults* known to be sensitive to peanuts.[1051] This may be cited as support for the ancient 'oils can't sensitise' myth. However, there are still measurable levels of peanut protein in even highly refined oil, enough to cause histamine release in studies.[1052] And anaphylaxis in infants.[1053] What is true of adults may not be true of infants. And in any case, TJ David calculated that to be 99.9 per cent sure that peanut oil would not cause a reaction in 99.9 per cent of peanut allergic patients, the study would need to be of 6905 peanut intolerant individuals.[1054] No one has done that study!

In addition, it seems unlikely to me that the commercial oil-refining process is universally infallible, or that cheaper oils are not used by at least some manufacturers of formula or

1044 Li J, Wang Y, Tang L, de Villiers WJ, et al. Dietary medium-chain triglycerides promote oral allergic sensitization and orally induced anaphylaxis to peanut protein in mice. *J Allergy Clin Immunol.* 2013 Feb; 131(2):442–50. DOI: 10.1016/j.jaci.2012.10.011. Epub 22 November 2012.

1045 ibid.

1046 David TJ. op. cit., p. 100.

1047 Hariharan K, Rao SV. Influence of partial replacement of butter fat with peanut oil (in infant formula) on erythrocyte fatty acids in infants. (PMID: 9475076) *Indian J Exp Biol*, 1997, 35(9):957–63. See also

1048 Moneret-Vautrin DA, Hatahet R, Kanny G. Risks of milk formulas containing peanut oil contaminated with peanut allergens in infants with atopic dermatitis. (PMID: 7951761) *Pediatr Allergy Immunol*, 1994, 5(3):184–8. DOI: 10.1111/j.1399 3038.1994.tb00236.x

1049 Hariharan K, Kurien S, Rao SV. Effect of supplementation of milk fat with peanut oil on blood lipids and lipoproteins in infants. (PMID: 8574857) *Int J Food Sci Nutr*, 1995; 46(4):309–17.

1050 Morris S, Simmer K, Gibson R. Utilization of docosahexaenoic acid from intravenous egg yolk phospholipid. (PMID: 10858022) *Lipids*, 2000, 35(4):383–8. DOI: 10.1007/s11745-000-535-9

1051 Hourihane JO, Bedwani SJ, Dean TP, Warner JO. Randomised, double blind, crossover challenge study of allergenicity of peanut oils in subjects allergic to peanuts. (PMID: 9133891) *BMJ*, 1997; 314(7087):1084–8. .

1052 Fraser op. cit., pp. 51–2.

1053 Moneret-Vauterin DA et al (1994) op. cit.

1054 David TJ. op cit., pp. 160–61.

creams. Price is always a consideration in mass manufacturing, and until recently the side effects were not being publicised. Fraser points out that it is not necessary to declare refined peanut oil on food labels in the USA because the FDA has classified it as Generally Recognised As Safe (GRAS). I don't think parents of peanut-sensitive children would be happy to test the quality of refining by exposing their children to foods in which peanut oil is present but not labelled. The Codex Alimentarius Committee on Food Labelling in 2000 made no decision about mandatory labelling of peanut oil in foods, although in 2004 the European Food Safety Authority created a guideline stating that – in Europe at least – all peanut oil, refined or not, must be noted on food labels.[1055] Hidden protein doses much too small to cause reactions in adults may be just what is needed to sensitise infants. (Especially perhaps, when injected in vitamin K doses soon after birth, or as an anonymous adjuvant in later vaccines, as peanut oil has been. Again, in the name of protecting trade secrets, CDC does not list all the ingredients in US vaccines.[1056] Protecting children should be more important!)

I suspect peanut oil might have been more common in US- than UK-made formulas, just from the commercial logic of constant US government protection and tariffs, higher national production volumes and lower transport costs of the 'all-American crop.' Past Australian-made formulas may also have used it quite commonly, since our peanut crop in Queensland was a reliable source, though prone to aflatoxin contamination[1057] and so diverted to stock feed at times. But infant formulas are global products, sold worldwide. And since no food safety authority has ever insisted on industry keeping long-term detailed records of what is used in every batch of formula, this can only be speculation. Labels tell parents some of what might be in there, not what actually is: that depends on price and availability.

Aflatoxins[1058] in peanuts, produced by moulds, are of concern in two ways – the levels that may be in foods consumed by humans, and secondly, the levels in the stockfeed of animals whose milk or meat humans consume. Unknown before the 1960s, the problem of mould toxins is a global concern because they survive processing and cause liver damage, probably liver cancer. Nations have very different standards. Reviewing 48 countries with established limits for total aflatoxins in food, Dohlman (2003) found that standards ranged from 0 to 50 parts per billion. The USA Food and Drug Administration established 20 ppb as the minimum acceptable level of aflatoxin in all foods other than milk, where it is 5ppb. The European Union has limits of up to 5ppb for cereals, nuts and grains as well as milk, but extremely low limits for infant foods, and limits on stockfeed as well. Milk production in warm wet areas increases the risk of mould toxins in the milk, and every nation needs to inspect both its local product and any imports of milk, along with its stockfeed and imports

---

1055 *EFSA Journal*, 2004,133:1–9.

1056 http://www.cdc.gov/vaccines/pubs/pinkbook/downloads/appendices/b/excipient-table-2.pdf

1057 I cannot now cite a reference, but I have a clear memory that one year, in the late 1970s or early 1980s, when aflatoxin levels in the Queensland peanut crop were found to be higher than allowable limits, Australia's food authorities solved the problem by raising the allowed limit! Otherwise virtually all the crop would have gone into stock feed. Aflatoxin researchers speaking at an ALCA-Vic Branch conference in the 1990s advised not eating commercially-reared chicken livers in paté. Chicken livers concentrate aflatoxins found in chicken feed, which is where peanuts unfit for human consumption can end up.

1058 An online resource with good links to follow is http://www.foodsafetywatch.org/factsheets/aflatoxins/

of stockfeed. How feasible is that in many less developed nations? And if the imported milk or the stock feed is heavily contaminated with aflatoxins, how safe is the formula produced from that milk? Again, the major formula producers have the resources to monitor aflatoxin levels in milk they receive, but does every formula maker?

Does every infant formula company keep detailed records of ingredients in each batch of the product for decades? Of each ingredient in each vitamin or fat pre-mix supplied by other sources for inclusion in the formula? Given the constant global pressure applied to the USFDA and FSANZ (the Food Standards Authority of Australia and New Zealand) and EFSA (European Food Safety Authority) to reduce the 'regulatory burden', I suspect not. An industry-friendly change to older Australian labelling laws now allows industry simply to state 'vegetable oils' on its labels, with no further details. Peanuts could just be one of several 'vegetable oils' in use, although I would hope the allergen labelling provisions would mean that its use would have to be declared in small print on the can. Coincidentally or not, this labelling change roughly coincided with industry's inclusion of the new fungal and algal oils. (Fungi and algae are 'vegetable', in the sense that they are neither animal nor mineral.) I suggest parents boycott any formulas that do not give full source details of the fats they *might* contain. Half a loaf is better than none.

Fraser[1059] has reviewed the highly plausible role of peanut oil and other ingredients used in multiple vaccines in creating the current peanut allergy epidemic. This book is well worth reading for its overview of the uniquely Western peanut allergy problem, now spreading into precisely those Asian populations adopting both artificial feeding and Western multiple vaccines. At one point Fraser asks, 'if digestive failure was to blame, what would cause an abrupt increase in this kind of bowel dysfunction in children just in these certain countries at the same time?' Similarly, Blaser asked 'Could there be one underlying cause fueling all these parallel increases' (in immune related disorders). Fraser thinks peanut oil exposure, Blaser the disappearing microbiota. What links these? Infant formula is the obvious candidate, and perhaps the epigenetic changes inherited from the previous generation of badly mixed-fed or formula-fed mothers. And perhaps within infant formula, the medium chain triglycerides, those MCTs mentioned earlier, have a special role to play in fostering allergy – along with other factors.

And there is one more obvious question rarely asked and not yet answered so far as I can see. Is peanut allergy a direct consequence of artificial formulas? Consider this next parapgraph, excerpted from an authoritative overview.[1060]

Cross-Reactivity with Other Foods

> Peanut belongs to the plant family Leguminosae. The legume family also includes soybeans, peas, lima beans, green beans, other beans, chickpeas, and lentils. The fact that they are low in fat, contain no cholesterol, and are high in protein, folate, potassium, iron, and magnesium has contributed to their widespread consumption in the North

---

1059 Fraser H. op. cit.

1060 Al-Ahmed N,1 Shirina Alsowaidi S, Vadas P. Peanut Allergy: An Overview. *Allergy Asthma Clin Immunol.* 2008; 4(4): 139–143. DOI: 10.1186/1710–1492-4-4-139.

American diet. *[And, as I noted much earlier, the fact that soy oil and soy protein is cheap explains its appearance in infant formula and foods since the 1920s.]* Barnett and colleagues demonstrated a high rate of cross-reactivity between peanut and legumes when they screened sera from 40 patients with peanut allergy against 10 other legumes..There was demonstrable IgE binding to multiple legumes in 38% of patients ... Cosensitization to tree nuts is also common, although the cross-reacting proteins are not yet known. The rate of coallergy varies from 2.5% in one survey to as high as approximately one-third of peanut-allergic patients *[Palm and coconut oils are tree oils.]* There is a high degree of co-sensitization with seeds... *[And cottonseed, sesame and sunflower are seed oils. All in infant formulas.]*

So is peanut allergy the result of a century of infant exposure to these proteins and oils in formula, setting up the potential for cross reaction? Soy in particular seems a likely suspect when the Avon Longitudinal Study found that peanut allergy was independently associated with two things: intake of soy milk and soy formula,[1061] and use of skin preparations containing peanut oil, probably to relieve the rash resulting from exposure to cows' milk formula, (which in the UK usually precedes the use of soy) and then soy formula. The group stated that 'There was no evidence of prenatal sensitization from the maternal diet, and peanut-specific IgE was not detectable in the cord blood.' Thus the problem is created postnatally. Thus they concluded that

> Sensitization to peanut protein may occur in children through the application of peanut oil to inflamed skin. The association with soy protein could arise from cross-sensitization through common epitopes. Confirmation of these risk factors in future studies could lead to new strategies to prevent sensitization in infants who are at risk for subsequent peanut allergy.[1062]

Even without rashes, the infant skin is so delicate that greater absorption of antigens via skin contact might be expected. (The outer layer is only .01-.05mm thick, while in adults it ranges from 0.1–0.9mm, ten, twenty, even ninety times thicker.) So why is breastfeeding blamed so readily, infant formula not investigated? and why isn't the use of peanut oil in skin preparations and vaccines outlawed?

## Contaminants and GE foods in fats and oils

Scare stories about breastmilk contamination are legion. And it is true that women's bodies, like the environment they inhabit, are polluted by a wide range of chemicals. But contaminants of infant formula fats can also be legion. Almost any process or container or ingredient can contribute something unwanted, sometimes something not even considered. Lead, cadmium, aluminium, hexane, beetles, pesticides – not what we think of as formula ingredients! This is discussed further in the Chapter 3.9 Unavoidable contaminants.

1061 Heppell UM, Sissons JW, Pedersen HE. A comparison of the antigenicity of soya-bean based infant formulas. *Br J Nutr.* 1987; 58: 393–403.
1062 Lack G, Fox D, Northstone K, Golding J. Factors associated with the development of peanut allergy in childhood. (PMID:12637607) *NEJM* 2003, 348(11):977–985 DOI: 10.1056/NEJMoa013536.

Formula fats are a great vehicle for picking up and storing fat-soluble chemicals from plastics, for example, and even the lining of metal formula cans will contribute some chemicals to the powder in the tin. And those fats are going into a body to build a brain and nervous system. Consider the life history of the fats and oils used: corn, or soy, or cottonseed oil, for example, may carry some of the many pesticides used on those crops; milk-derived ingredients reflect the cows' exposure, and so on. When you are dealing with allergic families, what is in the milk fats can be part of the problem. Sometimes, for example, cream from King Island in Bass Strait may be tolerated with only minor symptoms, whereas cream from Gippsland causes reactions. There are differences in the cows themselves, the grasses and weeds the cows eat, and in their exposure to petrochemical residues from coal-burning power stations, which perhaps explains that difference in reactions.[1063] Stock feed concerns would be raised if hen egg yolks or fish oils are used as sources of long-chain polyunsaturated fatty acids (LCPUFAs) for infant formulas. Many patents suggest they have been so used and will continue to be (without always being noted on the label, of course). What the hen is fed is reflected in her eggs. And as hens get older, the fatty acid composition of the egg changes.[1064] What the farmed fish eats and swims in is reflected in its oils. And once the cow starts eating novel foods like palm kernel wastes,[1065] there will be changes in the composition of the fats in her milk. All formula ingredients reflect their environment, just as the mother's diet does.[1066] Quite apart from allergy and environmental issues, this raises interesting questions about the cost of quality control in making infant formula. (So much cheaper and better to educate and feed a breastfeeding mother!)

# Genetic engineering and pesticide residues in oils

Selective breeding is a traditional form of genetic modification that few people have problems with, as the gene pool manipulated is natural to the organism. At one level, genetic engineering is simply using more sophisticated tools, and more precise knowledge of how to achieve a desired result, only sometimes by tinkering with a wide range of organisms that could not naturally interbreed. The problem is that we cannot know what the undesired results will be until they appear, and it may be too late to close the Pandora's box we have unwittingly opened.[1067] The complexity of biological ecosystems deserves respect, as does the instinctive human concern about tampering with the natural world without there being a compelling need (other than to make money). 'First do no harm' is a basic principle. The risk-benefit analysis needs to include informed speculation as to possible adverse consequences.

The issue of genetic engineering and food is complex, and discussed later (see Chapter 3.14 Genetic engineering in infant formula). There are many dimensions (such as its potential

---

1063 An island with clean air and different grasses to the mainland, noted for quality dairy products. By contrast, Gippsland has major electricity generating plants and high rates of respiratory disease, made much worse in 2014 by a fire burning in the abandoned areas of the huge open-cut coal mine (privatised in the 1990s, then allegedly not covered with fireproof soil or clay, while the fire-fighting equipment was removed).

1064 Nielsen H. Hen age and fatty acid composition of egg yolk lipid, op. cit.

1065 Wikipedia reports that New Zealand palm kernel imports went from 0.4 tonnes in 1999 to 455 000 tonnes in 2007 and then to 1.1 million tonnes in 2008, one-quarter of the world's palm-based animal feed.

1066 But a mother's body processes and filters what goes into her milk, to varying degrees.

1067 It seems clear to me that this is the lesson we should take from using monkey kidneys to grow vaccines. See Cribb J. *The white death* (Scribe Books, 1996). The CDC excipients list shows some are still in use.

for increasing problems of antibiotic resistance) that I won't discuss fully, but recommend you read about in Marion Nestlé's brilliant books.[1068]

But much of the genetic engineering done to date is about creating pesticide resistance in food crops, so that crops survive drenching with pesticides better than competing weeds, at least for a generation or two. (Resistance will develop – that's how evolution works – as plants and their pests adapt, there are already reports of superweeds and rising doses of pesticides.[1069]) The idea that oils in our babies' food might come from crops that withstand pesticide doses lethal to hardy weeds is deeply unappealing. I was not surprised to read in *New Scientist* that 'Claims that eating GM maize gives rats tumours have provoked a storm in Europe.'[1070] The report has since been withdrawn amid great controversy, but I predict that as the doses of pesticides increase[1071] to kill the ever more resistant weeds, such reports will increase in coming decades. I hope I'm wrong.

With internationalisation of agricultural markets and formula manufacture, only industry's own quality controls may act as safeguards. Pesticide levels in Western food supplies have been dropping since the unregulated 1960s. The major formula manufacturers do have high quality standards, and presumably would buy organic or test suppliers' oils for pesticide residues. And in theory governments should be testing independently for residues.

However, at present there is a massive multiplication of small infant formula manufacturers or formula ingredient exporters[1072] seeking to cash in on developing countries' markets, especially Asia and Africa. The Internet allows them to sell formula direct to purchasers and onsellers globally. Who is responsible for quality testing these exports? Most countries don't even routinely test their formula imports, designed to be fed to their own children, much less their exports to anonymous children worldwide, in families with no avenue for legal redress if harm is done.[1073]

The infant formula industry knows full well that many people would like to be able to avoid GM or GE foods. America's biggest formula maker, Ross/Abbott, has an organic formula in its range, and niche products exist in other Anglophone countries.

The bottom line about GM in infant formula fats is this. All fungal and algal oils are produced by genetically-altered organisms. Any corn or soy oil in formula is likely to be from GM corn or soy unless a company has an active policy of supporting GM-free sources only. Given that these are relatively cheap oils thanks to America's generous farming subsidies, and

1068 A book for everyone's library is Nestle M. *Safe food: the politics of food safety* (University of California Press, 2009). The 2004 edition was titled *Safe food: bacteria, biotechnology and bioterrorism*.

1069 Washington State University (2 October 2012). 'Superweeds' linked to rising herbicide use in GM crops, study finds. *ScienceDaily*. Retrieved 10 January 2014, from http://www.sciencedaily.com / releases/2012/10/121002092839.htm

1070 *New Scientist* 29 September 2012, p. 5.

1071 Benbrook CM. Impacts of genetically engineered crops on pesticide use in the U.S. – the first sixteen years. *Envir Sci Europe*, 2012, 24:24. DOI: 10.1186/2190-4715-24-24.

1072 Kent G., op. cit., p. 21.

1073 Shamir R. Thiamine-deficient infant formula: what happened and what have we learned? *Ann Nutr Metab*, 2012, 60(3):185–7.

their cultivation for export in less developed countries, GM corn and soy are likely to be in virtually all infant formulas unless manufacturers take a lot of care to avoid this. So parents looking for GM-free or organic infant formulas will find their options very limited. Does this matter? We don't know. And given the politics, we are unlikely ever to know. Because once there is no comparative population of infants fed GM-free infant formula, no effects can be identified. That said, trying to isolate the outcomes of that one difference is probably impossible anyway, given that each batch of infant formula differs slightly from every other batch! What can't be cured may have to be endured – by those who are formula-fed. And since their parents can't change this, it probably is best for such parents to focus on the fact that no proof of harm has emerged to date, and hope that none ever will.

# Tropical oils: not GM, but allergenic

Other oils such as palm kernel oil (a tree nut) or palm olein, and coconut (the saturated 'tropical oils' that adults were taught to avoid as artery-clogging, but which may not be) may be less likely to come from GM sources. French allergists have reported a clear case of allergy to coconut oil,[1074] uncommon in this generation but perhaps a clue to a coming epidemic, as coconut oil has become ubiquitous in infant formula since the 1980s.

Cases of palm oil pollen allergy seem to be on record in Indonesia and Thailand,[1075] and this tree nut oil is banned in some schools attended by anaphylactic children[1076] as much for its allergy potential as for its connection with the destruction of orangutan habitat. (It somehow seems deeply sad that bottle-feeding parents may be unwittingly complicit in driving our mammalian cousins to extinction. And as palm-oil production moves to Africa, taking valuable agricultural land, more fellow human beings may also be driven to starvation.) While Unilever scientists[1077] may be reassuring about the allergenicity of oils, they concede that oils can cause reactions in some individuals. If your child suffers, it's no comfort that other people's don't.

Similac advertising criticises the use of palm oil, which Ross/Abbott doesn't use and its competitors do. Here (with my comments in square brackets) is a sample spruik:

> Bone mass increases at its fastest rate during the first year. That's why it is so important to give your baby the right amounts of key bone nutrients – such as calcium – from the very first day. [*True. Not true is the implied idea that a formula can give your baby the right amounts. In fact, the less formula and the more breastmilk preterms receive, the greater their adult whole body bone mass.*][1078]

---

1074 Couturier P, Basset-Sthème D, Navette N, Sainte-Laudy J. A case of coconut oil allergy in an infant: responsibility of 'maternalized' infant formulas. (PMID: 7702732) *Allergie et Immunologie*, 1994; 26(10):386–7.

1075 Baratawidjaja IR, Baratawidjaja PP, Darwis A, Soo-Hwee L et al. Prevalence of allergic sensitization to regional inhalants among allergic patients in Jakarta, Indonesia. (PMID: 10403003) *Asian Pac J Allergy Immunol*, 1999; 17(1):9–12.

1076 Steingraber, op. cit. p. 142–3. Lip balm often contains palm oil, and can cause reactions in sensitive children.

1077 Crevel RW, Kerkhoff MA, Koning MM. Allergenicity of refined vegetable oils. (PMID: 10722892) *Food Chem Toxicol*, 2000, 38(4):385–93. DOI: 10.1016/S0278-6915(99)00158-1.

1078 Fewtrell MS, Williams JE, Singhal A, Murgatroyd PR et al. Early diet and peak bone mass: 20 year follow-up of a randomized trial of early diet in infants born preterm. (PMID: 19306955) *Bone*, 2009; 45(1):142–9. DOI: 10.1016/j.bone.2009.03.657.

Calcium absorption is better without palm olein oil. Your baby's body needs to absorb calcium before her developing bones can use it. [*True, but incomplete. Calcium has many uses in the body, and is interactive with many other minerals in bone formation. And why does breastmilk for girls contain more calcium than breastmilk for boys?*[1079] *Should formula?*]

Palm olein oil, an ingredient in most baby formulas, allows fats to bind with calcium, resulting in decreased calcium absorption. [*But we still don't know that what is absorbed is the 'right' amount or not. Excesses are harmful just as deficiencies are. Binding calcium to fats might even be a good thing!*]

Similac® Advance® is the only leading formula brand with no palm olein oil, and it has been clinically shown to support greater* calcium absorption† for strong bones.

Similac would do better to point out that palm oil plantations are destroying orangutan habitats; at least that's a proven fact. Greater bone density because of their palm-oil-free fat blend is not. Bone density can be very complex. Getting too much calcium too soon may even mean lower peak bone mass by early adulthood. Greater calcium absorption, even if true, says nothing about bone strength. Bone is made from more than calcium. Does industry have the results of any bone density tests to show differences long term? If not, this is simply a ploy. If there are, where are the references?

It would be an interesting, if complex, project to track different formula fat blends for their health outcomes. The short- and long-term consequences for health and cholesterol metabolism seem to remain uncertain even now.

## Fat blends and brain problems

Of even greater concern is the possibility that in changing fat blends (and protein too) we have changed normal central nervous system and brain development. By the 1990s and since, the epidemic of what is now described as autistic spectrum disorders could no longer be denied. There are many possible explanations for this astonishing new level of child brain dysfunction, and I have no doubt that both genetic and environmental factors will be found. Research into biological markers has begun,[1080] but seemingly without awareness of infant nutrition as a variable needing to be explored precisely and in great detail. That this would be logical is surely suggested by those studies showing different structural growth, (see page 157) cognitive and developmental outcomes in artificially fed infants.

Some of this is discussed in the chapter on protein and elsewhere. But the brain is constructed using vast quantities of fats, and research is showing actual physical differences in white matter development in infants fed artificially.[1081] Frankly, as a parent I find that

---

1079 Hinde K. op. cit. http://www.abc.net.au/radionational/programs/healthreport/the-effect-of-breastfeeding-on-infants/5587144#transcript

1080 Walsh P, Elsabbagh M, Bolton P, Singh I. In search of biomarkers for autism: scientific, social and ethical challenges. (PMID: 21931335) *Nature Reviews. Neuroscience*, 2011, 12(10):603–12. DOI: 10.1038/nrn3113.

1081 Deoni SC, Dean DC 3rd, Piryatinksy I, O'Muircheartaigh J et al. op. cit; Isaacs EB, Fischl BR, Quinn BT, Chong WK et al. Impact of breast milk on intelligence quotient, brain size, and white matter development. (PMID: 20035247) *Pediatr Res*, 2010; 67(4):357–62.

scary, even while I recognise that the vast majority of humans fed artificially went on to be within a normal range of cognitive functioning – as defined in the twentieth century.

Why scary? Differences in brain white matter growth could well be linked to the multiplicity of emerging leukodystrophies (white matter disruption) that cause children with vulnerable genomes to regress, possibly due to the absence of breastmilk fats in the first two years of life, or indeed, the presence of cytotoxic free fatty acids from digested formula (see page 321), or to those traces of hexane and other chemicals used in the manufacture of additives like lutein (see page 475). Leukodystrophy is precisely the sort of subtle, emerging damage which Dr Neil Campbell predicted in the 1980s[1082] would eventually come to be recognised as the consequence of artificial feeding causing normal brain development to be warped ever so imperceptibly from birth. So too are some of autism's subtle brain anomalies.

Deoni et al used sophisticated imaging techniques to examine infant brain development. They examined the relationship between breastfeeding duration and white matter microstructure, and found that

> Breastfed children exhibited increased white matter development in later maturing frontal and association brain regions. Positive relationships between white matter microstructure and breastfeeding duration are also exhibited in several brain regions, that are anatomically consistent with observed improvements in cognitive and behavioral performance measures.

Earlier studies had shown

> increased white matter and sub-cortical gray matter volume, and parietal lobe cortical thickness, associated with IQ, in adolescents who were breastfed as infants compared to those who were exclusively formula-fed.

As Deoni et al. rightly said,

> While the mechanisms underlying these structural differences remain unclear, our findings provide new insight into the earliest developmental advantages associated with breastfeeding *[=risks associated with not breastfeeding]*, and support the hypothesis that breast milk constituents promote healthy neural growth and white matter development *[=and infant formula doesn't]*.[1083]

Those children who regress months down the track after developing normally to begin with may prove to be children who never had sufficient myelin laid down because they were fed a particular brand of formula with, say, excess trans-fats, or not enough of the fatty acids breastmilk would have supplied. Or fed a formula in which heat treatment was less than perfect and toxic changes occurred. Or children in whom inflammation destroyed inadequate levels of myelin, thanks to an inherited susceptibility. Or perhaps this also had to

---

1082 Neonatologist at the Royal Children's Hospital, Parkville, Dr Campbell lectured to students in a course I organised at Monash University for some years in the 1980s. His presentation on infant formula included this concern.
1083 Deoni et al., op. cit.

coincide with a microbiome that includes organisms producing toxins, a microbiome that would have been different if the gut had not been exposed to infant formula or antibiotics soon after birth. That may sound extreme, but remember, scientists have just noticed that infant formula can be cytotoxic – that is, cell-killing – in the infant gut.[1084] Until recently the idea that the products of digestion could be toxic (although the food before ingestion was deemed safe) would have seemed improbable. Now we realise that every child is an experiment of one, with so many interlocking variables that can influence development that it can be critical to get the early nutrition right. And all those different formulas can't all be right, especially when they are replacing mother's milk, nutrition tailor-made for the unique child in her or his environment, complete with stem cells to infiltrate and develop into functioning tisssue where needed.

Nor are the leukodystrophies the only possible candidates for concern when thinking about autoimmune or cognitive dysfunction. The huge increase in mood, behavioural and cognitive disorders among Western children has been remarkable to those of us who have lived long enough to see different generations of children. Yes, we can posit many sociocultural factors contributing to such ill health. But when these problems manifest in very young children, it seems eminently reasonable to ask just how much early infant diet contributes to cerebral disorder.

## What will we ever know about fats in formula?

One thing most parents won't ever know is just what fats they are feeding their child. Fat blends have always changed as supply and market forces dictated. Recognising this, formula labels are permitted to list a wide variety of fats that might be in the product, so as to facilitate companies using whatever fats are available cheaply in the world market when any batch is being made, without needing constantly to re-label the cans. (Such generic labelling makes life difficult for those with allergies, and for those who develop them!) Precisely when and how fats in formula have changed differs by company and product, and may not be anywhere on the public record[1085] – or even company records by now. They can differ between formulations of the same product: powder versus liquid, for example. We do know that peanut oil was used in some brands, as well as in widely used creams for mother and baby alike (see page 330).

Before moving on, stop for a moment and ask what can be done about the formula-fed children who missed out on both human cholesterol and omega-3 fats over decades. New is better, and even closer to breastmilk, but somehow magically, there were never any admissions of responsibility for adverse effects in past artificially fed infants. Yet over the 40–50 years in which artificially fed infants have lacked all omega-3 fats, and many have had no cholesterol in their infancy diet, problems such as dyslexia, ADHD, minimal brain damage syndromes, early-onset Alzheimers and much more, have all become more common, especially where breastmilk was lacking. Could fatty acid deficiency or distortion

---

1084 Penn AH, et al., op. cit.
1085 Some old paediatric texts contain information supplied by industry, but this may not be complete and is certainly not independently verified.

have contributed to some or all of these conditions? It must be just coincidence, surely, because after all, those older formulas were 'so close to breastmilk as to make no difference', weren't they? Many parents wouldn't have used them otherwise. Yet today adults find that omega-3 fats seem to help with cerebral problems such as depression[1086] and cholesterol is no longer seen as harmful in itself, but as a marker of inflammation ...

So was that old formula advertising false and misleading? And if it was, why was it not cause for prosecution? Is the new advertising misleading? And if it is, why is it allowed? Will advertising standards agencies in every country look into infant formula advertising as a priority?

My profound unease about so many aspects of formula fats and human central nervous system development is not irrational, even where, as I freely admit, the evidence to date is suggestive rather than conclusive. Which is the rational approach: to assume no harm because artificially fed infants look normal in the school playground, or to suspect that so many indications of deviance from human biological norms will have negative consequences? The absence of proof of harm is not proof of the absence of harm. It may simply be proof of the absence of thought or research or observation.

Scientists are still unsure in 2013 what the science reveals about the best fats for infants. As one world authority said in 2010,

> 'I don't believe that dairy fats have been looked at in a fair and logical manner, particularly given their range of nutrients. I was one of the proponents many years ago of saying we have got to get the dairy fats out of infant formulas and replace them with vegetable oils, and I think I was dead wrong about that. I think we need to do theq trials and look again at the relative benefits of dairy fats.'

He also suggested that cholesterol should be put back into formulas, and that the cholesterol hypothesis (its presence in the diet being causative of heart disease) was being questioned.[1087] Cholesterol may not be the leading villain causing vascular damage by inflammation; it is after all part of the body's response to inflammation caused by other factors such as turbulence in blood under high pressures, sugar with its cascade of hormonal responses, and stresses. (However, in excess cholesterol certainly blocks arteries, and causes heart attacks, whatever the process that triggers its deposition!)

If the world's leading scientists don't know exactly what fats should be in infant formula, and companies haven't yet included them, should industry be allowed to maintain the myth that their products nowadays are safe?

---

1086 Breggin P. *Your drug may be your problem. How and why to stop taking psychiatric medications* (da Capo Press, 2007); Kendall Tackett K. *Non-pharmacologic treatments for depression in new mothers* (Clinics in Human Lactation series no 1; Thomas Hale Publishing, 2001).
1087 Gibson RA, in Clemens Hernell & Michaelsen (eds) op. cit., p. 203.

# 3.7 Basic ingredients: Carbohydrates including FODMAPs

Carbohydrates: we think of sugars and starches, the latter being complexes of a large number of sugars (polysaccharides) which can be broken down by enzymes (amylases), heat, or acids. Sugars come in many forms: among them, monosaccharides (single sugars, like glucose) and disaccharides (two sugars combined, that can be split by enzymes). Milk also contains many other sugars, some linked together to form oligosaccharides (oligo means a few), some linked to fats (glycolipids) and to protein (glycoproteins); some are also linked to nucleotides (part of the non-protein nitrogen found in milk). All these sugars are present in varying quantities across species, and have many roles in both nutrition and health. Science is only now revealing the importance of some of these to feeding humans and their microbiota, and to gut health and disease. There are, for example, more than 200 oligosaccharides in human milk, more than any other mammal, and vastly more, in quantity and variety, than could ever safely or economically be put into infant formula. More on this later.

Lactose, a disaccharide, is the major carbohydrate of breastmilk. Lactose is made in the breast from glucose and galactose brought there by blood. Progesterone – produced through pregnancy – prevents lactose synthesis, and levels of progesterone drop after birth of the baby. This allows lactose production, and that in turn switches on full-scale milk production, sometimes referred to as Lactogenesis II. About 7 per cent of breastmilk is lactose, and it is the principal energy source for infants, breaking down again to galactose and glucose, which the infant body uses for about 40 per cent of its energy needs.

Within that infant body, its bacteria also have to be fed: breastmilk oligosaccharides, another major milk component, form a large part of their diet, and help determine bowel health and faecal characteristics. Breastmilk feeds the baby and the baby's microbiota, which in their turn help feed and protect the baby by breaking down other food substrates.

But carbohydrates have many functions in the body. They form part of body structures as well, from galactolipids in brain tissue to blood cells, where it is a carbohydrate-linked component that identifies the ABO blood types. Excess carbohydrates are converted to fat and stored against a time of famine. (In the days of wagon trains crossing the Rockies, latecomers could be trapped in a mountain pass for months, and it was reported that women were more likely to survive than stronger and leaner men, thanks in part to greater fat stores.) The liver also stores glycogen as a reserve of carbohydrates readily converted to release glucose.

Lactose is also the principal carbohydrate in cows' milk, although bovine milk has many other carbohydrates as well, not identical to human milk. Whenever whole cows' milk was the basis for infant formulas, infants obviously received lactose; where milk was diluted and water added, additional lactose (labelled milk sugar) was often added as well. This powdered lactose was sold in packets and was certainly not free of milk protein, although often assumed to be when used as a placebo in research studies evaluating cows' milk reactivity.[1088] Lactose could be recovered from the acid whey left over after cheese making, which contains about 5 per cent lactose. (Neutralising acid whey with sodium bicarbonate resulted in high sodium levels in formula, a problem identified by the 1960s and reduced by the 1980s. See Chapter 3.10)

Excess carbohydrate seemed unavoidable in early infant formulas. This is because the excess protein of cows' milk needed to be reduced by diluting the milk with water; but then the total caloric value had to be made to equal or exceed that of breastmilk, by adding fats and carbohydrates. This balancing act is performed differently with modern formulas, which can assemble different protein components from ingredients not available before 1970. But they must still add what are inevitably less bioavailable fats and carbohydrates in amounts that can survive a shelf life of up to two years from the assembling of the pre-existing ingredients into a canned powder, which is seen as the date of manufacture. (The ingredients themselves have usually been manufactured elsewhere, and unless quality control is good, may already be heat-damaged or ageing.) It is interesting to note that in 2013-2014 Abbott, the American market leader, is now reducing the total caloric value of its Similac formulas, from twenty to nineteen calories per ounce.[1089] It might not sound like much, but it's a five percent reduction in total dietary intake, and an admission that excess has consequences for infant weight gain. Companies may now compete to produce the leanest babies, which would not be advisable.

## Early formula carbohydrates

Early patent infant foods or formulas were often a mix of cows' milk and wheat flour with malt sugar (maltose) or table sugar (sucrose). The starch in wheat flour was difficult for babies to digest, although processing heat had improved its digestibility somewhat. Starch is broken down into dextrins; how far it is broken down determines the sweetness level of the dextrins produced, and the name they are given in food chemistry. It seemed sensible to break down starches before adding them to formula, as indigestion was inevitable when infants lack the enzymes needed to digest starch. A synthetic 'dextri-maltose' made from potato starch was an early US experimental addition, and was the first of many maltodextrins to be used, all synthesised from the starch of a variety of cereals and vegetables (wheat, potato, corn, tapioca, rice …). Maltodextrins are oligosaccharides, and can vary in sweetness, depending on how the base starch is refined. Above a certain degree of sweetness, maltodextrins are called glucose syrup, which is the basis of sugar solutions used in hospitals. Because highly refined, only a minuscule quantity of protein is likely to be present in maltodextrins, perhaps as little as .002 per cent, or 20 parts per billion, which is the standard below which there is no need for declaration of allergen content on European food labels. However, maltodextrins derived from wheat are not permitted in European infant formulas. Parents can't know the source of maltodextrins in American or Australian

1088 Both commercial grade and pharmaceutical grade lactose have been shown to contain proteins including known antigens; in fact milk protein may be the nucleus for lactose crystallisation. See David TJ, op. cit., p. 36.
1089 Read the details in this WIC circular: http://www.dphhs.mt.gov/wic/newsletters/2014/documents/FAQSimilacChange.pdf

infant formulas: in fact ingredient source labelling is much better on a local sweet wrapper than on local infant formula. Compare the two:

| Infant formula: | Marshmallows: |
|---|---|
| Lactose (milk), vegetable oils *[from ...??]*, enzymatically hydrolysed whey protein (milk), minerals [12 chemical names], maltodextrin *[from ...??]*, omega LCPUFAs (DHA from fish oil, AA from ??), vitamins *[13 listed]*, l- phenylalanine, L-histidine, L- tyrosine, choline bitartrite, acidity regulator (citric acid), taurine, inositol, nucleotides [4 listed], L-carnitine, culture (bifidus) *[what species and strain ??]*, antioxidant (ascorbyl palmitate). | 'Cane sugar, glucose syrup (from wheat), starch (from corn or tapioca), gelatin *[from?? beef probably]*, vegetable fat (from coconut), natural colouring (carmine), humectant (sorbitol), food acid (malic acid). |

How many neonatologists and paediatric allergists know that maltodextrin may be derived from wheat? Even if there are regulations mandating allergen labelling, they may be set at levels of detection too high (e.g., 10 mg/kg in Japan[1090]) to prevent reactions in people sensitive to smaller quantities – or they may never be policed. And the newborn gut may be sensitive to even the 20parts per billion allowed to be present without labelling maltodextrin as derived from wheat ...[1091]

Similarly, reactions to maltodextrins derived from corn may be possible. Corn syrup or corn syrup solids have been a basic staple of infant formula making, and may be the basis of glucose water in hospitals (or it might be rice or wheat or something altogether different). This ubiquitous 'sugar water', (sometimes dextrose) may have been less harmful to normal infant gut development and microbiome than infant formula was to be. It might also be less harmful to breastfeeding initiation: a 1986 study showed that using maltodextrin meant a greater volume of breastmilk ingested on day four, when compared with the use of formula supplements.[1092] That babies would be hungrier and breastfeed better when given sugar water than when fed formula seems self-evident, making the experiment hard to justify ethically. What was not explained is why so few infants were fed only breastmilk. Perhaps it can't be explained without acknowledging deficient hospital practices.

Sucrose too was used in early infant formula making, often as a replacement for lost lactose after the dilution of cows' milk with water. Sometimes called saccharose, sucrose is a mix of glucose and fructose. Sucrose itself, derived from sugar cane or sugar beets, was essential for the production of sweetened condensed milk, and in that form was fed to millions of children,

---

1090  Akiyama H, Imai T, Ebisawa M. Japan food allergen labeling regulation – history and evaluation. (PMID: 21504823) *Adv Food Nutr Res*, 2011; 62:139–71. DOI: 10.1016/B978-0-12-385989-1.00004-1.

1091  See the onlne Gluten-Free Dietitian newsletter and search for relevant information. E.g., maltodextrin http://www.glutenfreedietitian.com/newsletter/maltodextrin/

1092  Rosegger H. Maltodextrin in a 13 per cent solution as a supplement in the first 4 days of life in breast-fed mature newborn infants. Effect on drinking behavior, weight curve, blood picture, blood glucose and bilirubin (MED:3727591) *Wiener Klinische Wochenschrift*, 1986; 98(10):310–15.

especially when there was no refrigeration. At sufficient concentrations, sugar is a powerful preservative. And sugar can be an osmotic laxative as well: adding more fructose-containing sugar or prune juice was once the usual remedy for constipation in artificially fed infants.

## Sucrose scares

The carbohydrates in formula, like everything else, have altered over time. The 1970s and 1980s saw a general move away from added or included sucrose, partly due to graphic publicity about the growing epidemic of baby-bottle mouth syndrome (rotting front teeth requiring extraction, caused by sucking bottles laden with sugary milk formulas or infant 'teas').[1093] In Brisbane Australia up to 20 per cent of disadvantaged children under six were said to suffer from it. The UK Department of Health 1989 COMA (Committee on Medical Aspects and Nutrition Policy) report on tooth decay stated that simple sugars should not be added to bottle feeds, and by the 1990s German parents would win damages from Milupa, a formula maker which until 1992 produced and exported popular sugar-laden herbal teas for children.[1094]

This baby-bottle mouth syndrome, however, was soon re-labelled 'nursing caries' after a few cases of partially or even formerly breastfed children were found with extensive decay. The case reports had obvious defects: no mention of other diet in toddlers, for example.[1095] Despite this, ill-informed speculation soon began about the dangers of night-time breastfeeding, or breastfeeding past the age of tooth eruption, and some dentists advised against 'prolonged' breastfeeding, whatever that means.

This illustrates a constant feature of infant feeding history. The defence of artificial feeding has always included covert attacks on breastfeeding, to create or sustain a perception of roughly equivalent risk.[1096] Whenever breastfeeding is being shown to have indisputable benefits, or formula indisputable risks, it is not long before the waters are muddied by a riposte that creates doubt.[1097] The authors disprove nothing; they just want publicity for their views. They only have to create doubt for others to seize upon their unscientific opinions or statements with relief and suggest that breastfeeding 'extremists' have got it

---

1093 Brian Palmer is a dentist who has made a special study of the oral impacts of feeding. See his website, http://www.brianpalmerdds.com/ could be useful here. Relevant research can also be found at http://www.acsu.buffalo.edu/~andersh/research/caries.asp

1094 Lawyers claimed that in Germany alone over 100,000 children were affected. See (Australian Lactation Consultant Association) *ALCA News,* 1991; 2(2);35.

1095 There is a chapter on breastfeeding and dental health in *Breastfeeding matters*. See also the Lactation Resource Centre paper on this topic, available from the Australian Breastfeeding Association.

1096 There is a book to be written about the use of language in relation to infant feeding. The words used to discuss a range of infant feeding issues almost always convey a sense of the unnaturalness of anything but bottle-feeding. Americanisms all make the unnatural processes sound beneficial and normal for humans. Artificial or formula feeding? Dummies or pacifiers? Teats or nipples? Crying or fussing? Baby bottle caries or nursing caries? One has to wonder whether this is indicative of extensive marketing influence on the US vernacular. In a powerful and influential article Dianne Wiessinger has made this point, as I had in *Breastfeeding matters* a decade before. See Wiessinger D. Watch your language! *J Hum Lact*, 1996; 12:1–4. DOI:10.1177/089033449601200102. Online at http://www.motherchronicle.com/watchyourlanguage.html

1097 Two important books to read in this connection are Michaels D. *Doubt is their product: how industry's assault on science threatens your health* (Oxford University Press, 2008); and Nestle M. *Food politics* op. cit.

wrong.[1098] As if it is extreme to consider basic physiological mechanisms to be the human normal and deviations to be risks requiring proof of safety!

Corn allergy is very common in the United States, not surprisingly. When corn syrup solids have been in infant formulas for generations, I would expect to see such sensitivity. In the 1980s Wyeth cited the risk of corn allergy as the reason for instead using sucrose in its soy formulas, which were then the principal resort for those who failed to cope with bovine-based formulas.[1099] This was cleverly exploited in rival Mead Johnson advertising[1100] with dramatic bar graphs of sugar intake. Anti-sugar advertising worked, in the 1980s context of massive promotion of artificial sweeteners and campaigns against sugar by academics whose work was often sponsored by the industry making the artificial sweeteners.[1101] Sucrose became something to avoid; corn syrup solids and maltodextrin did not trigger the same parental anxiety as sucrose then did, even though it seems that maltodextrin causes the same sharp fall in oral pH as sucrose, increasing the risk of dental caries, especially in malnourished children.[1102]

The European Society for Paediatric Gastroenterology, Hepatology and Nutrition, (ESPGHAN), recently warned against the use of sugar in infant formula because of its adverse effects in children with fructose intolerance. This is a tiny minority of children: logically one would expect that ESPGHAN would warn against using any dairy products given how many more children have problems with those! But there presently is no realistic substitute for cows' milk in formula making. And like all such bodies, ESPGHAN works within industry-created assumptions. Had there been no profitable sugar substitute for industry to make formulas with, I would lay long odds that medical and government authorities alike would not be condemning sucrose. Its demonising has led to children being fed artificial sweeteners as safer, when that is very dubious indeed.

Since the 1980s, there has been such a major reduction in sucrose in all products for infant use, that when looking for oral rehydration solutions, for example, it is almost impossible to find one not laden with potentially reactive chemicals like aspartame[1103] and saccharin. Sucrose may rot your teeth, make you fat and increase your risk of diabetes or later heart disease, but it doesn't trigger headaches and seizures, as MIT scientists maintained before aspartame was approved in what many see as scandalous circumstances. Case reports

---

1098 The classic example of this – Barston S. *Bottled up* (University of California Press, 2012). See Bibliography.

1099 At this time a trial of soy formula was the usual treatment for distressed infants consuming cows' milk formula. It is still the case in some places, and is all that is available to parents who cannot access doctors willing to prescribe more expensive formulas.

1100 Promotional literature collected at International Childbirth Education Association (ICEA) Convention, June 1984, alleged that Wyeth-fed infants consumed up to 1.5 kg of sugar per month. On file.

1101 De la Pena C. *Empty Pleasures: the story of artificial sweeteners from Saccharin to Splenda.* (University of North Carolina Press 2010.) Ch. 6

1102 Johansson I, Lif Holgerson P. Milk and oral health. (PMID:21335990) Nestlé Nutr Workshop Ser Pediatr Program 2011, 67:55–66. Published as *Milk and milk products in human nutrition* (Karger/Nestec 2011) comment, p. 108. Available online at http://www.nestlenutrition-institute.org/Resources/Library/Free/workshop/BookNNIW67/Pages/booknniw67.aspx

1103 For an overview, discussing recent disturbing studies, see http://www.drbriffa.com/2012/11/13/aspartame-linked-with-cancer-in-humans/

indicate that sensitive people are still at cerebral risk.[1104] The demonising of cane sugar has reached absurd proportions when people will risk their brains to avoid it, especially as it seems that artificial sweeteners may in fact contribute to higher blood sugar levels[1105] and weight gain[1106] or even increase cancer risk – and a little sugar can be a useful part of home-made oral rehydration solutions. (See Book 3.) Equally, the scandal around the approval of aspartame casts doubt on the ability of regulatory agencies to protect public health when a major corporation has friends in government.[1107] While all major corporations try to have friends in high places in government and its agencies, some like Monsanto (who developed aspartame) have succeeded spectacularly!

## Corny solutions

Physical growth was the outcome investigated whenever formulas were changed. Fomon had found that 'Replacement of lactose with corn syrup solids appears to be of little nutritional consequence', while it was 'economically advantageous'.[1108] That is, cheaper for industry. So American formulas used corn syrup solids. Few parents had any idea of the processes that produced these innocent-sounding ingredients, starches and sugars, but they were better than lactose, it seemed. But the more processed the food, the more likely it is to have picked up some traces of the processing plant. Where did the mercury in recent Chinese infant formulas come from?[1109] High fructose corn syrup (HFCS) solids[1110] have been discovered to be mercury-contaminated, for example.

> Mercury cell chlor-alkali products are used to produce thousands of other products including food ingredients such as citric acid, sodium benzoate, and high fructose corn syrup. High fructose corn syrup is used in food products to enhance shelf life. A pilot study was conducted to determine if high fructose corn syrup contains mercury, a toxic metal historically used as an anti-microbial. High fructose corn syrup samples were collected

---

1104 Pisarik P, Kai D. Vestibulocochlear toxicity in a pair of siblings 15 years apart secondary to aspartame: two case reports. (PMID: 20126318); *Cases Journal*, 2009, 2:9237;Van den Eeden SK, Koepsell TD, Longstreth WT Jr, van Belle G, et al. Aspartame ingestion and headaches: a randomized crossover trial. (PMID: 7936222) *Neurology*, 1994, 44(10):1787–93.Walton RG, Hudak R, Green-Waite RJ. Adverse reactions to aspartame: double-blind challenge in patients from a vulnerable population. (PMID: 8373935) *Biological Psychiatry*, 1993, 34(1–2):13–17

1105 http://online.wsj.com/news/article_email/research-shows-zero-calorie-sweeteners-can-raise-blood-sugar-1410973201-lMyQjAxMTA0NzE3ODIxNDgwWj. See Professor Marion Nestle's take on this at http://www.foodpolitics.com/2014/09/do-artificial-sweeteners-cause-not-cure-glucose-intolerance/

1106 Yang Q. Gain weight by going diet? Artificial sweeteners and the neurobiology of sugar cravings. *Yale J Biol Med*, 2010; 83:101–8.

1107 http://www.rense.com/general33/legal.htm or Google 'Rumsfeld and aspartame and Monsanto' and the timeline is shocking: astonishing examples of what might be seen as corporate corruption in any underdeveloped nation. Start with http://www.huffingtonpost.com/robbie-gennet/donald-rumsfeld-and-the-s_b_805581.html. See also de la Pena, op. cit. Ch. 6.

1108 Fomon SJ (1974) p. 383. I could find no studies assessing brain development comparing a standard formula made using lactose with one using corn syrup solids.

1109 http://www.bbc.co.uk/news/world-asia-china-18456795 China's Yili recalls mercury-tainted baby formula milk.

1110 High fructose corn syrup (HFCS) is produced by catalysing dextrins with an enzyme that converts glucose to fructose. Corn syrup can be made sweeter than sucrose. Natural sucrose is more expensive than this by-product of vegetable starches. Hence corn syrup is used in countries like the US that subsidise corn production so that it is dirt cheap.

from three different manufacturers and analysed for total mercury. The samples were found to contain levels of mercury ranging from below a detection limit of 0.005 to 0.570 micrograms mercury per gram of high fructose corn syrup. Average daily consumption of high fructose corn syrup is about 50 grams per person in the United States. With respect to total mercury exposure, it may be necessary to account for this source of mercury in the diet of children and sensitive populations.[1111]

Was HFCS used in any infant formula globally? Industry says it isn't now, but labelling requirements rarely mandate detailed disclosure of the origin of ingredients.

The controversies about various forms of sugar and artificial sweeteners will continue for decades yet. As a recent review says,

> Both controversy and confusion exist concerning fructose, sucrose, and high-fructose corn syrup (HFCS) with respect to their metabolism and health effects. These concerns have often been fueled [sic] by speculation based on limited data or animal studies. In retrospect, recent controversies arose when a scientific commentary was published suggesting a possible unique link between HFCS consumption and obesity. Since then, a broad scientific consensus has emerged that there are no metabolic or endocrine response differences between HFCS and sucrose related to obesity or any other adverse health outcome. This equivalence is not surprising given that both of these sugars contain approximately equal amounts of fructose and glucose, contain the same number of calories, possess the same level of sweetness, and are absorbed identically through the gastrointestinal tract ...

There is a link between fructose, HFCS, sucrose or any other sugar and increased risk of heart disease, metabolic syndrome, or fatty infiltration of the liver or muscle; how strong the link remains in dispute with different studies using different methodologies arriving at different conclusions.[1112] Which seems to be saying that HFCS may be no worse than sucrose, not that both may be harmless!

What is *not* in dispute is that breastfeeding mothers do not have to worry about this particular issue, as over millions of years breastmilk has not deviated from supplying lactose and other complex sugars that optimise development. Yet perhaps the single most damaging hospital practice in the period from 1960 onwards will prove to have been that of giving almost every baby, breastfed or not, industry-supplied 'sugar water', a 10 per cent dextrose solution, and/or a few feeds of cows' milk formula. And few studies seem to have looked at the implications of this still common use of sugar water for the programming of glycaemic control. Have I missed seeing them in my decades of reading the infant feeding literature? Or are they perhaps 'company data on file'? Or non-existent? There would be no need for speculation about some risks if all the company-funded science was in the public arena, and was conclusive or convincing.

1111 Dufault R, LeBlanc B, Schnoll R, Cornett C et al. Mercury from chlor-alkali plants: measured concentrations in food product sugar. *Environ Health.* 26 January 2009; 8:2.
1112 Rippe JM, Angelopoulos TJ. Sucrose, high-fructose corn syrup, and fructose, their metabolism and potential health effects: what do we really know? (PMID: 23493540) *Adv Nutr* 2013; 4(2):236–45. DOI: 10.3945/an.112.002824

# Lactose intolerance

But what about lactose intolerance? The 1980s growing parental awareness of milk-induced 'allergy' – pointing directly at hospital-supplied infant formulas as the cause – may have helped companies frame the ever-increasing problem of infant gut distress as due to 'lactose intolerance' (a problem digesting a sugar rather than an allergy in the strict sense). This diagnosis was popularised at the same time as industry was sourcing new materials to create new formulas that they claim result in a more normal infant gut microbiome.

For industry, the good thing about the diagnosis of lactose intolerance was that it can occur in both breastfed and artificially fed infants, and industry could replace lactose in formulas. (Other sugars were cheaper and had names that meant many people did not recognise as sugars.) Infant symptoms might well abate as the amount of lactose in the gut dropped. But the real problem to be diagnosed was not its symptom (lactose intolerance), but the cause of the gut damage that allowed lactose intolerance to develop. That cause could be microbial or antigenic, or both, in young infants. A disturbed gut can mean maldigestion; adding in different carbohydrates or pre-digesting proteins to formulas might help. So perhaps most importantly, categorising infant distress as 'lactose intolerance' resulted in the creation of a new range of value-added cows' milk or soy-based products, which some doctors could and did prescribe to all and sundry, breastfed or bottle fed. These were the misleadingly labelled Lactose Free or LF infant formulas promoted as panaceas in the 1980s and 1990s.

Companies produced literature educating health professionals to try eliminating lactose, and if symptoms abated, this was proof that the problem was an enzyme deficiency in the baby (i.e., not the fault of the formula). Industry conceded that a minority of babies would not improve and that these might be allergic to cows' milk, especially if their parents were. (Again, parental defect, not the result of the infant's own formula exposure, or the parents' exposure in the previous generation.) Hundreds if not thousands of 'colicky' breastfed babies were tried on a LF formula, and if their symptoms abated they ended up weaned from the breast. Mothers were convinced there was something wrong with their milk or their baby's ability to digest lactose. Some mothers told of being advised to avoid lactose, and so going off milk products; when their babies improved they were sure the diagnosis was right, never suspecting that the underlying problem was not the sugar but the protein in cows' milk. Some babies failed to improve when mothers avoided only milk but ate – on dietetic advice – low-lactose dairy products like hard cheeses or some yoghurts; it proved hard to get those mothers to consider the possibility of cows' milk protein allergy. Diagnosing a symptom while ignoring its cause is always a recipe for further damage. And it could be argued that the more severe forms of gut disease becoming ever more common nowadays, such as food protein induced enterocolitis, the non-IgE form of food allergy, are a legacy of such early misdiagnosis and neglect of parental concerns. See further Book 3.

# Carbohydrates feeding bowel bugs

Carbohydrates feed both the growing infant and his or her microbiome. This has been known since 1886, when Escherich published a monograph on the relationship between intestinal bacteria and the physiology of digestion in the infant.[1113] This research established him as the leading bacteriologist in paediatrics.

Gut bacteria need food, and in breaking it down to feed themselves, produce compounds that feed other bacteria and the growing infant, and prevent dangerous bacteria from thriving. Oligosaccharides are complex carbohydrates used by the body for this purpose. The more than 200 breastmilk oligosaccharides are not readily digested in the small intestine and appear to, instead, have probiotic activities that promote the growth of the harmless bacteria Bifidobacterium bifidum, as well as other anti-infective properties.[1114]

Breastmilk oligosaccharides in fact prevent respiratory pathogens like H. influenzae and S. pneumoniae from infecting cells in the mouth and throat, and also prevent some bacteria, like enteropathogenic E. coli and Campylobacter jejuni from attaching to the gut surface, preventing diarrhoea. Some oligosaccharides are absorbed and excreted in the breastfed baby's urine, their absence probably helping to account for the higher incidence of urinary tract infections in infants not being breastfed. Studies into other systemic effects of these complex sugars are continuing.

After almost a century of basic scientific work[1115] on these milk components, by the 1990s industry was trying to emulate the presence and activity of these sugars in infant formulas, and so healthworkers and parents began to be inundated with talk of prebiotics, inulin,[1116] FOS and GOS (fructo- or galacto-oligosaccharides) and their benefits. Of course, so far it has not been possible to copy the oligosaccharides in milk, and to do so would be very expensive. What formula manufacturers do instead is to try to find other sources of oligosaccharides, which are much less complex and much less diverse.[1117]

A review chapter on this topic[1118] included a figure illustrating some structural differences between breastmilk and formula oligosaccharides, included here as it makes the point visually.

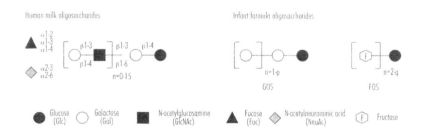

Figure 3-7-1 Some structural differences between oligosaccharides

1113  Robertson AF. Reflections on errors in neonatology. op. cit.
1114  Hale TW, Hartmann PEH op. cit., p. 67.
1115  Kunz C. *Historical aspects of human milk oligosaccharides.* Adv Nutr. May 2012; 3(3):430S–9S. Published online 4 May 2012. DOI: 10.3945/an.111.001776 PMCID: PMC3649480.
1116  This particular carbohydrate was one which many bacteria could not metabolise, yet it is in many formulas.
1117  Hernell O. *Discussion in Clemens,* Hernell, Michaelsen op. cit. p. 27.
1118  Bode L. Human Milk oligosaccharides and their beneficial effects. Ch. 30 In Zibadi, Watson, Preedy op. cit.

Structure always affects function. Which means that the oligosaccharides and mixtures used are not the same as breastmilk, will not have the same effects, and perhaps not be as safe. Anything that has the power to do good has the power to do harm. An adult anaphylactic reaction to inulin is already on record.[1119] Inulin might not be the first suspect in a case of infant anaphylaxis. Put into an infant body with a different microbiome, some oligosaccharides may cause problems, so proof of safety is essential. And if they produce no good effects, they are simply increasing prices for no benefit.

One thing is certain. Formula oligosaccharides are not the same as breastmilk oligosaccharides. The presence and relative abundance of 200+ oligosaccharides in mother's milk is genetically determined, related to blood type, and determined by the mother's Secretor and Lewis type. And all 200 or more have a multitude of specific tasks to perform, some interactively. In human milk oligosaccharides change over time; in formula they do not. Soon after birth neutral or acidic human milk oligosaccharides abound, but by 2–3 months postpartum this has changed to a personalised oligosaccharide profile, which lasts until other foods are introduced. Oligosaccharides are metabolised in the infant gut, and those in infant faeces reflect what is in milk. By contrast, blood group specific oligosaccharides are absent from the faeces of formula-fed infants.[1120] The oligosaccharides added to infant formula are in fact 'structurally different from human milk oligosaccharides, and they are likely not to be able to mimic all the beneficial and highly structure-specific effects of HMO.'[1121]

What difference that makes we don't know. In fact, it won't be for some time that we can say for sure that GOS, FOS, inulin and their few friends in formula are doing more good than harm. Why? Because even if trials had shown crystal clear benefit – which they haven't – population-wide studies (with exclusively breastfed control groups) would be needed to see what the health outcomes are in any population. Trial results are not sufficient by themselves, because trials are always done only in healthy children, best able to cope with a new product, and unlikely to confuse results. What of those who are less healthy, born early, or just vulnerable genetically?

And might there be second-generation effects if these food derivatives are given to children in this generation, and they develop sensitivities to particular oligosaccharides? Some have: already one study has described five cases, ranging from five to thirty-eight years of age, who developed 'an unusual form of IgE-mediated anaphylaxis triggered by low-molecular-weight oligosaccharides'[1122]

Those were not the milk proteins or long-chain oligosaccharides in supplemented cows' milk formula. But to me, the fact that any oligosaccharides can trigger immune reactions should mean that no one presumes safety. Yet industry added these compounds to formulas

---

1119 Franck P, Moneret-Vautrin DA, Morisset M, Kanny G et al. Anaphylactic reaction to inulin: first identification of specific IgEs to an inulin protein compound. (PMID:15650313) *Int Arch All Immunol* 2005; 136(2):155–58.
1120 Albrecht S et al. Gastrointestinal metabolization of human milk oligosaccharides In Zibadi et al, op. cit., p. 296.
1121 Bode L. In Zibadi et al, op. cit., p. 516.
1122 Chiang WC, Huang CH, Llanora GV, Gerez I, et al. Anaphylaxis to cows' milk formula containing short-chain galacto-oligosaccharide. (PMID: 23102546) *J Allergy Clin Immunol*, 2012; 130(6):1361–7.

sold in Australia without prior regulatory approval, although they were not permitted ingredients for Australian infant formula according to Standard 2.9.1. In July 2007 the New South Wales Food Authority prosecuted Nutricia for adding prebiotics without seeking approval from FSANZ after submitting evidence of safety – and for making health claims on labels. The action was later dropped as FSANZ did its own evaluation and in January 2009 amended the Infant Formula Standard 2.9.1 to allow the addition.[1123] All too often that's how innovation in formulas proceeds.

To date no obvious problems have arisen from the addition, so far as I was able to discover. However, it has taken decades for problems with gluten and peanuts and, above all, milk to be recognised as manifesting population-wide, and to influence infant formula composition.[1124] And only very recently has the question been raised[1125] as to whether the rising rate of gluten intolerance is not in fact is due to the chemical load carried by cereals subjected to pre-harvest applications of the herbicide glyphosate.[1126] Others consider gluten intolerance likely to be intolerance of cereals' fermentable carbohydrates – such as oligosaccharides and disaccharides.[1127] The possible suspects are legion.

Scientists are now debating the contribution of FODMAPs to many gut disorders: FODMAPs being the unwieldy acronym for Fermentable Oligosaccharides, Disaccharides, Monosaccharides and Polyols.[1128] (Inulin is one.) Safety information for any new additions to formula could be generated over time by that 'extensive post-market surveillance' that agencies like the USFDA politely request industry to provide – but no industry regulator requires; none has been published.

Meanwhile, the formula marketing goes on, with implied benefits of FOS and GOS and inulin well ahead of the scientific proof. Stay tuned to the scientific literature, and don't believe all you hear from industry. After all, at the 2012 Scientific Conference of the Australasian Society of Allergy and Clinical Immunology (ASCIA), one of the speakers was quoted as saying, 'For the last 20 years we have been trying to create carbohydrates to add to infant formula that can mimic those found in breastmilk. We haven't been able to do it yet.'[1129]

1123 http://www.foodauthority.nsw.gov.au/news/news-may-09-nswfa-resolves-prosecution-nutricia/#. U482GRZbrG4

1124 The revised Codex Infant Formula Standard states that 'all ingredients and additives shall be gluten-free.' They weren't in the past!

1125 Samsel A, Seneff S. Glyphosate, pathways to modern diseases II: Celiac sprue and gluten intolerance. *Interdiscip Toxicol.* 2013; 6(4): 159–84. DOI: 10.2478/intox-2013-0026 Online: www.intertox.sav.sk & www.versita.com/it

1126 Agriculture Department, Alberta Canada. Desiccation or pre harvest glyphosate application: FAQ. See http://www1.agric.gov.ab.ca/$department/deptdocs.nsf/all/faq7206. Sprayed crops are approved for animal feed, and there is a mention that maltsters reject such crops, possibly because they interfere with fermentation. But no discussion of implications for the use of such cereal crops as human foods.

1127 Biesiekierski JR, Peters SL, Newnham ED, Rosella O et al. No effects of gluten in patients with self-reported non-celiac gluten sensit-ivity after dietary reduction of fermentable, poorly absorbed, short-chain carbohydrates. (PMID:23648697) *Gastroenterol* 2013, 145(2):320–8.e1–3.

1128 Muir JG, Gibson PR. The Low FODMAP Diet for Treatment of Irritable Bowel Syndrome and Other Gastrointestinal Disorders.(PMID:23935555) *Gastroenterol Hepatol (N Y)* 2013, 9(7):450–52

1129 Prof. Johan Garssen, quoted in *Sydney Morning Herald* 7 September 2012, p. 2. www.smh.com.au

Not easy to do it, when breastmilk oligosaccharides – which have been proved to be protective – vary between women. How significant are differences in maternal blood groups to the outcomes? There are already suggestions that this may be relevant.[1130]

There are indications that some prebiotic mixtures do alter some stool characteristics in adults. Oligosaccharides and other prebiotics might be beneficial for artificially fed infants, already on unnatural diets. Anything that improves their bowel microbiome and gut function without reducing nutrient absorption would be a good thing, and might, repeat might, prevent or reduce allergic symptoms. However, to date there is no consistent evidence to support the value or usefulness of such additives, and no consistent global policy about their addition to the diet of very young infants. For more about prebiotics, probiotics and synbiotics (the two mixed together) go to page 467.

## An internal brewery? What food for bugs?

It needs to be remembered always that the breastfed baby's microbiome is different from top to toe. It is not only in the colon that this difference can have an effect. The different microbiome and gut pH (degree of acidity) of the artificially fed infant may allow bacteria to reproduce, so that where formulas were not acidified, 'many very premature infants empty formulas with a large bacterial contamination from their stomach, even if the formula was sterile when fed.'[1131] This can sometimes facilitate an auto-brewery syndrome[1132] impossible in breastfed infants with greater gut acidity. Incredible as this sounds, the high pH (too alkaline) can result in some gut bacteria and fungi producing alcohol by fermenting infant formula sugars. This is not routinely mentioned to bottle-feeding parents, as it is thought to be extremely rare. It has been reported to date only in infants subjected to surgery, but might perhaps occur in some infants exposed to acid-suppressing medication such as antacids, along with antibiotics altering gut bacteria. Bivin and Heinen questioned whether this syndrome might contribute to some cases of unexplained infant death. Using over-the counter acid-suppressants, or keeping refluxing babies for long periods on proton-pump inhibiters, seems unwise, to say the least. Any tinkering with any infant's finely balanced digestive system needs to be taken seriously and all possible side effects considered broadly, without tunnel vision focussed on reducing one symptom.

But concern about infant ingestion of alcohol has focussed heavily on the breastfeeding mother. Certainly the poorer metabolism of alcohol by young infants means that binge-drinking, and heavy or frequent consumption of alcohol is harmful, but science simply does not justify a total ban on the occasional drink (preferably just after a breastfeed). The mother's milk alcohol content will match her blood alcohol, and will decline at much the

1130  Blank D, Dotz V, Geyer R, Kunz C. Human milk oligosaccharides and Lewis blood group: individual high-throughput sample profiling to enhance conclusions from functional studies. (PMID: 22585923) *Adv Nutr*, 2012; 3(3):440s–9s.

1131  Carrion V, Egan E. Gastric pH and quantitative bacterial colonization of the stomach in neonates <1250gms. *Ped Res* 1988, abstract 1675; Carrion V, Egan EA. Prevention of neonatal necrotizing enterocolitis. (PMID:2246712) *J Pediatr Gastroenterol Nutr* 1990, 11(3):317–23.

1132  Bivin WS, Heinen BN. Production of ethanol from infant food formulas by common yeasts. *J Applied Bacteriol* 1985; 58:355–7. DOI:10.1111/j.1365-2672.1985.tb01473.x.

same rate, so that globally authorities say that a one standard drink is of little concern. How much .05 per cent milk would a baby need to consume to be affected, when infant medications routinely contained up to 5 per cent alcohol until a voluntary agreement in the 1990s?[1133] Banning even light occasional alcohol intake during lactation is simply another needless restriction that discourages normal breastfeeding durations of many months, if not years. Many baby boomer mothers like myself cheerfully imbibed low moderate amounts while breastfeeding for years, and still produced brilliant children! We may all be better off without the calories and the alcohol, but there is no scientific justification for a complete ban on drinking while lactating. More discriminating guidance is needed, as a recent Slate article[1134] sensibly argues.

Bacteria will utilise whatever foods they are given. Not all infant formula companies have added novel foods (like FOS and GOS) for gut bugs. Some waited, just as some waited to see outcomes before adding nucleotides (see page 463). The marketing advantage goes to the early-bird company because of the parental assumption that 'they [those mythical omniscient independent regulators] wouldn't let them do it if it wasn't safe, would they?' But intelligent and experienced industry scientists know better than healthworkers and parents that changing any one ingredient in infant formula can have unpredicted consequences. And apparent safety, avoidance of obvious harms, can only be proved or disproved in the end by use in large numbers of infants, non-English speaking ones first, usually. Yes, unwitting guinea pigs, our bottle-fed children.

But all things considered, are the changes to formula involving foods for gut bacteria an improvement? After all the reading I've done, I don't know. Nor, I think, does anyone else. The evidence for safety and efficacy of these many different products remains confused and confusing. Those multiple novel products being put into formulas come from a wide variety of sources, so each requires individual study. There seems to be a consensus developing that some make a formula-fed baby's poo more like a breastfed baby's. But there is no way companies can match the multitude of different oligosaccharides and other carbohydrates in women's milk, mixes which can vary with their blood group.

In fact, concern has even been expressed about the amounts and effects of the large quantities of carbohydrate found in formulas for older infants and children. Undigested carbohydrate can be the basis of osmotic diarrhoea, after all, and diarrhoea kills many children and wastes many more. In fact any such special products for older children are unnecessary, as the World Health Assembly asserted in 1986 and has been repeated endlessly since. An excellent online review of these products can be found at First Steps Nutrition Trust, a superb UK nutritional resource. Said the authors:

> The use of milk-based 'growing-up' formula does not bring additional value to a balanced diet in meeting the nutritional requirements of young children in the European Union. EFSA's scientific experts could identify 'no unique role' for young-child formula (commonly

1133 http://www.medicine.virginia.edu/clinical/departments/pediatrics/education/pharm-news/1995-2000/199609.pdf
1134 http://www.slate.com/articles/double_x/the_kids/2014/12/breast_feeding_and_alcohol_it_s_fine_to_drink_while_nursing.html

called 'growing-up formula') in the diet of young children (those aged 1–3), concluding that it is no more effective in providing nutrients than other foods that constitute the normal diet of young children.[1135]

Personally, I am finding that there are other dangers in these growing up milks. As I finish this book I have been dealing with the parents of an allergic two-year-old boy, who was not eating much food – but bottle-drinking daily at least three litres of fluid, over a litre of Stage 3 formula, and considerably more than a litre of plain water. The day after all such formula was stopped as part of a milk elimination diet, he started eating family food. And stopped waking drenched in sweat at night, and began to calm down and speak better. Symptoms of allergy are not always the classic obvious ones, as Figure 4-1-1 on page 562 makes clear.

## Conclusions about carbohydrates?

Like proteins and fats, the carbohydrates in breastmilk and those in infant formula are light years apart. Yes, not to be feeding babies wheat flour is certainly progress, though we are living with the inherited consequences of having done so. But there are still just as many unanswered questions about the best possible ingredients and how they can be put together without introducing other problems. And the acid test of safety and efficacy is still real-time experimentation on infants whose lives and descendants will be affected by the experiment.

Yes, fewer children now die as the direct result of maldigestion of current formulas carefully made up and fed in hygienic circumstances, for which I am grateful. But worldwide, the existence of these products, and the dishonesty and secrecy about their problems, undermines breastfeeding. *In absolute numbers, more children than ever die and are malnourished as a result of artificial feeding.* What should be the priority in human research? Further tweaking an unnatural product few families worldwide can afford, or getting breastmilk into babies? How comfortable are formula industry shareholders and employees, when many more than a million babies die every year for lack of breastfeeding? There is no doubt that the assiduously-cultivated industry myth of formula safety and virtual equivalence to breastmilk causes those deaths. Remember, 'Anyone who, ignorantly or lightly, causes a baby to be fed on unsuitable milk, may be guilty of that child's death.'[1136] It's still true. Think about that, budding authors, or obstetricians, before ignorantly or lightly advising mothers that nowadays formulas are so good that breastfeeding really doesn't make much difference for affluent women like you. And think about whether you want to be responsible for the increased health risks for those mothers themselves. Even one child orphaned because a mother bottle-fed is too many.

---

1135 Crawley H Westland S. *Fortified milks for children: a worldwide review of fortified milks marketed for children over 1 year of age.* First Steps Nutrition Trust, June 2013. Online at http://www.firststepsnutrition.org/newpages/fortified_milks_for_children.html

1136 Dr. Cicely Williams, Singapore: Milk and Murder speech 1939. op. cit.

# 3.8 Additives – intended and unintended

In the twentieth century, physical growth (weight and height, not so often head cirumference) was the test of a satisfactory formula, and more than sufficient protein, fat and carbohydrate ensured such growth. In most cases the base ingredients used to make formula contained a wide range and ample supply of trace minerals and vitamins, so that the importance of the right amount of any minor ingredient was not recognised until cases of deficiency or excess were identified, sometimes by accident. The potential for harm of excess mineral intakes is now being discussed much more widely.[1137]

In every chapter of this book there are references to ingredients added to, or subtracted from, or altered in, infant formula: taurine in the protein chapter, omega-3 fats in the fats chapter, lactose in the carbohydrate chapter, nucleotides in the marketing chapters, for example.

In this chapter I will highlight just a few of the deliberate and/or necessary additions to the infant formula recipe that were widely discussed and used in marketing campaigns. No doubt other changes were made behind the scenes as market prices rose or awareness grew of less than desirable side effects: sodium levels were lowered, and carrageenan, for example, largely disappeared from infant foods without any public fanfare. There has been very little by brand attack marketing, like that advertisement damning sucrose in a competitor's formula, or corn products as potentially allergenic and sugar as better! Naturally enough, when something risky is taken out, there is less publicity than when something (possibly) beneficial is added. I have yet to see a company advertising that their formula has the lowest arsenic, lead or radioactivity levels of all brands, even though one company must have that honour. Industry groups would surely think such marketing damaging to the reputation of all formulas, even if it benefitted one brand temporarily. So this is more often a tale of additions and alterations than subtractions.

## Vitamins

Additions to the basic ingredients in formula recipes began early in the twentieth century. The discovery of vitamins[1138] triggered many changes. Cows' milk is low in vitamin C. The occurrence of scurvy due to vitamin C deficiency in formulas resulted in fresh orange juice becoming part of children's diets. The makers of SMA created a spray-dried orange juice/lactose mix to try to prevent scurvy; later, vitamin C would routinely be added to all infant formula, although processing heat would inactivate much of it. Carotene had been added in 1933 after vitamin A was recognised as affecting vision. These were among the first additives to the self-styled 'complete' patent foods.

---

1137 Molska A, Gutowska I, Baranowska-Bosiacka I, Noceń I et al. The content of elements in infant formulas and drinks against mineral requirements of children. (PMID:24706326) *Biol Trace Element Res* 2014, 158(3):422-427 DOI: 10.1007/s12011-014-9947-1

1138 Apple RD. *Vitamania: vitamins in American culture* (Rutgers University Press, 1996); Valenze op. cit.

As noted earlier, rickets (skeletal deformities due to vitamin D deficiency and calcium malabsorption) had become common in artificially fed infants in the early twentieth century. 'Sun baths' were prescribed for all babies, and putting babies out in the sunshine and fresh air[1139] in a pram or cradle became a norm for baby care, sometimes carried to absurd lengths. In addition, cod-liver oil was universally recommended for infants once it was recognised as being rich in vitamin A and D. Synthetic vitamin D was added to evaporated milk and milk powders, and these milks were irradiated during manufacture by exposure to ultra-violet light as a way of increasing vitamin D content. As noted earlier, cottonseed and linseed oil were also irradiated and used in formulas.

Most major infant formula makers had used irradiation to increase vitamin D levels, but for some reason mention of irradiation of formulas had disappeared by the 1950s. It may be that a better or cheaper vitamin D analogue was available, or that the experience of the atomic age suggested that this was not a selling point. The word 'radiation' was no longer evocative of the shining sun, but of Hiroshima and Nagasaki. Or perhaps it was the increasing understanding that irradiation creates unpredictable, damaging metabolites and affects the nutrient values of some ingredients. I have found no public explanation. Nestlé's Vi-Lactogen just disappeared from sale in Australia,[1140] and advertisements no longer mentioned irradiation.

Ironically, recognition of vitamin D deficiency problems was to lead to so much fortification of infant foods that the reverse problem of hypercalcaemia emerged by the late 1940s.[1141] Problems of calcified kidneys[1142] due to excess calcium intake and absorption would recur with the use of 'fortifiers' from the 1980s: Wharton cautioned that 'Vomiting and constipation should always arouse suspicion of hypercalcemia'. Does it? Reassurance should not be sought from the label on the can. One 1992 study found, for example, that where vitamin D is concerned, seven of ten US formulas contained more than double the amount stated, and one contained over four times as much. As the authors said,

> Milk and infant-formula preparations rarely contain the amount of vitamin D stated on the label and may be either under-fortified or over-fortified. Since both under-fortification and over-fortification are hazardous, better monitoring of the fortification process is needed.[1143]

What country routinely monitors what is in the cans imported or produced domestically? Independent monitors of formula additives also need to be aware of how the additive has been created. Recently a product combining bovine beta-lactoglobulin and vitamin D3 has been shown to be effective in making vitamin D more bioavailable. Great. But there was no

---

1139 They were right about fresh air being beneficial and reducing disease. See *Swain F.* Fresh air and sunshine: the forgotten antibiotics. New Scientist 2013; 220 (2947): 34-37 And vitamin D research has shown sunshine to be important.

1140 So too Nestlé's Pelargon, an acidified formula made for use in warm climates, which met with consumer resistance because it smelt 'off', but which in some ways was probably more digestible and microbially safer.

1141 Wharton BA, Darke SJ. Infantile hypercalemia, in Jelliffe EFP & Jelliffe DB, op. cit., pp. 397–404

1142 Woolridge M, cited in *ALCA News*, 1992; 3(2):2

1143 Holick MF, Shao Q, Liu WW et al.. The vitamin D content of fortified milk and infant formula. (PMID: 1313548) *N Engl J Med*, 1992; 326(18):1178–81

discussion of the allergy risk this poses if the product label simply includes 'vitD3' and not 'contains milk protein'.[1144] Parents should not have to have a degree in food technology to identify the source of the ingredients in baby food!

Vitamins are among the ingredients that are affected by prolonged storage during the shelf life of the product, generally up to about two years. As with protein, 'overages' are added to ensure that enough is present for that whole period. In 2008 a study outlined the actual amounts in the can compared with the label, and measured the decline at different temperatures, in two different formulations. They found

> higher vitamin A (140 per cent and 139 per cent), vitamin E (109 per cent and 198 per cent) and vitamin C (167 per cent and 118 per cent), but lower iron (65.0 per cent and 65.3 per cent) and selenium (72.9 per cent and 79.4 per cent) than the amounts declared on the label ... As expected, all the studied vitamins showed decreases during storage, and these decreases were higher in formulas stored at 40 °C. The losses of vitamin A at 40 °C after 18 months of storage were 27.5 per cent in IF-A and 29 per cent in IF-B, while vitamin E losses under the same conditions were 23.1 per cent and 28.1 per cent, and vitamin C losses under the same conditions were 28.4 per cent and 48.6 per cent. All these losses justify the over-fortification of the aforementioned vitamins.[1145]

What you see on the label is never precisely what is being fed. And storing infant formula in a cool place is important to its ingredients. It would be interesting to repeat this study on cans bought in the open-air stores where I saw it being sold in Nigeria and Pakistan, for example.

Most other vitamins have also proved problematic at some time over the infant formula experiment. Some examples on the public record follow.

## Vitamin K

Vitamin K was added after acute bleeding episodes in infants fed early casein hydrolysates like Nutramigen after antibiotics; more recently, a study revealed that some infants fed newer hypoallergenic formulas are also at increased risk of severe haemorrhages (compared with infants breastfed or fed regular infant formula).[1146] Preterm infants can have with blood levels of Vitamin K up to 100 times those in adults, ten to twenty times those found in formula-fed infants, which are many times higher than those in breastfed infants. While no harm has yet been identified, such an excessive intake is indeed 'worthy of further study', to quote a doyen of American paediatrics.[1147]

---

1144 Diarrassouba F, Garrait G, Remondetto G, Alvarez P, et al. Increased stability and protease resistance of the β-lactoglobulin/vitamin D3 complex. *Food Chem.* 15 February 2014; 145:646–52. DOI: 10.1016/j. foodchem.2013.08.075. Epub 28 August 2013

1145 Chávez-Servín JL, Castellote AI, Rivero M, López-Sabater MC. Analysis of vitamins A, E and C, iron and selenium contents in infant milk-based powdered formula during full shelf life. *Food Chem*, 2008; 107(3):1187–1197. DOI: 10.1016/j.foodchem.2007.09.048

1146 van Hasselt PM, de Vries W, de Vries E, Kok K, et al. Hydrolysed formula is a risk factor for vitamin K deficiency in infants with unrecognised cholestasis. (PMID: 21057325) *J Pediatr Gastroenterol Nutr* 2010; 51(6):773–6.

1147 Greer FR. Vitamin K the basics – what's new? (PMID: 20116943) *Early Hum Dev*, 2010; 86 Suppl 1:43–7

## Folic acid and vitamin C

Megaloblastic anaemia resulted from formula with low folic acid and vitamin C levels.

## Vitamin A and vitamin D

Vitamin A excess and vitamin D deficiency were found in a formula due to human error: one task omitted and one repeated during processing, and the mandated compositional checks not done.[1148]

## Iodine

Cases of goitre from early soy formulas led to iodine being added. There are still concerns about thyroid development.

## Vitamin B6

Overheating led to B6-deficient formula brain-damaging babies, so that heat-stable pyridoxine was added in 1953; litigation resulted in confidential settlements. This problem recurred in 1982, when Wyeth was forced to recall SMA, which had been on the market for a month before independent testing revealed the deficiency.[1149] Too high a temperature on the processing line destroys this vitamin, and only an independent audit revealed that a newly constructed processing line was reaching too high a temperature. The company had argued that FDA inspection was not necessary as the product was being made for export; fortunately for non-American children, including perhaps some Australians, the FDA disagreed, inspected, and found the fault.

## Vitamin B1 (thiamine)

Vitamin B1 (thiamine) deficiency in an imported German formula was discovered only after children became ill. From this Israeli report, there are now four deaths on record, and more than twenty cases of severe brain damage. Shamir concluded that:

> The fact that 3 infants had to die and more than 10 be admitted to hospitals before a common denominator could be established calls into question the ability of apparent history of safe use to be used as a valid tool. It is not conceivable that small differences in growth, cognitive development and later risk of disease could be detected with this approach.[1150]

An 'apparent history of safe use' could be summarised as the assumption of safety in formula that has been on the market for a long time. In fact, the only regulatory indicator for US-made formula safety and efficacy is its ability to keep babies alive and support normal infant growth, measured as weight gain.[1151] (The opposite of normal physical growth is defined

---

1148 Stehlin D. Faulty Premix Prompts Infant Formula Recall. *FDA Consumer*; May 1, 1986.
1149 http://www.nytimes.com/1982/03/12/us/fda-asks-wyeth-to-recall-infant-food-short-on-vitamin.html
1150 Shamir R. Thiamine deficient infant formula: what happened and what have we learned? *Ann Nutr Metab*, 2012; 60 (3) 185–7
1151 Bier, DM. Safety standards in infant nutrition: a US perspective. *Ann Nutr Metabol*, 2012, 60(3):192–5

by the FDA as 'not gaining weight'[1152] – surely a little simplistic in the age of obesity.) How many more deaths and damaged brains linked to formula go unnoticed? It had been known for years that breastfed babies' heads grew bigger on average than formula-fed babies' heads, reflecting more brain growth, but even that measurement was not included in safety and efficacy infant formula studies: just weight gain and sometimes height.

It is simply not possible to chart all the many problems and recalls of infant formula in any one country or any decade. There is no central global registry, and no vested interest in keeping such records or even making the problem public in the first place. (It would be a useful service – and one would think a task for a group such as the World Alliance for Breastfeeding Action, or indeed, the International Pediatric Association.) The Syntex problem in Chapter 3.8. The drive to regulation: health concerns, is just one of many incidents; the difference was that the babies affected belonged to highly educated and vocal parents who made the matter public. My earlier book, *Breastfeeding matters*, contains a partial list of problems and recalls, the tip of a very large iceberg. The website of NABA, the North American Breastfeeding Alliance, contains some others.

In one of the few cases on record where this affected a cluster (and so was noticed) of preterm babies, infant formula caused 'unexpectedly high renal net acid excretion', and 'unintended high differences in mineral contents [of the formula] were discovered'. The formula being used varied from amounts on the label. The problem was noticed because the babies were being laboratory-tested. Were parents told about this? Are the infants being followed to see if there are long-term effects on renal health? Who pays if there are: the hospital that fed the formula, or the company that made it? The authors of that study concluded:

> The production of infant formulas needs to be more closely monitored to avoid marked deviation of the mineral content in individual lots from the concentrations shown on the can.[1153]

Indeed it does. After this twenty-first century episode, Israel classified infant formula as a product to be sampled and tested regularly by government agencies.[1154] Would that every country did the same, as problems can be batch-specific. And labels need to be understood, not as precise statements about what analysis will show is in the can, but as a general outline of what would probably be there if the base ingredients did not deviate too widely from the expected template for such ingredients, and if there had been no human or machine error in preparation not picked up by company analyses of batch lots, and if storage conditions had been adhered to post-production....

As I outlined in the earlier part of this book, it is now accepted that there are long-term effects of early infant feeding and its programming of metabolic responses. As you read about

---

1152  Draft Minutes of the FDA Food Advisory Committee Meeting on Infant Formula, April 2002, p.10. Online at
http://www.fda.gov/ohrms/dockets/ac/02/minutes/3852m1-draft.pdf

1153  Tolle HG, Manz F, Diekmann L, et al. Effect on renal net acid excretion of various mineral contents in three lots of a common preterm formula. *J Trace Elem Electrol Hlth Dis*, 1991; 5:235–8. See also Remer T, van Eyll B, Tölle HG, Manz F. Contents and batch-dependent variations of mineral substances in milk formula for premature infants and possible effects on renal acid burden. (PMID:2079941) *Monatsschr Kinderheilkd* 1990, 138(10):658-63

1154  Shamir, op. cit.

omissions discovered and defects rectified – here and elsewhere in this book – consider what this means for citizens today. People artificially fed before 1933 may be more likely to have developed sight problems due to vitamin A deficiency. While many will have died, these are our current eighty to ninety year olds. Do their degenerative sight problems relate to their 'perfect' infant formulas? Similarly, how much of their osteoporosis relates to dietary vitamin D deficiency as artificially fed infants, or their kidney disease to excess mineral loads?

# Metals in milk: iron

Minerals in milk have been like vitamins, a process of addition and subtraction. Many trace elements come to us in our diet and we need them all; an excess or deficiency can have major effects.

Up until the 1970s there had been epidemics of iron deficiency anaemia in not-breastfed infants, especially if they were fed on whole cows' milk for any length of time in the first year of life. Iron deficiency anaemia was rightly a major concern for paediatricians. This was one of the first major differences between cows' milk and the newer patent formulas. Industry used the threat of anaemia to expand their market share, to oust older formulations and to replace cows' milk in the diet of the bottle-fed infant.

Adding iron to infant formula was not simple. Wyeth's SMA was available with the option of added iron from 1942; in 1959 some was added to Similac. However, the iron compounds initially added were not universally popular. Some iron compounds interacted with other ingredients, created off tastes, or were not bioavailable to the baby's body. Off tastes and interactions reduced product shelf life and undermined consumer confidence.[1155] When in 1967 the American Academy of Pediatrics Committee on Nutrition (AAP CON) made its first recommendation about the nutrient composition of infant formula, it suggested 17 vitamins and minerals; with iron at 1mg/100kcal (6.7mg/L) in iron-fortified formula, and less than one-sixth of that for low-iron formula, the market-leading choice.[1156] In 1971 the use of iron-fortified formula (at 6-7mg/L) was recommended by the AAP Committee on Nutrition, and sales of iron-fortified formula rose from just seventeen per cent to thirty-seven percent in the next two years.[1157] In 1976 the AAP CON would increase this to between six and twelve mg/L, with infants thought to be at risk of iron deficiency to get the higher doses.[1158] Did this encourage infection and the deadly NEC among preterm infants?

Medicinal iron drops and elixirs had been in use, and were thought to have many adverse side effects such as constipation, diarrhoea and vomiting. Companies produced formulas with added iron and without it. Through the century there had been much debate about which iron compounds, in what doses, could be safely added to formula to prevent iron deficiency, but without causing problems like zinc deficiency or disorders of copper

1155 Packard VS. *Human Milk and Infant Formula*. (Academic Press 1982) p. 164-5. "Of all nutrient additives, iron has to be the most irksome."
1156 AAP CON. Proposed changes in FDA regulations concerning formula products and vitamin-mineral dietary supplements. *Pediatrics* 1967; 40: 916
1157 Fomon (1974) op. cit. p. 313.
1158 AAP CON. Iron Supplementation of infants. *Pediatrics* 1976; 58:765-8

metabolism, or fostering infection, or even damaging cognitive development. All these essential minerals compete for absorption, and too much of one can lead to too little of another, with occasional devastating effects. A 1983 independent analysis of then-current infant formulas showed a very wide range of ratios between key minerals. For example, zinc ranged from .1mg/L to 13.5mg/L of infant formula, while the ratios of zinc to iron ranged from 0.02 to 40. (The zinc:iron ratio in breastmilk ranged from 2.5 to 10.)

Those getting only formula with the .02 zinc:iron ratio could have been at risk of zinc deficiency-induced disease and iron overload; the opposite is true for those drinking only formula with a zinc:iron ratio of 40. In every decade there needs to be such analysis of the actual content of infant formula, not just an acceptance of label-stated figures.

Anaemia in artificially-fed infants continued to be a problem. In 1978 the AAP reviewed its recommendation after studies suggested iron was producing a gut environment favouring infection, and again urged the use of the iron fortified formula to prevent anaemia. This concern about anaemia, a common American childhood disease, underlay the AAP suggestion to introduce iron-rich solid foods at no later than 4 months of age, undermining breastfeeding.

In 1980 the AAP CON set 4 months as the appropriate time for introducing other foods to milk-fed infants, a recommendation analysed in Appendix 3. In the 1980s, reams of advertising material descended upon health professionals and parents alike, about iron deficiency harming infant mental development. This message came not only from the formula industry, but also babyfood manufacturers, fortifying their first superfine cereals –then often gluten containing- with iron. Gerber and friends urged solids from three months or ten pounds bodyweight, whichever came sooner. The irony was that some of the recommended weaning foods, like pureed pears, chelated (bound) iron[1159] so that "... addition of a supplemental food to the diet of the breast-fed infant impairs the bioavailability of the iron from human milk." No wonder some partially-breastfed babies could be found with low iron levels after weeks of babymush feeding!

It is worth repeating here that a major cause of infant iron deficiency is early (before 3 minutes) cord clamping. This counter-intuitive practice deprives the baby of nutrients that all other baby mammals are given: the umbilical cord does not separate until it has delivered its blood to the offspring. Now the cord often delivers the baby's blood to a private blood bank, while a delay of just two minutes means an increase in iron bodystores at 6 months of 27-47mg.[1160] As Jelliffe said so well in 1978, "early clamping has the same effect as a haemorrhage from the umbilical stump."[1161] Why is it still happening? Doctors unaware of the advantages of bilrubin (see page 79) seem to fear jaundice quite unreasonably.[1162]

1159 Oski FA, Landaw SA Inhibition of iron absorption from human milk by baby food. (PMID:7377151) *Am J Dis Child* 1980, 134(5):459-460.

1160 Chaparro CM, Nuefeld LM, Alavez GT, Cedillo RE et al. Effect of timing of umbilical cord-clamping on iron status in Mexican infants: a RCT. *Lancet* 2006; 367: 1997-2004.

1161 Jelliffe, *Human Milk in the Modern World* op cit p. 47

1162 Watchko JF. Vigintiphobia revisited. *Pediatrics* 2005; 115(6):1747-1753. (PMID:15930239)

For breastfed infants there never was, and still is not, a scientific basis to these 3-4 month recommendations (See Book 3, chapter 7.). Even with exclusive breastfeeding to 9 months, only a minority of infants had sub-clinical evidence of iron deficiency,[1163] and there is simply no risk for the normal infant who is exclusively breastfed to 6 months of age.[1164] Even exclusive breastfeeding to 9 months will affect only a minority of children.[1165] But if you had asked any Western health professional in the 1970s and 1980s when solids should be introduced to breastfed babies, and why, "the risk of iron deficiency by 4 months" would have been given as the answer. It still is by some who should know better!

Where iron is concerned, it would be a safe bet that in 2014 some health professionals believe two things:

- breastfed infants are at increased risk of iron deficiency and so of cognitive damage, and
- high-iron formulas prevent cognitive deficits in children.

Neither is true. In fact, high-iron formulas may cause cognitive deficits as well as increase infection risks. In 2008 the results of a ten-year randomised controlled trial in almost 500 children indicated that 12 mg/L formula (cf. 2.3 mg/L) is associated with significant cognitive deficit (an 11 point IQ difference) at the age of ten. Said the authors:

> The randomized trial design suggests a causal relation between the 12 mg/L iron-fortified formula and poorer developmental outcome at 10 years ... The results raise the possibility that long-term development is adversely affected in iron-sufficient infants who receive formula fortified with iron at the level commonly used in the United States.[1166]

This supported earlier work by Dewey et al[1167] which showed that routine iron supplementation of breastfed infants could have negative effects on linear growth and head circumference: the mechanism might be damage by unbound iron. They found

> ... evidence that iron-mediated free radical formation is involved in brain damage in neonates and that non-protein bound iron is a highly significant early predictor of later neurodevelopmental outcomes. It has been shown that recombinant human lactoferrin added to formula or human milk attenuates, and iron present in infant formula, increases;

---

1163 McMillan JA, Landaw SA, Oski FA Iron sufficiency in breast-fed infants and the availability of iron from human milk. (PMID:989894) *Pediatrics* 1976, 58(5):686-691.

1164 Lucas A. *Infant feeding: the facts.* (OUP 2007) p. An exception would be, for instance, if the child had lost blood for some reason, or had been extremely preterm. But for normal term solely breastfed infants, the risk is virtually non-existent.

1165 Siimes MA, Salmenpera L, Perheentupa J. Exclusive breastfeeding for 9 months: risk of iron deficiency. *J Pediatr* 1984; 104 (2): 196-199

1166 B, Castillo M, Clark KM, Smith JB Iron-fortified vs low-iron infant formula: developmental outcome at 10 years. *Arch Pediatr Adolesc Med*, 2012, 166(3):208–15. http://www.medscape.org/viewarticle/574363

1167 Dewey KG, Domellof M, Cohen RJ, et al. Iron supplementation affects growth and morbidity of breastfed infants: results of a trial in Sweden and Honduras. *J Nutr*, 2002; 132:3249–55. See also Lönnerdal B, Kelleher SL. Iron metabolism in infants and children. *Food and Nutrition Bulletin*, 2007; 28 (3), S491–499

iron-mediated free radical formation and lipid peroxidation. There is direct evidence of an antioxidant action of human milk.[1168]

Even earlier studies had shown that adding iron to infant formula influenced the development of the gut microbiome, away from that of the breastfed infant's pattern of dominant bifidobacteria.[1169]

Breastmilk contains very little iron, just the right amount, because its absorption by the baby (its bioavailability) is dramatically increased by breastmilk's metal-transport protein, lactoferrin. Too much iron can be as bad as too little, because too much encourages bacterial overgrowth. Human bodies therefore regulate the amount of iron taken up, via a newly discovered regulator called hepcidin. 'Hepcidin assesses both iron need and the threat of infection, and makes a physiological judgement as to when it is safe to absorb iron.'

The following 'News Article' appears on the Nestlé Nutrition Website:

> Prof. Andrew Prentice (MRC International Nutrition Group at the London School of Hygiene and Tropical Medicine in the UK, and MRC Keneba in the Gambia) shared new findings related to iron deficiency. Iron deficiency in utero and in the first postnatal years can have long-term effects on children's development, especially in relation to the brain. Since the human species has evolved to succeed on the basis of a large and complex brain, any deficits in cognitive ability contribute strongly to reductions in the 'human capital' of nations, as well as harming the individual. Therefore iron status is an important component in programming for a healthy life. In developed countries, iron deficiency is generally uncommon because of easy access to animal foods and food fortification. But the picture is very different in developing countries where multiple factors such as helminth infections, malaria, gut damage and poor diets contribute to creating very high levels of iron deficiency.
>
> For decades it was assumed that young children are poorly equipped to physiologically absorb enough iron and therefore need to be given large bolus doses of easily absorbed iron. Numerous studies have recently shown that this strategy has caused an increase in infections and severe adverse events because iron feeds potential pathogens and encourages their growth. The new findings reveal that young children in highly infectious environments are actively excluding iron so that it does not increase their risk of infection. This process is orchestrated by the new discovery of a master regulator of iron metabolism called hepcidin. Hepcidin assesses both iron need and the threat of infection, and makes a physiological judgment as to when it is safe to absorb iron. These insights suggest a complete revision of our approaches to combating iron deficiency.[1170]

In short, the excess iron in infant formula may be part of the reason for higher infection rates in artificially-fed children. And perhaps iron supplementation in pregnancy needs to be re-

---

1168 Sullivan JL. Cognitive development: breast-milk benefit vs infant formula hazard. *Arch Gen Psychiatry*, 2008; 65(12):1456. Downloaded from www.archgenpsychiatry.com at Northwestern University, 24 April 2012
1169 Balmer SE, Scott PH, Wharton BA. Diet and faecal flora in the newborn: lactoferrin. *Arch Dis Child* 1989; 64(12):1685-1690.
1170 Downloaded from http://www.nestlenutrition-institute.org/News/Pages/New-insights-suggest-a-complete-revision-of-approaches-to-combating-iron-deficiency-Pre-and-post-natal-nutrition.aspx News posted 24 February 2014. I have not seen it reported widely elsewhere!

evaluated? After all, levels are lower because of the increase in plasma volume: is this an advantageous adaptation or a risk? Does it influence the bacterial colonisation of the placenta?

Label-declared formula iron levels in the 1980s ranged from less than one to over twelve mg/L, with the usual range of variation inevitable when making a complicated product with a long shelf life. A 1983 study found that the actual range of iron in infant formulas then on sale was from zero to 57.5mg/L.[1171] The range of iron currently allowed (in 2013) in first infant formula is still one to twenty mg/L in the USA,[1172] two to eight mg/L in Europe,[1173] three to thirteen in the UK.[1174] The current Codex Alimentarius level is a minimum of 3mg/L with a note that upper levels may need to be set by national authorities.[1175] European infant formula iron levels has long been around 4–7 mg/L, which is probably more than sufficient for normal infants.

In 1999 eminent scientist Bo Lönnerdal said:

> We have the old dilemma about what is a low-iron formula. What was a low-iron formula 10 years ago is not a low-iron formula today, because in the United States the manufacturers are adding more and more iron to "low-iron" formulas. So even a low-iron formula is now an iron-fortified formula. I certainly think that there should be iron in formulas, but what level should be used will vary under different conditions. I would say that in most developed countries a level of about 2 mg/L would be satisfactory, and I consider that to be an iron-fortified rather than a low-iron formula. That is a 10-fold or 1000 per cent higher iron level than in breast milk, and if there are differences in absorption, that should certainly compensate for them. [1176]

It should be noted that WIC-approved iron-fortified formula has to contain at least 10 mg/L.[1177] This means that WIC mandates five times what Lönnerdal suggests, which makes it fifty-fold or 5000 per cent higher than breastmilk! The top end of the US-allowed range would thus be a hundred fold what breastmilk supplies. Does that affect the predominantly disadvantaged children WIC serves? If and when iron levels are further revised, I suspect that there will be no concerted media releases to tell the world about such an improvement to infant formula. Why not? Because to point out the obvious – that for decades iron-replete children fed the

---

1171 Lönnerdal B, Keen CL, Ohtake M, Tamura T. Iron, zinc, copper, and manganese in infant formulas. *Am J Dis Child* 1983; 137(5):433-437. (PMID:6846270)

1172 US Code 350a, section 412 can be tracked down via http://www.fda.gov/Food/GuidanceRegulation/ GuidanceDocumentsRegulatoryInformation/InfantFormula/default.htm; or try direct at http://www.ecfr. gov/cgi-bin/text-idx?c=ecfr;sid=5af2a35de1ba3464af55f53e369fd570;rgn=div6;view=text;node=21%3A2.0.1. 1.7.4;idno=21;cc=ecfr

1173 Commission Directive 2006/141/EC of 22 December 2006 on infant formulae and follow-on formulae and amending Directive 1999/21/EC. Text at http://eur-lex.europa.eu/legal-content/en/ALL/;jsessionid=lpgvTC shSCvPP26dhfGFPmn7mvcpL1jjvyvl2dp4dvT5K4pLgFYp!-17543456?uri=CELEX:32006L0141

1174 The most convenient place to access UK infant formula information is via Crawley H, Westland S. op cit. Online at http://www.firststepsnutrition.org/newpages/Infants/infant_feeding_infant_milks_UK.html

1175 www.codexalimentarius.org/input/download/standards/.../CXS_072e.pdf. This looks like deference to pressure not to make regulations that could interfere with any manufacturer's trade.

1176 Lönnerdal B. Effect of nutrition on microbial flora: the role of lactoferrin, iron and nucleotides. In Hanson L, Yolken RH. op. cit., p. 201.

1177 Kent G. WIC's promotion of infant formula in the United States *Int Breastfeed J* 2006, 1:8 DOI:10.1186/1746-4358-1-8

highest-dose iron formulas may have been harmed, and that dosing vulnerable children with iron supplements may have contributed to lower IQ and devastating infections – would undermine confidence in formula, distress bottle-feeding parents, and perhaps start some lawsuits. Compare such discretion with the global headlines about the theoretical – or should I say imaginary? – risks of not getting more iron into breastfed babies before six months of age. And the lack of concerted international action about early cord clamping, that recent unscientific obstetric procedure robbing babies of needed blood iron. See page 590)

In fact as late as 2010, the American Academy of Pediatrics (AAP) Committee on Nutrition issued a statement recommending universal iron supplementation of four-month-old exclusively breastfed babies, basing their prejudicial statement on a study of mixed-fed babies,[1178] and reflecting industry promotional materials about iron since the 1980s. The AAP Committee on Nutrition could perhaps pay more careful attention to the problems of artificial feeding, and leave breastfeeding issues to the AAP Section on Breastfeeding, which promptly and publicly dissented from its statement.[1179] Happily, the parties were later reconciled, and an excellent statement on breastfeeding finally resulted in 2012.[1180] Given the AAP's interdependence with major formula companies, it is not surprising that change takes time, no matter how committed the AAP may be to optimal child health. I would be surprised if a survey of the membership revealed awareness of the manifold risks of artificial feeding, or comfort with the idea that parents need to be informed of such risks. (But I'd be happy to be proved wrong!)

One other incident indicative of the problems of global trade deserves inclusion. By the 1980s, the American choice of infant formula was 1 mg/L (or even less) in low-iron formulas, or a minimum of 6mg/L up to 12-13 mg/L in iron-fortified formulas.[1181] In 1984 Australia set an Infant Formula standard requiring a minimum of 3mg/L of iron. US-based formula companies were bringing into Australia formulas made overseas, then as now. The level of iron in one infant formula was below the minimum limit.[1182]

No official inspection or paediatric authority revealed this deficit. It was discovered only because a concerned competitor (making formula in Australia to the regulated standard)

---

1178 A recent plain English overview of iron and the breastfed infant is Tawia S. Iron and exclusive breastfeeding. *Breastfeeding Review*, 2012; 20:35–47.

1179 Schanler RJ and the AAP Section on Breastfeeding. Concerns with universal iron supplementation of breastfeeding infants. *Pediatrics*, 2011; 127:e1097

1180 Feldman-Winter L. The AAP updates its policy on breastfeeding and reaches consensus on recommended duration of exclusive breastfeeding. (PMID: 22526337) *J Hum Lact*, 2012; 28(2):116–17. See American Academy of Pediatrics, Section on Breastfeeding. Policy statement: breastfeeding and the use of human milk. *Pediatrics*. 2012;129[3]:e827–e841. Available at: www.pediatrics.org/content/129/ 3/e827.full

1181 Fomon's classic text, *Infant Nutrition*, recorded specific US infant formula composition in 1967, but by 1974 was providing "a more general treatment" and referring those needing specific information to annual editions of the Physicians' Desk Reference, to which I have not had access.

1182 *ALCA News*, 1991; 2(2); 6. In the next edition a letter from Mead Johnson's Australian General Manager advised that their hospital RTF bottles of formula would contain 'either .3mg iron or 1.2 mg iron per 100 ml, and health professionals will make the choice on which they consider more appropriate.' *ALCA News*, 1991; 2(3):13. That's three or twelve milligrams per litre. Australian low iron formulas contained more than US low-iron formulas.

notified regulatory authorities.[1183] One company 'dobbing in' another for any breach of regulations is said to be a rare event in an industry that knows that the companies united can rarely be defeated. There was no penalty for this, and it was never widely publicised. Knowledge of such events is probably rarer than the events themselves. I suspect that such breaches of existing recommendations and regulations could happen anywhere that there are no regular detailed analyses of imported products. An international database with whistleblower protection would almost certainly uncover others, as formula makers multiply, in the rush to profit from Asia's move to bottle feeding.

In 2014 the final word has yet to be said about what iron, and how much, is good for which infants. But perspectives have changed.[1184] Too much is just as bad as too little, perhaps even worse for infants already iron-replete.

# Ups and downs: selenium, chromium, molybdenum as examples

### Selenium

Selenium is an essential trace mineral present in breastmilk at about 15–20 mcg/L, and up to 45 mcg in some areas with high selenium soils. Selenium was originally not added to infant formulas, but some occurred naturally in base ingredients, so that an industry researcher estimated that infant formula contained roughly 2–13 mcg/L[1185] throughout the twentieth century. (Although this has varied widely.) This relative deficiency compared to human milk was noted back in the 1970s, when it was shown that formula-fed infants' blood levels of selenium were lower than their cord blood levels had been, while breastfed babies blood levels were higher than their cord blood levels: in other words, breastfed babies were gaining selenium, and formula-fed babies were using up their stores. The selenium content of one Finnish formula was as low as 3–5 mcg/L. This is of concern as selenium is linked to heart health and protection against heavy metals and cancer. In 1982 a paper had noted that three-month-old formula-fed infants still had lower levels than breastfed infants.[1186]

Back in 1985 a Ross scientist made it clear that selenium posed a particularly difficult problem, because

> "in animals there is a narrow range between deficient and toxic levels of selenium. Also, research studies will have to be conducted to determine the appropriate form of selenium for use in infant formula if selenium fortification is deemed appropriate."

In 1989 it was stated that 'Since selenium deficiency has been associated with two diseases of childhood, prudence dictates that the concentration of selenium in infant formula be

---

1183 Personal communication with regulatory authorities at the time; confirmed by an industry source.

1184 Quinn EA. Too much of a good thing: evolutionary perspectives on infant formula fortification in the United States and its effects on infant health. (PMID:24142500) *Am J Hum Biol* 2014; 26(1):10-17. **DOI:** 10.1002/ajhb.22476

1185 McSweeney et al., in Park and Haenlein op. cit. p. 465

1186 Smith AM, Picciano MF, Milner JA. Selenium intakes and status of human milk and formula fed infants. (PMID: 7064903) *Am J Clin Nutr* 1982; 35(3):521–6.

standardised' and a range of 10–45 mcg be permitted; an upper as well as lower limit because excess selenium can be damaging.[1187]

So in 1989 the US National Research Council set a recommended intake of 10–40 mcg for infants up to six months. A range of 10–35 mcg/L was suggested by the Expert Panel of the Life Sciences Research Office (LSRO)[1188] of the American Society for Nutritional Sciences in 1998, and an estimated daily intake allowance was set at 10 mcg/day. Formula makers may have added some selenium after hearing it had been declared an essential nutrient. However, this was entirely voluntary, and levels could vary.[1189]

In 1997 a study of twenty-four formulas (mostly made in Europe) on sale in Saudi Arabia showed wide variation: a range from 22–74 mcg/L. (Not only stage two formulas were at the top end of the range.)[1190] In 2004 a study of formulas on sale in Spain was published. The authors began by saying,

> The selenium content of infant formulae varies as a result of differences in the amount of intrinsic selenium compounds. Manufacturers have been gradually changing the protein profile of infant formulae to reflect human milk contents more closely. Because of these variations in infant formula composition and their potential impact on selenium content, this trace element was analysed with regard to the different protein sources.

According to their results,

> on an overall view, infants fed on the studied infant formulae have an intake between basal and normative requirements. This might be considered as providing an adequate selenium supply. However, the intake of selenium provided by several formulae included in this research did not reach the RDA [recommended daily allowance] for the first month of neonate life.[1191]

A 2008 study[1192] stated that 'The optimal form and dose of selenium supplementation required to achieve indicators of selenium status equivalent to those in breastfed infants are unclear.' They went on to experiment with supplemented formulas, and suggested 18 mcg/L. The UK specified a minimum of one and maximum of 9mcg/L in its 2007 Infant Formula and Follow On Formula Regulations. And in April 2013, the US The Food and Drug Administration (FDA) finally proposed

---

1187 Levander OA. Upper limit of selenium in infant formulas. (PMID: 2693651) *J Nutr* 1989; 119(12 Suppl):1869-72; discussion 1873.

1188 The Executive Summary of the LRSO Report is online and is a useful reference for anyone wanting to understand the rationale for USFDA regulations relating to infant formula. See Raiten DJ, Talbot JM, Waters JH. Executive Summary for the Report: *Assessment of Nutrient Requirements for Infant Formulas.* http://jn.nutrition.org/content/128/11/suppl/DC1. Downloaded 4 January 2014

1189 Dorner K, Schneider K, Sievers E et al. Selenium balances in young infants fed or breastmilk or adapted formula. *J Trace Elem Electrolytes Health* 1990; 4: 37-40

1190 Al-Saleh I, Al-Doush I. Selenium levels in infant milk formula. *BioMetals*, 1997; 10:299–302

1191 Navarro-Blasco I, Alvarez-Galindo JI. Selenium content of Spanish infant formulae and human milk: influence of protein matrix, interactions with other trace elements and estimation of dietary intake by infants. (PMID: 15139390) *J Trace Elem Med Biol* 2004; 17(4):277-289DOI: 10.1016/S0946-672X(04)80030-0

1192 Daniels L, Gibson RA, Simmer K, Van Dael P, et al. Selenium status of term infants fed selenium-supplemented formula in a randomized dose-response trial. *Am J Clin Nutr* 2008; 88(1):70–6

Chapter 3: Infant formula, past, present and future
3.8 Additives – intended and unintended
| 365

to amend the regulations on nutrient specifications and labeling for infant formula to add the mineral selenium to the list of required nutrients and to establish minimum and maximum levels of selenium in infant formula.[1193]

The proposed range is 2–7 mcg/100kcal, or roughly 13–40 mcg/L. Industry has now been asked to comment about whether this is achievable on a regular basis, given the variability in the ingredients going into formula. The Codex Standard requires a minimum of one microgram/100kcals, which works out to around 7 mcg/L. Their "guidance upper limit" is nine times that, or around 60mcg/L, which seems excessive, but may reflect formulas already on sale in Europe.

So over three decades another defect of infant formula has been identified and subsequently corrected by mandatory supplementation. But what were the consequences of the lack over the century? And are you surprised that industry did not widely advertise this new addition? "Now with added selenium to correct a longstanding deficiency" doesn't sound so great.

I agree with the UK's Scientific Advisory Committee on Nutrition:

> If an ingredient is unequivocally beneficial as demonstrated by independent review of scientific data it would be unethical to withhold it for commercial reasons. Rather it should be made a required ingredient of infant formula in order to reduce existing risks associated with artificial feeding. To do otherwise is not in the best interests of children, and fails to recognise the crucial distinction between these products and other foods. [1194]

## Chromium

Chromium and selenium are similar stories, except that the problem is one of excess rather than deficiency. Chromium is essential for maintaining normal glucose metabolism: too much or too little is detrimental. In the 1980s Belgian researchers showed that three-month-old exclusively breastfed infants consumed just one-tenth of a microgram per day, and infants fed cow's milk five times more, or half a microgram, but 'the exclusive use of commercial infant formulas resulted in an intake of 2 up to 10 micrograms chromium a day.' That's twenty to one hundred times more than breastfed babies. Two decades later, Spanish researchers reporting on their analysis of 104 formulas discussed 'the influence of the type of container used, the impact of industrial process from different manufacturers and the physical state (powder and liquid formulae) on chromium levels.' Infant formulas still contain more chromium than human milk. Just as with aluminium, the highest levels are in the most processed types of formula: hypoallergenics, lactose-free, and pre-term formulas, and soy-based formula. (In other words, in formulas for infants with problems: great.) The researchers called on manufacturers 'to make continued efforts to routinely monitor chromium levels, particularly for specialised and pre-term formulae' and to declare

1193 https://www.federalregister.gov/articles/2013/04/16/2013-08855/infant-formula-the-addition-of-minimum-and-maximum-levels-of-selenium-to-infant-formula-and-related

1194 http://www.sacn.gov.uk/reports_position_statements/position_statements/infant_formula_and_follow-on_formula_draft_regulations_-_september_2007.html

chromium levels on labels.[1195] That the formula doses did not exceed a theoretical upper safety limit set by an American self-styled "leading trade association for dietary supplement manufacturers" does not entirely reassure me... Codex Alimentarius has not addressed the problem: no doubt in twenty years time there will have been some independent global regulation of chromium in formula. The EU has set a minimum of 1mcg/100kcal, or 6-7mcg/L, with a recommended maximum of 60mcg/L. There is no FDA specification for chromium in US infant formula. Yet.

## Molybdenum

The story is similar again for molybdenum, another trace mineral present in excess in infant formula. Methods for ascertaining levels in formula are being developed. In 2011 Canadian food scientists bought samples of all types of powdered formula available in North America, and assayed them to determine the molybdenum content. This ranged from 15.4 to 80.3 mcg/L, while the breastmilk range was 1.5 to 9.5 mcg/L. There was eight to nine times more in formula than breastmilk if the means of each were compared. As they went on to say, 'High Mo intake may pose health risks, despite lower bioavailability of Mo from formula compared with HM [human milk].'[1196] Yes, it might. Come back in twenty years.....

I could go on filling pages with details like this, showing just how different formula now is from formula then, and how all of it is now, and always was, radically different from breastmilk. Choose any ingredient and do a PubMed search yourself if you're interested, though you may find it frustratingly difficult or expensive to access many of the most interesting articles. There is a lengthy series of journal articles to be written here, which should be informed by an assumption of the risks of excessive deviations from that  human norm.

## For better or worse

**But the single important thing to remember is that all these nutrients are interactive in one body, interacting with one another and with the gut microbiome.** Infant body systems need to determine their use and absorption, and have to cope with deficiencies and eliminate any excesses. So even if industry could get the ingredients just right, and that's impossible, there would still be different outcomes. A deficiency or excess of just one can have a domino effect that alters much more than the predicted outcome. Too much iron: too little zinc or copper, for example. Too little chromium: poorer management of carbohydrates. When it comes to feeding babies, millions of years of human evolution – or God if you prefer – have done a better job than 150 years of biochemists. The World Health Organization said in 2002, 'Infants who are not breastfed ... constitute a risk group.'[1197] Formula advocates might want to deny that reality, but their denial doesn't change facts.

1195 Sola-Larrañaga C, Navarro-Blasco I. Chromium content in different kinds of Spanish infant formulae and estimation of dietary intake by infants fed on reconstituted powder formulae. (PMID: 17071518) *Food Addit Contam.* 2006, 23(11):1157–68. DOI: 10.1080/02652030600812956

1196 Abramovich M, Miller A, Yang H, Friel JK. Molybdenum content of Canadian and US infant formulas. (PMID: 21279467) *Biol Trace Elem Res*, 2011; 143(2):844–53.DOI: 10.1007/s12011-010-8950-4

1197 Paragraph 19 of the WHO/UNICEF *Global strategy for infant and young child feeding* (2003) is available for download at http://www.who.int/nutrition/publications/infantfeeding/9241562218/en/index.html

# 3.9 Unavoidable contaminants

Dr Lewis Barness said in 1981, 'When using a formula, no matter how good, one must beware of possible missing ingredients.'[1198] True. No one has said that 'When using an infant formula, one must beware of possible damaging inclusions.' But that's also true, so I'm saying it now!

Infant formula is the product of a real world and a host of manufacturing environments. The more complex it becomes, the greater the number of industrial environments the ingredients are exposed to. A worn axle in a Danish gearbox, and oil seeped out into 1100 tons of milk powder over a period *of almost 6 months* in 2002. It was contaminated with fine iron particles and oil that caused the milk powder to be a greyish shade, which a customer in Thailand finally noticed in the finished product. [1199] (Great quality control there!) Sometimes the solution is hardly ideal: make sure that the machinery oil used in food manufacture is food grade so that if it gets into the babyfood (as it did in the UK in 2000) it is not a toxic substance that an alert mother can smell and report to the local authorities, as one did.[1200] (And what effect does adding even an edible machine oil have on the fatty acid makeup of formula and baby?) Stoke on Trent Council confirmed that tests revealed "a toxic substance" in the can of Heinz babyfood. How many other mothers did not smell the babyfood before feeding it to their child? Another mother who did, in the late 1990s, caused a recall of over 190,000 cans of what was supposed to be a soy formula but in fact was Vanilla Sustacal.[1201]

Contamination has taken and will always take many forms, many invisible, and is difficult to avoid in the real world. It is a risk for both breastfed and formula-fed babies. In some cases the risk may be small, but has been publicised in ways that discourage breastfeeding, with no acknowledgement that the risk exists and is usually greater for any alternatives to breastmilk. In others the degree of risk remains unknown. While Danish authorities reassured customers that the six-month contamination of that milk powder was not a health risk, infant formula was recalled in Thailand, China and the Philippines.

In this book I can discuss only some contaminants, here and in other chapters where they are relevant. Heavy metals are among the most concerning, because as late as 1983 it was possible for an expert to write:

> A health risk to infants from the intake of heavy metals via bottled food cannot be excluded... the effect on children has thus far been excluded from discussions of safety margins or limits on intake.. This age groups has also been excluded from studies determining

---

1198 Barness L. Letter to the editor – reply to Ganelin RS. *Pediatrics*, 1981; 67:166
1199 Judge D. Switching to food-grade lubricants provides safety solution. *Machinery Lubrication* July 2005. Online at http://www.machinerylubrication.com/Read/774/food-grade-lubricants-safety
1200 Ibid.
1201 Lodato P, op.cit.

acceptable daily intake values for other substances. Paradoxically, such studies often contain a comment that children are particularly sensitive to these substances.[1202]

While there has been some progress since then, the children of the 1980s are the parents producing children today. They deserve to know just how unprotected they may have been as infants, as there may well be consequences for their children.

## Metals in milk: lead

Some metals in infant formula are benign, necessary for human life. The 1980s also saw a growing awareness of some contributed by processing and packaging contaminants. Lead, cadmium, aluminium, and other heavy metals were found in some formulas, and industry became aware that industrial processing always leaves traces.[1203] In 2014 Codex re-visited the issue of lead[1204] in infant formula, halving the allowable levels to 0.01mg/kg in ready to use formula. That's .01mg/L, 10 micrograms per litre, 10parts perbillion

This lead hazard to infants had existed for many decades. Particularly high lead levels in liquid infant formula (50–500 mcg per litre)[1205] arose from the lead seams and solder. (In 1979, over 90 per cent of all US-produced cans used lead solder, according to the National Food Processors' Association.[1206] As noted elsewhere (as noted earlier), in the USA most infant formula by 1970 was sold either as ready-to-feed liquid and concentrates. Adding water to dilute the infant formula concentrates could also add more lead (see page 370). Once these levels were known, infant formula manufacturers tried more thorough washing of formula cans, then plastic coatings on cans,[1207] before phasing out the use of lead-soldered cans for liquid feeds.[1208] The USFDA obliged industry by allowing a ten-year phase out, with a generous 40ppb maximum lead exposure level.[1209] Many companies solved the problem under the decade allowed them, so that by 1982 it was reported that levels were only 10–20 per cent of what they had been when the problem was first uncovered,[1210] and

1202 Hildebrandt EG, Schmidt E. *Health Evaluation of Heavy Metals in Infant Formula and Junior Food.* (Springer-Verlag Berlin/NY 1983)

1203 Dabeka RW. Survey of lead, cadmium, cobalt and nickel in infant formulas and evaporated milks and estimation of dietary intakes of the elements by infants 0–12 months old. *Sci Total Environ*, 1989; 89:279–89. PubMed.

1204 Harrison-Dunn AR. UN tightens regulation on lead in infant formula and arsenic in rice. *Dairy Reporter* July 14, 2014; online at http://www.dairyreporter.com/Regulation-Safety/UN-regulation-infant-formula-lead-and-rice-arsenic

1205 Walker B. Lead content of milk and infant formula. *J Food Prot*, 1980; 43(30:178–9; see also the September 1980 issue of *Food Chemical News*

1206 Reported in *Food Chemical News* 2 July 1990, p. 52

1207 Which would contribute other chemicals, see Chapter

1208 Fomon SJ. Reflections on infant feeding in the 1970s and 1980s. *Am J Clin Nutr*, 1987; 46:171–82

1209 Dabeka R, Fouquet A, Belisle S, Turcotte S. Lead, Cadmium and aluminum in Canadian infant formulae, oral electrolytes and glucose solutions. *Food Addit Contam Part A*, 2011; 28(6):744–53. Published online, 31 May 2011. DOI: 10.1080/19393210.2011.571795

1210 Jelinek CF. Levels of lead in the United States food supply. (PMID: 7118801) *J Assoc Off Analyt Chem*, 1982; 65(4):942–46

deaths from lead poisoning were becoming rarer.[1211] Which means of course that some pre-1970s infants must have been seriously harmed!

There was a well-documented sharp rise in American child deaths from lead poisoning[1212] from the 1920s onwards, which parallels the rising use of lead-soldered cans of evaporated milk for infant feeding. This could be yet more unrecognised collateral damage, the tip of the toxic iceberg of lead damage via artificial substitutes for breastmilk. Undoubtedly lead paint also contributed. More rarely, so did lead nipple shields: the makers described how the 'nipple will be bathed in a solution of lead' – very anti-microbial, but also very unhealthy for babies,[1213] though the advertising says the reverse.

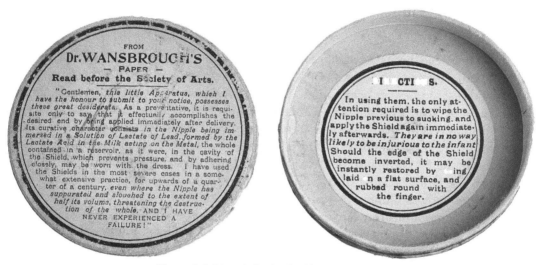

Figure 3-9-1 Lead nipple shield instructions

It is perhaps typical of America's blind spot about infant feeding that the latter two causes are noted in Warren's prize-winning history of lead, but the role of artificial feeding – the major source[1214] of constant and ongoing infant lead exposure– is not even hinted at. The longstanding fact of lead from can solder in foods that were infants' sole daily diets goes unnoted.[1215] Yet that surge in lead poisoning deaths was uniquely North American. In countries where powdered formula was the norm, not liquid, no such dramatic increase was recorded. It cannot be attributed to the use of leaded petrol, which began in 1941, but increased only in the 1950s. The problem had begun decades before that, and there was

1211 Warren C. *Brush with death: a social history of lead poisoning* (Johns Hopkins University Press, 2000) A fact attributed to the 'phase-down of leaded gasoline'. Yet Warren attributed the rise in deaths to the use of lead paints, not gasoline. In my view canning technology better fits the time frame and exposure profile.

1212 ibid., p. 137. Many deaths from lead poisoning were never diagnosed as such, as the symptoms were varied and convulsions often attributed to other causes, such as meningitis or influenza.

1213 Dr Mavis Gunther told me of her struggle to get rid of these from the wards of her London hospital: though they had been condemned, some midwives kept hiddden supplies which they surreptitiously used: then as now there were power struggles between doctors and other staff.

1214 Dabeka RW, McKenzie AD. Lead and cadmium levels in commercial infant foods and dietary intake by infants 0-1 year old. (PMID:3396737) *Food Addit Contam* 1988; 5(3):333-342

1215 Warren C, op. cit.

no notable increase in child deaths from lead poisoning when leaded petrol use increased markedly. Lead contamination was also surely relevant both to contemporary US concerns about declining IQ, and to lifelong cognitive capacity, as lead is a cumulative toxin. Some of those lead-exposed 1950s babies are now early Alzheimer's cases.

Lead in paint was finally outlawed in the United States only in 1977, after the paint industry had changed to using cheaper ingredients, although neighbouring Canada had banned it in the1920s.[1216] But lead paint persists everywhere in the built environment, as a risk to children and renovators alike. Yet there has been almost no paediatric death from lead poisoning[1217] since the time that lead solder was removed from liquid infant formula and evaporated milk cans, in the mid to late 1970s. (Can-making had moved to using plasticised linings that instead leached into formulas a substance known as BPA (see page 301) another chemical which would cause great controversy before it too was finally removed).

The allowable lead limits have since been lowered drastically; in fact in 2003 the US Environmental Protection Agency (EPA) declared lead to be 'a potent neurotoxin for which no safety threshold has yet been found'. Yet a 2004 congressional hearing documents that the problem persists: Washington DC had been horrified to learn that in the twenty-first century lead levels in drinking water were above mandated standards, and some parents able to afford testing found their children to have blood levels well above the theoretically acceptable limits.[1218] Washington DC is a predominantly black city with a substantial number of low-income families. How many families are low-income because their cognitive and earning potential was blunted by lead and copper decades or a generation before? Being low-income compounds the damage done to children exposed to lead where, and while, the official tolerance limits were so high and regulatory agencies so slack. There must be adults still struggling with the consequences, who most probably have no idea of the cause of their brain dysfunction and susceptibility to illness.

All artificially fed babies of families living with neighbourhood lead pipes are certainly still at risk from their water supply: a small sample of Boston homes found that

> Two of the 40 samples (5 per cent [95 per cent CI: 2.0, 18.2 per cent]) had lead concentrations above 15 micrograms/L, the current action level for safe water according to the Environmental Protection Agency. The two samples with lead concentrations of 17 and 70 micrograms/L were prepared using cold tap water (water run for 5 and 30 sec, respectively) drawn from the plumbing of houses greater than 20 years old.[1219]

And two Canadian infants are recorded as suffering lead poisoning because of the solder in the kettles used to boil water: another unsuspected and avoidable hazard of artificial

1216 Graef JW, Shannon M. Would breast-feeding decrease risks of lead intoxication? *Pediatrics*, 1992; 90 (1):132

1217 Other than a child known to eat lead paint chips. And not all parents permitted their children to gnaw on painted surfaces!

1218 Detection of lead in the DC drinking water system. Hearing before the Sub-Committee on Fisheries, Wildlife, and Water of the Committee on Environment and Public Works, US Senate 108th Congress, second session April 7, 2004. Available online www.gpo.gov/fdsys/pkg/CHRG.../html/CHRG-108shrg94604.html

1219 Baum CR, Shannon MW. The lead concentration of reconstituted infant formula. (PMID: 9204097) *J Toxicol Clin Toxicol*, 1997, 35(4):371–5

feeding.[1220] Lead glazes on pottery and lead crystal glasses are other potential sources of lead intake.

The problem of contaminated drinking water in developed countries is not isolated to America, of course. As recently as 2012, a child in Port Pirie, South Australia, died of lead poisoning simply because her mother made up the day's infant formula first thing every morning, after the house water had stood in lead pipes overnight.[1221] Sydney researchers showed significant levels in older houses, due no doubt to older plumbing supplying them. They said:

> It would appear that unless the infant consumed 100 per cent of first flush water at lead concentrations of approximately 100 micrograms/L, the blood lead would not exceed the recommended 'level of concern'. However, if more than 500 ml of first flush water was consumed in drinks and formulae, then the blood lead could easily exceed the recommended level. Likewise, a pregnant mother could be at risk of consuming considerably more than the 0.5l/day first flush water of the concentrations measured, or throughout the day, if the system were not fully flushed.[1222]

Household water supplies should not be assumed to be safe when a baby's brain is at stake. In America a 13 month old infant was lead-intoxicated because the "first draw" water contained 130parts per billion of lead; the clinicians reporting this stated flatly that

> "Whenever infants are fed powdered formula, consideration should be given to analysis of the home tap water."1223

After all, some infants routinely consume a litre or more of formula per day, not just 500 ml, for months. That could add up to brain damage if lead is at such concentrations. In any location where smelters are emitting fumes containing lead (as in South Australia's Port Pirie), town water and child blood lead levels need to be monitored: blood levels as low as 5mcg/dL put children at risk of intellectual deficits and behavioural problems, and in Port Pirie in 2012, 23.5 per cent of children up to four years old had blood lead levels above 10mcg/dL.[1224]

In Washington in 1975, when the then-accepted risk level was set at 30mcg per day, the range of lead in infant formula was 50-500micrograms per litre, while breastfed babies' range of lead intake was zero to 25micrograms. Appallingly, an EPA report makes it clear that the problem in Washington DC had not been solved by 2003, almost twenty years later. Residents were advised as follows:

---

1220  Ng R, Martin DJ. Lead poisoning from lead-soldered electric kettles. (PMID: 837317) *Canadian Medical Association Journal*, 1977, 116(5):508–9, 512

1221  http://www.abc.net.au/news/2012-05-24/blood-lead-levels-port-pirie/4030402

1222  Gulson BL, James M, Giblin AM, Sheehan A, Mitchell P. Maintenance of elevated lead levels in drinking water from occasional use and potential impact on blood leads in children. (PMID: 9372633) *Sci Total E*1997, 205(2–3):271–5. DOI: 10.1016/S0048-9697(97)00198-8.

1223  Shannon M, Graef JW. Lead intoxication from lead-contaminated water used to reconstitute infant formula. *Clin Pediatr* 1989; 28:380-382.

1224  http://theconversation.edu.au/lead-poisoning-of-port-pirie-children-a-long-history-of-looking-the-other-way-8296

Because the source of lead found in drinking water is from lead service lines or household plumbing, levels are highest after water has been sitting in the pipes for a period of 6 hours or more. All District of Columbia consumers should use cold water for drinking or cooking, as hot water will contain higher levels of lead. Cold water should be heated on the stove for drinking or cooking.

For homes with non-lead service lines, flush water lines that have not been used for 6 hours or more by running the cold water (flush) for 60 seconds prior to using the water from a faucet for drinking or cooking; periodically remove and clean the strainer/aerator device on your faucet to remove debris.

In addition, if consumers believe they have a lead service line *[lead piping from the mains to your house; do you know what your hidden pipes are made of? And the mains in your street?]*, the following actions should be taken:

Draw water for drinking or cooking after another high water use activity such as bathing or washing your clothes so that a total of at least 10 minutes of flushing has occurred. (The large amount of water used will flush significant amounts of water from your home's pipes.)

Flush the faucet from which drinking water will be drawn by running the cold water tap for 60 seconds prior to use. Collect drinking water in a clean container and store in the refrigerator for use during the day.

Boston and other US city water supplies have similar warnings on their websites, and specifically advise that artificially fed infants are at risk; remediation programs exist that are designed to replace fittings that might be leaching lead. As noted earlier, lead levels in children have dropped since lead was removed from petrol, but any lead exposure is still a problem. Additionally, parents should be warned that old paint contains high lead levels. If renovating, they would do well to seal over old paint rather than to strip it back, thereby creating fine dust. Childcare centres may also need to be considered.

The First National Environmental Health Survey of Child Care Centers was conducted in licensed child-care centres that serve children under the age of six (DHUD, 2003). An estimated 14 200 or 14 per cent of licensed child-care centres have significant lead-based paint hazards. Centres in older buildings are more likely to have significant lead and asbestos hazards than those in newer buildings. In the United States, day-care centres where the majority of children are African American are likely to have significantly higher lead exposures and exposure to allergens than those where a majority of the children are Caucasian.

Water is only one route of exposure for children, but infants consume more by bodyweight than any other family member, at a time of maximum vulnerability, which makes safe drinking water essential. While most developed countries claim (naturally) that their water supplies present no problems, parents would do well to take sensible precautions. Some towns still have lead and asbestos cement piping, and who knows what is in their replacements? It may be fair enough not to be too worried about adult intakes, and the breastfeeding mother can generally relax knowing that her body acts to filter out many chemicals before they reach her milk, but a bottle-fed infant is like the dialysis patient, much more dependent on a pure water supply.

## Metals in milk: copper

Copper in small quantities has always been known to be necessary for humans, and so all infant formula has regulated amounts. Codex Alimentarius, the European Union (EU), and the UK all specify a minimum of 235mcg/L, and the US 400mcg/L; the EU and UK's maximal amount is 670mcg/L while the US has no maxima - and so Codex has a mere GUL (guidance upper limit) of 1200mcg/L. A 1983 study found that the range in infant formulas then on sale was from 10 to 2140mcg/L.[1225]

Problems arise when copper intake is excessive. All metals can present a problem in drinking water used for infant formula. In a new development in 1990s suburban Melbourne Australia, green water (due to high copper levels) required replacement water supplies to be home delivered. High copper levels are also a threat to health, which is why water from hot taps (which flows through copper piping) should never be used for drinking or cooking. Where water is acid, more copper will leach from pipes. A German case report of a boy (breastfed for just four weeks then bottle fed) with liver cirrhosis[1226] at thirteen months makes it clear that the combination of copper pipes and acidic water can harm even children in wealthy nations. In fact, ten years ago WHO set in train a review of copper levels for drinking water, which had been based only on the occurrence of acute gut disturbances, after

> 'Recent studies in rabbits have suggested a link between copper in drinking-water and Alzheimer disease. Levels in the rabbits' drinking water were well below the current WHO guideline of 2 mg/litre, based on acute gastrointestinal effects; however, it has not been established whether rabbits are an appropriate model. In addition, a communication received by WHO Headquarters suggested the need to review the guideline value and text on copper with regard to toxicity in the preparation of formula for bottle-fed infants.'[1227]

I haven't found the results of this review as yet.

## Metals in milk: aluminium, manganese

Lead and copper are not the only metals of potential concern for infants consuming infant formula. Shockingly high levels of aluminium have been found for decades in the most highly processed formulas, those for preterm and sick infants – up to 40 times that in breastmilk. A study published online in 2010 said very bluntly,

---

1225 Lönnerdal B, Keen CL, Ohtake M, Tamura T. op. cit.

1226 Bent S, Böhm K. Copper-induced liver cirrhosis in a 13-month-old boy. (PMID: 8527884) *Gesundheitswesen* 1995; 57(10):667–9

1227 www.who.int/entity/water_sanitation_health/dwq/chemicals/copper/en See WHO (2003) *Copper in drinking-water. Background document for preparation of WHO Guidelines for drinking-water quality.* http://www.who.int/water_sanitation_health/dwq/chemicals/copper.pdf?ua=1 Geneva, World Health Organization (WHO/SDE/WSH/03.04/88). To find the latest statements, search the WHO site for Chemical hazards in drinking-water – copper: www.who.int/entity/water_sanitation_health/dwq/chemicals/copper/en

There has been a long and significant history documenting the contamination of infant formulas by aluminium [3–9] and consequent health effects in children [10–13]. Through these and other publications manufacturers of infant formulas have been made fully aware of the potentially compounded issue of both the contamination by aluminium and the heightened vulnerability, from the point of view of a newborn's developing physiology, of infants fed such formulas. There have been similar warnings over several decades in relation to aluminium toxicity and parenteral [intravenous] nutrition of preterm and term infants [14–17]. To these ends the expectation would be that the aluminium content of current infant formulas would at the very least be historically low and at best would be as low as might be achieved for a processed product. We have tested this premise and we have found that the aluminium content of a range of branded infant formulas remains too high ...

The aluminium content of infant formulas measured herein are not significantly different to historical values and this lack of improvement in lowering their content suggests either that the manufacturers are not monitoring the aluminium content of their products or that the manufacturers are not concerned at these levels of contamination ...

It is clear that aluminium in infant formulas is a significant component of early life exposure to this ubiquitous contaminant and as such every effort should be made by manufacturers to reduce the aluminium content of these products to an achievable practical minimum while at the same time manufacturers should be compelled to indicate the level of contamination by aluminium on the packaged product ...

Infant formulas are integral to the nutritional requirements of preterm and term infants. While it has been known for decades that infant formulas are contaminated with significant amounts of aluminium there is little evidence that manufacturers consider this to be a health issue. Aluminium is non-essential [25] and is linked to human disease [22]. There is evidence of both immediate and delayed toxicity in infants, and especially preterm infants, exposed to aluminium, and it is our contention that there is still too much aluminium in infant formulas.[1228]

Researchers at the University of Keele also thought so, when they "discovered levels exceeding the European recommendation for drinking water in some of the country's most popular products."[1229] though everyone instantly moved to reassure parents that the doses in UK formulas were below levels of concern about toxicity. But that's almost beside the point when dealing with any mineral given to young babies: the concern is about how traces may affect long term development and how traces accumulate over a lifetime. When aluminium can be used in municipal water supplies, the bottlefed child is at risk.

If it were easy to prevent or remove the aluminium, the formula companies would have done it by now. Obviously it can't be done. But again, whenever health professionals urge mothers to use fortifiers to adulterate their breastmilk for prems, or suggest infant formula, is this contamination taken into consideration?

---

1228 Burrell SA, Exley C. There is (still) too much aluminium in infant formulas (MED:20807425) BMC *Pediatrics*, 2010, 10:63. DOI: 10.1186/1471-2431-10-63
1229 Astley M. Danone, BSNA, FSA attempt to dispel infant formula aluminium contamination concerns. *Dairy Reporter* 11 October 2013.

So-called fortifiers and highly processed, complicated formulas are the most likely to contain significant levels of minerals like aluminium. Much formula nowadays is assembled from a global menu of previously created dairy product fractions and vitamin pre-mixes and so on, rather than being created from whole milk. I have been told that the processing environment needed to fractionate milk or to produce multi-mixes of vitamins and minerals will contribute traces, including aluminium, as will the formula manufacturing environment. One American recall in the 1980s was due to defective vitamin pre-mix not well-enough checked by the recipient formula company. Soy formula is often singled out in discussions of aluminium contamination, because soybeans absorb aluminium from soils. For more on soy formula, (see page 38) Preterm and exempt infant formulas absorb metals from the manufacturing environments. And when many brands of formula are actually packaged in foils containing aluminium, this may contribute to the problem.

Manganese is another metal that soybeans tend to concentrate from soil. There can be several hundred times more manganese[1230] in formula than in breastmilk, even two thousand times.[1231] How safe is that for even six months' intake, when manganese is neurotoxic in excess, and suspected of being a factor in neurological disorders. A review in 2013 identified one pathway for such damage ('inhibition of DNA-damage-induced poly (ADP-ribosylation in human astrocytes by exposure-relevant Mn concentrations', if you need to know) and concluded that 'in terms of Mn [Manganese] the existing guidelines for infant formula, but also drinking water, should be critically reconsidered'[1232] (see page 376). And enforced, perhaps?

Yes, manganese is essential and in the infant formula regulations everywhere. Codex and the UK both specify a minimum of 6-7mcg/L; the US minimum is five times that at 33mcg/L. The UK's maximal amount is 1000mcg/L while the US has no maxima - and so Codex has a mere GUL (guidance upper limit) of 1200mcg/L. A 1983 study found that the range in infant formulas then on sale was from zero to 7800mcg/L.[1233]

As I looked for the evidence on which these wide ranges were based, I found the following 1985 statement by the Director of Paediatric Nutrition Research at Ross Laboratories. It left me breathless:

> The requirement for manganese is not known. The minimum of 5mcg/100kcal (33mcg/L) was used because it was the level found in milk-based formulas. The result of choosing the former mean level of milk-based formulas as the new minimum standard was that formula manufacturers had to supplement their formulas with manganese to ensure their products met this standard. The manganese level in human milk is very low, approximately 1.5mcg/100kcal.[1234] (10mcg/L)

1230 Ljung K, Palm B, Grandér M, Vahter M. High concentrations of essential and toxic elements in infant formula and infant foods – a matter of concern. *Food Chemistry*, 2011; 127(3):943–51
1231 *Food Chemical News* November 2, 1981, p. 2
1232 Bornhorst J, Meyer S, Weber T, Böker C, et al. Molecular mechanisms of Mn induced neurotoxicity: RONS generation, genotoxicity, and DNA-damage response. *Molec Nutr Food Research* 2013; 57(7):1255–69. DOI: 10.1002/mnfr.201200758
1233 Lönnerdal B, Keen CL, Ohtake M, Tamura T. Op cit.
1234 Benson JD. Nutrient Guidelines for Infant Formula. In AOAC *Proceedings* 1985, op. cit., p. 308-9.

How many other nutrient levels for infant formula were determined by accepting that *the level found in older outdated infant formula is the necessary minimum*? When will America update its Infant Formula Act regulations? When the industry tells the FDA that it can comply with the globally-accepted minima and maxima, perhaps?

## What water can add

Then, what about the drinking water used for making up powdered formula? Water quality for infant formula is a huge issue. First there is the simple fact that water supplies across any country can vary enormously. One sixth of America's water comes from groundwater and private wells. This can be enormously variable in quality and contaminants.

Most people are aware that fluoride levels vary between districts, but so do many other chemicals, if authorities care enough to do careful regional assays to find out. In Denmark, for example, levels of iodine obtained from fifty-five different locations varied more than a hundredfold, from less than 1 to 139 mcg/L. Similarly, the levels in the infant formulas they tested – made up with demineralised water – varied fourfold, from 37 to 138 mcg/L. As they said,

> Hence the final iodine content would depend heavily on the source of water used for preparation. We found that iodine in tap water was a major determinant of regional differences in iodine intake in Denmark. Changes in water supply and possibly water purification methods may influence the population iodine intake level and the occurrence of thyroid disorders.[1235]

Why do these formulas' iodine content vary so widely? Possibly dairy disinfectants such as iodophors [iodine-based sanitisers]. But water is of course used in formula manufacture: some processes start with rehydrating milk-derived powder, and so the quality of that water is important. And all equipment and containers are washed with water, and so on. Then in liquid feeds, the company uses local water to create the product, controlling the quality of that water. (There have been examples of water from contaminated wells[1236] being used by industry in the past, and no doubt the industry is more careful in these days of greater pollution and increased awareness.) The EU and UK regulations specify a range of 67 to 335mcg/L in formula, while Codex mandates a minimum of 67mcg/L and a GUL of 402 mcg/L, and the US Infant Formula Act allows a range of 34 -502 mcg/L.

But then parents do have to use their local water to reconstitute powder formula into a feed. Any excess of minerals or chemicals will add to the mandated excess[1237] in the formula powder. Water quality at every stage is important. Local water can be lacking in essential

---

1235 Pedersen, KM, Laurberg, P et al. Iodine in drinking water varies by more than 100-fold in Denmark. Importance for iodine content of infant formulas. *Eur J Endocrinol*, 1999; 140 (5):400–3

1236 *Food Chem News* 28 November 1983, p. 29

1237 Formula by design always contains more of almost everything than breastmilk, simply because what is there is less bioavailable, and has to last for the shelf-life of the product.

minerals, or over-mineralised,[1238] or contaminated, whether with arsenic (discussed in a later chapter in relation to rice; see page 523), jet fuel or residues from shale gas extraction. Perchlorate is a by-product of the petrochemical industry that harms thyroid development. It has been found in major brands, including US ones.[1239] Such contamination means that some water should not be used for infants. Pity families using wells in areas being mined for coal seam gas, or where mining or animal wastes are being stored, as they consider how to assess whether their groundwater has been affected. As of course it will be sooner or later. Clay pans crack when earth moves; piping leaks as it rusts out...

By way of response to concerns about water quality, the International Formula Council passed on the FDA suggestion that parents use bottled water,[1240] as though such water is risk-free and affordable! Bottled water could be as good as tap water, or it could be more contaminated, it may add more minerals, and it comes in plastic, which inevitably leaves residues. What is more, even seven litres a week – no allowance for washing, etc., – adds to the household bills considerably.

Further, one writer[1241] has pointed out that what formula-fed infants consume relative to their bodyweight is the equivalent of a 70 kg adult drinking 7 litres a day. Quality of water surely matters more to bottle-fed babies than any other person. Yet many discussions of water quality have considered the amount of contamination in tap water that could affect the breastfed baby, whose usually lower daily intake is filtered by his or her mother's body, barely mentioning the bottle-fed child consuming perhaps a litre of such water per day. Don't bottle-fed babies matter? Is it more important not to upset their parents than to protect the babies? The answer to that question perhaps depends on the fact that it is parents, not babies, who have purchasing power.

In fact, the quality of water being used for infant formula reconstitution remains a literal minefield of potential risks, despite anodyne reassurances from governments. More bore water than ever before is being sourced for municipal supplies, after the drought in south-east Australia showed how easily major cities could run out of adequate supplies. The controversial practice of 'fracking', forcing water laden with toxic chemicals into the ground to retrieve gas, will almost inevitably increase contamination risks to groundwater supplies – as well as lock away millions of gallons (per well), in fact billions[1242] of gallons of scarce drinking water underground up to a mile or more below the water table, where

---

1238 Fluoride remains controversial for many. An objective overview of concerns can be found in Cheng KK, Chalmers I, Sheldon TA. Adding fluoride to water supplies. *BMJ* 2007; 335: 699-702. The Cochrane review on this has been widely misquoted.
1239 Schier JG, Wolkin AF, Valentin-Blasini L, Belson MG et al. Perchlorate exposure from infant formula and comparisons with the perchlorate reference dose. (PMID: 19293845) *J Expo Sci Environ Epidemiol,* 2010; 20(3):281–7.
1240 http://www.infantformula.org/news-room/press-releases-and-statements/infant-formula-and-perchlorate
1241 Jelliffe & Jelliffe op. cit., p.97.
1242 Goldenberg S. *Fracking is depleting water supplies in America's driest areas, report shows.* Online at http://www.theguardian.com/environment/2014/feb/05/fracking-water-america-drought-oil-gas?CMP=ema_632

it may never be retrievable.[1243] As noted on page 524, mining wastes have already caused concerns about New Zealand dairy products, and Fonterra has been forced to act to limit the potential damage to its market share, and also discard 150,000 litres of milk from cows grazing on contaminated pastures.

Local pipe networks and household plumbing can include lead, asbestos cement, and plastics, all of which can leach chemicals. In the Iwantja Australian Aboriginal community, piping newly installed in 1999 was decommissioned after only six months, when lead was found to be leaching into the water from the plastic pipes.[1244] Any bottle-fed babies and young children would have been adversely affected, but this is unlikely to be noted on the child's health record, which has no space for recording potential environmental exposures. I'd encourage parents to add such details, and seek recompense for any children with learning difficulties..

Recently there has been widespread concern about the discovery in water supplies of perfluorooctanoic acid or PFOA,[1245] a persistent chemical that even in low doses is considered dangerous, because it accumulates in the blood and is slow to degrade. While this may well contaminate breastmilk, the dose for the formula-fed child would be far greater. As is the dose of lithium and boron,[1246] or indeed virtually any chemical authorities care to test for. While women worry about breastmilk passing on chemicals to their babies, as indeed they may have reason to at times, they forget that their adult bodies usually act as filters and de-toxifiers as well as immune and nutritional support systems. Their formula-fed baby would be on his or her own, and drinking close to a litre each day of unfiltered water and variable formula. Obviously bottle-feeding parents who can afford to do so should buy a top quality water filter, and make sure it is well-serviced, as filters too can be a source of contamination.

Those of us who have lived long enough have experienced many problems with water quality due to both climatic variability and human error. Many country towns have water supplies of varying quality; rainwater tanks have multiple problems (city dwellers are advised not to use them for drinking water, while country folk depend on them); water supplies get contaminated by chemicals; chlorophenols formed during disinfection treatments can

---

1243 And is in any case poisonous, loaded with toxic chemicals, so that retrieving and cleaning it would be impossibly expensive. Read Ch. 10 in Steingraber's *Raising Elijah*, op. cit., for an excellent exposé of just what fracking means. She talks of a million or more gallons of water per wellhead per year being permanently lost, and as much needing to be stored in safe depositories above ground, so contaminated that it would be toxic to soil and water and life. Already in America leaks from storage sites have poisoned water supplies. And in Australia ground water has been contaminated with arsenic and uranium: http://www.smh.com.au/environment/santos-coal-seam-gas-project-contaminating-aquifer-in-use-after-two-years-20140310-34h9f.html

1244 Willis E, Pearce M, Jenkin T, Wadham B, McCarthy, C. Indigenous engagement with modernity: domestic water supply, risk and reflexive modernization. *TASA Conference, University of Western Australia & Murdoch University, 4–7 December 2006.* Online at http://www.tasa.org.au/conferences/conferencepapers06/papers/Indigenous%20issues,race,%20ethnicity%20and%20migration/Willis,etal.pdf.

1245 Post GB, Cohn PD, Cooper KR Perfluorooctanoic acid (PFOA), an emerging drinking water contaminant: A critical review of recent literature. (PMID: 22560884 *Environmental Research*, 2012; 116:93–117

1246 Harari F, Ronco AM, Concha G, Llanos M etal. Early-life exposure to lithium and boron from drinking water. (PMID: 23017911) *Reprod Toxicol* 2012; 34(4):552–60

be hazardous; run-off from grazed areas can lead to nitrate and giardia problems ... the list is endless. For more about the problem of safe water for artificial feeding in Australia, read John Archer's books,[1247] and the definitive Nestlé text on water for bottling.[1248] But these risks are today small, compared with the risks faced by those who have no access to sanitation or water-treatment plants, for whom artificial feeding is often lethal. And they may come to seem trivial in future, if the coal seam gas industry is allowed to go ahead: let's hope enough farmers lock the gates![1249]

Water poses many risks, some large, some small, and all mostly unknown to parents who are so trusting about the safety of their municipal water supply for infant feeding. I was shocked to be told that when certain procedures are undertaken by water authorities, advance notice is given to all those known to be reliant on renal dialysis machines, as the excess chemical load could damage the machines' sensitive filtration systems. No advance notice is given to the parents of babies with sensitive filtration systems, in a nation where kidney disease has increased exponentially over the twentieth century. Nor does anyone suggest they check their water reticulation supply for lead or copper or asbestos cement piping, often found in older areas where water authorities have not had the resources to renew the infrastructure. In some cases the problem is the tap housing itself, and this can readily be fixed, but plumbing work is not cheap. Again, the brains and bodies of rich people's babies will be better protected than those of the poor. Another piece of the poverty trap?

## Radiation by-products

Radioactivity was another unrecognised additive to, or contaminant of, both breastmilk (widely reported) and infant formula (rarely publicised) in the postwar period. Although few Americans seem conscious of it, nuclear testing had caused widespread and unpredictable fallout right across their country, and killed many workers in the industry.[1250] Only many decades later was any compensation made available.

According to the US National Cancer Institute in 1992, about 150 million curies of radioactive iodine was released in open air from nuclear testing in Nevada, causing heavy contamination of the nation's milk supplies from the early 1950s to the early 1960s. At the time of open-air testing, millions of children were drinking this contaminated milk. Estimates of relative cancer risk due to this fallout have since been published, [1251] but secrecy surrounded the issue at the time.

Should radioactivity in milk have been a national concern? After the ratification of the Limited Test Ban Treaty in 1963, the US Food and Drug Administration established 'Protective Action Guides' for Iodine-131 that triggered removal of dairy products from

1247 Archer J. *The water you drink* (1996); *On the water front: making your water safe to drink* (1991), both from Pure Water Press, Sydney

1248 Dege N (ed). *Technology of bottled water*. Wiley-Blackwell 2011

1249 Lock the Gate Alliance is a national movement in Australia by landowners who want to refuse access to their property for coal seam gas mining. Their website is www.lockthegates.org.au.

1250 Michaels D. *Doubt is their product*. op. cit. Chapter 16 discusses the nuclear industry and its workers.

1251 Alvarez R. Nuclear testing and the rise of thyroid cancers. *Institute of Policy Studies*. 15 October 2012. http://www.ips-dc.org/articles/nuclear_testing_and_the_rise_of_thyroid_cancers#.UAY_KLeoH6s.email

human consumption following nuclear accidents. Had these limits been in place during the open-air nuclear testing in the 1950s and early 1960s, the NCI study indicates that milk supplies would have had to be removed from the markets for months at a time. The NCI admitted in testimony before the US Congress in 1998, after an investigation by the US Senate Governmental Affairs Committee, that it had suppressed this study for five years. The NCI also conceded this may have caused as many as 212,000 excess thyroid cancers[1252] ... not to mention leukaemia and other cancers.

Russian nuclear tests, and British nuclear testing in Australia and the Pacific, ended in 1963, but in places had created long-lasting contamination. Britain monitored radiation levels around its civilian nuclear power plants and advised against eating seafood from nearby shores. Accidents such as those at Three Mile Island and the Savannah River weapons plant[1253] in America and others in Russia added to the radiation burden and were documented as contaminating milk, river water, and local produce. French nuclear testing in the Pacific continued until 1974 despite widespread concern about radioactivity in the food chain. Even socially conservative groups like Australia's Nursing Mothers' Association were moved to protest strongly[1254] against fallout from French nuclear weapons testing contaminating breastmilk.

As a Reuters report said,

> Radiation is dangerous because it can cause changes or mutations in DNA, which may then go on to cause cancer. While the human body can repair DNA changes or damage, a person is only safe if the repair process happens faster than the time it takes for the damaged or mutated DNA material to replicate.

> Most experts agree that growing children and fetuses are most at risk because their cells divide at a faster rate than adults.

> They also consume more cows' milk than adults, putting them at further risk, said a Japanese scientist who treated victims of the atom bomb explosion in Hiroshima.

> 'Cows are like vacuum cleaners, picking up radioactive iodine that lands over a wide area of pasture, and then those particles very easily are concentrated and pass into the milk,' said the expert, who declined to be identified.

> 'This was what happened in Chernobyl, and unfortunately, information about the risk had not been supplied to parents.'[1255]

---

1252 ibid.
1253 Gould JA, Goldman BA. *Deadly deceit: low-level radiation, high level cover-up* (Four Walls Eight Windows, 1990). Infant morbidity and mortality rates are also discussed in relation to local nuclear power stations and their operation. Noted in *Food Chemical News* 21 May 1990 p. 50.
1254 Barnard J, Twigg K. *Nursing mums: a history of the Australian Breastfeeding Association 1964–2014* (ABA 2012) pp. 107–8
1255 See the Reuters website at:: http://www.reuters.com/article/2011/03/15/us-japan-nuclear-health-idUSTRE72E2JF20110315. Retrieved 27 March 2013

Just as it was not in America, despite American nuclear testing creating perhaps twenty times the fallout estimated to have been released by the Chernobyl nuclear accident. In fact, the Chernobyl explosions in 1986 caused widespread radioactive fallout across Europe, which affected pastures in formula-making countries such as France, Germany and Ireland. One reason Australian and New Zealand milk is sought for formula-making seems to be that the southern hemisphere and its grazing pastures have to date been seen as cleaner, less contaminated, at least since British and French and American nuclear testing ended.

Fortunately some of the radioactive particles created are relatively short-lived. Others are not. There were few reports of independent tests for radioactivity on milk products, although after Chernobyl, infant formula products exported to the Philippines contained measurable amounts of radiation, and were rejected. Similarly in 1993 it was reported in the *Weekend Australian* that radioactive Lithuanian milk caused Bangladesh to order the return of Dutch formula.[1256] (Australia did not test imports from the same sources. So there was no radioactivity? Authorities will never see what they don't want to look for.)

As late as December 2011 infant formula was recalled in Japan due to the discovery of radioactive caesium in the product, probably due to the Fukushima accident.[1257] It was suggested that radioactivity was introduced by the hot air used to spray-dry milk powder (as bacteria can be) but of course the radioactivity could also have come from any of the many foodstuffs used in industrial formula manufacture. Caesium, for example, has a half-life of thirty years, which means that in thirty years half of what was present will have decayed away, while the other half remains. And is dangerous.

Fomon in 1974 reported that Strontium 90 (half-life 29 years) accumulates in cows' milk, and in formulas made from cows' milk; and that if a pregnant woman is exposed, by fallout or by diet, Strontium 90 is deposited in her baby's growing bones.[1258] A mother's milk contains only about one-tenth of the Strontium 90 in her diet. Studies by leading UK scientists in the 1960s indicated that breastfeeding mobilises Strontium 90 from the baby's bones, allowing it to be excreted, and so reduces the overall infant body burden.[1259] A breastfed baby's levels of radioactive contamination decline; a formula-fed baby's remain higher. An American study of teeth showed that the longer the baby breastfed, the lower the level of Strontium 90.[1260]

---

1256 18–19 September 1993; cited in *ALCA News*, 1993; 4(3):95. Such reports rarely give company names. The product was sent to several countries; only Bangladesh was noted as returning it, perhaps because the others did not test imports for radioactivity.

1257 Caesium found in formula by Japan's Meiji. *Reuters.* 6 December 2011. http://www.medscape.com/viewarticle/754925

1258 Fomon SJ (1974), op. cit., p. 395-6.

1259 Harrison GE, Sutton A, Shepherd H, Widdowson EM. Strontium balance in breast-fed babies. (PMID:14275943) *Br J Nutr*, 1965; 19:111–17.; Widdowson EM, McCance RA, Harrison GE, Sutton A. Effect of giving phosphate supplements to breast-fed babies on absorption and excretion of calcium, strontium, magnesium, and phosphorus. (PMID:14066845) *Lancet*, 1963; 2(7320):1250–1

1260 Rosenthal HL, Austin S, O'Neill S, Takeuchi K et al. Incorporation of fallout Strontium 90 in deciduous incisors and fetal bone. *Nature* 1964; 203: 615.

Breastfeeding reduces cancer risks for both mother and child by this and other means, such as the cells , p. 395-6hat trigger apoptosis (programmed cell death) in cancer cells.[1261] Those cells have since been shown to make multi-drug resistant bacteria once again sensitive to antibiotics[1262] and capable of being killed: another story that was not widely reported but caused great excitement for those worried about MRSA (methicillin-resistant Staphylococcus aureus)! What would the publicity have been for an industry-produced 'novel antimicrobial adjuvant with the potential to increase the clinical usefulness of antibiotics against drug-resistant strains of S. aureus'? And what price would parents pay for a patented product that could mobilise some of the radioactivity from their baby's bones?

## Chemical pollution of breastmilk and formula

Contamination of infant foods has been a hot topic, generating concern globally. Toxic chemicals are by now ubiquitous in the environment. Which of course means that humans are contaminated, and so breastmilk will be. Parents hear a great deal about breastmilk contamination, and very little about formula contamination – why?

Environmental groups wanting to draw attention to the degradation of the environment will often dramatise the inescapable and widely reported fact of pesticides in breastmilk in attention-grabbing press releases. They seem unaware that Governments test breastmilk mostly because it is an easily accessible source of human body fat, where many toxic chemicals accumulate, and so can help assess overall exposures of humans, the top of the global food chain. Information about breastmilk contamination is thus more readily available, free, than data about levels of contamination in infant formulas. There is also no legal risk in slandering breastmilk, while telling damaging truths about formula might upset some very wealthy interests with expensive lawyers on staff. (Something I am conscious of.)

Some environmental groups also seem to share the popular myths that infant formula has always been highly regulated and inspected, and is less contaminated than breastmilk. Smoking mothers in particular have been made to feel that their milk is dirty and dangerous stuff. Some environmentalists fail to realise that cows are subject to contamination from many sources of agricultural and veterinary chemicals. *Modern Meat*[1263] told of automatic sprays of pesticide as cows went in and out of milking parlours, for example. What pesticides? Did milk buyers know about this practice? Who tested for them? What cleaning products? Commonly used iodophor disinfectants led to high levels of iodine in milk, an inadvertent public health benefit reducing rates of goitre; although since the 1980s the dairy industry has worked to reduce what became at times excessive levels, which caused thyroid

1261 Rammer P, Groth-Pedersen L, Kirkegaard T, Daugaard M et al. BAMLET activates a lysosomal cell death program in cancer cells. (PMID: 20053771) *Mol Cancer Ther* 2010, 9(1):24–32. DOI: 10.1158/1535-7163.MCT-09-0559

1262 Marks LR, Clementi EA, Hakansson AP. Sensitization of *Staphylococcus aureus* to methicillin and other antibiotics in vitro and in vivo in the presence of HAMLET. PLoS One, 2013; 8(5): e63158. DOI:10.1371/journal.pone.0063158

1263 Schell O. *Modern Meat*. Random House, 1984

disease.[1264] Perhaps the biggest companies infallibly conduct the batteries of tests needed to ensure the milk they use in formula is not affected by such chemicals – but it's certain that many formula producers globally could not afford to do so. The reality of independent government testing is described in Chapter 3.10 .

There are many possible avenues of contamination of cows' milk, and some of those contaminate mothers' milk. For most of the twentieth century the dioxins in human mothers' milk came from the bleached paperboard[1265] used in cartons of cows' milk drunk by those mothers on medical advice! Throughout the 1980s *Food Chemical News* documented some of the difficulties of ensuring cows' milk is free from contamination from stock feed – issues included both the presence of aflatoxins in feed and the use of gentian violet in feed[1266] to prevent moulds proliferating – and sulfamethazine residues[1267] and penicillin were also of concern when found in milk, penicillin triggering eczema in one case on record.[1268] But the multiple routes of exposure to contaminants are best summarised in this diagram, based on a chapter in the book aptly titled *The health hazards of milk.*[1269]

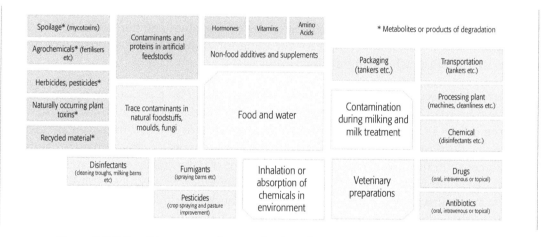

Figure 3-9-2 Possible sources of contamination of cows' milk © Catherine Horsfall.

Natural pastures too, can pose problems. Rohrbach reported in 1925 on seven infants whose symptoms disappeared when the cows' feed was changed, in one case from hillside grazing to meadowland. He always enquired about bovine diet, and had "great satisfaction in observing many a seriously sick infant become normal in a short period if the offending

1264 *Dunsmore DG, Wheeler SM. Iodophors and iodine in dairy products 8: the total industry situation. Aust J Dairy Tech 1992; 32(4)*

1265 Ryan JJ, Shewchuk C, Lau BPY, Sun WF. Polychlorinated dibenzo-p-dioxins and polychlorinated dibenzofurans in Canadian bleached paperboard milk containers (1988–1989) and their transfer to fluid milk . *J Agric Food Chem*, 1992; 40(5):919–923. DOI: 10.1021/jf00017a045

1266 This was the concern that ultimately led to gentian violet becoming hard to source in Australia, though it can still be bought over the counter in America and many other countries.

1267 *Food Chemical News*, multiple entries in 1988; check the index of this rarely held journal.

1268 David TJ. *Food and food additive intolerance in childhood.* (Blackwell Scientific Publications 1993) p. 40. Diagram by Catherine Horsfall.

1269 Freed DLJ. (ed) *Health hazards of milk* (Bailliere-Tindall 1984)

food was eliminated from the diet given to the dairy cattle."[1270] When smallholders had a house cow, this awareness of bovine diet was common.

Once the cows are milked, much more processing lies ahead before infant formula reaches babies. Even now, many people still seem not to realise that all industrial processes will leave traces in the resulting product. The more processing, inevitably the more contamination, even though companies doubtless work hard to keep it down. Only recently an industry audit of the chemicals which contact processed food was undertaken. It was reported that many chemicals of concern (COCs)[1271] were in use, many "classified as carcinogenic, mutagenic or reprotoxic. Others are considered to interfere with the hormone system, so called endocrine disruptors. A third group of chemicals is considered persistent and bioaccumulative." The problem needed to be addressed by industry.

Pesticide contamination of breastmilk is of real concern, not so much to the individual child, but because of what it says about Western use of dangerous chemicals in our environment. But unless the mother is so heavily contaminated as to be toxic, it is no reason to formula-feed. To swap a *possible* risk for *certain* harms is not good decision-making. The most brilliant writing on this topic comes from Sandra Steingraber, and her books *Having Faith* and *Raising Elijah* should be compulsory reading for all health professionals, politicians, and envirnmentalists who denigrate breastmilk.

Mothers still perceive chemical pollution of breastmilk to be a serious risk, even though the levels recorded in all milk have dropped steadily over decades, as awareness has grown. Research in one severe contamination problem referred to as The Firemaster Incident[1272] showed that despite what were very extreme exposures of breastfeeding women to chemicals likely to cause brain insult, their children were not disadvantaged when compared with formula-fed children not exposed to the local contamination.[1273] (Which I think means they were harmed – just no more than they would have been if formula-fed! But then I consider breastfed babies the human norm, not the bottle-fed ones.) Infants exposed to high levels in utero were not so fortunate, showing evidence of developmental damage. There is a qualitative difference between being exposed in utero and postpartum, and breastmilk provides many mitigating factors the pregnancy woman's body cannot.

What do international experts say about this issue of environmental pollution and infant health? It is an issue of concern, but they never advise artificial feeding as the solution. Rather, they find that breastfeeding reduces the harms. Read the following excerpt from an authoritative report created within the framework of the Inter-Organization Programme for the Sound Management of Chemicals (IOMC):

---

1270 David op cit., p. 40.

1271 Geueke B, Wagner CC, Muncke J. Food contact substances and chemicals of concern: a comparison of inventories. *Food Addit Contam Part A Chem Anal Control Expo Risk Assess*. 2014;31(8):1438-50. doi: 10.1080/19440049.2014.931600. Epub 2014 Jul 7. Report and summary at http://www.foodpackagingforum. org/news/hazardous-substances-in-food-contact

1272 Chen E. *PBB: an American tragedy* (Prentice Hall, 1979). See also Jelliffe, *Adverse effects of foods*, op cit., ch. 11.

1273 Gladen BC, Rogan WJ, Hardy P, Thullen J, et al. Development after exposure to polychlorinated biphenyls and dichlorodiphenyl dichloroethene transplacentally and through human milk. (PMID: 3142988) *J Pediatr*, 1988; 113(6):991–5

Studies of newborns suggest that lower levels of PCB exposure can affect a number of newborn behaviours. Exposed infants are more likely to exhibit signs that are consistent with immaturity of the central nervous system (e.g. increased startle response, abnormal reflexes) (Rogan et al., 1986; Huisman et al., 1995). In a longitudinal investigation in the United States of infants born to mothers who consumed fish contaminated with low-level PCBs, investigators found early recognition memory deficits in exposed infants, poorer scores on a preschool IQ test, and reduced verbal IQ and reading comprehension at 11 years of age (Jacobson & Jacobson, 2002a,b). The authors also found that adverse effects of developmental PCB exposure were observed less frequently in breastfed infants, suggesting a protective influence of breastfeeding on the behavioural development of exposed infants [my emphasis]. Further studies of this cohort at 11 years of age have found evidence of increased impulsivity as well as deficits in concentration and working memory in exposed children (Jacobson & Jacobson, 2003). Again, adverse effects were primarily seen in subjects who had not been breastfed [my emphasis]. A study from the Netherlands found that prenatal PCB exposure was related to longer and more variable reaction times in childhood, suggesting persistent deficits in basic cognitive processes (Vreugdenhil et al., 2004). Although these studies and others provide significant evidence of a relation between low-level PCB exposure and intellectual impairment, some studies have not observed such effects, and the relationship between PCB exposure and deficits in childhood cognition remains controversial (Gladen & Rogan, 1991; Gray et al., 2005) [1274]

Women worried about possible breastmilk contamination can take some control of this problem. They can have some idea of their own level of risk by assessing their lifetime exposure, and they can find out by testing if they feel that they have real reason to be concerned. They can reduce their risk by using fewer toxic chemicals within their own environments, getting rid of environmental tobacco smoke, and sourcing less contaminated food and water. They can take comfort in the studies that show so many positive factors in breastmilk that help their infant develop normally. By contrast, mothers feeding artificially have no knowledge of, or control over, contamination risks in infant formulas that originate in multiple food sources mostly in another country or countries. Nor can most control the purity of the water supplies needed to make formula, much less the feeding equipment. And any contaminants that challenge a bottle-feeding baby will not have been passed through an adult body and detoxifying liver before reaching the baby in breastmilk, an advantage the breastfeeding baby has!

Media reporting of risks has much to do with perception of risk. Headlines that might worry bottle-feeding mothers were not acceptable for much of the twentieth century, and sometimes strange things appeared in papers. One *Lancet* letter reported that microwaving cows' milk formula resulted in the formation of neurotoxic peptides formed from bovine protein.[1275] Somehow, this resulted in warnings on the front page of a Melbourne paper of the dangers of microwaving breastmilk. Yet the *Lancet* letter did not address breastmilk; breastmilk contains

---

1274 Environmental Health Criteria 237, *Principles for evaluating health risks in children associated with exposure to chemicals* (WHO 2006) p. 76 published jointly by WHO, UN Environment Programme, and the ILO. Online http://www.who.int/ipcs/publications/ ehc/ehc237.pdf
1275 Lubec G, Wolf C, Bartosh B. Amino acid isomerisation and microwave exposure. *Lancet*, 1989; 2(8676):1392–3

less total protein, not to mention different proteins; and breastfeeding mothers provide most of their milk warm and freshly made from a breast, not a microwaved bottle!

And infant exposure comes in many ways, to many chemicals. The IOMC went on to say:

> It is important to take into account the fact that ... the number of environmental chemicals that might affect the neurological development of children is increasing. Recently, cognitive effects have been shown for environmental tobacco smoke (Yolton et al., 2005), arsenic (Calderón et al., 2001; Wasserman et al., 2004), manganese (Wasserman et al., 2006), and some mixtures of arsenic and manganese (Wright et al., 2006).[1276]

As they said, ' based on the numerous advantages of breastfeeding, the benefits in the majority of cases by far exceed the potential risk (Kacew, 1992; Pronczuk et al., 2004).'[1277] Once people know more about the risks of artificial feeding of all kinds, including modern infant formula, that conclusion will be a no-brainer.

There is an important book to be written about toxic chemicals and infant feeding. Yes, major companies take pains to produce infant formula with as few toxic chemicals as humanly possible, and sometimes the levels of particular contaminants in infant formula can be lower than the levels in breastmilk. That is almost irrelevant in the balance of risks to infants. No one can test for every possible contaminant: note how Fonterra resolved the problem of the cost of testing for some ingredients of fracking waste (see page 524) disposed of in New Zealand fields. But such wastes will spread via water soil and air at different rates. How wide a margin of exclusion will be needed over time? And how will they check what any dairy farmer has done on his fields? it will not be in his interest to disclose the truth if asked, and some may not know what was done on newly-bought farms. Will Fonterra's existing tests for contaminants spot all of the many possible agricultural and mining chemicals? If so, why exclude any farmer's milk without testing? If not, how will they exclude contamination via groundwater?

No infant feeding product, breastmilk included, will be completely untainted by the environment. But no one tests for a chemical that should not be there, which is why melamine (and before it, boric acid and many other adulterants) could do so much harm to infants, as well as to dogs and other animals via feedstock. (Just recently another scandal surfaced about its use in calf feeds.) .There has been a double standard about what is said in print and on air, especially in mainstream media, which I am consciously ignoring for much of this book. But its existence is at the heart of parental ignorance about formula feeding. Articles about the (relatively minor) risks of a mother's less than totally ideal diet far outnumber articles about the diet of the cows that produce milk ending up as infant formula. But what about that bovine diet?

---

1276 *Environmental Health Criteria* 237, op. cit., p. 35
1277 ibid.

# Stock feed and contamination

Formula companies clearly have a strong vested interest in ensuring access to large supplies of high-grade milk. Securing these, even educating farmers about improving herd and milk quality, have always been important for major milk producers, as we saw in the very early days of evaporated milks. Yet what cows are fed is another issue not commonly considered in infant formula discussions. Where milk is concerned, the marketing image is of contented cows freely grazing on nutrient-rich pastures and producing perfect natural organic milk. The vast quantities of milk needed for global formula production annually could never be sourced from such idyllic scenes of free-ranging animals. Australia and New Zealand are unusual in having large herds of pasture-fed cows, but in fact a huge amount of lot feeding still goes on. And even when cows have access to pasture, their diet is supplemented in many different ways to increase ever-higher milk yields and to prevent disease. Just as with human mothers, what mother cow is exposed to and eats is reflected in her milk.

Cows are fed a wide range of products that can include not only cereals such as barley, wheat, corn, and so on, but also agricultural residues and crops deemed not fit for human consumption - such as those perhaps mould-toxin-laden peanuts, and 'rendered by-product' – animal protein sources from feathers to fats to faeces – chicken poo is particularly high in nitrogen! The future of stock feed is likely to involve the use of insects and bacteria as protein sources, going by recent industry news releases.[1278] Newspaper mixed with molasses can present problems if all staples are not first removed, but cows can digest cellulose, and the toxicity of the inks is not great enough to damage the short-lived cow, though traces will be found in her milk. Had cows not become unknowing carnivores, the problem of mad cow disease might never have surfaced: it was consuming scrapie-infected carcasses which almost certainly allowed the inter-species leap of prion diseases, and the devastating spread of brain-wasting Creutzfeldt-Jacob Disease, or CJD.[1279]

The importance of stock feed to human health is increasingly recognised by global authorities. WHO and FAO, the world health and agriculture arms of the UN, have organised a special conference on this topic for mid 2015. Even grass-fed animals can be at risk. In clean green New Zealand in 2014, 17 cows died of lead poisoning and 100 were destroyed after being allowed to graze fodder beet in a paddock leased by a gun club, and so lead-contaminated.[1280]

---

1278 Byrne J. 'Bacteria beats insects and algae hands down,' Nutrinsic CEO talks up new feed protein source from factory wastewater. *Feed Navigator,* 01-Aug-2014. http://www.feednavigator.com/Suppliers/Bacteria-beats-insects-and-algae-hands-down-Nutrinsic-CEO-talks-up-new-feed-protein-source-from-factory-wastewater.

1279 Cooke J. *Cannibals, cows and the CJD catastrophe* (Random House, 2000); Powell D, Leiss W. *Mad cows and mother's milk* (McGill-Queen's University Press, 1997)

1280 Cows' deaths on Southland farm linked to lead poisoning. *The Southland Times*, updated 6/9/2014. Online at Stuff.co.nz. © Fairfax Media.

DairyNZ has issued an advisory for southern dairy farmers after cows had become sick and in some cases died after grazing on swede crops. DairyNZ Southland/South Otago regional leader Richard Kyte said in the advisory to farmers the issue was only with swede crops and appeared to be widespread throughout Southland. Autopsies undertaken by local vet practices had, in some cases, shown severe liver damage and occasionally kidney damage, associated with the death. Further blood testing on some affected animals - which included all ages and classes of stock - had shown significantly elevated liver enzymes and compromised kidney function. (*Southland Times* © Fairfax Media)

The cow deaths prompted the investigation; were these cows being milked before they died? Not all companies would routinely test for lead in the milk of pasture-fed cows! (See also fracking wastes, page 524)

Let's be clear: this is not a reason to avoid NZ milk products. Such problems can occur anywhere; NZ has the capacity to notice and deal with them. The point being made is that EVEN in a clean green country like NZ, what cows eat affects their milk, and infant formula is made from cows' milk, about which parents have no knowledge. Animal fodder, natural or industrial, creates certain risks - which are entirely avoidable if the baby is breastfed. Among those are the risk of exposure to important and unknown allergens.

A stock-feed company's computer is programmed to create the 'least cost ration' from the variety of available inputs whose theoretical nutritional value and cost are known. So long as the final mix meets the theoretical calculated dietary needs of the cow, the product is deemed suitable. Obviously this means what cows eat varies with the price of commodities. So what is sampled in cows' milk varies. So it is almost impossible to know what antigens may persist in the milk, through a variety of processing techniques, into infant formula.

Yet when dealing with allergic families, what is in the milk they consume is a part of the problem. Sometimes, as I note elsewhere, cream from King Island in Bass Strait[1281] may be tolerated with only minor symptoms, whereas cream elsewhere causes reactions. Milk is not all the same, in cows or in people.

In the 1980s American allergy sufferers were importing Australian lamb as a low-allergen meat.[1282] Our sheep were not (then) corn or grain fed, unlike most US animals, so were safe for those allergic to corn and wheat. Animals live in our polluted environment, just as humans do, and their milk and meat reflects all that they are exposed to and eat, just like humans. Why was America the country where corn allergy was so severe that meat had to be imported? Why do Chinese parents hear so little about cows' diet, but so much about the breastfeeding mother's?

---

1281 op. cit. See page 331.
1282 Prof. John W Gerrard, personal communication.

# Stock feeds and allergy?

It seems reasonable to me that stock feeds may also be implicated in the rise of allergy to milk, perhaps together with that change in antigen intake via whey-dominant formulas discussed previously. It also seems reasonable to assume that if health professionals were unaware that the mammal mother's diet affects what her baby eats, so might be even the most careful of infant formula manufacturers.

But do manufacturers know what the cows have been eating? How far back does quality control go? If companies import milk fractions and other multi-mix ingredients internationally, and assemble infant formulas in another country (as some do) how possible is this? Is it likely that such companies always investigate or control the rations fed to make the milk itself?[1283] In the chapter on fats (see Chapter 3.6) I mentioned some of the changes stockfeed can produce in animals, whether fish or hens or cows. I also mentioned the concerns about mould toxins which can be found not only in peanuts, but maize (corn) and any other cereals fed to animals, sometimes because they are deemed unfit for human consumption due to moulds! Experts are concerned about complex cocktails of moulds reducing animal productivity;[1284] I am concerned about the persistence of mould toxins in their meat and milk. What is more, animals routinely eat foods humans would not: maggots may soon be on their menu.[1285] That could make interesting changes to their microbiome, surely.

And there is another concern: the use of antibiotics as growth promoters in animals. Very recently indeed, a study showed that the allowable level of a certain antibiotic in hen feed resulted in levels of the chemical in eggs that greatly exceeded notional safety limits for humans, and a call was made to reduce the maximum tolerable intake in the stock feed.[1286] But reducing the dose may lead to further problems of microbial resistance, of course. And ending antibiotics in animal feed seems light years away, even though there is increasing consensus that animal use is probably the single largest cause of the rise of the superbugs (multiply-resistant strains of pathogens that will see human epidemics return.) Global appeals for changes to agricultural practices are increasing.[1287] Denmark has significantly reduced the problem of multiply-resistant organisms by controlling non-veterinary use.[1288] Dairy factories do test for antibiotic residues, as these can seriously affect the use of the milk in say, cheese-making. But if all farmers willingly adhered to the suggested withholding

---

1283  Major companies do attempt to control milk *source*; I recommend mothers choose any needed infant formula only from a major company.

1284  Byrne J. 'We have seen complex cocktails in feedstuffs' - EU feed safety expert says mycotoxin legislation not strong enough. *Feed Navigator 10*-Jul-2014. http://www.feednavigator.com/Regulation/We-have-seen-complex-cocktails-in-feedstuffs-EU-feed-safety-expert-says-mycotoxin-legislation-not-strong-enough

1285  Byrne J. Insects and algae top the line-up in future feed ingredients for pigs. *Feed Navigator* 11-Jul-2014. http://www.feednavigator.com/R-D/Insects-and-algae-top-the-line-up-in-future-feed-ingredients-for-pigs

1286  Olejnik M, Szprengier-Juszkiewicz T, Jedziniak P. Semduramicin in eggs – incompatibility of feed and food maximum levels. *Food Chem.* 15 April 2014; 149:178–82. DOI: 10.1016/j.foodchem.2013.10.091.

1287  Haenlein O. Conference calls for responsible use of livestock antibiotics *Global Meat News.* Oct 3, 2014 http://www.globalmeatnews.com/Industry-Markets/Conference-calls-for-responsible-use-of-livestock-antibiotics

1288  Levy S. Reduced Antibiotic Use In Livestock: How Denmark Tackled Resistance. *Environ Health Perspect.* 2014;122(6); see also http://www.pewtrusts.org/en/research-and-analysis/issue-briefs/2010/11/01/avoiding-antibiotic-resistance-denmarks-ban-on-growth-promoting-antibiotics-in-food-animals

periods of 9-10 days in some cases, there would be little need for the antibiotics given to a mastitic or injured cow to include, as they do, tell-tale dyes that show up in milk. And the infant gut may be sensitive to even trace levels of antibiotics.

Some will dismiss this concern about intakes from stock feed as scaremongering, while being all too ready to tell human mothers that what they eat is reflected in their breastmilk, described by some as "toxic waste"(= not scaremongering?). Mothers can know a good deal about what they eat; and some can choose less polluted options. They cannot know what was eaten by the cows that gave the milk to make their baby's formula. Yet their fear of the results of inadequate human diet – a fear fostered by formula-can wording, formula advocates and some myopic environmentalists– leads some women to trust formula as safer for their baby.

In the early days when formula was still getting established, advertisements often claimed closeness to the milk of "healthy well-nourished women," quietly implying that the milk of poorly nourished women could be deficient. Women got the subliminal message and even well-nourished women still worry about whether their milk is good enough when their diet is not perfect (as it never is). The reality is that babies have thrived and will thrive on the milk of poorly nourished women, as long as the woman's body can make *enough* milk. If this were not so, there would be no population problem on the planet, for in many places under-nutrition is, and possibly always has been, endemic among women. Lactation, that fundamental human survival mechanism, is remarkably resilient. We would do better to feed mothers (and clean up the environment) than to fear their ability to feed their babies, making sure there is no obvious interference with milk production and transfer.[1289]

## Microbial contamination of formula products

Besides stockfeed, there is yet another invisible influence on cows milk, and thus formula. What microbes is the milk providing? What microbes survive or are added duirng industrial processing? No one can see bacterial loads or viruses or fungal spores! This was touched on earlier, but deserves further consideration. Complete sterility is impossible except in terminally sterilised liquid formulas. Contaminated before the can of powder is opened, and more contaminated afterwards: over the century, few parents realised that this was and is a risk for infant formula. Yet a 2008 review said,

> Powdered infant formula is not sterile and may be intrinsically contaminated [i.e., already contaminated before you open the can] with pathogens, such as Salmonella enterica, that can cause serious illness in infants. In recent years, at least 6 outbreaks of Salmonella infection in infants that have been linked to the consumption of powdered infant formula have been reported. Many of these outbreaks were identified because the Salmonella strains were unique in some way (e.g., a rare serotype) and a well-established Salmonella surveillance network, supported by laboratories capable of serotyping isolates, was in place. [*These infections are easily missed when those conditions don't exist ... or are denied*

---

1289  That so many western women have difficulty establishing and enjoying breastfeeding is tragic but not incurable, once it is accepted that this matters to the whole human race (not just the mother and baby, who rate very low on many societies' real operative priorities).

*as being due to the formula if the home environment contains a common strain.*] Another common feature of the outbreaks was the low level of salmonellae detected in the implicated formula (salmonellae may be missed in routine testing). 1290

The authors went on to say in science-speak that these recent multi-country outbreaks are likely to be the tip of a rather large and often unnoticed iceberg.[1291] It astonishes me that there are bloggers online who seriously assert that modern infant formula has never killed a baby in America or Australia or wherever! Of course some[1292] have a vested interest in saying so, but it really is outrageously ignorant and irresponsible. Cicely Williams would consider such bloggers complicit in infant deaths – and I do in maternal deaths as well.

Nor is Salmonella the only concern. A recent Chinese study[1293] found Staphylococcus aureus in both formula (over 11 per cent of those sampled) and baby rice cereals. There were multiple strains, over 80 per cent of which were antibiotic-resistant and contained multiple toxin genes. What is found usually depends on the willingness to look.

A 1988 study assessing 141 major formula brands from thirty-five countries – using the limited technology of the time– had found that over 50 per cent had low levels of organisms including Enterobacter spp, Citrobacter spp, E. coli, Klebsiella spp, and Hafnia alvei.[1294] That high contamination rate was recorded despite the fact that then current sampling methods were not very likely to detect pathogens, as they are not evenly distributed throughout the product![1295] And in 1988 health professional students were shocked when I taught them that powdered formula could never be sterile.

Formulas have also contained Clostridium botulinum, the anaerobic bacteria whose toxins can cause botulism, since linked with regressive autism. Recently a new Botulinum toxin has been identified in the faeces of an infected infant, so deadly that a mere 2 billionths of a gram will kill an adult.[1296] The possible presence of spores of Clostridium botulinum has led to a still current and much publicised ban on honey for children under twelve months old.[1297]

1290  Cahill SM, Wachsmuth IK, Costarrica Mde L, Ben Embarek PK. Powdered infant formula as a source of Salmonella infection in infants. (PMID: 18171262) *Clin Infect Dis,* 2008; 46(2):268–73. DOI: 10.1086/524737
1291  ibid.
1292  Such as those who could not breastfeed their own children, or who are involved in selling infant formula, for example. Check the CV of all those who comment, particularly the most emotive and obnoxious: one I checked turned out to be a pharmacy owner, a salient fact she failed to declare, instead noting her connection with a reputable association she did not in any way formally represent.
1293  Wang X, Meng J, Zhang J, Zhou T et al. Characterization of *Staphylococcus aureus* isolated from powdered infant formula milk and infant rice cereal in China. *Internat J Food Microbiol,* 2012; 153(1–20:142–7. http://dx.doi.org/10.1016/j.ijfoodmicro.2011.10.030
1294  Muytjens HL, Roelofs-Willemse H, Jaspar GH Quality of powdered substitutes for breast milk with regard to members of the family Enterobacteriaceae. (PMID: 3284901) *J Clin Microbiol,* 1988; 26(4):743–6
1295  Cetinkaya E, Joseph S, Ayhan K, Forsythe SJ. Comparison of methods for the microbiological identification and profiling of Cronobacter species from ingredients used in the preparation of infant formula. (PMID: 23089182) *Molec Cellular Probes,* 2012; 27(1):60-64. DOI: 10.1016/j.mcp.2012.10.003
1296  Mackenzie D. New botox super-toxin has its details censored. *New Scientist* 14 October 2013; citing *J Infect Dis* article, DOI: 10.1093/infdis/jit528
1297  Smith JK, Burns S, Cunningham S, Freeman J, et al. The hazards of honey: infantile botulism. *BMJ Case Reports,* 2010; 2010:239–42. (PMID: 22778374) DOI: 10.1136/bcr.05.2010.3038.

Whether contracted from formula[1298] – which parents rarely hear about – or from honey – which parents are warned about[1299] – botulism can be lethal.[1300] Once infected, artificially fed infants are more likely to be severely affected or to die than breastfed babies,[1301] who are almost protected by a different microbiome, and maternal provision of relevant immune factors in milk. (I rejoiced to hear contemporary icon P!nk describe herself in August 2013 as a walking antibiotic! That segment of the conversation was not included in the online text report of the interview – why not?)

Infant formula is in fact globally accepted as one of the vectors for Clostridial organisms,[1302] ubiquitous in soil and dust around the world, though fortunately only some species, such as C. botulinum and C. tetanii are both neurotoxic and lethal. Cases of botulism were often diagnosed as cot death, as the toxin is so fast acting and powerful in the conditions provided by an artificially fed infant's body. A vaccine to treat infected infants was due to be available in 1991, but the outbreak of the Bush Senior Gulf War meant supplies were restricted to the US Army (for protection from those mythical weapons of mass destruction). Supplies for infected American children became available only in 1992.[1303] Priorities.

After yet another formula recall in 2002, manufacturers had to consider as a matter of urgency both how to prevent formula powder inoculation with anaerobic bacterial or fungal spores, and how to prevent microbial growth in that powder (once thought impossible). Another bacterium, Enterobacter sakazakii, in 2007 renamed Cronobacter sakazakii, provoked more serious study once it was realised that some strains were able to survive in a desiccated state in the tin for more than two years, pretty much the whole shelf life of formula, and yet still multiply when water was added.[1304] Deaths from E. (or C.) sakazakii were first noted in the US in the 1980s, and in December 2011 US authorities were investigating the source of such infections in three formula-fed babies, one of whom died.[1305] This bacterial species is almost everywhere: eight of nine food factories, forty percent of locations (including air filters)

1298 Barash JR, Hsia JK, Arnon. SS Presence of soil-dwelling clostridia in commercial powdered infant formulas. (PMID:20004414) *J Pediatr* 2010;156(3):402–408. DOI: 10.1016/j.jpeds.2009.09.072

1299 Hoarau G, Pelloux I, Gayot A, Wroblewski I, Popoff MR, Mazuet C, Maurin M, Croizé J. Two cases of type A infant botulism in Grenoble, France: no honey for infants. (PMID: 22159905) *Eur J Pediatr*, 2012; 171(3):589–91. DOI: 10.1007/s00431-011-1649-5

1300 http://www.infantbotulism.org/parent/prevention.php. Among hospitalised patients, the mean age at onset of infant botulism in formula-fed infants (7.6 weeks) was significantly younger and approximately half that of breast-fed infants (13.8 weeks, by which time solids may be a vector). In addition, those who stopped breathing and died at home were *all* formula-fed.

1301 *Arnon SS, Damus K, Thompson B, Midura TF, et al. Protective role of human milk against sudden death from infant botulism. (PMID: 7038077) J Pediatr 1982; 100(4):568–73.*

1302 Barash JR, et al., op. cit.

1303 Schwarz PJ, Amnon SS: Botulism immune globulin for infant botulism arrives – one year and a Gulf War later. *West J Med* 1991;156:197–8. I hope no child died from botulism in 1991 who might have been saved: additional collateral damage indeed.

1304 Osaili T, Forsythe S. Desiccation resistance and persistence of Cronobacter species in infant formula. (PMID: 19720413) *Internat J Food Microbiol*, 2009; 136(2):214–20

1305 Officials search for source of bacteria that caused baby's death updated 23 December 2011 http://www.cnn.com/2011/12/23/health/missouri-infant-infection/index.html

sampled in an infant formula plant, twenty seven percent of kitchen locations, including sinks, counters, refrigerator door handles and interiors.[1306]

## Controlling contamination

Recently researchers discovered that Shigella,[1307] Salmonella[1308] and Cholera[1309] could grow in reconstituted formula. Research has also found mould toxins (ochratoxins and aflatoxins, known carcinogens) in infant formulas.[1310] Parents must take seriously the label advice to keep opened formula cans in a cool place, as moulds can grow readily in powdered formula kept at room temperatures. Aflatoxin levels have in fact been shown to increase over time in cans opened and re-sealed.[1311] I suggest that in warm homes or in hot climates opened formula cans should be carefully re-sealed (by clean washed hands) and stored in the refrigerator.

These overdue studies prompted action to reduce the risk (it cannot be eliminated, though there are hopes that adding other bacteria to the formula may help). International efforts resulted in high-level meetings and improved guidelines for infant formula manufacturers. The Codex Alimentarius Working Group Meeting on Infant Formulae in May 2006 considered adding a chapter, 'Control measures for safe preparation of formula' to its draft Code of Hygienic Practice. The following wording was agreed 'Powdered infant formula is not a sterile product and may be contaminated with pathogens that can cause serious illness. Correct preparation and handling reduces the risk of illness.' (But the risk remains.)

Sterility is an impractical goal in the real world. Even clinically controlled Special Care Nurseries can find that infants are colonised by serious pathogens: the recent Melbourne case where over thirty babies proved positive for Vancomycin Resistant Enterobacter (VRE) makes that point for the doubtful.[1312] The best protection is prevention of microbial growth, which involves breastfeeding plus 'soap and water and common sense'.[1313] Bottle-feeding parents are advised to make up formula and feed it immediately, one bottle at a time. Consumption immediately after preparation decreases the risk, as it reduces the time for bacterial multiplication. But making up a single feed each time also increases the inconvenience and stress of artificial feeding, and may not be adopted by any but the most

1306 Alvarez-Ordonez A, Ruiz L, Prieto M, Jordan K. Cronobacter Spp and infant formula. In Preedy V et al, op. cit., p. 380.

1307 Day JB, Sharma D, Siddique N, Hao YY, et al. Survival of *Salmonella typhi* and *Shigella dysenteriae* in dehydrated infant formula. (PMID: 22417504) *J Food Sci* 2011; 76(6):M324–8.

1308 Wu FM, Beuchat LR, Doyle MP, Mintz ED, et al. Survival and growth of *Shigella flexneri, Salmonella enterica serovar enteritidis,* and *Vibrio cholerae O1* in reconstituted infant formula. (PMID: 12224592) *Am J Trop Med Hyg,* 2002; 66(6):782–6.

1309 ibid.

1310 Meucci V, Razzuoli E, Soldani G, Massart F. Mycotoxin detection in infant formula milks in Italy. (PMID: 19787514) *Food Addit Contamin,* 2010; 27(1):64–71

1311 Akşit S, Caglayan S, Yaprak I, Kansoy S. Aflatoxin: is it a neglected threat for formula-fed infants? (PMID: 9124050) *Acta Paediatr Jpn,* 1997; 39(1):34–6

1312 http://www.canberratimes.com.au/national/greatest-threat-to-health-of-humanity-just-decades-away-20131227-2zzfh.html?skin=text-only

1313 The title of an excellent book: see Bibliography.

conscientious of parents with plenty of time to spare, or else scrupulously careful substitute carers.

Giving *the advice* to make up one feed at a time absolves companies and health authorities from legal (if not moral) responsibility for the inevitable damage that will occur, shifting legal responsibility for harm onto the carer. Companies do warn that misuse of the product is dangerous: once they've said 'make each bottle and feed it immediately', if parents don't do so, they have misused it. And the companies state that their product is *safe only if made up in accordance with their instructions*. So the advice to feed made-up formula immediately protects the company – not the parents or the child. Experience suggests – and industry knows - that many parents will still make up twenty-four-hour supplies once a day, not a bottle every time the baby needs it. (How convenient is artificial feeding if you have to do that?!) Even health authorities are sucked into the trap of adding advice about storage of made-up formula, a habit which parents correctly interpret as tacit approval: "they wouldn't tell us to do that if it was really dangerous, would they?" And of course, most of the time it is safe enough in ideal conditions: but not all the time.

Warnings that protect the baby – by clearly informing parents of the existence of the risk of bacterial growth in formula – but which threaten the company's profits, are not so readily agreed to. I proposed to FSANZ (Food Standards Australia and New Zealand) a new warning for formula labels as follows:

> Infant formula is not a sterile product, and cannot provide many important breastmilk factors. Whether considering formula feeding from birth, or changing over to infant formula, first discuss your situation with a health professional, so that you can make an informed decision and minimise the risks.

This would replace the irrelevant Breast-is-best warning that industry has subverted so cleverly. It would be great if a major formula-producing nation, perhaps New Zealand or Ireland, or even one major manufacturer, would take the lead with such a warning, giving parents important knowledge they currently lack, and protecting babies. Meanwhile, I keep hoping that industry bodies – those that assert that they support breastfeeding – will voluntarily do something to show that they give a toss for more than the bottom line. Manufacturers' associations could voluntarily agree on such a warning. It also protects them, after all. And they do claim to be ethical bodies concerned about infant health. Of course, the health professionals consulted would need to know how to minimise the risks, and educate parents about this, which many currently do not.

## Progress in reducing bacterial risks at last

After a series of international meetings and discussion papers and consideration, WHO Geneva produced some important advice materials about reducing the risks of formula-feeding. WHO declared on its website that powdered infant formula is not sterile, and mandated extreme care in preparation, both at home and in institutions.[1314]

---

1314 http://www.who.int/foodsafety/publications/micro/pif2007/en/index.html

Much more attention in the UK has been paid to the reality of infant formula preparation and storage. The UK government[1315] and UNICEF UK[1316] lead the Anglophone world in providing literature for parents that actually gives them evidence-based information. Both mandate making up infant formula as WHO suggested, with water no cooler than 70º Celsius.[1317] This is hot enough to kill some serious pathogens in the powder – though it may well kill any added probiotics too. And as IFM, the International Association of Infant Food Manufacturers, stated "the high temperature will also activate spores of the natural flora contained in infant formula. This includes B. cereus..[that] may be naturally present at low levels. Such activation can lead to rapid growth.."[1318] Thus it is very important for formula to be cooled quickly, the baby fed immediately, and any remnants discarded.

Shockingly, in the same month that ten-day-old Avery Cornett died in Missouri from an apparent bacterial infection,[1319] draft Australian Infant Feeding Guidelines were circulated which ignored WHO's evidence-based global recommendations, and instead cited the submission from Australia's infant formula manufacturers, the Infant Nutrition Council, which wanted lukewarm water used. Possibly for good reason: hot water can make infant formula hard to mix, or alter its nutrient content, and so result in a brand new cluster of infants affected by deficiencies of nutrients damaged by heat. If hot water causes clumping of powder, pathogens may not be destroyed but protected, said IFM. IFM also pointed out that such heat could "affect essential micronutrients such as amino acids, polyunsaturated fatty acids and other ingredients. It may also lead to reactions causing blockage of lysine, precipitation of mineral salts or proteins, fat separation or the formation of unwanted components."[1320]  Such possibilities are rarely openly discussed, as they might affect consumer confidence in the product. We have to hope that government food safety agencies are actively researching the consequences, rather than waiting for enough babies to be affected for harms to become obvious. Meanwhile, the bottom line is that there are risks whatever temperature of water is used, but fortunately most healthy babies can cope with this level of contamination, or formula feeding would never have become entrenched in western society as it has. (Again, this is no consolation to the rare family whose baby suffers, but true.)

In the end, the final Australian Guidelines adopted the WHO advice, as the UK government has done, despite the practical difficulties this entails for parents, and the losses for industry

---

1315  http://www.orderline.dh.gov.uk/ecom_dh/public/saleproduct.jsf?catalogueCode=2900017; http://www.unicef.org.uk/Documents/Baby_Friendly/Leaflets/4/guide_to_bottle_feeding.pdf

1316  http://www.unicef.org.uk/BabyFriendly/Resources/Resources-for-parents/A-guide-to-infant-formula-for-parents-who-are-bottle-feeding/ There is a health professional guide as well.

1317  This is still debated by some as impractical: Davanzo R, Giurici N, Demarini S. Hot water and preparation of infant formula: how hot does it have to be to be safe? *J Pediatr Gastroent Nutr*:, 2010; 50 (3):352–353. DOI: 10.1097/MPG.0b013e31819f65b1

1318  IFM. Position on the WHO Guidelines for reconstitution of infant formulas at temperatures of 70*C. February 2007. in 2014 no longer on the  IFM website, and membership of IFM seems to have changed since then as well. A history of formula manufacturers' associations could be interesting.

1319  http://bangordailynews.com/2011/12/28/health/bacteria-tied-to-babys-death-linked-to-formula-since-1980s/

1320  IFM, op.cit..

if parents realise that probiotics and enzymes and bioactive proteins may not survive such temperatures and therefore are not worth paying for.

The risk of scalding infants with hot water was also sometimes cited as a reason not to follow the WHO guidelines. IFM noted that "such incidents have occurred irrespective of warning and information provided to caregivers", and saw this as a major public health issue. It remains one of the totally avoidable risks of bottle feeding. But in fact the risk of inadvertent scalding is greatest with bottles heated in microwave ovens – which neither industry nor health authority vociferously campaigns against, perhaps because microwaving is so much part of the convenience society. Parents know that they have used hot water to make up a feed, and will allow it to cool. Not all parents know that a bubble of intense heat can exist within a seemingly cool-to-touch bottle of microwaved milk. And such bubbles have literally burned holes in sensitive mouths.

Why am I concerned about these temperature issues? Everyone has seen mothers in warm shopping centres and sunny parks pull out a bottle of readymade infant formula, and watched tired, grizzly babies clutching such bottles and sucking off and on for hours. If these bottles were prepared with tepid water, as industry labels suggest, any bacteria will have begun to grow from the moment they were made. If bacterial population doubling times are around ten minutes, after two hours and twenty minutes just one hundred bacteria – a trivial number – have become 1.2 million.[1321]

When babies like Avery die, it is common for industry to announce that tests were done and no pathogens were found in the formula. Recent studies have shown why. Unless sampling is extremely carefully done, using different techniques than those usually employed, bugs are easily missed.[1322] Sampling 300 g of a batch of many kilograms is really needle in a haystack testing. One recent batch recalled was 19 tonnes, of which 3 tonnes was deemed to be affected. Formula is made on a large scale!

And who benefits from being told that the bug was found in the formula? Should parents rely on the integrity of a commercial firm that stands to lose millions if it admits to this problem? A firm with a fiduciary duty to make money for shareholders? Can parents rely on government agents who see their role as reassuring the public that formula is safe? In one notorious PCB (polychlorinated biphenyl) contamination case,[1323] farmers resorted to splitting samples in two, then paying for independent testing of one half while submitting the other half for State Agriculture Department tests. Guess which half told them what the

---

1321 Wassenaar, TM. Op cit., p. 5

1322 Jongenburger I, Reij MW, Boer EP, Gorris LG et al. Actual distribution of Cronobacter spp. in industrial batches of powdered infant formula and consequences for performance of sampling strategies. (PMID: 21893361) *Internat J Food Microbiol* 2011; 151(1):62–9; Cahill SM, Wachsmuth IK, Costarrica M de L et al. Powdered infant formula as a source of Salmonella infection in infants. (PMID: 18171262) *ClinInfect Dis* 2008; 46(2):268–73. Perhaps especially novel ones found only in infant formula production areas: cf. Popp A, Cleenwerck I, Iversen C, De Vos P et al. *Pantoea gaviniae* sp. nov. and *Pantoea calida* sp. nov., isolated from infant formula and an infant formula production environment. (PMID: 20061487) *Internat J System Evol Microbiol*, 2010; 60(Pt 12):2786–92

1323 The Firemaster Incident. See Jelliffe. *Adverse effects of foods*, op. cit.

problem was? Not the one tested by the official government agency, the de facto servant of big moneyed interests, not citizens.

Certainly the infant deaths in the US, UK, France and Israel have led to manufacturers reducing the level of bacterial contamination in formula, but however small, in the real world a risk remains.[1324] Yet instructions on some cans have not changed: tepid water is suggested for formula-making in 2013. Industry warrants its products as safe if used as they direct, despite the fact that many parents cannot or do not follow the instructions about safety on the tin.[1325] As I said earlier, any misuse of the product relieves industry of responsibility for the outcome. Will parents following guidelines created by the World Health Organization and endorsed by national governments be deemed 'misuse' by industry? Will industry lobby to get those guidelines revised? I suppose it is some progress that in February 2014 the USA at long last adopted specific regulations about allowable levels of microbial contamination of infant formula, which many countries had done decades before.

## GAS, NOT GRAS?

When formula contains pathogens, there can sometimes be a clear and traceable connection between infection and illness, if enough trouble is taken with testing. Links between other ingredients of infant formula and potential harm are harder to prove. Some other ingredients used for decades are later suspected of causing problems. For example, carrageenan, a seaweed-derived ingredient used as a stabilising agent in liquid formula and some baby foods, was finally deemed a possible carcinogen and its use in formula – though not in some other foods – discontinued in the 1990s. Questions about the safety of carrageenan in formula had been raised decades before. If a carcinogen, it may have contributed to the higher rates of cancer in artificially fed infants, although many other mechanisms are also possible, and probably all interact with vulnerable genomes. But no one would ever be able to prove that carrageenan was a causative factor, precisely because of this complexity. And in 2014, after substantial lobbying, it was deemed safe enough to be allowed back into infant formula.

Carrageenan had once been on the US FDA's much-misunderstood GRAS (Generally Regarded As Safe) list.[1326] GRAS was an arbitrary category created in 1958 when Congress passed an amendment to the Federal Food, Drug, and Cosmetic Act (FD&C Act) to regulate additives to food. It is not a list of chemicals known to be safe, but of those exempted from safety testing – because before 1958 they had been in use and were presumed to be safe.

1324 Australia's 1990s actions on issues such as food labelling of GM and irradiated products, and infant formula itself, often seem to favour industry over health. Nor was any strong action taken to protect Australia's food crops from contamination by patented GM strains, which will doubtless become an issue when industry chooses to make it one. Secrecy about sites, and failure to quarantine adequately, probably means that some farmers might get a shock if they try to market their crops as GM-free. As happened with rBST, the synthetic bovine growth hormone, government will almost certainly side with industry and put an impossible burden of proof on those who seek to sell the unaltered product.

1325 Labiner-Wolfe J, Fein SB, Shealy KR. Infant formula-handling education and safety. (PMID: 18829836) *Pediatrics*, 2008; 122 Suppl 2:s85–90

1326 http://www.fda.gov/Food/FoodIngredientsPackaging/GenerallyRecognizedasSafeGRAS/ucm083022.htm; http://www.naturalproductsinsider.com/news/2011/08/gras-v-food-additive-v-dietary-ingredient.aspx

GAS – Governmentally Assumed Safe – would be the more accurate designation. What parents don't understand is what Marion Nestle calls

"a shocking gap in FDA regulatory authority over GRAS determinations.

Manufacturers get to decide whether food additives are safe or not.

Manufacturers get to decide whether to bother to tell the FDA the additives are in the food supply, and even if they do,

Manufacturers get to decide who sits on the panels that review the evidence for safety."[1327]

# Who really knows what baby is getting to drink?

Another concern is unexpected variability of infant formula. Some problems have resulted from the vitamin pre-mix supplied for addition to the formula, made by another firm altogether. No doubt it was a shock for some infant formula companies to discover that a company marketing oils for use in formula had not realised that encapsulating the oils with milk and soy proteins could be a problem (see page 318). It was a shock to me that infant formula producers didn't realise this about the oils, and put them into formulas likely to be fed to allergic children. Some manufacturers added fluoride or used fluoride-containing water in manufacture, without considering the infant's total potential intake in fluoridated areas: by 1992 Australia's Dental Health Committee of the NHMRC was recommending its removal, if need be by legislation.[1328]

Then there are the variables of hiccups in manufacturing, or human error in processing, and of course the multiple variables of scoops, caregiver practice, and water, mentioned earlier.[1329] As I've said before and doubtless will need to say again, if any healthworker needs to know precisely what a sick child's real intake is, the actual formula being drunk would need to be analysed. The label figures and calculations made from them are approximations.

All of which makes a tragic joke of what many mothers (and healthcare workers) say they like most about infant formula: 'You can see what they are getting.'

All anyone bottle-feeding can see is that their child consumes *x amount of a white liquid*. They cannot see what that liquid is. It has been flour and water in the past, and in poor communities it may still be! It has been dairy whiteners/coffee creamers in the US, causing cases of protein-calorie malnutrition in California in the past[1330] and Laos in the present.[1331] Recently it has been adulterated with detergent: scientists have just developed a rapid screening test for detergent detection, because 'Reports of infant milk formula adulteration

---

1327  http://www.foodpolitics.com/tag/GRAS

1328  Health Forum, September 1992 p. 28. Cited in *ALCA News*, 1993; 4(1): 33

1329  Renfrew MJ, Ansell P, Macleod KL. Formula feed preparation: helping reduce the risks; a systematic review. (PMID: 14500301) Free resource. *Arch Dis Child*, 2003, 88(10):855–8. Health Forum, September 1992 p. 28. Cited in *ALCA News*, 1993; 4(1):33

1330  Sinatra FR, Merritt RJ. Iatrogenic kwashiorkor in infants. *Am J Dis Child* 1981; 135: 21-23

1331  Barennes H, Andriatahina T, Latthaphasavang V, Anderson M et al. Misperceptions and misuse of Bear Brand coffee creamer as infant food: national cross sectional survey of consumers and paediatricians in Laos. *BMJ* 2008, 337:a1379(PMID:18782843) Free full text article

by detergent powders as economic frauds and poisoning incidents are common, as detergents are readily available and are inexpensive household items.'[1332] And melamine, which made headlines only after many thousands of babies were permanently affected. The possibility of such gross substitutions may be rare, but they are on record. Parents do well to smell, and to taste, whatever white liquids they intend to feed their babies, and to monitor every new can they open. We can all smell sour milk, but unless we learn the normal smell of each infant formula we may not detect a can that has the wrong product in it, or has spent too long in the heat, during transport or while on display in the shop window. Not everyone takes seriously the industry advice to store formula cans in a cool place.

You can see what they are getting? Looks can be deceptive. It is on record that New Guinean mothers observed wealthier expatriate mothers feeding orange juice to their older thriving (breastfed) babies, and copied this by mixing orange clay with water to feed by the magic bottle. Hey, it looked the same, and they could see what the baby was getting! New Guinea banned feeding bottles in 1978 after such problems emerged.

## So what can parents really see when a baby is bottle-fed?

*Is the baby getting a formula too high in protein and iron, too low in long chain polyunsaturates and lacking selenium?* No one saw that in the 1980s, but it was true then, and probably mostly still is.

*Is the baby getting a formula designed for an average baby, when she is not average?* Probably. Who has an average baby?

*Is the formula too low in sodium of the first week of life, too high in sodium for the second month?* By comparison with breastmilk, yes.

*Is the formula too dilute or over-strength, not exactly what the manufacturer says it will be if exactly the right amount of water is added?* Very likely: precision is impossible.

*Is the formula contaminated with heavy metals, with waterborne solvents, to a significant degree?* We hope not, but how can we know?

*Should the formula fat mixes and proteins levels be different in the first month from mixes in the second or third month?* Breastmilk certainly varies as neurological growth needs do.

*What microbes is baby ingesting with his formula, and what will be their effects on his microbiome and gut health?* Breastfed babies will be sharing their mother's microbiome and her immune system.

---

1332 Tay M, Fang G, Chia PL, Li SF. Rapid screening for detection and differentiation of detergent powder adulteration in infant milk formula by LC-MS. *Forensic Sci Int.* 2013; 232(1–3):32–9. DOI: 10.1016/j. forsciint.2013.06.013. Epub 2013 Jul 27

We need to be constantly aware that what little we know about excesses and deficiencies, contaminations and consequences, from any place or time, is not the result of careful, organised, independent after-sales monitoring by health authorities.

It is not the result of regular scheduled self-reporting by industry to government agencies.

It is the result of *haphazard discovery and parental reporting*, with even a sick infant's formula rarely checked by doctors either for nutritional or microbiological problems.

In the twentieth century many regulatory authorities left infant formula quality control to the companies, and most still do, though an annual inspection of the plant is said to occur in the USA. Most countries had no regulations until quite recently, or did not – or do not – enforce what I see as the very inadequate regulations that were developed within parameters acceptable to industry, and which did not apply to specialty formulas anyway.

But don't despair! For all that, millions of people are still alive who were fed even formulas now considered deeply deficient. Some might not have survived without infant formula, in societies that make breastfeeding difficult to impossible. Virtually everyone born in western countries since 1960 has been exposed to formulas since changed many times. They survived. Few have any idea of the association between their infant feeding history and any subsequent problems, whether immune dysfunction or cerebral difficulties.

That the vast majority of those exposed to infant formula did survive this uncontrolled experimentation is not proof that infant formulas were or are totally trustworthy, much less 'perfect mixtures of science and love.' That babies fed infant formula grow up and function well enough to pass for normal, now even to define normal, is, to me, simply proof of humankind's astonishing omnivore adaptability.

Anyone made anxious by my recital of the harsh realities needs to focus on human capability and brain plasticity, which together allow us to address and remedy many of the deficits that infant formula dysnutrition creates for our children. Responsive parenting, love[1333], a good education, with adequate food, shelter and clean water, can make a huge difference to those who get off to a bad start by missing out on breastfeeding and its obligatory skin to skin contact. And recognising that our children's gut and immune system and cognitive development *have inevitably been affected* allows us to consider ways of remedying any problems created. Accepting and dealing with reality is always preferable to pig-headed denial of uncomfortable facts. Bottle-fed and bottle feeding parents have every reason to be distressed and angry about these realities. However understandable the urge might be, shooting the messenger will not change them. Promoting and enabling the only true mix of science and love, mother's own milk, for our children and our grandchildren, is the only safe way forward.

---

1333 Oliver James's *How not to f\*\*\* them up* (2010) and *Love Bombing* (2012) are helpful here.

# 3.10 The drive to regulation: health and trade concerns

## The growth of knowledge about infant feeding

In the 1970s-1980s there was little understanding of lactation, and so high rates of breastfeeding problems. Advice about how to help mothers and babies was dreadful. When I taught the first Australian course on infant feeding for healthworkers in the 1980s, it seemed a semi-miraculous revelation for midwives to understand that babies breastfeed rather than nipple-suck;[1334] and it was heresy to insist that mastitis means inflammation, and was most often not an infection needing antibiotics. Both ideas, and many other heresies, are now taken for granted. As for contemporary pediatric and nursing textbooks, I used their photos and diagrams as illustrations of what not to do when helping mothers. (It was quite routine for see teaching photos and diagrams which, if imitated, resulted in ineffective feeding, compressed and fissured nipples, and maternal back soreness as well. And one hospital video in wide circulation actually illustrated – inadvertently – how to produce mastitis by bruising the breast when hand expressing.)

Infant feeding information for mother and healthworker alike was still supplied by the formula industry, and not questioned by most health professionals. The world's largest pioneer mother support group, La Leche League, deserves great credit for seeing the importance of certifying basic professional competence in lactation management, and investing thousands of dollars in setting up what would become the International Board of Lactation Consultant Examiners in 1985. This was the first group to see lactation as a specialty worthy of study, and in time the availability of lactation consultants would make a difference to hospital practice. For at this time, even when research had validated maternal resistance to formula-based schedules and restrictions on breastfeeding,[1335] responsive and flexible feeding had still not been adopted in clinical practice. Fortunate women were able to call on family networks or women friends or a supportive midwife to get help with breastfeeding problems, and some simply got on with breastfeeding a baby who knew how to breastfeed, as most would if put near a naked breast soon after birth.[1336] But for many women in the 1970s and 1980s breastfeeding was a huge struggle because the help needed wasn't available, and their desire to continue breastfeeding was often seen as odd – or even perverse in some cases, once the baby was more than a few months old.

But the 1980s would also see a growing scientific realisation of the many protective and immunomodulatory capacities of breastmilk, which revived global interest in

---

1334 Health professionals who deal with new mothers and don't know the difference need education about lactation immediately. There are many worthwhile online courses.

1335 Salariya EM, Easton PM, Cater JI. Duration of breast-feeding after early initiation and frequent feeding. (PMID: 82695) *Lancet*, 1978, 2(8100):1141–3.; Cruse P, Yudkin P, Baum JD. Establishing demand feeding in hospital. (PMID: 626524) Free resource *Arch Dis Child*, 1978, 53(1):76–8

1336 Widström AM, Lilja G, Aaltomaa-Michalias P, Dahllöf A et al. Newborn behaviour to locate the breast when skin-to-skin: a possible method for enabling early self-regulation. (PMID:20712833) *Acta Paediatr* 2011; 100(1):79-85

breastfeeding as seriously protective for infants and mothers. This followed earlier articles by immunologists like Lars Hanson, nutritionists like Leif Hambraeus, and paediatric allergists like John Gerrard, along with the publication of the Jelliffes' superb and ground-breaking 1978 book, *Human milk in the modern world*,[1337] which summarised what was then currently known, and had galvanised its (regrettably few) readers, myself included (though for me, the most important book had been Mavis Gunther's *Infant feeding*, published in 1970). Dr Ruth Lawrence's *Breastfeeding: a Guide for the Medical Profession*, and a small book by Professor GJ Ebrahim of the Institute of Child Health at the University of London[1338] were also influential internationally, as were my own books. The International Society for Research into Human Milk and Lactation (ISRHML) was formed in 1984, and their published conference proceedings[1339] serve as an expensive record of the emerging frontiers of scientific research in this field. In 2012 ISRHML outlined what they see as some of the more important questions still to be researched and answered.[1340] (The Academy of Breastfeeding Medicine[1341] was set up in 1993 by pioneer physicians well aware of the need to educate their colleagues about infant feeding; many of the founding members had been actively supportive and involved with La Leche League and the creation of IBLCE and ILCA in the 1980s, and recognised that a doctors-only group was also needed.)

The 1980s would also see the beginnings of research using better definitions of breastfeeding which showed that being formula-fed increased the risk of disease and death in infants even in developed nations. Parents began to hear the message that breastfeeding wasn't just good for bonding, it was good for survival and long-term health, for both mother and baby alike.

That realisation had the potential, rightly advertised by some wealthy vested interest group, to cause the bottom to drop out of the formula market. Families might demand hospital and social arrangements that would make it possible for women to succeed at breastfeeding. Regrettably, there is no such vested interest group, short of another Gates Foundation, that wants to save children in this most cost-effective and practical way, independently of Big Pharma. It would take a very brave individual with very deep pockets to adopt this cause. (Oprah, where are you?) National governments could save billions,[1342] but this would require a bi-partisan policy that involved offending important businesses with cash to donate to election campaigns: how likely is that, when bi-partisanship cannot be achieved over ever more obvious global threats with overwhelming international scientific consensus on the need for action?

---

1337 Jelliffe DB, Jelliffe EFP. *Human milk in the modern world* op. cit.

1338 Ebrahim GJ, op. cit.

1339 Regrettably published only in very expensive volumes that limit the circulation of the important research they contain. It is to be hoped ISHRML will make them available on their website. These volumes chart the growth of scientific progress in infant feeding and to some degree, lactation knowledge.

1340 Neville MC, Anderson SM, McManaman JL, Badger TM, et al. Lactation and neonatal nutrition: defining and refining the critical questions. (PMID: 22752723) *J Mammary Gland Biol Neoplasia*, 2012; 17(2):167–88

1341 http://www.bfmed.org/Resources/Protocols.aspx

1342 The US would save something like $13 billion annually if 90 per cent of children were fed to six months. See Bartick M, Reinhold A. The burden of suboptimal breastfeeding in the United States: a pediatric cost analysis. *Pediatrics*, 2010;125(5):e1048–56

Still, the information that began to reach elite parents by the 1980s had the potential to seriously derail the use of infant formula via a grassroots rebellion, if infant formula could not at least plausibly claim to match breastmilk in some key areas of infant health and development. However convenient or even necessary it may be to leave one's children in the care of others, few parents are prepared to do so if they know that this will be damaging. Had anyone in 1950 known how significant breastmilk was to normal development and immune health, it is highly unlikely that any patent infant formula offered for sale would have succeeded. In my experience, it is a tiny minority of parents who choose advertised convenience over their children's health. Industry saw the challenge, and responded brilliantly, as outlined in Chapter 3.11.

# Improving infant formula

By the 1980s, scientists and doctors alike had more tools both to identify and rectify problems of infant formula. New developments in food technology began to provide many more ingredients to manipulate in the quest for the perfect infant formula. There seems to be worldwide consensus in the scientific community that, overall, 1980s formula changes were a major step forward, and significantly reduced the inevitable harms of artificial feeding. The period since the 1980s has been an era of constant change in formula products, but with slightly different emphases in both product development and marketing.

Improvements of infant formula content were usually the result of some observed damage in children being formula-fed. Occasionally identifying a formula problem led to real and rapid improvements, and saved lives. The problem had to be both common and obvious, like rickets and scurvy, to be seen and addressed, in those cases by adding vitamins A, D and C. (Less common problems could be thought to be a defect of the child or fault of the parent.) The most obvious and widespread example of formula defect was the issue of the excessive renal solute loads of most early infant formulas.

# Decreasing renal solute load and hypernatraemia

There had been similar problems, with too much or too little nutrient in infant blood. In many countries, for example, the high-phosphate levels of early infant formula triggered infantile convulsions in late winter or early spring, as babies became hypocalcaemic or hypomagnesaemic.[1343] However, they did so only if born of mothers vitamin D deficient during pregnancy, thanks to the lack of sunlight exposure. This should be a warning for modern mothers who are not exposed to enough sunlight to ensure adequate vitamin D intakes, now thought to be important in the prevention of allergy as well.[1344]

---

1343 That is, they had too little calcium or magnesium in their blood. Professor Forrester Cockburn, in Crowther et al, op.cit. p. 54.

1344 The role of vitamin D in the causation of allergy (sometimes referred to as the Vitamin D hypothesis) is not discussed at any length in this book, as it does not seem to be the currently dominant explanation globally. However, maternal vitamin D deficiency is a plausible contributory factor in immune dysfunction and even adult disease.. For more on this, check out: Martineau A, Jolliffe D. "Vitamin D and Human Health: from the Gamete to the Grave": Report on a meeting held at Queen Mary University of London, 23rd–25th April 2014. (PMCID:PMC4113768) Free full text article *Nutrients*. Jul 2014; 6(7): 2759–2919. Published online Jul 22, 2014. doi: 10.3390/nu6072759

But in every country from the 1920s onwards babies had convulsed, suffered brain damage, and even died due to hypernatraemia (too much sodium in the blood, as a result of wrong mineral ratios and excess protein in infant diet, along with too little water). This was being widely discussed by the 1950s and 1960s in relation to infant formula. But starting with cows' milk as the base protein, it was difficult to get enough of some essential amino acids without also giving too much total protein and minerals. Improvements became possible once filtration techniques allowed demineralised whey to be used in formula making (see page 260). But up until the 1970s older casein-dominant formulas based on cows' milk were still in use, and protein levels in formulas were still too high. Most children coped well enough, although so far as I could discover, no one has investigated the links with later adult renal disease. But the margin of safety was too small under conditions when their water intake was inadequate to infant needs: hot weather, fever, simple fluid restriction, or over-concentrated feeds. (Parents mistaking liquid concentrate formulas for ready to feed liquid formula[1345] could be fatal; as could mis-labelling of those liquid concentrates, which famously did occur, the latest being in 1996.[1346])

These high solute formulas were clinically toxic in conditions where body water loss increased, such as diarrhoea, vomitting, excessive sweating. As Wharton said, clinical toxicity can be widespread but unrecognised: 'it may take some years for the problem to be apparent and a few more for it to be tackled effectively.'[1347] Not so effectively as to eliminate the problem universally, however. Fomon states that

> ... even at the end of the century, infant formula regulations permitted the marketing of formulas with undesirably high potential renal solute load. In 1998, an Expert Panel recommended to the Food and Drug Administration (FDA) that infant formulas provide a potential renal solute load ... no greater than 33 mOsm/100 kcal ... the FDA took no immediate action on this recommendation.[1348]

That issue has been ongoing since 1960 at least! Pioneering UK researcher Dr Mavis Gunther wrote a book for parents, *Infant Feeding*, published in 1970, in which she publicly expressed her concern about the high infant renal solute loads (the burden on kidneys) of artificial formulas, and the link with epidemics of convulsions due to hypernatraemia, seen in many bottle fed infants in hot weather. Before the paperback edition was available, industry had acted to reduce sodium levels.

Fortunately the major formula companies had been reducing the renal solute load, and most formulas from the 1980s were better than their predecessors, though still much higher than breastmilk's renal solute load, at the time quoted as around 79 mOsm per litre,[1349] compared with the proposed 220mOsm per litre).

---

1345 The add-water symbols manufacturers used were "shown to be understandable to major percentage of the non-English-reading parents to whom they were shown." Gelardi R. IFC Perspectives, in AOAC op. cit p. 12.
1346 http://www.nytimes.com/1996/08/25/us/carnation-recalls-a-mislabeled-baby-food.html See also http://www.naba-breastfeeding.org/images/Formula%20Recalls-W.pdf
1347 Wharton BA. An approach to setting maxima in infant formulas. *J Nutr*, 1989; 119:1768–72
1348 Fomon SJ. Infant feeding in the 20th century, op. cit. A useful overview from an industry pioneer.
1349 Zeigler EE, Fomon SJ. Fluid intake, renal solute load and water balance in infancy. *J Ped*, 1971; 71:561–8

This reduction in renal solute load was not just tinkering: it saved lives in Britain, America and Australia and every country where babies were artificially fed. As Wharton said in 1989:

> Mortality from gastroenteritis also fell considerably after 1974. This reduction was almost certainly related to the marked reduction in hypernatremia that had occurred. Severe metabolic disturbance (particularly hypernatremia) now occurs much less frequently – now about 1 per cent in some series compared with up to 30 per cent prior to 1974. There seems little doubt that this is due to reductions in protein and electrolyte content of formulas, and hence renal solute load.[1350]

Why a reduction in child deaths after 1974? Concern amongst UK health professionals about declining breastfeeding rates and the prevalence of both hypercalcaemia (excess calcium in the blood as a result of wrong mineral ratios in diet) and hypernatraemia (excess sodium) had led a 1973 Department of Health Working Party to review and advise on infant feeding practice. This resulted in the important 1974 report, *Present day practice in infant feeding*. This 1974 report led to a major change away from the old powdered cows' milk fortified with iron and a few vitamins (National Dried Milk), to the wholesale UK adoption of the new 'complete' and 'humanised' infant formulas with lower protein and mineral levels.[1351] Infant feeding was part of the reason for a dramatic overall lowering of mineral levels in UK infant formulas.[1352] And fewer babies died or were brain-damaged. Or to put it another way, as late as the 1970s, after one hundred years of artificial formulas, many normal term babies had died needlessly from gastroenteritis, which it is highly likely they would not have suffered from had they been breastfed. How many had died in each country in that hundred years? Do formula advocates know that this happened on this scale, and does still happen in even the richest countries?

## UK Guidelines

Further reformulations of UK formula were recommended or supported by a 1980 Department of Health and Social Security (DHSS) document, *Artificial feeds for the young infant,* which followed the 1977 DHSS report, *The composition of mature human milk.* These were guidelines which all UK manufacturers were asked nicely to observe: the 1980 'regulations' became UK law only in 1995. By which time they were in need of updating, and the UK was by then part of the European Economic Community (EEC) or European Union (EU).

In the 1970s neither the US nor Australia had such detailed 'guidelines', much less any real regulation of infant formula. As noted in earlier chapters, protein and mineral levels were excessive by modern standards, and this was not an easy problem to identify or solve. As a formula industry technologist wrote in 1982,

---

1350 Wharton, *J Nutr,* 1989, op. cit. p. 1771
1351 The UK Department of Health and Social Security (DHSS) also commissioned national surveys by Office of Population, Census and Statistics, *Infant feeding 1975* and *Infant feeding 1980*. These surveys have continued at five-year intervals and provide valuable information not available in other countries.
1352 Gunther M. *Infant feeding* (Methuen, 1974; Penguin, 1978). Dr Gunther told me that the threat of publishing comparative figures in the paperback edition of her book hastened the changes by some manufacturers.

A recent survey indicated some rather wide variations in the level of certain mineral and trace mineral components of infant formula. Both excessively high and excessively low concentrations of given mineral elements were reported for some products. A number of factors could be responsible. In general, consistent standardisation would have to take into account variations in initial concentration in formula ingredients and the influence in dairy-based products of feed, medications, and udder health. In addition, technologies of protein separation and refinement may add to or deplete from these components more or less of a variety of minerals and trace minerals. Quality control would require a rather exact accounting prior to fortification, if indeed fortification is needed.[1353]

I have not seen studies investigating 'excessively high or low mineral levels' as a likely cause of the rising rates of renal problems in Western societies over the century. Kidney disease has created the need for huge numbers of dialysis machines to serve communities notable for artificial feeding, such as urban Indigenous Australians in the postwar period. Why is it that renal specialists fail to see the connections?

## Towards US regulation

Formula companies then and now made and marketed products as they saw fit, without more than minimal oversight. (And medical researchers, trusting infant formula, rarely factored type of feeding into their search for causes of disease.) In the US in 1980 there were in fact 'only two [legal] requirements for the manufacture of baby formula: (1) the formula must be manufactured under sanitary conditions, and (2) the label must reflect what is in the can.'[1354] There were few compositional standards or required quality control procedures,[1355] although in 1941 some federal labelling requirements and minimum amounts for four vitamins had been specified. Previous attempts at regulation had in fact failed. In 1962, after B6 deficiency problems causing brain damage, the FDA had attempted to develop regulations. They were never enacted, although in 1971 after further debate, a list of suggested minimum requirements for protein, fat including linoleic acid, seventeen vitamins and minerals created controversy. (No upper limits were suggested. Specifying a maximum would make industry's task much more complicated than making sure a minimum was present for the shelf-life of the product.) The FDA commissioned the AAP to give advice, and of course the AAP worked with its industry partners to provide it.

The American Academy of Pediatrics (AAP) Committee on Nutrition had been responsible for most suggestions re American infant formula composition. In 1967[1356] they had proposed the list of 17 ingredients the FDA adopted in 1971. In 1974 they devised a revised outline for formula composition which contained minima for some thirty-two nutrients.[1357] It was

---

1353 Packard V. *Human milk and infant formula* (Academic Press, 1982). pp. 154–5.

1354 Laskin CR, Pilot LJ. Defective infant formula: the Neo-Mull-Soy/Cho-Free Incident, in Moss HA, Hess R, Swift CF. *Early intervention programs for infants* (The Haworth Press, Inc, 1982) vol 1, pp. 97–106

1355 Laskin CR, Pilot LJ. Defective infant formula: the Neo-Mull-Soy/CHO-Free incident. In (eds) Moss, Sweet, Swift. *Early intervention programs for infants* (Haworth Press, 1982) pp. 97–106

1356 AAP CON. Proposed changes in the FDA regulations concerning formula products and vitamin-mineral dietary supplements for infants. *Pediatrics* 1967; 40:916.

1357 AAP CON. Commentary on breastfeeding and infant formulas, including proposed standards for formulas. *Pediatrics* 1976; 57:278.

reported in 1979 that there were still just seventeen of these in current formulas.[1358] What industry did was its own business. And business was ever more influential. 1977 was the year the US FDA "decided to overturn a rule in place since 1938 that had required the clear marking of all packages containing substitute ingredients with the word "imitation".[1359]

## The Syntex disaster and the Infant Formula Act of 1980

So in 1978–79, when Syntex, a US formula company, tried to lower its various formulas' high sodium levels by removing salt, many infants were harmed. In taking out the sodium Syntex had also taken out the chloride. Hypochloraemia (too little chloride, essential for humans) damaged infants fed that formula over some time. There was less severe brain damage in infants fed a variety of formula or previously breastfed.[1360] It was believed by parent advocates that chloride levels had already been too low before this removal, as some damaged children pre-date the known period of deficiency.

A successful media campaign (including an appearance on the US TV program 60 Minutes) by parents of damaged infants resulted in 60 000 letters – and the 1980 Infant Formula Act. As a US Food and Drug Administration (FDA) director said,

> As a result of clear public concern and, to some extent, professional consensus, an Act was passed which, in many respects, clarified FDA's authority to establish minimum requirements for infant formula and to provide for the assurance of the quality of these formulas. Nevertheless in spite of the fact that one of the major problems in dealing with the Syntex situation was control of the recall of these formulas, the bill as finally passed did not contain mandatory recall authority for the Agency, but rather gave the Agency authority to regulate the recall only after the company had begun such a recall voluntarily. In other words, at the moment of truth, the Congress could not bring itself to give to the Agency all of the authority it needed at the expense of corporate freedom of action.[1361]

## Regulation or self-regulation?

No regulations were included in the Act. The US Congressional Act had mandated the USFDA to create stringent regulations controlling formula composition and quality. However, it would be 1982 before any draft quality control regulations emerged from an embattled FDA, which the incoming Reagan administration[1362] stripped of 450 staff.[1363]

---

1358 *Food Chemical News* 5 November 1979, p. 41

1359 de la Pena,. op. cit., p. 182.

1360 *Biochemistry of milk and milk products* (Royal Society of Chemistry, 1994), p. 99

1361 Forbes AL, Miller SA. FDA's perspectives on infant formula. In Association of Official Analytical Chemists. *Production, regulation and analysis of infant formula.* Proceedings of a Topical Conference, Virginia, 14–16 May 1985

1362 Cost-cutting national governments usually allege that the civil service is overstaffed, and sack needed staff in key agenicies as a way of reducing oversight or regulation of the vested interests that have supported their election campaigns. They then outsource oversight, often by absurdly expensive contracts, to groups that will not uncover awkward facts, or whose reports can be kept confidential. Or as is currently being proposed in Australia, they devolve authority to states or regions, ensuring either massive duplication of functions, or an inability to fund them properly, or both.

1363 *Food Chemical News,* 15 March 1982, p. 51

The FDA wrote such regulations, and ran into the brick wall of industry resistance, complaints about the cost of compliance, and insistence on the need to exempt some formulas from the content regulations. Meanwhile, an election brought Ronald Reagan to power, and with him figures from a very well-connected industry lobby. (That lobby ensured that in 1981 the USA was the sole dissenting vote against the adoption of the International Code or Marketing of Breastmilk Substitutes (see page 412). In December 1982 a coalition of consumer groups took legal action. They charged that the Republican Reagan administration (known to be pressuring the FDA) had violated the Infant Formula Act of 1980 'in yielding to pressure from the $550 million dollar a year infant formula industry.' The contemporary account in an expensive industry news journal, *Food Chemical News,* records the extent to which industry was allowed to write its own quality control regulations.[1364]

> In the interim, other problems with formula had emerged, including a major recall of B6-deficient Wyeth formulas.[1365] A senior FDA officials was optimistic - Since the passage of the Infant Formula Act, the Agency is aware of four instances where infant formulas were manufactured and distributed in interstate commerce with nutrient deficiencies or overages [*a nicer word than excesses*]. As long as these nutrient deficiencies are identified prior to children becoming ill, it is my opinion that these laws and regulations [*not finalised until 1985*] are working.[1366]

Why did the FDA Director think that? What follows is an absolutely true statement taken for granted by industry and regulators alike, but not understood by most parents. Read it carefully.

> It is not possible to manufacture this volume of product without some mistakes occurring in their manufacture. It is not possible to legislate perfection in production or anything else. [1367]

Indeed it is not. But do parents know that? Caveat emptor – buyer beware! Congress eventually passed additional regulations specifically for infant formula in 1986. As an official briefing paper later said,

> In passing the 1980 Infant Formula Act and its 1986 amendments, Congress recognized infant formulas as a special category of foods that, because there is no margin for error in ensuring the healthy growth and development of infants, requires more regulation than other types of foods. Regulation of infant formulas involves both general safety provisions of the act and additional requirements specific to infant formulas (e.g., CGMPs *[Current Good Manufacturing Practices]*, quality control procedures, nutrient levels and analysis, and quality factors).[1368]

But as that paper went on to say,

---

1364 *Food Chemical News* 6 December 1982, pp. 15–17
1365 *Food Chemical News,* 15 March 1982, pp. 47–8
1366 Forbes AL, Miller SA. op. cit. p. 6
1367 ibid.
1368 Briefing information B1 for the 18–19 November 2002 FDA Food Advisory Committee Meeting on Infant Formula. Downloaded from http://www.fda.gov/OHRMS/DOCKETS/ac/02/briefing/3852b1_01.pdf

For most of the requirements specific to infant formula, manufacturers ***must provide assurances*** that the requirements have been met for each 'new' product (including marketed products in which a major change has occurred) prior to marketing.[1369]

In short, while standards were set, US industry was (and still is) largely trusted to meet them. For example, the Act prescribes detailed audits – by the company itself. Reports of any of the regular audits prescribed by the Act need not be sent to the FDA –this requirement of the Act involves simply sending a form letter advising that audits have been done. Of course, audit records require skilled staff to check them and perhaps order more tests, and the FDA had lost those hundreds of staff. However, any FDA file of any such audits would be an independent historical record that could prove incredibly valuable over time. No such archive will ever exist unless the regulations are changed. If industry has done the detailed audit, why not file it with the FDA? US formula industry records have to be kept for just a year after the expiry date of the batch; other countries lack even such a minimal requirement. Will audit records held only by the company all be destroyed? What is the point of them, if they are simply in-house checks never checked by a government authority, which simply lends its credibility to industry?

This remarkable trust in formula manufacturers extends to the process of adding new ingredients to formulas. Industry is simply obliged to notify the FDA that it is adding new ingredients, providing supporting documentation, just ninety days before it markets the new product– then it can go ahead without any need for FDA approval.

In fact, technically the FDA does not approve any infant formula or infant formula changes, or always carry out independent testing, as parents blithely (but perfectly reasonably) suppose. FDA simply asks industry

- to state on the record 90 days before the formula goes onto the market that industry believes it is safe,
- to file post-market reports on any problems; and –perhaps, if budgets permit –
- to facilitate an annual inspection, including of consumer complaints.

FDA may do more in certain cases, but it is not obliged to. Although it has been proposed in committee meetings, there is no official website like Medwatch 'Your FDA gateway for clinically important safety information and reporting serious problems with human medical products' where professionals and the community can give feedback to the FDA. It could be reasonably argued that the USFDA does more to protect the American infant formula industry from criticism than it does to protect infants from American infant formula.

Infant formula is a food and not a medical product; it needs its own online open-access reporting site, Formulawatch. Do parents or professionals believe that the USFDA maintains strict control, independently scrutinises, and then approves, every infant formula marketed in the United States? If so, they are utterly deluded. It would require big budgets for any regulatory agency to maintain an independent staff capable of doing the detailed

---

1369 ibid.

investigations needed to assess all aspects of every infant formula and its outcomes. Much of the oversight in every country, including America,  comes from people involved with industry, sharing its assumptions, and dependent on it for research funding. Some rotate into and out of government and industry jobs at critical times.[1370] Most quality assessment and certification of manufacturing sites has been farmed out to private entities, as in Ireland, not conducted by independent public servants. There is very little completely independent expertise about infant formula in the world, especially in countries where government does not fund any such research.

This is not to imply that all industry-associated researchers are stooges incapable of independent thought or criticism: they would be of little use to industry if so. However, there is an entirely human tendency not to bite the hand that feeds you, and a tacit awareness that going public with industry-damaging information (rather than quietly informing industry and getting a research grant to solve the problem, say) could result in legal, professional or other reprisals, as such information undermines the market. Sanford Miller, FDA Director, was frank about that issue too:

> Whenever a recall is initiated, whenever a problem is identified, the FDA and industry in particular are recipients of consumer criticism, and consumer confidence in the product and the system is lost.[1371]

True again. More alarming to me was what followed that comment:

> It is our responsibility to restore this confidence so that parents throughout the US will not be wondering, as they are now, if the product they are feeding their infant is indeed complete and wholesome.[1372]

## The role of a regulatory agency

How loudly does it need to be said: the role of a regulatory agency is not identify with the regulated, and seek to restore public confidence in risky products. That is the job of industry PR departments. The role of a regulatory agency is not to assure consumers of the completeness and wholesomeness of commercial products that are second-rate by comparison with an alternative available to virtually all parents. If those 1980s formulas had been truly wholesome, there would have been no damaged children. If they had been truly complete, there would have been no need for further deletions or additions, soon to follow! They were neither.

The role of a regulatory agency is to prevent unsafe products reaching the market by stringent regulation and frequent inspection, and to prevent consumers being misled into thinking inherently risky products are totally safe. It is to actively monitor hazardous products in

---

1370  In the 1980s struggle for US regulations, the FDA is said to 'have relied on a purportedly independent economic analysis" –prepared by Dr Dennis L. Heuring, the author of Mead Johnson's objections. Heuring had left Mead Johnson to work for a new firm, then reported as returning to Mead Johnson. (*Food Chemical News*, December 6, 1982, p. 16. Marion Nestle discusses "the revolving door" in her excellent food politics blog.

1371  Forbes, Miller, op. cit. p. 6

1372  ibid.

Chapter 3: Infant formula, past, present and future | 411
3.10 The drive to regulation: health and trade concerns

the market and assess the cost-benefit of continued marketing or market removal. Infant formula is a hazardous product. It would be interesting for a scholar to compare FDA's concerns and actions about the very much smaller and less important issue of raw milk, with its concerns about infant formula!

'Restoring confidence' can be rationalised by the industry-agreeable belief that telling unpleasant truths about formula will alarm and upset parents dependent on it for their children. Yes, it will. And that new awareness can help prevent future problems. US and global regulatory actions are white-anted by the sometimes-unacknowledged belief that, as one FDA official said to me, 'We have to reassure parents that formula is safe, because American society depends on bottle-feeding.'[1373]

Indeed it does. That could change. American society depended on slavery until it was recognised as morally wrong and detrimental to the whole of society, however much it enriched the elite. The role of health regulators is to protect the health of children, and that cannot be done by suppressing inconvenient truths about artificial feeding, no matter how dependent Western society has become on the ability to separate mothers from their young infants.

In the US, since the Reagan era of the 1980s, there has been strong political interference in the regulation of health issues that might have an impact on industry profits. Doctrinaire neo-conservatives everywhere oppose regulation as a source of needless cost – though in fact regulation can save both business and society far greater costs.[1374] That new 1980s head of the FDA, Sanford Miller, was an industry consultant who continued to accept industry honoraria while in office, a practice later made illegal; he believed in industry self-regulation. Marion Nestle and others have documented the way in which industry personnel influence decisions relating to food and chemicals alike, and rotate in and out of industry and government employment.[1375] Expensive industry-oriented journals like *Food Chemical News* recorded the triumph of ideology-driven politicians over science-based regulators.

## UK developments

The very different UK (and formerly Australian) perception of healthcare as both a right of citizens, and a duty of government, has meant that the National Health Service provided employment opportunities not then dependent on industry money. This may have allowed greater independence of thought by regulators than evinced by Sanford Miller's comments.

---

1373 Conversation at FDA Office in Washington, 1985. Recorded in *Breastfeeding matters*, 1985. This was the result of a discussion explaining why a *Pediatrics* article entitled Problems with human milk and infant formula, not only omitted various infant formula recalls after 1979, and exaggerated the risks of breastfeeding, but also included the published work of other authors without what I saw as adequate attribution. The article was part of the *Report of the Taskforce on the assessment of the scientific evidence relating to infant-feeding practices and infant health*. Supplement to *Pediatrics* 1984; 74 (2). AI wrote to Pediatrics about this, and have the reply on file.

1374 See Hilts PJ. *Protecting America's health: the FDA, business and 100 years of regulation* (Alfred Knopf NY, 2003). Ch. 14 et seq.

1375 Nestle M. *Food politics* op. cit.

As I read the literature, the UK government, among Anglophone governments, had clearly taken the lead on infant feeding issues in the 1970s and 1980s, partly thanks to some key paediatricians, midwives, obstetricians and scientists[1376] more aware of the importance of breastfeeding,[1377] and less in thrall to private industry and their dependents, wealthy elites.

Independent data collection had begun in the UK from 1970. Where a government provides free healthcare, it has a vested interest in reducing costs[1378], which means identifying causes of ill health via data collection. In the US at that time only Ross Laboratories' infant feeding data was available, and that was collected only from mothers with telephones (i.e. relatively affluent families). When any government fails to collect relevant data, it can ignore a national problem or even deny that one exists. WHO has tried to persuade governments to keep standardised data on breastfeeding, using reliable sources and agreed definitions, but the global picture remains incomplete. Since the 1990s US states have begun to collect data on infant feeding rates, and CDC (Centers for Disease Control and Prevention) to collate it, so the scale of US problems is becoming clearer.

## Codex and Standards

The infant formula trade was a global one, with products made in one country being exported widely. Regulation in any one country had the potential to make exports and imports of this or any other foodstuff complicated or impossible. This was felt strongly in Europe, where many small countries had foodstuffs circulating widely, and attempts were made to harmonise definitions, standards, labelling, methods of analysis and more. In 1963 the World Health Organization (WHO), and FAO, the UN Food and Agriculture Organisation, had collaborated to create the Codex Alimentarius (Food Code) Commission, whose task was to develop 'harmonized international food standards, guidelines and codes of practice to protect the health of the consumers and ensure fair practices in the food trade.'[1379] In 1976, amid growing global concern about infant formula and its marketing, the UN's Codex Alimentarius Commission made a set of recommendations about infant formula composition. This would be formalised as Standard 72-1981, and is discussed further on page 415.

## The International Code

Meanwhile, WHO was working with UNICEF to attempt to control marketing for a trade endangering infant health. Throught the century there had been notable medical critics of infant formula marketing, from Dr Cicely Williams in the 1930s to Derrick (Dick) and Patrice Jelliffe from the late 1960s. Worldwide pressure from concerned health professionals and Christian misssionaries led to multiple expressions of concern in the World Health Assembly from 1974 onwards, when the 27th WHA condemned the "the mistaken idea caused by misleading sales promotions that breastfeeding is inferior to feeding with

---

1376 People such as Ben Mepham, Malcolm Peaker, Roger Short, Sylvia Rumball, Margit Hamosh, David Baum, Lars Hanson, Peter Hartmann, and Miriam Labbok, for example.
1377 Crowther et al, op.cit.
1378 This helps explain why Scandinavian countries were so generous with parental leave! See page 128.
1379 http://www.codexalimentarius.org/about-codex/codex-timeline

manufactured breast-milk substitutes."[1380] The Catholic religious order, the Sisters of the Precious Blood, sued Bristol Myers (Mead Johnson) in 1975. US Senate Hearings were held in May 1978. Senator Edward Kennedy then wrote to the WHO Director General, Dr Halfdan Mahler, asking for a conference including both industry and its critics, to create 'a uniform code of ethics acceptable to all infant formula manufacturers'. This led to an historic Joint WHO/UNICEF Meeting on Infant and Young Child feeding, in Geneva in October 1979, and the formation of the International Babyfood Action Network (IBFAN). Eventually, after much debate and global consultation and compromise, the International Code of Marketing of Breastmilk Substitutes, approved by the World Health Assembly in 1981, as a voluntary recommendation to world governments. While the United States initially was the only nation to vote against the Code in 1981, in the May 1994 World Health Assembly the USA endorsed it.[1381]

The stated aim of the Code was

> to contribute to the provision of safe and adequate nutrition for infants, by the protection and promotion of breast-feeding, and by ensuring the proper use of breast-milk substitutes, when these are necessary, on the basis of adequate information and through appropriate marketing and distribution.[1382]

The WHO Code (as it became known) prohibited the advertising to the general public of any breastmilk substitute or other product within the scope of the Code. A breastmilk substitute was 'any food being marketed or otherwise presented as a partial or total replacement for breast milk, whether or not suitable for that purpose'.[1383]

The Code applies to

> the marketing, and practices related thereto, of the following products: breast-milk substitutes, including infant formula; other milk products, foods and beverages, including bottlefed complementary foods, when marketed or otherwise represented to be suitable, with or without modification, for use as a partial or total replacement of breast milk; feeding bottles and teats. It also applies to their quality and availability, and to information concerning their use.[1384]

In the diverse infant feeding industry, only the infant formula manufacturers would pay much attention to the Code, as they were its principal targets. In Australia the Commonwealth Health Department and industry produced a voluntary code by 1983 without reference to industry critics or breastfeeding advocates alike: it banned expensive direct-to-consumer advertising, freeing up more money for other forms of marketing. And it did nothing about industry's perhaps most pernicious form of marketing: the supply of infant formula to hospitals, which

1380 cited in Jelliffe & Jelliffe, *Human Milk*. op cit., p. 325.

1381 Wirpsa L. Formula Giants Pursue 3rd World Market; U.S. Switches, Agrees to Back WHO Code on Breast Milk Substitutes. *National Catholic Reporter* 1994; 30 p. 31

1382 Shubber S. *The WHO international code of marketing of breast-milk substitutes: history and analysis* (Pinter & Martin, 2011)

1383 International Code of Marketing of Breast Milk Substitutes (WHO, 1981). http://www.who.int/nutrition/publications/code_english.pdf

1384 ibid.

then passed it on to mothers. For more on this see page 503. In America the International Code was ignored. In the UK, which had endorsed it, little was done initially to implement it.

Thanks to the International Baby Food Action Network (IBFAN) it is clear that many, probably all, manufacturers and distributors continue to violate provisions of the Code to the present day.[1385] It is also worth noting that many manufacturers of feeding bottles and teats, and purveyors of complementary baby foods – all covered by the Code – have blithely ignored this international public health initiative in the pursuit of ever greater profit. It is also clear that governments have considered implementation of the Code to mean very different things. One interesting comparative review of this was commissioned from the NHMRC Clinical Trials Unit at the University of Sydney, by the Australian government, and is available on line.[1386]

Quite obviously, it is never in industry's own interest to make products that can be quickly shown to be harmful or deficient, as this can cost them megadollars. Most major companies do the best they (currently) can to avoid harm, and find ways to accommodate new regulations, after making sure they help to shape such regulations into an acceptable form. But every serious attempt to create better standards for infant formula or its use will run into tactical obstruction and delay, if that change will inconvenience a powerful vested interest. Not all governments have the ability to control multibillion-dollar national companies, and even fewer have the courage to try. Those that do try can find their democratic decisions to protect their people's health corrupted, subverted, defied or undermined by those with profits to lose, as when the Philippines banned infant formula advertising in 2006.[1387] (The companies, led by Mead Johnson, challenged this ban as infringing their freedom to trade; the Philipppines Supreme Court initially granted a restraining order which prevented enforcement of the ban, but in 2007 upheld the right of the national government to regulate the promotion of infant formula within its borders. Similarly, on behalf of the industry, the US Embassy in Vietnam tried to stop advertising bans in another sovereign state – and failed.[1388]) Even if defeated, such legal challenges consume scarce resources, so some countries try to avoid any such conflict by engaging with industry and compromising. The threat of referral to the World Trade Organisation has been used in the past to achieve such ends. At the very least, legal challenges ensure delay in enforcement, by which time the company may have new strategies in place. (In Australia any Code-violating advertising campaign could have run its course before the responsible body came to any conclusion

1385 Brady JP. Marketing breast milk substitutes: problems and perils throughout the world. Arch Dis Child, 2012; 97(6):529–32. (PMID: 22419779). Allain A. *Fighting an old battle in a new world: how IBFAN monitors the baby food market.* ( Development Dialogue, 2005) The International Code Documentation Centre (ICDC) issues reports on industry marketing by region and globally. See http://www.ibfan.org/code-publications.html, and NABA's website:http://www.nababreastfeeding.org/

1386 NHMRC Clinical Trials Centre University of Sydney. *An international comparison study into the implementation of the who code and other breastfeeding initiatives.* Final Report. http://www.health.gov.au/internet/main/ publishing.nsf/Content/1C29E44FE6BB3C4DCA257BF0001BDBC5/$File/111027%20Final%20Report.pdf

1387 Conde CH. Breast-feeding: A Philippine battleground. *NY Times* Tuesday, July 17, 2007. Downloaded October 21, 2014. http://www.nytimes.com/2007/07/17/world/asia/17iht-phils.1.6692639.html

1388 Astley M. *Dairy Reporter* July 25, 2012. http://www.dairyreporter.com/Regulation-Safety/US-urged-Vietnam-to-reconsider-infant-formula-advertising-ban

about it!) How the Code would be interpreted by industry was to lead to yet other battles: see page 496 in relation to Follow On Formulas (FOFs).

# Setting compositional standards

Early formula standards were largely written around existing products, and reflected the inadequate knowledge of the times. A sketchy timeline of some key events is included at th end of this chapter. America's Infant Formula Act of 1980 – which possibly would never have come about without the support of Senator Al Gore, from Tennessee - did not get its accompanying nutrient regulations finalised for years, and microbiological standards were not set for decades.

A first global infant formula standard, Codex Standard 72-1981, based on 1970s knowledge about infant feeding, had been set by the Codex Alimentarius Commission in 1976 and was not substantially amended before 2007.[1389] But it has always been up to national governments to adopt the Codex suggestions as law or to set whatever other limits they wished to. Codex was and is a voluntary advisory standard for infant formula that initially served to legitimise virtually all the then current brands of infant formula, so generous were its provisions. The focus on facilitating trade sometimes seemed to dominate the concern for public health.

So the first global Codex Standard for infant formula was widely seen as a minimum standard, written with wide ranges of permitted ingredients. Modern formulas would meet or improve on it over time. While minimum amounts of some ingredients are specified, there were few upper limits on ingredients, even though some ingredients could be toxic in excess, and an excess of any could have consequences for the infant's use of other ingredients. Upper limits involve more quality control and cost to industry than minima. Industry generally has resisted the creation and publication of maxima. An industry source in the 1990s said that for some ingredients it is hard to not have excesses soon after manufacture, if the minimum levels are still to be there by the end of the specified shelf-life. Perhaps shortening the shelf life would address that, but it would also increase formula costs.

In the early 2000s attempts were made in the Codex Alimentarius Commission (hereafter Codex) to develop a new international standard for infant formula. A great deal of preparatory work was done before the Codex Committee on Nutrition and Foods for Special Dietary Uses (CCNFSDU) met in 2005.[1390] The USA again argued that any standard should be wide enough to include all its current formula, and that maxima, or definite upper limits on ingredients, should be imposed only on ingredients already proven to be toxic in excess. This was a position that was successfully argued when Australia had tried to set maxima in its Infant Formula Standard in the 1990s. Other countries wanted more binding upper limits. The Codex Committee eventually resolved this by setting maximal values (MVs) only on those few ingredients known to be toxic in excess, and non-binding GUL (guidance upper limits) on other ingredients not yet known to be toxic in excess.[1391]

---

1389 http://www.codexalimentarius.org/standards/list-of-standards/en/?no_cache=1
1390 http://espghan.med.up.pt/position_papers/con_23.pdf
1391 The Infant Formula Standard 72–1981 can be downloaded from http://www.codexalimentarius.org/ committees-and-task-forces/en/?provide=committeeDetail&idList=11 Once there, click on related standards and see what documents are available.

As should be obvious, guidance limits are just suggestions, with no regulatory power. From what extensive database are they derived?

> Specifications for the currently permitted maximum amounts of micronutrients in formulae were generally calculated as three to five times the minimum amounts established at the time, took into account established history of apparent safe use (Codex Stan 72-1981, Codex Stan 156-1987, the Directive 2006/141/EC, and the SCF (2003a)), and were not based on scientific evidence for adverse effects *owing to the lack of such evidence for most nutrients.*

In short, they are derived by reasonable guesswork, in the complete absence of evidence other than infant survival and growth. That lack of evidence can be seen as reassuring: by the 1980s quite a number of micronutrients that are damaging in excess amounts had already been identified and remedied. The Panel noted that there is no evidence of adverse effects of others, but goes on to say two important things:

Firstly, that while there is no evidence of harm, there is no research evidence of safety either:

> there are no studies available which were designed to investigate the short or long-term health consequences of consumption of formulae containing the currently permitted maximum amounts of micronutrients in IF/FOF.

And secondly, that some ingredients may exceed the declared upper limits for older children, although infants may have different tolerances, which could be higher or lower:

> The Panel acknowledges that the scientific data available to derive ULs for infants remain scarce for most micronutrients and only for vitamin D a UL for infants could be set (EFSA NDA Panel, 2012b). For magnesium, zinc, selenium, iodine, molybdenum, vitamin A, niacin, vitamin B6 and folic acid, ULs for children aged one to three years have been established (SCF, 2000b, 2000c, 2000d, 2000g, 2001a, 2002b, 2002d, 2002a, 2002c). Assuming an energy intake from formula of 500 kcal/day (average of the AR for energy of boys and girls aged three to four months), regular consumption of a formula by an infant containing the currently permitted maximum amounts of zinc, iodine, vitamin A and folate (if the whole amount is provided in the form of folic acid) would imply that the ULs would be exceeded for these nutrients. Assuming an energy intake from formula of 700 kcal/ day (highest observed mean energy intakes in infants below six months of age), intakes of selenium would also exceed the UL. The Panel acknowledges that the ULs used in this estimation were those derived for young children and there is considerable uncertainty with respect to the extrapolation to infants.[1392]

That second point is a bit worrying. A lack of evidence of either harm or safety proves nothing one way or the other when the issue has not been researched.

So parents who want to use formula, as their child's sole diet from birth especially, need to know that *regulators really don't know what the upper limits of formula ingredients should be,*

---

1392 EFSA Panel Draft Opinion 2014, op. cit., p. 70.

*that there are very few independent investigations, and that where the impact of infant formula is concerned, each child is an experiment of one.*

Where formula use is avoidable, parents may prefer not to take any risk, however small. Where formula use is unavoidable, parents can instead focus on the idea that few obvious harms from unregulated upper limits have emerged, but keep a minimal awareness that a child's problem could be due to excesses – or indeed, deficiencies..

Industry can breach GULs with impunity, or take their time to comply, and cannot be held accountable, other than in the court of public opinion – if authorities want to use that power and risk the displeasure of powerful lobbies. In many countries, including Australia, no independent body will actively and routinely check and enforce compositional standards, instead accepting assurances that the companies can be trusted to get every single batch right. (So if no one ever looks, we can all assume there never is a problem. Looking might have uncovered the melamine problem in China months earlier – though it is alleged that even this gross contamination was known about six weeks before any action was taken.[1393]) In the USA, formula manufacturing facilities are subject to yearly inspection, a token gesture of oversight, but better than nothing. However, these inspections are not publicly reported, there are few sanctions, and with the cutbacks in every governmental budget, it is unlikely that there are enough staff to do frequent inspections. What is more, industry has even argued that plants making formula for export should be exempt from inspection, though fortunately the US FDA disagreed on that. Insisting on such an inspection revealed a temperature control problem that would produced brain-damaging B6-deficient formula. And what of a factory that makes only Toddler formula and other "exempt" formula –like the alphabet soup varieties, the AR, and LFs and HAs and EHFs and so on?

In 1980s Australia, the process of trying to persuade the infant formula industry to implement the International Code of Marketing of Breastmilk Substitutes[1394] proceeded in fits and starts, initially with no public consultation. The first edition of Australia's *Guidelines on Infant Feeding for Health Professionals* was published in 1984 under the auspices of the NHMRC, the result of 1981 submissions [1395] criticising health professional practice and industry marketing. Work on the Australian Standard for Infant Formula, referred to as

1393 http://www.stuff.co.nz/business/710852/Fonterras-melamine-response-too-late
1394 http://www.who.int/nutrition/publications/infantfeeding/9241541601/en/
1395 For the record, my NHMRC submission (initially requested by NMAA) and the book *Food for thought, a parent's guide to food intolerance* (Alma Publications, 1982), may have sparked this development. Both began as formal Nursing Mothers' Association of Australia (NMAA) projects, and had been developed through NMAA networks, including the Maryborough Victoria group. A change of leadership meant that NMAA hastily put together a separate, much weaker, submission to the NHMRC, and backed away from a book that recorded their own members' experiences. Such are the vagaries of life! It may have been relevant that a key NMAA figure seemed to me to be in denial about her offspring's quite obviously food-related behavioural issues ...*Food for Thought* sold more than 30,000 copies in Australia, the UK and Japan, and enabled me to travel to research *Breastfeeding matters*. Those trips resulted in much productive work and my involvement in the formation and internationalisation of both the International Lactation Consultant Association (ILCA) and the International Board of Lactation Consultant Examiners (IBLCE). A negative or painful life event often has a positive and unpredicted outcome, which can seem providential.

Standard R7 had been ongoing since 1977 and was not finalised until 1988[1396]; five years later the process of revising it began, and 2000 Standard 2.9.1 was gazetted. Revision was similarly delayed by, among other things, industry objections that any new Standard could be a restraint of trade if more stringent than the Codex Alimentarius Standard.

But there has been little sense of urgency about infant feeding in Australia. Rather, it seemed to me that there was astonishing smugness that our rates were so much better than those of our allies. There was implicit trust in infant formula as good enough and safe enough. That complacency was widely shared, even by women whose breastfed babies moved on to infant formula without immediately obvious problems.[1397] Industry was well aware that promoting breastfeeding (in a society where it would fail) was the best way to ensure infant formula use: Abbott's Vice President, WD Smart, said in 1981 to investors that

> 'the growth of breastfeeding has been good for the infant formula business ... Our research shows that many breastfeeding mothers eventually use more infant formula than those mothers who start their infants on our products.'[1398]

That was undoubtedly true in the 1980s. A breastfed start meant greater tolerance of the formula for many babies later switched on to it, and educated mothers could afford and were quick to take up the modern 'humanised' formulas, as convenient supplements or substitutes. These women pioneered formula use till 12 months, in many cases supported by health professionals convinced that the new modern formulas were so much better and more convenient. Public breastfeeding in the 1980s was still very problematic even in Australia, while in the UK and US it could be very difficult indeed. Some mothers, who had used formula without incident for the first child after breastfeeding through difficulties like nipple pain, even started a subsequent child on formula from birth. (Many I met regretted that decision. The child artificially fed from birth had many more problems than his sibling, even when the formula was the same, because of the effects of early programming.)

The 1970s onwards was the period in which many educated advantaged women returned to breastfeeding, but women in this demographic were also the de facto leaders in the uptake of the 'modern' formulas, just as their equivalents had been in the 1940s and earlier. All too often intelligent (but uninformed) women are the vocal, even offensively aggressive, defenders of an industry that has persuaded them that its products are the virtual equivalent of women's milk - and not only necessary but better than breastfeeding. It is easier to communicate with industry scientists and salesmen than it is to communicate with some women who might well be termed bottle bullies, as the names they call breastfeeding advocates are deeply hurtful (as well as utterly inappropriate).

---

1396  R7 was obsolete before it began, and calls for revision led the National Food Authority to publish a full assessment report and call for submissions in 1995. See  http://www.foodstandards.gov.au/code/proposals/documents/P93%20Full%20Assesment%20Report.pdf
1397  Or perhaps I should say diagnosed problems, as some problems seemed obvious to others!
1398  Smart WD. Transcript of Abbott Laboratories Investor Seminar, 4 June 1981 (copy on file)

# Enforcement and inspection

Most parents are ignorant of just how poorly regulated infant formula has been, and how little has gone into the enforcement of even minimal theoretical standards in the past. It may well be the most regulated food product in the world, as industry claims, but regulation is useless without enforcement. And enforcement is useless without penalties and publicity. When there are few public reports of inspection processes, we tend to think that all is perfect: they wouldn't be careless with such a critical product, would they? But was that always the reality? And is that the reality even today?

Was that the reality? In the 1980s I was told that formulas made in New Zealand were concocted in batches to the different company recipes twice a year, some in the same manufacturing facility. Brand batches of powder were discharged into large plastic bales to be transported elsewhere for decanting into tins and labelling. Bales could split, and piles of formula sat on the floor amid evidence of vermin infestation. My informant, an industry insider, saw staff shovel the top of the pile back into the bales before sealing it up for transport. This was the 1980s. And babies survived, though such contaminated formula was almost bound to have been implicated in some illness, perhaps meningitis, where few think that food could be the problem.

As the importance of the infant formula market began to be appreciated, the New Zealand government helped fund a state of the art production facility which addressed the obvious hazards of this type of production. The merging of the New Zealand Dairy Board with the two largest New Zealand dairy co-operatives via the formation of Fonterra in 2001 created a virtual monopoly, controlling over 95 per cent of the New Zealand raw milk market, for which it sets prices.[1399] After the global adoption of the international Hazard Awareness Critical Control Points or HACCP protocols, such gross safety breaches should have been eliminated by the major formula manufacturers. But there are many smaller players making infant formula and its ingredients in the world today, in New Zealand and elsewhere, and in some countries precious little critical and independent regulation or inspection, especially of products being exported.

I have no reason to doubt that major food companies with their own production facilities take care to source high-quality and clean milk, or multiple ingredients, and to process formula as hygienically as possible – a process that has improved dramatically over time. I also have no doubt that any such systems are not infallible, as the US scandal over genetically modified Starlink corn illustrated.[1400] Or that little gecko! (see Figure 2-11-1 on page 179) Regular independent monitoring of production needs to be the general rule – and penalties for breaches should include mandatory publication of the problems encountered.

---

1399 State sponsored and subsidised enterprises are seen as beneficial when they generate markets and profits for owners, self-funded unions as dangerous when they create collective bargaining power and wage increases for workers.

1400 Nestle M. *Safe food: bacteria, biotechnology and bioterrorism* (University of California Press, 2003). See also the Report on Agricultural Biotechnology by the Federation of American Scientists (FAS) at http://www.fas. org/biosecurity/education/dualuse-agriculture/2.-agricultural-biotechnology/starlink-corn.html ; Bucchini L, Goldman LR. Starlink Corn: A Risk Analysis *Environ Health Perspect* 2002; 110:5–13. Online 10 December 2001 http://ehpnet1.niehs.nih.gov/docs/2002/110p5-13bucchini/abstract.html

In 2006 the EU Directive on Infant Formulae and Follow-On Formulae had been adopted, and was made law in the following year by some European Union countries, the UK and Ireland included. The EU conducts global inspections of foodstuffs to be imported into its member countries, as does the United States; but the EU publishes the reports of such inspections for all the world to access, while I have found no such reports of US inspections. Interestingly, in 2007 the EU conducted independent inspections of formula-producing facilities in its member states.

As the 2007 EU Annual Report says, "A new inspection series concerning official controls over infant formulae, follow-on formulae, cereal-based food and baby food started in 2007. In preparation of the inspection series a questionnaire had been sent to all Member States in 2006 to gather information on different aspects of official controls in this sector. Based on the responses, a number of Member States were selected for inspection, four of which were visited in 2007: Ireland, Czech Republic, France and Poland." [1401]

Problems were found in all four countries. The findings of the Irish investigation are perhaps particularly important in the Anglophone world, as Ireland has become the low-tax home of both US and European companies producing massive quantities of infant formula for global export. In fact Ireland produces almost a sixth of ALL the world's infant formula, much of it for export to countries like Australia, outside the scope of EU regulations. The *Irish Times* tells the story:

A report by inspectors from the Commission's Food and Veterinary Office finds evidence of poor hygiene, lax controls, gaps in official supervision, and a failure by State agencies to follow important EU regulations at Irish-based baby food and formula manufacturing plants.

In one plant they found that raw milk containing antibiotic inhibitors was being dumped into the sewerage system.

In another factory manufacturing infant formula they found dusty and dirty paper bags in the pre-dump storage area. *[And these, containing ingredients, were not cleaned before the contents were dumped into the formula-making process. Shades of NZ in the 1980s! see page 419]*

Ireland is the largest producer of infant formula in the world, accounting for some 15 per cent of total production. Much of this is exported outside the EU. However, according to the report, infant and follow-on formula being *exported outside the EU* is not controlled for its composition or tested for pesticide residues or contaminants.

Product sold within the EU is subject to random sampling, but at a low frequency. Just six samples have been officially tested for pesticide residues since 2003. The report, based on an inspection carried out of the five Irish plants in September 2007, says there is a low level of compliance with labelling requirements, with just four infant formula products out of 19 and none of the follow-on products studied complying with the regulations.

---

1401 *EU Food and Veterinary Commission AnnuaL Report 2007*. http://ec.europa.eu/food/fvo/annualreports/ ann_rep_2007_en.pdf p. 4

The Food Safety Authority of Ireland (FSAI) is responsible for the enforcement of food legislation but it has contracted work in this area to the Department of Agriculture and the Health Service Executive (HSE). However, the HSE has not been given the powers to enforce three key EU regulations, the inspectors found, while the department has been exempted from enforcing legislation on infant formula and follow-on formula.

"FSAI oversight over the agencies did not effectively address gaps in official supervision over the evaluated sector," the report states. Moreover, the FSAI was aware of some of these gaps in official supervision for a number of years."

Testing for pesticides and contaminants focuses on shop products and does not specifically target the food businesses involved, according to the report. Some of the laboratories used for analysis were not accredited, and there were shortcomings with regard to the registration and approval of establishments.

The report also criticises the department for allowing manufacturers "unacceptable time-frames" to take corrective action when they are found not to be complying with regulations, "in particular for non-compliance which poses a potential risk to public health".

Responding to the report, the FSAI undertook to audit official controls in the sector and address any gaps identified. The Department of Health said it would transpose EU regulations in the area into Irish law, and the Department of Agriculture said it would examine procedures and carry out more tests.[1402]

The full Report and Ireland's responses to it can be accessed on the web.[1403] (No such transparency is possible in many countries where quality control is industry's business and is kept very much in house.)

But consider this report of practice in the Emerald Isle source of 15% or more of the world's infant formula .

- Just six samples of formula tested for pesticides in four years, and those possibly by a laboratory not accredited for the purpose!
- Dirty bags of ingredients coming from other factories, not even wiped before the contents are tipped into the mix! Any wonder that it has been difficult to avoid contamination of formula with fungal spores?
- Private non-accredited and outsourced laboratories doing such critical work when negative results might cause them to lose repeat business?

Reflexive avoidance of infant formula products labelled made in Ireland might be tempting, but it would not be sensible. At least Ireland is subject to some independent oversight by the EU Food and Veterinary Commission, even it that seems token. What do we know

---

1402 Cullen P. *Irish Times* July 7, 2008. http://www.irishtimes.com/news/ireland-criticised-over-controls-on-making-baby-food-1.943169. © Irish Times.
1403 http://ec.europa.eu/food/fvo/rep_details_en.cfm?rep_id=1977

about regulations and inspections anywhere else? Even if regulations exist, how frequently, and what are the results of inspections?

Many countries, like Ireland and New Zealand and the USA, exempt export formula from compliance with national compositional regulations, saying instead that they should comply with regulations of the countries they are going to. Which may explain why it makes economic sense for a US or European company to produce formula in Ireland or Singapore or New Zealand and ship it to Australia or China or the UK- perhaps especially now that China is tightening its regulations for formula made in China.

In Australia much infant formula is made for export. Under the old Standard R7 all exports had to comply with Australian Standard 2.9.1. In a recent industry meeting I asked whether it is now legal for non-compliant infant formula to be exported from Australia, and was told by local manufacturers that it does not have to meet Australian standards, only the standards of the importing country. New Zealand, another major dairy producer, does not require exports to comply with our joint domestic standard, Standard 2.9.1. In 2014 China has required formula importers to register, and imports to meet higher standards of disclosure,[1404] partly to deal with the widespread problem of poor quality, counterfeiting and false labelling of infant formula reaching China from what has been said to be over 3000 importers. And 2014 testing showed that Heinz formula imported from Australia contained more Vitamin B2 and less B5 than its labels declared, while in Hong Kong tests showed that two Japanese brands, Morinaga and Wakodo, were iodine deficient.[1405] What is happening in other Asian countries?

I believe that the more often, the more independently, and the more thoroughly countries test, the more anomalies and breaches they are likely to uncover in the infant formula trade. Government agencies may see it as their role to reassure parents, and governments don't want to upset major industries or spend money on legal contests all the way to the WTO. Thus it is not surprising that they leave quality control to the industry itself, with only token inspection, often outsourced to private business. It sometimes seems that the purpose of government regulation is not really to prevent or identify problems, but simply to support industry sales at home and abroad by reassuring potential purchasers. Wilful blindness and words on paper protect no one.

I hope this overview will spur readers to find out what is happening in their own countries, and to record that for global comparison. Perhaps WABA, the World Alliance for Breastfeeding Action, could undertake such a project.

---

1404 http://www.dairyreporter.com/Regulation-Safety/NZ-infant-formula-exporters-have-actions-to-undertake-to-meet-Chinese-standards?nocount

1405 http://www.dairyreporter.com/Regulation-Safety/China-Are-imports-to-blame-for-latest-infant-formula-problems

## Formula for export from the USA

Persons responsible for the manufacture or distribution of infant formula produced in the United States for distribution outside of the United States must register with FDA in accordance with section 412(c)(1) of the act. (See 61 FR 36154.) This section requires persons responsible for the manufacture or distribution of infant formula to register with FDA the name of the responsible person and their place of business, the name of the manufacturer, the manufacturer's place of business, and all establishments at which the manufacturer intends to produce the new infant formula. However, pursuant to section 801(e) of the act, infant formula manufactured for export is exempt from the act's adulteration and misbranding provisions, if the infant formula:

- accords to the specifications of the foreign purchaser,

- is not in conflict with the laws of the country to which it is intended for export,

- is labeled on the outside of the shipping package that it is intended for export, and is not sold or offered for sale in domestic commerce.[1406]

A US formula is adulterated if it does not comply with the nutrient regulations. A US-made formula labelled for export is not. So an American formula bought outside the United States may be very different from one bought within the United States. How many countries to which the formula is exported have any laws about infant formula? Or any capacity to develop them? Who checks that the formula accords with those laws or even the Codex minimum standard, not mentioned anywhere? To me, this says the US government, like Australia and New Zealand, recognises no ethical responsibility to children outside the United States. We have to hope, therefore, that all US companies cashing in on the white gold rush don't supply any overseas purchaser with goods that would be deemed unfit for American children. (And if they are fit, why can't they be sold in America?)

Regulation of infant formulas and their marketing is the subject for more than one book. Infant formula sales are booming worldwide, up another $5 billion in 2013, the fastest growing product in 'functional foods', the fastest growing food category.[1407] Remember that the total world market in 1980 was around $2 billion with 25% of that in North America thanks to government subsidies. It is globally already over $30 billion (see Figure 3-13-3

---

1406 http://www.fda.gov/Food/GuidanceRegulation/GuidanceDocumentsRegulatoryInformation/InfantFormula/ucm136118.htm

1407 Starling S. *World's fastest growing functional food in 2013? Infant formula (by a mile)*. Nutraingredients.com, 30 October 2013, http://www.nutraingredients.com/Consumer-Trends/World-s-fastest-growing-functional-food-in-2013-Infant-formula-by-a-mile. Also at http://www.dairyreporter.com/Markets/World-s-fastest-growing-functional-food-in-2013-Infant-formula-by-a-mile

on page 494.), in the estimated $50 billion babyfoods market,[1408] Perhaps 70% of that $30 billion is first stage formula. Not surprisingly, every company competes hard for a share of one of the most lucrative value-adding businesses ever created, with profit margins noted of 14-15% by one company. Given the margins on infant formula, it was predictable that some sections of industry would seek to evade any restraints on marketing that might decrease company growth and profits. It was also predictable that where one led, others would follow, to protect their share of a lucrative pie. And it is utterly predictable that the result is more death and disability and inherited disease. Who cares?

The international community has moved over time towards better regulation of infant dietary foods. A partial outline of some key events is below, for reference purposes. This will be expanded on the website at some stage. [1409][1410]

| Regulation of Infant Formula | |
|---|---|
| 1941 | US FDA required labelling declaration of can contents, and minima for iron, Vitamins A, B₁, C, and D. |
| 1967 | (US) AAP CoN: sets nutrient requirements for 17 vitamins and minerals; iron1mg/100kcal |
| 1971 | USFDA accepts AAP CoN recommendations – as *guidance* for industry. FDA iron minimum reduced to .15mg/100kcal (1mg/L) low iron formula, 6-7mg/L for iron-fortified. 17 nutrients specified. |
| 1971 | (US) AAP CoN recommends iron-fortified formula (80% US sales not) |
| 1974 | WHO noted decline in breastfeeding, World Health Assembly urged member countries to take action: WHA 27.43 |
| 1974 | UK DHSS COMA report Present Day Practice in Infant Feeding, first of what would be important 5-yearly reports. |
| 1976 | UN/FAO Codex Alimentarius Commission statement on infant feeding; first Codex Alimentarius infant formula guidelines - 60-70kcal/100ml; protein 1.8-3grams/100kcal (12-18g/L); 33 nutrients specified |
| 1976 | (US) AAP CoN expands recommended contents to 29 items; iron. |
| 1977 | UK report on Composition of Mature Human Milk |
| 1977 | Australia: NHMRC begins consideration of a standard for infant formula, a process that takes 11 years |
| 1977 | Scientific Committee on Food of the ESPGAN (Stockholm) Recommendations for the composition of an Adapted Formula |

1408 It is surprisingly difficult to get details of global and national infant formula sales (without spending around fifteen thousand US dollars to buy a global Euromonitor report, or A$20,000 to get an Australian report) Many bodies, even publicly funded ones like Dairy Australia, consider this confidential or sensitive information, even when all that is requested is the total value and volume of sales, with no market share data. A number of sources say that China is roughly 25% of global sales, and that the value in China is $13.3billion, so $50 billion may well be true. I am sure the industry will set me straight on this once the question is raised, though they have been reluctant to help when asked, so this may be amended.

1409 AAP CON Proposed changes in FDA regulations concerning formula products and vitamin-mineral dietary supplements for infants. Pediatrics 1967; *40: 916*

1410 http://www.foodstandards.gov.au/code/proposals/documents/P93%20Full%20Assessment%20Report.pdf

| | |
|---|---|
| 1978 | Syntex omission of chloride from formulas, parent campaign |
| 1978 | US Congressional Hearings |
| 1979 | WHO/ UNICEF meeting on infant and young child feeding |
| 1980 | UK DHSS guidance on Composition of Artificial Feeds |
| 1980 | US Infant Formula Act : regulations not till 1985, |
| 1981 | WHO International Code of Marketing of Breast Milk Substitutes. America opposed. |
| 1982 | Australian Dietary Guidelines had Promotion of breastfeeding as first guideline; later demoted as not universally applicable! |
| 1983 | Scientific Committee on Food of the ESPGAN. Report on the essential requirements for infant formulae... |
| 1984 | NHMRC Guidelines for Healthworkers |
| 1984 | IFM set up, replacing ICIFI |
| 1985 | Creation of the International Code Documentation Centre (ICDC) |
| 1985 | (US) FDA finalises some regulations for 1980 Infant Formula Act. 29 nutrients; 60-70kcal/100ml; protein 1.8-4.5g/100kcal; 60-70kcal/100ml |
| 1988 | Australia: National Food Authority Standard R7 – Infant Formula gazetted; work began 1977 after Codex. |
| 1989 | Council of Europe formed; European Union (EU) created |
| 1989 | Joint WHO/UNICEF statement- Protecting Promoting and Supporting Breastfeeding; the special role of maternity services. Spelt out the Ten     Steps to Successful Breastfeeding |
| 1990 | UNICEF/WHO Innocenti Declaration on Protection Promotion and Support of Breastfeeding |
| 1991 | James Grant (UNICEF) speech at IPA meeting in Turkey: creation of global Baby Friendly Hospital Initiative begins |
| 1991 | First EU Directive on IF and FOF adopted; specified composition, labeling |
| 1991 | Australia's National Food Authority created, responsible for Standards |
| 1992 | Safety of carrageenan questioned in UK; EU SCF 1994 |
| 1993 | National Food Authority initiated a review of Standard R7. Proposal P93 to create a Standard for Infant Formula begins its torturous eleven year progress to become Standard 2.9.1 |
| 1994 | USA endorses the International Code |
| 1995 | UK FIF and FOF regulations made law |
| 1996 | ANZ Treaty; Agreement to harmonise Food Standards Code. NFA 1996 NFA becomes ANZFA, Australia and New Zealand Food Authority. |
| 2002 | ANZFA becomes FSANZ, Food Standards Australia and New Zealand. Australian Infant Formula Standard R7 replaced by Standard 2.9.1 |
| 2003 | EU Scientific Committee on Food report on essentials for IF and FOF |
| 2006 | EU Directive 2006/141/EC on FIF and FOF based on SCF Report and lobbying/consultation: allows novel ingredients |

| 2007 | EU Inspections of manufacturing sites in four countries reveal very few industry safety checks |
|------|-----------------------------------------------------------------------------------------------|
| 2007 | UK Infant Formula and Follow-On Formula Regulations, legislating EU Directive |
| 2007 | Australia/NZ Food Standards Code, Standard 2.9.1; ongoing revision |
| 2012 | Australia Infant Feeding Guidelines for Healthworkers<br>Call for input into revision of Infant Formula Standard 2.9.1 (ongoing) |
| 2013 | EU regulations on advertising and health claims |
| 2013 | FDA regulates microbial contaminants in formula, considers selenium supplementation of US formulas |
| 2014 | EFSA NDA Draft Opinion: call for input into formula composition standard |

Figure 3-10-1 Some key dates in formula regulation.

# 3.11 The 1980s: bettering breastmilk

In the 1980s the use of infant formula worldwide was given a massive boost by a combination of new products and new infectious challenges, both of which made breastmilk seem far from perfect, and allowed people to consider that infant formula perhaps even better than breastmilk.

## 'Fortifying' breastmilk

The 1980s saw massive global marketing of a product called 'Human Milk Fortifier', developed by Mead Johnson, and soon other competitors. These have been mentioned previously (see index), but deserve a more detailed discussion, as they were significant in many ways.

In the mid 1990s I saw at first hand a premature baby whose paediatrician was so concerned to avoid formula exposure (because of the family allergy history) that the baby was kept longer than usual on parenteral (tube) feeding. The young midwife brought her taut-gut, tense, miserable baby to a course I was conducting. She apologised in advance for the noise the baby might make. I offered to wear the baby upright in a sling while teaching, as the least disruptive option for everyone especially the fatigued mother. The baby was clearly very uncomfortable, but constant patting and adjusting and movement against my non-lactating body kept her quiet enough, while modelling the sling's use (and the need to learn multi-tasking) was educative for some students.

Given the baby's behaviour and feel, I asked whether the baby had been exposed to cows' milk. No, said the mother. She told the group of the strong bilateral family 'allergy' history and the paediatrician's decision. So they never 'fortified' your milk? 'Oh yes, but it was the *human* milk fortifier', said this intelligent midwife mother. Imagine her fury when I told her what was in that fortifier. The class was shocked, as was her paediatrician when she spoke to him. So we discussed what to do for this sensitised breastfed baby. Three weeks later, back for the second session of the course, the baby was charming, relaxed and happy, snoozing peaceably beside her mother in a bassinet- a different child within days of the mother dropping the last remnants of milk from her diet. The happy, no-longer-stressed mother told the class that if she had a drop of milk in her tea, the screaming started again. I have never had a more convincing class assistant!

Well, one swallow doesn't make a summer, as they say, but is anyone looking for the flocks of swallows? I keep seeing them, and so do other experienced lactation consultants. The mechanisms that affected that midwife and her baby are the same in many other people, and many are deceived as she was. In late 2013 as I wrote I was helping a mother of a preterm baby in a major teaching hospital. She told me that the baby of every other mother she met in that NICU over five weeks has been given either fortifier or bovine formula or both; she was the only one to escape bottles of cows' milk in some form, and felt under enormous pressures to conform to the usual procedures. Some donated milk saw her through a very difficult patch as she recovered from dramatic blood loss necessitating multiple transfusions.

It helped enormously that her own mother had breastfed and was an articulate professional. The result: an easy baby, eating, sleeping and growing well. And a happy mother, relieved to escape without infant gut distress.

That baby did need more milk than the compromised mother could supply; fortunately she had a lactating neighbour. I have no trouble conceding that some nutritional supplements may be necessary for abnormal, very preterm, or extremely low birth-weight infants who are being mother-fed, especially where the mother has difficulty establishing lactation - usually for iatrogenic reasons. But ideally all supplements would be, or be developed from, human milk, so as to reduce metabolic and immunological risks; and their introduction would be independently tested for benefit and side effects. 1980s Scandinavian studies showed that preterms of 31-36 weeks fed pooled expressed and mother's own milk at intakes of 185 and 200mL/kg/day postnatal achieved weight gains comparable to intra-uterine growth with no signs of metabolic distress,[1411] and that such gains could also be achieved in VLBW infants with intakes of ultra-filtrated and freeze-dried donor milk at 110kcal/kg/24hrs and protein intake of up to 3.5g/kg/24 hrs, again with no biochemical problems or necrotisng enterocolitis.[1412] Those studies might have led to widespread women's milkbanking and use of adapted donor milk for preterms, tailored around the carefully-fostered mother's own milk supply.

Instead, the 1980s onwards saw bovine milk-based products in almost universal use in major hospitals, with parents feeling they had no option but to 'fortify' the mother's own milk, whatever its composition[1413] (rarely known and certainly not routinely tested, despite the risks of adding an imprecise amount to an unknown quantity). Many paediatricians still keep breastmilk-fed prems on the lower intake volumes suitable for gut-damaging infant formula, then order fortifiers added to breastmilk, rather than increasing intake volumes to those suggested by the Academy of Breastfeeding Medicine. The goal was to increase weight gain, as many units aimed to achieve intra-uterine rates of growth. (After birth, in a more stressful and demanding environment than the womb, such growth rates may not be optimal - or even possible for many children, though as with other forms of animal force-feeding, infants can be made to gain weight.) It was also to avoid devastating bone fragility by adding additional minerals intended to increase bone density.

While they may increase weight gain, and in some cases temporarily thicken bone, there are risks to using any such synthetic and unnatural products as cows-milk based fortifiers. Like the thickening starches added to formulas, fortifiers can greatly increase the osmolality of breastmilk (or formula) to which they are added, and increase gastric emptying time and the risk of infections, including NEC.[1414] As one review article stated, 'Addition of mineral and vitamin supplements to small volumes of milk can increase osmolality significantly and should

1411 Jarvenpaa AL, Raiha NCR, Rassin DK, Gaull GE. Preterm infants attain intrauterine weight gain. *Acta Paed Scand* 1983; 72 (2) 239-243

1412 Hagelberg S, Lindblad BS, Lundsjo A et al. The protein tolerance of VLBW infants fed human milk protein-enriched mothers' milk. *Acta Paediatr Scand* 1982; 71 (4):597-601.

1413 de Halleux V, Rigo J Variability in human milk composition: benefit of individualized fortification in very-low-birth-weight infants.(PMID:23824725) *Am J Clin Nutr* 2013, 98(2):529s-35s

1414 Lucas A, Fewtrell MS, Morley R, Lucas PJ et al.Randomized outcome trial of human milk fortification and developmental outcome in preterm infants.(PMID:8694013) *Am J Clin Nutr* 1996, 64(2):142-151.

be avoided if possible'.[1415] Higher mineral loads can also result in the formation of concretions called lactobezoars that can block the gut and require surgical removal.[1416] There are concerns too about the impact of oxidative stress, and the effect of the fortifier on the nutrient and immune components of the breastmilk it is added to.[1417] And in the long run bone density is as good or better in the infants not getting fortifiers, which may affect later osteoporosis rates.

Can we justify the use of cows' milk based products in milk-allergic populations when it costs more and harms infants?[1418] Such products must also influence the composition of gut flora, away from the normal healthy breastmilk-created template, with incalculable consequences. There is by 2014 a growing realisation that the harms associated with prematurity can be reduced by avoiding exposure to bovine protein, instead providing adequate intakes of solely human-milk based products and mothers' own fresh breastmilk, while dramatically reducing infant stress and energy needs by Kangaroo Care[1419] (see page 120). The "use of donor human milk from milk banks is currently becoming an accepted standard of practice for feeding preterm infants" even though pasteurised milk is damaged; fresh human milk is qualitatively better than heat-treated.

## What's in a name?

Yet first consider the name, 'human milk fortifier' – in my view a brilliantly deceptive term. Words do matter, as my readers may have noticed. The term 'human milk fortifiers' has become a damaging generic term, which makes interpreting research results difficult. Do a PubMed search for 'human milk fortifiers' and you will not know if the outcomes described in abstracts relate to

- bovine protein additives,
- hydrolysed protein additives,
- elemental products,
- mineral or vitamin additives,
- human-milk-derived additives, or
- whole human milk concentrates .

Look at the following table:

---

1415  De Curtis M, Candusso M, Pieltain C, Rigo J Effect of fortification on the osmolality of human milk. *Arch Dis Child* 1999; 81:F141-3; Pearson F, Johnson MJ, Leaf AA. Milk osmolality: does it matter? (PMID: 21930688) *Arch Dis Child*, 2013; 98(2):F166–9. DOI: 10.1136/adc.2011.300492

1416  Stanger J, Zwicker K, Albersheim S, Murphy JJ 3rd. Human milk fortifier: an occult cause of bowel obstruction in extremely premature neonates. (PMID:24851756) *J Pediatr* Surg 2014; 49(5):724-726.

1417  Hossain Z, Diehl-JonesW, Mackay D, ChiuA et al. Human mik fortifiers and the premature infant. In Preedy et al, op.cit., ch 18

1418  Ganapathy V, Hay JW, Kim JH. Costs of necrotizing enterocolitis and cost-effectiveness of exclusively human milk-based products in feeding extremely premature infants. (PMID: 21718117) *Breastfeed Med,* 2012, 7(1):29–37

1419  One prem baby who dropped from 2800 to 2600grams at 36 weeks  was 2700 at discharge (37 weeks) and 4700grams by 3 weeks postdate; skin contact and exclusive human milk feeding put her on the 75th centile in weight or full-term infants, and 90th in length.

| Recommended dose | Liquid multi-component HMFs | | | Powdered multi-component HMFs | | | | |
|---|---|---|---|---|---|---|---|---|
| | Similac Natural Care, Abbott Laboratories Abbott Park, II — 100 ml (dilute 1:1 with human milk) | Prolact +4 HMF Prolacta Bioscience — 20 ml (add to 80 ml human milk) | Enfamil HMF Acidified Liquid (4 pk) Mead Johnson — 4×5 ml vials added to 100 ml human milk | Similac HMF (4 pk), Abbott Laboratories Abbott Park, II — 3.6 g/100 ml human milk | SMA/S-26 HMF Pfizer Nutrition — 4 g/100 ml human milk | Nutriprem Cow and Gate — 4.4 g/100 ml human milk | Enfamil HMF, Mead Johnson — 3.8 g/100 ml human milk | PreNAN FM85 HMF, Nestle Laboratories — 5 g/100 ml human milk |
| Energy, kcal | 40.5 | 29.4 | 30 | 14 | 14.6 | 16 | 14 | 17 |
| Carbohydrate, g | 4.3 | 1.8 | 1.2 | 1.8 | 2.4 | 2.8 | 2.7 | 3.3 |
| Protein, g | 1.1 | 1.2 | 2.2 | 1 | 1 | 1.2 | 0.7 | 1 |
| Lipids, g | 2.2 | 1.8 | 2.3 | 0.36 | 0.16 | 0 | 0.1 | 0.02 |
| Calcium, mM | 2.135 | 2.57 | 2.89 | 2.92 | 2.25 | 1.65 | 2.25 | 1.87 |
| Phosphorus, mM | 1.518 | 1.74 | 2.03 | 2.16 | 1.49 | 1.23 | 1.45 | 1.45 |
| Magnesium, mM | 0.205 | 0.19 | 0.076 | 0.29 | 0.12 | 0.21 | 0.04 | 0.16 |
| Sodium, mM | 0.75 | 1.6 | 1.2 | 0.65 | 0.8 | 1.57 | 0.3 | 1.13 |
| Chloride, mM | 0.95 | 0.8 | 0.8 | 1.07 | 0.5 | 0.73 | 0.5 | 0.65 |
| Potassium, mM | 1.35 | 0.64 | 1.15 | 1.62 | 0.7 | 0.61 | 0.4 | 1.69 |
| Iron, mg | 0.15 | 0.1 | 1.76 | 0.35 | - | 0 | 0 | - |
| Zinc, µg | 610 | 700 | 960 | 1000 | 260 | 600 | 710 | 900 |
| Copper, µg | 101.5 | 63.4 | 60 | 170 | - | 36 | 60 | 50 |
| Manganese, µg | 4.9 | 12 | 10 | 7.2 | 4.6 | 8.2 | 4.7 | 6.3 |
| Vitamin A, IU | 504 | 61.2 | 1160 | 620 | 270 | 232 | 950 | 355 |
| Vitamin E, IU | 1.6 | 0.4 | 5,6 | 3.2 | 3 | 2.6 | 4.6 | 4 |
| Vitamin K, µg | 5 | 0.2 | 5.7 | 8.3 | 11 | 6.4 | 4.4 | 8 |
| Vitamin D, IU | 61 | 26 | 188 | 120 | 304 | 200 | 210 | 152 |
| Vitamin C, mg | 15 | 0.2 | 15.2 | 25 | 40 | 12 | 11.6 | 17.5 |
| Vitamin $B_1$, µg | 100 | 4 | 184 | 233 | 233 | 132 | 150 | 150 |
| Vitamin $B_2$, µg | 250 | 15 | 260 | 417 | 260 | 174 | 210 | 200 |
| Vitamin $B_6$, µg | 100 | 4.1 | 140 | 211 | 260 | 112 | 110 | 130 |
| Vitamin $B_{12}$, µg | 0.225 | 0.1 | 0.64 | 0.64 | 0.3 | 0.2 | 0.18 | 0.11 |
| Niacin, mg | 2 | 0.05 | 3.7 | 3.57 | 3.6 | 2.4 | 3 | 1.5 |
| Folic acid, µg | 15 | 5.4 | 31 | 23 | 30 | 30 | 25 | 40 |
| Biotin, µg | 15 | - | 3.4 | 26 | 1.5 | 2.6 | 2.7 | 3.5 |
| Pantothenic acid, mg | 0.77 | 0.07 | 0.9 | 1.5 | 0.9 | 0.76 | 0.73 | 0.7 |

Figure 3-11-1 Composition of so-called fortifiers added to women's milk (© Wageningen Academic Publishers)

These very different options, with very different risks, are covered by the one term of 'human milk fortifier'. At the very least the generic term for products deemed necessary for addition to breastmilk for babies under 1500 g should be changed to a neutral one, such as 'additives for human milk'. Differing greatly between countries and brands, as the table above[1420] makes clear, the recipes included corn syrup solids (sometimes called glucose

---

1420 Hossain Z, Diehl-Jones W, MacKay D. *Human milk fortifiers and the premature infant*. In Zibadi, Watson and Preedy, op. cit., p. 430. © Wageningen Academic Publishers

syrup), bovine whey, bovine casein, trace minerals and vitamins. Adulterating breastmilk with any of these could be relied upon to *make breastmilk more like formula*, in both parental perception and infant outcomes. 'Fortifying' breastmilk with foreign proteins may make for faster growth, but in fact weakens its ability to protect against infection and allergy.

Mead Johnson's 'human milk fortifier' was not the first such commercial adulterant for expressed human milk: Wyeth had introduced a 'fortifier' to Australia in 1981, and Ross had produced Similac Natural Care, a liquid 'fortifier', in 1985. (Language again: what is 'natural' or 'caring' about adding these industrial powders to breastmilk?) But at least in Australia in the late 20th century, Mead Johnson's was the most actively marketed product in this class. It was promoted to key hospital-based neonatologists and paediatricians only too ready to believe women's milk inadequate. Its initial high cost per sachet would plummet to 25 cents (or $1 per 100 ml breastmilk) after Nestlé Australia in 1992 introduced a (38 cents/100 ml) fortifier, named FM85. This was probably a better product in that it contained hydrolysed protein - and was not misleadingly named.[1421]

The names given to products seem to me to say something about a company's intentions and ethics. A name can be anonymous, instantly recognisable to those who need to use it, but giving no subliminal message such as 'your milk isn't strong enough for your very tiny precious baby, it has to be fortified. Women's milk is weak, and commercial mixes are strong and reliable'. If Mead Johnson didn't intend their product's name, 'Human Milk Fortifier', to give those messages (as I believe it does), or to mislead the allergic (as it certainly does), why not prove their bona fides by renaming it, now they know it is seen to be undermining women's confidence in their milk, and has harmed more than one baby, to my certain knowledge? Or better still, why not discontinue corn-laden bovine-based supplements altogether, now their risks have been demonstrated, when better products are readily available?

I cannot believe that the company was unaware of those subliminal messages of the name, or the powerful modelling effect of using such products for the smallest sickest babies in the most high-tech section of a modern hospital, endorsed by leading paediatricians. Health authorities and paediatricians are equally at fault in not subjecting such products to intense critical scrutiny before allowing them to be used everywhere without agreed protocols and scientific justification for every inclusion in the mixture. In 1995 the Australian Lactation Consultants' Association (ALCA) and the Mercy Hospital for Women in Melbourne organised a two-day conference, 'Breastmilk and special care nurseries: problems and opportunities'. Dr Andrew Watkins, staff neonatologist at the Mercy, presented the results of a survey he had sent to all directors of high level neonatology units in Australia, addressing 'issues surrounding the use of human milk fortifiers, timing and treatment of feeds used, nutritional supplements, and the use of stored or banked breastmilk'. As his paper said, nineteen of the twenty Australian units responded. 'The most striking feature of the responses was the wide variety of practice in many areas ... There is a particularly wide

---

diversity in the area of breastmilk fortification.'[1422] In short, when it came to feeding prem babies, doctors were doing different things for differing lengths of time and in response to different clinical indications. No agreed protocol existed, and side effects were common. Another expert presented a paper showing inter alia that 'commercial fortifiers are poorly tolerated and their clinical benefits marginal'.[1423] What was more, the team of which she was part had written that

> "The addition of nutrients of unproven value to breast milk at considerable cost requires urgent investigation, especially considering the lack of any national regulations for human milk fortifiers. For example, it would seem more scientific to investigate the need for trace elements before routine supplementation begins."1424

The conference was shocked by these clear revelations of uncontrolled experimentation. An expert in human tissue matters, Law Professor Suzie Linden-Laufer, had been invited to listen and respond to any obvious legal liability and ethical issues. She had anticipated focussing on concerns about consent issues and the use of donor human milk. Instead, she began her task as rapporteur by expressing shock at the wide diversity of practice in relation to fortifiers. She then pointed out that any person adding anything to any woman's milk was manufacturing a new product, which must be done under the strict legal requirements of Good Manufacturing Practice codes, and for which he or she becomes personally responsible in law. She went on to say that in medico-legal defence cases, protection is conferred by being able to show that what was done is standard practice among one's peers; but that it seemed there was no such standard practice to appeal to in the case of 'fortifying' breastmilk. The eminent neonatologist chair later commented to me privately that given the legal liability problems, it seemed that only exclusive maternal breastmilk and breastfeeding was legally safe; his take-home message from the conference was that his staff had better work harder to facilitate maternal breastfeeding and breastmilk supply. Yes indeed.

Some assume that 'human milk fortifier' has saved many lives. Perhaps it has, though there is little evidence of that. To me it seems certain that the uncritical and experimental use of cows' milk based fortifiers from the 1980s has caused deaths and injury (meningitis, sepsis, surgery, brain damage) that might not have occurred otherwise. I was told by one neonatologist of a paediatrician whose excess fortification practices had led to four children with gut damage being transferred to the Royal Children's Hospital for surgery to excise dying sections of gut; two would end up as nutritional cripples. In the ALCA/Mercy Hospital conference, invited UK expert Dr. Andrew Whitelaw described how the combination of commercial fortifier and mother's milk caused calcified infant kidneys, so that a completely calcium-free formula had to be prescribed; the child could not be breastfed. Who is responsible for the harm to that child, and his/her children and grandchildren?

---

1422 Watkins A. Australian Lactation Consultants Association, Proceedings, *Breastmilk and special care nurseries: problems and opportunities.* Melbourne: Dept of Paediatrics, Mercy Hospital for Women (1995) Melbourne, Australia.

1423 Dr Karen Simmer, part of an Adelaide team which had expressed their disillusion with some commercial fortifiers in print- see Metcalf R, Dilena B, Gibson R, Marshall P et al. How appropriate are commercially available human milk fortifiers? *J Pediatr Child Health* 1994; 30: 350-5.

1424 Ibid.

No one talks openly about such things to parents. The proof of harm to babies is not only in case reports in the medical literature, with its discussion of an old syndrome of gut obstruction revived.[1425] Proof is also in the better outcomes now being obtained by exclusive human milk feeding and lacto-engineering, and the development of fortifiers that are truly *human milk fortifiers*, being made from human milk. These are logical scientific developments. I consider that the existence of unregulated, under-examined and uncritically accepted commercial products delayed those better outcomes. Bovine-based human milk fortifiers were and are a marketing and commercial success, but it seems reasonable for me to think that they have harmed more babies than they have helped.

What of neurodevelopmental outcomes, though? Surely we have proof that these extra nutrients have helped preterm, low-birth-weight (LBW) and small for gestational age (SGA) infants? A global team expert in this area, led by Professor Maria Makrides, has reviewed the evidence in a Nestlé Workshop, which can be accessed and read online. Here I will simply quote its aims and conclusions.

> A comprehensive literature search was undertaken to identify systematic reviews of RCTs [random controlled trials] or RCTs including postnatal protein-energy, micronutrient or LC-PUFA supplementation in LBW infants and reported neurodevelopmental outcomes. LBW infants have well-documented cognitive deficits compared with their term, normal-birthweight counterparts. While it makes logical sense that at least part of these cognitive deficits may be explained by nutritional deprivation and that nutritional enrichment may improve the longer-term neurodevelopmental outcomes of LBW children, *few studies have been able to support this hypothesis. (my emphasis)*

So no, we don't have such proof, and we don't know yet what we should be doing about supplements. Makrides goes on to say, quite rightly, that

> the lack of support for the hypothesis linking nutritional supplementation and neurodevelopmental outcome is largely because the available studies were too small or had methodological shortcomings, limiting their ability to draw robust conclusions. Further large-scale rigorously designed intervention trials, with long-term neurodevelopment follow-up, are required to determine the optimal nutritional supplements and the timing of their administration to LBW infants.

Personally I hope those studies will rigorously compare outcomes where the products used are solely mother's own whole milk plus human milk products (preferably not heat-treated), and formulas and products that are non-human in origin. And as Professor Alan Lucas said in a later review, "This is what you're doing to premature babies when you feed them in neonatal intensive care: you're totally changing their biology for life."[1426]

---

1425 Wales JK, Milford D, Okorie NM. Milk bolus obstruction secondary to the early introduction of a premature baby milk formula: an old syndrome re-emerging in a new population. *Eur J Pediatr* 1989; 148: 676-8; Koletzko B, Tangermann R, von Kries R et al. Intestinal milk-bolus obstruction in formula-fed premature infants given high doses of calcium. *J Pediatr Gastroent Nutr* 1988; 7: 548-53.
1426 Lucas A, Morley R, Isaacs E. Nutrition and mental development. *Nutr Rev* 2001; 59 (8): S24-S33.

Although they tolerate breastmilk sooner than they tolerate artificial feeds, small sick babies are sometimes tube fed before they can be fed orally. Parenteral feeds also cause microbiomic disturbance, and sometimes serious infections. In the UK in June 2014 one baby has died and 14 have developed septicaemia[1427] from a feed containing Bacillus Cereus, a common milk contaminant, whose spores can be activated at temperatures of 65-75 degrees Celsius, and can grow at temperatures as low as 6 degrees. It has been the cause of many cases of meningitis and septiceaemia in the past.[1428]

## Impacts on research of formula exposure of breastfed children

It is important to record the use of all fortifiers and other supplements. Given what we know about the infant microbiome, no child given even one dose can be classified for research purposes as exclusively breastfed. And research matters. Poor-quality research had led to a widespread belief by the 1980s that breastfeeding wasn't really important to prevent sickness or death in countries with clean water supplies and sanitation: even breastfeeding advocates could bolster this idea inadvertently by talking as though only coloured babies in other countries were at risk of death from artificial feeding. Poor research explains why breastfeeding was for so long promoted in affluent nations as being about warm and fuzzy things like feelings and bonding, not about protecting children's lives and development.

In the 1980s, research was still failing to use exclusively breastfed infants as a control group, or even to disaggregate breastfed and bottle-fed. This flawed research, largely funded by industry, inevitably favoured the null hypothesis[1429] (that there was little difference between children who were breastfed and not breastfed.) It continued even after some of the studies by Peter Howie et al[1430] showed that any artificial feeding increased disease rates in affluent Western children, that exclusive breastfeeding from birth was protective. Those were really important studies. As James Akré has noted,

> In discussions with the principal investigator in 1989, prior to publication, and again in 2007, Dr Howie confirmed that this study was the first to satisfy droves of even the most sceptical observers that investigators had indeed finally managed to tease apart the impact of breastfeeding for even 13 weeks on infection and hospitalisation rates vs. the usual confounding socioeconomic variables in a high-income environment. The full text is available here http://www.ncbi.nlm.nih.gov/pmc/articles/PMC1661904/.

---

1427 Stones M. Baby death linked to contaminated feed. June 6, 2014. http://www.foodmanufacture.co.uk/Food-Safety/Baby-death-linked-to-suspected-food-drip-contamination

1428 Lequin MH, Vewrmeulen JR, van Elburg RM, Barkhof F et al. Bacillus cereus Meningoencephalitis in Preterm Infants: Neuroimaging Characteristics. *AJNR* 2005 26: 2137-2143. http://www.ajnr.org/content/26/8/2137.full

1429 An early critique of the literature was Auerbach KG, Renfrew MJ, Minchin MK. Infant feeding comparisons: a hazard to infant health. *J Hum Lact,* 1991; 7 (2):63–71. Dr Miriam Labbok has done sterling work on this issue: search by her name in Pub Med.

1430 Howie PW, Forsyth JS, Ogston SA, et al: Protective effect of breastfeeding against infection. *Br Med J*, 1990; 300(6716):11–16

These results in turn should be seen in the light of two factors: (a) the extremely low rates of breastfeeding prevalence and duration in Scotland during the period (1985–1989); and (b) the mass of information generated and validated since then, particularly with respect to the impact of following the World Health Organization's global public health recommendation that infants be exclusively breastfed for the first six months of life to achieve optimal growth, development and health.[1431]

Or even to survive. Formula-related deaths were finally beginning to be noticed in wealthy nations. Some were from infant formula contaminated by Salmonella, Klebsiella, and Enterobacter sakazakii (later renamed Cronobacter). These are discussed in Chapter 3.7 Unintended contaminants.

Microbial contamination of infant formula before the baby drinks it is unavoidable, given its conditions of manufacture and use. The most that can be done is to reduce or sometimes eliminate the worst of these microbes, the harmful ones classified as pathogens. Awareness and control of this aspect of risk has no doubt improved enormously over the century, both in factories and at home. The cost of a recall due to any microbial contaminants above the allowed levels can be phenomenal. In 2013 the recall of infant formulas, including Fonterra-supplied whey protein concentrate (contaminated with Clostridium sporogenes, mis-identified as Clostridium botulinum), has not only cost Fonterra, but also resulted in a demand for €200 million in damages from Danone, the second largest global infant formula manufacturer.[1432]

Companies have every reason to try to prevent such mishaps. But nothing can eliminate the risk entirely when a strange food is given to an immature organism: the very immaturity of the bottle-fed infant creates risk. That same degree of risk does not exist in an immature baby being breastfed, who is being constantly supplied with so many different factors that help the immature body better manage both microbial risk and other stressors, such as too much or too little of any nutrient. And in addition, many specific components of

---

1431 Just for the record, so that my children will know my trips away were worth what it cost them ... I travelled by train from London to Scotland in 1983 solely to speak to Dr Peter Howie about the lack of an exclusively breastfed control group in his research. I arrived to be told that he had double-booked– and so would now give me just 10 minutes as a French obstetrician was visiting. With no time to mess about, I spoke more forcefully than was politic, and his response was equally emphatic: exclusive breastfeeding would make no difference in any 'developed' nation. I left that meeting furious that he would arrogantly dismiss a biologically plausible idea – I had talked about the proven effects on gut flora – without testing it. Being a self-respecting Australian mother, I had said so in no uncertain terms! Years later I smiled to read his research, the first to show clearly that exclusive breastfeeding was indeed different from mixed feeding in developed nations. My time and money had not been wasted after all. The moral of the story: any individual can make a difference! A good scientist will test your idea, sometimes just to be sure that you are wrong (I could tell several similar stories, one about lactose and colic ...) Of course, you may indeed *be* wrong. Or you may be right! You might even be acknowledged, but don't hold your breath for that. The joy is in the achievement, not the recognition (but historians do like recording relevant facts).

1432 Astley M. Fonterra, Danone in talks to resolve WPC botulism dispute. *Dairy Reporter.co*, 2 October 2013. Check out this story at the website, http://www.dairyreporter.com [http://www.dairyreporter.com/ Manufacturers/Fonterra-Danone-in-talks-to-resolve-WPC-botulism-dispute.[?]

breastmilk, such as the newly-discovered protein called neuregulin-4 (NRG4)[1433], may be protective against the intestinal destruction caused in NEC. Lack of breastmilk's protection, nutrient imbalances and microbial exposures and cytotoxic products of fat digestion (see page 321) probably combined in creating what I see as another classic example of infant formula's global and often fatal collateral damage: the twentieth century NICU epidemic of necrotising enterocolitis (NEC).

## The NEC epidemic: 'a disease of medical progress'?[1434]

Preterm babies are well known to be at greater risk of devastating, often fatal, NEC (necrotising enterocolitis),[1435] which is so clearly linked to formula-feeding that in 1994 Dr Nils Raiha stated that

> "In Finland and Sweden there is not a single preterm baby who has not been fed exclusively on human milk. We would consider it unethical to give formula." 1436

Dr. Thomas Cone's admirable *History of the care and feeding of the premature infant,* carefully charts the emergence of NEC (necrotising enterocolitis) as a major cause of serious illness and death. By 1985 Cone reported that at least 1100 US infants died each year from NEC, and discussed whether the disease was due to the progress that kept more babies alive long enough to contract it. NEC prevalence had increased throughout the twentieth century, accompanying the rise of perinatal infant formula exposure for preterms, but American writers seemed able to overlook that fact.

Deprived of normal necessary gut protection and development, up to 7 per cent of Anglophone Western premature babies, including some being 'breastfed,' developed what could be described as gut gangrene: parts of the bowel died, and began to decompose. Surgery was needed to cut out the dead areas and re-connect the remaining healthy gut. The death rate from NEC was up to thirty per cent, while those who survived were often nutritional cripples for life, after bowel surgery created short gut syndromes. So 1–2 per cent of all preterm babies given infant formula were dying, many needlessly. For VLBW

1433 McElroy SJ, Castle SL, Bernard JK, Almohazey D et al. The ErbB4 ligand neuregulin-4 protects against experimental necrotizing enterocolitis. (PMID:25216938) *Am J Pathol* 2014, 184(10):2768-2778. DOI: 10.1016/j.ajpath.2014.06.015; Frey MR, Brent Polk D. ErbB receptors and their growth factor ligands in pediatric intestinal inflammation. (PMID:24402051) Free full text article *Pediatr Res* 2014, 75(1-2):127-132. DOI: 10.1038/pr.2013.210; onine report Breast milk may be protective against devastating intestinal disorder: http://www.sciencenewsline.com/articles/2014090913220004.html

1434 Cone TE. *History of the care and feeding of the premature infant* (Little Brown & Co, 1985) Ch. 7

1435 Sullivan S, Schanler RJ, Kim JH, Patel AL et al. An exclusively human milk-based diet is associated with a lower rate of necrotising enterocolitis than a diet of human milk and bovine milk-based products. (PMID:20036378) *J Pediatr* 2010, 156(4):562-7.e.  Both diet and body stores do affect the composition of maternal breastmilk fat, but do not determine it.

1436 Raiha NCR.(ed) *Protein metabolism during Infancy.* (Raven/Nestle 1994) p. 102. Nestle Nutrition Institute Workshop Series. Vol 33, online at http://www.nestlenutrition-institute.org/resources/library/Pages/default.aspx

babies, those with a birthweight of less than 1500gms, the incidence of NEC was up to 15 percent. [1437]

NEC can occur (rarely) no matter how babies are fed, if they have been subjected to serious stresses or damage before feeding is initiated. As better technology allowed more babies to survive, more babies would live to develop NEC. Both those facts helped explain the surge so that parents considered the death unavoidable. But parents were not told – and many doctors were not aware either – that where human milk alone was used for preterm infants, as in some Scandinavian or East German special care units, or hospitals that had active milk banks and informed paediatricians, NEC rates were as low as .05 per cent and occurred only in very damaged children. The rate rose wherever an established milk bank closed, as in Vancouver Canada. Even in 1991, when WHO's *Infant feeding: the physiological basis* was published, NEC deaths were not openly acknowledged as formula-related deaths. There had even been in-house debate over whether this major WHO text should note that NEC was related to artificial feeding.[1438] James Akre and I argued strongly that it should be. The decision to do so was soon justified: shortly afterwards, the definitive Lucas et al. study was published, showing that NEC was up to twenty times more common in formula-fed babies, even when compared with babies given a combination of breastmilk and formula. (The analysis made no comparison between exclusively women's-milk-fed infants and solely formula fed infants.) Read the abstract:

> In a prospective multicentre study on 926 preterm infants formally assigned to their early diet, necrotising enterocolitis developed in 51 (5.5%). Mortality was 26% in stringently confirmed cases. In exclusively formula-fed babies confirmed disease was 6–10 times more common than in those fed breast milk alone and 3 times more common than in those who received formula plus breast milk. Pasteurised donor milk seemed to be as protective as raw maternal milk. Among babies born at more than 30 weeks' gestation confirmed necrotising enterocolitis was rare in those whose diet included breast milk; it was 20 times more common in those fed formula only ... In formula-fed but not breast-milk-fed infants, delayed enteral feeding was associated with a lower frequency of necrotising enterocolitis. With the fall in the use of breast milk in British neonatal units, exclusive formula feeding could account for an estimated 500 extra cases of necrotising enterocolitis each year. About 100 of these infants would die.[1439] Just look at their data, in the table below, re-typed from the *Lancet* article:

---

1437  Kliegman RM. Neonatal necrotizing enterocolitis: bridging the basic science with the clinical disease. (PMID:2231220 *J Pediatr* 1990, 117(5):833-835

1438  Akre (ed.) op. cit., p. 32.  I was a paid consultant on this project, and the inclusion of this information about NEC resulted from a trip to Scandinavia, where I discussed NEC with Rolf Lindemann of Ulleval Sjukhuset. I came away astounded that such vital information was not being widely publicised. Scandinavian researchers had long been bemused by the high rates of NEC elsewhere. It was on that trip that I first stated to a medical audience that if breastmilk was needed for normal growth and development, logically they should regard the growth and development of artificially fed infants as abnormal.

1439  Lucas A, Cole TJ. Breast milk and neonatal necrotising enterocolitis. *Lancet,* 1990; 336(8730):1519–23 (PMID: 1979363)

| Gestation | All cases | | Confirmed cases | |
|---|---|---|---|---|
| | Formula only | Human milk* | Formula only | Human milk* |
| 25-27 wk | 7/35 (20%) | 13/83 (16%) | 5/35 (14%) | 7/83 (8%) |
| 28-30 wk | 7/83 (8%) | 11/231 (5%) | 5/83 (6%) | 6/231 (3%) |
| 31-33 wk | 6/75 (8%) | 3/263 (1%) | 3/75 (4%) | 1/263 (0.4%) |
| 34-36 wk | 4/43 (9%) | 0/113 (0%) | 4/43 (9%) | 0/113 (0%) |
| *Breast milk alone or in combination with formula. | | | | |

Figure 3-11-2 Gestation and frequency of NEC in babies fed some human milk or solely on formula. Data from *Lancet* 1990; 336(8730):1519–23.

A later study evaluating the Mead Johnson 'fortifying' product found "some evidence that infection and NEC could be increased with human milk fortification," suggesting "a need for postmarketing surveillance with this type of product" and a need to "further define potential adverse consequences as well as potential outcome benefits."[1440] That was published in 1996, more than a decade after the products had been introduced into many hospitals by those who thought breastmilk needed fortifying, and who assumed the safety of any industrial product rather than use women's milk.

Many parents still grieve for babies who died needlessly as Western NICUs used formula and bovine fortifiers instead of breastmilk and human-milk-derived products. It is true, of course, that NEC will (rarely) kill some babies no matter how they are fed, or even if not fed orally all, especially among the smallest and sickest who have been oxygen-deprived. Understandably, parents of damaged or dead babies do not want to hear that breastmilk or breastfeeding might have prevented the death or damage, when it is too late to do anything about the matter.

But every neonatologist and paediatric nurse surely has a moral and legal duty to reduce or avoid risks in this population of at-risk babies. And that means making sure parents understand ahead of time that mother's milk and *human milk derived* additives are especially important to these babies, and should not be contaminated after production, or adulterated by adding bovine protein mixes[1441] which reduce the likelihood of the baby establishing a normal microbiome.[1442] Regrettably, as noted earlier, adulteration and contamination of breastmilk have become almost routine in some countries, like Australia. In one study comparing determinants of breastfeeding at discharge from hospital in 2002/2003 with those reported for 1992/1993, the strongest predictor in both studies for a woman to be not exclusively breastfeeding at hospital discharge was having an infant who had been admitted to the special care nursery after delivery.[1443] Indeed, it is almost routine for studies citing

---

1440 Lucas A, Fewtrell MS, Morley R, Lucas PJ et al. Randomized outcome trial of human milk fortification and developmental outcome in preterm infants.(PMID:8694013) *Am J Clin Nutr* 1996, 64(2):142-151. (PMID:8694013)

1441 Sullivan S, Schanler RJ, Kim JH, Patel AL, et al. An exclusively human milk-based diet is associated with a lower rate of necrotizing enterocolitis than a diet of human milk and bovine milk-based products. (PMID: 20036378) *J Pediatr*, 2010; 156(4):562–7.e1.

1442 Heine WE. Protein source and microflora. In Hanson LA, Yolken L op. cit p. 186

1443 Scott JA, Binns CW, Graham KI, Oddy WH. Temporal changes in the determinants of breastfeeding initiation. *Birth* 2006; 33(1):37-45. DOI: 10.1111/j.0730-7659.2006.00072.x

the advantages of breastfeeding for infants, even ELBW ones, to mention a breastfeeding rate at discharge that I see as shameful.[1444]

Others, however, have got the message. The fact that exclusive human milk use reduces not only neonatal sepsis but also NICU costs will help bring about needed change.[1445] And the recent study showing that formula can cause gut damage even when not microbially contaminated, simply because of the free fatty acids formed during digestion,[1446] adds further urgency to this message.

The formula companies probably know the time is coming when only human milk products will be considered safe in NICUs. Ross, Abbott's formula arm, has created a co-promotional arrangement with Prolacta Bioscience Inc, 'the pioneer in standardized human milk-based nutritional products for premature infants'. Which is to say, the first commercial operation selling products made from women's donated milk.[1447] This privately owned company should recoup its investment fairly swiftly, now that one American state, Kentucky, has virtually mandated that only human milk be used in neonatal intensive care nurseries (NICUs).[1448] In the USA a second commercial milk bank is also now providing such products.

Such expensive and sophisticated human milk products may well be useful, and certainly will save money by preventing serious illness and decreasing length of stay in NICUs.[1449] But they are not always necessary either. Comparatively simple methods of lacto-engineering and milk banking can ensure that premature babies grow well and healthy on human milk alone, even when the mothers supplying the milk come from disadvantaged communities. In 1991 Dr Rolf Lindemann demonstrated how he routinely freeze-dried around 30 litres of donor breastmilk, and added some of that whole-milk powder concentrate to mothers' own milk if extra calories were needed; NEC was almost non-existent at Ullevål Sjukhuset in Oslo, where he worked. (I had never before visited a hospital where all the babies were so peacefully asleep.) Dr Paula Meier in Chicago pioneered the use of maternal 'creamatocrit' (percentage of cream) to make individual breastmilk formulas for preterms ... She was working with predominantly disadvantaged urban mothers, who proved capable of feeding their preterm babies unique blends of their own mother's milk, with the support of the

1444 Vohr BR, Poindexter BB, Dusick AM, McKinley LT et al. Beneficial effects of breast milk in the ICU on the developmental outcome of ELBW infants at 18 months of age. *Pediatrics* 2006; 118 (1) e115 -e123. doi: 10.1542/peds.2005-2382) doi 10.1542/peds.2005-2382

1445 Chapman D. Human milk dose in the first month is inversely associated with sepsis and NICU costs. *J Hum Lact*, 2013; 29(3):339–40

1446 Penn AH et al. Op cit.

1447 http://www.prolacta.com

1448 http://www.marketwatch.com/story/prolacta-praises-landmark-legislation-in-kentucky-mandating-human-milk-diet-for-preemies-in-jeopardy-of-intestinal-disease-2013-05-07

1449 Cristofalo EA, Schanler RJ, Blanco Sullivan S, et al. Randomized trial of exclusive human milk versus preterm formula diets in extremely premature infants. *J Pediatr* 2013; 163(6):1592–5

Mothers' Milk Club[1450] Meier created at Chicago's Rush Presbyterian Hospital.[1451] Informally many mothers have done simple lacto-engineering, using more cream for energy and sparing protein for growth needs.[1452] Dividing breastmilk into two lots, letting it stand, then skimming cream from one lot and adding it to the other: a simple process that can have dramatic effects on catch-up growth, and has been used successfully when fluid-restricted diets are imposed, eg, on an infant needing cardiac surgery.

In 1980s Japan, Professor Tsuyoshi Matsumura's unit mandated that every mother would provide breastmilk for her preterm infant, and thanks to strong medical support, and provision of free Kaneson breast pumps, each did.

Where there is no spare breastmilk, infants still do not have to be exposed to alien proteins. Indian doctors trialled the use of a mix of protein-sparing food oil and sugar fed by teaspoon to babies needing some extra calories, with no apparent gut problems emerging, unlike those when babies were fed alien protein.[1453] Such cheap (1-2US cents) and empowering initiatives have been too little recognised and publicised; they are omitted from consideration wherever the safety of industrial additives is assumed, and there is no vested interest to publicise them. Others are described in Chapter 5 of WHO's *Infant feeding, the physiological basis*, cited elsewhere.

But one of the leading American university hospitals is now achieving excellent growth in small sick babies by doing what was done a hundred years ago: giving them more cream. Breastmilk fat is being added to the diet of preterm tiny (750-1250gm) infants at Baylor College of Medicine Texas Children's Hospital.[1454]

Such initiatives need to be developed wherever preterm babies – or indeed newborns in general – are cared for. The case for donor human milk being preferable to infant formula is now established beyond doubt. In August 2013 WHO released a statement that makes this clear. It is available online[1455] and should be posted on noticeboards in every hospital.

> Every year, more than 20 million infants are born weighing less than 2500 g – over 96% of them in developing countries. These low-birth-weight infants are at increased risk of neonatal morbidity and mortality.

---

1450 Check out www.rushmothersmilkclub.com/ Mothers are capable of being milk technicians! Meier PP, Engstrom J, Murtaugh MA, Vasan U et al. Mothers' milk feedings in the NICU: accuracy of the creamatocrit technique. *J Perinatol* 2002; 22: 646-649.

1451 Meier PP, Engstrom J, Patel AL, Jegier BJ, et al. Improving the use of human milk during and after the NICU stay. *Clin Perinatol* 2010; 37(1):217–45. DOI: 10.1016/j.clp.2010.01.013. Free online: http://www.ncbi.nlm.nih.gov/pmc/articles/PMC2859690/

1452 I have known cases where the mother enriched her own milk with cream from donated milk and resolved jaundice rapidly, rather than using the infant formula that staff were threatening to give her baby, product of an allergic family. It helped that she had a lawyer partner.

1453 Singhania RU, Bansal A, Sharma JN. Fortified high calorie milk for optimal growth of VLBW babies. *J Trop Pediatr* 1989; 35: 77-81. These were 28-36 week babies of 1000-1750gms.

1454 Pathak D. Human milk fat improves the growth of small preterm infants. Baylor College of Medicine News, August 15, 2014. https://www.bcm.edu/news/pediatrics/human-milk-fat-helps-premature-infants-grow

1455 www.who.int/elena/titles/donormilk_infants/en/index.html

WHO recommends that low-birth-weight infants should be fed mother's own milk. When a mother's own breast milk is not available, the alternatives are either expressed breast milk from a donor mother or formula milk. Available evidence shows that compared with formula, donor human milk is associated with lower incidence of the severe gut disorder 'necrotising enterocolitis' and other infections during the initial hospital stay after birth.

WHO recommends that low-birth-weight infants who cannot be fed mother's own milk should be fed donor human milk in settings where safe and affordable milk banking facilities are available or can be set up.

Similarly, in 2013 ESPGHAN issued a statement[1456] confirming breastmilk as the feeding of choice for preterms, with mothers' own the best option.

If Brazil can support forty-six milk banks, why have wealthier nations had so few? The numbers are increasing and becoming more organised; even a Mothers Milk Co-op has been created.[1457] It is obviously not a question of resources, but of priorities and awareness.

Some have called the NEC epidemic of the 20th century "a disease of medical progress." I consider the NEC epidemic to be a disease of medical neglect of, and disrespect for, women's milk. I hope that greater public awareness of the scale of the deaths leads to greater accountability in future.

Figure 3-11-3 Breastfeeding rates in Europe[1458]

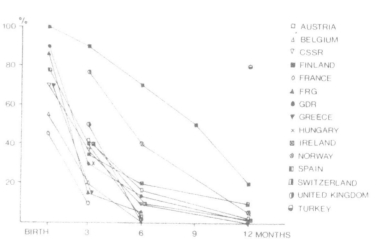

But doctors were not alone in discounting the value of women's milk by the 1980s. The value of breastfeeding was simply not understood except by those deemed to be crusaders and fanatics, perhaps even religiously motivated or with covert anti-feminist agendas. Breastfeeding rates had risen but were low everywhere, even in Europe, (see above) though campaigns involving changes in hospital practices and ongoing mother support could make a big difference: in 1972 only seven per cent of Finnish mothers breastfed to 6 months, and by 1983 the figure was around 70 per cent. [1459]

1456 ESPGHAN Committee on Nutrition: Arslanoglu S, Corpeleijn W, Moro G, Braegger C et al. Donor Human Milk for Preterm Infants: Current Evidence and Research Directions *J Pediatr Gastroent Nutr* 2013; 57 (4) 535-542. doi: 10.1097/MPG.0b013e3182a3af0a

1457 http://www.mothersmilk.coop/about

1458 Ballabriga A, Rey J. *Weaning Why, What and When*. Raven Press/Nestec 1984. p. 131.© Nestlé. Used with permission from Nestlé.

1459 Verrronen P in Jelliffe and Jelliffe, *Programmes to promote breastfeeding*. (OUP 1988)

But why, thirty years later, do so many hospitals still make little effort to see that preterm babies are solely breastfed with only donor milk or human-milk-derived additives, when the costs of illness are so high and can be lowered by the use of human milk alone, while growth can be fostered by skin contact?

Is this a legacy of the late 20th century marketing of 'fortifiers', which provided quick fixes that rapidly came to seem normative? Or is it the result of the distrust of human milk which developed in the 1980s, thanks to the way new immune challenges affected public perception of breastmilk? The first of these challenges was the emerging allergy plague; the second, viral transmission through breastmilk. Both combined to erode confidence in women's milk.

## The allergy plague emerges

Breastfeeding provides many complex forms of immune support for the infant, and modulates the development of the immune system[1460] for life and into the next generation. Yet by the 1980s, breastfeeding was becoming more like formula feeding, in that it was being associated more and more often with distressed and eczematous babies. The placid contented normal breastfed baby was becoming rarer; infant 'colic' was commonplace and even expected. Observant mothers began to talk about how their milk was affecting their baby's health and happiness. Sneered at by some as suffering from 'the muesli-belt syndrome', intelligent Anglophone mothers saw the connections with maternal or infant diet, and rejected the then current 'infant temperament' theory for distressed babies who were failing to thrive or developing other symptoms.

Previously, blaming the baby ('Some babies are difficult, and you've just got one of those, Mrs Jones') had alternated with blaming the mother. Both patronising putdowns are a common substitute for taking a detailed history. In the first half of the twentieth century, infant and child distress had been ascribed to the 'ignorant or incompetent mother', or 'cold mother'. Confident educated women of the late 1970s and early 1980s were also given what could be called the 'maladjusted mother' explanation. 'Mrs Jones, you are [too old/too young/too educated/too uneducated/too travelled/too untravelled/too experienced/too inexperienced] to settle into enjoying the dreadful restrictions of being at home with a baby. The baby senses this and cries, because you are not relaxed. Relax and your screaming baby will stop.' Confident women responded, 'Show us how to stop the baby screaming, and we'll relax!' Less confident women accepted a diagnosis of depression, and took the happy pills increasingly offered, retreating into drugs and distancing themselves from the distressing reality of their unhappy babies.[1461] Or else, in order to stay sane, they found ways to leave their babies with other carers, or dosed them with sweetened barbiturate mixtures, sedating antihistamines, and medications containing alcohol.

---

1460  Belderbos ME, Houben ML, Van Bleek GM, Schuliff L et al. Breastfeeding modulates neonatal innate immune responses: a prospective birth cohort study. *Ped Allergy Immunol* 2012; 23: 65-74

1461  I remember a wonderful 1970s paper which I cannot now locate entitled: "My doctor gives me pills to put him out of my misery." I have often cited the title and always get wry smiles and positive affirmation from mothers.

In fact, in 1977, amid much hilarity in a mothers' group I hosted, we discovered that none of us, from eighteen to forty-two, from high school drop-out to senior academic, were the right age or background or life experience to be having a baby. Obviously, if our medical advisers were to be believed, teen or post-menopausal pregnancy was what nature intended. Both are now increasing, but the babies still cry ... Perhaps Western women simply shouldn't have babies? This did remind me of a theme uncovered when I researched some nursing history: men hypothesizing that education made women unfit to mothers... because educated women's babies seemed then to do worse than those of the (breastfeeding never mentioned) poor.

What was also shared in my 1970s mothers' group was the reality that our babies cried hardest when they got too much cows' milk in their diet, either from us via breastfeeding, or in their weaning food, religiously introduced at four months in those days. To give credit where it's due, it was a radiologist, mother of baby Richard,[1462] who first made this connection, which all of us found incredible at first, so brainwashed were we about cows' milk. This started me reading. Having written a book on the history of the Victorian Nursing Council,[1463] I knew where the medical libraries were. And when I moved to the country in 1978, I made time to write. Over a hundred mothers responded to a 1979 article in the *NMAA Newsletter* sharing the idea that cows' milk exposure was the cause of infant misery; years of correspondence ensued as my three children grew. UK and US research about infant food intolerance and 'allergy', and the writings of Dr Claire Isbister in Australia, supported mothers' heretical findings. I collated experience and research in my book *Food for thought: a parent's guide to food intolerance*.[1464] This went through 20,000 copies in the decade from 1982. A significant number of Australian mothers soon discovered that their children's health and behavioural problems related to food intake.

Mothers in Australia, New Zealand, and the UK created self-help groups for parents of crying babies, infant 'allergy', and autism. All came to see infant diet as causative of both physical and behavioural symptoms in their children, and diet change as helpful, as NMAA mothers had done. In almost every case colicky infants had been formula-exposed soon after birth, then began crying ten to twenty-one days later. Where this was not the case, invariably the mother herself had been bottle-fed, and often the baby had been super-active in utero (see page 625). Parents who needed to do something about their children's problems with cows' milk often found pharmacists more helpful than their doctor. Was the reluctance to address diet due to a desire to protect parents from possible guilt feelings? Or simply reaction against a new concern and reluctance to take lengthy and tedious detailed histories, keep records, and offer dietary support? How much more important than ongoing diet is the pioneer diet that sets up gut function initially? (Remember the discussion of the Milk Hypothesis earlier in Book One.)

---

1462 I hope you read this and get back in touch: would love to know how things went from Fitzroy days.
1463 Minchin, MK. *Revolutions and rosewater: a history of the Victorian Nursing Council 1923–1973* (VNC 1977)
1464 Minchin MK. *Food for thought* op. cit.

## Mental functioning and allergy

Though ignored by many doctors in the 1980s, symptoms of allergy – whether to cows' milk or soy – can be cerebral: behavioural and psychological disturbances. In the period from 1950 onwards, cerebral dysfunction seems to have dramatically increased in affluent formula-feeding nations. The incidence and diagnosis of Attention Deficit Hyperactivity Disorder (ADHD) has risen steadily since the 1970s, when Australian parents were blamed for their child's behaviour, or told they were seeing a problem where none existed. MBD or Minimal Brain Damage was a term used in the 1980s to describe children who were 'just not right', couldn't concentrate, and had learning difficulties or odd behavioural problems and traits. Minimal for whom? It disrupted lives and relationships, in my experience. A mothers' group in the UK in the 1970s called Allergy Induced Autism (AIA) first charted regressive autism emerging after the weaning of breastfed children. Such parents of autistic children first pioneered the gluten/casein-free diets that seem to bring varying improvement – in some cases full recovery- for many children. The Hyperactive Children's Support and Action Group (HACSAG) helped thousands of families see their children's problems as diet-related, as did the Allergy Awareness Association (AAA). In Australia, a farsighted specialist, Colin Little, helped allergy sufferers set up AESSRA, the Allergy and Environmental Sensitivity Support and Research Association. All took seriously what pioneering Dr Richard Mackarness had found in his psychiatric patients: that diet and environmental exposures profoundly affected mental functioning.[1465] All were initially considered heterodox and a deviant minority. Their concerns are now mainstream, thirty years later. The complex and interlocking mechanisms are now being unravelled.[1466] And every teacher I talk to now has such damaged children in her class.

By the 1990s and since, the epidemic of what is now described as autism spectrum disorders can no longer be denied. There are many possible explanations for this astonishing new level of child brain dysfunction. Research into biological markers has begun,[1467] but seemingly without widespread awareness of infant nutrition as a variable needing to be explored *precisely and in great detail*. That this would be logical is surely suggested by those studies showing astounding 20-30% differences in white matter development in infants fed artificially,[1468] and disorganised patches in the cerebral neocortex.[1469]

Of course in even raising these connections I run the risk of being classified as a nincompoop[1470] by journalists who feel free to make sweeping assertions and derogatory comments without bothering to cite any research, simply dismissing what others say. Perhaps they should read everything that's out there, talk to parents of allergic children and

---

1465 Mackarness R. *Not all in the mind* (Pan, 1975)

1466 Cryn J, Dinan T. A light on psychobiotics. *New Scientist* 25 January 2014, pp. 28–9

1467 Walsh P, Elsabbagh M, Bolton P, Singh I. In search of biomarkers for autism: scientific, social and ethical challenges. (PMID: 21931335) *Nature Reviews. Neuroscience*, 2011, 12(10):603–12. DOI: 10.1038/nrn3113

1468 Deoni et al., op. cit.; Isaacs EB, et al. op. cit. Read about this at *Science* Daily, June 6, 2013. http://www.sciencedaily.com/releases/2013/06/130606141148.html

1469 Stoner R, Chow ML, Boyle MP, Sunkin SM et al. Patches of Disorganization in the Neocortex of Children with Autism. *N Engl J Med* 2014; 370:1209-1219March 27, 2014. DOI: 10.1056/NEJMoa1307491

1470 Kluger J. Got Credibility? Then You're Not PETA. *Time*, May 30, 2014. http://time.com/2798480/peta-autism-got-milk/

the children themselves, check out Ellen Bolte's video (see page 165), before dismissing ideas that are uncomfortable, but which may offer hope to parents dealing with cerebrally-disturbed children. For in fact world experts on allergy now freely include disorders like autism, schizophrenia, depression, and other 'mental health' concerns, even those common in the elderly, in their lists of possible outcomes of inflammation and allergy, including food allergy.

In North America there had been numerous pioneering doctors who had been writing for parents with these issues for decades: John Gerrard, Doris Rapp, Lendon Smith, William Rea ... and in the UK John Soothill, Maurice Lessof, Jonathan Brostoff, Andrew Cant and others. Pioneering dieticians like Joan Breakey[1471] in Queensland and GPs like Dr Vicki von Witt in Tasmania, along with nutrition pioneers like Dr Ian Brighthope and Robert Buist, and specialists like Dr Colin Little and Dr Robert Loblay, all deserve Australian recognition. Being vocal at this time took moral courage. But conviction was easy to come by, as clinical experience showed that the suggested dietary (and increasingly environmental) changes made a huge difference to desperate families. In the UK, the Royal College of Physicians of London and British Nutrition Foundation (RCPL & BNF) Report[1472] in 1984 had been very significant in getting some medical and scientific recognition of the problems of food allergy and intolerance, which are not all classic immune reactions.[1473] The chief author of that Report, Professor Maurice Lessof, encouraged my involvement in the medical allergy world of the time.

## Industry and Allergy

Industry knew perfectly well that the problem of infant allergy was exploding: their advertising exploited the fact. 13% of children would have problems with regular formula, said Mead Johnson as it introduced its more expensive 'exempt' formula, Olac. Industry had been busy for decades trying to create less allergenic formulas. Industry has to stay ahead to be able to mould the discussion to sell its products. The growing parental awareness of milk-induced 'allergy' – pointing directly at hospital-supplied infant formulas as the cause – may have helped companies to frame the problem of infant gut distress as due to 'lactose intolerance' (a problem digesting a sugar rather than an allergy in the strict sense), at the same time as they were sourcing new materials to create new, perhaps less reactive, formulas (see 3.5.3 Carbohydrates and oligosaccharide).

Soy allergy used to be rare, and is now common, after generations of infant exposure to soy oil and lecithin in cows' milk formulas. Milk allergy used to be rare and is now endemic. Cows' milk allergic children once tolerated goats' milk, and now many react to it with anaphylactic shock. Donkey milk is now being trialled; the Pope remembers drinking it as

---

1471  Breakey J. *Are you food sensitive?* See her website, *www.foodintolerancepro.com*; other books and resources are available.

1472  Lessof M (ed). *Food intolerance and food aversion* (RCPL/BNF, 1984)

1473  Jyonouchi H. Non-IgE mediated food allergy. (PMID:18782024) *Inflamm Allergy Drug Targets* 2008, 7(3):173-180

a child. Camel milk, sheep milk, horse milk, you name it: all are being discussed as possible food sources for infants;[1474] as is pea protein.

But I'd lay long odds that any food used the way that cows' milk has been used since the 1930s will cause identical problems three generations down the track. To develop a normal immune system, human infants need human milk, it's as simple and as difficult as that. Not synthetic industrial products, or milk of other mammals, but milk made by women, preferably their own mothers, or an allo-mother. Once, it was understood that breastmilk was unquestionably best for babies. And exclusive breastfeeding is still the basis for minimising harms of allergy introduced into Western populations, as Book 3 makes clear.

But industry in the 1980s also received a major boost to the standing of infant formula from an unexpected source, one which would seriously undermine public confidence in all natural bodily fluids, including, and perhaps especially, breastmilk. Viral diseases proved to be transmissible via body fluids.

## Viral disease and breastfeeding: HIV

This major public health threat almost certainly slowed the resurgence of breastfeeding in the 1980s. Fear of HIV/AIDS and other viruses led to widespread milk bank closures. Yet the soon-proven transmission of HIV through semen used for artificial insemination did not cause sperm banks to close.[1475] There is no adequate artificial substitute for either of those vital body fluids, but one was seen as indispensable, and the other as risky and readily replaced. Objectively, that is a drastic misperception: more global deaths, disease, and environmental degradation result from the lack of women's milk than result from any shortage of men's sperm!

## The first reported cases of breastmilk transmission of HIV

If a breast of any HIV-positive woman had been in the baby's mouth, many leapt to unwarranted conclusions that, if made about a uniquely *male* bodily fluid, would not have been tolerated.[1476] For example, the first 1980s sensational case of so-called breastmilk transmission was a child of a mother who had been transfused with HIV-positive blood after surgical delivery and blood loss. At that time in Australia such postnatal maternal illness almost invariably meant that the child was comp-fed in hospital, and so had an abnormal gut microbiome at the very time the mother would have been seroconverting.[1477] The child

---

1474 cf. Park and Haenlein, op. cit.

1475 Tyler JP, Dobler KJ, Driscoll GL, Stewart GJ. The impact of AIDS on artificial insemination by donor. (PMID: 3542178) *Clin Reprod Fertil,* 1986; 4(5):305–17. Ziegler JB, Cooper DA, Johnson RO, Gold J. Postnatal transmission of AIDS-associated retrovirus from mother to infant. (PMID: 2858746) *Lancet,* 1985; 1(8434):896–8

1476 Initial reports of infection via AI were challenged in ways that reports of infection via breastfeeding were not. Similarly, some studies concerned about infant infection focussed more on protecting infants from breastfeeding than on ending male-preferred sexual practices making maternal infection more likely, such as so-called 'dry' intercourse, which increases rates of all STDs in women but is not loudly condemned.

1477 Ziegler JB, Cooper DA, Johnson RO, Gold J. Postnatal transmission of AIDS-associated retrovirus from mother to infant. (PMID:2858746) *Lancet,* 1985; 1(8434):896–8

continued to get some formula even after hospital discharge, because by six weeks he/she had been fully weaned by a mother struggling to recover both from the birth and her unrecognised HIV seroconversion. By three months severe eczema was present (as in so many other bottle-fed children), along with that abnormal gut microbiota. Impetigo and iron-responsive anaemia also are on record.

Thus a seroconverting mother cared for a baby with a dodgy gut, low immunity, and multiple areas of damaged skin for thirteen months before the blood donor's status was known. Recipients of his blood (including this mother) were then tested. Both the mother and her toddler were HIV-positive.[1478]

This Ziegler et al report, often cited as "the first proven case of breastmilk transmission", **did not** in fact categorically blame breastfeeding, noting "some other form of close contact" might be responsible. But what route of transmission was widely assumed and publicised? Breastfeeding. Not gut damage due to early comp feeding, or mixed feeding leading to early weaning, or skin damage due to eczema and impetigo, or other blood or intimate contact. *Without any discussion of the fact that this was not and had never been an exclusively breastfed child,* this case was widely accepted as the first proven case of breastfeeding transmission.

And perhaps it wasn't. The context needs to be understood. At the time strenuous efforts were being made to deny the possibility of transmission by other routes, for fear of rampant homophobia. Since this time there have been many documented cases of 'casual' transmission: from a sibling whose bite did not break the skin[1479], from dentistry, from contact other than sexual, and in babies completely formula-fed from birth. Today, it is accepted that 10 per cent of paediatric HIV is *not* caused by mother-to-child transmission (MTCT) during pregnancy, birth or breastfeeding;[1480] we know that babies fully artificially fed from birth can acquire HIV postnatally. Pregnancy and birth pose the greater dangers, while any activities that expose an infant to the blood of any person with high viral titres are also recognised as dangerous. So am I the only mother ever to have had a nose bleed, or cut a finger peeling vegies, or had a scrape gardening or from little fingernails or the cat, and who did not remove all trace of blood when caring for a small child? I don't think so. My children have bled on me and I on them. If their skin had been damaged as that child's was, and I infected with a blood-borne disease, I might well have infected them. (As I wrote this chapter, my now-adult daughter was covered in blood helping a bike-rider hit by a car. Blood happens! And she did not rush to find protective clothing before helping.)

We also know now that exclusive breastfeeding might well have meant a very different outcome for this first unfortunate Australian child, as children exposed while breastfeeding

---

1478  ibid.

1479  Cocchi P, Cocchi C, Weinbreack P, Loustad V. Postnatal transmission of HIV infection. *Lancet* 1988; 331 (8583) i: 482. doi:10.1016/S0140-6736(88)91284-6

1480  However, this is usually phrased in a slightly different way, e.g., 'An estimated 430,000 children were newly infected with HIV in 2008, over 90% of them through mother-to-child transmission (MTCT).' WHO, 2010 document on PMTCT and strategic visions 2010–15, http://www.who.int/hiv/pub/mtct/strategic_vision.pdf) p. 6

have now been shown to develop antibodies to HIV,[1481] just as other mammals do. (Antibodies will not be totally protective, for HIV or any other disease, of course.) Exclusive breastfeeding for 6 months has been shown to reduce the risk of infection.[1482]

## Response to the first cases

In the 1980s many people, including health professionals and childcare workers, became almost terrified of women's milk. At least two infant formula companies distributed videos publicising the idea of breastfeeding as a means of HIV transmission. Though of course they were not trying to take breastfeeding's share of the infant feeding 'market,' just helpfully educating health professionals about infant feeding. (Industry claims this as its responsibility – though health authorities should disagree.) Breastfeeding by HIV-positive women was simply banned in developed countries, without any ongoing research into morbidity and mortality outcomes. That was possible only because formula was *presumed to be safer* for all children of HIV-positive mothers.

It definitely was not for some. Any infants born already HIV-positive – at that time the estimate was roughly one in four - were certainly harmed by this presumption, having a poorer quality of life and dying sooner. Researchers were well aware that they were in effect 'writing off' some children,[1483] if those I spoke to in the 1980s were typical. Unlike adults, quality of life was not a consideration for infants, and those babies already positive were not worth worrying about - HIV-infected infants were seen as doomed, although healthy survivors were later reported. This could have been predicted by anyone who respected breastmilk, since shown to contain "a soluble Toll-like receptor 2 (STLR2) [which can] significantly inhibit HIV-1 infection and inflammation.'[1484]

This helps explain why infants who acquire HIV via breastfeeding are at lower risk of early death than those who acquire it perinatally by other routes of exposure.[1485] And is part of the reason why

1481 Moussa S, Jenabian MA, Gody JC, Léal J, et al. Adaptive HIV-specific B cell-derived humoral immune defenses of the intestinal mucosa in children exposed to HIV via breast-feeding (PMCID:PMC3660449) *PLoS One,* 2013; 8(5):e63408 http://www.ncbi.nlm.nih.gov/pmc/articles/PMC3660449/pdf/pone.0063408.pdf

1482 Humphrey JH. The risks of not breastfeeding. *J Acquir Immune Defic Syndrome* 2010; 53 (1):1-4.

1483 One researcher 'justified' this by saying that these babies would die anyway, while to admit the possibility of damaged skin transmission meant that gay men might become social pariahs. I understood his views – LGBTQ people faced horrendous discrimination in the 1980s – but was not impressed by his care for infants, as he clearly *assumed* that infected infants would die, while I wondered if, with the help of exclusive breastfeeding, infected infants might become healthy immunised survivors who could help humanity deal with a new threat. I also thought that the quality of infant and maternal lives mattered, however short or long those lives might be. Knowing little about breastfeeding, he apparently saw no quality of life issue for women and children, while thinking quality of life and continued sexual functioning very important for his mostly male adult clientele. In my view, such tunnel vision facilitated 20 years of bad policy in relation to AIDS and infant feeding: policy that killed women and children.

1484 Henrick BM, Nag K, Yao XD, Drannik AG et al. Milk matters: soluble Toll-like receptor 2 (sTLR2) in breast milk significantly inhibits HIV-1 infection and inflammation. (PMID:22792230) Free full text article *PLoS One* 2012; 7(7):e40138

1485 Becquet R, Marston M, Dabis F, Moulton LH, et al. Children who acquire HIV infection perinatally are at higher risk of early death than those acquiring infection through breastmilk: a meta-analysis. (PMID:22383946) Free full text article *PLoS One* 2012; 7(2):e28510

"The majority of infants who breastfeed from their HIV-positive mothers remain uninfected despite constant and repeated exposure to virus over weeks to years. This phenomenon is not fully understood but has been closely linked to innate factors in breast milk (BM)."[1486]

No one heard that message in the mid 1980s. Instead, there was a rush to provide infant formula. So many babies would die needlessly in the next two decades. It is hard to overestimate the damage this all scaremongering and reflexive advice against breastfeeding did to public perceptions of breastfeeding and the growing advocacy movements. Some people were even frightened of bottled breastmilk contained in work fridges!

The US CDC led this mad 1980s rush to ban breastfeeding by HIV-positive women.[1487] This had serious spill-over effects on breastfeeding even by HIV-negative mothers, who once again heard prestigious health and aid agencies supporting artificial feeding as safe. (A CDC scientist even stated that "Artificial feeding is of no risk to the infant."[1488]) For in any situation where a significant number of heterosexual men are infected, and women have too little power to insist on safe sex, even the HIV-negative woman might be infected the next time she had sex. And since she could not know, or protect herself, she got the (dangerously wrong) message to protect her baby by not breastfeeding, and instead using 'replacement feeding.' Industry helped governments and aid agencies provide supplies of infant formula. By 1997 massive trials of 'replacement feeding' had started, another marker of western ignorance about breastmilk. As Kuhn would later write:

> It is unclear why there was any debate about whether replacement feeding is "safe" for HIV-infected women. Decades of paediatric research has documented the beneficial effects of breastfeeding for maternal and child health. Despite this substantial evidence base, evidence-based medicine proponents demanded that studies document whether breastfeeding or replacement feeding was the better choice for HIV-infected women. Randomised and unrandomised studies were done in several different settings with remarkably similar results.[1489]

Those results predictably were higher infant morbidity, poorer growth and – not at all surprisingly –more child deaths than maternal breastfeeding by HIV-positive women would have permitted.[1490] Dying young from diarrhoea or pneumonia thanks to artificial feeding is hardly a gain, though it reduces death rates from other AIDS-related illnesses! Yet some of these trials curiously measured only HIV infection rates as outcomes. Kuhn also notes that the (ineffective) policy of replacing breastfeeding to protect infants could be seen as delaying the (effective) policy of introducing antiretroviral therapy for pregnant

---

1486 Henrick et al, op. cit.

1487 Center for Disease Control. Current trends recommendations for assisting in the prevention of perinatal transmission of human t-lymphotropic virus type III/lymphadenopathy-associated virus and acquired immunodeficiency syndrome. *Morbidity and Mortality Weekly Report* 1985;34:721-6,731-2.

1488 Rogers MF. Breastfeeding and HIV infection. *Lancet* 1987; ii: 1278.

1489 Kuhn L. Breastfeeding and HIV transmission. In Zibadi et al, op. cit., p. 677.

1490 Humphrey JH. The risks of not breastfeeding. *J Acquir Immune Defic Syndrome* 2010; 53 (1):1-4; Kagaayi J, Gray RH, Brahmbhatt H, Kigozi G, Nalugoda F, et al. Survival of infants born to HIV-positive mothers, by feeding modality, in Rakai, Uganda. *PLoS ONE*, 2008; 3(12): e3877. DOI:10.1371/journal.pone.0003877; see also Coutsoudis A, Coovadia HM & Wilfert CM, HIV, infant feeding and more perils for poor people: new WHO guidelines encourage review of formula milk policies, *Bulletin of the World Health Organization*, 2008; 86:210–14

and breastfeeding women, so that *the assumption that replacement feeding would be safe for infants also killed women.*[1491]

As always, new technology was a factor in the ban: polymerase chain reaction (PCR) testing enabled the magnification of any viral fragments, so that viral traces were found in milk. For those ignorant about breastmilk, any virus trace in milk equalled serious health risk. However, viral traces in milk can be expected, given the immunising role of the breast discussed in Book 1. Whether the viral fragments found were infecting, or protecting, babies was not initially investigated.

It is very possible, indeed likely, that high virus loads from a seriously immunodeficient woman in the end stages of AIDS can infect and lead to disease and death. It is also quite likely that lower doses from a healthier mother with low virus loads do not, but importantly may prime the immune system in ways that can be passed on to the next generation.

Think about that. Retroviruses are not always fatal. Many mammals, from cats to monkeys, co-exist with retroviruses. It seems as though few people have asked whether the adaptation of humankind to living with retroviruses *depends on the creation of healthy survivors and immunised offspring*, in which breastfeeding must play an important and central role. I have said this since the 1980s, and to HIV professionals, to no avail. I was therefore delighted to see a recent study that showed that in our primate relatives, mucosal immunisation of the lactating female results in strong immune responses in milk, 'and may be a useful strategy to interrupt postnatal HIV-1 transmission.'[1492] At last!

It would take time for breastfeeding promotion to recover from this reflexive 1980s paranoia about infection via breastmilk. Some people haven't got over it yet, not realising that breastmilk inactivates many viruses such as Hepatitis C,[1493] and enhances the clearance of Hep B antigen in infected infants, reducing the incidence of chronic hepatitis and the number of lifelong carriers of the disease.[1494]

Forbidding breastfeeding was more draconian and damaging than forbidding all sexual contact for the HIV-positive, which none of the HIV researchers would have dreamt of doing: instead, they looked for ways of making sex safe. Why? Because sex is an important human activity – and breastfeeding just wasn't seen that way in the 1980s by the US CDC and such bodies. Assumptions and prejudices drove policy, not science and rational thinking. When finally the science was available, it became clear that

---

1491 Kuhn, op. cit., p. 683.

1492 I was told that they had not submitted such findings for publication, as it had to be a mistake. I thought not. And later research indicates breastmilk does attack HIV. See Fouda GG, Amos JD, Wilks AB, Pollara J, et al. Mucosal immunization of lactating female rhesus monkeys with a transmitted/founder HIV-1 envelope induces strong Env-specific IgA antibody responses in breast milk. (PMID: 23596289) *J Virol* 2013, 87(12): 6986–99.

1493 Pfaender S, Heyden J, Friesland M, Ciesek S et al. Inactivation of hepatitis C virus infectivity by human breast milk. (PMID:24068703) *J Infect Dis* 2013, 208(12):1943-1952

1494 Breastfeeding enhances the clearance of HbsAG in infants wwith hep B virus infection. Vajro P, Fontanella A, Avelllino N. *Gastroenterology* 1985; 88:1702. This abstract was followed by Vajro P, Fontanella A. Breastfeeding and hepatitis B. *JPGN* 1991; 12(1): 141.

studies are consistent in reporting these remarkably low rates of breastfeeding-associated transmission despite the HIV-exposed child ingesting many liters of virus-containing milk over many months (Richardson 2003)[1495]

In the absence of any anti-retroviral therapy, infant infection rates are thought to be around 10% in utero, 10% during birth, and 10-15% from breastfeeding, so that in total, about two-thirds of children born to HIV-infected mothers escape infection, and will be the base from which human adaptation proceeds. Formula fed children negative at birth can also become infected postpartum, so breastmilk is not the only way in which postpartum infection occurs. Infection risks are greatest when maternal viral levels are highest, during initial infection and end-stage disease. Keeping mothers safe from infection is the best way to protect infants – and prevent them from becoming orphans. Those who care about babies might spare a thought for their mothers!

## Learning from past mistakes

That already low rate of transmission via breastfeeding can be dramatically reduced. Subsequent long-overdue studies have shown that mother-to-child transmission of HIV can be almost eliminated by strategies that protect both infant health and also provide contraceptive benefits and allow the mother's body to recover, while protecting her against disease long-term.[1496] The rate of MTCT of HIV through breastfeeding has been reported to be under 1 per cent in nine studies where mothers received adequate antiretroviral therapy (ART) and exclusively breastfed.[1497] (Those few infected were said to have neglected their medication.) For a course of action that harms the mother and baby – as denial of breastfeeding or early weaning can do – to be considered ethical care, the alternatives need to be shown to be worse for her and/or the baby. Clearly breastfeeding while on ART (and developing those anti-HIV antibodies[1498]) is not worse, but better, for the baby.

Thus by 2005–06, the WHO-recommended course of action had become ART in pregnancy and lactation, as well as for the infant while breastfed, together with exclusive breastfeeding to around six months, and abrupt weaning (with care to avoid mastitis)[1499] thereafter; weaning not to formula but to suitable mixes made from nutritious family foods.[1500] The default assumption *should always have been* that ending breastfeeding at 6 months needed

1495  Kuhn L, op. cit, p. 677.

1496  Kuhn L, Maternal and infant health is protected by antiretroviral drug strategies that preserve breastfeeding by HIV-positive women. *S African Journal of HIV Medicine*, March 2012, pp. 6–13

1497  Morrison P, Greiner T, Israel-Ballard K, Informed choice in infant feeding decisions can be supported for HIV-infected women even in industrialized countries, *AIDS*, 2011, 25:1807–11 e-pub ahead of print *AIDS*, 1 August 2011, final version 24 September 2011, (PMID: 21811145) http://www.ncbi.nlm.nih.gov/pubmed/21811145)

1498  Mabuka J, Nduati R, Odem-Davis K, Peterson D et al. HIV-specific antibodies capable of ADCC are common in breastmilk and are associated with reduced risk of transmission in women with high viral loads. (PMID:22719248) Free full text article *PLoS Pathog* 2012; 8(6):e1002739

1499  Lunney KM, Iliff P, Mutasa K, Ntozini R. Associations between breast milk viral load, mastitis, exclusive breast-feeding, and postnatal transmission of HIV. (PMID:20121424) *Clin Infect Dis* 2010; 50(5):762-769.

1500  WHO, UNICEF, UNAIDS, UNFPA 2007, *HIV and infant feeding, update: based on the technical consultation held on behalf of the Inter-agency Task Team (IATT) on Prevention of HIV Infection in Pregnant Women, Mothers and their Infants, Geneva, Switzerland, 25–27 October 2006* http://whqlibdoc.who.int/publications/2007/9789241595964_eng.pdf Accessed 24 April 2013

to be proved safe. Instead, the policy of abrupt weaning at 6 months was prescribed before studies were done as to health outcomes for mother and child. Breastfeeding wasn't seen as sufficiently important for mother or child after six months of age. Later research then showed that *without* breastmilk after six months of age, more babies died of malnutrition and disease than died from HIV acquired in the second six months of life via breastfeeding.[1501] Not a good outcome, and again, the result of assumptions that breastmilk doesn't matter that much. We live in a mad world when the biological norm has to be proved safe and its synthetic substitutes are assumed to be.

## Current WHO recommendation

So by 2012 the WHO recommendation had become ART for all HIV-positive mothers from the time of diagnosis, and continued for life, resulting in an undetectable viral load. Child survival HIV-free is enhanced by breastfeeding exclusively for six months and continued until twelve months with normal weaning foods. However, if any HIV-positive mother cannot find another source of milk or enough food to safely wean, it is recommended that she continue breastfeeding for the normal time, i.e., up to two years or beyond,[1502] while continuing to take antiretroviral drugs, which help keep *her and her baby* healthy. (And which are being made available cheaply in low-income countries.)

And guess what? A recent study showed no transmission from mothers who received and were adherent to their ART for twelve months, and who exclusively breastfed their babies for six months, and then continued to breastfeed with other foods and liquids (as per usual) for the following six months.[1503] By 2012 proof of the value of breastfeeding is so strong that breastfeeding is recommended even if the impoverished or inaccessible mother cannot access ART.[1504] And the possibility of transmission of the disease to children by means other than the mother has been clearly demonstrated over time.

National and sub-national authorities are now tasked with providing mothers with clear recommendations about the safest way to feed their babies, rather than simply encouraging

1501 The many references for this statement can all be found in WABA's HIV Kit, *Understanding international policy on HIV and breastfeeding: a comprehensive resource*, released 3 December 2012, which has its own dedicated website at www.hivbreastfeeding.org. The morbidity/mortality studies of breastfeeding vs formula-feeding are listed at Section 3. They are taken mostly, but not exclusively, from the latest WHO HIV and IF guidance, which is also a good resource listing the various individual studies, see WHO 2010. *Guidelines on HIV and infant feeding 2010: principles and recommendations for infant feeding in the context of HIV and a summary of evidence.* Free online: http://whqlibdoc.who.int/publications/2010/9789241599535_eng.pdf?ua=1. http://www.who.int/child_adolescent_health/documents/9789241599535/en/index.html

1502 ibid.

1503 Ngoma M, Raha A, Elong A, Pilon R, et al. *Interim results of HIV transmission rates using a Lopinavir/Ritonavir based regimen and the New WHO Breast Feeding Guidelines for PMTCT of HIV.* Presented at the International Congress of Antimicrobial Agents and Chemotherapy (ICAAC) Chicago Il, 2011.

1504 For the most up-to-date interpretation, read together: WHO 2010 *Guidelines on HIV and infant feeding.* op. cit. *Plus* the Programmatic Update: http://www.who.int/child_adolescent_health/documents/9789241599535/en/index.html. *Use of antiretroviral drugs for treating pregnant women and preventing HIV in infants, Executive Summary*, April 2012, available at http://whqlibdoc.who.int/hq/2012/WHO_HIV_2012.8_eng.pdf

them to choose so-called replacement feeding.[1505] This means that health authorities are now responsible for giving accurate guidance on *the risks of all options*, *then supporting the mother's decision.* Yet most Western countries, including Australia, have not changed their paranoid position of advising *all* HIV-positive women not to breastfeed. Once again those with little knowledge of lactation assume that replacement feeding is safe without doing the long-term studies to assess relative risks of death and long-term disease created by replacement feeding. A baby dying from meningitis or SUDI or NEC or pneumonia or liver disease[1506] is just as dead as one who dies from HIV-related infections. And a baby's risk of dying from any of those cause (and others) is greater if not exclusively breastfed from birth to 6 months. Is that information HIV+ women are given? Who has the right to choose?

## What choices in 2014?

Only a minority of the world's women can exercise any real choice in this devastating situation. Women need to be educated and assertive to exercise any choice other than blind obedience to medical authority. Not to choose but just to obey blindly is one choice that often leads to regrets.

Personally, I suspect that any decision about whether, and for how long, to breastfeed will ultimately be made as much from gut instinct, as from the most recent scientific data. And frankly, so it should be. Emotionally, some HIV-positive women couldn't possibly breastfeed, and shouldn't be pushed to, whatever the risks. Equally, for others, not breastfeeding would cause huge emotional trauma, and have serious social consequences. By what divine right does anyone tell a mother what to do when either course could lead to harm for her child or herself? I knew of one brave UK mother who chose to breastfeed, with the full support of a wide range of health professionals who respected her decision; she did not continue all that long. But I suspect she will not be the only one to make that decision as awareness grows of the deficiencies of infant formula.

For there is much more to infant feeding than giving milk. Breastfeeding carries strong family, marital, cultural and traditional significance, as well as being crucial to child survival. Charities or medical authorities that dogmatically assert that HIV-positive women *should or should not* breastfeed are an utter disgrace. Whatever any HIV-positive mother does, she will be plagued by doubts and uncertainties about whether her feeding choice was the best one she could make. No woman should be denied the right to decide what is best for her and her child in her unique situation. For good or ill, we all get to live with the consequences of our decisions; we all need support, not condemnation, from those who may have made different decisions. Whatever a well-informed HIV+ mother decides will be the best decision for her and her child, but perhaps not for her sister or her friend. Given current research, we can support all HIV-positive mothers in their struggle to do what is best.

---

1505 IATT (Interagency Task Team), WHO, UNICEF Toolkit, *Expanding and simplifying treatment for pregnant women living with HIV: managing the transition to option B/B+,* March 2013, available at www.emtct-iatt.org/ toolkit/ (accessed 8 April 2013)

1506 Udall JN Jr, Dixon M, Newman AP, Wright JA et al. Liver disease in alpha 1-antitrypsin deficiency. A retrospective analysis of the influence of early breast- vs bottle-feeding. (PMID:3872949) *JAMA* 1985; 253(18):2679-2682

If we cared about HIV-positive women and their babies, one of the choices available to them could be sources of HIV-negative milk. This is likely to be an excellent option for a mother who felt she simply could not have her baby to breast, wondering if she was transmitting a deadly disease, but who also knows that her baby's quality and length of life will be worse if fed industrial milks. (Prolacta provides some processed human milk,[1507] a tiny drop in an ocean of need.)

But another mother might not want such processed donor milk, if she believed that her own fresh milk could possibly be a source of unique protective factors that immunised, rather than infected, so that her child could be one of the healthy survivors who will help create human immunity to this new plague. Informed choice – like universal access to antiretrovirals and care for the quality of life – can indeed be supported worldwide, and should be respected.[1508] Sadly, for many HIV-positive women since 1980 no such choice has been available, and no such support provided.

In fact it seems to me quite possible that only healthy breastfed survivors will enable the human race to adapt to living with both retroviruses or other new disease threats still to emerge. Scientists have found components of breastmilk that kill retroviruses. When in Washington in 1985, I was told of one laboratory's frustration with breastmilk: after spiking breastmilk samples with live HIV to see if it would grow, they found no trace of the virus by the time they looked for signs of replication. Later studies confirmed this.[1509] As I noted earlier, babies exposed to HIV via breastmilk do mount immune responses that may be critically important not just to them as individuals, but to the human species.[1510] The authors of the study concluded that

> The intestinal mucosa of children exposed to HIV by breast-feeding produces HIV-specific antibodies harbouring in vitro [i.e., in the laboratory] major functional properties against HIV. These observations lay the conceptual basis for the design of a prophylactic vaccine against HIV in exposed children. *[Mimic what's in breastmilk and we may have a vaccine!]*

And of course, these observations support WHO's current position of six month's exclusive breastfeeding by mothers on medications that keep virus levels low. Artificial feeding harms and impoverishes families and communities worldwide: it may threaten human survival if it prevents an adequate global response to such new infectious challenges. An immune system modulated wrongly by artificial feeding might be handicapped in dealing with such new global threats as bird flu, compared with an immune system modulated by breastfeeding.

---

1507  See http://www.breastmilkproject.org/give-milk/
1508  Morrison P, Israel-Ballard K, Greiner T. Informed choice in infant feeding decisions can be supported for HIV-infected women even in industrialized countries. *AIDS* 2011, 25:1807–11. Pamela has also contributed substantially to the indispensable 2012 World Alliance for Breastfeeding Action (WABA) research paper, *HIV & breastfeeding*, available online from WABA at http://waba.org.my/whatwedo/hcp/ihiv.htm#kit. Her writing can be downloaded from another useful website. Check out http://www.anotherlook.org/position.php
1509  Orloff SL, Wallingford JC, McDougal JS. Inactivation of human immunodeficiency virus type 1 in human milk: effects of intrinsic factors in human milk and of pasteurization. *J Hum Lact*, 1993; 9(1):13–17
1510  Moussa S, Jenabian MA, Gody JC, Léal J, et al. op. cit.

## Help or hindrance

Will this message that breastmilk may hold the key to human adaptation to new threats reach the wider world? I despair when I read:

> ... Ross students worked as business consultants to Rwandan government and healthcare organizations on a project that aimed to reduce mother-to-child HIV transmission and stimulate entrepreneurship and manufacturing in Rwanda. The assignment: Assess the country's capabilities to produce infant formula, which for children whose mothers are HIV-positive is safer than breast milk. The project was sponsored by the Clinton Foundation's HIV/AIDS Initiative ... Working with a team of teaching assistants from Rwanda's Kigali Institute of Science and Technology, the Ross team researched consumer needs, including interviewing 30 mothers; assessed local sourcing, production, packaging and distribution capabilities; and analyzed the financial feasibility of producing infant formula in Rwanda. The students found that the production of infant formula for the health market in Rwanda would be feasible if certain business conditions were met.[1511]

Let's imagine that this developing nation could afford to produce and maintain a state-of-the-art industry that produced formula with only as much contamination as that made in developed nations. Imagine too – a giant stretch of the imagination, this – that the University of Michigan, which sent these first-year Ross Business School students, agrees to underwrite the gift of infant formula to all those who want it. Even so, the product, however clean or free, will still kill more babies than will die from HIV contracted via breastmilk. Why is that not blindingly obvious? Or don't we care about how black babies die, so long as they are not HIV carriers? Their deaths certainly solve that problem!

## Viral disease and breastfeeding: HTLV-1

The second viral boost for infant formula in the 1980s was the earliest identified human retrovirus, HTLV-1 (human T-cell lymphotrophic virus). Japanese researchers had discovered that, like HIV, this was transmitted sexually and via blood, and could be transmitted by breastmilk. As a retrovirus, HTLV-1 compromises the immune system and allows serious disease to develop. It is a less serious threat than HIV, and less often fatal. But about 5 per cent of those infected[1512] do develop some rare but very nasty diseases, including cancer which typically appears in mid-life.

Because breastmilk has been assumed to be readily replaceable by formula, public health authorities (especially in Japan) have tested women for HTLV-1 in areas of high prevalence, and told all those who test positive not to breastfeed. In the next hundred years this will certainly reduce the incidence of those few rare diseases. It will equally certainly increase the incidence of many other diseases linked to the absence of breastmilk and the presence of formula in any child's diet – in the whole population and in future generations.

---

1511 *Dividend,* Fall 2006, p. 38-39. http://www.bus.umich.edu/kresgelibrary/resources/dividend/2006-fall-dividend.pdf.

1512  cf. the National Centre of Human Retrovirology website: http://www.htlv1.eu/htlv_one.html

Leukaemia researchers surely have an obligation to look at (for example) total cancers in both mother and child over their lifetime before concluding that they have done any good even for the 5 per cent saved from these particular cancers (adult T-cell leukaemia and lymphoma). We know that the 95 per cent who were not breastfed and who were never going to get such cancers are at greater risk of many diseases, including more common reproductive tract cancers. They have been put at risk for no purpose -especially when formula feeding does not totally eliminate the risk of HTLV-1 infection in any case. Read the following abstract:

> ... we conducted a prospective study to investigate the seroconversion rate among children born to HTLV-I carrier mothers on two highly HTLV-I-endemic islands where 8% of pregnant women carry HTLV-I. Between 1985 to 1991, 428 pregnant women were found to be positive against anti-HTLV-I antibody and were advised not to breast-feed their newborn babies. Among them, 212 women (50%) accepted this advice and the other mothers proceeded to breast-feed. Results were obtained from 277 children born to HTLV-I carrier mothers and were followed up until more than 30 months of age. When the seroconversion rate was analyzed by feeding manner, short-term breast-feeders (< or = 6 months) showed a statistically significant lower seroconversion rate than long-term breast-feeders (2/51; 3.9% vs. 13/64; 20.3%, p < 0.05). On the other hand, four out of 162 bottle-fed children (2.5%) became positive. It is hypothesized that maternal HTLV-I antibody may protect babies from HTLV-I infection through breast milk during the first 6 months.[1513]

So four of 162 (2.5 per cent) fully bottle-fed infants seroconverted, showing that they had been exposed to the virus. No prizes for seeing that if those children had been breastfed, breastfeeding would have been deemed to be the mode of transmission. How were these formula-fed children infected? The supposedly 'infected-due to-breastfeeding' children may have been at risk from that same mode of transmission, whatever it was.

And it is clear that formula-fed children who were not infected at birth do become infected later: another study found that all of four seropositive infected children who were formula-fed had been PCR-negative in their cord blood, while five whose cord blood had been seropositive 'gave no evidence of infection' later on. As they said, 'The results are not consistent with intrauterine infection, but suggest the presence of a perinatal or postnatal infection route *other than through breast milk*.'[1514]

In the Tadazaki et al. study above, just two out of fifty-one children (3.9 per cent) who were breastfed up to six months seroconverted - and may never develop disease as a result, while being at reduced risk of other cancers and diseases. For the two breastfed children who seroconverted, no mention was made of possible contributory factors like gut damage from early exposure to formula or other foods under six months; there was no discussion of exclusive breastfeeding versus partial breastfeeding, and almost all those mothers have reduced their children's risk of multiple diseases. Were the forty-nine mothers who ignored

1513 Takezaki T, Tajima K, Ito M, Ito S, Kinoshita K, Tachibana K, Matsushita Y. Short-term breast-feeding may reduce the risk of vertical transmission of HTLV-I. (PMID: 9209298). *Leukemia*, 1997, 11 Suppl 3:60–2
1514 Kawase K, Katamine S, Moriuchi R, Miyamoto T, et al. Maternal transmission of HTLV-1 other than through breast milk: discrepancy between the polymerase chain reaction positivity of cord blood samples for HTLV-1 and the subsequent seropositivity of individuals. (PMID: 1429208) *Jpn J Cancer Res*, 1992, 83(9):968–77

medical advice (and whose babies never seroconverted) congratulated for trusting their instinct to breastfeed?

But then, why are we worried about seroconversion at all, if 95 per cent of those exposed to HTLV1 will go through life without developing related disease? Seroconversion is generally a Good Thing. We vaccinate repeatedly to be sure of seroconversion happening. Seroconversion is a marker of exposure and immune response, as in vaccination, providing protection to be passed on.

I found more questions than there seem to be answers in the literature I could access. Skip over this next section, if you are not that interested in HTLV1, because frankly, the rest of this chapter just adds to our consciousness of what we don't know. Is breastfeeding over past Japanese generations the reason why the disease rates from HTLV-1 infection are now so low? Will more of these not-breastfed children later acquire HTLV-1 from blood or sexual activity as adults, and without any breastmilk exposure or vaccination, will this be more serious or more rapidly fatal in more than 5 per cent of them? Is the low seroconversion rate and even lower disease rate a marker of human adaptation to living with the virus, just as cats and monkeys have evolved to live with retroviruses?

So 20 per cent or thirteen out of sixty-four children breastfed past six months seroconverted, perhaps because of factors as well as, or other than, breastfeeding. (Toddler scrapes and cuts were being treated by infected mothers, and remember, formula-fed babies are also seroconverting months later. Are these thirteen children now immune, or infected and diseased? If the statistics given for whole populations apply, 5 per cent of 20 per cent – or 1 per cent – of children breastfed past six months by infected mothers are at risk of those serious cancers. That has to be balanced against all their other increased risks if they are not breastfed.

Using percentages with these small numbers can be misleading and proves nothing. We need to consider in detail the six out of the 277 mothers – four bottle feeders and two breastfeeders – whose infants seroconverted under six months postpartum. What was different about them from all those other mothers whose seronegative infants did not become positive under six months? Was this a lag from pregnancy exposure of the six infants? (One website suggests a 4 per cent rate for seroconversion postpartum: in what population of babies, how fed?) What was different about these babies? Was there any social transmission via damaged skin – of the mother (bloody nipples, infant oral thrush) or the infant – allergy producing infant dermatitis and maternal skin damage involving bleeding, after cuts peeling vegetables or gardening? What formula did the four bottle-feeding mothers use? Was it one whose fats are cytotoxic when digested? Did these babies' formula contain other pathogens, or their diet ingredients, making colonisation by HTLV-1 more likely? If the virus 'is not passed person to person by coughing, sneezing, cuddling or other social contact', do we just assume the formula-fed children were in fact infected in utero or during birth? If so, why didn't more breastfed children show up positive: did breastfeeding in the first six months reduce the number rather than add to it?

And what about the 151 children for whom no reports are given? Only 212 of 428 accepted the advice not to breastfeed, which means that 216 did breastfeed. Information is given about 115 of 216 breastfed and 162 of 212 bottle-fed infants. Those 101 breastfed infants and fifty formula-fed infants who are missing: were they healthier and not available for follow up, or sicker? Were they breastfed differently or mixed-fed from birth? What would they add to the picture? Was there any difference in infant mortality, hospital admissions,[1515] allergic disease, you name it in these cohorts? Are they being followed up to see at what price a small reduction in a nasty virus has been purchased?

The researchers concluded that short-term breastfeeding might be a good idea. But what about the longer term? Why did so few breastfed babies seroconvert when the breast seems designed to expose babies to manageable doses in order to trigger seroconversion and with it protection? Does breastfeeding make the difference to seroconversion, and is that seroconversion helpful to the human population in general, with established immunity rates for 95 per cent while risking 5 per cent? Once the human population loses its adaptation to HTLV-1, will the virulence of the virus increase in human populations? Globally, colonisation brought new respiratory viruses that wiped out indigenous populations not previously exposed to them. Will the dermatitis more common in artificially fed children exacerbate risks of social transmission? Are we sure it is a good thing we do when we eradicate HTLV-1 exposure and seroconversion in childhood, when small bodies are protected by breastmilk with maternal antibodies? These are questions whose answers we need to know before taking the serious step of advocating a total dietary substitution.

Or, if that childhood seroconversion is responsible for more harm than good, and the 20 per cent in this study is representative of the cumulative incidence of breastfeeding by a HTLV-1 positive mother, are there significant modifiable risk factors associated with long-term breastfeeding? While it is important that allergic infants are introduced to a wider diet while still being breastfed, is the reverse true for these children at risk? Should we advise mothers to freeze their milk for giving to children during the introduction of solids, as we know that freeze-thawing[1516] kills HTLV-1 of carrier mothers? Should we suggest that intermediate step WHO did for HIV (and has since abandoned) of exclusive breastfeeding to six months then rapid weaning with care to avoid mastitis for the mothers?

## The take home message about HTLV1

I hope there is lifelong follow-up of this experiment in banning breastfeeding. Survivors may be able to teach us much. The advice not to breastfeed given to them so confidently in the 1980s may be changed, a step at a time, just as HIV advice has been since researchers looked at outcomes more widely than simply the rate of proven seroconversion to a specific virus. So if you deal with a HTLV-1 positive mother, make sure that she has the knowledge and the power to make an informed choice, and support that choice, as for the mother with

1515 Tarrant M, Kwok MK, Lam TH, Leung GM, Schooling CM. Breast-feeding and childhood hospitalizations for infections. (PMID: 20864890) *Epidemiology* 2010; 21(6):847–54
1516 Ando Y, Ekuni Y, Matsumoto Y, Nakano S, Saito K, Kakimoto K, Tanigawa T, Kawa M, Toyama T. Long-term serological outcome of infants who received frozen-thawed milk from human T-lymphotropic virus type-I positive mothers. (PMID: 15566458) *J Obstet Gynaecol Res* 2004, 30(6):436–8

the much more deadly retrovirus, HIV. Playing God is not part of any health professional's role or duty of care.

It is hard to overestimate the boost the HIV/HTLV issues gave to artificial feeding, and the extent of the setback it gave to breastfeeding promotion worldwide. Infant formula suddenly looked better than breastmilk, safer, and more reliable. It emboldened the formula promoters. Breastmilk became a risky product while formula looked safe. Absurdly.

## Modernity and prudery

These links with serious disease meant that people had a reason to feel breastmilk was icky stuff.[1517] Another factor that needs to be mentioned briefly is the issue of dominant western cultural attitudes to breasts.[1518] In modern America until recently, the idea that a mother – or for that matter, a child – might enjoy breastfeeding was somehow obscene, a fact that is absurdly ironic in a culture where physical pleasure is so idolised. Breasts were depicted as big boys' toys, nothing to do with babies. Women who breastfed a child for longer than a few months could be accused of deviant tendencies, if not sexual abuse.[1519] Some lost their children to social welfare agencies because the length of breastfeeding was seen as abnormal.[1520] Another family was accused of possessing child porn simply because of breastfeeding photos, and their children removed to foster care for months.[1521] Breasts were never seen in public use feeding babies: in some states this was lewd behaviour and even illegal. Not until March 1993 would Florida pioneer legislation explicitly (a) protecting the right of any woman to breastfeed anywhere she otherwise had a right to be and (b) declaring that breastfeeding did not fall under restrictions governing lewd behaviour.[1522]

The B word, 'breast', was snigger fodder, and women were urged to breastfeed "discreetly" so as not to give offence. Many women could not contemplate going out socially while their baby was still breastfeeding: at my first 6-week postnatal checkup, a Greek mother told me in tears that her failure-to-thrive baby hated his bottle, but she wasn't able to breastfeed. Seeing her ample bosom, I enquired why not? 'Because I can't spend my life in the bedroom', was the answer. She wept as I put Philip to the breast in the waiting room. My husband would never allow that, she said. And I thought, thank God I waited till I was thirty to have this child, and no one will ever tell me where or when or how to feed him!

Where lip service was still widely paid to the idea that breastfeeding is best, as in Commonwealth Anglophone countries, it was bottle-feeding mothers who sometimes felt

---

1517 Breastmilk as polluted and polluting is discussed in Mavis Kirkham's book, *Exploring The Dirty Side Of Women's Health* (Routledge 2007). Oddly, formula's many links with disease do not result in similar treatment, though cows mik still does at times.

1518 Again, there are excellent discussions of this elsewhere.

1519 Many of these cases are mentioned in Rodriguez-Garcia op cit. Denise Perrigo was deprived of her three year old daughter for almost a year.

1520 Kedrowski KM, Lipscomb ME. *Breastfeeding Rights in the United States.* (Greenwood Press 2008)

1521 http://www.dallasobserver.com/2003-04-17/news/1-hour-arrest/full/

1522 Today, most US states have adopted similar legislation http://www.ncsl.org/issues-research/health/breastfeeding-state-laws.aspx. As James Akré said, the only thing worse than adopting such legislation is the necessity to do so.

defensive. But so did breastfeeding mothers. Elite Australian women created the "Nursing Mothers Association" – "breastfeeding mothers" would be controversial – even though the word 'nursing' was confusing, not normally used for breastfeeding in Australia, but for a profession, or more general care of invalids. Breastfeeding women too felt defensive, and needed support groups both to help them establish breastfeeding, or to maintain their resolve to breastfeed longer than the norm, in a bottle-dominated culture. Breastfeeding in public could be confronting; some people objected, and some tried to interfere and request mothers to leave the premises, or use the toilets! Breastfeeding for three months or so was applauded; to six months, perhaps even nine, was odd but OK. But breastfeeding solely without any formula, breastfeeding beyond 12 months – these were and in places still are weird and deviant behaviours.

Mothers who breastfed longer in small communities were talked about as odd: I certainly was. I had to explain to my two-year old that in a small country town we couldn't always just sit down and feed anywhere, because so many people had never been breastfed, "and it made them feel all twisted and sad inside to see us enjoying ourselves, because they had missed out on all that lovely cuddling. So as not to make them feel bad I would feed him back home; he was so big now that it would be awkward anyway without a comfy chair." (To which he responded hopefully: We could lie down on the grass? I laughed out loud at the thought of how that would go down with some of the locals!)

That was laidback rural Australia, where breastfeeding was unusual but approved of... in small doses for little babies in wraps with no hint of a nipple, puh-lease! It had to be much more difficult in BabyBottleLand, the USA. At least I was never arrested for breaking any laws about public decency! (Though I would have been in the States: no nursing aprons for me!)

Of course all these negatives about breastfeeding were broadcast in medical journals to health professionals worldwide, and publicised to parents. Thanks to these negatives, and the positive and persuasive marketing of infant formula, many countries in the 1980s experienced an increase in overall infant formula feeding, even where breastfeeding initiation was increasing. The sales figures kept going up. Breastfeeding duration declined as formula feeding duration increased. In countries with the means and the will to monitor this, such as Kenya, huge rises in infant mortality would be recorded as a result.[1523] This would draw the world's attention to the problems of suitable complementary feeding for children after the first six months of life. But even when this is discussed, breastmilk and formula feeding are still treated as identical interchangeable activities, when they are not.

Why do modern parents - unlike all previous generations- believe that they are? The answer is not hard to find on the web.

---

1523 Wafula SW, Ikamari LD, K'Oyugi BO. In search for an explanation to the upsurge in infant mortality in Kenya during the 1988–2003 period. (PMID: 22708542) *BMC Public Health* 2012, 12:441. The infant death rate rose from 59 to 78 per thousand births. Shorter breastfeeding duration was seen as a key cause.

- In May 2014, the Mead Johnson website says, under "Choosing to Formula-Feed" There are many reasons a mother may decide formula feeding is the best option for providing her child with the basic nutrition requirements needed for proper growth and development. .....

- According to a recent study, most new mothers (9 out of 10 actually) use formula at some point during baby's first year. So you're not alone, not by a long shot.

- According to a recent study, most new mothers **(9 out of 10, actually)** use formula at some point during their baby's first year. So you're not alone, not by a long shot.."

Normalising bottle feeding again. Framing it as "the best option", no risks involved, "proper growth and development" guaranteed. Appealing to women's need to control their own lives. And sliding over the fact that most of the ten do not choose, but are forced to use, infant formula, thanks in large part to the mythology industry maintains.

This is not a matter of choice between equivalent options, as we are brainwashed to think. It is a choice between the normal and the abnormal. We can be grateful that prostheses exist, but never consider them as good as normal limbs; we do not suggest using prostheses except when truly needed, and are always working to improve them. So we accept that formula exists and is sometimes needed, but understand that it should never be chosen over better alternatives which we should be constantly striving to make available. After all, losing a limb does not alter the normal development of our children or grandchildren. Not being breastfed does.

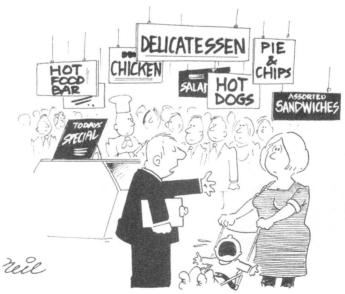

"Feed a baby in here? Out of the question!"

Figure 3-11-4 An appropriate place to breastfeed? Image © Neil Matterson. From *Is he biting again?* (Marion Books, 1984) p. 81

# 3.12 Making or marketing immunity?

By the late 1980s and 1990s, formula was coming to be considered by many health professionals, and much of the general public, to be almost equivalent to breastmilk in terms of its nutritional composition. Perfect nutritionally, or at least 'so close as to make no difference'. But discoveries in immunology had created a reviving interest in breastmilk, at that time still synonymous with breastfeeding. (Soon this would no longer be true, as breastmilk morphed into a product quite often available by bottle.)[1524] Even in their own advertising the companies now conceded that breastmilk contained important 'antibodies' that 'perfect' formula didn't– and they all ramped up research into immune factors capable of being added to infant formula. Added, preferably before too many parents became aware that infant formula in this regard was a good deal less than 'the perfect mix of science and love'.

The delaying tactic meanwhile was to reiterate the old mantra that of course these antibodies in breastmilk –no mention of hormones, enzymes, nerve growth factor, or transfer factors, just antibodies - were really important in 'developing' countries, but made little difference in countries where water was clean and medication available. 'Antibodies' weren't necessary for normal health and function. All formula labels emphasised that only the *misuse* of the product could make babies ill. Yet soon properly designed research was beginning to show that *any* use of the product, however carefully prepared, could increase illness in children; and that infant formula is both a risk factor and a vector for infection.

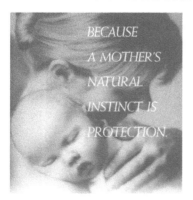

Figure 3-12-1 Scientific and factual or still playing the fear card?

Industry simply cannot allow a public perception to develop globally that formula is deficient, lacking anything very important in breastmilk – though of course it always had and still does. The discovery of thousands of new distinct immune and bioactive factors in breastmilk has provided many options for industry to commercialise, so that companies could claim to be providing immune protection for babies too. Industry well understood that *being thought to* provide immune protection was all that was needed for marketing purposes. The proof that their selected additives provided any such thing has been a long time coming, and even in 2014 a Draft Opinion makes it clear that there's little to show for the money spent on what the EFSA Panel on Dietetic Products, Nutrition and Allergies (EFSA NDA) characterises as poor quality research.[1525] But after the nutrition-focussed marketing of the 1980s, industry

---

1524 The history of breast pumps and their effects since the 1980s is complex. Obviously they facilitate women continuing to breastfeed in some circumstances, and are useful for many women. They also facilitate milk sharing. But it can be argued that they undermine breastfeeding and reduce any societal pressure to allow women to be with their infants for at least six or more months after birth. They make the milk more valuable than the breast/body/woman that provides it, and facilitate commercial exploitation of women and women's milk. This too is a subject for a detailed examination – but not in this book.

1525 EFSA NDAS http://www.efsa.europa.eu/en/consultations/call/140424.pdf *Essential composition of infant and follow-on formula – draft for public consultation*. EFSA Panel on Dietetic Products, Nutrition and Allergies. doi 10.2903/j.efsa.20xx.NNNN

moved on to immune-focussed marketing in the 1990s. One company's four-page spread full of baby images[1526] asked "Is his immune system functioning as well as it could?" The truthful answer to which is: "No, not if he is formula-fed." Their marketing implied that the answer would be yes, if their nucleotide-containing formulas were used. Ironically, one of the images used to advertise this was of a cute smiling child that most experienced clinicians might immediately suspect of being allergic.

Advertising works to grow the business, by addressing parents' concerns, even if the research doesn't prove that formula has the benefits it claims. Parents' feeding choices are based on beliefs, not facts.

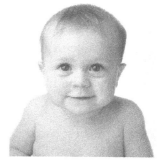

That infant formula is completely safe is one such belief – or few mothers would choose infant formula, because – as the industry tells us in the above image, so factually and scientifically, not at all emotionally – "a mother's natural instinct is protection."

Figure 3-12-2 Panda eyes?

## Nucleotides

One of the first campaigns to insinuate that infant formula had protective properties revolved around the addition of nucleotides. Involved in making RNA and DNA, and in enzyme reactions, these were the first overtly immune-related infant formula additives in the 1990s. Added to Japanese formula in 1965, in the 1980s these were trialled in the UK, where researchers found that they discouraged the growth of bifidobacteria, and encouraged the growth of E. coli in the neonatal gut;[1527] and also in Spain, where researchers lodged a European patent application.[1528]  Other US company research was done in Mexico. Ross Abbott added them to US formula in 1989, at a level of 33mg/L. They could do so, because the additives used were on the FDA GRAS list, being used in other foodstuffs.

Breastmilk contains many nucleotides, all interactive, and present in milk in doses influenced by circadian rhythms. Industry added just five synthetic ones, with – of course – none of the other interactive immunomodulatory factors of breastmilk. This was then advertised in language that can be paraphrased as:

- breastmilk confers immunity
- nucleotides occur naturally in breastmilk
- nucleotides help maintain a baby's immune system
- our formulas are now fortified with nucleotides.

---

1526  The 'panda eyes' typical of allergy, shown above, represent perhaps inadvertent truth in advertising.

1527  Balmer SE, Harvey LS, Wharton BA Diet and faecal flora in the newborn: nucleotides. (PMID:2696432) *Arch Dis Child* 1994; 70: F137-140.

1528  It ought to be mandatory for authors of scientific articles accepted for publication to declare their interest in patents or shares or other potential avenues of reward when writing about infant formula developments. Some journals require this nowadays.

What would you conclude? At the very least, this implicit but faulty[1529] syllogism allows an inference of safety and efficacy to be drawn. (Which is why such language has since been explicitly warned against in the 2013 UK DH (Department of Health) *Guidance Notes on the UK Infant Formula regulations.*[1530]) Around the world media reported that "Infant formula bridges the gap with breast milk."[1531] Companies did not state in black and white that the small amount of five nucleotides in formula provides the immune protection of the much larger quantity of thirteen or more nucleotides in breastmilk. They did not claim that the four or five they added had been *proved* to provide *any* actual immune protection. But it seems likely that parents thought they did, hearing that "infants who are not breastfed can now enjoy the benefits of mother's milk." The smartest advertising allows its targets to believe something which, if stated plainly, could be successfully prosecuted as false and misleading.

In fact, the best commentary on the addition of nucleotides that I saw came from a manual for sales reps provided by another US company, on how to respond to Wyeth's new formula with nucleotides.[1532]

Do not discuss the new SMA formulation unless a physician or nurse asks you about it. Keep your focus on selling [Their products!]

If a doctor or nurse asks you about SMA with nucleotides, try to keep the discussion short. Too much discussion on your part may make the SMA reformulation seem more important than it is. You may want to suggest the physician ask the Wyeth representative one or more of the following questions:

° If nucleotides stimulate the immune system, how did Wyeth's studies determine whether or not they also stimulate increased allergic reactions?

° Only one study is mentioned, and that only as an abstract. Is there a confirming study available?

° When will Wyeth conduct studies to learn more of the long term implications of hyperstimulating an infant's immune system.

Wyeth's addition of nucleotides to SMA is primarily an attempt to get more promotional attention. Remember that Wyeth was unable to show any benefits from adding nucleotides, nor that infants' current diet is deficient in regards to nucleotides. Keep your efforts focused on selling your products, and the proven benefits they provide.

We'll provide you more information as it becomes available.

Figure 3-12-3 Advising industry reps about handling a competitor's additive

Ironically, not long after, still with no proof that any immune effect of nucleotides would be beneficial, that second company was selling formula with added nucleotides. I guess they

---

1529 This implies that there is no other aspect of breastmilk that has a beneficial effect; or that combines with the nucleotides to enable their beneficial effect, and that any combination of just five of thirteen interactive nucleotides will have the same effect, despite the different effect of infant formula on gut bacteria.

1530 This detailed Guidance is online at https://www.gov.uk/government/uploads/system/uploads/attachment_data/file/204314/Infant_formula_guidance_2013_-_final_6_March.pdf

1531 *Drug Topics*, February 5, 1990, p. 36.

1532 Company literature on file, collected in the USA in the 1990s

discovered that their competitor's sales had improved because their formula was believed to provide 'immune protection' ...

Marketing is perfectly happy to assert benefits long before population exposure reveals any, or rules out risks. There is still very little evidence that the few nucleotides in infant formula in the doses that infants get[1533] make any major difference to the infant's risk of infection. The EFSA NDA Panel in 2014 stated that "taking into account the lack of convincing evidence for a benefit for the addition of nucleotides to IF and/or FOF, the Panel considers the addition of nucleotides to be unnecessary." This conclusion was reached despite the fact that some effects on responses to immunization had led one group[1534] to state that "Available evidence suggests a positive benefit of ribonucleotide-supplemented formulas on infant health without any risk."

In fact, adding synthetic nucleotides to infant formula may be quite unnecessary. Intake via food is not the only source for infants. The liver makes nucleotides, and additionally all infants have access to nucleotides as the breakdown product of body cells. An exchange recorded in an industry-funded colloquium makes that clear.

> Dr Brunser: One of the main problems when one reviews the few publications on the effect of nucleotides in infants is that very few of these studies have controlled the nucleotide intake from other sources. That raises in my mind a doubt that I've always had and that I've never been able to resolve. Surely, the nucleotides liberated from desquamated epithelial cells from the mouth, esophagus, stomach, and small intestine are an adequate supply?

> Dr Lönnerdal: That's what I tried to convey. I said there was no indication that there was any limitation in supply in the first place.[1535]

In short, they're not necessary? Whether five added nucleotides make any significant difference to infant health is still unclear, though they may have some immune effects, heightening vaccination responses,[1536] for example. But they have certainly made a difference to public perception of infant formula as 'immunoprotective'. Look at the results of some US surveys in the box on the next page.

Products containing 'immunoshield' or 'immunofortis' mixes undermine breastfeeding's chief claim to superiority, that it is genuinely bioactive and immunoprotective. The hype

---

1533 In 1996 the amount included was increased to 72mg/L in some formulas. Schaller JP, Kuchan MJ, Thomas DL, Cordle CT et al.Effect of dietary ribonucleotides on infant immune status. Part 1: Humoral responses. (PMID:15496604) *Pediatr Res* 2004, 56(6):883-890. DOI: 10.1203/01. PDR.0000145576.42115.5CM. Variations in types and amounts make by brand comparison studies important.

1534 Gutiérrez-Castrellón P1, Mora-Magaña I, Díaz-García L, Jiménez-Gutiérrez C, et al. Immune response to nucleotide-supplemented infant formulae: systematic review and meta-analysis. *Br J Nutr.* 2007; 98 Suppl 1:S64-7.

1535 Hanson LA, Yolken RH. op. cit., p. 199. A conclusion reiterated in another Nestle workshop: Clemens Hernell and Michaelsen (2011) op. cit. p.28. "...if you look at nucleotides and read the literature, it's very hard to say yes, they are beneficial, they do have a health consequence."

1536 Schaller JP1, Buck RH, Rueda R. Ribonucleotides: conditionally essential nutrients shown to enhance immune function and reduce diarrheal disease in infants. *Semin Fetal Neonatal Med.* 2007 Feb;12(1):35-44. Epub 2006 Nov 30. "This chapter intends to summarize an area of pediatric nutrition that has yielded both enlightening evidence and seemingly contradictory data."

## Is breastfeeding healthier? Is formula harmful?

With so much advertising focussed on promises of IQ gains, and immune protection, have American public perceptions of formula changed? The US CDC commissioned some surveys which make interesting reading: they are online at http://www.cdc.gov/breastfeeding/data/healthstyles_survey/index.htm. Some of the questions asked boiled down to:

## Is breastfeeding healthier? Is formula as good?

Consistently respondents are willing to concede that *infant formula is not as good as breastmilk*, though one in five think it is by 2013.

1999  14% yes, 52% no        2005  28% yes 43% no        2013  20% yes 48% no.

In 1999, two-thirds agreed that *Breastfeeding is healthier*. But by 2013 only a quarter thought so, and third thought it isn't any healthier.

1999  67% yes 7% no        2005  21% yes 46% no        2013  25% yes 35% no

## But does formula increase the chance of sickness?

1999 22% said yes and 41% no

Asking about any link between infant formula and specific diseases was even more interesting.

| Diarrhea? | Ear infection? | Diabetes? |
|---|---|---|
| 2004  6% yes  66% no | 2003 18% yes, 48% no | 2003  4% yes, 63% no |
| 2005  7% yes 61% no | 2005  20% yes, 45% no | |

| Respiratory disease? | Overweight? |
|---|---|
| 2003  18% yes  42% no | 2003  7% yes  57% no |
| 2004  17% yes  47% no | 2004  7% yes   63% no |
| 2005  19% yes  48% no | 2005  10% yes  58% no |
| 2013  11% yes  43% no | |

Not even one in five would agree that infant formula could cause any specific sickness; by 2013 only one in four thinks breastfeeding is healthier than infant formula, down from two-thirds in 1999.

Although in 1999 roughly half pay lip service to the idea that infant formula is not as good as breastmilk, by 2013 one in five believe that it is.

about immune protection also justified a price increase, and also persuaded some parents not to buy cheaper formulas that lacked nucleotides. The price of premium formulas went up. Considerably. These new additives are definitely proven to be value-adding for industry, but not as yet for infants.[1537] The same seems to be true for the next starter in the race to provide immune protection: the biotics.

# Baby biotics

'Prebiotics' are food sources for 'good' bacteria (like Lactobacillus and Bifidobacteria). There are many prebiotics, or good-bug foods, including oligosaccharides, or complex sugars (the FOS, GOS and inulin on current labels). These are discussed in the chapter on carbohydrates in formula. 'Probiotics' are the bugs themselves, generally species that form a large part of the breastfed infant's microbiome, such as the Lactobacillus and Bifidus species and strains. Synbiotics are a mix of the two.

The importance for immune function of creating and maintaining a healthy microbiome is now accepted. By the 1990s, largely due to widespread marketing of yoghurts, and live bacterial supplements of a variety of Lactobacillus strains, popular awareness of the importance of bowel and gut flora to immune function had increased. Gastrointestinal flora directly influences health,[1538] and that flora can be altered by probiotic consumption. Probiotics may be suggested for adults when antibiotics have been prescribed; some suggest them as a way of restoring a better bowel flora. (Others dispute that they would be of any use, as stomach acid could destroy live bacteria, and existing microbes will resist their invasion.) It is generally accepted that as one review put it, "Probiotics are safe but lack evidence on benefit from long-term use."[1539]

As discussed in Book 1, the microbiota of artificially fed infants deviates considerably from that of breastfed infants. Research into immune components to be added to formula has focussed on prebiotics and probiotics that might reduce the differences, and perhaps improve outcomes. Both prebiotics and probiotics have been added to some infant formulas, in varying amounts and combinations, manufactured from varying substrates, and patented by different companies. Experiments with such bacteria and their preferred foods have been going on for decades, in fact.[1540] Breastmilk of course is rich in both the bugs and their foods, and this has been the basis of formula companies' research.[1541] However, the possibility of harm cannot be totally excluded.[1542] Even 'good' bacteria can

1537 Wu T-C, Chen P-H. Nucelotides and nucleosides in human milk: a perspective from Taiwan. In Zibadi et al, op. cit, ch.28.

1538 Agostoni C, Axelsson I, Braegger C, Goulet O, et al. Probiotic bacteria in dietetic products for infants: a commentary by the ESPGHAN Committee on Nutrition. (PMID:15085012) *J Pediatr Gastroenterol Nutr* 2004, 38(4):365-374.

1539 Lombard MJ, Labuschagne I. Prebiotic, probiotic and symbiotic (sic) use in infant formula. In Preedy V et al, op.cit., p. 305.

1540 Saavedra JM. Microbes to fight microbes: a not-so-novel approach to controlling diarrheal disease. *J Pediatr Gastroenterol Nutr*, 1995; 21:125–9

1541 Kunz C. Historical aspects of human milk oligosaccharides. (PMID: 22585922) *Adv Nutr.* 2 012, 3(3):430S-9S] DOI: 10.3945/an.111.001776

1542 Vahabnezhad E, Mochon AB, Wozniak LJ, Ziring DA. *Lactobacillus bacteremia* associated with probiotic use in a pediatric patient with ulcerative colitis. (PMID: 23426446) *J Clin Gastroenterol* 2013; 47(5):437–9

make you ill under certain circumstances![1543] And putting such bacteria into infant formula is pointless if WHO Guidelines about infant formula preparation are followed: water at 70 degrees Celsius kills bacteria, pathogenic or patented.

Prebiotics simply encourage the growth of certain bacteria already in the gut. Probiotics are live bacteria, with their own inherent survival mechanisms and adaptive strategies. Probiotics have been discussed and fed cautiously as far back as 1912 in cases of infant enterocolitis,[1544] when early acidified milk formula was soured by Streptococcus lactis. It had been known since 1900 that the gut flora of breastfed infants was different from that of those artificially fed,[1545] so logically the effects of adding new bacteria may differ between breastfed and artificially fed infants. What works well for a breastfed child may have different effects in a child exposed to bovine proteins. As the European Society for Paediatric Gastroenterology, Hepatology and Nutrition (ESPGHAN) Committee on Nutrition said recently,

> Infant formulae are increasingly being supplemented with probiotics, prebiotics, or synbiotics despite uncertainties regarding their efficacy ... At present, there is insufficient data to recommend the routine use of probiotic- and/or prebiotic-supplemented formulae.[1546]

And the EFSA NDA in April 2014

> notes that evidence available on beneficial effects of IF or FOF supplemented with "probiotics" and "synbiotics" on infant health mainly comes from single studies and studies with methodological limitations or it is inconsistent across the few studies that are comparable. Therefore, the Panel considers that there is insufficient information to draw conclusions on beneficial effects on infant health of "probiotics" added to IF and FOF and even less in the case of synbiotics. There is no evidence to raise concerns about the safety of the tested "probiotics" or "synbiotics". Taking into account the lack of convincing evidence for a benefit of the addition of "probiotics" or "synbiotics" to IF and/or FOF, the Panel considers that the addition of "probiotics" and/or "synbiotics" to IF or FOF is not necessary.[1547]

All the same, some of these products are permitted in infant formula: to ban them in any country could lead to trade wars and legal action, which no government wants. Europe permitted their addition, through what seems to me a liberal reading of Directive 2006/141/EC, which allows the addition to infant formula of food ingredients "shown to be suitable for infants through a systematic review of the available data or, when necessary, by appropriate studies (Article 5 and 6)."

1543 Lombard MJ, Labuschagne I, op. cit., p.316.

1544 Clock, RO. Intestinal implantation of the bacillus lactis bulgaricus in certain intestinal conditions of infants, with report of cases. *Journal of the American Medical Association* (JAMA), 29 June 1912

1545 Tissier H. *Récherches sur la flore intestinale des nourrissons* (Callé et cie, Paris, 1900)

1546 ESPGHAN Committee on Nutrition. Supplementation of infant formula with probiotics and/or prebiotics: a systematic review and comment. *J Pediatr Gastroenterol Nutr* 2011; 52(2):238–50 Online at http://www.espghan.med.up.pt/position_papers/JPGN_CoN_Infant_formula_probotics_prebiotics.pdf

1547 EFSA NDA Draft Opinion op. cit.

Are these biotics "suitable for infants"? That is, for ALL infants? Not all bacterial products are equally safe, reliable or effective. When ingested in infant formula, can they displace long-established existing flora? Results from a study using one particular patented strain of bacteria at a particular dose under particular conditions do not apply to all other related strains of bacteria, doses and conditions. As with any related-but-different organisms, bacterial or viral strains can be very different one from another. Even authors who find that there is some small apparently positive effect of prebiotics agree that "the impact of the microbiota induced by breastfeeding is still superior to probiotic prophylaxis."[1548]

Further, living organisms are capable of mutating and behaving differently under different conditions, in response to other organisms and the nutrients available in their environment. What began as a safe bug might pick up some nasty traits from some other organism: this has happened in vaccinated chickens, and wiped out flocks.[1549] Just as each of us is unique, so is our microbiome, the mix of living things we host internally. There are many times more bacteria in our bodies than our own cells. So getting this right may prove tricky.[1550] Some bacteria in the gut can cause sepsis, blood-borne infection.[1551] Will the virulence of any introduced microbe increase, and cause disease? Or antibiotic resistance? Can we rely on the quality control mechanisms of the suppliers of the bacterial strains used? There might well be casualties. The EFSA NDA noted that there was no evidence of any safety concerns with what seems like a very significant caveat:

> It has been generally concluded that currently evaluated "probiotic"-supplemented IF do not raise safety concerns with regard to growth or other adverse effects, although in many studies adverse events were inconsistently reported (Azad et al., (2013) and further evaluations of safety in long-term studies are needed (Braegger et al., 2011).[1552]

It is concluded that they are safe but there have been adverse events? In many studies? Among the casualties almost certainly will be allergic children, as an independent study found that 'Probiotic compounds may contain hidden allergens of food and may not be safe for subjects with allergy to cow's milk or hen's egg.' This study looked at

> Labels of probiotics commercially available in Spain ... to assess their content of cow's milk or hen's egg ... No label advertised about egg content, eight labels warned about lactose, lactic acid or cow's milk, one label claimed to be milk-free, and two gave no information. Cow's milk proteins were detected, by at least one lab technique, in 10/11 probiotics ... Hen's egg white proteins were detected in 3/11 probiotics.[1553]

1548 West CE, Gothefors L, Granström M, Käyhty H et al. Effects of feeding probiotics during weaning on infections and antibody responses to diphtheria, tetanus and Hib vaccines. (PMID:18086218) *Pediatr Allergy Immunol* 2008, 19(1):53-60.

1549 Kupferschmidt K. Chicken vaccines combine to produce deadly virus. *Science Now*. 12 July 2012. http://news. sciencemag.org/sciencenow/2012/07/chicken-vaccines-combine-to-prod.html

1550 Shanahan F. A commentary on the safety of probiotics. (PMID: 23101692) *Gastroenterol Clin Nth Amer* 2012, 41(4):869–76

1551 Carl MA, Ndao IM, Springman AC, Manning SD et al. Sepsis From the Gut: The Enteric Habitat of Bacteria That Cause Late-Onset Neonatal Bloodstream Infections. (PMID:24647013) *Clin Infect Dis* 2014

1552 EFSA NDA op. cit

1553 Martín-Muñoz MF, Fortuni M, Caminoa M, Belver T, Quirce S, Caballero T. Anaphylactic reaction to probiotics. Cow 's milk and hen's egg allergens in probiotic compounds. *Pediatr Allergy Immunol* 2012:00

So ten of eleven products exposed allergic children – for whom probiotic supplementation is being considered – to unlabelled bovine allergens capable of producing anaphylaxis, life-threatening allergic reactions - and two of those ten were not labelled as containing milk products. Three contained egg proteins as well. Is this the case worldwide? Will labels disclose in what culture media these bugs were grown, and what traces they carry with them? That hasn't happened in the past with other formula ingredients like the fungal and algal oils and peanut oil. How detailed will labelling regulations need to be? Again, do the potential gains justify the risks? Plaintiffs in ten suits in New Jersey, California and Washington allege that US infant formula company Gerber (since 2007 a Nestlé subsidiary)

> ... markets its infant products containing so-called probiotic and prebiotic bacteria [sic] as healthier than other baby food, but that there is no reliable scientific data to back up those claims. In fact, scientists cannot say for sure whether increasing one type of bacteria in the human intestine may in fact be harmful, the plaintiffs say.[1554]

What will be the outcome of these 2012 US class actions alleging that such infant formula is not as healthy as is being claimed? We don't know. If the decision is unfavourable to industry there will surely be an appeal.

What we do know for sure is that fresh (not heat-damaged) breastmilk facilitates a favourable microbiome; formula doesn't. And in very small preterm babies it seems that certain patented bugs may help prevent serious gut damage and with it death. A 2011 Cochrane Review of studies found that the use of *[particular patented]* probiotics reduces the occurrence of NEC and death in premature infants born less than 1500 grams. There is insufficient data with regard to the benefits and potential adverse effects in the most at risk infants less than 1000 grams at birth.[1555]

A 2012 review was more cautious but basically agreed.[1556]

Neonatologists who have investigated this are convinced that any risk to small sick preterm babies is outweighed by the benefits.[1557] Their clinical expertise and experience has to be respected, but they do all need to document the outcomes of their practices carefully, as this may prove to be another error of judgment. Do probiotics reduce such the risk of NEC and death and lifelong harms as well as human milk feeding does? Are they simply a distraction from the need to ensure human milk availability for all preterms, when Scandinavian neonatologists consider this the priority and formula use unethical? (For more on NEC go back to page 436.) And long-term follow-up of those same children may reveal that even

---

1554 *Law 360*, 12 September 2012. Gerber urges MDL Panel to consolidate baby formula suits. Online at www.law360.com/articles/379446

1555 http://summaries.cochrane.org/CD005496/probiotics-for-prevention-of-necrotizing-enterocolitis-in-preterm-infants

1556 Mihatsch WA, Braegger CP, Decsi T, Kolacek S et al. Critical systematic review of the level of evidence for routine use of probiotics for reduction of mortality and prevention of necrotizing enterocolitis and sepsis in preterm infants. (PMID: 21996513) *Clinical Nutrition* 2012, 31(1):6–15

1557 Deshpande GC, Rao SC, Keil AD, Patole SK Evidence-based guidelines for use of probiotics in preterm neonates. (PMID: 21806843) *BMC Medicine* 2011; 9:92

this benefit comes at a price. (Preterm survivors are known to have many problems later in childhood in which nutrition may be a contributing factor.)

If those small sick babies were to be given their own mother's fresh breastmilk, or organisms cultured from that milk, they would be at less risk, and not need to take their chances with commercially produced probiotics. A wide variety of friendly bacteria, including Lactobacillus species, will reach the baby via the placenta, then birthing (through vaginal flora), and then breastfeeding.[1558] Investigating and managing the mother's flora might be a priority, as well as encouraging as much skin-to-skin contact and breastfeeding as humanly possible. A trial is said to be investigating the benefits of inoculating babies born surgically with flora from the mother's skin and vagina; anecdotal reports suggest that some parents are not waiting for the results of any trial, but doing this themselves, which could be hazardous. Vaginal flora after a normal birth would perhaps be influenced by the placental microbiome, so perhaps this too needs consideration in any trials.

Logic suggests to me that mothers might be fed safe and effective probiotics during pregnancy and lactation, especially if prescribed antibiotics (say for Strep B); that if preterm delivery is anticipated, vaginal pessaries of probiotics might be used; but that probiotics need to be considered postpartum only if infants are exposed to substances that compromise gut flora, such as infant formulas. Why? Because breastfed infants are getting their prebiotics and probiotics at the breast. At the very least we could find out what the breastfeeding mother's synbiotic mix is, before rushing to displace it, and not measuring the result!

Perhaps all artificially fed babies should be supplemented, as their distorted microbiomes are more favourable to disease. But with what? Some formulas now are already including both prebiotics and probiotics: should these 'synbiotic' mixes be allowed ahead of proof of safety, efficacy, or benefit? And how might they interact with any medically prescribed strains? Do they survive making up formula with water at 70 degrees? A great deal of research is underway at present, and certainty may emerge over the next few decades – from the experience of babies being experimented with over that time. And trade journals report in 2014 that the potential health benefits of synbiotics may be limited because many combinations simply don't enhance the survival and growth of their associated bacteria.[1559]

But how do companies apply any information gathered from research? Some optimistic researchers attempted to answer that question by asking the companies. Their study also explored

1558 Martín V, Maldonado-Barragán A, Moles L, Rodriguez-Baños M, del Campo R, Fernández L, Rodríguez JM, Jiménez E. Sharing of bacterial strains between breast milk and infant feces. *J Hum Lact* February 2012 28:36–44. DOI: 10.1177/0890334411424729

1559 Harrison-Dunn A-R. Synbiotic gut health benefits limited, say researchers. *Dairy Reporter,* 18-Jul-2014. http://www.dairyreporter.com/R-D/Synbiotic-prebiotic-probiotic-gut-health-benefits-limited Citing Adebola OO, Corcoran O, Morgan WA. Synbiotics: the impact of potential prebiotics inulin, lactulose and lactobionic acid on the survival and growth of lactobacilli probiotics. *J Funct Foods* 2014; 10: 75-84. DOI:10.1016/j.jff.2014.05.010

"what happens after the clinical trials using infant formula are completed, data is published or remains unpublished; the effectiveness and type of medium the formula manufacturers use to educate consumers on probiotic, prebiotic or synbiotic infant formula."

What did they find out? Nothing. Not a single one of twenty-five companies was willing to answer their questions. So much for post-market surveillance! Read the reasons given. The researchers concluded that greater transparency is needed.[1560] Amen to that.

Much of that infant feeding research is done without reference to breastfed babies, when company scientists see their task as checking whether an additive to a formula changes its performance when compared to the same formula without that additive. (As earlier noted, partial or initial breastfeeding is often involved, and may influence the results without any apparent attempt to quantify this.[1561] So too might the type of infant formula used, if excess iron is present.)

Of course, commercial logic suggests that, instead of careful long term research subjected to independent critique, what we will see almost immediately is the targeting of affluent mothers (mostly breastfeeders) to buy probiotics their babies are less likely to need, while artificially fed babies of (mostly poorer) mothers are ignored unless a formula company can create a safe, cheap, affordable product. And then some of those disadvantaged mothers will spend money they cannot afford, on products their babies would not need, if both had been helped to breastfeed.

So, what did I conclude after reading so much about all this?

- Probiotics and prebiotics may prove to be an advance or a mistake.
- Or an advance for some babies and a mistake for others.
- Or some items and strains may provide a benefit, and some of them may be a disaster.
- Or pre- and probiotics may make no difference at all to infant mortality except in very small preterm babies, but perhaps reduce morbidity.
- Or they may increase morbidity, as unexpected interactions with other gut microbes occur, and create new resistant strains of pathogens.

Any of these outcomes are still possible. And probably others I haven't thought about. An overview of probiotics and prebiotics can be read on the American Academy of Paediatrics website.[1562] At present the consensus seems to be that any benefit to term infants is unproven, as is safety (other than not immediately displaying toxicity). And scientists are

---

1560 Mugambi M. Young T, Blaauw R,]. Application of evidence on probiotics, prebiotics and synbiotics by food industry: a descriptive study. *BMC Research Notes* 2014, 7:754 doi:10.1186/1756-0500-7-754

1561 For example, the study that enrolled children aged three to twenty-four months, including some who were breastfed twice a day, and excluding those with a history of allergy or diarrhoea or malabsorption: what does this tell us about the safety of a product when fed from birth to less healthy, never-breastfed children? Nothing. Saavedra JM, Abi-Hanna A, Moore N, Yolken RH. Long-term consumption of infant formulas containing live probiotic bacteria: tolerance and safety. (PMID: 14749232) *Am J Clin Nutr* 2004; 79(2):261–7.

1562 Thomas DW, Greer FR. Probiotics and prebiotics. *Pediatrics* 2010; 126(6);1217–31. (DOI: 10.1542/peds.2010-2548); downloadable: http://pediatrics.aappublications.org/content/126/6/1217.full.pdf+html

aware of the inadequacies of the research that has gone into trying to sort out the value of these additives. As Szajewska summarised, in an article well worth reading,

> In 2011, the Committee on Nutrition of the European Society for Paediatric Gastroenterology, Hepatology and Nutrition systematically reviewed published evidence on the safety and health effects of the administration of formulae supplemented with probiotics and/or prebiotics compared with unsupplemented formulae. The document could serve as an example of problems relating to the choice and definition of outcomes assessing the addition of new ingredients to infant formulae. The studies were often too small with insufficient power to identify relevant effects, and the follow-up periods in the trials were too short. The clinical outcomes, even those relating to the same domain (eg, gastrointestinal infections) differed. Even if the same outcomes were measured, the definitions of the outcomes were heterogeneous, often not widely agreed upon, or just lacking. The use of inappropriate outcome measures and/or their definitions may result in misleading conclusions. It may also lead to an overestimation or underestimation of potential benefits of the intervention or fail to reveal any potential benefits. There is a need for well-designed and carefully conducted randomized controlled trials, with relevant inclusion/exclusion criteria and adequate sample sizes. These studies should use validated clinical outcome measures.[1563]

Amen, alleluia! Just don't hold your breath while waiting. And don't expect industry to wait till we have such results before marketing the things.

## Benefits to industry

The sad fact is that even if the outcome of population-based studies were to show that these live bacterial products are harmful, and they had to be withdrawn, all this experimentation with immune factors might still have been financially worthwhile investments for industry. Why? Because making claims about providing immune shields, or immunoprotection, has helped grow the multi-billion dollar world market for infant formula. For many parents, the marketing of baby biotics has created the illusion that formulas now provide immune protection, just like breastmilk. And so Wyeth was worth $12 billion to Nestlé in 2012. If things should go wrong and recalls are needed, they can be very costly — the beetle recall in 2010 is said to have cost Abbott $100million.[1564] But industry may escape any serious consequences by restructuring, going bankrupt, or persuading governments to bail them out and provide immunity from legal liability. The brand name can be changed or maintained with new owners. Profits for the unscrupulous and greedy are generally greater than the risks in a capitalist society – and the profits go to people who think they don't share the risk.

---

1563 Szajewska H. Supplementation of infant formula with probiotics/prebiotics: lessons learned with regard to documenting outcomes. (PMID: 22955362) *J Clin Gastroent* 2012, 46 Suppl:S67–8. DOI: 10.1097/ MCG.0b013e3182647a49

1564 Harrington R. Abbott infant formula recall to cost US $100m. *Food Production Daily,* 29-9-2010. http://www. foodproductiondaily.com/Safety-Regulation/Abbott-infant-formula-recall-to-cost-US-100m Downloaded 20/11/2010

Cynical comment? Ordinary ethical humans would respond instinctively to this idea that 'Of course no company executives really think like that!' Being raised a moral human, I used to think that way as well. I have my reasons for no longer doing so. Read David Michael[1565] and Marion Nestle[1566] and George Kent.[1567] I guarantee you will see this as plausible rational strategy in the real world of money matters. (A world often insulated from the everyday lived reality of ordinary families, and in some ways deeply alien and amoral.) A company's primary legal obligation is to benefit its shareholders, not the consumers of their products. Greedy bastards can rationalise anything, as the global financial crisis surely taught us: having helped to bring it about, the super rich are even richer for it.[1568]

The quality and independence of research, and the regulatory oversight of the manufacture of live organisms being fed to infants, is critical in a world where people can behave as Michael outlines. But (as I've said repeatedly, because it is true in every aspect of infant nutrition) even after decades of breastfeeding advocates pointing this out, there still seem to be too few studies that look at **infants fully artificially fed from birth** and compare them with infants **fed only breastmilk from birth** for at least four months, preferably six, controlling for any antibiotic exposure or family history of allergy - as well as other confounders in both groups. Short-term trials that include infants breastfed for some days or weeks before being formula-fed make it impossible to draw conclusions about which factors have what effects. In some studies such children are defined as breastfed, in others, as formula-fed!

Where prebiotics and probiotics are concerned, caveat emptor (buyer beware!) indeed. History suggests to me that another new infant formula promising reduced infection rates will lead to less breastmilk feeding, not more. I hope I am wrong. Market data suggests I'm not. From US$7.9billion in 2005[1569], babyfood sales are expected to be worth $55 billion by 2015, up almost $20billion from 2010 –according to one source[1570], anyway. Another says a mere $30 billion for infant formula in 2014, up five billion from the previous year. How reliable these figures are is uncertain; what is certain is that it is appalling so much money is being made from replacing breastmilk and family foods.

A detailed account of infant formula markets is available only to those with deep pockets, so there's another book for someone else to research and write. The table on page 494 summarise what I have been able to find with my now very restricted means.

---

1565  Michaels D. *Doubt is their product* op. cit.

1566  Nestle M. *Food politics* op. cit.

1567  Kent G. *Regulating infant formula* (Hale Publishing, 2010)

1568  http://www.smh.com.au/business/richest-85-boast-same-wealth-as-half-the-world-20140120-314vk.html

1569  Kaminis M. A growing boost for baby formula. *Business Week* Jan 11 2005. Online at http://www.businessweek.com/stories/2005-01-10/a-growing-boost-for-baby-formula

1570  http://www.statista.com/topics/1218/baby-food-market/

Chapter 3: Infant formula, past, present and future
3.12 Making or marketing immunity?

| 475

# Addition and subtraction: improving infant formulas or profits?

Ever since infant formula was first manufactured, there has been constant pressure to add something new that competitors did not yet have. Parents scrutinise formula labels, looking to see what one might have that another didn't. Parents assume that any new additive has been proved to be both necessary and *totally safe*, not simply a better marketing ploy.

Few stop to think about the process whereby an industrial supply of a specific ingredient has been formulated, and the possibility that more may mean more traces of possibly undesirable chemicals used in manufacture, like the hexane traces in fatty acids. Industrially-produced lutein for use in infant formula, widely touted but not proven beneficial for infant eyes, is extracted from marigolds using hexane. (Although in theory both forms of lutein are equally acccessible to the baby, in practice the lutein uptake from breastmilk is almost 5 times greater than from infant formula.[1571]) Lycopene production involves toluene, a neurotoxic benzene derivative. Taurine production necessitates the use of carcinogenic sulphuric acid. And as noted earlier, traces are likely to be present, and have not been proved harmless to infants.

Yet the marketing of each new additive usually says that the new addition makes our product more like/ or closer to breastmilk, even before there is proof of either safety or efficacy, simply limited proof of no overt or immediate toxicity. (Which is not at all the same thing.)

# Would organic formula be better?

Some educated parents (who can afford to) look for organic products for their young children, in the hope of minimising the body burden of agricultural chemicals. But organic formulas can still contain problematic ingredients, despite the best efforts of national organic bodies. Some of these are unable to prevail with regulators when the infant formula industry is concerned. Read the eye-opening account online about American organic infant formulas.[1572]

Organic means different things in different countries. Industry sees organics as a value-adding growth opportunity. However, expansion could be limited as there may not be enough genuinely organic product to use in manufacture. Definitions of organic may change to accommodate the increased demand, as has happened with Martek's oils, thanks to an intervention by a senior administrator who is said to have overturned the considered decision of USDA staff after a chat with Martek's lawyer.[1573] The EU has clearer standards and seems to enforce them better than in the USA. Globally, organic infant formula is

1571 Lipkie TE, Banavara D, Shah B, Morrow AL, et al. Caco-2 accumulation of lutein is greater from human milk than from infant formula despite similar bioaccessibility. (PMID:24975441) *Mol Nutr Food Res* 2014; 58(10):2014-2022. DOI: 10.1002/mnfr.201400126

1572 Vallaeys C. How to find the safest organic infant formula http://www.cornucopia.org/2013/12/find-safest-organic-infant-formula/

1573 http://www.cornucopia.org/2009/10/dangerous-hype-infant-formula-companies-claim-they-can-make-babies-smarter/

another topic for specialist investigation and reporting. Global standards will eventually emerge from the pressure of consumer advocacy, but are likely to be watered down so as to allow the major players to fit in their products. Abbott's Organic Similac, containing Martek oils, quickly cornered over 30% of US organics sales. The leading organic formula brand, Nature's One, does not use these GM oils. It is a stretch indeed to consider such oils either natural or organic as parents understand those terms.

All this tinkering with additives and subtractives adds costs to the consumer. As Hernell was to warn,

> New ingredients, some with potent biological activities and produced with new techniques, are likely to be expensive and they may also confer a safety risk. Moreover, even a proven biological activity may not necessarily confer a health benefit on the recipient infant. Therefore it is – and will be even more so in the future – extremely important to rigorously ascertain safety and efficacy before formulas with such ingredients are launched on the market, and the cost-benefit must be considered for formulas intended for infants at large.[1574]

Hear hear! But Hernell went on to conclude, 'and particularly for formulas intended for infants in low-income countries.' I disagree, since poverty is global. And so is wealth: Asian purchases are creating scarcity of infant formulas in all high-income countries, because the prices there are so much higher for premium products. A product that sells for around twenty Euro or less can be sold in China for thirty, even forty to fifty Euro per can. Why wouldn't companies sell as much in China as possible?[1575]

Respected nutrition researcher Professor Bo Lönnerdal (of UC Davis) said in a Nestlé symposium,

> Even in the USA, and within the state of California, the price issue is a relevant one. We have a significant population of poor people in the state, and as soon as the price of infant formula is raised, they will go to evaporated cows' milk or whole cows' milk because it is much cheaper. This is something we do not want to see happening. There is no way you can add a highly-enriched alpha-lactalbumin fraction to regular term formula without increasing the price.[1576]

Lönnerdal was right about that. Infant formula prices have risen steeply since 1994, and that was before much of the new advances. Who is monitoring the effects among those who cannot access taxpayer-funded bottle-feeding via WIC? Some American parents are certainly watering down infant formula to make it stretch.[1577] If, in the effort to reduce formula-induced obesity, the total caloric value of infant formula is reduced by ten to fifteen percent from 67kcal/100mL to just 60kcal/100mL, a greater volume of infant formula will be needed

1574 Hernell O. in Clemens Hernell & Michaelsen (eds) op. cit. p. 23
1575 This price gap explains why so many families have been shipping formula overseas to relatives and friends or setting up small import businesses, or simply smuggling the stuff whre import limits have been set.
1576 Discussion in Raiha, N (ed) *Protein metabolism during infancy,* op. cit., p. 131
1577 Ackerman S. 'Liquid gold' for babies coveted by moms, thieves. *The Tampa Tribune,* 3 December 2008. http://tbo.com/news/metro/2008/dec/03/na-babies-needs-strain-food-banks-ar-120878/ (accessed 19/8/2013)

by some babies.[1578] Which mean higher costs. Dilution will then pose even greater risks of protein-calorie deficiency.

A recent *New Scientist* article about America's hidden epidemic of the diseases of poverty makes shocking reading.[1579] So too do any statistics about the health of Indigenous peoples in Australia.[1580] Rural peasants in Asia are not the only poor at risk. Disadvantaged people in every country are further disadvantaged by artificial feeding. Both the lack of breastfeeding, and the presence of infant formula, interact with some of the many adverse factors that cluster in disadvantaged groups, and exaggerate health, educational, and financial inequalities, for people with fewer resources for remediation. This topic is a book in itself, for someone else to write. So artificial feeding is an important issue, not just for public health and the environment, but for everyone concerned with social justice. [1581] Which is why the marketing of those 'perfect' infant formulas has been a political as well as public health issue. It astonishes me when apparently highly intelligent, well-educated western women loudly defend their own (undoubted) freedom to choose infant formula, without apparently seeing any of the ramifications of their behaviour and advocacy of this inferior choice for the wider world and its most vulnerable humans. Privilege comes with responsibilities to more than one's own small circle of other privileged families. And even that circle is not immune from pervasive, sometimes serious, even disastrous, consequences for a minority. No one should choose infant formula for their child. And no one should be forced by circumstances to feed artificial milks. It's that important.

---

1578 One trial has shown that babies will up-regulate their intakes (drink more) of the 60kcal/100mL formula. See Timby N, Domellöf E, Hernell O, Lönnerdal B, Domellöf M Neurodevelopment, nutrition, and growth until 12 mo of age in infants fed a low-energy, low-protein formula supplemented with bovine milk fat globule membranes: a randomized controlled trial. (PMID:24500150) *Am J Clin Nutr;* 2014, 99(4):860-868 **DOI:** 10.3945/ajcn.113.064295 That will be good for business, but for obesity? Another experiment.

1579 http://www.newscientist.com/article/mg22029473.200-americas-hidden-epidemic-of-tropical-diseases. html?full=true#.Ur-p8KV15uY

1580 http://www.healthinfonet.ecu.edu.au/health-facts/summary

1581 Roberts TJ, Carnahan E, Gakidou E. Can breastfeeding promote child health equity? A comprehensive analysis of breastfeeding patterns across the developing world and what we can learn from them.(PMID:24305597) Free full text article *BMC Med* 2013, 11:254

# 3.13 Selling the stuff, or marketing matters

There is simply no room in this book – which focuses mainly on what babies drink and its effects – for a full and fair analysis of the growth of the infant formula market and its players. What follows in this chapter is just one selection of some industry marketing issues. It is as much a witness statement as reportage, being coloured by my (entirely self-funded) involvement with these issues since the 1970s. It covers firstly, some background both about culture, infant formula marketing and attempts to restrict it, secondly, an outline record of the rise of back-marketing and brands; thirdly, the decline in developed nations of in-hospital marketing; and finally looks briefly at the dangerous new/old strategy of deliberately marketing formula products as supplements to breastfeeding. (This latter strategy being ably assisted, indeed encouraged, by those same intelligent formula advocates who seem to me to care only for others like themselves and their feelings.) The Bibliography provides resources to look more deeply into these and other aspects of infant formula marketing.

## The infant feeding culture

Marketing works within a culture. By the 1980s, America had normalised artificial feeding to an extent unknown in history. British culture overtly approved of breastfeeding, just made it seem impossibly awkward. In the United States, and countries influenced by US culture, breastfeeding mothers had long been feeling unbelievably defensive. La Leche League founders had chosen Spanish to avoid giving offence by using the B(reast) word, by then as culturally uncouth as the F word (see Modernity and prudery on page 459). Baby bottles were quintessentially American, symbols of modernity. Any basic health message that breast is best was socially invisible, while infant feeding bottles were ubiquitous - as toys, as containers, on cards, as balloons to give to parents of newborns, on the cover of magazines, everywhere. Sentimentally cute depictions of infants and older children and even animals with baby bottles were rampant. It was as though American adults, as children, had so bonded with their infant feeding bottle that they enjoyed and responded to constant reminders of the object of their affection, and the comfort it gave them. Ironically, baby bottles themselves were - and remain? Obscenely dangerous in the absence of any relevant safety regulations: moulded objects in every shape and size, from baseballs to bears, all impossible to clean; vectors of disease, similar to the old murder bottles that France (but not America) had banned in 1912. (See Figure 3-2-1 on page 215)

Broad social changes since 1970 are beyond the scope of this history. But the almost-mandatory return of women to the paid workforce after childbirth, and the explosion of commercial childcare, among others, have had a huge effect on infant formula use and the possibility of breastfeeding. Women have always worked and breastfed, but factory work in the early industrial revolution was one of the forces that drove artificial feeding.[1582] Where women are educated, motivated and have access to appropriate workplace arrangements, working women can continue to breastfeed and express their milk when at work, although

---

1582 Hewitt M. *Wives and Mothers in Victorian Industry* (Rockliff, London 1958) 1830s factory workers returned to mills days after birth, babies in care from 5.30am to the evening.

this is a huge added pressure some will find demanding or unmanageable.[1583] However, the reality of most paid work for women, and most paid childcare, means an early demise of breastfeeding for many.

This issue of breastfeeding and the women's paid employment is complex and I am doing no more than touching on it, and on the question of attitudes to breastmilk and breastfeeding in this era. But as I mentioned earlier, an excellent article indicts the failure of feminists to support this quintessentially female work of breastfeeding, and sets out strategies for change.[1584] A large section of my library is taken up by books discussing social and political constraints on breastfeeding.[1585]

ch of what is written might be re-thought if the writers considered infant formula an unacceptable risk to the life and health of the coming generations. I hope this book will influence some of my feminist sisters to think again, and like Sandra Steingraber and Jacqueline Wolf, write as though formula feeding is an unknowable risk, not a comfortable fallback substitute facilitating modern life. As Amy Koerber said, "I hope we could all agree that all women should live in a world where it is possible for mothers who so desire to adopt the behaviours that medicine currently recommends as most supportive of mothers' and infants' health."[1586] But while women should, they *don't* live in such a world and won't, until we make it so.

And they certainly didn't live in such a world in the 1980s when I began teaching Australia's first Infant Feeding course for health professionals. (Yes, there was a session on making artificial feeding safer and more enjoyable for the baby and mother alike.) What follows was part of the very first presentation...exaggerated, but the students knew exactly what I was saying, even adding to my original list. This was the reality of breastfeeding promotion and support in the mid twentieth century, a reality still for many people. People may have paid lip service to the idea that Breast is Best, but their attitudes ensured that too few babies did just that.

# Of course breast is best...

## For the mother who is not

- ✓ on drugs
- ✓ drinking alcohol
- ✓ smoking
- ✓ contaminated by pesticides
- ✓ at risk of viral disease
- ✓ infected

1583  Berggren J. *Working Without Weaning* (Hale Publishing 2010)
1584  Wolf J H (2006) op cit
1585  Hall Smith P, Hausman BL, Labbok M. *Beyond Health, Beyond Choice. Breastfeeding Constraints and Realities.* Rutgers University Press 2012. Among others.
1586  Koerber A. *Breast or ? Contemporary controversies in infant-feeding policy and practice.* (University of South Carolina Press 2013) p. 146.

- ✓ depressed
- ✓ feverish
- ✓ in the paid workforce
- ✓ averse to it
- ✓ too old
- ✓ too young
- ✓ too tired
- ✓ too ill (diabetes, mastitis, epilepsy..)
- ✓ too socially active
- ✓ too physically active
- ✓ too fair-skinned
- ✓ too ethnic
- ✓ too disadvantaged
- ✓ too handicapped (clefts, Down Syndrome..)
- ✓ too selfish
- ✓ too anxious
- ✓ too unintelligent
- ✓ too dirty
- ✓ too fat
- ✓ too thin
- ✓ allergic

[***To which we might now add*** of an unfavourable maternal genotype]

AND who does not mind:

- ➲ physical pain and serious discomfort
- ➲ droopy boobs
- ➲ overweight
- ➲ fatigue
- ➲ being used as a dummy
- ➲ being subject to her baby's *demands*
- ➲ being tied down
- ➲ having no sex life
- ➲ excluding her partner from equal care

ALWAYS PROVIDED THAT  her baby is not:

- ▪ too big
- ▪ too small
- ▪ preterm
- ▪ overdue
- ▪ jaundiced

- dysmature
- too sick
- too lethargic
- too weak
- too strong
- too irritable
- too handicapped
- too new
- too old (at 3, 6, 9, 12months)
- gaining too little
- gaining too much
- at risk of
  - infection
  - hypoglycaemia
  - jaundice
  - dehydration
  - becoming too dependent
  - waking at night for feeds
  - lactose intolerance
  - having GI/skin/other symptoms due to her milk
- adopted
- suffering from inherited enzyme deficiencies

AND that her milk is not

- too scanty
- too abundant
- too low in protein
- too high in lactose
- too fatty
- too weak
- too thin
- too thick
- too contaminated
- too allergenic
- lacking ingredients a-z...

*Breast is best, just not for everybody....or was that anybody?*

## Background: Marketing wars and the scale of the battle

Marketing explains how we got to that absurd position. Marketing also explains how American infant formula achieved global dominance in many places outside America. Chetley  stated that of the top fifteen global marketing agencies in 1979, fourteen were American.  American marketing skill rapidly reduced the market share of older brands entrenched in Australia and the UK, as we have seen. The USA was the mid 20th-century world leader in formula feeding rates, and the most valuable single market, thanks above all to US government policies and subsidies. In the second half of the 20th century,  US taxpayers paid billions of dollars to make formula-feeding affordable and normal in the world's then-dominant economy. Earlier United States Department of Agriculture (USDA) food aid programs had expanded to deal with the huge surpluses that post-war large-scale agriculture was creating, using cheap oil and water, and American technological know-how. Within a few decades, the USDA became the world's biggest buyer and distributor of infant formula. By 1979 American infants were consuming a quarter of the total world infant formula production.

> The growth of the US infant formula market has been rapid since 1980.
>
> In 1979 US sales were US$ 500million, of a $2billion global market;
>
> By 1981 US sales rose to US $700 million; while in 1983 the global market was US$3.3billion
>
> By 1989 US sales were $1.6 billion of a $5billion global market
>
> By 2010 US sales were $6.6billion of a $25.2 billion global infant formula market.
>
> One projection for 2015 was a global infant formula market of $35-$40 billion dollars.

Currently between 58 and 67% of all infant formula used in the United States is paid for by US government food programs.

The issue of US market change and its impact on company market share, the price of formula, and worldwide industry re-structuring and consolidation, deserves detailed historical investigation beyond the purposes of this narrative. But I think it important to sketch a little of both the degree to which the US taxpayer has subsidised artificial feeding, and also the way ownership of those corporate beneficiaries of the public purse has changed over time.

## US Brand Wars 1980s

Until the 1980s, the US infant formula market had been dominated by a few large US firms, US pharmaceutical giants Abbott/Ross and Bristol Myers/Mead Johnson, together with American Home Products/Wyeth.  Americans have always tended to support US brands over foreign interlopers. (Such chauvinism is not uniquely American: in Paris I heard a French paediatrician denounce the scandalous inadequacies of American formulas – and go on to talk of how safe French formulas are by comparison. Maybe. It didn't prevent

Salmonella contamination of French formula! Or deaths from sepsis caused by unidentified bacteria in drip feeds in December 2013. Where is the historian of infant feeding in France?)

How had the US companies kept out major competitors, preventing Borden, Gerber, Baker/BeechNut and others from succeeding with past infant formula launches? As noted earlier in this history (see page 226), from their inception they had strong ties with the US medical profession. They were not seen as selling foods, but as feeding infants. They positioned themselves as trusted colleagues, in the cause of infant health. Ross/Abbott, the market leader, provided a huge range of products and the technology needed to deliver them to patients. Mead Johnson was similarly helpful.

Some American professionals I talked with in the 1980s and 1990s had the utmost faith that Ross/Abbott and Mead Johnson/Bristol Myers would never market their products unethically, or undermine breastfeeding. Many blindly trusted Ross as the sole source of data on infant feeding modes, prevalence and duration. They thought me rude to challenge the data, and extreme to object to Mead Johnson buying the right to use Beatrix Potter's Peter Rabbit for marketing purposes. Some were hugely offended when I maintained that US marketing strategies were just as bad, or even worse than, any European company, and were undermining breastfeeding globally. They did not want to hear that in Australia at that time, I saw American companies' marketing practices as much worse than those of Nestlé Australia, so that I could not support helping the US companies by reviving the boycott we had organised in Australia some years before.

How did Nestlé get past this problem of disastrous PR and re-establish itself in baby feeding in the USA? They went native, buying an American brand. Carnation was once the provider of much of the evaporated milk that 80% of US babies drank in 1960, and was trusted and familiar and American. Nestlé moved to enter the lucrative taxpayer-funded US infant formula market, by purchasing this American icon in 1985. In so doing, Nestlé challenged the American oligopoly.

All these US companies (and other minor players, past and present) engaged in massive marketing campaigns. But in the USA, the American companies had concentrated most of their marketing endeavours on indirect marketing: medical detailing, funding professional bodies and advertising to health professionals, lavishly supporting the healthcare professional industry with gifts, scholarships, entertainment and treats of all descriptions, as well as contacting every mother through those professional channels, with free gifts and incentives. This was clever and cost-effective, as it used the credibility of the institutions and individuals giving the products to parents, hospitals, doctors, nurses. Hospital discharge gift packs for mothers (containing free formula or coupons or advertising for formula as well as other items) could be elaborate and expensive, and were good strategy: even in the 21st century, after decades of discussion about this marketing, mothers who did not receive a gift pack (and 90% in this study did) were twice as likely to exclusively breastfeed at 6 months. Television and print advertising was both expensive and unnecessary for companies already dominating the market. Parents remained blithely unaware of the reality that companies were influencing professional decisions by such spending, and that the cost of the products they bought included such gifts. (When told about this, some angrily denounced it as deeply corrupt behaviour; in 2014 Italian authorities are investigating it as just that. )

Nestle tried to break into that medical marketing chain by offering a different and perhaps better product. Their formula Good Start was the first of the partially hydrolysed less-allergenic whey formulas, which all would make claims of being better/gentler/kinder for babies. It was the equivalent of Nan HA in Europe and Australia and other HA (hypo-allergenic) brands. In a country noted for allergic disease, it captured an initial 4% of the US market. Older formulas making such claims had been casein-based for the most part, and no one objected to their claims of hypo-allergenicity. US companies objected to Nestlé's claims, however, and the FDA contracted the American Academy of Pediatrics (AAP)to assess the claims of hypoallergenicity being made for this formula.

Astonishingly to me, on the Committee the AAP set up were representatives of Ross/Abbott and Mead Johnson, a clear indication of the unexamined closeness between all American parties. Nestlé/Carnation's request for similar representation on the committee was denied, although as they said, with some justice, that

> It is simply untenable from a fairness and appearance standpoint for a FDA-sponsored committee addressing a subject with significant regulatory and competitive implications to include the two major companies that occupy 90% of the market share and to exclude a new entrant.

It was also time-wasting when some questions they may have had about the formula needed to answered by the company making the product! But seeking advice from competitors about a rival's product was seen as perfectly appropriate by the AAP. And perhaps there was no unaligned expertise available!

As that behaviour seems to suggest, Carnation/Nestlé was to a large extent locked out of the usual American health-care-industry route to reach parents. Initially, Carnation had advertised

> "...Good Start H.A. only to the healthcare community as a pleasant-tasting infant formula for routine use that has the added benefit of being a nutritionally complete, reasonably priced, hypoallergenic alternative to soy-based or cows' milk-based formulas."

A policy of staid press releases featuring credible professionals soon morphed into the other obvious marketing avenues industry had always used to penetrate new markets. The US companies lobbied their health professional allies to try to prevent Carnation using television and print advertising direct to consumers, although this was what had earlier won Wyeth its market in the UK. In July 1989 Carnation began such advertising, a year after it had given the FDA the usual 90day notification of its intention to market the new formulas. (Nestle had ended such advertising in Australia before 1980.) Mead Johnson, while condemning such advertising, did a deal to provide babyfood company Gerber with infant formula - which was then advertised direct to the public in a 1989 multi-million dollar TV campaign funded by Mead Johnson, which claimed that "Nothing comes closer to your own milk than Gerber Baby formula." (Hmmm...does nothing really come closer? That's a bit worrying!) Gerber also produced a post 6 months formula to compete with the second stage Carnation/Nestlé product, called Good Nature. Coincidentally or not, FDA and AAP interventions had delayed the launch by almost a year, allowing time for this American riposte.

The AAP denounced both Nestlé and Gerber – but not Mead Johnson - for direct to consumer advertising. I suspect that this was not entirely because it could undermine breastfeeding – supplying formula in hospitals did that far more directly, and the AAP was not attempting to end that practice just then! As Dr Laurence Finberg was to say of direct to consumer advertising, many US paediatricians "see this as diminishing breastfeeding, as undermining their role, and as a means of diverting profits from supporting pediatric education and research into direct advertising costs."

The AAP had been dependent on large donations of industry money, which had helped to build its headquarters, and subsidised AAP costs for every US paediatrician.  AAP refused Carnation/Nestlé donations because of the direct-to-consumer advertising in the US, while continuing to ignore the US companies' direct-to-consumer marketing, mailouts, access to hospital discharge lists, and free gifts to parents. In addition, while AAP condemned the Gerber campaign, it did not refuse support from Mead Johnson/Bristol Myers, whose product was being advertised to parents via television: "If it doesn't come from you, shouldn't it come from Gerber?"

Federal Trade Commission investigators would later conclude that the purpose of opposition to direct-to-consumer advertising was to prevent Nestle entering the market. It is hard not to see the initial AAP/FDA response as both self-interested  and helping out the US companies who had funded the AAP for so long. The AAP could have done far more to protect, promote and support breastfeeding in the 1980s, if child health was its primary concern. The NY Times reported that in the period 1983-1991, industry gave some US$8.3 million to the AAP alone.  While this may not have corrupted individuals, the system was corrupt. In that freewheeling time the US market grew from roughly half a billion dollars in 1972 to $1.6 billion in 1989, according to Oski.

The US Department of Agriculture (USDA) had long been responsible for the distribution or destruction of surplus food, the product of taxpayer-subsidised large-scale agriculture. Originally USDA's Food Stamp programme was created to help in that effort, and the 1972 Women Infants and Children programme (WIC) prioritised needy mothers and children. But the formula industry has largely been allowed to set the terms of its co-operation. From the 1960s to the 1980s industry charged WIC virtually full retail prices for infant formula, with some huge increases over that time.

Testifying before a Senate Antitrust Subcommittee hearing last spring, Robert Greenstein, executive director of the Center for Budget and PolicyPriorities, said that "from December 1979 to December 1989, the wholesale prices charged by (Mead Johnson, Ross Laboratories, and Wyeth Laboratories) for milk-based infant formula increased at least 145 percent. During the same period... overall food prices rose 51 percent. ...

Infant formula was consuming a third of the entire WIC budget. WIC's payments for infant formula had to be reined in. Cost containment measures had to be put in place, and state by state they were. The WIC programme shifted in 1989 to a mandated tender process for exclusive supply rights. This would be the catalyst for major market changes. The new competition to cut costs opened up new US marketing opportunity for Nestlé. Nestlé tendered for the WIC market at well below the previous high prices paid by the USDA, as did some other smaller players in the market. In some states WIC was soon effectively paying less than a fifth of the pre-tender prices. However, the Nestlé boycott was revived just at this time, and a bid in some states could fail: an involved lactation consultant proudly told me she had ensured Nestlé was seen as an unacceptable choice for her WIC programme, and was surprised when I asked, "Did you evaluate which formula was better for babies?" Revival of the Nestle Boycott had again focussed attention on that brand and not on artificial feeding itself. American Home Products, makers of Wyeth, with 20% of global sales and annual sales of $5 billion, were notionally included in this new campaign, but very little was ever heard about them.

Wholesale targeting of any one or two infant formula companies worldwide, regardless of which company's practices are actually worst in any given country, or (even more importantly) *worst for any baby*, changes little more than the pockets into which the profits flow. It supports the efforts of all the other formula companies' marketing gurus, whose job it is to increase their company's market share. It is not the job of breastfeeding advocates to help any infant formula marketer, and even Baby Milk Action (formerly Baby Milk Action Coalition, now IBFAN UK), which derives some of its income from sales of Nestlé Boycott items, rightly exempts infant formula from its list of Nestle boycott targets. Choice of infant formula should be based first on nutritional science, not politics. (And there are plenty of other Nestlé products to choose for political purposes!)

It would seem that the US companies were not delighted by the idea of open competition and cost containment, as at least one major US company initially refused to tender for any WIC contract. In one State no bids were received. Yet the fact both of Nestlé competition and overall lower prices, and Wyeth's eagerness to increase its market share through greater access to WIC clients, forced the Big Two, Abbott/Ross and Mead Johnson, both to agree to bid, and to lower their prices by as much as 85% of the retail price.[1587] A detailed study found evidence that in states where there were two other competitors tendering, those two reluctant giants offered higher rebates than when they were competing solely against each other.[1588]

1587 Betson S. Impact of the WIC Program on the Infant Formula Market. Final Report for Grant Award 43-3AEM-
    3-80107 Online at http://www3.nd.edu/~dbetson/research/documents/WICImpactonPrices.pdf
1588 Betson S, op.cit.

Nestlé also flexed its considerable muscle in 1993 when it took legal action, alleging a price-fixing conspiracy of the AAP and American formula companies.[1589] Predictably, Nestlé lost the case against the AAP. But it seemed to me that by acting thus, Nestle was really serving notice that the cosy relationship between health professional groups and American formula companies was restricting competition, affecting market share, and that the game had to change. Nestlé is still a minor player in the US compared to Ross or Mead Johnson, but even a small slice of a huge and very rich pie is worth having!

Other political and economic developments were also to spark or support the process of change in the popular use of infant formula. Some were market forces. Changes happen quickly, where there is money to be made from the move. The system of rebates that WIC adopted had meant an initial drop in profits for US formula companies; unbelievably, companies ended up with perhaps 15% of what had previously been charged.[1590] (That says something to me about profit margins!) To compensate, retail prices of formula rose. As economic times grew ever more difficult, price became an ever more significant influence on choice, and so sales of powdered formula rose. (In no other Anglophone country had ready-to-feed ever been affordable.)

In the 1990s, for the first time, US store-brand powder formulas emerged, and began to take a small but growing share of the market, thanks to their lower cost. Often beaten by Ross and Mead Johnson for WIC tenders, Wyeth initially manufactured many of these store-brand formulas for large chains like Wal-Mart. Increasingly involved in birth infant feeding and vaccine production after the 1986 US National Childhood Vaccine Injury Act made this attractive for industry,[1591] in 1996 Wyeth stopped selling infant formula under its own name in the US market, and shifted its focus to the growth markets elsewhere. SMA was to disappear from the US market. Wyeth in America continued to produce 'house brand' formula, and formula for export. In 1999 Wyeth was bought by another major drug manufacturer, Schering. Wyeth had by then invested in formula manufacturing plants in low-tax Ireland and Singapore, and sold its American plants to PBM Nutritionals LLC, which had been contracted to make Wyeth product since 1997. PBM continues to make store-brand formulas, and in 2012 is even exporting one, AdvancedKare, to be sold through the Discount Drugstore chain in Australia.[1592] (This seems to be basically the old S26 formula, though of course it cannot be marketed as such.) US store brands are generally much less expensive than Wyeth's old SMA/S26, and around half the price of Mead Johnson's Enfalac+ or Lipil, and less-educated parents think that means they are not as good as a brand name.

---

1589 McCarthy M. USA: Nestlé sues American Academy of Pediatrics. *Lancet* 1993; 341(8859): 1526. doi:10.1016/0140-6736(93)90650

1590 Oliviera V. *Winner takes (almost) all. How WIC affects the infant formula market.* Downloaded from http://www.ers.usda.gov/AmberWaves/September11/Features/InfantFormulaMarket.htm

1591 By the end of 1984 Wyeth was the only US vaccine manufacturer; to ensure supplies Congress created a no-fault compensation scheme funded by a levy on each dose, with families of injured children offered payouts. See College of Physicians of Philadelphia: a history of vaccines. Online at http://www.historyofvaccines.org/content/articles/vaccine-injury-compensation-programs

1592 What does it say about profit margins and economies of scale if imported tins of 'Gold' formula can be sold for $4-$5 less than formula made in Australia?

Mead Johnson advertising of its added LCPUFA brands had suggested that PBM's formulas lacked important ingredients for eyes, showing blurry images of a yellow duck resolving to clarity. PBM has fought and won three lawsuits against Mead Johnson; in 2012 a US$35 million dollar court award was upheld.[1593] Another class action suit was brought by a mother who bought their formula because she believed that it contained nutrients not in other cheaper formulas. While not admitting fault, Mead Johnson has agreed to repay $12million to parents who bought Enfamil between October 13, 2005 and March 31, 2010.[1594] It remains to be seen whether those amounts are sufficient to stop effective, if unscrupulous, advertising, and also whether PBM or another smaller company can afford to keep paying legal fees to pursue such cases. (Note too, that the prosecution was not the result of independent regulatory oversight, but of an injured competitor's complaint.) Such behaviour makes immediate sanctions imperative: regulators need the power to cause advertising to be put on hold while the case is adjudicated, as a process that takes months allows a contested campaign to conclude successfully. After which a company can say sorry, get a slap on the wrist, and write off its costs as tax deduction.

Perhaps the 1990s US formula market shake-up would have occurred anyway, for other reasons. But knowing there were hungry under-bidders willing to slash grossly inflated prices certainly helped create change in the industry. Wyeth moved on, and Nestle established its 4% beachhead. The American giants Ross Laboratories/Abbott Ross and Mead Johnson, so long enmeshed with the US medical professions, have continued to hold the greatest share of the taxpayer-subsidised US formula market: in 2008 Abbott/Ross (Similac) held 43% and Mead Johnson (Enfamil) 40%, with Nestlé having achieved only 15%.[1595]

The late 1980s ferment caused the State of Florida to set the Federal Trade Commission looking at the issue of price-fixing by the three major US infant formula manufacturers. Abbott would settle this case in 1996 at a cost of $32.5 million,[1596] and Bristol Myers/ Mead Johnson for $31.8million.[1597] By 2014 price-fixing concerns have been expressed by China[1598] and Saudi Arabia[1599] and substantial price-reductions achieved. Other countries like Australia do little to investigate, much less control, costs to parents, who are always willing to pay for what they think is the very best formula, the most expensive.

---

1593 PBM News: *Store Brand Baby Formula Wins a Final Round in Court.* www.pbmproducts.com/press. aspx?ID=317. Oliviera V. *Winner takes (almost) all. How WIC affects the infant formula market.* Downloaded from http://www.ers.usda.gov/AmberWaves/September 11/Features/InfantFormulaMarket.htm

1594 http://www.browardbulldog.org/2011/04/weston-mom's-lawsuit-alleging-false-advertising-by enfamil-leads-to-12-million-settlement. April 25, 2011 report by Gehrke-White D.

1595 Oliveira, Victor, Elizabeth Frazão, and David Smallwood. *Rising Infant Formula Costs to the WIC Program: Recent Trends in Rebates and Wholesale Prices,* ERR-93, U.S. Department of Agriculture, Economic Research Service, February 2010

1596 http://www.apnewsarchive.com/1996/Abbott-Laboratories-to-Pay-$32-5-Million-in-Price-Fixing-Suit/id-b7a42ad50de81d3e926ce5d34e2420be

1597 http://articles.latimes.com/1996-09-05/business/fi-40631_1_infant-formula-market

1598 http://www.abc.net.au/news/2013-08-08/an-china-fines-formula-firms-24us108-million-for-price-fixing/4872452

1599 http://www.dairyreporter.com/Manufacturers/Nestle-working-with-Saudi-officials-to-harmonize-formula-prices; Abouh-Alsam R. May 25, 2014. Of expensive infant formula. http://www.arabnews.com/news/576421

Just as hospitals were, WIC has been a key factor in parental brand choice in the USA. As noted earlier (see page 324) legislation in 2004 removed WIC's ability to determine which formulas it wanted from a tendering company; companies could decide what formula they offered to WIC, at what price, provided the formula met the specifications for WIC use. If companies offered only the most expensive or novel brands, WIC had no choice but to become the inadvertent marketer of such products, without proof of the many advertising claims. In every state, WIC acceptance of any infant formula tender means massive increases in sales of the chosen brand (see figure below). Thus WIC also helps industry sell expensive infant formula.

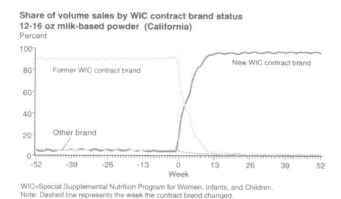

Share of volume sales by WIC contract brand status
12-16 oz milk-based powder (California)
Percent

WIC=Special Supplemental Nutrition Program for Women, Infants, and Children.
Note: Dashed line represents the week the contract brand changed.

Source: USDA, Economic Research Service calculations based on Nielsen supermarket scanner-based data.

Figure 3-13-1 Effect of WIC on brand sales.[1600]

Two-thirds of all US formula is bought through the WIC programme. This has flow-on effects: if the US norm becomes formula with particular additives, the rest of the world will most likely follow, as it did with whey-dominant formulas from the 1970s.

Companies claimed to be justified in charging a great deal more for infant formula, not because of the WIC rebate system, but because of the new additives – such as nucleotides and fatty acids– that were now going into formula. Attempts as late as 2010 to study the new ingredients objectively were stymied by high-powered industry lobbyists who used the old slanders, that this was a ploy being pushed by "lactivists who want to force women to continue breastfeeding".[1601] It was, rather, a plea from the better-informed for independent knowledge about products that might help or harm babies. This perfectly reasonable request was defeated despite the 2009 discovery that L-carnitine, added with great fanfare in the 1990s, "significantly promotes the growth of Listeria"[1602] so that "addition of carnitine to baby formula may pose a potential food safety risk", another unpredicted and unexpected outcome. If enough babies suffer – and are known about – perhaps independent research will happen.

In fact, every new additive, however trivial it may seem, can have effects on other ingredients and creates the potential for new and unexpected problems. Experienced company scientists are the only ones who know just how tricky it can be to change just one thing. Thus rigorous long-term independent study (not simple reliance on industry's own

1600 http://www.ers.usda.gov/media/121286/err124.pdf Accessed October 14, 2014.

1601 Lanny Davis, Martek lobbyist New York Times Dec 2010 . See also Molly M. Ginty. Infant-Formula Companies Milk U.S. Food Program. *WeNews* Monday, November 7, 2011 Source URL (retrieved on 2012-05-11 19:26): http://womensenews.org/story/reproductive-health/111106/infant-formula-companies-milk-us-food-program

1602 Sleator RD, Banville N, Hill C Carnitine enhances the growth of Listeria monocytogenes in infant formula at 7 degrees C. (PMID:19610343) *J Food Protect* 2009; 72(6):1293-5.

"post-marketing surveillance") is warranted, and indeed overdue if we care about bottle-fed babies as well as their mothers. Are those derided as 'lactivists' the only people who do?

WIC now relies on rebates from infant formula sales while promoting breastfeeding. (Theoretically WIC could run out of money to support breastfeeding if too successful in its efforts!) In some areas of the USA, WIC has indeed become a force for promoting breastfeeding. It has been reported that

> Policy changes, training of front-line WIC staff, and participant education, have influenced issuance rates of WIC food packages. In California, the issuance rates of packages that include formula have significantly decreased and the rate for those that include no formula has significantly increased.[1603]

Good news indeed, as WIC serves some of those who most need to breastfeed for socio-economic reasons, and whose children are at highest risk for ill-health and early childhood obesity.[1604] (By as young as 24 months infants predominantly fed formula for the first 6 months have two and a half times the risk of being obese, as their usually bottle-fed parents have been before them.) For WIC to stop supplying formula would probably lead to catastrophic rates of ilness among America's poor, but it is hard to see how to end this vast endorsement of infant formula.

## Consequences for poor families everywhere

Even WIC families that are bottle-feeding will pay more for the formula they buy. Once a family's monthly formula allowance runs out, families must buy that brand of formula on the retail market at the increased prices where the companies recoup foregone profit on WIC sales. Non-WIC families do pay more for infant formula as a consequence.[1605] Formula can cost families $100–$300 per month, up to a quarter of their projected income.[1606] "Despite generic formula being less expensive when replacing WIC-supplied brand name formula that runs out, more than three-quarters of the families in the study would not consider it. Half of the families incorrectly thought generic/storebrand formula was not nutritionally equivalent."[1607] It is not surprising that parents might think so, as buying the most expensive is equated with buying the best. Governments and health professional organisations could and should run educational campaigns informing parents that generics are indeed equivalent, and brand names can be over-priced: but the major players might be very unhappy if they did.

---

1603 Whaley SE, Koleilat M, Whaley M, Gomez J, et al. .Impact of policy changes on infant feeding decisions among low-income women participating in the Special Supplemental Nutrition Program for Women, Infants, and Children. (PMID:23078467) *Am J Public Health* 2012; 102(12):2269-2273.

1604 Gibbs BG, Forste R. Socioeconomic status, infant feeding practices and early childhood obesity. (PMID:23554385) *Pediatr Obes* 2013. DOI: 10.1111/j.2047-6310.2013.00155.x

1605 Oliviera V, Prell M. Sharing the economic burden. *Amber Waves* 2004. Online at http://www.ers.usda.gov/amber-waves/2004-september/sharing-the-economic-burden-who-pays-for-wics-infant-formula.aspx#.VDPoHb6PA20

1606 Burkhardt MC, Beck AF, Kahn RS, Klein MD. Are our babies hungry? Food insecurity among infants in urban clinics. *Clinical Pediatrics*. 2012;51(3):238-243.

1607 Ibid.

Not all poor American families can ever access WIC. It is a state by state programme, and its budgets are limited. Unlike Australian or UK or European welfare programmes, it is not a universal entitlement, but a privilege for whatever limited number of people a particular state can afford to subsidise. An official Report stated that in 2003 perhaps 20% of eligible families would not have access to WIC benefits[1608] because the programmes lack funds to serve them. Many American families must be going hungry in hard times because of their dependence on artificial feeding. Some of those will be using the older solutions, evaporated and fresh milk, inappropriately, and without access to the practical knowledge that made this safe enough to seem acceptable up until the 1960s.

In fact, a recent Cincinnati study showed that perhaps a third of all families lucky enough to be enrolled in WIC clinics were "food-insecure" or worried about getting enough to eat.[1609] And yes, they were "stretching" any WIC-provided formula. The maximum monthly amount of infant formula WIC gives families vouchers for is 128 dry ounces of powder, 403 fluid ounces of liquid concentrate, or 806 fluid ounces of ready-to-feed infant formula. To make it last the month, parents added too much water,[1610] leading to infant malnutrition, even water intoxication.[1611] The long-standing problem of hunger in America has not gone away, and grinding poverty is not confined to 'developing' nations, but exists in every country without an adequate social welfare safety net. What is the cost of a damaged brain or retarded growth?

Studies such as this, looking at parental beliefs about formula, and the reality of infant feeding by the poor in affluent nations, are rare. Poverty is sometimes not even named by Western authorities as a critical risk factor for infant feeding and infant mortality. Instead various ethnic or racial groups are linked to higher morbidity or mortality.[1612] Parental ethnicity or race is not what puts an infant at greater risk; in some situations traditional cultures are protective.[1613] Inequality, disadvantage, lack of education: all are words used to avoid naming poverty and the lack of necessary food, shelter and services in so-called "developed" countries like America.

The high price paid by USDA WIC programme for infant formula had once acted as a massive industry subsidy to the retail price of US formula, allowing quart cans of liquid formulas to be a realistic choice for many families. That changed. The once-usual ready-to-feed products became uneconomic. By 2000 80% of US formula sales were of powder. Childhood malnutrition, sickness and even death rates may well have risen among poor US

---

1608  US General Accounting Office. Food assistance potential to serve more WIC infants by reducing formula cost. www.gao.gov/products/GAO-03-331

1609  Burkhardt MC, Beck AF, Kahn RS et al, op. cit.

1610  http://www.cincinnatichildrens.org/news/release/2012/formula-stretching-01-17-2012/

1611  Keating JP, Schears GJ, Dodge PR. Oral water intoxication in infants. An American epidemic. (PMID:1877579) *Am J Dis Child* 1991; 145(9):985-990.

1612  EJ Heisler. *The* U.S. Infant Mortality Rate, *2012 www.fas.org/sgp/crs/misc/R41378.pdf*. Deaths of black infants are over 30% of the total, although blacks are just 16% of the population. The Black rate is 12.7 per thousand, the Native American rate is 8.7, the white 5.7, compared with all races 6.6. There is a strong correlation with short interbirth intervals- and no mention of breastfeeding as a factor in that, or other relevant areas.

1613  Small MF. *Our Babies, Ourselves. How biology and culture shape the way we parent.* (Anchor Books, 1998). See also  http://www.kathydettwyler.org/detbooks.html

families using even adequate supplies of powdered infant formula rather than the previously cheap ready-to-feed liquid formulas. It is difficult to reconstitute powder safely (see page 216). I know of no studies investigating relative infant morbidity and mortality rates among disadvantaged Americans (of whatever ethnic origin) using powdered formula, while living in urban or rural slum conditions, where access to power, clean water and sterilisation is problematic or non-existent. And what do the many homeless American families do?

Widespread use of usually sterile liquid formula had meant that some US authorities never emphasized boiling the water used for infant feeding, as British authorities always have. Formula companies can blame local water and parental hygiene standards for any sickness caused by infant feeding. They do not advertise that powdered infant formula is not sterile, might be contaminated or manufactured incorrectly, and cannot be safely used by many people: many of those with disabilities, or living in adverse social conditions. Most deaths due to infant feeding are likely to go unrecorded as such, unless the fault is obviously the carer's. Not boiling water for infant feeding increases risks, as WHO has made clear. To investigate this could be an eye opener in times of recession. What poor mother can spend a quarter of her income on infant formula, wherever she lives? How many living on the scandalously low American minimum wage lack facilities to feed infant formula as safely as possible?

This issue is now being seen as a serious consumer concern by at least some groups. After the 2010 Abbott recall of 5 million cans of Similac (due to contaminating beetles and larvae) *Consumer's Digest* published an article about infant formula[1614] which makes interesting reading. First it points out that in June 2011 there were still no FDA regulations defining Good Manufacturing Practice and infant formula quality (regulations which were promised in 1996). *Consumer's Digest* went on to argue that new additives enable disproportionate cost increases, which buyers must cover.

It also states that in 2004, the Institute of Medicine (IOM), which is a division of the US National Academy of Sciences, published the results of a 2-year study (commissioned by FDA) which concluded that current guidelines and regulations are insufficient for evaluating the safety of the new class of ingredients[1615] that mimic the properties of breast milk.

IOM wanted feeding trials to continue for at least 6 months. The current standard is 120 days, or just under four months. And many such short trials are of mixed feeding: i.e., babies being classed as "formula-fed" were breastfed for days or even up to three weeks, before swapping to formula; while babies being classed as "breastfed" are given bovine formula in hospital or after discharge, but continue to get some breastmilk. I can find no published trials in which infants are fed only one formula from birth to six months of age. We have no idea what that means for infant health and development.

---

1614 Elton C. Hard to Swallow: the truth about infant formula. *Consumer's Digest* June 2011 www.consumersdigest. com/health/hard-to-swallow

1615 Institute of Medicine, National Academy of Sciences. *Infant Formula: Evaluating the Safety of New Ingredients* (National Academy of Sciences Press 2004). Notably fungal and algal oils and prebiotics and probiotics and so on.

When I first visited the United States in the early 1980s, I was confronted by a truly perverse souvenir: the 'Red Indian' mother and her baby trapped inside a baby bottle, sometimes complete with coloured candy and always a teat. (Never nipple!) Given the harm done to First Nations in America and worldwide by the destruction of traditional indigenous infant care practices and food sources, this made me angry. It has been documented[1616] that many problems of infant feeding are greater among America's native peoples, immigrants, blacks and migrant workers, and the substantially worse infant mortality rates for such groups testify to the damage. So do the lifelong morbidity rates. In every country, rich or poor, it is the dispossessed and marginalised who will suffer most from the harms done by artificial feeding. And taxpayers are funding those harms, at home and abroad. When will it stop? A country that spends so much on arms and space exploration and infant formula has absolutely no excuse for an infant mortality rate 50% higher than the OECD average.[1617]

It has to be acknowledged that since the 1990s the US Surgeon General and US health and welfare authorities and groups such as the American Academy of Pediatrics and the Academy of Breastfeeding Medicine have taken many important steps in attempting to promote and support breastfeeding. But as I see it, these pale into insignificance beside the massive structural and cultural support America provides for artificial feeding. It would take a full-scale investigation of industrial, agricultural and social welfare policies in every state to begin to identify taxpayer contributions to the welfare of the formula industry, beginning with the cheap base products it uses, milk, soy and corn. I suspect that no other country in history has done, and still does, so much to protect, promote and support formula-feeding.

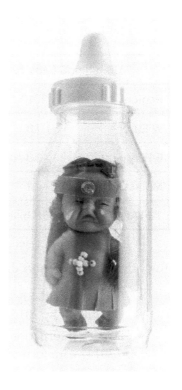

Figure 3-13-2 Weeping child in feeding bottle

## Growing the world market

It is not only in America that this American (and Dutch and French and Kiwi and German and Swiss and Australian...) dysnutritional pressure affects poor children. There have been many other significant changes in the world infant formula market since the 1990s. Western countries are seen as mature markets, where initial breastfeeding is on the increase, and growth is largely limited to extending the market into older infants, formerly breastfed. Whether companies realise it or not, this is a safer long-term strategy, as any food will do

1616  Salisbury l, Blackwell A. Public Advocates Inc. *Petition to Alleviate Domestic Infant Formula Misuse and Provide informed Infant Feeding Choice.* June 1981. See online discussion of this important document: Leslye E. Orlolf, Citizen Petitioning of Federal Administrative Agencies - Domestic Infant Formula Misuse: A Case Study, 12 *Golden Gate University Law Review.* (1982).http://digitalcommons.law.ggu.edu/ggulrev/vol12/iss3/4
1617  EJ Heisler. Op. cit.

less harm to a baby that starts out breastfed (which might be why such babies are so often used in formula studies, tather than babies formual-fed from birth.)

Profit in developed country markets comes from these additional sales along with steep price increases. Increases are justified as due to the new ingredients being added and marketed as important to infant health (although not so important that the company immediately stops producing its 'classic' older formulas, as we have seen!)

What of the global market? A market analysis firm, Statista, published the following data for this table of world babyfood market sales in 2010 and projected growth to 2015.

| US billion$ baby food market sales according to Statista (www.statista.com) | | | | | |
|---|---|---|---|---|---|
| Region | 2010 | 2015 | Asia Pacific | 13.4 | 24.5 |
| W Europe | 7.8 | 8.4 | N America | 6.6 | 7.6 |
| E Europe | 2.9 | 6.2 | Latin America | 3.6 | 4.6 |
| M East/Africa | 2.1 | 3.3 | Australasia | .4 | .4 |
| TOTAL 2010 | $36.8 billion (25.2 formula) | | TOTAL 2015 | $55 billion ($35-$40) (EST.) | |

Figure 3-13-3 The global babyfood market 2010-2015

But other sources report different global market figures:

- Gira Consultancy - $29 billion global infant formula sales in 2012, to rise to $35billion by 2016.
- Zenith International - 7% growth rate for $50billion infant nutrition market (2014) with formula perhaps two-thirds of that;
- Dairy Reporter - $5billion increase in infant formula sales in 2013 alone
- Reuters - China formula sales $17billion by 2017

Average annual growth of the infant formula market in the period 2006-2011 has been 6%. China is 26% of the world market, up from 15% in 2006. In 2009 Asia was responsible for more than half of the world sales. All the biggest growth markets are in poorer areas of the world: India, China, Asia and Latin America generally. Danish vegetable-oil company AAK, an ingredients suplier, has online[1618] an image of the 6% average annual growth in the period 2007-2010, by region. Asia grew by 19%, Africa 9%, Eastern Europe and Latin America by 5%, Oceania by 4%, Europe by only 2%, while North America dropped by 6%.

So every area of the world except North America grew, with the fastest increases in Asia and Africa. Companies have shifted production facilities and resources towards servicing those areas, hence the new plants in Singapore, Vietnam, China, Mexico. Asia and Latin America are fast growing markets, as company annual reports and investment strategies make clear. Yet

1618 Lidefelt J-O. Infant Nutrition presentation, p. 5. Downloaded 19/9/2014 http://www.aak.com/Global/Investor/Infant%20Nutrition%20presentation%20111115.pdf

industry leaders must know that the lack of breastfeeding in such areas will cause enormous harm and millions of deaths. It could be argued that the formula pioneers knew not what they did. That cannot be said today for any infant formula company scientist, director, or investor. Infant formula (instead of breastmilk) is harming more babies than ever.

Wyeth's history (see box) illustrates the international nature of formula markets. The brand *name* persists globally, because it is trusted by parents who have used the product, even when the product changes, and the name is owned by various other entities. Production sites change to wherever in the world is best suited for low-cost production and distribution into growing markets. Tax breaks help in relocation decisions, so taxpayers subsidise a public health risk to their infants.

### Wyeth's Metamorphosis

After selling manufacturing facilities to PBM Nutritionals in the USA, Wyeth (Schering-owned after 1999) did not go out of infant formula making. They continued to make product in the USA for export, and set up plants in Ireland and Singapore and Mexico to manufacture formula for sale in the new growth markets of eastern Europe and Asia. After company re-structuring, Wyeth was bought by Pfizer in 2009 for $68 billion and a nutrition unit created. The ultimate irony came in 2012 when Pfizer's nutrition unit was bought by Nestlé, so that SMA in the UK became a Nestlé brand!

A 2013 online investor seminar outlined Nestle plans for Wyeth Nutrition, to be maintained as a distinct embedded division within the Nestle portfolio. But SMA will not be a Nestle product in some other countries, and the brand may even disappear in them. In both Mexico and Australia, for example, national competition laws[1619] have caused Nestle to sell off the Wyeth infant formula business in that region. Wyeth's SMA and S26, with Australian sales revenue of AUD$83million in 2012, were sold in April 2013 for USD$215million to a South African company, Aspen Pharmaceuticals, which currently makes Infacare brand formulas. The Wyeth-Nestlé-now-Aspen brands SMA and S-26[1620] will continue to be made in Singapore – by Nestle for Aspen – for a few years, only until they can be transitioned to other sources of supply and manufacturing facilities in South Africa.[1621] Nestle retained the Wyeth Singapore manufacturing plant and Wyeth's Hong Kong business, strengthening its reach into the lucrative Asian market.

Nestlé acquired Pfizer's Wyeth despite stiff competition from Danone (France). Nestlé and Danone are two international food giants with tremendous reach and capacity for vertical integration of production, as both produce many types of milk products globally. Danone has recently been criticised for blatant undermining of breastfeeding in Turkey, using the old strategies of the 1960s, aligning their formula with breastmilk and pushing their product

---

1619 http://www.accc.gov.au/media-release/accc-to-not-oppose-acquisition-by-nestlé-of-pfizer-nutrition

1620 But what's in a name? The UK once-Wyeth's whey-dominant SMA was always Wyeth Australia's S-26, with SMA in Australia being a casein-dominant product...if you're confused, so was I and so were many mothers! Bottom line here: S-26 and SMA will mean different things and be made by different companies and factories worldwide. But the no-longer-Wyeth brands won't just disappear immediately. Travellers beware!

1621 http://www.dairyreporter.com/Manufacturers/Nestle-agrees-to-licence-out-Pfizer-infant-nutrition-brands-in-Australia-Southern-Africa; http://www.aspenpharma.com.au/news/article/index/id/67/

as a suitable supplement for breastfeeding women who have insufficient milk.[1622] Danone has similarly been expanding its ownership of milk production facilities and formula companies worldwide.

Mead Johnson's story is similar. Changes of ownership. Production in Mexico, the Philippines and China. Persistence of known brand names but with altered recipes. A trusted brand name influences infant formula recommendations and decisions, and gathers the support of grandmothers who brought a child up on that brandname, though not that formula.

## Marketing new products, and evading the International Code?

Infant formula use has expanded world-wide, on a phenomenal scale. In the 1980s and since, profit in the infant formula market has come from new sources: an increasing variety of types of formulas among them. When the International Code of Marketing of Breast Milk Substitutes (hereafter the Code) was being drafted around 1980, infant formula was 'a product suitable as the sole diet for an infant' for just four to six months, with contemporary advice being to introduce other foods by four months. Cows' milk was eaten from around four months in yoghurts and custards and cheese, as part of the weaning diet. Babies drank milk from six months and were eating family foods by twelve months. Once it was realised that many infants drinking only whole cows' milk (or the earlier iron-deficient infant formulas) with poor quality weaning foods became iron-deficient under twelve months, the duration of iron-fortified formula use was extended to twelve months. The timing of this varied from country to country.

After the Code restricted advertising of breastmilk substitutes,[1623] more formula companies launched new products, which they called not infant formula, but follow-on formula (FOF) (discussed in Chapter 3.5 Basic Ingredients: Protein and its problems). Industry claimed that these were not covered by the Code. In fact, these products are breastmilk substitutes,[1624] as the normal course of lactation recommended by WHO is 'into the second year and beyond'. Industry refused to accept this, basically arguing that:

---

1622  http://www.independent.co.uk/news/uk/home-news/exclusive-after-nestl-now-breast-milk-scandal-strikes-aptamil-manufacturer-danone-8679226.html Plus http://babymilkaction.org/pressrelease/pressrelease28jun13

1623  In *The politics of breastfeeding*, Gabrielle Palmer argues that the companies created these milks 'to avoid marketing restrictions' (Pinter and Martin, 2009) p. 273. While this may be so, it seems clear that industry would always have tried to expand product sales beyond the four to six months envisaged in the WHO documents, for purely commercial reasons. Abbott/Ross's 'Advance' had been launched in 1971, after all, and since the 1960s there had been a change of formula at 3-4 months in some countries. With the benefit of hindsight, it is unfortunate that this was not noticed by industry critics in the late 1970s, and this obvious tactic blocked when the code was being drafted.

1624  The UK Scientific Advisory Committee on Nutrition (SACN) has stated that the even newer 'goodnight milks' – milk with cereals added – are breastmilk substitutes: see http://www.sacn.gov.uk/pdfs/final_sacn_statement_on_good_night_milks.pdf

- no mother breastfed her baby past six months (and at this stage very few did in Western countries),

- so follow-on formulas were not either breastmilk substitutes or infant formulas in fact, or by definition,

- so they could advertise these new products widely in parent and professional journals if they wanted to pay to do so. And they did!

As noted earlier, in America the healthcare and welfare systems were the main marketing channels for infant formula. Advertising in professional journals and conferences was a massive revenue source for professional associations; this money would not be available for such associations if buying advertising space on TV or in parent magazines. As Rima Apple documents, doctors had always disapproved of industry advertising direct to consumers: mothers might not consult doctors about infant feeding if all the information they needed was freely available.[1625] Interestingly, the American Academy of Pediatrics (AAP) initially saw no purpose for FOFs and supported the use of first formulas for twelve months. This was perhaps a welcome sign of growing independence, as its industry sponsors were marketing FOFs globally. However in America there was no need to alter marketing practices, as the USA was the sole nation to vote against the Code in 1981, and some American companies insisted that the Code only applied in developing countries.

Coincidentally or not, after 1981 most global formula companies moved to develop new FOFs or rebrand old post-six months formulas (usually the old casein-dominants), so that 'infant formula' was now labelled 'Brand X1' and the so-called 'follow on formula' was labelled 'Brand X2'. In 1986 the World Health Assembly declared these 'follow-ons' unnecessary,[1626] but few health professionals openly condemned them, though some paediatricians argued that they were potentially hazardous and confusing as well as unnecessary.[1627] As indeed they still are. But thanks to industry's longstanding links with professional groups worldwide, dieticians, home economists, doctors and midwives alike have allowed industry to get away with this by mostly ignoring the issue, and the parental confusion it created.

Some breastfeeding advocates of the time accepted industry's terminology of FOFs (follow-on formulas), while insisting that such products fit the definition of breastmilk substitutes, whether first infant formula (FIF) or FOF. Industry disagreed worldwide, and went on its merry way, advertising the FOF2, and with it, their FIF1. This is a recognised marketing strategy: variously described as back marketing, or brand marketing by association, or cross marketing.

Virtually all the American and European companies now have stage two and three milk drinks; some have a stage four. Just to make things more complicated, some stage twos are

---

1625 Greer FR, Apple RD. Physicians, formula companies, and advertising: a historical perspective. *Am J Dis Child*, 1991;145:282–6. See also Apple RD. *Mothers and medicine: a social history of infant feeding, 1890–1950* (University of Wisconsin Press, 1987)

1626 World Health Assembly (WHA) Resolution 39.28, 16 May 1986. The text (of this and all relevant WHA resolutions) can be found in Shubber S, op. cit., pp. 262–3.

1627 The UK Guidance Notes referred to earlier make a point of trying to prevent such confusion, widely acknowledged as a serious problem.

FIFS, usually casein-dominant, and some are FOFS, incomplete milk drinks, not suitable for under six months. Their obvious visual and linguistic connection to stage one FIFs means that some parents consider them to be suitable as sole foods, or use them with a bare minimum of other foods, rather than using them as the supplements to a good varied diet which industry describes them as in the fine print on the cans.

But then, such confusion is hardly surprising when industry has varied recipes for FOFs. When in 1989 Wyeth Australia recalled S-26 cans that had been inadvertently filled with S-26 Progress, their letter to pharmacists stated that "the feeding of S-26 Progress instead of S-26 infant formula does not present a hazard to the health of the baby."[1628] If suitable for infants, it is an infant formula. If not, it is a hazard. Wyeth was maintaining that Progress was *not* an infant formula for Code purposes.....

Talking to mothers in 2012, I found that parents and healthworkers alike do not understand that it could be unsafe to feed any FOF to three- to six-month-old babies *as the major or sole diet,* because stage two FOFs are **by definition** quite unsuitable as a whole diet. Stage two FOFs can lack specific nutrients. Some have had even more protein and calories than FIFS,[1629] because the volume to be consumed was less, and there were no global nutrient standards for FOFs. The use of more protein/calorie dense Stage 2 formulas may have accelerated infant formula's contribution to the dramatic rise in obesity: an increase has seen since their merchandising began in the 1980s. They do not provide all the micronutrients that should be coming to a child from a good varied family diet. FOFs are 'foodstuffs intended for particular nutritional use by infants when appropriate complementary feeding is introduced, and constituting the principal liquid element in a progressively diversified diet.'[1630] (In fact breastmilk should always the principal liquid element in infant diet, and after that water, which is found in foods as well as formulas!)

Are FOFS nowadays researched and regulated? That depends on the company and the country. These products are intended for use *as part of a mixed diet* so deficiency problems in the infant should be rare. But being part of a mixed diet means also that they are less likely to be seen as the source of any problem or infection. They may not be subject to the same testing and inspection regimes as 'infant formula' from birth.[1631] Which makes it additionally risky to give them to infants under six months, or to rely heavily on them from six to twelve months, as some parents do. Parents of infants under six months need to read labels very carefully and choose from those stating that they *can be fed from birth.* (None should be labelled 'suitable from birth.' Parents could rightly claim to have been misled by such a government-approved label, whenever the product proves unsuitable for their particular baby.)

---

1628 Robertson JA. Important Notice. November 9, 1989. On file.
1629 Some were formulated at ESPGHAN's suggestion so as to provide a daily protein intake of 15 g in just 500 ml, the recommended volume intake when given to weaned infants on protein-poor diets. That's 30 g/L, excessive and perhaps obesogenic for those getting adequate protein from complementary foods, and potentially useful only for those least able to afford to buy the product, where protein is scarce!
1630 European Commission Directive 2006/141/EC. http://www.babyfeedinglawgroup.org.uk/thelaw/eudirective
1631 Bier, DM. Safety standards in infant nutrition: a US perspective. *Ann Nutr Metabol* 2012, 60(3):192–5. US Requirements for Infant Formulas can be found online at http://www.fda.gov/RegulatoryInformation/Legislation/FederalFoodDrugandCosmeticActFDCAct/FDCActChapterIVFood/ucm107864.htm

Marketing of the stage two or 'follow-on' products has been brilliantly done, with themes and product names that play into parents' natural desire to see their babies 'progress' 'forward' or 'advance'. That makes their misuse more likely, as parents can be notoriously competitive about their baby's progress.

Stage three (i.e., post twelve months or Toddler or young child) formulas now emphasize the idea of 'nutritional insurance'. That implies to me that they contain everything a toddler might lack in his diet, which *by definition* they do not. Heavy reliance could lead to excess intakes of some nutrients, or cause deficiency that a varied diet guards against. They can cost parents almost as much as the stage two and stage one formulas. Yet they are less expensive compositionally: highly refined alpha-lactalbumin and other such forms of protein in Stage 1or even sometimes Stage 2 formulas are considerably dearer than less refined milk ingredients, and other additives and trace elements need not be present in Stage 3 as well. They could also condition children to prefer bland and sweet foods, as a considerable amount and variety of sugars are used. Regular (full-fat) cows' milk itself is a suitable food for non-allergic children of this age, and is both cheaper and probably less cariogenic, for starters. The First Steps Nutrition website makes clear the differences: see their online monograph, *Fortified Milks for Children.* [1632] (And if you use it, please support them with a donation!)

One FOF was advertised on YouTube in 2013 as being for 'when you move on from breastfeeding'. How misleading, when almost all mothers 'move on' or give up breastfeeding well under twelve months, and many under three months! What is true of some FOFs is certainly true of Toddler Formula: they are generally TOTALLY unsuitable as sole diet for infants, and by definition are not an infant formula, but a filled milk drink.[1633] Although work is progressing on a standard for so-called FOFs, the EU has no plans to set a standard for Toddler/Stage 3 milk drinks. They are simply another food product in a very diverse diet (we hope). In fact the EU calls them *drinks for the young child*, not formula at all: there is no industry-accepted formula for them.

Yet these young child drinks *are* frequently talked about as infant formula, baby formula, not as a completely different filled milk product for older children. Anyone who doubts this should check out online coverage of the March 2014 scandal in which China accused an Australian company, OZDairy, of tampering with the expiry date on its "baby formula"

---

1632 Crawley H, Westland S. *Fortified milks for children* (First Steps Nutrition Trust June 2013) http://www. firststepsnutrition.org/newpages/fortified_milks_for_children.html

1633 There is one exception to this statement. The Columbus Ohio producer of Nature's One, a formula sold as suitable for infants, labels its product as a Toddler formula, saying that it does so because it wants to encourage mothers to breastfeed for 12 months. A reply to a FAQ recommends it for use by children over 12 months. But the company knows that the product is being used as an infant formula, and says that while it meets AAP 2014 nutrient content guidelines for infant formula and the US Infant Formula standard, it is "not regarded by the USFDA as an infant formula." (correspondence 10/5/2014) The product seems to be a classic 82:18 casein-dominant whole cows' milk based formula using organic ingredients. Enquiries reveal that it is a 70kcal formula with 17g/L protein. The Toddler label may or may not have regulatory consequences: under the International Code it is clearly an infant formula, since the makers represent it as able to be used to supplement or replace breastmilk. The potential for confusion seems real. It is hoped that US parents do not get the idea that Toddler formulas in general are safe for infants under 12months!

cans: the cans are clearly marked 3, but the owner, the reporter, the discussants, Australian and Chinese alike, talked about these filled milks for children aged one to three years, as baby formula, infant formula.[1634]

A recent independent scientific review[1635] commissioned by the European Food Safety Authority -available online- makes it clear that such formulations offer no special benefits. Analysis of the different themes and contents or marketing, and the emotive images and language used, would put paid to any idea that these products sell because they are scientific. Almost all formula marketing plays on emotions rather than provides accurate and complete information. The M in the UK SMA logo (2010) resembled a love heart, or could even be mistaken for an abstract breastfeeding mother. Talk of nutritional insurance subtly implies that babies need protection from inadequate family food intake.

From the beginning formula advertising played on women's fears that their baby might be harmed by their actions or even their diet. (See Appendix II) As one ad man said frankly:

> Advertising deals in open sores...Fear. Greed. Anger. Hostility. You name the dwarfs and we (the admen) play on every one. We play on all the emotions and on all the problems."[1636]

Yet any breastfeeding promotion that plays on parental emotions is bitterly condemned as unkind, and as just trying to make non-breastfeeders feel bad. That constant double standard ensures formula's continued growth. If health authorities ever employed professional marketers and allowed them to use normal industry tactics to defend breastfeeding against its inferior competitors, very few parents would *choose* to bottle-feed. Which is why the US National Breastfeeding Campaign, developed by advertising experts, could not be allowed to proceed, and lobbying politicians saved industry's bacon. (Discussed in Appendix 2.)

Breastfeeding advocates handicap their cause by trying always to be "objective" and "not give offence." Of course there is a need for dispassionate discourse. There is also a far greater need for informed but passionate advocacy and truth-telling. Passion has power that generates change: look at how a small number of assertive women (mostly unable to breastfeed) have changed the public discourse about infant feeding. Hard-working volunteers are blithely abused as 'Nazis' and 'lactivists' by formula-feeding fans who truly use fascist tactics, with impunity. These help to silence the sensitive, who find verbal abuse painful, and don't want to upset anyone. Their hostile language contributes to breastfeeding failure, by making some mothers afraid to ask for needed help with breastfeeding in case they might be bullied by monsters of insensitivity, rather than – as is more usual - helped by other kind-hearted women who've succeeded despite difficulty (known as breastfeeding

---

1634  See the video http://www.abc.net.au/lateline/content/2014/s3967052.htm Or read the *China Daily* account., talking of mislabelled infant formula!! http://www.chinadaily.com.cn/china/2014-04/03/content_17401720. htm

1635  Tijhuis, EL Doets, M Vonk Noordegraaf-Schouten; Extensive literature search and review as preparatory work for the evaluation of the essential composition of infant and follow-on formulae and growing-up milk. EFSA supporting publication 2014:EN-551, 448 pp. www.efsa.europa.eu/publications . Online at http://www.efsa. europa.eu/en/supporting/doc/551e.pdf

1636  Gold P. *Advertising politics and American culture, from salesmanship to therapy*. Paragon House (May 1987) p. 119.

counsellors). Formula feeding fans need to read this book and think again about the damage they may be responsible for, when women who listen to them 'choose' formula believing it to be safe for baby and themselves. I wouldn't want that on my conscience!

Many Western mothers now use FOFs or toddler milk products at some point, even those who can't afford to waste money that could be better spent on fresh foods, including dairy products. As that FDA official said in another context, 'society depends on bottle-feeding'. So over the last thirty years mothers have gone from buying infant formula for maybe four to six months, to buying a variety of heavily-marketed white liquid products for at least one year, and sometimes two or more. The sight of many older children still sucking on bottles is now so common as to sadden the heart of orthodontists (or gladden the cynical ones, since it creates remedial work[1637]). By contrast, the sight of older children breastfeeding remains rare, and is always controversial – persuading even some breastfeeding mothers to resort to breast pumps and use bottles or cups to feed breastmilk to their children when in public. (Cups are intrinsically safer, and WHO recommends their use.)[1638] And the AAP 2005 Statement endorsed breastfeeding beyond two years.

UK Stage One and Stage Two products are analysed in the excellent publication *Infant milks in the UK: a practical guide for health professionals.* Dr Helen Crawley did an admirable job putting this together for the Caroline Walker Trust, and has now set up an independent First Steps Nutrition Trust with its own website,[1639] where the updated version can be found and downloaded. Similarly a publication examining the Stage Three products is available: *Fortified milks for children* which concludes that

> " There is little evidence that fortified milks are a necessary addition to the diets of healthy children over the age of one year. The high sugar content and potential over-supply of micronutrients also provide a product that could potentially be harmful if consumed in large amounts by some children. The use of novel ingredients which are not tested and which have no proven efficacy should be questioned....Fortified milks are an example of an unnecessary product designed to make profit and heavily marketed without evidence to substantiate claims made. If parents and carers spent the same amount of money on local diverse foods that would provide most children with the nutrients they need. [1640]

Would that every country had such a national document online for parents and health professionals to consult. I find it surprising that international and national associations of dietitians have not seen this as an important aspect of their role – though a truly independent and critical document might harm their access to industry funding, which can be important to such organisations.

---

1637 Labbok MH, Hendershot GE. Does breast-feeding protect against malocclusion? An analysis of the 1981 Child Health Supplement to the National Health Interview Survey. (PMID: 3452360) *Am J Prev Med,* 1987, 3(4):227–32

1638 Perhaps they are less likely to cause problems with later breastfeeding by preterms, but they result in greater losses, and so less certainty about infant intake. Experience has taught midwives the need to ensure that it is not the bib that is being filled with milk. Lang S. *Breastfeeding special care babies,* (Bailliere Tindall, 2002).

1639 First Steps Nutrition Trust: *www.firststepsnutrition.org*

1640 Crawley H, Westland S. *Fortified milks for children* (First Steps Nutrition Trust June 2013) p. 74.

Such work by well-informed independent nutritionists is long overdue. Real harm is being done by those who do not carefully control the language about, and marketing of, all milk drinks for children, restricting the term Infant Formula to guess what – products for infants, persons under 12 months of age. Why don't leading authorities clearly say that infant formula is a product for infants till 12 months of age; and that other milk drinks are not "formulas" of any kind, but simply milk drinks with added and probably unnecessary supplements? All later milks –whether Stage 3 or labelled as Stage 2 for after 6 months - need to be completely separated verbally, visually, and commercially from infant formulas to be fed from birth. Consider the damage if infants are fed solely a Toddler milk drink, thanks to advertising chicanery (or any manufacturer's ignorance that the product he makes is NOT an infant formula). Would we tolerate such misleading advertising in any other field? To pass off –incidentally or deliberately - a Toddler milk-based drink as an infant formula is simply criminal. The reverse, however, is perplexing: a US manufacturer labelling as a Toddler Formula what is clearly an infant formula in composition and use. I hope the USFDA will address this anomaly!

## So what is infant formula? Australia, NZ, America and the Code

In Australia, responsibility for implementation of the International Code was handed over to the Trades Practices Commission from the Health Department in 1989. Consultation finally took place to determine what Australia would do 'to implement the Code in conformity with Australian law', the mandate given by the minister. Certain companies were clearly prepared to fight for the definition of breastmilk substitutes applying only to FIFs, and to fight for the right to advertise FOFs. A meeting was set up to reach consensus about an Australian industry agreement. At this meeting I pointed out that under Australian law, the definition of an infant was 'a person of less than twelve months of age', so that an 'infant formula' was, necessarily in Australian law, any such product for a baby less than twelve months old. This made any discussion of the FOFs unnecessary, no matter how the International Code was interpreted. Fortunately the experienced government bureaucrats agreed. So while we breastfeeding advocates present in the meeting had to concede the use of some simple non-pictorial price advertising (so as not to breach competition law under the Australian Trade Practices Act), industry had to swallow the fact that in Australia there would be no clever back-marketing in parents' magazines of any infant formula product for a baby under twelve months of age. That resolved the immediate Australian battle.

But as usual, industry won the war. If companies could not directly advertise a second tier product, they would create and advertise a third. By 1991 Wyeth was marketing a milk-based product for children over twelve months, Wyeth KindiVite,[1641] being advertised as nutritional insurance for fussy eaters. In Australia this 'toddler' drink would soon be rebranded as S-26 Toddler, then S-26 3. Obviously S-26 3 implies the existence of S-26 2 and

---

1641 Aktavite was a well-known Australian icon: a crunchy chocolate flavoured cereal-based vitamin-enriched tonic food, first created in 1915 by the Nicholas company of Aspro fame, and known to all Australians. Wyeth's 'Kindivite' introduced the idea of a tonic food for toddlers, but without risking S-26 name brand damage if it should fail to take in the market. Once the market was established, the name changed to S-26 3 or S-26 Toddler.

S-26 1, and so advertises their availability, to anyone who can count. The other companies soon followed their lead.

No health authority at this time took regulatory or even cautionary action about this obvious strategy of marketing infant formula by association[1642] with even less necessary filled milks for older children.[1643] And forewarned, the infant formula industry in New Zealand was able to push through in that country's regulatory system a different definition of 'infant formula', one which means 'stage two' infant formulas (FOFs) can be advertised there, and were, relentlessly, on TV as well as in magazines. Just as stage three drinks are in Australia. Experience suggests that breastfeeding advocates[1644] were right to declare the promotion of FOFs to be stealth marketing of infant formula.

American companies had pioneered this move, at least in Australia. This was odd when the US definition of infant formula covers the child to twelve months.

> The Federal Food, Drug, and Cosmetic Act (FFDCA) defines infant formula as "a food which purports to be or is represented for special dietary use solely as a food for infants by reason of its simulation of human milk or its suitability as a complete or partial substitute for human milk" (FFDCA 201(z)). FDA regulations define infants as persons not more than 12 months old (Title 21, Code of Federal Regulations 21 CFR 105.3(e)).[1645]

When in 1988 Nestlé introduced to the USA not only Good Start – a complete infant formula – but also Good Nature, a FOF, the FDA insisted that both were infant formulas and must comply with the infant formula regulations. Nestlé argued that Good Nature was intended as a complementary weaning formula, to no avail. So all the US companies acknowledged their Stage 2 products – Follow Ons in NZ - to be infant formulas in America, yet disowned them as such in another country where this meant they could be advertised. Go figure. What does that say to you? That politics and money are more important than science, perhaps?

We need to be very clear about what is and is not a first infant formula (FIF) able to be fed to babies from birth, because a new challenge is coming: "staging" within infant formula, by variation of the amino acid profile, thanks to the dairy industry providing new blends of proteins to manufacturers.[1646]  (see page 538)

# Decline of an old marketing strategy?

As described earlier in this book, supplying free or low-cost infant formula to maternity facilities and other health professional outlets was the key marketing strategy used with great effect in Anglophone countries from 1959 onwards. Wherever direct to consumer

---

1642  Berry NJ, Jones S, Iverson D. It's all formula to me: women's understandings of toddler milk ads. *Breastfeed Rev*. March 2010; 18(1): 21–30
1643  *Infant milks*, op. cit.
1644  Berry NJ et al, op. cit.
1645  See Guidance for Industry: Frequently Asked Questions about FDA's Regulation of Infant Formula: http://www.fda.gov/Food/GuidanceComplianceRegulatoryInformation/GuidanceDocuments/InfantFormula/ucm056524.htm
1646  Mullaney L. op.cit.

advertising had largely ceased, as in Australia from 1983 (before the Follow-On Formula back-marketing campaigns), the key marketing strategy had been providing hospitals and child health clinics with free supplies of formula. These 'gifts' – indirectly from taxpayers and formula-feeding parents – were condemned repeatedly by international agencies like UNICEF and WHO and breastfeeding advocates everywhere.

Giving free samples and supplies to every maternity hospital or clinic that wanted them was an expensive exercise. But the first company to cease unilaterally would lose market share, as customer brand loyalty was so high. To end free and low-cost supplies would require a negotiated cessation by all parties. I suspect that this is why in 1991 Nestlé Australia – whose executives wanted to end free supplies – supported breastfeeding activists' call for industry regulation.[1647] At the time, it is doubtful whether the government would have acted had the whole of industry been obdurate, and some parts certainly seemed to be. Breastfeeding advocates had been calling for regulation of these supplies ever since the International Code was adopted by the World Health Assembly in 1981!

Simple economics made this a sensible strategy for Nestlé in Australia. Over the 1980s Nestlé had lost considerable market share to the more aggressive un-boycotted American companies marketing in Australia, especially Wyeth, just as older UK formula had lost out in the 1950s thanks to Wyeth's pioneering use of TV advertising. Wyeth had invested in local plant for formula making, and was becoming the clear leader in sales and marketing, although Mead Johnson was gaining considerable market share too.[1648] Nestlé marketing had been more constrained – in Australia at least – by the stated company policy of supporting the WHO Code worldwide; its top Australian executives included fathers of breastfed babies, who strongly endorsed the superiority of breastfeeding. So importantly, Nestlé in Australia stood to benefit from the creation of a more level playing field by government action to rein in the most blatant (and effective) marketing tactics of the other companies, notably Wyeth and Mead Johnson. With unity among consumer advocates, and a breach of industry solidarity by Nestlé, government was emboldened to facilitate discussions to end all such free and low-cost supplies. And did so, as noted earlier.

This was of course a financial benefit to industry. The free-supplies strategy was expensive, but no one company could stop while others persisted. With several changes of ownership since then, and emerging new players who have not even joined the Australian industry body or signed on to the 1992 Agreement, it will be interesting to see if this moratorium continues. By now, with International Board Certified Lactation Consultants[1649] in most hospitals, it should be difficult to get free supplies into hospitals. Even so, anecdotal feedback

---

1647 Nestlé White Paper, *Infant feeding in Australia*, July 1991, informed the Federal Health Department that Nestlé was resigning from the weak 1983 Australian industry Voluntary Code of Conduct, and urged state and national authorities both to implement the WHO code in full and end the provision of free and low-cost supplies in all areas of the healthcare system. Correspondence on file, my archives.

1648 Pharmacy wholesalers produced annual reports that documented these changes of market share.

1649 IBCLCs have been accredited after passing an international fully professional examination set by IBLCE, the International Board of Lactation Consultant Examiners. They must be re-accredited every five years, sitting the examination itself every ten years. See the IBLCE website for more information.

suggests to me that the modelling effect of infant formula in some hospitals continues to be strong – and not fully appreciated by staff.

It has taken another twenty years, but even in formula's heartland, the USA, the practice of hospitals supplying free formula giveaways to new mothers is now being challenged, and perhaps declining.[1650] Public Citizen, a consumer organisation, has created a petition with over 18,000 signatures, demanding an end to such sampling.[1651] And in the US, once a movement starts, it can gain momentum relatively quickly. 'As of 2011, nearly half of about 2,600 hospitals in a survey by the Centers for Disease Control and Prevention had stopped giving formula samples to breast-feeding mothers, up from a quarter in 2007.'[1652] (The survey did not ask about distributing samples to non-nursing mothers, which means hospitals model and endorse formula products.)

Recently, twenty-four hospitals in Oklahoma agreed to a ban on such samples of formula and allied products,[1653] and Massachusetts became the second state, after Rhode Island, in which all hospitals halted free samples.[1654] In New York City, Mayor Michael R. Bloomberg started the 'Latch On NYC' campaign,[1655] urging hospitals to stop giveaways and monitor formula like other medical supplies, stored in locked cabinets and accounted for when mothers have medical needs or request it; twenty-eight of forty hospitals have agreed.[1656]

America has certainly taken the lead from Australia in relation to hospital practices, with national action to promote truly exclusive breastmilk feeding in US hospitals.[1657] On 30 November 2012, the Joint Commission (which accredits US hospitals) announced that a new Perinatal Care Core Measure set would become mandatory for all hospitals with 1100 or more births per year, effective 1 January 2014. One of the core measures is exclusive breastmilk feeding. The US Breastfeeding Coalition (USBC) toolkit, *Implementing the joint commission perinatal care core measure on exclusive breast milk feeding*[1658] covers this, and an article in the *Journal of Human Lactation*[1659] explores the implications. In any facility where

1650 Belluck P. Hospitals ditch formula samples to promote breastfeeding. *NY Times*, 15 October 2012

1651 http://action.citizen.org/p/dia/action/public/?action_KEY=10062

1652 US Department of Health and Human Services, Centers for Disease Control and Prevention. *CDC National Survey of Maternity Care Practices in Infant Nutrition and Care (mPINC)* 2009. Table 5.2a: Distribution of infant formula discharge packs by facility type, size, NICU level, and region. Retrieved 14 February 2012, from http://www.cdc.gov/breastfeeding/data/mpinc/data/2009/tables5_1a-5_2a.htm

1653 http://www.ok.gov/health/Organization/Office_of_Communications/News_Releases/2012_News_Releases/Hospitals_Encourage_Breastfeeding_by_Not_Giving_Formula_Bags.html

1654 http://www.bostonglobe.com/lifestyle/health-wellness/2012/07/12/all-massachusetts-maternity-hospitals-now-ban-infant-formula-gift-bags/6MociHyPZH76Un3EfNsIUO/story.html

1655 http://www.nyc.gov/html/doh/html/pr2012/pr013-12.shtml

1656 ibid.

1657 http://www.usbreastfeeding.org/HealthCare/HospitalMaternityCenterPractices/ToolkitImplementingTJCCoreMeasure/tabid/184/Default.aspx

1658 Go to the US Breastfeeding Committee website to download this. http://www.usbreastfeeding.org/HealthCare/HospitalMaternityCenterPractices/ToolkitImplementingTJCCoreMeasure/tabid/184/Default.aspx

1659 Feldman-Winter L, Douglass-Bright A, Bartick MC, Matranga J. The new mandate from the joint commission on the perinatal care core measure of exclusive breast milk feeding: implications for practice and implementation in the United States. (PMID: 23599268) *J Hum Lact* 2013; 29(3):291–5

exclusive breastfeeding is practised, the amount of formula used drops dramatically, and the cost of formula supply is not an issue.

Free supplies to healthcare facilities and samples to parents had been for almost five decades very cost-effective marketing strategies.[1660] Industry will adapt to their loss in affluent Anglophone countries. But some still object to the restriction. The International Formula Council does so on the interesting grounds that giving such samples is not a breach of the International Code of Marketing of Breastmilk Substitutes. Why? Because America has not made the Code into law so it can't be broken in America. If the report outlining their statement[1661] is accurate, they seem to be saying that an International Code does not exist unless America says it does. The Code says sampling is a forbidden practice. To give samples breaches the Code. Simple, really.

In affluent countries and communities I would expect to see more concentration on direct communication with parents via baby clubs and websites[1662] and other more immediate forms of contact such as apps, and also the direct or indirect subsidising of highly vocal formula advocates, women especially. The tactics outlined by Michaels[1663] have worked well for all industries that have employed them to date.

But in the developing markets of Asia and Africa and the Middle East it seems that free and low-cost supplies and samples and gift packs to mothers and even bribery of health professionals are continuing,[1664] even increasing, as the companies seek to cement relationships with healthcare facilities trusted by locals. Reports of bribes and free supplies come from countries where people are adopting that potent symbol of affluence and modernity, infant formula. A Reuters Special Report on China clearly indicates that this occurs there, despite a 1995 Chinese regulation "designed to ensure the impartiality of physicians and protect the health of newborns. It bars hospital personnel from promoting infant formula to the families of babies younger than six months, except in the rare cases when a woman has insufficient breast milk or cannot breastfeed for medical reasons." But the Report records violations by major companies.

> "Visitors to the maternity ward at Hangzhou Tianmushan Hospital in eastern China were greeted with banners from Mead Johnson that read: "Healthy babies, happy mothers" and "Give baby the best start in life!"

It must be a marketer's dream scenario, to have health authorities discouraging breastfeeding by giving out free formula. It worked well in the USA with hospitals and WIC, why wouldn't it influence people everywhere? That fact alone speaks volumes about the sincerity of any infant formula company's hand on heart avowal of their desire to support breastfeeding. So too does

---

1660  http://www.usbreastfeeding.org/NewsInfo/PositionStatements/tabid/227/Default.aspx
1661  Astley M. US hospital infant formula samples not a violation of the Code. http://www.dairyreporter.com/Manufacturers/US-hospital-formula-sample-giveaways-not-violation-of-WHO-Code
1662  The UK DH Guidance Notes referred to earlier cover these areas of marketing.
1663  Michaels D. Op cit.
1664  The International Code Documentation Centre (ICDC) based in Malaysia provides numerous examples of marketing practices ranging from outright bribery to price-fixing to gifts of formula to parents,...Go to http://www.ibfan-icdc.org/ and browse.

the apparent indifference and apathy of some health professionals and their associations to harms outside their national borders, or to indigenous groups within those borders.

I consider it vitally important for industry critics to be fair in their analysis, or they may simply change market shares, benefitting other companies and not affecting the overall market. Baby Milk Action, which serves as the secretariat for the UK Baby Feeding Law Group (BFLG), facilitated an UK coalition of groups concerned with infant feeding, and so created a body capable of commanding wide respect for an even-handed approach to law enforcement by all the formula companies, not just selected ones. The Baby Feeding Law Group website[1665] set out the International Code, the relevant UK law and regulations, encouraged reports on violations from those in the field, and published these and regular reports on company action; it was successful in getting the industry-funded Advertising Standards Authority to make judgements regarding breaches of UK law, regulations, and official guidance. However, there is  a need for national coalitions that go beyond legal concerns.

Most of the recent progress in the United States built on the work of many such groups and individuals over decades. But significant national change has accelerated with the formation in 2008 of the United States Breastfeeding Committee (USBC), a nationally representative coalition of many non-profit groups, which annually hosts a conference that draws together representatives of the state coalitions (most states now have such committees), tribal groups, and the more than 40 professional and consumer member groups, along with non-voting government agencies, under its umbrella of a comprehensive action plan.[1666] Without such a national advocacy body, US progress would be as it has been in other countries like Australia, piecemeal and easily subverted, dependent on key individuals and specific funding events, rather than making steady progress overall.

A smaller coalition had been created in Australia when after doing in-service education for their staff, I helped Greg Thompson of World Vision organise a meeting in Canberra in June 1990 from which ACOIF, the Australian Coalition for Optimal Infant Feeding emerged. Initially a loose coalition and later an incorporated association, ACOIF included World Vision, ALCA (the Australian Lactation Consultants' Association), NMAA/ABA,  ACA (Australian Consumers Association), Save the Children, Community Aid Abroad and other overseas aid groups, all urging the government both to implement the International Code and end free supplies of formula in healthcare facilities.[1667] This development came after the Health Department handed responsibility for the International Code to the Trades Practices Commission, or TPC. In 1989 the TPC had called a series of meetings and asked for input into Australia's implementation of the Code, as consumer criticism had continued unabated since the weak 1983 Code that the Health Department had created with industry.

The creation of Australia's Advisory Panel on the Marketing in Australia of Infant Formula (APMAIF), established in 1992, was largely the result of concerted action by ACOIF and

1665 http://www.babyfeedinglawgroup.org.uk
1666 http://www.usbreastfeeding.org/Portals/0/USBC-Strategic-Plan-2009-2013.pdf
1667 *ALCA News*, August 1990; 1: 11-16.

its member organisations and individuals. So too was the ending of free supplies of infant formula to health facilities, and sampling to parents, noted earlier. It helped enormously that the initial Chair of APMAIF was a committed and well-informed doctor with experience in developing countries, who appreciated the importance of breastfeeding to health. APMAIF was initially effective, providing illustrated reports of wrongdoing, and even getting the Health Minister to name a recalcitrant company in the Federal Parliament. (This was said to have infuriated the company, but brought a change in their marketing.) For a very few years, companies were being held to account and full details of the breaches published (belatedly) in APMAIF reports. All of which shows what even a limited coalition can achieve in a short time.

But Howard government industry-friendly changes to the Panel's composition in the mid 1990s were to mean that APMAIF evolved from its early public health advocacy role to being a shelter for industry from relevant consumer protection law. Meanwhile ACOIF was hampered by internal politicking, and in 1996 incorporated to create a more formal structure, trying to ensure that it could act despite persistent minority disagreement, and broaden an envisaged coalition of national organisations. As the Baby-Friendly Hospital Initiative took off in Australia,[1668] observance of the Code by hospitals became a part of its remit. Initially BFHI was envisaged and created as just such a wide-ranging national coalition, with ACOIF's most active members heavily involved with BFHI; so ACOIF was finally wound up in 2001.

But in fact since UNICEF Australia handed sole control of BFHI to the Australian College of Midwives, there has been no active Australian umbrella group concerned with infant feeding issues. One is sorely needed,[1669] as the 1991 Innocenti Declaration had made plain. Seeing the weekly Wednesday Wire from the US Breastfeeding Committee[1670] makes me wish Australian organisations could once again see the value of working together within an umbrella group, and commit some resources to developing one. But even the most effective advocacy groups can be subverted by individuals and organisations pushing personal agendas: as the saying goes, 'Self-interest makes fools of us all.'[1671]

Breastfeeding had stayed on the Australian political agenda largely thanks to the passion of the Australian Breastfeeding Association and lactation consultants, now organised in the trans-Tasman group LCANZ (Lactation Consultants of Australia and New Zealand.) Under the Rudd/Gillard Labour government, whose Health Minister Nicola Roxon was strongly supportive, a national breastfeeding strategic plan[1672] was drafted in 2009. However, this largely recognised what was being done, provided some support for existing groups, but

---

1668  In February 1992, I brought the Global BFHI documents back from Nigeria where I had led the pilot
assessment of hospitals for UNICEF NY. BFHI is now owned and managed by the Australian College of
Midwives. This has been chronicled in *Breastfeeding Matters*.

1669  An outline history of ACOIF, BFHI and ALCA to 1998 is covered in *Breastfeeding Matters*; further changes
to BFHI are outlined in a monograph *From Collaboration to Control: BFHI in Australia 1991-2001* - lodged in
Australian libraries of record in Canberra and Melbourne and the ABA Lactation Resource Centre.

1670  To subscribe to the Weekly Wednesday Wire, go to http://org2.salsalabs.com/o/5162/signup_page/sign-up

1671  There is more about this in the 1998 edition of *Breastfeeding matters*, and it would be a good subject for a
doctoral thesis. I would be happy to provide all the contemporary documentation to a serious scholar.

1672  http://www.health.gov.au/internet/main/publishing.nsf/
Content/6FD59347DD67ED8FCA257BF0001CFD1E/$File/Breastfeeding_strat1015.pdf

did not result in a truly national working coalition such as the USBC to continue the work. Government relies on on handpicked groups of academics, sporadically consulted. In Australia in 2013-2014 there seemed to be some signs of a revival of interest in political action, sparked inter alia by the writing of a key economic researcher Dr. Julie Smith. She and her co-author summarise how the Code issues have developed to the present:

> In 2007, the Commonwealth Parliament House of Representatives Standing Committee on Health and Ageing considered evidence on the effects of commercial marketing on breastfeeding decisions. Its Best Start report concluded that full implementation of the World Health Organization International Code of Marketing of Breast-milkSubstitutes (WHO Code) was needed to increase breastfeeding to adequate levels in Australia (Recommendation 22). However, the National Breastfeeding Strategy agreed by Australian Health Ministers in November 2010 stated that breastfeeding protection including restrictions on marketing of infant formula was one of several "complex issues that do not lend themselves to immediate solutions" (p. 24). In late 2011, the federal Department of Health and Ageing commissioned a study on the implementation of the WHO Code in Australia including the effectiveness of the MAIF Agreement in achieving its aims. In July 2013, the consultant's report was released. It recommended no change to the voluntary industry self-regulatory model, no change to the scope of the MAIF, and no extension of MAIF to formulas marketed for toddlers. Instead the report recommended 'consideration' of restricting labelling of toddler milk drinks so consumers could distinguish these from infant formula, but this was ruled out by the Department in releasing the report. That is, five years on, no significant action has been taken, nor now seems likely to be taken, to implement the 2007 recommendation of the Australian Parliamentary Committee that the WHO Code be fully implemented in Australia. [1673]

Seven years ago now. Australia really should tackle this "complex issue" which theoretically Australia has been committed to since the 1980s. Paradoxically, it may even be helpful that our new prime minister has just abolished APMAIF as unnecessary. That could be a Good Thing. APMAIF had become a toothless tiger (perhaps a tamed pussycat would be more accurate), which had no power to ensure industry compliance. Some companies are allowed to market in Australia products within the scope of the International Code without even a notional commitment to abide by the Industry Agreement, the Australian Government's mechanism for implementing the Code. Now APMAIF has gone, the infant formula industry, without the protection of any special body, should now be held accountable under the overarching provisions of Australia's Competition and Consumer Act 2010 (formerly the Trades Practices Act 1974), which prohibits and punishes false and misleading advertising and deceptive conduct, and can impose penalties of millions of dollars. APMAIF had no such powers, and relied on naming and shaming, in a process that could be endlessly delayed by industry. And previously the ACCC (Australian Competition and Consumer Commission) had simply referred on to APMAIF any complaints they received about the infant formula industry. Very little happened. Complacency reigns supreme. However, given the nature of the current Abbott government, it is probably more likely that the ACCC will lose its powers than extend them to deal with infant formula

---

1673  Smith J, Blake M. Infant food marketing strategies undermine effective regulation of breast-milk substitutes: trends in print advertising in Australia, 1950–2010. *ANZ J Publ Hlth* 2013; 37(4):337–44

marketing. And that industry will be allowed to revert to self-regulation without sanctions: in 2014 those covertly considering this issue failed to consult even those with longstanding track record of engagement, such as former APMAIF and ACOIF chairs and consumer representatives.

By contrast, it seems to me, as an outsider looking in, that the United States of America is beginning to take breastfeeding seriously as a public health issue, and might soon leave Australia in its wake. The US CDC has been empowered to collect relevant data, and since 2007 CDC has been publishing annual *Breastfeeding Report Cards* for the nation. In their first report, they said:

> One goal of the Centers for Disease Control and Prevention (CDC) is to improve the health of mothers and their children. One way to reach this goal is to encourage breast-feeding, which has many benefits for infants and children. People from all walks of life play a part in reaching this goal. When health care professionals, legislators, employers, business owners, and community and family members work together, their efforts can increase the number of women who breastfeed their babies and the number of months that they breastfeed them. The *Breastfeeding Report Card — United States, 2007* is an important tool for spotting ways to increase breastfeeding nationwide. It gives states information on how breastfeeding is being promoted within a given state. It also makes it possible to compare states* across the country.[1674]

Nothing like this exists in Australia, though sporadic data collection has occurred. CDC went on to talk about the importance of every US state working in a dedicated and co-ordinated way to protect, promote and support breastfeeding.

- State agencies responsible for public health and welfare of women and children include the state health department, WIC program, and Early Intervention program. They help ensure that breastfeeding is included in public programs and services that affect women and infants. FTEs [*that's fulltime equivalent staff*] dedicated to the protection, promotion, and support of breastfeeding are needed to develop and implement breastfeeding interventions.

- A statewide coalition dedicated to breastfeeding represents a basic level of community support for breastfeeding. State breastfeeding coalitions differ between states in terms of what they do and how they do it. What they have in common is an understanding of the need for community members who can be agents of change locally. The coalition members make the case to their community for the importance of breastfeeding.

- State coalitions with a Web site have an effective way to communicate. On their Web site, they can share information with existing coalition members and also recruit new members interested in the issues related to breastfeeding. Coalition Web sites are also an excellent way to reach community members who want quality breastfeeding information and online support.[1675]

---

1674 Read the 2007 Report Card and the basis for it at the website: http://www.cdc.gov/breastfeeding/data/reportcard/reportcard2007.htm
1675 http://www.cdc.gov/breastfeeding/data/reportcard.htm

The strength of the US movement to promote breastfeeding is that it is supported at the highest levels. Michelle Obama has made better US nutrition her crusade, and as a former breastfeeding mother, is not afraid of including breastfeeding as part of that agenda. (Perhaps Margie Abbott might like to take a leaf from her book.) The White House TaskForce on the Prevention of Childhood Obesity promotes breastfeeding as a preventive factor.[1676]

I hope I am right in sensing some momentum shift in US infant feeding policy and practice, and a significant increase in awareness of harms. America's can-do spirit can make real change happen quickly. I hope too that in this instance, America might begin to take a lead globally in an attempt to undo some of the collateral damage it has caused world-wide. American politicians like Senators Edward Kennedy and Al Gore Jnr. were important in getting the issue into the world arena. Where is the new American champion of infants? This is the very bedrock of health.

Concerted and strong political advocacy and action is needed everywhere, despite understandable concerns about this upsetting bottle-feeding parents. (SIDS prevention campaigns surely upset parents whose babies died, but they are still necessary.) The formula industry's long-standing and close links with, and funding of, health professional groups has helped to shield infant formula from intelligent scrutiny. I hope that the sleeping giants of paediatrics and obstetrics are finally waking to their overlooked responsibilities, being encouraged by statements like the following from Professors Charlotte Wright and Tony Waterston:

> If breastfeeding, with all its benefits, is to be established as a majority activity, we paediatricians must learn to recognise the elaborate web woven around us by formula manufacturers, which currently ensures our goodwill and support for a product that we may acknowledge, but would mostly not wish to actively promote. Fifty years ago nearly everyone, including doctors, smoked and it was perceived to be a necessary and inescapable part of our culture. Now it is unimaginable that we would smoke in front of our patients or accept gifts from cigarette manufacturers. It is time for a similar shift to take place with respect to formula milk. Just because many mothers currently choose to bottle feed their infants and a tiny number of infants cannot be breast fed, it does not mean we should be seen to be endorsing *a product that causes net damage to the health of children.* The time has come for paediatricians to recognise the influence of IFMCs, shake off their silken chains, and become truly uncompromised advocates for breast feeding and against the hazards of formula milk.[1677]

World obstetric authorities need to acknowledge how their practices undermine breastfeeding. No man, within a few days of major abdominal surgery, and while still on analgesics and antibiotics, would take on a stressful new job that involved repeated heavy lifting and carrying. Unnecessary caesareans impose that reality on far too many women. Keeping mothers and babies drug-free and in skin-to-skin contact from the moment of birth can make a huge difference both to breastfeeding success and to infant microbiomes.

---

1676 http://www.whitehouse.gov/the-press-office/childhood-obesity-task-force-unveils-action-plan-solving-problem-childhood-obesity-

1677 Wright CM, Waterston AJR. Relationships between paediatricians and infant formula milk companies. *Arch Dis Child* 2006. 91383–385.385

Obstetricians need to examine their consciences – and make changes - wherever they do not both encourage and facilitate natural birthing, family-centered postpartum care, and exclusive breastfeeding. They also need to pay attention to studies evaluating the outcomes of inoculating the surgically-born infant with vaginal flora via gauze swabs.[1678] It would be wise for them to do so. As Blaser says,

> One day the parents of a child who has developed a problem attributed to an elective C-section – maybe obesity or juvenile diabetes or autism – will sue the doctor and hospital for malpractice. Currently the fear of being sued is for *not* doing something….Soon there will be the fear of getting sued because of unnecessary and unjustified actions."[1679]

Breastfeeding advocates are not attacking formula-feeding parents when they condemn industry  marketing practices. They are acting as advocates for all parents and infants: preventing industry from marketing its products unethically is most important to those parents who decide to formula-feed. Only when the truth about industry products is freely available can parents make choices based on what seems to them to be the most suitable and least harmful of those available in any country. And in the post 1980s Greed is Good world, industry cannot be trusted to sacrifice profit on the altar of full disclosure. (Not that it ever could be.)

## Targeted marketing: formulas for supplementation of breastfed babies

So in the USA breastfeeding is strongly supported by the White House, and data collection routinely collected by the CDC. This probably helps explain the emergence of so much recent industry advertising aimed at positioning the use of infant formula as a way to continue breastfeeding. (Truly, the Abbott website said  that 8 out of  10 mothers agreed that feeding their babies Similac helped them to breastfeed longer.[1680])  It seems to be American companies which have pioneered this recent revival of the older "formula for supplementation" strategy that had existed for a century before Mead Johnson used those images of Mrs Rabbit bottle feeding a baby rabbit while Peter stood by her side with a sippy cup.  Is it proof of the companies' deep desire to promote breastfeeding? Perhaps. It *is* the best way to ensure that real differences between breastfed and formula-fed children are blurred in research findings, now that more subtle tools like MRIs and immune investigations are uncovering physical biological differences between the groups.

I can also see the PR value of companies marketing an infant formula for breastfeeding mothers to use to supplement. The formula is just another infant formula, but the marketing positions the company as Good Guys wanting to support and help 'moms who choose to supplement' now that the healthcare professions are seeing breastfeeding as important. Yet industry must know that supplementing undermines milk production. So how do they sell this 'new' 'helpful' formula?

---

1678 Blaser MJ op cit., p. 208.
1679 Ibid, p. 209.
1680 https://similac.com/baby-formula/similac-for-supplementation. Source: Abbott Nutrition, data on file 2013

Using Abbott as an example makes it clear. Their website says:

> "Similac For Supplementation is the first Similac formula designed for breastfeeding moms who choose to supplement. It has more prebiotics than any other Similac formula, along with the same benefits as Similac Advance. Some moms may notice changes in stool patterns when introducing formula to a breastfeeding routine, and studies have shown that prebiotics produce softer stools more like those of breastfed infants. 8 out of 10 moms who supplemented with formula agreed it helped them continue to breastfeed."[1681]

This is really a bit odd. All breastfeeding mothers – other than those who are blind, have no sense of smell, and who employ nannies to deal with nappy changes - will notice stool changes when formula is introduced. The nappies stink, where before they did not. But why *more prebiotics* than in their regular formula? To compete with breastmilk prebiotics and probiotics? To make more work for the infant digestive system? To overload the normal quota of digestive enzymes supplied by both breastmilk and the baby's body?

When there is precious little evidence that the prebiotic doses in formula offer any real benefit to healthy term babies, why do this? To justify increased costs? To subtly imply that breastmilk lacks their super-duper prebiotics and probiotics and so mothers *should* supplement, as a matter of 'nutritional insurance', one of the phrases industry popularised in relation to Toddler formulas. Surely Abbott could have created a formula *without any added biotics* for a breastfed baby, unless there will be almost no breastmilk going into the child? And double the dose for the formula fed? While baby is getting breastmilk there is absolutely no need to worry about adding bacteria and food for bacteria because breastmilk does a better job than industry can ever do in that regard.

But industry will invent new ways to coax naïve healthworkers to use their influence with parents to promote a particular brand. Abbott, like its rivals, knows perfectly well that breastfeeding is a far better strategy for gut health, and that breastfeeding is now formula's chief competitor, no longer evaporated milk or whole cows milk. Eliminating the use of the latter products was industry's 1960s rationale to justify advertising infant formula to parents, even though by the mid 1960s there was almost no such products in use and by 1970 they were gone. It's interesting that fifty years later, as breastfeeding initiation rates rise, Abbott chooses to create a product that, if used, will decrease the duration of breastfeeding and increase the risks of infant feeding for mother and child alike, making breastfed babies more like formula-fed ones. Mixed feeding is the way to maximise industry profits and minimise industry risks.

Look a little closer too, at some subliminal PR messages I hear in this short statement.

- Mothers *"choose to supplement."* (Not are forced to by social structures and expectations such as those Abbott creates; choice is an act of adult self-determination, and sensible women like our "StrongMoms"[1682] choose to mix breast and bottle feeding.)

- Mothers will give their child *"the benefits of Similac"* if they supplement with this formula. (Infant formula only has benefits, never risks, and only the meanest of mothers refuse to *benefit* their child.)

- Introduce formula into your breastfeeding *routine*. (Routines are normal, and determined by mothers, who vary them as they choose. Mothers who feed responsively and fully are abnormal; babies are a management problem, not persons in a relationship.)

- Prebiotics produce *softer* stools (Gentle, caring, "comfort" formula makes *softer* stools for babies.... Does that word mean looser, runnier, sloppier, more liquid, than breastmilk stools? This emotive language is appealing, and indeed sometimes accurate: the stools of diarrhoea, more common in formula-fed and allergic infants, are soft - but hardly desirable.)

- *More* probiotics than for formula-fed babies. (Why? Does this imply breastfed babies need ingredients to soften their stools? In fact constipation is relatively common in *formula-fed* babies.)

- Supplementing helps mothers breastfeed *longer*. (Breastfeeding duration is more important than ensuring *complete* breastfeeding to around 6 months and *continued* breastfeeding while introducing other foods. After all, just one breastfeed a day means mothers may be classed as breastfeeding in some research. )

Reading on in this website is instructive as to the likely outcomes of using Similac for supplementation. Abott advises that mothers who breastfeed directly have no way to measure what their babies get (more undermining), and suggests that mothers

> Try to feed 2 ounces of baby formula at a time to see how much your baby will eat. You might discover at first that your baby will eat more or less than that amount every two to three hours. As your baby gets older, he might be able to eat more in one feeding, and eat less frequently.

Helpfully, they add that formula is available in premeasured 2-ounce bottles that do not require any mixing. (After all, they are targeting the advantaged breastfeeding mother, who can afford ready-to-feed types.) Nowhere do they say that if you feed your baby 60mL of formula every 2-3 hours, your milk supply will rapidly dwindle by as much as 60mL every 2-3 hours.

The website continues with other advice. If your baby does refuse the breast, try feeding him when he is sleepy. (Which may ensure he falls asleep after his 60-90mL of formula, without breastfeeding well. Babies fed by bottle may refuse the breast if not hungry, a fact nowhere mentioned.) And when milk supply does fall, they recommend pumping to boost supply, not cutting back on formula intake. So now the new mother is breastfeeding,

---

1682 The title of the online club Abbott has set up for mothers. Women don't need industry to tell them they are strong. And it seems to me a cynical attempt to play on mothers' insecurities.

pumping *and* bottle-feeding, a huge time burden. Guess what happens next? The incentive just to use the 'gentle' powder is likely to be considerable.

Other companies are pushing formula for supplementation of the breastfeeding infant, even though the World Health Organization and every credible paediatric authority is urging exclusive breastfeeding from birth on the basis of good science.

This is targeted advertising at its canniest. Marketing budgets can be bigger than research and development budgets, which says much about priorities and the purpose of this industry. Unless countries like China and Vietnam and India take drastic steps now to curb the growth of artificial feeding, they will repeat the disasters of the twentieth century in the twenty-first, just as affluent nations are beginning to count the multiple and intolerable costs. It is probably already too late to do more than reduce the scale of the disasters they face, if the Chinese State Television (CCTV) report saying that 70% of Chinese children receive infant formula is correct.[1683] Certainly breastfeeding has dwindled in this last decade:

> Government surveys show a low breastfeeding rate - just 28 percent of Chinese women were exclusively breastfeeding at six months as of 2008, down from 51 percent in 2003. Independent researchers suggest the real figure is much lower. One study published in the *Journal of Health, Population and Nutrition* in 2010 found exclusive breastfeeding rates at six months in parts of China were as low as 0.2 percent.)[1684]

Infant formula's damage is not confined to obvious disease. As an eminent researcher into the roots of violence in society has said, infant formula

> may be the single worst invention of the twentieth century, as it deprives the infant/child of not only essential physical nutrients but also the essential sensory-emotional nutrients that can only be obtained at the breast of the mother -touch, movement, smell and taste of the mother's body – that forms the foundation for intimacy, pleasure and love of mother and of women throughout adulthood.[1685]

It is not a coincidence that rates of maternal abuse and neglect are higher when infants are not happily breastfed.[1686] How much of the worst aspects of western culture has its roots in the loss of such intangibles, and the unbreakable bonds they create? Does the developing world really want to duplicate western attachment disorders and their cultural consequences? Surely we must emphasize to women who cannot breastfeed –for whatever reason - the need for frequent and deeply intimate physical contact, for their own sake as well as their baby's?

---

1683 Cited in ICDC Public Statement on Danone/Dumex Bribery scandal. http://www.ibfan-icdc.org/index.php/alerts/2013-12-18-10-44-32

1684 Harney A. op cit.

1685 Prescott JW. Nurturant versus non-nurturant environments and the failure of the environment of evolutionary adaptedeness. In Narvaez D, Panksepp J, Score AN, Gleason TR (eds) *Evolution, early experience and human development* (Oxford University Press, 2013) p. 427

1686 Strathearn L, Mamun AA, Najman JM, O'Callaghan MJ. Does breastfeeding protect against substantiated child abuse and neglect? A 15-year cohort study.(PMID:19171613) Free full text article *Pediatrics* 2009;123(2):483-493. DOI: 10.1542/peds.2007-3546 Read the rest of this corpus of work.

For there are things we cannot measure about the value of breastfeeding. Bottle feeding mothers love their babies no less than breastfeeding mothers –how can anyone measure love? – but I do think that breastfeeding creates a unique learning environment that helps women adjust to motherhood. Yes, the hormones help, and all those other physical differences. But as Marni Jackson said:

> Breastfeeding is an unsentimental metaphor for how love works, in a way. You don't decide how much or how deeply to love – you respond to the beloved with joy exactly as much as they want. In all our efforts to demystify motherhood and free women from their identification with the life-force, we risk overlooking the amazing integrity of the female body and its power. Breastfeeding is above all a relationship.[1687]

All infant feeding should be made the basis for such a relationship and responsive parenting style, instead of a competition to push independence on the child. Dr Pamela Douglas has written a wonderful description [1688] of how to bottle feed carefully and responsively, a process which demands at least as much as time and attention, and often much more than, breastfeeding.

Of course the ad men recognise that infant feeding is deeply emotional. Providing food is an expression of love, whether that food is breastmilk or an expensive substitute. Women who love their babies feed them; food is love made tangible, and so for some, the more expensive the food the greater the proof of love. Industry exploits this. How else can we explain the proliferation of heart shapes and love images and doting mothers in formula logos and marketing? It may be that the mother's love helps the bottle fed child ovecome the deficiencies of its artificial feed, for love does indeed help babies grow.

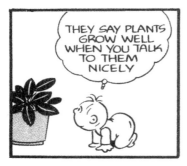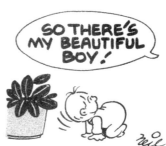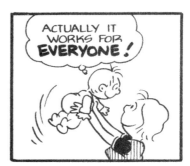

Figure 3-13-4 Love makes babies grow. Image © Neil Matterson.
From *Sleepless Nights*. (Marion Books 1988).

---

1687 Marni Jackson. *The Mother Zone: love sex and laundry in the modern family* ( Henry Holt 1992)
1688 Douglas P. *The discontented little baby book.* (Uni of Queensland Press 2014)

# 3.14 Genetic engineering and infant formula: inevitable?

Infant formula production and marketing faces many challenges. One major issue is ensuring a cheap reliable supply of the ingredients for its products. Naturally grown food is expensive, and often transport costs are prohibitive, while volume of supply can be uncertain. The growing demand for infant formula risks impoverishing the world and damaging the environment on a scale never before seen. Industry growth has been phenomenal as globalisation brings infant formula to communities that once routinely breastfed. To date many people have been reluctant, sometimes irrationally so, to eat what they know to be genetically-modified (GM) or genetically-engineered (GE) food. But with infant formula the use of such foodstuffs seems to me unavoidable.

## Genetically engineered ingredients

GE (genetically engineered) oilseed crops will inevitably find their way into formula, where they have not already. Many current infant formula fat blends contain oils from other genetically modified (GM) oil crops such as corn and soy, and very few formulas are made from certified organic ingredients. Industrial-scale Western agriculture is now so dependent on both genetic engineering and synthetic chemical use, including pesticides, that a completely non-GM organic formula, in which all ingredients are sourced and verified as such, would be prohibitively expensive. It would probably be impractical on the scale that big manufacturers produce infant formula.

In fact in May 2011, formula manufacturers admitted they cannot guarantee their products are completely GM free, although they had 'chosen not to source GM ingredients for infant formulas, and used third-party certifiers to trace ingredients from seed to product.'[1689]

While one company did claim on its website that

> We follow a strict policy of using only non-genetically modified (GMO) ingredients in our infant formulas. All suppliers of soy or maize-based ingredients provide either identity-preserved certification or polymerase chain reaction (PCR) testing that is conducted independently and renewed on a biennial basis, to meet regulatory requirements.[1690]

in their submission to the Australian Senate inquiry into GM labelling of foods, the Infant Formula Council says that

1689 Infant Nutrition Council Submission 11 February 2011. Senate Community Affairs Committee Inquiry into the Food Standards Amendment (Truth in Labelling – Genetically Modified Material) Bill 2010 Go to https://senate.aph.gov.au/submissions/comittees/viewdocument.aspx?..and look for the Infant Nutrition Coucnil submission, a document labelled *in response gm material bill 2011.pdf* For an overbiew of the Australian situaiton see http://www.daff.gov.au/__data/assets/pdf_file/0020/2132354/Doc_25.pdf ?
1690 Australia: Wyeth Nutrition dismisses GMO baby formula claims 28 September 2010. Since Wyeth has been sold by Pfizer, this disclaimer is no longer on the Pfizer website. It can be read at www.flex-news-food.com/console/PageViewer.aspx?page=32453

Globally, regulators and health authorities, however, acknowledge that products grown without genetic modification, such as soy or maize, may unintentionally contain traces of genetically modified organisms. This may be due to cross-pollination during cultivation, harvesting, storage, transport or processing despite all rigorous processes that farmers and ingredient suppliers put into place.[1691]

The manufacturers told the inquiry that GM tests of a soy-based infant formula by two laboratories[1692] gave conflicting results 'due to the limitations of the analytical method', and claimed that it was 'due to these limitations that a "zero" threshold is unrealistic and unworkable'.[1693]

## Genetic engineering of new ingredients

Having discovered over a century of experimentation and rising allergy rates that foreign proteins fed to infants can cause health and growth problems, scientists are now trying to produce human proteins for use in infant formula, using recombinant gene technology. What is the stated justification for using gene technology in developing human proteins to add to infant formula?

> Human milk provides proteins that benefit newborn infants. They not only provide amino acids, but also facilitate the absorption of nutrients, stimulate growth and development of the intestine, modulate immune function, and aid in the digestion of other nutrients. Breastfed infants have a lower prevalence of infections than formula-fed infants. Since many women in industrialized countries choose not to breastfeed, and an increasing proportion of women in developing countries are advised not to breastfeed because of the risk of HIV transmission, incorporation of recombinant human milk proteins into infant foods is likely to be beneficial.[1694]

Well, that statement is now badly out of date about the latest HIV advice (see page 452), and maternal 'choice' is a dubious concept when there are no workable alternatives and mothers know too little about what they are 'choosing'. A more recent article by the same author outlines the implications of breastmilk's bioactive proteins for infant formula composition.[1695] This really boils down to saying 'babies should get breastmilk because of its unique factors, but won't; and as a well-paid researcher I believe that adding genetically engineered human proteins to our current mixtures will be beneficial.' Will it?

Will a few novel manufactured bioactive ingredients bearing traces of their production media work just like the hundreds of interactive proteins in breastmilk's complex mixture,

---

1691 ibid.

1692 http://www.foodstandards.gov.au/scienceandeducation/monitoringandsurveillance/foodsurveillance/surveyofgminsoybased5068.cfm

1693 Bita N. No guarantee formula GM-free *The Australian*, 2 May 2011. http://www.theaustralian.com.au/news/nation/no-guarantee-formula-gm-free/story-e6frg6nf-1226048014303

1694 Lönnerdal B. Recombinant human milk proteins in Rigo J, Ziegler EE. *Protein and energy requirements in infancy and childhood* (Nestlé Nutrition Workshop Series Pediatr Program, vol. 58, pp. 207–17, published online and by Nestec Ltd., Vevey/S. Karger AG, Basel, © 2006. DOI: 10.1159/000095064

1695 Lönnerdal B. Infant formula and infant nutrition: bioactive proteins of human milk and implications for composition of infant formulas. (PMID:24452231) *Am J Clin Nutr* 2014, 99(3):712s-7s DOI: 10.3945/ajcn.113.071993

- in differently-designed formulas
- with other animal/vegetable proteins
- and different fat and carbohydrate mixtures
- in formula-fed babies' different bodies
- despite formula-fed babies' different microbiomes?

Frankly, that all seems extremely unlikely. In the end, benefit or harm can only be proved or disproved by experimenting on thousands of infants, as the scientists well understand. To date their attempts have not produced a great deal of proven benefit to babies. But they have dramatically increased the cost of formula and, worldwide, it is predominantly poor families who bear that burden, along with taxpayers in some countries. And it is poor families who will be forced either to use cheaper alternatives, or to skimp on other necessities.

## Animals as manufacturing sites

As parents realise that the bioactive factors in breastmilk are indeed important, finding ways to supply such factors in infant formula is the only way industry can keep claiming to be closer than ever to breastmilk. For marketing purposes, only small quantities are needed for each can, but it takes a great deal to put even a little in billions of cans. Early experiments focussed on trying to get other mammals to produce human proteins in their milk. That raises many questions. Is the production process itself ethical? If using animals such as cows, what are the side effects for the animals?

> In a certain number of cases, the recombinant proteins produced in [bovine] milk have deleterious effects on the mammary gland function or in the animals themselves. This comes independently from ectopic expression of the transgenes and from the transfer of the recombinant proteins from milk to blood.[1696]

In short, the animal's immune system reacts to the foreign proteins, as you might expect, generating damaging inflammation. How much pain and suffering does this cause? Any human mother who has had mastitis would know that the cow suffers! And if mastitis is caused, what antibiotics will be used to treat it? Sulfamethazine has been found in US milk.[1697] Can this suffering be justified?

How will this unwanted damage to expensive animals be dealt with?

> One possibility to eliminate or reduce these side-effects may be to use systems inducible by an exogenous molecule such as tetracycline, allowing the transgene to be expressed only during lactation and strictly in the mammary gland.[1698]

Am I reading this right? That seems to be saying that the new chemical will be produced only during lactation and only in the udder, when tetracycline is administered. For the whole duration of lactation? What dose of this powerful antibiotic is envisaged, how is

---

1696 Houdebine LM. Transgenic animal bioreactors. (PMID: 11131009) *Transgenic Res* 2000; 9(4–5):305–20
1697 *Food Chemical News* May 2 1988, p. 2
1698 ibid.

it delivered, do residues persist? What could that mean for bacterial drug resistance or adverse effects on the microbiome of the recipient child? Is this something that will affect other drug interactions? In the cow or the consumer? What does the future hold? Will it be the rosy prospect researchers with a vested interest outline?

> The available techniques to produce pharmaceutical proteins in milk can be used as well to optimize milk composition of farm animals, to add nutriceuticals in milk and potentially to reduce or even eliminate some mammary infectious diseases.[1699]

Wait a minute. To eliminate udder infectious diseases? Does that mean that the tetracycline used as a marker will be present in the udder (and so the milk) in sufficient quantity to be activly antibiotic for the months of lactation?

If so, trace amounts will transfer with the 'pharmaceutical protein' and affect infant gut immune function.

If fed with substances that act as adjuvants, like vaccines, will those traces create hypersensitivity and lead to allergic reactions, when the drugs are prescribed to fight infection?

Will they accelerate disease resistance and create new super-pathogens?

Enthusiasm for exchanging mammalian proteins has declined in the wake of transplant-related infections, Mad Cow Disease, and the possibility of transferring undetectable threats like viruses and prions – the agents for the devastating Creutzfeldt-Jacob disease. Notice the weasel word 'may' when a scientist writes:

> Among the biological contaminants potentially present in the recombinant proteins prepared from transgenic animals, prions are certainly those raising the major concern. The selection of animals chosen to generate transgenics on one hand and the elimination of the potentially contaminated animals, thanks to recently defined quite sensitive tests may reduce the risk to an extremely low level.[1700]

This scientist knows the risk cannot be eliminated totally. How very reassuring, when we are dealing with infectious agents that may not cause overt disease for years or even decades, and other disease agents not yet discovered perhaps. There have always been people who decide that profit to them outweighs risk to others, even infants. How else can we explain marketing that knowingly undermines breastfeeding?

Animal biofactories might also contribute viruses, as early vaccines did. Once, no one thought viruses could transfer between species as readily as they now are known to do. Their capacity to mutate, develop resistance, and increase in virulence is increasingly well documented. It has happened in chicken guts, and killed flocks.[1701] Will it happen in infant

---

1699  Houbedine et al., ibid.
1700  ibid.
1701  Kupferschmidt K. Chicken vaccines combine to produce deadly virus. *Science Now*. 12 July 2012. http://news.
       sciencemag.org/sciencenow/2012/07/chicken-vaccines-combine-to-prod.html

guts? We have no way of knowing ahead of it happening, just as chicken farmers never knew before their flock sickened. Reliably bioactive milk from the daughters of Hermann the genetically engineered bull seems to me like, well, a whole lotta bull, to use an apt Australianism. Mammals are risky biofactories.

They are also expensive ones. The logical alternative is industrially produced ingredients made by cheap and prolific life forms. As noted earlier, genetically modified fungi and algae are currently producing the omega-3 oils previously lacking in infant formula. And an enzyme from genetically modified fungus, Candida antarctica, will remodel hazelnut oil for that purpose. Yum, I can't wait to try it. Naturally that enzyme won't have any trace of its parent fungus, and that Candida won't have anything in common with other Candida species that have recently emerged as important causes of septicaemia showing high resistance to anti-fungal treatments – or they wouldn't be doing this, would they?

## Finding a lactoferrin factory

Gene technology can transform not only animals, but plants, bacteria, eggs, and much more into 'bioreactors', mini factories for making large quantities of commercially valuable additives quite cheaply. To take one example: lactoferrin (a metal-transporting protein found in breastmilk, mentioned earlier) is absent from infant formula. This is yet another way in which the protein of infant formula is and always has been deficient (i.e., not the same as protein in breastmilk) and this could have been discussed in Chapter 3.6, Basic Ingredients: Protein and its problems. However, with specific proteins needing to be industrially manufactured to exist on a commercial scale, it makes sense to discuss this here, in relation to genetic engineering.

Lactoferrin (a metal-binding protein; see page 360) and other breastmilk transfer factors had been the research focus of 1970s infant formula manufacturers, driven by increased awareness of the poor bioavailability of nutrients in formula. Bovine lactoferrin extracted from cows' milk was added to some experimental UK formula, but this did not get scaled up to commercial levels. I was told at the time by a senior lactoferrin researcher that bovine lactoferrin in formula might well take up available minerals, but then not release them to infant body receptors for use,[1702] depriving the infant of minerals, rather than increasing their bioavailability. Subtle differences in receptor sites could make a difference to infant uptake.

Research has continued ever since, as a PubMed search for lactoferrin and infant formula will quickly reveal. In a Nestlé Nutrition webinar[1703] it is stated that bovine lactoferrin added to infant formula did not improve iron status, although another study seems to suggest that

---

1702  Discussion with Dr Sylvia Rumball in New Zealand, 1987
1703  Hernell O. *Human milk versus cow's milk and the evolution of infant formula* Presented at: 67th Nestlé Nutrition Institute Workshop, Marrakech. Accessed 3 December 2012. In this video Hernell ends with a caution that any change to infant formula can result in unexpected and very negative outcomes. http://www.nestlenutrition-institute.org/resources/online-conferences/Pages/OnlineConferences.aspx

in a preterm infant population it reduced the incidence of severe infection, or sepsis[1704] (perhaps because less formula iron was available to the gut bacteria now known to cause sepsis[1705]?) Overall, trials of bovine lactoferrin in formula have shown no clear health benefit and some companies are moving away from using bovine lactoferrin to trying recombinant human lactoferrin. It seems that alien proteins don't work in babies the way human ones do. But will even human lactoferrin work the same way in infant formula, a very different mix?

Any lactoferrin in infant formula may, or may not, be a useful addition in nutrition terms. It will certainly be useful in marketing terms, as every new additive generates new profit possibilities. Bovine lactoferrin powder is being trialled in other forms for older children with diarrhoea, with some apparent success, and as the price is now around $1000 per ton, cows' milk factories are working to produce ever larger quantities.[1706] If the addition to infant formula goes ahead, expect to hear much about the fact that lactoferrin is important in breastmilk, and little about either its bovine beginnings or, if a human analogue, any genetic engineering or biofactory producing it.

There is however, another good commercial reason to add lactoferrin to infant formula. The oxidation of fats –especially those newly–added less-saturated fats- in infant formula itself  is increased by the presence of iron and copper. Lactoferrin in the formula might reduce the risk of rancidity and extend shelf-life.[1707] But perhaps it might also mean too little unbound iron left for the baby by the ned of thecan's shelf-life?

Work continues on how to secure a reliable supply of lactoferrin and other potential additives on a commercial scale, and in novel forms able to be patented. Recombinant technology allows ownership of these human-plant proteins, while the use of natural proteins may not. Some companies are said to be trying to create human lactoferrin (and lysozyme) in rice, for use as an alternative to antibiotics in poultry diets. Again, this uncontrolled industrial search for profit may have unconsidered side effects: if the chickens eat human proteins, then allergic pregnant humans eat the chickens or their eggs, is there any chance that intolerance to the human protein may be created in mother or baby? If no labelling law demands that animals eating GM-sourced food be identified, will those pregnant women need to avoid all egg protein, as now many avoid milk protein, for the sake of the baby? Whose responsibility is it to monitor industry's efforts to make novel products that may have a harmful effect on human health? Is there an independent Taskforce looking at these concerns?

1704 Manzoni P, Rinaldi M, Cattani S, Pugni L, et al. Bovine lactoferrin supplementation for prevention of late-onset sepsis in very low-birth-weight neonates: a randomized trial. (PMID: 19809023) *JAMA* 2009, 302(13):1421–8.

1705 Carl MA, Ndao IM, Springman AC, Manning SD et al. Sepsis From the Gut: The Enteric Habitat of Bacteria That Cause Late-Onset Neonatal Bloodstream Infections. (PMID:24647013) *Clin Infect Dis* 2014; press release http://news.wustl.edu/news/Pages/26660.aspx

1706 McAloon C. Golden ingredient fuelling interest in processor. ABC Rural, November 20, 2013. http://www.abc.net.au/news/2013-11-20/nrn-lactoferrin/5104848

1707 Saphier A, Silberstein T. Lipid peroxidation of infant milk formula. In Preedy, op.cit., p. 251-2.

## Plants and microbes as factories

Much of this research has been done in plants of various types, including algae and fungi for those omega-3 fats (see A fishy tale of fungi and algae and eggs on page 315). Using plants as bioreactors can also have problems.

> Loss of foreign protein as a result of biological and physical processes such as proteolytic destruction and irreversible surface adsorption can occur in plants and plant culture systems.[1708]

In plain English, animals and plants defend themselves against foreign materials, and this could change the amount or even the character of the foreign protein being produced. Plants produce a variety of defence chemicals, some of which are now used as pesticides or repellents: the daisy family is the source of pyrethrin compounds. Will any defence chemicals persist in the final product? Will this defence evolve over generations? Will they affect infant health?

In the end, costs of manufacture in the different 'bioreactors' – surely unlikely to include bacteria when the product is destined for infant formula? – and costs of purification will strongly influence and perhaps determine the outcome. Scientists are aware of the potential for reaction if known allergens are included. But some seem less aware than others that chosen plants can have other problems. Consider this statement:

> ' ... we are expressing human milk proteins known to have anti-infective activity in rice [sic]. Since rice is a normal constituent of the diet of infants and children, limited purification of the proteins is required.[1709]

Excuse me? Since when has rice been a normal constituent of human milk, the only normal diet for human infants in the first months of life? Have we learned nothing from the Western experience of exposing infants to wheat and milk and soy proteins in the first infant formulas? How safe is universal infant exposure to rice?

## Of rice and men and mining

Rice is not the totally harmless food implied in that statement. Food scientists have had reason to be concerned about levels of arsenic found in rice products:

> ... food can be a significant source of arsenic to an individual, especially if their diet is rice-based. Infants are particularly susceptible to dietary exposure, since many first foods contain rice and infants have a low body mass.[1710]

In fact, rice naturally accumulates inorganic arsenic, the dangerous form that disrupts cell metabolism, from ground water and the soil. And there are some US infant formulas

---

1708 Lönnerdal B. Human milk proteins: key components for the biological activity of human milk. (PMID: 15384564) *Adv Exper Med Biol* 2004; 554:11–25
1709 ibid.
1710 Jackson BP, Taylor VF, Punshon T, Cottingham KL. Arsenic concentration and speciation in infant formulas and first foods. (PMID: 22701232) *Pure and Applied Chemistry.* 2012; 84(2):215–23

which use organic brown rice syrup as a sweetener. This contains about 60 ppb of arsenic, compared with the US EPA's standard for drinking water of not more than 10 ppb,[1711] a level too low to permit in-field testing, and so hard to police without dedicated resources. Ten parts per billion is the equivalent of 10 micrograms per litre. Only a little, but arsenic accumulates. Bengalis eating rice with more than 0.2 mg/kg of arsenic (but not otherwise exposed to arsenic) have recently been shown to have chromosomal damage:[1712] alterations to chromosomes.

Arsenic is already a serious problem for infant feeding (and adults) in areas of the world where the water supply contains high levels: areas of the USA, the Asian sub-continent, Hungary, Vietnam, China, Argentina, Chile, Taiwan, and Mongolia included.[1713] Even in Finnish infant foods in 2013 there is enough to cause concern.[1714] Will arsenic be in the mix of unknown chemicals flowing back for disposal or above ground storage from the controversial – and to me insane[1715] – practice of fracking, exploding deep layers of rock to liberate gas, "shattering the bedrock of our nation in order to bring methane out of the earth, consuming enormous quantities of precious fresh water to do, without any clear idea of the health and environmental consequences."?[1716] We cannot know – industry's chemical mixes are protected proprietary secrets. (But both arsenic and uranium came back to pollute groundwater in Australia: see What water can add on page 376)

Fracking (and other techniques of coal seam gas extraction) worldwide adds new impetus to the longstanding need for constant and frequent community monitoring of ground water supplies: 'not only for arsenic, but also for manganese, fluoride, pesticides, other chemicals and pathogens.'[1717] And not only the water, but the food grown with it. This process will now need to include looking for those chemicals that are known to be used in fracking: 'acids, rust and scale inhibitors, pesticides to kill microbes ... gelling agents, petroleum distillates, glycol ethers, formaldehyde, and toluene.'[1718] Water will bring unknown compounds and micro-organisms that until now had been safely trapped in subterranean rock; about half of the chemical-laden water injected into the smashed rock layers will be returned to the surface to be disposed of somewhere ... Will the coal-seam gas industry be made to pay for a vast futures fund under government control, for the long-term monitoring and disposal of its wastes and the harms they will cause? Already concern has been expressed about

1711  Blum, D. On rice and arsenic, http://blogs.plos.org/speakeasyscience/2012/02/21, reprinted in *Sensitivity matters*, Allergy and Environmental Sensitivity Support and Research Association (AESSRA) no 71; March 2012, pp. 12–13

1712  Banerjee M, Banerjee N, Bhattacharjee P, Mondal D et al. *Scientific Reports* 3, DOI:10.1038/srep02195

1713  Chowdhury AM. Arsenic crisis in Bangladesh. *Scientific American* August 2004; pp. 71–5

1714  Rintala EM, Ekholm P, Koivisto P, Peltonen K, et al. The intake of inorganic arsenic from long grain rice and rice-based baby food in Finland – low safety margin warrants follow up. *Food Chem.* 1 May 2014;150:199–205. DOI: 10.1016/j.foodchem.2013.10.155. Epub 2013 Nov 4 PMID: 24360440

1715  Areas fracked also become earthquake-prone over time, as ground settles and water finds new pathways. Such seismic disturbance could have incalculable consequences, perhaps triggering larger faults, or causing the collapse of old mines and the development of sink holes in areas some distance from the fracking. The extent of which MUST be independently mapped. Ellsworth WL. Injection-induced earthquakes. *Science* 12 July 2013; 1225942 DOI:10.1126/science.1225942

1716  Steingraber S. *Raising Elijah,* op. cit., p. 270

1717  Chowdhury op. cit.

1718  ibid.

Chapter 3: Infant formula, past, present and future
3.14 Genetic engineering and infant formula: inevitable?

| 525

such waste products spread under New Zealand dairy pastures,[1719] following on from Sri Lanka's concerns about the use of dicyandiamide (DCD) on pastures.[1720] In New Zealand, the major dairy co-op Fonterra has said that testing for just some likely contaminants would cost them NZ$80,000 per annum, and so Fonterra will not accept milk from any more farms where fracking wastes are spread. This practice is ironically called 'land-farming', and could put an end to dairy farming on the affected pastures, as farmers may find it hard to get Fonterra contracts renewed if their milk proved to be contaminated. Do those Fonterra-banned farmers sell their milk locally, or to less fussy formula producers? Who records where these wastes are being or have been spread, who tells the next buyer of that land what is under his pasture? And who pays the costs of clean-ups and compensates residents for the stench created when Fonterra disposed of 150,000 litres of fracking-contaminated milk along with 3 million litres of excess buttermilk? The local Council waste disposal site was so overwhelmed by the task that residents have had to endure months of stench as the product rots away; the Council could be fined up to $600,000; Fonterra also faces charges to which it has pleaded not guilty[1721]– and residents are complaining of health problems. Clearly not understanding the likely outcome (Fonterra should have been able to tell them!) the Council gave permission for this dumping, akin to the "Lake of buttermilk"[1722] elsewhere. Said the Council official: "We were trying to do the right thing by helping Fonterra find an environmentally acceptable solution for an exceptional circumstance. But we got it wrong."[1723] People do get things wrong, in well-informed, technologically-advanced, affluent societies. Mining wastes make getting it wrong a very dangerous business. And expensive, not for the polluters, but for the ratepayer and taxpayer and affected humans.

Plants, including rice, need to grow in safe soils, because they will take up what the soil supplies. Soils are accumulating chemicals of all sorts from animal feedstuffs and medications where slurries are spread on the land as fertiliser. Water is accumulating human use chemicals too, and rice is a water-thirsty crop. I'd like to see very thorough purification of any rice used as a bioreactor for making human proteins. Before the human immune system was explored, few realised how tiny are the traces that it can detect. Nineteenth-century scientists thought wheat was a safe component of the human infant diet, remember, and fed it to newborns, and Western generations a hundred years later have reaped a harvest of serious gluten intolerances and allergy. Rice allergy is already relatively common in Japan compared with Australia, say, probably because rice is a frequently consumed staple there.

So far as I know, however, it was not traditional to feed newborn babies rice in hospitals, while Japanese mothers continued to consume rice during both pregnancy and long periods of lactation, increasing the chances of infant tolerance. How many generations might it

1719 Astley M. Fonterra 'confident' that oil and fracking waste no threat to dairy safety. *Dairy Reporter,* 5 June 2013. http://www.dairyreporter.com/Regulation-Safety/Fonterra-confident-that-oil-and-fracking-waste-no-threat-to-product-safety See also 19 June.

1720 http://www.dairyreporter.com/Regulation-Safety/Fonterra-attempts-to-pour-water-on-Sri-Lankan-DCD-concerns. DCD is used on pastures to try to prevent nitrate, a by-product of fertilisers, reaching waterways.

1721 http://www.radionz.co.nz/news/regional/255999/fonterra-denies-role-in-buttermilk-stink

1722 http://www.dairyreporter.com/Manufacturers/Fonterra-disposal-practices-probed-over-Lake-of-Buttermilk-concerns

1723 Harper L. Legal stink lingers over milk saga. *Taranaki Daily News,* 12/09/2014 Online at Harper L. stuff.co.nz

take before rice proteins are as problematic as wheat, if we are to feed newborn babies the protein traces that immunologists consider most likely to stimulate reactions and not suppress them? Already Australian research 'highlights the emerging importance of rice, a food commonly thought to be "hypoallergenic", as a significant trigger of FPIES [food protein-induced enterocolitis syndrome].' FPIES is just one form of severe gut damage, with bleeding from the bowel one of its symptoms; a disease of formula-fed babies. (It has not been documented in any fully breastfed child.) Has rice become a major allergen *because* industry re-formulated first infant cereals (like Farex) in the last few decades, substituting rice for what was once wheat, and so babies have been exposed to rice younger than they once were in Anglophone societies? Did everyone even notice this significant change in babyfoods, when the brandname stayed the same? I discovered it only by reading revised labels. Say the researchers:

> Paediatricians should be aware that rice not only has the potential to cause FPIES, but that such reactions tend be more severe than those caused by cow's milk/soy.[1724]

And there would be traces of rice in formula products with added rice-made-human proteins, even if purification is as thorough as humanly possible on an industrial scale. How much more so, if only 'limited purification' is carried out because industry once again assumes the neonatal gut can tolerate alien proteins? How catastrophic would it be for Asia in fifty or one hundred years if rice allergy took off the way milk allergy and gluten intolerance has in the West, after decades of feeding wheat and milk to newborns? Scientists and industry need to think about how they use rice, and experiment through generations before assuming safety.

## How pure is pure?

I once asked an eminent biochemist just how pure it is possible to make any product manufactured industrially on a commercial scale. His response: 'Everything carries traces of where it has come from.'[1725] (Fans of forensic detective stories should know that!) And of course some of those traces will not be benign. That we do know. I have long been concerned about the amount of cows' milk protein that may contaminate commercial lactose, used as a placebo in some milk allergy trials, and present in some inhalant medications puffed into the lungs of milk-allergic asthmatics, as well as in anti-histamine tablets swallowed by allergy sufferers. After all, a tiny amount contaminating soy formula caused anaphylaxis in one nine-month-old child,[1726] and my adult son reacts to lactose containing medications. An extreme case, but how many more reactions have never been investigated thoroughly

---

1724 Mehr SS, Kakakios AM, Kemp AS. Rice: a common and severe cause of food protein-induced enterocolitis syndrome. (PMID: 18957470) *Arch Dis Child* 2009;94(3):220–3. Professor Peter Hartmann, in conversation some years ago.

1725 Professor Peter Hartmann, in conversation some years ago.

1726 Levin ME, Motala C, Lopata AL. Anaphylaxis in a milk-allergic child after ingestion of soy formula cross-contaminated with cows' milk protein. (PMID: 16264012) *Pediatrics* 2005, 116(5):1223–5. 'This case demonstrates that trace quantities of cow's milk protein can elicit severe systemic reactions in highly milk-allergic individuals. This infant ingested the equivalent of 0.4 ml of cow's milk from the soy formula as documented by an immunoassay for beta-lactoglobulin. This highlights the ease with which cross-contamination can occur during food processing and reinforces the need for better quality control.'

enough to pinpoint the cause? A mere whiff of pavlova mix precipitated anaphylaxis[1727] in some egg-allergic children; I once knew a child so sensitive that his skin reacted with allergic wheals whenever his mother broke an egg in an adjoining room. How many molecules or osmyls[1728] of airborne egg was that? Airborne antigens can also trigger antibody formation in milk[1729], and such tiny traces can cause allergic reactions. I was told that American airlines stopped serving peanuts as snacks because air-conditioning can circulate enough antigen to cause anaphylactic reactions in the very sensitive. The dose is one that others can't even smell. People allergic to fish can have symptoms triggered by walking past a shop cooking it.[1730] Licking the wrapping from which rice-cakes had been removed triggered FPIES in one child.[1731]

Where in the world nowadays are field crops grown on the industrial scale needed for formula-making without exposure to contaminants from fertilisers and pesticides and diesel and other agricultural chemicals and organisms? Fungi and algae and bacteria can be grown in dedicated factories like the Martek plants. Even then, the processing contributes contaminants, it would seem.

Lactoferrin is by no means the only breastmilk protein being researched for addition to formula. Lysozyme is another, an enzyme that attacks bacteria, including gram-positive pathogens like Streptococci and Bacilli. But the human body only needs a little. High lysozyme blood levels (produced by some cancers) can lead to kidney failure and low blood potassium. As always, there is an interactive balance to be kept. Not too much, not too little. How much is too much, and how much too little, for each individual baby? Will renal specialists be made aware that sick babies might be given formula with excess lysozyme?

Other enzymes are also being targeted for production in bioreactors, in the hope of improving digestion, creating some of the by-products that naturally develop in the breastfed infant. Bile salt stimulated lipase (BSSL) is one such, and recombinant human BSSL (rhBSSL) is already being trialled in animals, with unexpected side effects. Hernell[1732] described how mice bred to lack BSSL responded to administration of human-derived BSSL. Unexpectedly, this caused crippling collagen-induced arthritis. He spoke of this as a lesson for researchers 'to expect the unexpected' when adding or subtracting anything from such complex heat-labile food for infants. As he said, many of the bioactives being researched, like BSSL, are found not only in milk, but also in blood and other tissues; they have multiple functions. The crippling arthritis showed that BSSL is involved in inflammatory processes in some way. Knowing that, I would not want any child of mine

1727 Kemp AS, Van Asperen PP, Douglas J. Anaphylaxis caused by inhaled pavlova mix in egg-sensitive children. (PMID: 3200200) *Med J Aust*, 1988; 149(11–12):712–13.

1728 Urbach E. Odors (osmyls) as allergenic agents. *J Allergy* 1942; 13(4): 387-396. http://dx.doi.org/10.1016/S0021-8707(42)90297-1

1729 Casas R, Böttcher MF, Duchén K, Björkstén B. Detection of IgA antibodies to cat, beta-lactoglobulin, and ovalbumin allergens in human milk. (PMID:10856160) *J Allergy Clin Immunol* 2000; 105(6 pt 1):1236-1240.

1730 David TJ. *Food and food additive intolerance in childhood.* (Blackwell Scientific Publications, 1993)

1731 Mane SK, Hollister ME, Bahna SL. Food protein-induced enterocolitis syndrome to trivial oral mucosal contact. *Eur J Pediatr* 2013; doi: 10.1007/s00431-013-2051-2.

1732 Hernell op. cit

to be swallowing synthetic or natural BSSL in any food other than breastmilk, where it is supplied with all the anti-inflammatory and regulatory extras needed to prevent harms.

There will be many more such scientific experiments to discover some new additive for infant formula. I personally think that this is because each company must latch on to some new gimmick to make itself competitive and justify price rises. Collaboration in research and decision-making about additives, under a strict regulatory framework with independent expertise, might be better for babies. If these new additives are safe and valuable, they should be added to all formulas. If they are not, they should not be advertised as important. Advertising has an effect. On page 466 you can see that in 2005, the number of survey respondents who agreed with the statement that infant formula was as good as breastmilk was over 28%;[1733] in 1999 that figure had been just 14%. Just two years after the USFDA allowed the addition of DHA and ARA to American formulas, advertising had persuaded them, not experience.

The unregulated multiplication of infant formulas simply conceals and confuses outcomes; it makes true informed choice of a brand almost impossible. It also adds immensely to costs, as well as risks, or so it seems to me. Where will the leadership come from to challenge this? Are the world's child advocates asleep? Or are international paediatric bodies too involved in these processes, too uncritical about scientific progress, to question them?

## Concerns about recombinant additives to formula

Obviously, genetic engineering is just a tool, which can be put to good or bad use. The development of recombinant human insulin has been a major scientific success. That however, was a needed solution to a common, devastating disease – one which could have been less common with universal breastfeeding. Human insulin replaced animal-derived products that created greater risks to human health, so whatever its problems, it is an enormous benefit. Similarly, there are risks in using recombinant genes as therapy. But if this treats a lethal condition like leukodystrophy or SCID (Severe Combined Immune Deficiency), the benefits may outweigh the risks, even outweigh any unexpected adverse outcomes in the process of developing such new technologies.[1734]

Genetic engineering, well designed and done, well-regulated, not controlled by immoral profiteers, may solve many global problems. Opposition to all genetic engineering of foodstuffs is simply unintelligent: issues need to be judged case by case. So, for example, to reduce preventable blindness, I would support planting free Golden Rice[1735] in areas of high vitamin A deficiency. I do not support the planting of patented herbicide-resistant strains of any crop that simply increases company profits, while leading to increased pesticide use, resistant weeds, and higher food prices.

---

1733 http://www.cdc.gov/breastfeeding/data/healthstyles_survey/survey_2013.htm
1734 Geddes L. Nowhere to hide for faulty genes. *New Scientist* 2013 Nov 2, pp. 8–9.
1735 While Greenpeace campaigns against this, the founder of Greenpeace thinks that their doing so is immoral. See Coghlan A. Embattled grains. *New Scientist* 2 November 2013, pp. 30–1

So it has to be said: it is possible that the addition to infant formula of recombinant or genetically engineered lactoferrin and lysozyme and BSSL and other human milk fractions will reduce current harms of infant formulas. Reputable scientists think so, and I'm in no position to contradict them, whatever my concerns about risk might be. In thirty years this may be seen as a triumph like human insulin.

But *when it is not necessary*, or *before any real benefit has been shown*, using such novel recombinant food additives in formulas for every infant raises many issues. How similar to the natural protein expressed in human milk can any transgenic protein be? (It will not be identical.) How will processing affect it? How will adding one protein affect the naturally balanced uptake of others? What contaminants of the manufacturing process will also be added inadvertently or deliberately, and how significant might this be given daily intakes of up to a litre in early infancy? How can a recombinant product be standardised, and who will regulate and routinely inspect this? What levels are safe or risky? What are the risks or benefits of each component transferred along with the desired protein? How will the recombinant protein behave when fed to infants in a radically different mixture from human milk? Will it make any difference, and will that difference be for good or ill? Is the possible benefit worth the cost? Whose babies will be the latest guinea pigs? (Non-American ones if past practice tells us anything.[1736]) Will their parents be fully informed about the experimental nature of the new additives? Will their mothers be persuaded by free formula to forego or to shorten the duration of breastfeeding? Who will monitor harms other than those envisaged as potential outcomes by the scientists? How long should such studies run, when effects might not be manifest until adulthood?

All these new additives and technologies raise legitimate concerns. I hope regulators insist on proof of safety across the wide range of potential concerns. I hope they do not accept assertions of non-toxicity by a company hoping to make more billions from formula sales with an ingredient that they have already added in some other country, because they think it is safe enough to do so, and that country has no regulations to prevent them. And I would hope that no study in any country, whatever its legal system, includes any baby who could have been breastfed.

## Recombinant growth hormone and infant formula

The genetic engineering revolution may affect the growth and fertility of artificially fed infants and weaned children in a more indirect way: the use of genetically engineered cow growth hormone, or recombinant bovine somatotropin (rBST). The Monsanto-patented growth hormone boosts milk yields, but also is said to increase the rate of bovine mastitis – and so increases the risk of debris, pus, and/or antibiotic residues in the milk collected,

---

1736  Senator Al Gore stated that he had been told American companies always 'pre-tested their formula on infants outside of the US'. *Food Chemical News* 5 November 1979, p. 41. Do they still? Judging by published research, Spain seems to test many products of other EU nations. Should it be mandatory for formulas to be tested in the country of manufacture or at least to include a similar number of nationals as any other country?

while shortening the lives of the cows.[1737] In addition, the milk of rBST-treated cows contains elevated amounts of IGF-1, which, as described earlier, is under suspicion of causing lifelong metabolic changes to body functioning, and higher rates of non-communicable diseases.[1738] USFDA reports say that rBST is safe, and that it will not harm anyone, that the small quantity of extra IGF-1 in bovine milk will not have a detrimental effect. All the same, a significant body of people would prefer not to have it in their milk!

Pasteurisation does not destroy IGF-1. Perhaps the heavy processing of infant formula does. While it is stated to be denatured by acid in the stomach, artificially fed infants' gastric pH is markedly higher (i.e., less acid) than normal, which has many consequences. And young babies do absorb and respond to hormones in their diet, growing at a rate never to be achieved again in life. The FDA logic may be unassailable – if one can infallibly extrapolate from rat studies to babies. But there is an instinctive aversion to the idea of any unnecessary meddling with the milk babies will drink. Many Americans dislike the idea of recombinant growth hormones grown by bug biofactories in the milk they see as quintessentially 'nature's perfect food.'[1739] They have voted with their wallets, sourcing milk from dairies willing to resist the tide towards greater profits[1740] at the expense of animal well-being.[1741]

The Wikipedia account of this struggle is worth reading.[1742] Millions of dollars have been spent in lobbying and trying to prevent labelling that would enable customers to choose milk from non-treated herds. The USFDA insists that any labels must say that the milk from treated cows is nature-identical, the same as milk made by non rBST-treated cows, and safe.

Consumer resistance had won a small victory, although rBST milk is still approved for use in America by the FDA and indeed may be in use in any country where there are no regulations requiring disclosure on labelling. It is approved for use in many countries.[1743] However, the European Union, Canada, Israel, Australia and New Zealand had banned use of rBST on herds within their territories, on the grounds of its effects on animal health. Infant formula made from milk produced in those areas will be rBST-free, although Canada has allowed the import of US rBST milk for processing into cheese. And Canadians will not be told that the cheese was made from rBST milk. Is the exclusion of rBST milk from infant formula worldwide? Is this being monitored? Formula is made in many countries and exported worldwide; the milk used to make it is imported and exported and there is no requirement to state country of origin of all ingredients. If rBST milk is significantly cheaper

1737 Woodford, K. op. cit., p. 200, says 'It is widely accepted among agriculturalists and veterinarians that the very high cow replacement rates on American dairy farms are associated with the use of rbST, which reduces the productive lives of cows because of more udder infections, reduced fertility and increased lameness. But the practice of injecting rbST continues because of the increased milk production, and in essence is economically driven.'

1738 Michaelsen KF, Larnkjær A, Mølgaard C Amount and quality of dietary proteins during the first two years of life in relation to NCD risk in adulthood. (PMID: 22770749) *Nutr Metab Cardiovasc Dis* 2012; 22(10):781–6

1739 DuPuis EM. *Nature's perfect food: how milk became America's drink* (NY University Press, 2002)

1740 Telesca J. Organic milk sales surged in 2011. *Supermarket News* 2011 http://supermarketnews.com/dairy/organic-milk-sales-surged-2011#ixzz2PInr2Jtt

1741 Mackenzie D. Doubts over animal health delay milk hormone. *New Scientist* 18 February 1992, p. 9

1742 http://en.wikipedia.org/wiki/Bovine_somatotropin. Read November 2012. Wikipedia entries are extremely malleable – it is always interesting to review changes/previous versions of any controversial article.

1743 http://ansci.cornell.edu/bauman/envir_impact/rbst_booklet.html Accessed. August 12, 2013

to produce, I feel sure that it will find its way into world milk supplies somehow. And as more and more of that milk supply goes into infant formula, it will take a lot of money and time to keep rBST milk out of formula. No doubt national authorities, as usual under pressure from industry, will set a standard that allows the inclusion of just the amounts of rBST likely to be there. That way there is no (perceived) problem!

Meanwhile, Monsanto in 2008 announced that it would divest its rBST product and operations; at the time of writing the brand is owned by Elanco Animal Health, a division of Eli Lilly and Company.[1744]

## The impossible dream: avoiding GM and GE

Avoidance of GM or GE ingredients is presently impossible, and that is not likely to change. Western government authorities, heavily influenced by industry lobbying, have refused to accede to consumer requests that all GM or GE sourced food be clearly labelled as such. Even organic foods may be contaminated: the US National Organics Standards Board very controversially judged Martek oils to be allowable additives.[1745] True organic producers have worked hard for years to recondition soil, to avoid all contamination and GM-sourced seed. They cannot label their products as GM-free if even PCR-magnified minuscule traces of accidental contamination could be shown: way below the limits of what would now trigger label declaration. Company strategies of national and global planting and crop handling have made cross-contamination of agricultural products like cereals and oil seeds almost unavoidable.

It would be a foolhardy producer who labelled his product GM-free without costly testing. Any large corporation with deep pockets (and a vested interest in making farmers dependent on the chemical inputs that produce higher yields) would find the cost of such testing no bother if a smaller competitor was gaining too much market share by implying that a GM-free option was available. The tiniest unintentional trace would ruin the competitor. So those who try to avoid GM inputs are handicapped by government regulation.

Such an absolute standard is not applied to labelling of food that does contain GM traces. Regulators specifically allow companies not to declare the presence of GM materials or sources provided that the amount present does not exceed a certain percentage, 1 per cent in Australia, seemingly calculated in response to industry's need to include the material and still avoid informing customers. So if the label is silent about the issue, it tells the buyer nothing: the product might have GM materials in it, or it might not. (This is not the only place such helpful flexibility is accorded industry, at the expense of the consumer's desire to know what they are ingesting; the official Australian definition of 'no added sugar' allowed juice producers to add up to 4 per cent sucrose and multiple sources of fructose without label acknowledgment, duping parents trying to avoid 'sugar' in juice. And note that the once-mandatory in Australia obligation to detail on the label likely formula fat sources has been removed.)

---

1744 Monsanto press release, at http://monsanto.mediaroom.com/index.php?s=27632&item=76980
1745 Go to http://www.cornucopia.org/replacing-mother-infant-formula-report/ and follow the links.

Europe has held out longest on this issue of GM product in food. The GM-free label is used in Europe, and labels can give information about processing. Cold-pressed GM-free oil from European sources has been available in Australia, and I buy it as a matter of principle. The option of choosing cold-pressed oils in glass containers reduces some contamination risks from oils, such as the excess of oestrogen mimics outgassing from plastics, but does not come cheap. Efforts to 'harmonise international trade', dominated by the US, seem to include strenuous efforts to end all such possibilities of informed consumer choice.

Infant formula already does contain products derived using biotechnology; in future it is likely to include more rather than less. "Organic" formula needs to be carefully investigated, not only for its organic pedigree, but also for the compositional requirements it meets. The biggest selling organic formula used by American infants of all ages is Nature's One Toddler Formula. A 70kcal/100mL casein-dominant formula with 18grams of protein per litre, this may suit some infants and not others. It will certainly stimulate growth, having so much protein. But because it calls itself a Toddler formula, it is exempt under FDA regulations, as are many specialty formulas. But because it calls itself a Toddler formula, it was exempt under FDA regulations, as are many specialty formulas. How much of this tinkering with both technology and definitions is done because it is best for infant health? or best for industry profits? Cows' milk feeds industry and investors better than it feeds women's babies - or for that matter, most farmers.

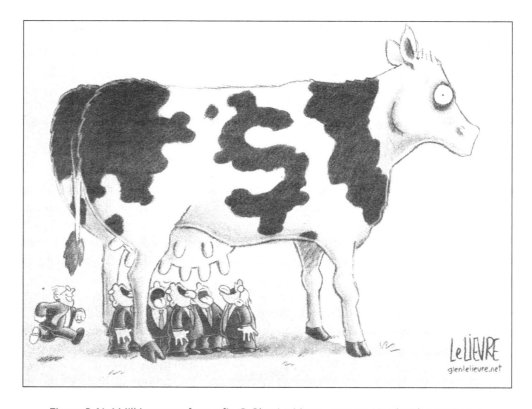

Figure 3-14-1 Milking cows for profit. © Glen Le Lievre cartoon. Used with permission.

# 3.15 Infant formula in the twenty-first century

The last decades of the 20th century saw considerable growth in scientific awareness of the risks of infant formula, and of the bioactive nature of breastmilk and breastfeeding. Many scientists speak and write as though the value of this new knowledge is not to persuade any government to re-structure society to enable breastfeeding, but solely to help to make more highly modified, value-added infant formula, which of course then can be sold for more money.[1746] As I've outlined earlier, industry researchers have made some frank admissions about the impossibility of the once-stated goal of infant formula makers, which was to attain chemical identity with breastmilk. But because they, like FDA staffers, cannot conceive of a world without the widespread use of infant formula, the now accepted new goal is to attempt to match breastmilk's effects on the recipient infant, or "breastfeeding performance".[1747]

Early 20th century doctors heard from the inventor of certified milk that all the newborn animals fed the milk of another species "were inferior to the breastfed animals, both at the time of the experiment and afterwards."[1748] Prized stud animals are so valuable that breeders will go to great lengths to find sources of species-specific colostrum and milk if a valued animal dies giving birth. Humans have been the only animals to adopt the milk of another species as normative, and then to expect their young to be normal. We are only now beginning to understand how differently the formula-fed child may express the potential of its genome if that child is not fed normally, that is, breastfed.

Despite this, or perhaps because of it, some researchers have argued that formula-fed children need only to be compared with one another, not with a control breastfed group. Such persons obviously consider that current formulas are good enough to be the controls against which new ones should be judged, and some may even try to argue, yet again, that their formula could be better than breastfeeding. No generation has a monopoly on hubris. In the 21st century, having better research parameters and definitions is essential. Yet in 2014, I read a study in which "Breastfed was defined as >80% of feeds consisting of breast milk at both points; formula-fed was defined as >80% of feeds consisting of formula milk at both points."[1749] (The points were a mean of 13 days and 6-12 weeks. How long might the follow-up need to be?)

There are bound to be other market-driven new infant formula developments. Industry is more aware than its customers both of the problems of its products and how to deal with

1746 Jensen E, Labbok M. Unintended consequences of the WIC formula rebate program on infant feeding outcomes: will the new food packages be enough? (PMID:21034164) *Breastfeed Med* 2011; 6(3):145-149. Hydrolysates can cost over $100 for 400gm can, compared with around $25 for a 900gm can of regular formula. Can that be justified?

1747 Hernell O. Human Milk and evolution of Infant Formulas. In Clemens, Hernell and Michaelsen op cit. p.21. This is now a truism, accepted by industry and scientists alike.

1748 Wolf JH, *Don't Kill Your Baby* op cit p.76.

1749 Gale C, Thomas EL, Jeffries S, Durighel G et al. Adiposity and hepatic lipid in healthy full-term, breastfed, and formula-fed human infants: a prospective short-term longitudinal cohort study. (PMID:24572562) *Am J Clin Nutr* 2014, 99(5):1034-1040 DOI: 10.3945/ajcn.113.080200.

them. Over the last few decades it has begun to address some of its more obvious practical problems: better packaging design removing infant formula from contact with lead and phthalates, for example, and building in a shelf to level off scoops without compacting the powder, along with providing a place for the scoop in the tin lid. The difficult issue of scoop accuracy with powder is also being addressed in a novel way by Japan's Meiji Company, which has patented packaging powder into standardised cubes[1750], to be dissolved in water, and by the Babynes system, previously mentioned. But those are peripheral concerns, compared with the issue of infant formula compositional recipes.

Here too change is certain. Lowering the total caloric value and the protein content of infant formula seems likely, indeed is already happening. While ignorant formula advocates might claim the link with obesity is unproven, this change is being justified by industry as meaning that some babies may be less likely to become obese. Others may well drink greater volumes of formula to meet their growth needs. (Both outcomes being good for industry.) One might think that less protein being used would make formula cheaper. On the contrary, the price rises that accompany formula changes are sometimes camouflaged by reducing volume in the can from a litre to 900 to 800 grams without lowering the price proportionately- or in the past, not even changing can size, just selling a little more gas and a little less powder.

Additionally, as flagged earlier in the chapters on ingredients, there may be new bioactive additives[1751], like fractions of the milk fat globule membrane (MFGM) lost when vegetable oils replaced milk fat because they were cheaper. One trial suggests that adding back the MFGM may reduce the cognitive losses of formula-fed infants.[1752] Or osteopontin might improve bone mineralisation. These changes are discussed later. But what are the realities of infant formula at the start of this new century?

## Measuring formula realities and processing effects

In 2007 the Codex Alimentarius Commission was finally able to revise what had always been defined as a minimum Standard for infant formula. Industry took this standard seriously, and set to work to assess how their formulas stacked up against the new standard. The first co-operative survey of levels of nutrients in infant formulas was conducted by several global manufacturers. They found that

> Whereas formulas met proposed minimum levels of all nutrients, 15 nutrients were identified whose levels were likely to exceed the proposed MV or GUL: vitamins A and K, thiamine, riboflavin, niacin, vitamin B6, folic acid, vitamin B12, vitamin C, iron, copper, manganese, potassium and iodine. Of nutrients with an MV, only levels of vitamin A in some batches exceeded the maximum; no batch contained levels previously reported in the literature to be associated with adverse effects. There were several nutrients with GULs for

1750 http://www.dairyreporter.com/Manufacturers/Asia-would-be-nice-next-step-for-infant-formula-cube-Meiji?nocount
1751 Lönnerdal B. Infant formula and infant nutrition: bioactive proteins of human milk and implications for composition of infant formulas. (PMID:24452231) *Am J Clin Nutr* 2014; 99(3):712S-7S DOI: 10.3945/ajcn.113.071993
1752 Timby N et al, op. cit.

which there were batches that exceeded the suggested upper limit. Data for some nutrients showed considerable variability, which related to form (liquid vs. powder), inherent levels of nutrients in formula ingredients, protein source, nutrient stability, analytical variability and effects of process, package and container size.[1753]

Hardly confidence-inspiring to see all those variables and variations in a product supposed to be exactly what a human baby needs, that perfect mix of science and love ...with so many variants on hearts and breasts woven into its logos.

'Effects of process, package and container size' are concerns that will have to be more fully explored in the twenty-first century. Heat treatment is needed to reduce contamination and ensure reasonable shelf life. Formulas, being complex mixtures of ingredients sourced around the globe, are

> ... more prone to thermally induced degradation reactions than regular milk products. Degradation reactions observed during milk processing comprise lactosylation yielding the Amadori product lactulosyllysine, the formation of advanced glycation end products (AGEs), and protein-free sugar degradation products, as well as protein or lipid oxidation ... Most studies confirm a higher degree of damage in infant formulas compared to regular milk products. Differences between various types of infant formulas, such as liquid, powdered or hypoallergenic formulas depend on the analyzed markers and brands ... [1754]

In fact, the more processed the formula, the greater the risk of damage to the ingredients. Damage will of course affect how the nutrients work in infant bodies. Having only recently recognised some of these by-products, it is too soon for scientists to tell us exactly how they might affect infants. So less reassuringly, the authors add:

> The nutritional consequences of thermal degradation products in infant formulas are largely unknown.[1755]

Unknown, yes. But there are concerns. Concerns that they block lysine absorption, for example.[1756] And the exaggerated - oh, sorry, "augmented" – growth of formula-fed infants' kidneys is thought to be the result of exposure to both higher levels of protein,[1757] and also exposure to these advanced glycation end products, according to some scientists,[1758] one of whom went on to suggest avoidance wherever possible:

---

1753 MacLean WC, Van Dael P, Clemens R, Davies J, et al. Upper levels of nutrients in infant formulas: comparison of analytical data with the revised codex infant formula standard, *J Food Composit Anal* 2010; 23(1):44–53. DOI:10.1016/j.jfca.2009.07.008

1754 Pischetsrieder M, Henle T. Glycation products in infant formulas: chemical, analytical and physiological aspects. (PMID: 20953645). *Amino Acids* 2012, 42(4):1111–18. DOI: 10.1007/s00726-010-0775-0

1755 ibid.

1756 Gadoth A, Somers NL. Melamine adulteration of infant formula, health impacts and regulatory responses. in Preedy, op. cit.

1757 Schmidt IM, Damgaard In, Boisen KA, Mau C et al. Increased kidney growth in formula-fed versus breastfed infants. *Pediatr. Nephrol* 2004; 19: 1137-1144; Escribano J, Luque V, Ferre N, Zaragiza-Jordana M et al. Increased protein intake augments kidney volume and function in healthy infants. *Kidney Internat* 2011; 79: 783-790. DOI: 10.1038/ki.2010.499 "augments volume and function" or distorts, stresses, alters normal..?

1758 Sebekova K et al, in Preedy et al, op. cit., p. 435.

High dietary load with IFs-derived MRPS [Maillard Reaction Products, one of the AGEs] could be avoided by breastfeeding. Since the producers do not declare the contents of MRPs in IFs, and hydrolysed formulas contain generally much higher amounts of MRPS than the regular formulas, prescription of hydrolysed IFs should be carefully considered and chosen only in clinically-indicated cases.[1759]

Reassuringly, the authors of one study of heat damage go on to say:

A considerable portion of protein degradation products in infant formulas can be avoided when process parameters and the quality of the ingredients are carefully controlled.[1760]

As of course infant formula manufacturing always would be. Wouldn't it? We all know how infallibly large-scale industrial manufacturing processes will go on, with never any human error, or computer malfunction, or machine failure, or inadvertent contamination, or ingredient defect, or contamination, or can defect, or mislabelling... Every one of those problems can be documented for infant formula in the past, but will never happen again. Of course.

Oh dear. More work for scientists and perhaps risks for babies. The finding, cited earlier, that free fatty acids formed during digestion of infant formula can be cytotoxic indicates that changes to foodstuffs are not always helpful. Trans-fats are an example of thermally-induced changes, and no one thinks they are healthy, even if they were listed as GRAS, by the USFDA. (And industry is opposing their removal from that GRAS list.[1761])

Heat and other processing damage to foodstuffs create risks, even when the product is human milk. I hope those heat-damaged ingredients and the new compounds produced will be the subject of a lot of careful independent study. But I wouldn't volunteer any of my grandchildren as the guinea pigs meanwhile. Artificial feeding is still a lottery, even though nowadays fewer of the losers die. While we are beginning to understand that genetic vulnerabilities contribute to the risk of damage, we are no closer to being able to predict or know the risks to any infant exposed to infant formula at any particular age.

And what I see as new risk factors keep on being added to the infant formula equation. Bacteria, food for bacteria, and new bioactive and inert ingredients from a variety of sources, including those produced by new technologies, which have never before existed. They may do good for some babies. But they add new risks, the extent of which can only be evaluated in retrospect. Remember always that these changes are to infant formulas that were the 'perfect mix of science and love' ... In the chapters that follow I can only dip into some aspects of what future infant formula developments will be or may include.

---

1759  Ibid. p. 423.
1760  Pischetsrieder M, Henle T. op. cit.
1761  http://www.foodpolitics.com/2014/03/food-companies-want-to-hang-onto-trans-fats/

# So new additives for infant formula?

While infant formula is used in affluent countries, there will always be a new frontier in research. Why? Because science is still discovering new things about what is in women's milk, and how that milk works in human bodies. As a recent overview article said, breastmilk is

> ... widely accepted to be a unique product believed to contain biological factors involved in the regulation of newborn optimal growth including brain when compared to milk-formula milks.

The author went on to say that there is growing evidence that infant formula lacks or is deficient in

> neuro-oxidative stress biomarkers, neurotrophic proteins and calcium binding proteins, known to be involved in a cascade of events leading to brain, cardiac and vascular development/damage.

> The article looks as some selected biomarkers such as: i) neurotrophic factors such as Activin A; ii) calcium binding protein such as S100B and, iii) heat shock protein known to be involved in oxidative stress response (namely hemeoxygenase-1, HO-1 or HO-1 or heat shock protein 32, HSP32). [1762]

As I've outlined earlier, any and all of these and other alphabet soup candidates may be extracted from milk or characterised and synthesised in biofactories, and then become candidates for inclusion in formula. But the more complex their effects in human milk and infants, the greater the risk that harm will result from adding them in an alien mix of nutrients to be metabolised by an infant subject to very different epigenetic pressures through artificial feeding. It is impossible to predict with certainty the results of these ever-changing experiments. Except that infant formula will become ever more expensive, perhaps to the point where governments have to pay for it, or else a dual-class system will emerge, with poor babies getting basic formulas and rich babies premium brands.

And it is not clear which babies will be the winners in that lottery. For instance, the osteopontin to be added to Asian formulas might indeed have an effect on bone. But when I read about its many involvements in the immune system and possibly control/stimulation of cancer cells[1763] I wondered how it could be determined what dose was safe enough to experiment with, and whether a different dose from that in breastmilk, or the lack of some other breastmilk controls, or the presence in formula of other potentiating factors, might mean a new epidemic of problems could arise. Ingredients powerful enough to have any effects may have effects we don't want, and only feeding them to many thousands babies will let us know.....Not my grandchildren, thank you.

---

1762 Serpero LD, Frigiola A, Gazzolo D. Human Milk And Formulae: Neurotrophic And New Biological Factors. *Early Hum Dev* 2012; 88 S1:S9–12. DOI: 10.1016/J.Earlhumdev.2011.12.021

1763 Pérez-Hernández AI, Catalán V, Gómez-Ambrosi J, Rodríguez A et al. Mechanisms linking excess adiposity and carcinogenesis promotion. *Endocrinol* (Lausanne). 2014; 5: 65. Free online. http://www.ncbi.nlm.nih.gov/pmc/articles/PMC4013474/

# Different formula stages under six months?

Another possibility flagged in some discussions has been the old/new idea of making different formulas for different ages: the first formula from birth to two months, when infants have some quite specific needs slightly different from the later period; the second formula from two months on. Perhaps they'll make them FIFa and FIFb so as not to be forced to re-number the current Stage 2 (post-six-months-mostly) FOFs?  Breastmilk of course changes all the time, in response to the baby's inputs and needs. No doubt the advertising will say that staging makes formula more like breastfeeding. This is in some ways a re-run of the old practice of whey-dominants to three months and casein-dominant after, just with different mixes reflecting more knowledge about average infant needs. (Except that no baby is average, each is unique.)

However, a US patent application[1764] does give some interesting insights into the logic behind this new development. The researchers who helped send neonatology down the track of nutrient-enriched formula for preterms in July 2011 applied for a patent for a lower-calorie formula for newborns. Having followed up the children, now teenagers, from those earlier studies, they found that those exposed to the enriched formulas have biological markers which suggest that they are at greater risk for cardiovascular disease and non-insulin dependent diabetes.[1765] The rapid growth due to enriched formula that was so valued then – and led to the rapid displacement of breastfeeding in many neonatal units – now looks like a potential long-term health hazard. So Singhal and Lucas are now proposing infant formula of between 25-50kcal per 100mL, down from the current 60-70kcal/100mL, for the first months of life, followed by 'conventional' formula from three months on. (Such under-nutrition of the formula-fed in the first three months may of course have other consequences only evident when the latest guinea-pigs reach adolescence.)

From the patent application:

> Disclosed are newborn infant formulas comprising fat, carbohydrate, and from 0.5 to 2.5 g of protein per 100 ml of formula, wherein the formula has a caloric density of from 25 to 50 kcal per 100 ml of formula. Also disclosed are methods of administering the infant formulas to provide newborns with optimal nutrition, to reduce the occurrence or extent of insulin resistance in an individual later in life, to reduce the occurrence or extent of atherosclerosis or coronary artery disease in an individual later in life, or combinations thereof, by feeding newborn infants the newborn infant formula described herein....

> Our prospective experimental study was designed to assess the influence of early nutrition on later cardiovascular risk factors. We found that adolescents born preterm who were randomized to a lower nutrient diet now recognized as sub optimal in terms of growth, had lower fasting 32-33 split proinsulin concentration, a marker of insulin resistance,

---

1764  United States Patent/ 8703173. Singhal A, Lucas A. Document Identifier US 20110262585 A1.  Go to http://patft.uspto.gov/netahtml/PTO/srchnum.htm and enter patent number in search box.

1765  Research from the 1970s into the link with early exposure to milk is reviewed in Dosch H-M, Becker DJ. Infant feeding and auto-immune diabetes. Chapter in Davis et al. *Integrating Population Outcomes, Biological Mechanisms And Research Methods In The Study Of Human Milk And Lactation.* (Kluwer Academic/Plenum Publishers 2002)

than those randomized to a nutrient rich diet. Further analysis suggested that these dietary effects, seen up to 16 years after dietary randomization, were likely to operate by influencing neonatal growth rate. We suggest therefore that a reduced early growth rate as a consequence of relative under nutrition programs a lower insulin resistance and, by inference, a lower propensity to non-insulin dependent diabetes mellitus.

Excerpts from US Patent Application 8703173

That's five to twenty-five grams of protein per litre in 250-500kcal/L formula. Meanwhile, Mead Johnson in America launched Enfamil Premium Newborn around 2010 as a formula for the first three months of life - but this is still a standard 20 calories per ounce formula. Once again, there will be confusion about what is appropriate as a first infant formula, if we have lower calorie formula as well as conventional ones.

There may be good scientific reasons for breaking up formula into even more stages. But its practical applications seem to me a nightmare, given that many parents want their babies to advance or progress on to the next stage as soon as possible, and the likely cost increases and differentials that could emerge between such formulas, and perhaps influence parental choices. It has been hard enough to get Stage 1 and Stage 2 (before and after six months) formulas clear to parents, as noted on page 274. Imagine another layer of confusion! Would the increased cost be worth any positive outcome for infants? Where is the social cost-benefit research?

Staging is already here for the elite in the form of the Babynes machine Nestle has produced (and sells in Hong Kong as a Wyeth product[1766]). Individual pods of formulas for the first, second, third to sixth month, and so on, are set up in pre-packaged single feed pods for immediate mixing with temperature controlled water and hygienic dispensing (so long as the machine is well maintained, of course.) The idea is attractive for the mega rich, but consider the resources used by such individual packaging of every feed and the waste the process creates!

# The use of nanotechnology

The rise of nanotechnology as a way of addressing food safety concerns will not have gone unnoticed by some of the world's largest manufacturers. The infant formula industry still faces many challenges in its task of making a product that is safe enough in every dimension, nutritional and microbiological. How nanotechnology will affect the infant formula product, or its safety and delivery, is a future concern for child health advocates to keep in mind. Just as with irradiation and genetic engineering, the impacts of nanotechnology on industrial food production are likely to be incremental, in small steps, as the issues are too easily manipulated and misrepresented on all sides. But the time to start reading about the possible future is now. The UK government's Food Standards Agency is a good place to start: http://www.food.gov.uk/policy-advice/nano/#Assessingnewfoodtechnologies.

1766 https://www.babynes.com.hk/hk-en/babynes-machine/machine-overview

Personally, I find it impossible to be blindly trusting of the billion dollar infant formula industry, given its history and the harm it continues to facilitate worldwide. There are many significant caveats about its products that in the end can only be proved or disproved by experimenting on thousands of infants, as the scientists and industry understand. In 2014 that European Food Safety Authority (EFSA) published a Draft Scientific Opinion stating that the addition of ingredients including fatty acids ARA and EPA, chromium, taurine, probiotics, and nucelotides should be considered "unnecessary" (for lack of evidence of benefit, though to be fair, there is also an absence of any evidence of harm to date). An industry group, Specialised Nutrition Europe, was disappointed that these ingredients were not instead labelled 'optional' because, and I quote, "it is only through their inclusion in formula and subsequent research that their presence can be proved to be beneficial."[1767]

There you have it. Industry needs lots of real-life babies to find out what formula ingredients do, if anything, for either good or ill. Industry understands that with every re-formulation, there may be unpredicted consequences, for good or ill, though the latter possibility is rarely mentioned to parents. Parents and healthworkers alike assume there has been positive proof of benefit to children before anything is added. Why wouldn't they, when advertising material says, above an image of the DNA double helix:

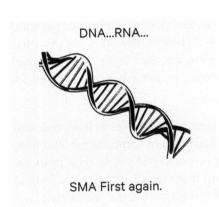

DNA...RNA...

SMA First again.

Then the blurb about what nucleotides might do followed. "Might" or "may" are enough to prevent allegations of false and misleading advertising. The addition of nucleotides made clear to me that proof of benefit to sales figures seems to be sufficient justification.

But if societies cannot support (or will not bother to support) the abundant lactation potential of women world-wide, and feed human babies human milk, then obviously infant formula, the deeply inferior substitute, should be developed to do as little damage as possible – which means genetic engineering of ingredients, nanotechnology, and new technologies as yet unheard of. Can the world afford this? Will this be cost-effective for human health, not just for industry profits? Not likely. But then one could argue that about coal seam gas extraction and many other noxious enterprises: those who profit have a vested interest in their continuance, even if it does cost us the earth, or the health of humanity. As always, poor people will suffer most. And as always, some parents will think only of how this issue affects them and their like in the here and now, worrying more about their feelings than the harm to women and children world-wide and into the future.

1767 Harrison-Dunn AR. SNE chips in on EFSA's draft opinion. *Dairy Reporter* June 17, 2014. http://www.dairyreporter.com/Regulation-Safety/SNE-EFSA-infant-formula-draft-opinion

# 3.16 Is matching breastmilk possible or necessary?

Why is any of this vast scientific enterprise necessary, when women make a far better product that poses far fewer risks to their infants, and provides major benefits for both women themselves[1768] and their children? Human milk could be much more widely available than it currently is, and even be used as medicine, not only for infants.[1769] And surely we know by now that matching breastmilk is simply not possible. Thousands of constantly-changing ingredients, all with specific functions, and all interactive: how can breastmilk ever be matched?

Bo Vahlquist, an eminent nutritionist, wrote in 1976:

> No doubt the formula industry will make every effort to produce new formulae which come closer, at least superficially, to human milk. But attempts to bridge the gap will remain futile since we are dealing here with such complex systems and such species-specific substances that even very costly models cannot be foreseen to reach the ideal model. Thus the new discoveries in the field of the species-specificity of human milk will serve to underline very strongly the uniqueness and biological superiority of this produce of Nature, and will provide new arguments for ardent action to retain the age-old breastfeeding tradition. We can be sure, too, that the discoveries of the last decade will not be the last in this context.[1770]

I believe (but cannot prove beyond all doubt) that both early exposure to infant formula, and lack of breastmilk, have been the major contributors to intergenerational amplification of food-related disease. Yes, assisted by other environmental and social changes, but still the one most fundamental distorting factor, because babies are constructed from what they eat, while other factors simply influence the construction.

If this is so, genetic engineering may mean that we are at the beginning of yet another cycle of clever scientists causing untold harm (with the very best of intentions: saving the lives of babies). At present, and for the immediate future, infant formula is a necessary evil. It is better than some of the much-worse evils, that range from starvation to naïve homemade formulas – on which, it must be said, some babies seem to thrive, as a minority always have on the most bizarre diets (such as 'perfect' infant formulas since discarded). But evil, because it is promoted as being so close as not to make much difference, and that belief causes both breastfeeding failure and global inertia about the many causes of that failure.

For feeding babies formulas simply need not be necessary in the long run. Lactation is in fact a powerful survival mechanism that is reliable, robust, and resilient. Women still have

---

1768 I am not covering the known and putative benefits of breastfeeding for women's health except in passing. But new discoveries are constantly being made, such as the greater risk for gall bladder disease in women who have not breastfed their children. Liu B, Beral V, Balkwill A, et al., Childbearing, breastfeeding, other reproductive factors and the subsequent risk of hospitalization for gallbladder disease. *Int J Epidemiol*, 2009; 38(1):312–18

1769 McGuire L. Ruth goes home: an adult's use of breastmilk. *Breastfeeding Review* 2012; 20 (3) 44–8. There are many documented uses for women's milk for the sick or elderly; in nineteenth-century Britain one Captain Ackerley 'employed lactating women to milk themselves and sold the milk to 'decrepit old men' to prolong their lives.' (Smith FB. *The people's health 1830–1910* (ANU Press, 1979) p. 339. One of the US Rockefellers is reported to have drunk human milk all his life; other notable cases are on record. A chapter on this topic is to be found in Ploss and Bartels, vol. 3, op.cit.

1770 International Pediatric Association (IPA) *Bulletin*, 1976; 5:45

breasts. Almost all breasts still lactate, despite unprecedented environmental challenges, unhelpful social attitudes to breasts, and modern forms of female mutilation willingly undertaken by those unaware of the importance of breastfeeding. Many women have always been capable of feeding more than one child.

There can be more than enough breastmilk in the world for all the world's children, if we choose to invest in human lactation rather than simply bovine, to structure society to meet human needs rather than greed. The rationale for so doing can be humanitarian or economic or both: Western societies and taxpayers stand to save billions in healthcare costs,[1771] at least as many billions as the formula companies pay out to their shareholders. The recent UK figure[1772] for some of those costs was substantial:

> Supporting mothers who are exclusively breast feeding at 1 week to continue breast feeding until 4 months can be expected to reduce the incidence of three childhood infectious diseases and save at least £11 million annually. Doubling the proportion of mothers currently breast feeding for 7-18 months in their lifetime is likely to reduce the incidence of maternal BC and save at least £31 million at 2009-2010 value.

If women's milk was rightly valued, milk banks would be recognised as safer than blood banks or sperm banks, and wet-nursing would become as well accepted as IVF.[1773] Milk banks decrease the use of infant formula.[1774]

Women worldwide are using global networking to share their milk, as they always have, with women who have too little.[1775] There would be more milk-sharing[1776] if women understood what infant formula actually has been and still is, a fallible and very imperfect product. Not bad, not evil, not poison; adequate for survival and even life-saving at times, but always at a price; definitely fallible, to be used – where necessary or unavoidable – with due caution, and awareness of the risks of both the product and the processes for procurement and feeding. In short, not "so close as to make no difference"! But seriously second-rate with incalculable - and certainly not calculated - consequences.

Infant formula is and always will be a distant poor substitute, of use in situations where the real thing is not available, or when enough good quality family food and water are not available in a suitable form. Yes, there are real risks to women sharing milk, and there are bound to be some

1771  Smith JP. Lost milk? Counting the economic value of breast milk in gross domestic product. *J Hum Lact*, 0890334413494827, first published on 12 July 2013

1772  Pokhrel S, Quigley MA, Fox-Rushby J, McCormick F et al. Potential economic impacts from improving breastfeeding rates in the UK. (PMID:25477310) Arch Dis Child 2014  DOI: 10.1136/archdischild-2014-306701

1773  Both raise ethical and practical problems, but are important for the health of a minority, and should be part of any modern health infrastructure. It could be argued that milk banking is the more important, as any society needs healthy babies more than it needs a greater number of babies.

1774  Utrera Torres MI, Lopez CM, Roman SV, Diaz CA et al. Does opening a milk bank in a neonatal unit change infant feeding practices. A before and after study. *Internat Breastfeed J* 2010; 5:4 http://www. internationalbreastfeedingjournal.com/content/5/1/4

1775  Akre JE, Gribble KD, Minchin M. Milk sharing: from private practice to public pursuit. (PMID: 21702986) Free resource. *Internat Breastfeed J* 2011, 6:8

1776  This raises problems that require careful solutions, but it is not an insuperable problem. Gribble KD, Hausman BL. Milk sharing and formula feeding: infant feeding risks in comparative perspective? (PMID: 22848324) Free resource *The Australasian Medical Journal* 2012, 5(5):275–83

problems over time. So parents need to make sensible, fully informed decisions about their personal cost-benefit ratios. But the real thing, mother's own milk, trumps any substitute.

Once this understanding spreads, breastfeeding may come to be seen as being as inevitable and necessary and ordinary as birthing. Both are common but incredible, almost miraculous, experiences that define us as humans. Both are demanding, but hugely rewarding, physiological experiences, whatever the extreme pain and grief they sometimes cause. Both are normal processes, but sometimes can go wrong and require specialist help for a good outcome. Those who want normal healthy children need to see the importance of both birth and breastfeeding in the process of creating such children. (Even when surrogates are used for gestating and birthing children, breastfeeding can be part of the equation for the non-birthing parents-to-be, and it has special rewards for adoptive parents. Induced lactation is indeed possible without having given birth, as traditional cultures understood. There is even a WHO monograph[1777] to consult!) Breastfeeding is the human norm; formula the recently introduced intervention, a shape shifter desperately trying to mimic what any woman's body can do better.

But as I wrote in *Breastfeeding Matters* three decades ago, formula will not disappear without major structural changes in society. So while it persists, it must be better regulated. Food is subject to much less regular critical independent oversight than drugs, but this is a very special food given at a time of unique vulnerability to adverse effects having lifelong consequences. All potentially bioactive components, and indeed infant formula itself, should be developed as medicines, tested on relevant mammals and adults in bodyweight related doses. Industry-funded studies in piglets and a handful of infants in non-English-speaking countries are not enough protection. No novel formula ingredient should be declared 'GRAS' (Generally Regarded as Safe) by the industry making money from them, or hidden from public view by industry-friendly labelling laws. Industry sells infant formula as a life-changing substance. it is, just not in the ways they cleverly suggest.

Once infant formula starts to make claims to act like a medicine, it should be regulated as such. Perhaps it is time for infant formula sales to be limited to outlets where there is some hope of professional advice on brand choice, and where education about safe use is possible. And if world scientists can get together to work on particle accelerators and finding the Higgs Boson, why can't there be a huge international not-for-profit effort to solve the problems preventing children from being breastfed or getting donor breastmilk, and also to create low-cost culturally appropriate alternatives for emergency use where breastmilk cannot be sourced? The results would be seen in the first generation, with huge cost savings to national budgets.

Research sponsored by industry and published openly adds immensely to our knowledge, as those who read it carefully know, despite the perhaps inevitable under-examined assumptions, areas of ignorance, and clear bias towards conclusions favourable to

---

1777 *Relactation: review of experience and recommendations for practice.* (WHO 1998) Online at www.who.int/ entity/maternal_child_adolescent/documents/who_chs_cah_98_14/en/

industry.[1778] I appreciate the high quality scientific resources that can be freely accessed via industry sites, most notably the Nestlé Nutrition Institute. But that doesn't mean that I am blind to the fact that Nestlé – like its competitors – is a profit-making business. It is hypocrisy to pretend that even the most scientific of industry institutes are purely philanthropic works, however excellent or useful they may be. Industry researches breastmilk in depth in order to make better saleable products, to avoid costly lawsuits, and to influence health professionals. Abbott, Nestlé, Danone, Mead Johnson and the rest are not philanthropic enterprises, whatever their origins and company mythology.

If infant formula manufacturers and their trade organisations like the Infant Nutrition Council or ISDI[1779] were really 'trusted partners' whose aim is to help health professionals save babies, they would create a global, completely independent foundation dedicated to protect, promote and support breastfeeding. They would provide it with a multi-million dollar endowment and annually contribute an amount equivalent to their current marketing budgets for infant formula. I challenge industry organisations to do so, or else to stop pretending that they are in business to save babies. Their marketing and their professional websites would not be tax-deductible if they did not assist companies in their prime raison d'etre, making profitable products, in part by ensuring that health professionals are on side with industry. They are in business to make money, and that they certainly do very well, at the expense of public health.

If such resources were available for the support, not of investors, but of breastfeeding, the world would be a different place. If formula companies told parents of the risks of formula, and had effective warnings on their labels, they might start to earn some respect and trust. Industry does know – or at least its scientists do – how far short of breastmilk their products are. Industry would be believed if they told parents that truth, whereas breastfeeding advocates are insulted as scaremongering (as I will be...sigh!). Industry has been, and is, believed even when it misleads and distorts and conceals the truth, as this history shows. Industry would be believed if it told the truth about its products and their inadequacies, discouraging artificial feeding. This book deliberately uses industry-funded literature, and published science available on industry sites, to make its point. I would lay long odds that a survey of industry scientists' families would reveal a high rate of breastfeeding!

At the highest levels, the global formula industry needs to accept responsibility, and make reparation, for the harm it has caused, both inadvertently and deliberately, over two centuries. When this all began, doctors and industry together were addressing a real problem as best they knew how, influenced by cultural assumptions about both women and food. We know much more now. I believe that to continue to be part of the problem is to be guilty of global child abuse, risking the future of humanity as epigenetic changes accumulate. Those who seek to profit from infant formula should take that thought on board. No doubt they are well-intentioned and accept the current societal myths of formula

---

1778 Bekelman JE, Li Y, Gross CP. Scope and impact of financial conflicts of interest in biomedical research: a systematic review. *JAMA* 2003; 289: 454-5. Their meta-analysis found industry sponsorship was associated with an OR of 3.6 (95%CI 2.63-4.91) in favour of a pro-industry conclusion. Surprise, surprise.

1779 ISDI is the industry lobby group for special dietary foods. It brings together national and international associations that are active in this food sector from more than 20 countries over 6 continents. check out the membership list.

safety and necessity. But what could be achieved if half a billion or a billion dollars went into supporting maternal breastfeeding and developing human milk resources, rather than vainly trying to match breastmilk, or to supply infant formula that replaces breastmilk?

Am I wasting my breath in appealing to the conscience of industry leaders? In asking them to consider giving up those many billions generated by harming children who would be better off breastfed? Is it a waste of time to beg them to consider protecting, promoting and supporting breastfeeding in deed, not weasel words? To refuse to expand into markets where they can do only harm? Probably, but it's worth a try.

For committed industry leaders and major companies could make a huge difference in a short time. The global infant formula industry is beyond the control of any one government: it simply re-locates to a more amenable jurisdiction if inconvenienced. Being a large part of the problem, industry does need to be part of the solution. And companies could be, if they took their own words seriously, and acted in the best interests of children.

But industry cannot be permitted to set the terms and timing of their co-operation. Governments have a mandate to protect their citizens. It is their responsibility to insist that corporate assaults on citizens via persuasive marketing campaigns and less healthy food options are as unlawful as an assault by an individual criminal.[1780] Democratic governments are meant to govern for the good of all, not just the rich. The United Nations needs to emphasize artificial feeding as a major global issue with ramifications for many other major global issues, from resources to environments to population concerns to climate change as well as to health. And national governments need to insist on intensive inspection, oversight and postmarket surveillance of all brands of infant formula as a necessary minimum, developing independent expertise not reliant on company funding, but paid for by a tax on company volume of sales including exports.

However, as I wrote in *Breastfeeding matters* in 1985, the infant formula industry by itself is not the sole or perhaps even the major, cause of breastfeeding decline, and industry blaming is often counter-productive. Industry reflects society, and both creates and responds to social needs. Bottle-feeding women defend industry precisely because women face problems for which industry offers practical solutions. (Poor solutions, and many women do not realise just how poor, or understand why such problems exist). Not only capitalist shareholders profit from industry's investment in infant feeding and its separation of women from their children's most basic needs. Even some breastfeeding advocates may be financially dependent on their actions against industry, which could make them as unconsciously conflicted as those who take money from industry more directly. Health professionals and their associations have benefitted from artificial feeding since it began, and many have failed in their duty of care to women and children, as well as their duty to advise industry and government objectively and authoritatively. Educated professionals and politicians of all varieties have allowed industry to control the education and marketing and regulation agendas. All of these people, as well

---

1780  Richter J. *Codes in context. TNC regulation in an era of dialogues and partnerships.* http://www.thecornerhouse.
org.uk/resource/codes/context

as ignorant and unscrupulous advertising agencies, have been fundamental to western acceptance of infant formula as safe, risk-free, and normal, being virtual breastmilk.

I choose to hope that, as elsewhere, there are good people in industry, and in science funded by industry, who genuinely want to use their knowledge and skills to help resolve the world's nutritional problems. I know that there are many within industry who think that is what they are doing when they sell infant formula, and I ask them read this and to think again. Of course there are also those within industry who just want to maximise profits – just as there are in other occupations, from medicine to marketing to media, law to legislating. Parents who want to have a baby without being inconvenienced by their offspring are part of the problem.  So are doctors who prescribe infant formula to fix a breastfeeding problem, politicians afraid to regulate industry or its marketing, anyone who makes mothers feel uncomfortable breastfeeding in public,  journalists who impugn the motives of breastfeeding advocates in inexcusably defamatory language... the list is endless .

Western society as it is currently constructed does indeed depend on artificial feeding, as that USFDA doctor said to me so reflexively all those years ago in Washington DC. The whole of society created this problem; it will take national and international leadership and industry co-operation to resolve it. Academic freedom, full disclosure of all research, quality well-funded research, open sharing of knowledge, and social structures that reward breastfeeding, even financially, are essential to that resolution.

Current knowledge about human milk[1781] needs to be understood in detail by all immunologists and public health workers and medical researchers. Industry is blindly reshaping human genomes via nutritional and microbial experimentation on babies. What is needed now, urgently, is far more international co-operative research into women's milk. Along with this, there needs to be scrutiny and regulation of infant formula at the highest levels, both fully funded so as to be utterly independent of industry money.

We already have in breastmilk the only perfect formula for any infant, a formula as individual as the mother-baby pair who jointly produce it. It is possible to concede that (rarely) this breastmilk formula might be imperfect, without accepting that industrial products would do better. Resources akin to those used to promote vaccination globally need to be given to the protection, promotion and support of breastfeeding and the safe supply of human milk to all children for at least the first months of life, when programming forces are strongest.

It took a co-operative international scientific effort to map the human genome. If infant formula is to continue to develop, it should also be as part of such a global effort. Allowing competing companies to conceal much of their research for commercial reasons is simply unconscionable. So is allowing companies to produce experimental or sub-standard formula for export into markets where other nations' children can serve as experimental subjects.  Governments might put a levy on every can, as has happened with vaccines

---

1781 This is such a rapidly expanding field that almost no text is fully current. An overview can be found in Rautava S, Walker WA. Academy of Breastfeeding Medicine founder's lecture 2008: Breastfeeding – an extrauterine link between mother and child.(PMID:19292608) Free resource *Breastfeed Med* 2009, 4(1):3–10.

in exchange for a no-fault indemnity plan. And price controls should prevent this being passed on to parents: in both Saudi Arabia and China government actions have reduced exorbitant costs. As bottle-fed children can be expected to use more health resources over a lifetime, it seems appropriate that the companies contribute substantially both to national healthcare systems and to global collaborative research.

However, I suspect that a world which independently assessed the cost of any such ethical non-profit development of better infant formula would very soon come to the conclusion that it was wasted time, money and effort, when women's lactational capacity has not been tapped. Stories abound of malnourished women in refugee camps feeding many more children than their own, and even of childless female volunteers in such places inducing lactation to save infant lives. Societies without modern global communications resources have in the past organised ways of getting breastmilk to children, in some cases with the assistance of the state, as when France had a system of wet-nursing bureaus, or large American hospitals employed uniformed wet-nurses to feed preterm infants, or hospitals everywhere had milkbanks for use not only by neonates. Human ingenuity and modern transport could make breastmilk available if this was seen as important. Every year brings a new crop of babies, and new decisions by new parents. And if it were to be seen as truly important, many more children would be mother-fed for much longer than they currently are, because society would make that possible and reward it –not simply exhort mothers to do it and make it difficult or impossible for them to do so. Which is the current state of play, well-described by Naomi Wolf.[1782]

What are the unavoidable problems of infant formula making? Among the obvious ones, how to source reliably,

- enough critical ingredients,
- at a cheap enough price,
- that formula remains affordable even without government subsidies.

Then there's what to do about

- the optimal quantity and quality of protein;
- types and interactions of fats and how to prevent these oxidising during commercial shelf-life;
- levels and interactions of vitamins and minerals;
- suitable carbohydrates and their gut effects;
- the multiple antigens in all ingredients and how to tame them;
- the effects of heat treatments and how to avoid damage to heat-sensitive ingredients like fats and vitamins;
- preventing contamination with pathogens or environmental chemicals; minimising the effects of processing equipment; maintaining quality over a commercially viable shelf-life....

---

1782 Wolf N. *Misconceptions: truth, lies and the unexpected on the journey to motherhood.*(Vintage 2002)

Industry knows how complex its task is, though parents currently do not. Though 700 million tonnes of milk are produced annually, simply getting enough of the raw materials can be difficult, so that there is now talk of a totally artificial/vegan cows' milk![1783] (No doubt major formula manufacturers know enough not to buy into such ideas, but will everyone?) While some manufacturers are privately critical of competitors using older plants or older technologies or cutting corners to harvest some profits from the "white gold rush," all are locking in raw material contracts with ever more dairy sources.[1784]

While this may mean more risk in the supply chain, probably most major manufacturers are performing to the *highest level possible with today's technology*. There's the rub. Exactly the same could be said of formula from 1880 till now: most of it was made as well as possible – *which is never perfectly or infallibly* – given the existing knowledge, food sources, and technology of the time. Only now are we aware that these formulas may have had profound effects on human growth and development: on eyesight, on coronary vascular disease, on obesity, on autoimmune disorders, on genetic material, on child and adult behaviour and mental health, and the rest. In 2050, when looking back from the vantage point of newer knowledge and technologies, it seems morally certain that adults fed 2012 formulas will be dismayed by what is seen as their distortion of normal development. As dismayed as parents of 2013 may well be by what I have outlined about the formulas they were fed decades ago, and those they feed their children today. Those distorted genomes and microbiomes recorded now will have had their effect by 2050. What effect, only time will tell.

As Kierkegaard said, 'Life can only be understood backwards, but it must be lived forwards.' Perhaps by 2050 industry will have created microbial mixes which undo the gut dysbiosis and the damage of Crohn's disease[1785] and other gastrointestinal illness; perhaps the peptides in formula will no longer distort normal arousal and sleep patterns in infants and SUDI will be as rare as it was before artificial feeding popularised tummy sleeping; perhaps the right balance of fats will have been created for brain and cardiovascular normalcy. Perhaps.

Or perhaps, with a few more generations of artificial feeding, the rates of infertility will be as high in humans as they were in Pottenger's cats by the fourth generation; perhaps cognitive damage will have been cumulative because of epigenetic changes, so that a significant sub-class of utterly uneducable or mentally damaged people exists; perhaps more adult diseases will now emerge in childhood; perhaps industry will have discovered that their chosen strains of bacteria cannot be controlled and new resistant pathogens will have emerged globally, spread by the multi-national formula trade. It would be safe to bet that there will still be problems, and that unanticipated problems of today's formulas will be known. It is not possible to eliminate risk from artificial feeding.

---

1783  Pandya R. Milk without the moo. *New Scientist* 28 June 2014, p. 28-29. The ersatz milk would contain just 6 major synthetic proteins, instead of hundreds, along with synthetic fat blends, sugars and minerals to taste. Yuk.

1784  http://www.dairyreporter.com/Manufacturers/Fonterra-and-Dairy-Crest-enter-infant-formula-ingredients-partnership/?

1785  A 1983 Scandinavian study found that "Crohn's disease patients were particularly over-represented among those with no or very short periods of breastfeeding." Bergstrand O, Hellers G. Breastfeeding during infancy in patients who later develop Crohn's disease. *Scand J Gastroenterol* 1983; 18 (7): 903-906.

Speaking of allergy research, Susan Prescott outlined the complexity of the work ahead:[1786]

> Just as there have been genetic studies looking for 'genome-wide associations' with disease, there also need to be 'environment-wide association' studies that go into similar depth. We need to be prepared to look in completely new direction and with new eyes. We need to be prepared to team up with mathematicians with serious computing power to look at these complex interactions. New discoveries have already challenged many past ideas, and produced many shifts in thinking. And we need to be prepared for more changes. We need to anticipate the dilemma of a factor that protects against one disease yet promotes another. Nothing is simple in any of the modern diseases that humanity now faces.

All that applies to the field of infant feeding research as well. And the allergists need to team up with experts in lactation and infant feeding. As I said more than three decades ago, paraphrasing Leif Hambraeus, artificial feeding is the largest uncontrolled in vivo experiment in human history. I should have said, ever changing series of in vivo experiments! Just how changing, and how uncontrolled, some readers may have found surprising, even shocking.

For infant formula is a shapeshifter, a product that morphs over time as its weaknesses are discovered, always able to dissociate itself from the errors in its past, and at the very same time, to use its length of existence to claim public trust. All that while, it has existed as if under a mantle of protection, exempt from serious challenge because it serves so many vested interests, maintaining a myth of moving only from perfection to perfection, closer and closer to the gold standard of human milk, its makers being motivated by care for children (why else the love hearts in logos?) Regulations belatedly written have allowed that flexibility for want of independent knowledge of what is really needed when breastmilk is not available.

For me, the single best argument for breastfeeding your own child is the reality of industrial infant formula feeding. The history of infant formula is the single best argument for the likelihood that this product has caused perhaps irreparable damage to human health through generations of dysnutrition. If I am right, immune disorder is just one formula outcome among many, nearly all harmful to humanity, even if profitable for global elites and convenient for industrialised societies in which mothers and children are not in reality valued, but exploited.

The truth about risks cannot be suppressed forever, no matter how hard vested interests will try. How great the risk is to any individual child is unknowable, but while women still lactate, it is an unncessary risk. And once enough ordinary people know enough about the reality of risks, change will happen. It can happen very quickly. Especially in any country like America, if there is leadership from the top, as now appears to be happening. Equally, it can be slowed by conservative industry-friendly governments which, for example, stop funding the important UK quinquennial survey of infant feeding practices, or as in Australia, make life more difficult for low-income families.

I *can* imagine that change, though I don't expect to live long enough to see it. But in my lifetime, lead has gone from most petrol and paint, and has been reduced in infant formula, at least in developed nations. Recently BPA has gone from bottles in western nations, despite being a

---

1786 Prescott S. op cit, p. 111.

trivial risk compared to infant formula. Public smoking is anathema. Yet I remember choking on smoke in US airports and planes in the 1980s, while wearing badges that said "Your rights end where my nose begins". Only thirty years later smokers and other addicts accept that their undoubted freedom to injure themselves does not include any right to harm others. In some countries those harmed have a legal right to redress from those responsible for the harms. Think about the implications. The asbestos industry closed its eyes and took the profits from an incredibly useful building material, but pigeons all come home to roost some day.

I am confident that we will see an end to misleading advertising which claims to be promoting the 'perfect mix of science and love', or which infers that formula is 'close to' breastmilk. Every change of ingredients documented in this book gives the lie to such advertising. Change has been touted as an improvement, even changes whose effects are still unknown. Commonsense could have told us that no one can improve on perfection, yet in every era companies have been allowed to claim to have a perfect product.

The most recent regulations stand as a partial and sometimes controversial record of what is now thought to be important to the normal growth of infants. *They are also mute testament to what has not been previously provided.* The many changes to infant formula over time are proof positive of some of the imperfections of the product sold to parents at the time as a 'perfect' and 'complete' food for infants, and make a mockery of those formula advertisements which ask for parents' trust because of their long track record. Brands have disappeared despite being 'perfect'...

I am confident that truthful advertisements previously suppressed (See Appendix 2), and others informing parents of the risks of artificial feeding, will eventually see the light of day. How can it not happen, knowing what such feeding is implicated in producing?[1787]

Risks of artificial feeding are real, and avoidable in the future. Whatever their current legacy of harm it does not need to be compounded, and it may be ameliorated. Truth cannot be forever suppressed.

And three very simple truths are:

- Parents want the best for their children
- That is not infant formula.
- Only women's breasts can provide babies with a perfect mix of science and love.

Mothers' Milk *really* matters.

---

1787 One valuable review of data up to 2006, which Wolf cites as evidence of harms in wealthy nations, is online at http://www.ahrq.gov/downloads/pub/evidence/pdf/brfout/brfout.pdf. But note that this was, as always, a very *conservative* partial and dated estimate: literature since then contradicts its finding that there is no observed effect on cognitive development, for example. And we know about stem cells in breastmilk now. And we know that breastmilk helps destroy antibiotic-resistant pathogens. And so much more! *All* such overviews by respectable authorities are *always* understatements. Meanwhile industry goes well outside proven science in marketing claims – with impunity. It seems to me that the bottle brigade has frightened some health authorities into saying no more than has already been proven beyond any doubt, regardless of basic science, human experience, or commonsense.

# BOOK 3

# Crying out for attention

From the clinical point of view, food intolerances are probably of much greater frequency and importance than classical food allergy, but many allergists avoid handling patients with food intolerances on the pretext that they do not have true allergies. Such allergists should be encouraged to broaden their outlook. But equally important is the fact that the information that those interested in food allergy have amassed is ignored by most of their specialist colleagues – paediatricians, physicians and psychiatrists alike. Children with ADHD are not placed on diets; patients with IBS [irritable bowel syndrome] are treated every which way, but rarely with elimination diets; those with migraine headaches are offered the latest painkiller but never, or hardly ever, is an attempt made to discover the food or foods that trigger the headache; dermatologists still lean heavily on topical steroids for the treatment of eczema; otolaryngologists (with the exception of a small group in the United States) prefer the knife and antihistamines to the sleuthing of the investigative allergist. There is a need for conventional allergists to take an interest in food intolerance, and for all allergists to educate the specialists and family physicians in the investigation and management of patients with food allergies and intolerances.

JW Gerrard, in Brostoff and Challacombe (eds) Food Allergies and Intolerances, (Saunders second edition 2002) p. 442

# Foreword

When, with my third baby in my arms, I first met Maureen Minchin in 1998 I was only just beginning to unravel the web of colicky, asthmatic, slow-growing allergic babies. I was astonished by how quickly Maureen was able to sum up my children's symptoms, and their causes. I'd been through the circuit of "not enough milk – give formula", steroids, creams, and medications. None of which worked. What she suggested did. I recognised that Maureen spoke my language, and what she said made sense.

Not much in has changed in the intervening years. In fact, some allergy symptoms have become so common as to be mistaken for normal. The child affected by allergies still goes unrecognised by many who should be helping families. Rarely is the mother supported to find and fix the underlying cause of her child's problems. Some health professionals even surmise that dietary changes "would be too much for the mother". Fashions in medication change rapidly. Children are prescribed steroids, puffers, antifungals, laxatives, analgesics and antacids. When they still can't sleep and are miserable after all that, they are conditioned to sleep at sleep schools. Mothers who have been through the mill recognise I am speaking their language when I joke that they have probably asked 5 different people about their child's condition, and have had more than 10 different opinions. Putting together the jigsaw puzzle seems insurmountable for so many parents, without any reliable guide. One mother, Kate Brian, sums it up.

"By the time I came across Maureen Minchin I was desperate, confused, angry, and frustrated with the advice I'd had to try to help my 8 month old breastfed baby's eczema and tummy cramps. Maureen encouraged me to treat the cause not the symptom. It was a relief to finally find someone who could not only sympathise with what I was going through, but actually provide some tried and tested advice that worked. She highlighted to me how important nutrition is for all stages of life, not just pregnancy and while breastfeeding. I now think carefully about where all my food comes from. I can't wait to get my hands on the new book. I hope every medical professional gets their hands on this book too – and reads it."

Since the 1980s Maureen Minchin has been a pivotal figure behind the scenes in the global field of human lactation and breastfeeding, and a powerful advocate for allergic families. She takes parental concerns seriously, because she knows that intervening early can help identify and resolve problems in all family members. Scientific evidence is always slow to trickle down to the community, hindered by the blinkered assumptions created by industry marketing, with the delay compounded by the power of industry to mould public health policy and influence health professionals. But the new field of epigenetics outlines mechanisms that explain what Maureen has been telling us for decades, that milk matters more than we have realised. Maureen Minchin has the powerful ability to cut through history, culture and science with fresh perspectives that make sense, and she speaks to health professionals and parents alike in a straightforward way. This book will be a revelation to the parents of the sensitive, allergic child, and is a must-read for all professionals working with parents and babies.

Barbara Glare BA, Dip Ed, IBCLC, Certificate 4 Counselling. ABA, Warrnambool Victoria

# CHAPTER 4

# Helping hyper-reactive babies

*Parents with a crying baby will head to this chapter first. So an introduction summarising the past two books, and some additional background, might be useful. Skip this if you are reading the book from front to back!* Here in summary is the relevant argument in the preceding chapters, encapsulated in this diagram and a couple of paragraphs.

We inherit more than genes. Because the eggs that will become us form in our grandmothers' wombs, we are affected by at least two gestations (our mothers' and our own) before being born. Then the next developmental stage begins, with exposure to ambient environmental influences, the greatest of which is postnatal nutrition. We are either breastfed or not, fully or not, and what we are fed affects us for the rest of our lives – and so, via their genes and their gestation, affects what our children inherit, too. Children are constructed from what they eat, in a process directed both by what they are genetically, and what they experience post-partum. There is nothing parents can do about the effects of their own gestation except acknowledge its possible impacts. There is a great deal parents can do about postnatal nutrition of children. Any artificial formula soon after birth can have lifelong consequences for some developing immune systems. We cannot predict how any one baby will deal with the odd 'comp feed', so it's a good idea to avoid them unless they are genuinely essential – which they rarely are. Most babies treated responsively and exclusively breastfed from birth will be normal happy babies, easy to love and loving. With an unfortunate combination of before and after birth exposures, any baby can have many problems, manifested by early distress and (sometimes subtle) symptoms. And parents of such distressed children will have major difficulties coping without a good deal of support.

What follows is meant to be a practical guide to preventing and dealing with a common problem, the young persistently crying baby. Some people believe such infant distress is normal. My firstborn colicky son (still allergic as an adult) was succeeded by far more peaceful children, despite my absolute terror that we would face a repeat of the endless sleepless nights his pain caused us – which was almost enough to put me off having subsequent children, and which meant that I lived in high anxiety, even fear,[1788] for the first months of my second child's life! Having had two calm and happy breastfed babies after that disastrous first, and having helped many families to do the same, I now see any infant distress as a sign that something is wrong. I believe that it is possible to find helpful solutions for distressed babies, or at least strategies for coping, that do not damage fundamental relationships and warp infant mental development towards insecurity and anxiety. (As all punitive, arbitrary, and unresponsive techniques inevitably do, if current neuroscience – and commonsense - can be trusted.)

I've been saying most of what follows for decades. Don't be surprised if some of it is very familiar. Nothing that I say is particularly complicated or even very original. It just puts together, sometimes in a different way, things that many people already know. The landscape is familiar territory, but the view can change. And it is knowledge which changes the view. Some of what follows is based as much on commonsense and experience as on the scientific literature, partly because that literature is deficient in a variety of ways, and partly because the evidence of individual parents is to me just as important. But all knowledge is fallible and this may well need revision in the light of further research and experience – in the new context that is emerging in the 21st century. In 2015 I will be setting up a website to allow me to advise parents of what I see as significant changes to any of this information.

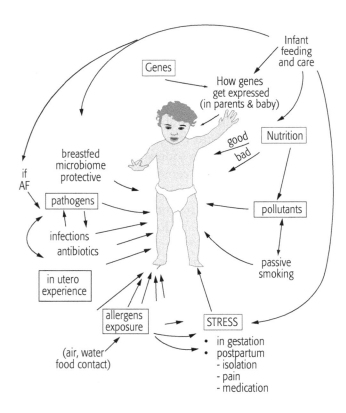

Figure 4-1-1 nfluences on the emergence of allergy symptoms

---

1788  I often wonder about the effects of my high cortisol levels on my second child, given what we are learning about cortisol in milk.

# 4.1  Allergies and your family

Knowledge about yourself comes first. Many parents with problem babies tell me that they are not allergic. So first answer the blank questionnaire for yourself and your family. This is also important if you are not a parent, but someone who wants to help others, as you then have some idea of how long it will take to do a proper history, and how many distractions it will generate. Allow two hours minimum, as there's quite a bit to think about. Some readers will quickly come to recognise that they themselves, or their families, have been, and even still are, affected by the allergy plague.

To do this thoroughly, get as much information as you can about your life and family health issues (yours and theirs) from any older family members (or friends) who knew you as a child. Some older relatives may exemplify the lifelong damage of not being breastfed, and their current health problems may prove to be relevant – the longer-term outcomes of neglected problems as children. It is quite common for grandmothers to discover a new level of personal health through this process of investigating a grandchild's problems.

But be warned – the issue of infant feeding rouses strong feelings. Some people (you included) may feel deeply about past breastfeeding failures; some may feel irrationally anxious or guilty.[1789] For some, this may be their first chance to talk about painful experiences, and it can take time before they can focus on solutions for the baby. Others may have mentally reworked their history substantially, for good or ill, so that their memories are inaccurate. There may be family documents that help recreate events that throw light on the family experience of allergy. Can you locate old hospital or health records and baby books? Photo albums? Letters describing you as a baby? They may all take on new significance .

Write all over this blank questionnaire as fully as possible, before moving on to consider my notes on each question, together with what you have written. Fill in your own replies first, so you won't be influenced by what is said in the later notes. However, if those notes jog new realisations, go back and add to what you've already written, in a different colour ink. Keep this document as a baseline record of what you knew when you started exploring the issue. You will learn more, and can add to it, as you live with the new awareness of diet as significant for your personal well-being.

---

1789 You can do much to relieve any guilt or shame you or they might feel, once you get past the first emotional reaction, so long as you are brave enough to persist with discussing the subject rationally. I recommend it. Once you raise these topics, the only way out is through: drawing back and agreeing to leave an elephant in the room creates worse ongoing problems and misunderstandings. (That doesn't mean you have to deal with it all at once. We're all different, and have to do things in our own time. It may be some time before you can talk it through. But don't give up on doing so. And don't confuse regret with guilt. See Appendix 2 On guilt and responsibility.)

# Are you allergic? A basic questionnaire

1.  What do you know about your birth and how you were fed as a baby? (When you were born, was the birth stressful?)

    ........................................................................................................................................

    Were you given antibiotics early in life?

    ........................................................................................................................................

    ☐  Don't know anything. (Ask, if possible.)
    ☐  Breastfed for ................................................................................ months.
    ☐  Exposed to formula in hospital

    What kind(s)?........................................................................................................

    When did you receive your first bottle?................................................................

    Regularly bottle-fed from ................................................................weeks/months

    Your early solid foods were ................................................................................

    When were they introduced? ........................................................weeks/months

    (Note here as much detail as you can, e.g., name of formula, what first foods, operative birth, maternal infection or illness, and other stresses from this early stage of life.)

2.  What has your mother, aunt or other relative said about you (an easy/difficult baby) or your food habits when you were young?

    ........................................................................................................................................

    ☐  Did you cry a lot?
    ☐  Did you sleep well? *

3.  What do you remember about liking or disliking foods as a child?

    ........................................................................................................................................

    ........................................................................................................................................

4.  Did you get free school milk and if yes, did you enjoy it?

5.  What do you know about your health as a child? Tick any that apply:

    ☐  Gut problems: colic, reflux/vomiting, constipation, diarrhoea, control problems

- ☐ Eczema, cradle cap, skin problems
- ☐ Asthma, croup, bronchitis, lower respiratory problems
- ☐ Hayfever, earaches, upper respiratory problems
- ☐ Fevers, night sweats
- ☐ Headaches, migraine, joint pains
- ☐ Bedwetting, urinary tract infections
- ☐ Learning difficulties
- ☐ Sleep difficulties, snoring[1790], night-waking, nightmares, night terrors
- ☐ Emotional mood swings, concentration and behaviour problems
- ☐ Do you experience these problems now?
  - ☐ Yes ☐ No ☐ Which? ...................................................................
  - ☐ Occasionally ☐ Often
  - ☐ Others? .............................................................................

6. Are you aware of 'allergy'/immune problems (diabetes, psoriasis, migraine ...) in:

   - ☐ yourself ..............................................................................

   - ☐ parents, siblings ....................................................................

   - ☐ your child's other parent ...........................................................

   - ☐ their family..........................................................................

   - ☐ older family members ................................................................

7. Were you smoked over as a child? (circle responses)

   ☐ Yes ☐ No ☐ Occasionally ☐ Often

8. Do you or those in your household smoke now? How often?

   - ☐ Actively ............................................................................

   - ☐ Passively...........................................................................

9. What if any non-human animals have shared your living space then and now?

   - ☐ As a child ..........................................................................

   - ☐ After childhood ....................................................................

   - ☐ Now ...............................................................................

---

1790 Brew BK, Marks GB, Almqvist C, Cistulli PA, et al. Breastfeeding and snoring: a birth cohort study. (PMCID:PMC3885662) *PloS one* 2014; 9(1):e84956 DOI: 10.1371/journal.pone.0084956

10. What if any medications do you use fairly frequently? (antihistamines, antacids, paracetamol, aspirin, ibuprofen, skin creams, nutrient supplements ...)

..................................................................................................................

..................................................................................................................

Why? ...............................................................................................................

..................................................................................................................

How many and what caffeine-containing drinks would you have daily?

..................................................................................................................

Any 'sugar-free' products? Protein supplements? If so, what?

..................................................................................................................

## About pregnancy (for mothers)

11. Did you have any problems conceiving this/any child?

12. How much cows' milk in any form (cheese, yoghurt, ice cream, milk, custard, etc.) do/did you have daily?

    ☐  None  ☐  Only a little  ☐  Not all that much  ☐  Lots*

13. On a scale of 1–10 (least to most liked), how much did you like plain milk during pregnancy?

    1        2        3        4        5        6        7        8        9        10

14. What three foods did you like most when pregnant?

..................................................................................................................

What three foods did you like least?

..................................................................................................................

15. When pregnant, did your food likes and dislikes change?

If so, how? .......................................................................................................

..................................................................................................................

..................................................................................................................

16. Did your eating habits change during pregnancy? If so, how?

Any food binges? ....................................................................................................

Aversions? ...............................................................................................................

What were your weight gains? ...............................................................................

17. What pregnancy-related symptoms have you been/were you aware of?

....................................................................................................................................

## Where you have siblings and/or other children

18. If you have siblings and/or other children, what ages are they now?

Siblings ....................................................................................................................

Children ...................................................................................................................

19. Were they 'easy' babies and toddlers?

Siblings ....................................................................................................................

Children ...................................................................................................................

20. Have they had any problems like those listed in question 5?

Siblings ....................................................................................................................

Children ...................................................................................................................

21. Have you or they noticed any consistent food likes or dislikes?

Siblings ....................................................................................................................

Children ...................................................................................................................

22. Have you or they thought any of these are associated with other symptoms? If so, which?

Siblings ....................................................................................................................

Children ...................................................................................................................

23. Have you or they taken any action to alter their diet?

Siblings ....................................................................................................................

Children ...........................................................................................................................................................

24. If yes, what did you or they do, at what age, and with what result?

Siblings ...........................................................................................................................................................

Children ...........................................................................................................................................................

## Other allergies than food

25. Make a note of any reactions you have observed to chemicals, pollens, dust, fragrances, cosmetics or environmental annoyances of any kind. They may also be relevant. Have you noticed any connection between symptoms and stages of your menstrual cycle?

...........................................................................................................................................................

...........................................................................................................................................................

...........................................................................................................................................................

...........................................................................................................................................................

...........................................................................................................................................................

...........................................................................................................................................................

Well done, you made it to the end! Jot down anything else you might be wondering about. Then let's move on to think about it all.

## Notes to help interpret the questionnaire
### Question 1 How you were fed under six months of age

These first questions are an attempt to identify early exposures to alien proteins, other nutrients and gut-altering substances, as well as early stresses, which make immune dysfunction and allergy much more likely because they affect gut development. Other chapters of the book explain this further.

If your mum says that you were 'breastfed', get more detail. What does that mean? For how long? When did she try you on the ubiquitous Farex/cereal/extra bottle? Or was it some other mix you were given? Some culturally determined food? When breastfeeding is seen as the ideal, some mothers will say they breastfed even if they did so only for the first days in hospital. Find out how soon you were given anything else.

Ask questions to jog memories about important details. If you were born in the era of hospital comp feeding, anytime from 1965 on in Australia, and 1950 or so in America, you can assume you were exposed to a bovine formula unless your mother took extraordinary steps to prevent this. So ask your mother these questions: How long did she stay in hospital? Were you separated from your mother for any length of time or overnight in hospital? For how many hours? (Any absence, especially of more than a couple of hours, often meant a comp feed was squeezed in. So if your mother says that you weren't interested in breastfeeding when brought back from the nursery, or slept a great deal in hospital, you were almost certainly fed formula.)

Why does this matter? If you were not exclusively breastfed by a mother who was exclusively breastfed, you are at greater risk of gut and immune problems. Ask your mother how much she knows about her own feeding as an infant.

### Question 2 Signs of gut distress in your infancy

Digestive distress is probably the most common cause of persistent inconsolable crying in the very young infant. Babies will cry when food is being regurgitated, perhaps burning the oesophagus, or rushed through the gut to produce loose green fermenting acid stools that scald bottoms, or just overfilling tummies so that bloated bellies feel like drums.

There are many causes of each of these symptoms, some just to do with feed efficiency and infant stress. But if such symptoms persist for weeks or months in otherwise well babies, they may be due to food hypersensitivity – and may disappear like magic with carefully targeted maternal diet change.

If you were a 'difficult baby', or you have one now, or your mother was one, the involvement of immune disorder is statistically more likely. A difficult baby is one who cries a lot, rarely sleeps, has many minor symptoms, as in Figure 4-2-1 on page 582

### Question 3-4 Foods you remember liking or disliking as a child.

Sometimes these are the foods that a young body instinctively 'knew' to avoid, or craved like an addict, because of their unrecognised effects. Both aversion and addiction can suggest sensitivity to those foods; people can move from one to the other over time.

Those who adored, and those who loathed, school milk may still have unrecognised problems with milk as an adult. If the taste of any unflavoured, relatively unaltered food, like milk, is offensive, and you like it only with lots of added salt (cheese) or sugar (ice cream) or other flavours (chocolate, vanilla) then it's a suspect food to consider as perhaps your problem. This applies to your parents as well.

### Question 5 Your health as a child

These and other symptoms of *possible* allergy can change over time or remain constant when exposed to different doses, or with adjuvant factors (things that assist) like smoke or mould or vaccinations. There are other explanations for each single symptom, but multiple and frequent symptoms are highly suggestive of environmental provocations such as allergy.

The allergic march describes the progression through infancy from eczema[1791] to asthma – same immune system, different symptoms as bodies and systems mature. One problem is that if Johnny has always been emotionally volatile as a result of exposures, the family may be unaware that he is reacting to allergens, and consider that's 'just Johnny' who's 'always been difficult'. It can be a huge shock to discover a person of a very different temperament and nature when Johnny ditches the allergens.

### Question 6 Family 'allergy'/ immune/endocrine problems

Many grandparents have asked me whether their middle-aged autoimmune problems are a likely logical outcome of years of untreated 'allergy'. In their children and grandchildren they see their past problems repeating, and now their immune system is attacking their own body. The allergic march may need to be extended and broadened as a concept, reaching from the cradle to the grave.

## The trouble with allergies

When you think allergies, you usually think itching, sneezing and wheezing. But allergies can affect your body in so many ways. Here are some of the many possible effects, both short- and long-term.

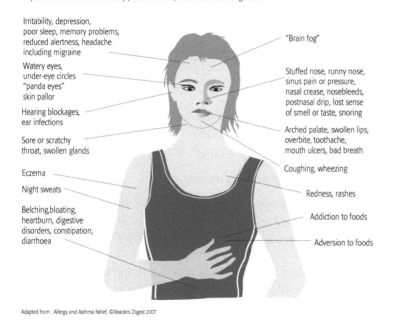

Irritability, depression, poor sleep, memory problems, reduced alertness, headache including migraine

Watery eyes, under-eye circles "panda eyes" skin pallor

Hearing blockages, ear infections

Sore or scratchy throat, swollen glands

Eczema

Night sweats

Belching, bloating, heartburn, digestive disorders, constipation, diarrhoea

"Brain fog"

Stuffed nose, runny nose, sinus pain or pressure, nasal crease, nosebleeds, postnasal drip, lost sense of smell or taste, snoring

Arched palate, swollen lips, overbite, toothache, mouth ulcers, bad breath

Coughing, wheezing

Redness, rashes

Addiction to foods

Adversion to foods

Adapted from : Allergy and Asthma Relief, ©Readers Digest 2007

Figure 4-1-1 Some symptoms that may stem from allergy

### Question 7-8 Environmental tobacco exposure

All and any smoke exposure – like cigarette smoke or diesel particulate in smog – or chemical exposure or detergent residue damaging mucosal surfaces, increases allergic risk. *But* smoking parents need to hear that while some tobacco compounds do transfer in breastmilk, bottle-fed babies of smokers get sicker and are hospitalised more often.

Ideally, breastfeed and don't smoke. However, as far as baby's health is concerned, it's better to breastfeed and smoke, than to feed artificially and smoke. So if you smoke, breastfeed, and also explore ways to reduce breastmilk contamination and your baby's exposure.[1792] .

1791  In solely-breastfed infants, eczema is the main risk factor for increasing sensitisation of infants, and itself a manifestation of active allergy. Flohr C, Perkin M, Logan K, Marrs T et al. Atopic dermatitis and disease severity are the main risk factors for food sensitization in exclusively breastfed infants.  (PMID:23867897) Free full text article *J Invest Dermatol* 2014, 134(2):345-350

1792  Minchin MK. Smoking and breastfeeding: an overview. *J Hum Lact* 1991; 7(4): 183-188

## Question 9 Exposure to other animals in childhood and now

The evidence around animal exposure and allergy is confused and confusing. As vets know all too well, a high proportion of those who live or work in close contact with any animal become sensitised to that animal sooner or later. As children we had cats and dogs, and I am moderately sensitive to both. I judge from personal experience that clean air is preferable to contaminated, and it is probably best that family animals do not share all living spaces, but spend a lot of time outdoors.

However, no one really knows. Short-haired pets that are washed regularly may even be beneficial. A recent Australian study suggested that pregnant women with pet dogs were less likely to have an allergic infant. On the other hand, animals that lick themselves and then their human carers are bound to be affecting human microbiomes, and perhaps not always for the better: animals can transfer some nasty pathogens. As well, animal microbiomes will be affected by the food they eat, and it is a reasonable bet that this includes antibiotic residues. So this question is simply gathering information that may or may not flag a common cause of reactions in the present.

Commonsense suggests never allowing animals to share bedding surfaces, and never leaving family pets alone with very small children – not just for reasons of allergy. Animals can resent recent intruders that monopolise attention once given to them, and many tragedies are on record.

## Question 10 Medications and other chemicals.

Some of these may do no harm if intake is moderate. However, all intakes powerful enough to have any positive effects can also cause side effects. Many contain lactose, which in turn will contain milk protein traces. GOS or galacto-oligosaccharides derive from milk: anything with lacto- or caso- in its name probably does. Protein supplements are often high-dose milk and soy proteins. Aspirin increases antigen uptake from the gut. Caffeine is a stimulant that affects some people adversely, and one that infants metabolise slowly, so it builds up in their system, affecting behaviour. Sugar-free sweeteners have a variety of undesirable side effects that many allergic families become aware of, such as worsening of gut symptoms or headaches. Reading the fine print and asking about all the ingredients is necessary and often illuminating. Some food allergy is just an intolerance of this sort of chemical overload.

# About Pregnancy (for mothers)

## Question 11 Fertility issues

Coincidence or not, the only breastfed children I have known to need seriously extended artificial or elemental diets for years were IVF babies created after multiple attempts, often in very slim mothers. A number of lactation consultants have agreed with this observation.

A gluten-free diet is often prescribed for women with infertility problems, so infertility in at least some women may be due to underlying allergy problems, or intolerance of those FODMAPs referred to earlier (see page 348). Infertility in animals can be a third or fourth generation result of poor nutrition, or a marker of contamination with pollutants or oestrogen analogues. And if infertile women were exposed early to bovine protein, that is likely to be one of many allergens. However, infertility is also linked with lacking sufficient body fat reserves: female athletes pared down to excessive leanness can stop menstruating altogether, as do many starved women in war and famine. Gaining some weight may be all that is necessary for conception, avoiding complex hormonal manipulations.

So a history of IVF *may* signal a greater likelihood of allergy being involved in the problem. But none of these factors is a determining cause so far as we know, and infertility has many causes: a fallopian tube blocked by past infection is perhaps less likely to be associated with immune consequences than, say, immune reactions against partner sperm.

A history of excessive weight gain in pregnancy, or overweight generally, has been associated in some studies with a higher risk of allergy.[1793] However, once again maternal obesity may be a carry-over from the mother's programming by infant formula in the previous generation, a second generation consequence of allergy.

### Question 12-14 Bovine protein intake and food likes and dislikes

12.     Either a lot or a little can suggest addiction or aversion.

13.     Milk during pregnancy can be significant for mother and child alike.

14.     Liked and disliked foods in pregnancy.

These three questions are only indicators – small red flags. If you either binged on or avoided some foods, it may be a sign of reactivity. Your reasons for disliking foods can be many and varied, and have little to do with adverse physical reactions. Your tolerance level and dose response can vary widely. But awareness of foods you like and dislike excessively during pregnancy can suggest caution with excess intakes. When breastfeeding, this awareness can help provide a logical starting point for dietary elimination, together with other clues.

### Question 15-16 Pregnancy foods and aversions

Great if you find yourself instinctively avoiding chemical-laden food, red wine, coffee, etcetera: your protective systems are working well. Not so good if you find yourself craving these! It would suggest that you are habituated to them and they may affect the baby you are gestating, especially if you are out of control and simply 'must have' some food often or in excess. Don't force yourself to eat 'good foods' like milk or egg or liver or fish, or cultural tonics, if they make you feel ill when you smell or taste them. Pregnancy nausea and vomiting can be linked to diet. Noses are above mouths to be used: learn to smell before you eat, and pay attention to how your body reacts. Some experience an immediate sense of nausea, or headache, triggered by the smell of foods they react to.

---

1793 Collado MC, Laitinen K, Salminen S, Isolauri E. Maternal weight and excessive weight gain during pregnancy modify the immunomodulatory potential of breast milk. (PMID:22453296) *Pediatr Res* 2012; 72(1):77-85

## Question 17 Pregnancy-related symptoms

Many pregnancy symptoms switch off instantly when diets change, and so do recurrent premenstrual migraines, for example. Hormonal changes can alter allergic symptoms and responses, as tolerance thresholds can vary over time. Puberty, pregnancy, lactation, menstruation, ovulation, menopause, times of emotional stress: all can affect symptom expression: migraines can appear reliably before each period, for example. Notice how your body works and record it, because it makes sense over time, and you won't always remember details ...

# Where you have siblings and/or other children
## Question 18 Siblings and/or other children

Adult siblings' problems often give clues to yours, and may disclose likely early feeding clues, if grandparents are not available or are reluctant to talk. They can also suggest genetic tendencies: an uncle with eczema or diabetes or coeliac disease may simply be a victim of his environment, but no allergist is surprised when certain allergy symptoms recur in families.

Some genes have been linked with allergy. But even sharing the same genes for particular problems does not mean those problems must emerge: nutrition and the environment affect gene expression, so those genes may be switched on in one child and off in another. Genomes are unique and so are their expressions. Siblings within any family can vary widely, as their whole experience of life is in fact very different from one another, both physically and emotionally, within an ever-changing family environment.

Short (under two years) interbirth intervals can leave some mothers relatively nutrient-depleted and more at risk of symptoms including depression, where there is a big diet link, so that a second child born very soon after the first may be affected by this. Omega-3 long chain polyunsaturated fatty acids (LCPUFAs), magnesium and zinc, vitamin D and B complex vitamins are reported as helpful, and there is some evidence that babies benefit. In any family, the firstborn usually has the best pantry to grow on – but equally, the first-born of a mother who loses a lot of weight post-partum can be exposed to the mother's lifetime load of contaminants to date, and will help reduce these both for subsequent babies and for the mother.[1794] The intra-uterine environment affects infant allergy risk: high total IgE levels at birth are predictive of 'allergy', though not determinant.

When mothers cannot replenish their nutrient stores between pregnancies, allergy symptoms seem to worsen with subsequent children and the  increasing maternal workload. So second and third children can be better or worse than the first, depending on such factors. Eggs, meat and fatty fish can supply useful nutrients for post-partum women. Optimal pre-conception and pregnancy nutrition is important in allergic families.

---

1794  For many, this conjures up fears of breastmilk poisoning babies, and the media loves this scare story. Not all maternal contaminants are taken up by the baby: much will have been detoxified and excreted by the mother. See Chapter 3.9 for discussion of pollutants.

Depression or a highly stressed pregnancy may result in sibling differences as well. The age of the mother and the sex and birth order of the child may also influence how inherited tendencies are expressed. A properly planned study of allergy in siblings would not hope to compare children as though the family environment was unchanged: that is comparing apples with oranges, when the study would also need to include details and analysis of a whole fruit salad of confounding factors.

### Question 19–24 Sibling/children intakes and symptoms

As adults with shared parentage, and even shared cells (see page 29), siblings' experiences with food can be of some – but limited – relevance and help provide clues as to where to begin. If you grew up together, your shared memories will help to provide more clues. One may remember the other hating oatmeal or loathing eggs at some point in time, for example.

It helps to know that other family members understand and do not see talk of allergy as hypochondria. It also helps to have people who can be trusted with your children's diets. But don't take that for granted: make sure anyone caring for your allergic child understands the consequences of dietary indiscretion, which are often delayed, so that the person feeding your child does not see the symptoms they trigger.

### Question 25 Other reactions

Food-sensitive people usually react to other environmental stressors, and vice versa: people sensitive to airborne allergens usually have some food sensitivities, in my experience. Thus if fragrances give you a headache, for example, or you feel your chest tightening when exposed to aerosols, it does suggest that there may be other stressors you react to, and chief among them is likely to be food.

Is this ringing any bells for you? Are you feeling that some of this describes you or your family? After completing the questionnaire, take time to consider whether allergy is likely in your case. These notes are just the tip of an iceberg, and the questionnaire is a simple preliminary exercise for you to gather background information *before* you consider the issues underlying your baby's misery.

Now, let's focus on the persistently crying young baby (who just might have a red umbilicus, which can a diagnostic sign of cows' milk protein intolerance[1795]).

---

1795  Iacono G, di Prima L, D'Amico D et al. The "red umbilicus": a diagnostic sign of cows' milk protein intolerance. *JPGN* 2006; 42: 531-534.

# 4.2 Dealing with a persistently miserable baby

*While there are many references to older children and adults, I am just focussing on the very early days of life, in the first year. Why? There are good books available for childhood and adult allergy; but above all, because at this age it is possible to intervene and prevent worse problems – of allergy and distorted relationships – emerging. (Or seem to prevent them: it's impossible to prove prevention of a non-occurrence! The proof is in the changed behaviours, emotions and sleep patterns before and after dietary changes. Unbelievers can always say that the passage of time is the sole explanation. Parents – who've usually tried a dozen things beforehand - don't believe them. Life will provide enough unexpected exposures to convince the family.)*

Babies can communicate, and crying is their most powerful means. The difference between life in the womb and outside is huge, and babies have a lot of adjusting to do. (So do even the best-prepared of parents, as every baby is unique.) It will take babies time to settle into their new reality, to feel secure in this bright, new, noisy, constantly-changing environment, to settle into sleep-wake patterns that leave them refreshed and happy to explore the new world. (It may also take varying quantities of the hormone rich 'night milk' science has just discovered to be slightly different from milk produced during the day.[1796]) Similarly, it will take parents time to adjust to the constant stimulus to their emotions, the re-centering of their lives, and inroads into their time and sleep, that even the happiest of babies creates.

There are many reasons why babies cry, and many skills parents have to learn to help them feel confident navigating this new world. It helps parents to have experienced mentors who can model humane ways of dealing with infant distress effectively, who can teach parents the 'mothercraft' skills of settling babies which many have never seen, not being part of large caring families from childhood onwards. (Not, I hasten to add, the bullying Mothercraft of some schools of rigid training, in which babies are treated in ways that animal welfare organisations would condemn for puppies or kittens!) However, while touching on some of those skills, this book will not go into detail about the many more than 'one hundred ways to stop the crying.'[1797] There are good books and websites out there that focus on palliative strategies, and I mention these in the Bibliography.

**This chapter deals with a sub-set of crying babies - principally babies whose sleep is disturbed and whose crying is erratic, persistent, prolonged, and heartbreaking:**

- who are either hyperactive before, and persistently miserable after birth, or
- who start screaming in the second or third week of life, and
    - who give many indications of gut discomfort,
    - who progressively develop other minor symptoms, like night sweats, cradle cap, or patches of rough dry skin
    - who do not respond more than briefly to mothercraft skills.

---

1796  I hope this doesn't start another irritating fad, as talk of foremilk and hind milk did. Remember if babies determine the timing and duration of their feeds, and are growing well on it, they will be getting what they need, whether that's day or night milk! (Or is that asleep and awake milk? Any differences between owls and larks?) This will vary between cultures and families.

1797  The title of Pinky McKay's helpful book for mothers of distressed infants. See bibliography.

These are babies likely to be allergic. Their parents instinctively think there must be something wrong: babies ought to be happy and healthy and growing when fed mother's milk, and they should sleep. I believe that parental instinct is sound. Even in conditions of poverty, most fully breastfed babies thrive (unless there is an overwhelming medical condition, of course) and they don't waste energy and valuable nutrients crying incessantly. Crying is a survival strategy, and babies are tough little survivors who cry for a reason. Babies rapidly stop crying once convinced by experience that their needs are being met in a timely way, and they then explore a whole repertoire of charming noises and behaviours that enchant their carers. Mothers of happily breastfed babies recognise the little waking-up noises that indicate it's soon going to be feed time, and get baby to the breast before he or she has any reason to sound distressing alarm calls. And so, well-fed, and happy, babies grow.

Growth and activity may falter after six months in poor communities, if adequate complementary foods are not available (see Chapter 6.5 What are 'good quality complementary foods'?) But young fully breastfed babies of poor families look a picture of plump, even roly-poly health. And they are contented, so that to hear a baby cry is unusual, a cause for concern or negative comment, and a cause for action.

People from traditional communities judge any parents to be shockingly neglectful if they ignore infant cries. An Australian father of four teaching in rural Laos in the 1990s was shocked to realise – on returning to an urban shopping mall in Thailand – that for many months he had not once heard a baby crying as they do in Western cultures, and he found the crying deeply distressing. In Australia he had learned to screen it out as usual. Another volunteer in Thailand said that the only babies she heard crying when in Thailand were babies of Westerners, who have been brainwashed to think crying normal. I suspect that will have changed as artificial feeding has increased in Asia! Doctors and magazines alike will hasten to reassure them that such misery is normal, the more usual it becomes. And affluent parents will escape the distressing noise by putting babies into the care of other people, who may find it equally distressing, but easier to ignore.

Of course there are many other cultural and environmental differences that help to explain the typical Western baby's misery. In countries like Laos few babies are left for long periods day or night without contact with a friendly human body. In conditions where being left alone is a risk to survival, all members of the family, even siblings, carry the infant around, and babies sleep with other people. They did so in Western communities until very recently: in cold British houses babies slept in servants' or family beds, while in poor dwellings everyone shared beds. (And yes, there were occasional overlying deaths, but not the epidemic of infant deaths artificial feeding would bring!) Being in arms or in contact with another living body has multiple positive benefits for infants.

But for the allergic breastfed baby, even being held constantly may not calm the crying. Usually I am called in to help mothers when a baby is crying inconsolably, or sleeping very poorly, and parents are at their wits' end. Sometimes I see an older child or parent so obviously allergic that before they speak I know the baby's misery is due to intergenerational allergy problems.[1798] But naturally, only going through the discovery process themselves will convince the parents.

# The abnormal usual Western baby

Babies have always cried when they need to, and always will. Intense and persistent infant crying is a universal language of distress. Only in the Westernised world of the nineteenth to twenty-first centuries has this sort of crying been classified as 'normal' infant behaviour. So brainwashed are we now that some parents express real concern about the placid plump breastfed baby who never cries – the child I consider normal. Yet I suspect that even today the majority of human beings alive on the planet know in their gut that intense and persistent distress is abnormal for an otherwise healthy child.

Infant crying affects all who have not been brainwashed into thinking of it as normal: watch how small children react even to a stranger's baby crying in the supermarket. We are programmed to respond to our offspring's distress; it takes conscious effort to ignore it. Normal crying quickly stops when you find the cause and fix it. I find that Western twentieth-century inconsolable and persistent crying does too, if we pay babies the respect they deserve and *take the time to find the cause*, rather than try to condition a baby to 'self-soothe' (or give up expecting comfort from others) by studied avoidance or control techniques.

I prefer finding causes to exposing the child to dubious solutions, from chemical-laden 'pacifiers' (rightly called dummies)[1799] to chemical sedation, whether by opioid peptides in cows' milk or misused antihistamines, analgesics, and anti-inflammatories, all with unpredictable impacts on struggling young bodies, certainly microbiomes, perhaps especially on kidneys and livers.

I prefer finding causes to going down the common but dangerous path of treating symptoms like reflux as stand-alone diagnoses, and prescribing powerful gut-altering medications that for some make matters worse.

I prefer finding causes to resorting to explanations involving maternal anxiety which, in the absence of any real ongoing help, only lead to mothers blaming themselves, being even more anxious, and becoming depressed. Mothers should be reassured that some anxiety is

---

1798 As I have grown older and more experienced, I have become capable of informing complete strangers that they don't have to suffer the miseries of an obviously hyperactive brain-scrambled child, and that they too are likely to lose symptoms if they sort out their child's physical problem. Then there are the adults who complain of their distressed gut or constant skin problems or tendency to come down with everything... I talk to them about 'allergy' too. One of my nonagenarian mother's carers was a woman whose story was an endless round of specialists, trying to sort out a huge variety of 'allergy'-related problems never diagnosed as such. A half-hour delay in her leaving Mum, while I took her through her dietary history, has led to dramatic improvements in her health and happiness. She tells me I was literally an answer to her prayer! People listen and identify; many of them make the effort to change; and those who do, seem to benefit. Because it's all common sense. And it often works. Try it!

1799 Again, notice how language is used to either encourage or discourage use of a product our distant ancestors never needed, when the breast was the universal 'pacifier'.

normal, even though it can become pathological. (And is manipulated by vested interests to sell unnecessary products as "nutritional insurance.")

I prefer finding causes of infant distress to parents hardening their hearts and thinking of their tiny babies as 'difficult' or temperamental *or manipulative*, which can do untold harm to family and social relationships. Many firstborns live with that burden for decades. More on that later.

So with this sub-set of crying babies, what's needed is a process that works through other likely explanations first, before considering whether allergy is involved. There are many things to keep in mind throughout the entire process, and other potential causes of distress to rule out. I found that such a process evolved from clinical practice, and it's summarised in the following table and spelt out in more detail below. But before we get to dealing with allergy, there are some other key factors to focus on.

*(Given the primary audience for this book, what follows is written as advice for the person assisting the family, hopefully a well-informed health professional. But of course many families do work through these issues for themselves, as I did, almost four decades ago now. And these factors are all interactive and interlocked, so need to be addressed simultaneously.)*

## First focus: resolving any breastfeeding problem

The first thing to do *always* is to identify and resolve any breastfeeding problems the mother is having. Her milk supply is crucial to her baby's health and growth; her health is important to her coping with a demanding baby. (And both are important to her own mental state, of course. Solving any breastfeeding problems usually reduces maternal anxiety, and improves confidence and mental well-being, often dramatically.)

Even if solving a breastfeeding problem like nipple pain doesn't stop the baby crying, if it helps the mother, it will help protect breastfeeding and prevent formula being introduced, and so almost certainly prevent more serious problems emerging. Besides, continued lactation maintains the mother in a favourable hormonal state that means she will feel better, sleep better, and be better able to cope with her distressed baby. The mother matters in her own right, not just because she affects the baby – but she does affect the baby as well, just as the baby affects her. So deal first with any immediate distress that threatens breastfeeding.

Asking about, and sometimes watching, feeds is essential: how often, how comfortable, how does baby behave before, during and after feeds, intervals between feeds, sleep-wake patterns; it all gives a picture that may suggest why baby is crying. Any good infant feeding consultant can interpret these behaviours. Any health professionals who can't, need to get educated, or to move out of work involving mothers and babies; without adequate knowledge of lactation, they are dangerously incompetent. My earlier book, *Breastfeeding matters*, deals with these issues, and a good reference text such as ABA's *Breastfeeding management in Australia* or Ruth Lawrence's *Breastfeeding: a guide for the medical profession* should be part of every professional library. Simple texts like Renfrew's

*Bestfeeding,* Nylander's *Becoming a mother,* or Welford's *Successful infant feeding* are helpful. And referring to the protocols on the website of the Academy of Breastfeeding Medicine would always be a useful starting point for doctors. (Go to www.breastfeeding.asn)

## Second focus: the need for support of parents, especially mothers

Many breastfeeding problems stem from the mother's perinatal experiences.[1800] Difficulties with breastfeeding can be the cause of maternal depression, due to both mental and physical impacts: and what sane person wouldn't become stressed and depressed when everything hurts, the baby is miserable, and restful sleep is non-existent?

Maintaining breastfeeding is paramount because that's the best treatment for an allergic baby, if this should prove to be one. It is also important to maternal physical and mental health. The interactions between mother and child are complex and definitely two-way traffic: giving up breastfeeding can lead to depression, even psychosis and maternal suicide,[1801] while depression can also lead to giving up breastfeeding. Giving up breastfeeding can sometimes seem attractive, meaning others can share the burden of night feeding, but often the baby's condition worsens when allergy is involved (sometimes not until a week or so has passed.) Sleep is a critical variable for parental coping and mood management. Minding a baby while a mother catches up on some sleep is an excellent preventive health strategy! So is education about safe co-sleeping - see page 577.

Finding out about the family's support networks is therefore important. An unsupported mother is more likely to become depressed and give up breastfeeding. *Sevrage* or weaning, the end of any breastfeeding, can be the start of a vicious cycle in which the depressed mother spirals downwards as her lactation-produced coping hormone levels drop, and as her baby's misery increases in response to both the loss of breastfeeding and the mother's depressed behaviour. *Not* to the mother's depressed mental state, per se – babies are not psychic mind-readers – but to the way the mother behaves and handles the baby. If she is depressed, she may withdraw, and want to avoid the baby, who is associated with her distress. Her own – or her partner's - handling may generate infant insecurity if movements are abrupt or rough, or they fail to speak or sing to the baby. Conversely, anxious parents may be intrusive and over-stimulatory, not recognising the cues the baby gives for needing rest and sleep. How people act can be different when they are depressed.

The distinction between being affected by parental *mood* and parental *behaviour* is a crucial one. To varying extents parents can control *what they do* if they know that their behaviour matters, even when they cannot control *how they feel*. Humans are not locked into expressing our feelings in our every action: up to the point where we lose touch with reality and are

1800  Humenick SS, Howell OS. Perinatal Experiences: The Association of Stress, Childbearing, Breastfeeding, and Early Mothering. *J Perinat Educ* 2003; 12(3): 16–41. doi: 10.1624/105812403X106937. PMCID: PMC1595161
1801  Reeves RR, Pinkofsky HB. Postpartum psychosis induced by bromocriptine and pseudoephedrine. (PMID:9267376) *J Fam Pract* 1997; 45(2):164-166; Iffy L, Lindenthal J, Szodi Z, Griffin W. Puerperal psychosis following ablaction with bromocriptine. (PMID:2516595) *Med Law* 1989; 8(2):171-174.

truly psychotic, we have a brain and some self-control. Yes, there are incredibly sensitive feedback loops between mothers and babies, and some we can't easily control, like levels of cortisol in milk. But parents can and do learn coping techniques if given even some support to do so. Most people manage to do just that *when they know they have to*. And people can grow stronger and more competent and confident by trying to do what they realise they must, and so discovering that they can. Consider what humans have survived in the twentieth century, and what refugees got through!

We need consciously to use such coping techniques even when this is a struggle; and not just as a noble sacrifice for the baby's sake (though this is a good enough reason by itself) but for our own sake. Self-discipline is needed by all parents, perhaps especially in societies where self-indulgence may be the prevailing cultural ethos, and parents are not getting the social support and endorsement and modelling needed to manage children humanely. While handling the baby, the parent who consciously makes her/himself act, as if calm and happy - with consciously gentle touch, controlled movements, steady breathing, and calm voice - may find that these positive actions help create positive emotions. Our feelings can influence our behaviour – and our behaviour can also influence our feelings. It is important to break negative feedback loops. And most people can, with empathetic support, and time out for reflection, meditation, yoga, sleep, venting with friends, whatever helps. (Because a reliable income is basic to parental mental well-being, health advocates ought also be advocates for social justice. )

Medications prescribed for depression can have complex effects[1802] and should never be prescribed lightly,[1803] whether or not a breastfed baby is involved.[1804] And thyroid problems should always be ruled out before other medications are considered. Breastfeeding is important in creating secure attachment bonds between mother and child, and in creating mutuality and sensitive responsiveness.[1805] Drugs that interfere with brain function have unpredictable consequences. Kathleen Kendall-Tackett has written an excellent monograph on depression in new mothers[1806] and another on non-pharmacologic treatments for depression.[1807] Wherever possible, the latter might be tried before heavy-duty psychoactive medication, needed for extreme psychosis.

Brilliant UK sociologist and feminist Ann Oakley once said something like, women are considered bad or mad when they are sad ... and talked of the harms done by trying to medicate people out of sadness when their lives are such as to make any sane person sad.

1802  Breggin P. Op. cit. A truly essential reference for those on psychiatric medication, or thinking of taking it.
1803  Reading Green A. *Saving Normal* (William Heinemann 2013) along with Peter Breggin's book will cure those who reach for medication too quickly.
1804  Buist A. Treating mental illness in lactating women. (PMID:11547266). *Medscape Womens Health* 2001; 6(2):3
1805  Tharner A, Luijk MP, Raat H, Ijzendoorn MH et al. *Breastfeeding and its relation to maternal sensitivity and infant attachment.* (PMID:22580735) *J Dev Behav Pediatr* 2012, 33(5):396-404.
1806  Kendall-Tackett K. *Depression in New Mothers: causes, consequences and treatment options.* (Routledge Paul, London 2010). Kendall-Tackett K. A new paradigm for depression in new mothers: the central role of inflammation and how breastfeeding and anti-inflammatory treatments protect maternal mental health. (PMID:17397549) Free full text article *Int Breastfeed J* 2007; 2:6.Open access article. See also Groer M, Kendall-Tackett K. *How Breastfeeding Protects Women's Health* op. cit.
1807  Kendall-Tackett K. *Non-pharmacologic treatments*, op. cit.

To feel happy when your life is a disaster is to be psychotic, out of touch with reality. Yet medication can sometimes be life saving, and there can be tragic outcomes if women fail to take medications they really need, as the death of one young mother attests. Read her story in this excellent open access journal, and weep.[1808] But drugs *alone* solve no problem.

*All* new mothers need – and deserve – social and emotional and practical support, and will suffer without it. Some vocal bottle-feeding parents seem to think that they alone have been unsupported, but they are dreaming: very few breastfeeding mothers get the support they need either, as the thirty per cent drop in breastfeeding rates in the first month makes clear to anyone interested. Rather than assailing those who try to help mothers breastfeed, women unable to breastfeed (for whatever reason) need to make common cause with those who want to change the society that ensured that they bottle-fed – and handed on unknown epigenetic changes to their descendants.

# Third focus: practical problems that can cause crying –other than allergy.

Even if the questionnaire suggests that parents are dealing with severe allergy issues, there are numerous other possible causes of distress to rule out or deal with. Doing so may reduce infant crying to the point where there is no need to consider allergy. The first seven of these points are not sequential; they can be tackled in any order and all at once.

### 1. Is baby crying because of too little breastmilk?

The best proof of adequate intake is adequate growth. Checking the child's growth across centile charts from birth is important. (However, we need to remember that some birth weights are artificially inflated by fluids absorbed during labour: some would argue that weight at 24 hours, when the extra fluid load has diminished, should be taken as the starting point for calculating gains or losses.[1809] That would reduce unnecessary concerns and comp feeds.)

Some miserable crying babies are just the hungry ones still active enough to protest, demanding more frequent, or longer, or more effective, feeds. Many mothers wrongly think that frequent feeding of young babies should not be necessary. It isn't – for *some* babies and mothers. It is when babies have small inelastic stomachs, or the mother has little breast

---

1808 Amir LH, *Ryan KM*, Jordan SE. Avoiding risk at what cost? putting use of medicines for breastfeeding women into perspective. *Int Breastfeed* J. 2012; 7(1):14. Epub ahead of print.; McDonald K, Amir LH, Davey MA Maternal bodies and medicines: a commentary on risk and decision-making of pregnant and breastfeeding women. (PMID:22168473) *BMC Public Health* 2011, 11 Suppl 5:S5. http://www.ncbi.nlm.nih.gov/pmc/articles/PMC3502159/

1809 Noel-Weiss J, Woodend AK, Groll DL Iatrogenic newborn weight loss: knowledge translation using a study protocol for your maternity setting. (PMID:21843331) *Int Breastfeed J* 2011, 6(1):10.; Noel-Weiss J, Woodend AK, Peterson WE et al. An observational study of associations among maternal fluids during parturition, neonatal output, and breastfed newborn weight loss. (PMID: 21843338) *Int Breastfeed J* 2011, 6:9.; Noel-Weiss J, Courant G, Woodend AK. Physiological weight loss in the breastfed neonate: a systematic review. *Open Med* 2008, 2(4):e99-e110.(PMID: 21602959)

storage capacity, which is not always easily judged by the size of the breast. A small tank needs refilling more often than a large one, but both can take you the same driving distance.

Ruling out hunger due to infrequent feeding, or too little milk being consumed, is easily done, and a first step. Often this is as simple as fixing the way the baby takes the breast, so that feeds are more effective, and baby then goes longer between feeds. Hungry babies stop crying and focus on feeding when they are being fed. They may not want to let go if they still feel hungry and have not got enough to feel satiated. They may let go, but search for the breast a short time later. If they want to feed, feed them.

If ineffective feeding has reduced mother's milk supply, increasing milk volume is easily done if parents (and those supporting them) understand the governing mechanisms and interactive feedback loops involved in milk production and regulation. The amount and rate of milk synthesis are both governed by the degree of breast emptying, with the breast sensitive to both internal pressure and a constituent that accumulates when and where the breast is not being well-drained.  If milk is not taken out, more milk will not be made after an interval, and gradually glandular tissue will regress. More frequent and more effective feeding increases supply;  all food from other sources reduces demand and so affects supply. The emptier the breast (it is never really empty), the faster the rate of milk synthesis and breast re-filling, and the more fat-rich the milk. So when the baby stays at the breast getting only small amounts, the caloric value of the milk may be higher. Milk from the second breast starts out more fat-rich than milk from the first, because the ejection reflex has squeezed some fat into the milk. So avoid one-breast feeding: always offer the second, and go back to the other side as many times as you like, provided that the baby has been allowed to finish the first breast and come off. One hint: warm the breast not being used to increase blood flow into it, and with that nutrients for milk making, to increase synthesis rates.

There's more to it all than this, of course. Any reliable breastfeeding literature will go through these issues: look online for that produced by breastfeeding mothers' support groups or a book like *Bestfeeding*, by experienced midwives.[1810] I intend to get my book *Breastfeeding Matters* updated and online, but it is still available in paperback. Ignore any advice linked to vested interests like formula companies, or stray online videos: one I spotted on YouTube, far from being helpful, is a recipe for agonisingly sore nipples. So too is an undiagnosed tongue-tie, not uncommon and easily remedied in a young baby, with more efficient feeding the usual outcome. Get help from an accredited breastfeeding counsellor or knowledgeable health professional.

## 2. Is baby crying because of too much breastmilk?

Equally, ruling out the chicken and egg situation of oversupply and excess infant intake is important. These babies are overfull, uncomfortably so, and cry. In the past they were probably diagnosed as 'overfed.' Over-feeding was seen as relatively common among breastfed babies in the first half of the 20th century, and led to restrictions and scheduled

---

1810  Renfrew M, Fisher C, Arms S. *Bestfeeding: getting breastfeeding right for you.* (Celestial Arts Press 2004)

feeds that often caused under-feeding! Nowadays some people talk about transient lactose overload. More on this in Chapter 5.1.

### 3. Is it something quite simple like a painful bottom or skin problems?

Sometimes other simple causes of infant irritability are overlooked.

- Being too hot can make anyone grumpy. Babies can be, swathed in layers of synthetic clothing and blankets. (See below, *4. Is it minor dehydration?*)

- Feeling cold can cause a baby to seek contact with breasts, which instinctively get warmer when baby needs warmth.[1811]

- Smoked-over babies are more likely to cry and be diagnosed with colic (and breastfeeding reduces the risk of colic).[1812]

- Tight nappies or sling straps can cause discomfort. Check for pressure marks, and be sure baby is held upright and can breathe well in the sling, not being compressed into a curve with chin on chest and airways and swallowing obstructed. Some slings can be unsafe.

- Sore gums can cause pain and irritability. Check for thrush, and teething.

- So can sore bottoms or any other irritated, itchy or crusted skin. Babies' skin is thinner than adult skin, and very sensitive. It is exposed to many chemicals, both applied and in fabrics. Even saliva with its food residues can cause irritation, as can the by-products of digestion in urine or poo. So a short digression about skin problems follows.

- Or it might be a minor pain. Take off all their clothes to ensure nothing is hurting them. One mother who did so found that her baby's toe was caught in some elastic of the babysuit she was wearing. Even a hair can become trapped around a digit and cause painful swelling.

- No one knows if babies can have headaches: more on that later.

## Skin problems: a practical aside

Reddened skin anywhere means inflammation. Wash with mild soap and water, then rinse off residues with clean water and dry gently, adding a very thin protective inert skin barrier like highly purified anhydrous lanolin. (I would have suggested old-fashioned white zinc cream – *not* the new invisible zinc creams with nanoparticles[1813] – except that it may contain castor seed or peanut oil and not be labelled as doing so. And while an occasional light smear is useful, some zinc cream does seem to dry out and leave residues, where pure lanolin does not.) Ultra refined lanolin is closer to human sebum than any other available option. Any petroleum-based product like Vaseline seems likely to do the job but also to

1811 Kimura C, Matsuoka M. Changes in breast skin temperature during the course of breastfeeding. (PMID:17293552) *J Hum Lact* 2007;23(1):60-69.

1812 Shenassa ED, Brown MJ. Maternal **smoking** and infantile gastrointestinal dysregulation: the case of **colic.** (PMID:15466076) *Pediatrics* 2004, 114(4):e497-505

1813 Too little is known about absorption and where these particles might end up with what effect for these to be used on infants, with their super-fine skin. See Cattaneo AG, Gornati R, Sabbioni E, Chiriva-Internati M et al. *Nanotechnology and human health: risks and benefits.*(PMID:21117037) *J Appl Toxicol* 2010, 30(8):730-744.

carry traces of its origins and processing. By contrast, ultra-purified lanolin has had wool alcohols and detergent and pesticide residues removed, and only the smallest smear is necessary. Cheaper unpurified lanolin-base products can be just as effective in reducing inflammation, but are unwise for infants: one paw-paw cream with a lanolin base was found to contain neurotoxic pesticide residues from sheep-dips, while tea-tree oil is a potent allergen in its own right.

An inert barrier cream will usually make a big difference, whether the inflammation is caused by chemicals or allergens. Using cortisone-containing creams also works wonders, but at a price: the risk of suppressed local immunity and greater risk of infection in the area. Steroids can be invaluable in allergic skin conditions but should never be used for minor problems. Skin microbiomes are like gut microbiomes, complex eco-systems that should be disturbed as little as possible. Broken or damaged skin provides opportunities for infection, usually by skin bacteria or fungi, which are entirely normal and naturally present in everyone, but harmful if they overgrow. They also increase the risk of sensitisation to food allergens.

Fungal infections such as *Candida* strains  (C. Albicans is commonly called thrush) can cause skin irritation. Dilute gentian violet (half a per cent to one per cent at most where available) can be useful though messy, if any fungal or bacterial infection has colonised damaged skin.[1814] As Dr Richard Goldbloom said,

> ... for many years before Nystatin strode onto the therapeutic stage, the sovereign remedy for oral thrush was 1% aqueous gentian viole tpainted in the infant's mouth. Cost: next to nothing. Efficacy: works like a charm ...Whenever the response of oral thrush to Nystatin has been less than stunning (not uncommon) I've reverted to my ancient violaceous ways with rapid, gratifying results.'[1815]

Though 2% gentian violet can cause skin damage, I've used this dilute purple paint for almost forty years. It works really well to clean up viral (chicken pox eg) lesions as well as fungal and bacterial problems. It can be bought over the counter in America, or in many other countries; it is only available in Australia on prescription, and via veterinarians.

Some mothers have found that expressed breastmilk is healing, while others have seen babies' skin react to antigens it contains. In seriously inflamed skin creases, a simple way of reducing inflammation can be to use a damp piece of plain, well-washed silk or very fine cotton to keep skin surfaces from touching, with a thin smear of ultrapurified lanolin to keep the cloth from adhering to any damaged skin. Moisten this well (preferably with chlorine-free water) before taking it off and replacing with a clean piece at each nappy change, if

---

1814 This can be purchased over the counter in many countries, the US and Singapore included. So when transiting via Changi, I always pick up some bottles. Knowledgeable GPs and pharmacists can also supply it, as can vets. It is excellent for any fungal, bacterial or viral skin infections, although hard to obtain in Australia after one US study showed that mice which ate it in chow for more than 75% of their lifespan developed more liver cancers than mice which ate it for less than 75%. How seriously to take that was evident when the FDA allowed confectionery manufacturers to go on using it in lollies/sweets, after banning it for occasional topical use by everyone... except surgeons, who use it to mark where they cut into skin!!

1815 *Pediatric Notes* 1997; 21: 6. Cited in *ALCA News*, 1997; 8 (1): 49.

the inflammation is in the genital area. In other areas, go by what seems reasonable. In hot weather this cloth will be changed more often than in cooler weather. (This works well for mothers with under-breast irritation or chafing too. It absorbs and dilutes chemicals and antigens in sweat and prevents skin chafing.)

## 4. Is it minor dehydration?

In Norway, I heard Dr Rolf Lindemann urge mothers to consider how easily babies can become overheated and thus fretful because they are slightly dehydrated and thirsty. (Dehydration can cause headaches in adults, perhaps also in children.) They are often warmly clad in hot interiors or prams, or swathed in unbreathing synthetic fabrics, or held in slings that restrict airflow and evaporation. He pointed out that instinctively swaying with babies helped to cool them by increasing evaporation, and recommended absorbent natural fibres (cotton, silk and fine wools) that breathe, along with reducing their clothing when baby is in a sling against an adult body, or taken from a cold place to a warm interior such as a heated shop or home. I have seen no research on bamboo fibre clothing for infants.

If a child has sweated excessively, so that clothes are wet with sweat but nappies dry, or urine is yellow rather than clear, and the mother finds a breastfeed isn't settling the child, a small drink of safe boiled and filtered water by teaspoon or cup can be indicated, and will do little harm. Unlike bottle-fed babies, breastfed babies absolutely don't need extra water even in the hottest climates[1816]. But if a sudden extreme water loss – such as being found saturated in sweat on an electric blanket, in one case I have known- causes thirst, a few mouthfuls of water can help immediately, as a mother's breastmilk supply takes a little while to respond. Of course any such babies should be at the breast as often as they wish, both to boost supply and to satisfy thirst. The breast is the best place for all grizzling babies, with breastfeeding rightly named as "stillen" in German.

## 5. Is it sensory deprivation?

Lack of physical contact with a known and comforting body can cause young babies to become distressed. Isolation of young infants is unnatural, not something humans could risk in the evolutionary environment or in conditions of poverty.[1817] Cuddles are comforting. And via oxytocin, cuddles evoke positive physical responses in stressed mothers as well. Slings are sanity savers for many parents. (However, they will not stop a baby with a serious gut-ache from crying.[1818]) Sleeping with your breastfed baby is normal and can be safe: check out the Mother-Baby Behavioral Sleep Laboratory, University of Notre Dame at www.cosleeping.nd.edu

---

1816 In August 1991 WHO Geneva's Control of Diarrhoeal Diseases Unit published an update: *Breastfeeding and the use of Water and Teas,* which concluded that such fluids were unnecessary and potentially harmful for the exclusively breastfed baby. Online at https://apps.who.int/chd/publications/newslet/update/updt-09.htm

1817 Babies left alone in slums are at risk of rat bites even today. And even in middle class homes the tragedy of animal bites does occur: in the UK both foxes and dogs have bitten babies in their own home. Animals can see a child as a tasty dinner.

1818 Barr RG, McMullan SJ, Spiess H, et al. Carrying as colic "therapy": a randomized controlled trial.'*Pediatrics*›1991;87(5):623-630

## 6. Is it over-stimulation?

Some babies can become overstressed by noise and sensation, and need quiet, calm handling, however noisy the environment. Parents need to recognise tired cues and allow babies to rest. Visitors need to respect the baby's biorhythms and not expect the child to be passed around like a toy for their entertainment. Slings that hold baby upright against parents' bodies can provide security, postural stability, and calm the child as he or she feels the familiar rhythms of a human body. When less distressed the baby can be left to sleep in safe, quiet familiar surroundings. We all know how grumpy we can become after broken sleep: either don't let other people disturb the sleeping baby, or else don't be surprised if this makes baby similarly grumpy because of disrupted biorhythms. Bodies set their own rhythms for sleep and waking, rest and activity, and not respecting these can cause distress. Every parent knows that after a big day out with no familiar pattern adhered to, some small babies are just overtired and need calm the next day. As well, it is impossible to know if a small baby or pre-verbal child has a headache. But no headache is improved by loud noise or rough handling and being joggled about.

## 7. Are there any unrecognised medical causes?

Despite medical oversight, there may be an undiagnosed painful problem, even an overlooked fracture from birth (it happens!), headache from muscle spasm in a tight neck or from meningitis, a urinary tract infection, an ear infection, or an invasive gut pathogen at work, even gut obstruction. Go back to the doctor if you feel something is wrong.

Parents should particularly note when the crying started in relation to any unusual event, such as administration of vaccines, perhaps especially live viruses going into the gut like rotavirus. (There are many parental reports of gut disturbance after that vaccine given at six weeks, not so many after oral polio vaccines. Some parents have become ill with rotavirus themselves, as live virus is clearly shed by the baby in its poo, just as the polio virus is shed. It is at least debateable whether a fully breastfed child needs that rotavirus vaccine at 6 weeks, but if a reaction occurs, it might be wise not to repeat the exposure.) There is more on vaccination in Chapter 2.6.

Ideally, any persistently unhappy baby will have been checked by an experienced child health nurse and a doctor, such medical causes of distress eliminated, and coping strategies that protect breastfeeding suggested. If that hasn't already happened, parents need to be encouraged to see their child health nurse or doctor. Almost all will have been to the doctor, in my experience, to be told that their baby is healthy and the distress is normal, because it is usual. (Again: those are not synonyms!

Last but certainly not least, a good paediatric physiotherapist, or even a gentle chiropractor or osteopath *experienced with babies* can also make a huge difference. Get the baby checked out, as structural problems are not uncommon. Signs of rigidity of posture or asymmetry in the baby – a head always turned to one side when lying down, for example – suggest this would be a good idea to check out. Many parents have found that simple adjustments and gentle exercises can dramatically improve feeding and infant comfort. Local breastfeeding counsellors or midwives often know of such practitioners through their contact with mothers.

# Finally, the elephant in our Western room: allergy

## 8. But first, is infant colic a headache, and not a gut ache?

The association of colic and parental migraine is real.[1819] Many colicky babies grow up to have migraine in adolescence and adulthood (though many don't.) [1820] Does that mean colic is an unrecognised headache? No. Infant colic is common parlance for a pain in the gut, assumed to be due to spasms of muscles in the gut wall. Associations can be real and have common causes, even if we don't know how to define those causes precisely. It is clear that both childhood and adult migraine, gut aches, and gut motility disorders can be caused by foods. Such gut aches – and migraines – respond quickly to the elimination of foods causing the problem, as well as to other gut-related remedies like anti-spasmodics. Parents who have lived with colicky babies know that a distended gut, motility changes and faecal output are all related to the baby's discomfort. Babies may also have a headache - how would we know? – but they certainly have gut distress, or colic in common parlance. Classifying colic as a headache –even if in some babies headaches may be present – is simply denying the evidence. It overlooks Great Ormond Street research which showed that

> **"93% of 88 children with severe frequent migraine recovered on oligoantigenic** diets; the causative foods were identified by sequential reintroduction, and the role of the foods provoking migraine was established by a double-blind controlled trial in 40 of the children. Most patients responded to several foods. Many foods were involved, suggesting an allergic rather than an idiosyncratic (metabolic) pathogenesis. **Associated symptoms which improved in addition to headache included abdominal pain**, behaviour disorder, fits, asthma, and eczema. In most of the patients in whom migraine was provoked by non-specific factors, such as blows to the head, exercise, and flashing lights, this provocation no longer occurred while they were on the diet."[1821]

The idea that colic is really a baby headache may be publicised by some very large drug companies marketing analgesics. Infant formula manufacturers not in the pharmacy business may not be so happy, as much of their high value sales comes from parents changing infant formulas in the hopes of finding one that causes less gut distress (and some do, or the whole extensively hydrolysed formula business would never have been so profitable!) Those companies have documented that such diet changes end the problem of colic for many infants. It seems reasonable to suppose that this relates to changes in the bodily organ most exposed to formula, the infant gut, not the infant cranium –although of course the gut-brain connection may mean that both are affected. On the other hand, the formula

---

1819 Gelfand AA, Thomas KC, Goadsby PJ. Before the headache: infant colic as an early life expression of migraine. *Neurology.* 2012;79(13):1392-1396.

1820 Romanello S, Spiri D, Marcuzzi E, Zanina A et al. Association Between Childhood Migraine and History of Infantile Colic *JAMA.* 2013;309(15):1607-1612. doi:10.1001/jama.2013.747.

1821 Egger J, Carter CM, Wilson J, Turner MW, Soothill JF. Is migraine food allergy? A double-blind controlled trial of oligoantigenic diet treatment. (PMID:6137694) *Lancet* 1983, 2(8355):865-869 DOI: 10.1016/S0140-6736(83)90866-8

industry may be glad of a putative cause for colic other than damage to the infant gut by foreign protein: it will be interesting to see their response.

Muddling these problems, colic and migraine headache, seems to me quite daft, and almost certainly dangerous. I dread the consequences of crying babies being dosed for weeks with potentially liver-toxic analgesic syrups, all laden with preservatives and artificial chemicals to make them palatable. These will certainly affect the gut microbiome. Many parents of allergic babies find that paediatric medicines cause digestive upsets: some are vomitted back, others trigger gut spasms.

## 9. Is colic gut distress, and if so, what causes it?

Only those who have never lived with colicky babies could imagine that the problem is all in infant heads, or that leaving tormented babies in quiet dark rooms without stimulation would resolve it. As far back as the 1980s, the allergy gurus at London's Great Ormond Street's Hospital for Sick Children were able to relieve severe gut inflammation with rectal bleeding and colitis in breastfed infants by identifying allergens in the mother's diet and eliminating them. They went on to 'suggest that food allergy is the major cause of colitis in infancy and that an exclusion diet is the treatment of choice.'[1822] Gut bleeding –now often labelled as FPIES - was in fact the high end of a spectrum of gut distress that extends back to colic, gut distress which 'is characterised by vigorous periodic crying episodes and bending up of the lower limbs, indicative of abdominal pain', about which Dr Donald Bentley went on to say, 'We have been impressed that if [breastfeeding] mothers of such babies remove all milk and dairy products from their diet, there is a sudden improvement in a high proportion of cases.'[1823] To discover that, it is necessary to eliminate milk for more than a few days and completely, which many doctors have never really supported mothers in doing. To paraphrase what Chesterton famously said about Christianity, the problem is not that bovine protein elimination has been tried and found wanting; the problem is that it has been found difficult and rarely tried. And also, that the problem is rarely JUST bovine protein allergy, but is much more complicated than that.

'Colic' was the traditional unspecific diagnosis for inconsolable episodic infant crying, given with assurances that it would disappear over time, as babies grow (see page 647 for the reason I suggest for that).When I am asked to help a family with a distressed breastfed baby, and preliminary phone calls establish the likelihood of allergy, I ask that both parents set aside two hours in which we will together investigate and talk through the strategy they can jointly choose to follow or reject, but which I think gives them the best chance of having a happy baby. Two hours goes very quickly. And there can be frequent follow-up discussions. Chapter 4.3 outlines a process for ascertaining whether the gut distress is caused by allergy.

Thanks partly to saturation industry marketing to health professionals, the old diagnosis of colic has largely been replaced by a diagnosis of gastro-oesophageal reflux (GOR) or gastro-

---

1822 Jenkins HR, Pincott JR, Soothill JF, Milla PJ, Harries JT. Food allergy: the major cause of infantile colitis. *Arch Dis Child* 1984; 59: 326-9.
1823 Bentley, Aubrey and Bentley, op. cit. p. 20.`

oesophageal reflux disease (GORD). The difference is purely one of symptom severity, not severity of the problem to the family. GORD was first invented and marketed as a diagnosis by an industry which wanted to sell antidotes, in the form of drugs or infant formulas. The diagnosis has greatly increased since the 1990s marketing campaigns by infant formula companies selling thickened brews (see page 288). In my view, GOR or GORD is a popular diagnosis by doctors because there are pharmaceuticals to prescribe and formulas to suggest, all of which are quicker than the painstaking investigation of allergy in mother and baby.

So many people do not know that allergy (as I have defined it for the purpose of this book) may be the principal cause of inconsolably crying babies. Most families do correctly identify gut or digestive problems as contributing to their child's misery, and others suspect allergy because it 'runs in the family'. (So too does migraine, sometimes.)  Parents have an unhappy baby, or a baby who is not thriving, or a baby who has developed inflamed skin. And who cries. And cries. And sleeps atrociously. And above all, the baby is a difficult feeder, going to the breast frequently because hungry, but then pulling off as the milk flows, and screaming, going back on again because still hungry, but pulling off because the milk seems to trigger inflammation as it flows. Breastfeeding mothers feel rejected and distressed by this behaviour, and need to be assured that changing *what is in their milk* (by changing their diet) will result in peaceful and satisfying breastfeeding. Formula feeding mothers need to be helped to change formulas appropriately. Instead, all too often they are still told to doubt the evidence of their own eyes and believe that this is just a mystery, probably psychosomatic, that food has nothing to do with infant crying. This undermines parental confidence that they can care for their children, disempowering them.

Using the questionnaire and sometimes just looking at the other family members allows me to judge whether or not the baby's problem is likely to be due to allergy. There are clear-cut facial signs in many cases, such as panda eyes set against ghostly skin, itchy dry patches of skin, nasal creases in older children, hectic 'rouge' patches on cheekbones. [1824] Babies who cry intensely and often have a variety of reasons for doing so. If the underlying problem is allergy, they will usually have  at least a few of the symptoms listed in this table from my second book, *Food for Thought*. Many of these symptoms persist past infancy, and are complicated by behavioural issues, so looking at older siblings can be instructive.

---

1824 Ibid.,

| GASTROINTESTINAL TRACT | RESPIRATORY TRACT | SKIN |
|---|---|---|
| Frequent possetting or regurgitation | Nasal stuffiness, mucus | Dry patches of skin, cracks |
| Vomiting, projectile vomiting | Sneezing | Cradle cap |
| Frequent loose stools - mucus | Coughing | 'Spots'; rashes |
| Windiness, excessive flatus | Nose-rubbing | Eczema |
| Diarrhoea | Unusual breathing | Hives, welts, swelling (eyes) |
| Constipation (uncommon in the full breast-fed) | Sniffing, snoring, etc. | Purpura |
| Stomach pains, bloating | Noisy breathing | Scratching or rubbing indicating itchiness |
| Colic | Hiccoughs | Sweatiness |
| Blood in stools | Recurrent croup | Redness around mouth, anus, or on cheeks |
| Poor appetite and weight gain | Recurrent bronchitis | Easy bruising |
| Feeding difficulties (breast-fed babe often refuses breast after couple of minutes and screams despite obvious hunger; also rejects bottles) | Frequent ear infections (or any, in the fully breast-fed) | |
| | Runny nose (clear at first) | |
| | Frequent 'colds' | |
| | Bad breath | **CIRCULATION** |
| | **GENITOURINARY TRACT** | Changes in pulse rate and regularity, palpitations |
| Mouth ulcers | Cystitis | Changes in temperature (usually slight fever) |
| | Vulvovaginitis | Changes in skin colour, especially around lips |
| | Haematuria | Anaemia, haemolysis |
| | Nephrosis | |

Figure 4-2-1 Common symptoms in infancy

As children get older, other seemingly unrelated problems may emerge, such as a lack of bladder control, or enuresis,[1825] headaches, abdominal pain, and behavioural problems. It is worth mentioning that if the latter symptoms occur in a child subject to epilepsy, a low-allergen diet may end both seizures and the other problems.[1826]

If one or both parents are allergic, or siblings have allergy symptoms, the next baby is *always* at increased risk of allergy. If the baby was extremely overactive *in utero,*[1827] it may have been sensitised there. In extreme overactivity Rapp included "vigorous kicking, prolonged hiccupping, mother's ribs bruised and sore, difficulty sleeping because of strong and frequent kicking (in some cases causing waves in a bath, or causing an object placed on the abdomen to fly across the room)." Any such evidence of probable intra-uterine sensitisation makes it critical for postnatal care to be optimal and breastfeeding or breastmilk to be exclusive from

1825 Egger J, Carter CH, Soothill JF, Wilson J. Effect of diet treatment on enuresis in children with migraine or hyperkinetic behavior. (PMID:1582098) *Clin Pediatr 1992,* 31(5):302-307. Classic studies too often overooked by those who believe irrelevant anything older than 5 years.
1826 Egger J, Carter CM, Soothill JF, Wilson J Oligoantigenic diet treatment of children with epilepsy and migraine. (PMID:2909707) *J Pediatr* 1989, 114(1):51-58 DOI: 10.1016/S0022-3476(89)80600-6
1827 Rapp D. *Is this your child?* (William Morrow 1993), p. 102.

birth, no non-human comp feeds. This is perfectly possible if you plan ahead, and enlist helpers to keep baby skin to skin. Knowing that you have access to supplies of human milk relieves anxiety and so makes the use of donor milk less likely to be needed. But there are some important things to remember before concluding that allergy is definitely the cause of any pre- or post-birth symptoms.

Because allergy causes symptoms that are common to many other conditions, it's important to rule out other explanations, which means always having a healthcare professional involved in the child's care.

Because allergy is complicated, it is important not to blithely suggest arbitrary trials that are likely to be unsuccessful. 'My doctor said to go off milk for three days and see what happens' is bad advice – it's not long enough, milk might not be the allergen (or the only allergen), and in some cases, going off an allergen makes people feel worse before they start feeling better after about five days. It can also change tolerance levels.

Because dealing with allergy is time-consuming and affects the whole family, it's important not to diagnose allergy where it doesn't exist, or over-diagnose.

Because allergy is life-changing, it is even more important not to under-diagnose- to miss diagnosing where allergy does exist. The consequence of under-diagnosis is ongoing and worsening immune disorder.

## Aversion and addiction: do doctors understand this?

Closely allied to a sensitivity to milk is an antipathy to it. This antipathy is an interesting phenomenon and warrants further study. It may be present at birth-we have seen it in newborns and even in a premature. Our data suggest that it is present in approximately one child in 20. It is as common in boys as in girls. Between infancy and parenthood, however, a significant proportion of girls (between one in four and one in five) develop a dislike or even a hatred of milk, so that among adults the antipathy is much more common among women than among men. ...The antipathy to milk is more common in milk-sensitive than in milk-insensitive families, but it cannot be equated with milk sensitivity, for we have been unable to demonstrate that those who dislike milk are necessarily sensitive to it. Nor can we say that the converse applies, namely that those who are fond of milk are never sensitive to it, for some milk-sensitive subjects are among those who are most addicted to it. Nevertheless the antipathy to milk sometimes appears to be a protective mechanism; some children with a persistent rhinorrhea and bronchitis who have always disliked milk, but who have been made to drink it by well-intentioned parents, remain free from respiratory problems when they are at last allowed to avoid the milk and dairy products they have previously tried to avoid.

Gerrard JW, Lubos M, Hardy LW et al Milk Allergy: Clinical Picture and Familial Incidence.
*Canad Med* Ass J 1967; 97: 780-785

# 4.3 Checking out allergy as a cause: a rough road map to start from with a distressed baby

This next chapter is about this sub-set of the inconsolable modern Western baby, who cannot be pacified by simple means such as those described above, whose crying is excessive and unpredictable and whose sleep – and his parents' – is disrupted. And also the unhappy irritable eczematous baby, being tormented by itching and pain. What follows summarises the route, roughly speaking:

Step 1 Get the history and reduce needless irritants

Step 2 Manage milk supply issues including lactose and fat intolerance

Step 3 Begin the allergy quest

Step 4 Decide on maternal diet elimination

Step 5 Eliminate the candidate food(s)

Step 6 The elimination diet

Step 7 Hospital-based allergy clinics

## Asking questions and reducing needless irritants

If allergy is to be investigated, taking a good history is always the first step. That's why I asked readers to complete the questionnaire earlier. Where a baby is involved, history taking includes details of birth and postnatal experiences, including stress, as there is a greater risk of allergy in infants subjected to stressful experiences (also a greater risk of medications as well, altering many aspects of metabolism). Understanding that allergy too can affect growth is also important.

Knowing exactly what baby has eaten and is eating is fundamental. There can be numerous concoctions being fed as well as breastmilk: drugs, herbal teas, water, formula, cereals. These confuse the issue. They can cause any number of gut effects. If the breastfed baby is under six months it is best, wherever possible, to get back to exclusive breastfeeding. (Of course if formula is 95 per cent of the child's diet it cannot just be eliminated in a snap! But top-ups and evening single feeds need to be eliminated, and the mother's milk supply built up again so that the baby is fully and solely breastfed, if at all possible. It usually is,[1828] where mothers are supported, and the mechanisms of making milk explained to them.)

---

1828 Where formula cannot be eliminated (because to do so would starve the baby) an extensively-hydrolysed-casein product can be substituted.

Meanwhile, the breastfeeding mother should stop consuming unnecessary substances that many mothers report are associated with infant irritability: excess caffeine,[1829] artificial sweeteners (especially aspartame[1830]), artificial colours, flavours and preservatives in foods. Diet drinks manage to combine many of these nasties – some of the most addicted women I have seen have got stuck on diet colas; withdrawal symptoms will be unpleasant for at least a week, but are temporary, though cravings can persist. Any oral contraceptives should be re-considered. Barrier methods of contraception may be needed, although if the mother is fully breastfeeding a baby under six months, and her menses have not returned, lactational amenorrhoea is at least as reliable as the oral contraceptive pill.[1831]

Ending mother and baby's exposure to environmental toxins such as smoke, pesticides, strong synthetic fragrances, bleach and detergent residues (common in feeding bottles) has been reported to reduce symptoms, and is in any case a sensible thing to do. At an Australian College of Allergy meeting I was told that one New South Wales allergy clinic always advised mothers of colicky bottle-fed babies to stop using hypochlorite bleaches for sterilising equipment; symptoms improved after a week of boiling bottles and dummies. Bleach metabolites could affect mucosal surfaces, decreasing protection against allergens and pathogens, and viruses can act as adjuvants to trigger allergic reactions. Babies can certainly taste chlorine traces, the taste of which can persist on plastic for a long time.

Similarly, look for strong indications of parents being anxious, over-stressed and depressed at this stage, and factor this into the advice being given. For some mothers, getting peer support and professional recognition of the strain they are under can be therapeutic in itself, a reassurance that they are not inadequate mothers, or coping worse than others would in the same situation. A demoralised mother will find it harder to take in and implement practical suggestions – not because she is uncaring or stupid, but because her brain is not functioning well amidst a deluge of stress hormones. Reassurance that feeling depressed is the appropriate, sane, normal human response to depressing situations, and that feelings will change as the situation does, can work wonders – without need for risky psychoactive drugs that can become a further problem for some. While serious cases at risk of self-harm, or harm to baby, may indeed need medication to restore a normal mental balance, women who are justifiably miserable would be psychotic (i.e., out of touch with reality) *not* to feel depressed and sad when their much-wanted baby is causing them to

---

1829  Tea and coffee and cola alone can each cause the most astonishing array of mental and physical effects: see Finn R, Newman Cohen H. 'Food Allergy': fact or fiction? *Lancet* 1978; 1(8061): 426-428. See also Finn's review in *J Roy Soc Med*. 1992; 85(9): 560–564. Cocoa is another source of caffeine, and Bentley notes that cocoa/chocolate can be linked to hyperactive behaviours.

1830  Many women consume this to excess when focused on losing weight. It may cause headaches and is suspected of causing seizures, but may in fact contribute to weight gain; it is also likely to be contaminating drinking water. Maher TJ, Wurtman RJ Possible neurologic effects of aspartame, a widely used food additive. (PMID:3319565) *Environmental Health Perspectives* 1987, 75:53-57.; Yang Q. Gain weight by "going diet?" Artificial sweeteners and the neurobiology of sugar cravings: *Neuroscience* 2010. (PMID:20589192) *The Yale Journal of Biology and Medicine* 2010, 83(2):101-108.; Lange FT, Scheurer M, Brauch HJ. Artificial sweeteners-a recently recognized class of emerging environmental contaminants: a review. (PMID:22543693) *Analy Bioanaly Chem* 2012, 403(9):2503-2518. De la Peña C. *Empty Pleasures. The Story of Artificial Sweeteners from Saccharin to Splenda*. (University of North Carolina Press 2010.) makes interesting reading.

1831  Short RV, Lewis PR, Renfree MB, Shaw G. Contraceptive effects of extended **lactational** amenorrhoea: beyond the Bellagio Consensus. (PMID:1672186) *Lancet* 1991; 337(8743):715-717.

be in pain, sleep-deprived and overwrought. And all medication has unpredictable side effects: read widely in the literature before using any. I particularly recommend Dr Peter Breggin's book, *Your drug may be your problem*[1832] as basic reading both for those using such medications and those considering doing so. Breggin was the expert whose advocacy got the USFDA to label these drugs as increasing violent tendencies and suicidality. Another book which charts how the pattern of widespread medication evolved is *Saving Normal*.[1833]

Similarly, food and drink chemicals can affect mothers' moods and behaviours, not just their babies'. The hyped-up caffeine junkie is just one example of chemicals affecting mood, and also physical behaviour.

The idea in this first step is to eliminate unnecessary biochemical exposures or stresses on baby and mother, and see if the problem resolves. That may be all that is needed to stop baby crying. And a happy baby is what tells us we're getting things right.

## Managing milk supply issues including lactose and fat intolerance

At the same time, feed management should be evaluated. Lact**ose** (milk sugar) in a baby's gut is broken down into glucose and galactose by the enzyme lact**ase**. When the amount of lactose exceeds the capacity of lactase to break it down, gut bacteria ferment the sugar, creating both acidity and gas, including hydrogen. Lactose intolerance caused simply by feed patterns is better referred to as lactose overload, and in breastfeeding babies it is common in the first months, before oversupply settles down. Usually it is due to a pattern of excessive snacking and topping-up at the breast, which means that a baby is constantly full but uncomfortable, so he feeds to relieve the discomfort, so he is constantly overfull. Then there is simply too much milk too fast for the baby's gut to digest all the lactose.

These are often very 'wet' babies: lots of liquid stools, lots of posseting and even vomiting, many with good weight gains, but unhappy. Some babies lose so much weight from the rapid passage of all food that they fail to thrive, although the mother often has a booming milk supply from all the stimulation, needing breast pads to mop up leakage. This is probably the origin of the old idea that some milk was too thin or not good quality. The quality of the milk is fine – it's just not being digested and absorbed, possibly because gut bacteria cannot cope with the consequences of excessive milk volume. Other babies gain well, but are uncomfortable and cry a lot. Symptoms of lactose overload in the breastfed baby can include a tight distended abdomen, like a little drum at times, but which softens when stools or wind are passed; and a sore bottom from acid scalds, along with expressions of pain and misery.

These symptoms of lactose intolerance can also be the result of infection or allergy, that damages the gut, flattening the little projections, the villi, where the enzyme is located. So lactose intolerance is really just a symptom, not a diagnosis. There are many causes:

1832 Breggin PR. op. cit.
1833 Green A. Op cit.

anything that damages the gut, like a parasite, a virus, bacterial infection. Live vaccines like rotavirus will sometimes set this going if maternal reports are accurate.

Taking out lactose, a vital ingredient of infant diet, is not a solution. It means putting in other sugars, which can cause other problems. Yet the very industry that popularised the use of cows' milk for infants – milk containing hundreds of proteins that can cause lactose intolerance among other damaging effects – has profited greatly from marketing both low-lactose formulas, and the idea that the problem is lactose. Using low-lactose formulas may indeed reduce some gut symptoms. But it can also delay diagnosis of the original cause of the gut damage: perhaps bovine protein 'allergy', or giardia in the water supply. The longer the cause goes undiagnosed, the more damage may be done.

Testing the baby's breath for hydrogen levels is one research tool to confirm the diagnosis of lactose intolerance in an artificially fed baby. But almost any breastfed baby will come up positive for any current test for 'lactose intolerance', due to the high lactose content of human milk. Babies don't have to have lactose overloaded to be positive on tests that are simply inappropriate for breastfed babies.[1834]

ABA's *Too much milk?* booklet[1835] has been helpful to many women. Breastfeeding counsellors and lactation consultants should know how to reduce milk oversupply by relatively simple adjustments of feeding patterns. They also know to prevent mastitis developing in an overfull breast. Doctors need to be aware of the excellent online Academy of Breastfeeding Medicine (ABM) Mastitis protocol.[1836]

Mastitis in an intact but very full breast often seems to be the result of milk leaking from ducts or glandular tissue into surrounding breast tissue, which activates the immune system. Longer intervals between feeds can generate high enough pressure to cause such leakage, leading to a pink inflamed area, often hard and sore, in the breast. Note that I said *intact* breast: meaning no breaks to skin of breast or nipple. Skin damage is likely to increase the risk of infection, but mastitis should always be taken seriously, even when it doesn't need antibiotics.[1837] Treatment needs to begin right away, and a doctor's visit is needed if this is the mother's first experience of mastitis. However, where there is no obvious infection, and the doctor does not advise that antibiotics be started immediately, it is usually safe to rest, feed, express, and generally drain the breast *well and often* for twenty-four hours, monitoring the progress of symptoms. If the problem is resolving without antibiotics, continuing that regime – described in all good breastfeeding manuals – may make antibiotics unnecessary. But if symptoms worsen, with areas of redness increasing, temperature rises and worsening symptoms, taking antibiotics *and continuing the same regime* will clear the breast. Without continued drainage of milk, pressure build-up is likely to lead to a recurrence as well as to reduce milk supply. I always suggest that where possible a breastfeeding mother has a script for antibiotics on hand, because the problem can become severe quite rapidly, and usually

---

1834  Joy Anderson RD, IBCLC: personal communication 2013
1835  see https://www.breastfeeding.asn.au/bf-info/common-concerns–mum/too-much-milk
1836  http://www.bfmed.org/Media/Files/Protocols/2014_Updated_Mastitis6.30.14.pdf ABM protocols are a good place to start with any breastfeeding problem requiring medical input, including care of the preterm infant.
1837  See Minchin M. *Breastfeeding Matters*, chapter on mastitis.

at a time when visiting a doctor is difficult. But after learning how to deal with mastitis, and to recognise early warning signs and likely risk factors, many mothers never need to do more than the self-help measures to bring it under control, as all those powerful anti-infective agents of milk are also working in her breast.

Getting milk supply into harmony with baby's needs results in a baby who drinks less by volume, but gets more cream and more calories, and whose previously acceptable or good growth may become startlingly good: 250-500gms in a week are not unknown (and are nothing to worry about). While the strategy for getting supply into balance with need is simple, it helps greatly if the mother has someone who can be with her for the twenty-four to forty-eight hours of patterned feeding it will usually take for her over-generous milk supply to reduce. The breast has evolved to establish a bountiful supply initially, but also to be able to down-regulate quickly, so as not to waste maternal nutrients. A pair of helping hands and a safe sling can ensure the process is swift and not traumatic for either mother or baby. And increasing the amount of cream baby drinks is possible if mother is expressing (see page 439). I have even had mothers stay with me for this time, or stayed overnight with them, when no other help was available. Of course that should be unnecessary, but in fact there is shamefully little community assistance available to most mothers.

Lactose overload is naturally less often seen by specialist gastroenterologists who are assessing mothers months down the track. Breastfed babies rarely get to specialists so young. If lactose intolerance is seen in older breastfed babies, it is more likely to be the result of a gut-damaging infection, than to be an artefact of feed management. But it can be both. And breastfeeding should not be stopped, or replaced by formulas. Remember, the mother's body actually ramps up production of protective factors in response to an infection in the child.[1838] When they have no real expertise in normal infant feeding, and are dealing with breastfed babies, hospital-based specialists should seek advice from International Board-Certified Lactation Consultants.

## Another older form of intolerance: 'fatty dyspepsia'?

Just as babies can take in more lactose than they have enzyme to digest, it was once common for those who were bottle-fed to take in more fat than they could readily digest. They lack the breastmilk enzymes like BSSL (bile-salt stimulated lipase) that help breastfed babies break down dietary fats. This problem was said to be more common when babies drank full-cream milk formulas, with butterfat, and the problem decreased with the use of more readily absorbed vegetable oils in formula. A typical pattern of sore bottom, illustrated in some books, was seen as diagnostic of fat overload, or fatty dyspepsia as it was sometimes called. It was not mentioned in connection with breastfed infants, so what is the connection?

A couple of years ago, a mother consulted me about her thriving, fully breastfed baby's creamy white, yes really white, poo. With her doctor we worried about liver disorders and

1838 Riskin A, Almog M, Peri R, Halasz K et al. Changes in immunomodulatory constituents of human milk in response to active infection in the nursing infant. (PMID:22258136) *Pediatr Res* 2012, 71(2):220-225

biliary atresia, these being the only diagnoses in modern medicine for such white faecal output. But when stumped by some new occurrence, I always go back through the early twentieth-century paediatric texts, to the era when baby poo was examined as carefully as oracles once inspected chicken gizzards. When I read about 'fatty dyspepsia' and its characteristic creamy white poo, I called the mother and told her about it, assuming that there must be some odd genetic quirk at work that produced fat intolerance like this. She promptly told me that she, a busy mother of three, had been 'living on chocolate for a week' – it was around Easter. I was sceptical that the effect could be so dramatic, but she changed her diet and the problem went away, never to recur. That baby is a sturdy thriving omnivorous three year old as I write this.

So for what the anecdote is worth, don't panic if you see white poo, but get it checked out. One visiting doctor said that he would not have believed it if he hadn't seen it: even in a children's hospital where he had worked, the liver-disordered children didn't manage such a colour. So white poo might just be fatty dyspepsia! Chocaholics beware ... It didn't trouble the baby greatly: she was a bit grumpier than usual, but completely unharmed by that dose of cocoa butter and the rest. Her weight gains were great!

## Beginning the allergy quest

Having ruled out lactose overload, we now have a solely breastfed baby who is still distressed and giving every sign of gut discomfort, or perhaps developing dry skin. This is the point where a baseline diary is helpful – ideally a one-week absolutely-no-cheating diary that records maternal intakes of anything, with infant sleep, stooling, and crying periods. Mothers need to talk this through with their breastfeeding consultant (formal or informal!) cum allergy adviser. They can be told that no one else needs to see their personal food diary, but that they do need to put everything down; it won't be inspected, but they mightn't see connections if they leave out their Tim Tams or vitamin supplements or chewing gum or alcoholic drinks. An infant baseline sleep and crying chart is essential if they want to be sure that any changes made are working, and when. But if mothers choose not to take the time to do all this recording, and to get to work on changing diet immediately, that's their decision.

The allergy questionnaire comes into use here. After completing it, mothers may have reason to suspect – more often than not these days – that food and chemical allergy or hypersensitivity may be the problem both for themselves and for any young breastfed baby gaining poorly or crying excessively. Mothers need to think about their pregnancy and lactation addictions and aversions, and the baby's exposure to alien proteins.

*Think before acting* is the motto. Realise that it's natural to resist any idea that requires changes of diet, and that change is always more difficult when stressed. From my experience, sorting out allergy issues is hard work, but the least work over the long run: so take the time to plan and do it right the first time. The extra work is only worthwhile if it will save time, money and sanity, and create infant – and so parental– happiness.

Many working with allergic people suggest nutrient supplementation. Some mothers could not face changing their diet have reported to me that these can help. Among those most often mentioned as beneficial are zinc, magnesium, omega-3 long chain polyunsaturated fatty acids (LCPUFAs)[1839] DHA and ARA, the whole complex of B vitamins, and perhaps vitamin D[1840] (which can be supplemented by simply getting enough sunlight on bare skin, though readers in sunny climates should get sun exposure at safe times of the day.) As well, maternal consumption of appropriate dairy-free probiotics (lactobacillus and bifidus strains for example) may be helpful.

There is some evidence to support most of these supplements, perhaps especially LCPUFA supplementation from plant[1841] sources. Probiotics (for the breastfeeding mother or bottle-fed child) look as though they may be helpful, as research has shown early differences in gut microbiota of babies that go on to be colicky.[1842] The problem is that we really don't know what probiotics in what doses, and what suits one person may not be ideal for another. Keep records of anything used. A little natural scepticism is always wise, as knowing what caused what is never simple, and the placebo effect is real – but extremely useful even so.

I always enquire about the quality of maternal diet (because the mother will suffer if her diet is poor). Changing hospital practices (fewer transfusions after blood loss, for example) and maternal lifestyles (less red meat consumption, low LC-PUFA intake) can mean mothers are more at risk of anaemia and depression post-partum, while the increasing use of psychiatric medication introduces new dangers to mother and baby alike. Babies born in some hospitals (where cord blood is so eagerly harvested for other purposes, such as stem cell research or private bloodbanking) are also more at risk of anaemia[1843] than those whose cord is clamped only after it has stopped pulsing, around two to three minutes after the birth.

New mothers also need high-quality protein, *not* protein supplements made from deconstructed cow's milk or industrially rendered soybeans, but eggs, animal meats or milks or carefully balanced vegetarian mixes. Egg yolks contain not only omega-3 fata but also choline, said to be deficient in many diets. The ratio of omega-3 to omega-6 fatty

---

1839 Jensen RG, Ferris AM, Lammi-Keefe CJ, Henderson RA et al. Possible alleviation of atopic eczema in a breastfed infant by maternal supplementation with a fish oil concentrate.(PMID:1517955) *J Pediatr Gastroenterol Nutr* 1992; 14(4):474-475; Makrides M. Dietary n-3 LC-PUFA during the perinatal period as a strategy to minimize childhood allergic disease. In Makrides M, Ochoa J, Szajewska H (eds). *The Importance of Immunonutrition* NNI Workshop Series vol 77, 2013

1840 Vuillermin PJ, Ponsonby AL, Kemp AS, Allen KJ. Potential links between the emerging risk factors for food allergy and vitamin D status.(PMID:23711121) *Clin Exp Allergy* 2013; 43(6):599-607.

1841 Linnamaa P, Nieminen K, Koulu L, Tuomasjukka S, et al. Black currant seed oil supplementation of mothers enhances IFN-γ and suppresses IL-4 production in breast milk. (PMID:23980846) *Pediatr Allergy Immunol* 2013; 24(6):562-566.

1842 de Weerth C, Fuentes S, de Vos WM. Crying in infants: On the possible role of intestinal microbiota in the development of colic. (PMID:23941920) *Gut Microbes* 2013, 4(5) '..we found that infants with colic showed lower microbiota diversity and stability than control infants in the first weeks of life. Colic/control differences in the abundance of certain bacteria were also found at 2 weeks. These microbial signatures possibly explain the colic phenotype.'

1843 Chaparro CM. Timing of umbilical cord clamping: effect on iron endowment of the newborn and later iron status. (PMID:22043880) *Nutr Rev* 2011, 69 Suppl 1:s30-6.

acids may well be important for mother and baby alike, although concern about this can be overdone. More omega-3 is needed where omega-6 intake is high, so lower the omega-6.

Short interbirth intervals are never good for mothers or babies, and even worse if a crying baby needs to be sorted out, so parents would be wise to find appropriate contraception methods as a matter of priority. The mother who gives up breastfeeding and instead uses formula is at greater risk of a new pregnancy, made more difficult by her allergy, and a second, often more difficult baby to deal with (especially if the problem is not yet identified and sorted).

Families are wise to avoid another pregnancy for at least a couple of years while dealing with this problem of possible allergy in an infant. Responsive parenting is not easy with an allergic child, and an allergic child places strains on all members of the family. A previous or subsequent child is often unavoidably short-changed at a critical time for development wherever parental resources are overstretched by the demands of an unwell child. Sometimes, as in my own case, it is only with the benefit of hindsight and input from adult children that we can see just how much strain – which is probably just as well! Read *Why love matters* by Sue Gerhardt,[1844] and Margot Sunderland's *The science of parenting*,[1845] and reflect on your own parents and parenting, and you'll realise how your own childhood has shaped the adult you, for good and ill.

## Deciding on maternal diet elimination

In discussing the questionnaire and any allergy diary, one or two major suspect foods usually emerge. I find that if the mother was artificially fed as a child, and her child was 'comp fed' after birth, the starting point might as well be cows' milk protein (CMP) elimination, because milk will be a major contributor to the problem, if not the whole cause. (The older the child is when allergy is diagnosed, the greater the number of likely allergens, as the gut struggled to deal appropriately with the damage done by the first. When we realised that our four-year-old son was allergic to milk, we discovered that he reacted to several of the foods used as first solids as well: beef, banana, honey, wheat, peanut, among others. Even now the smell of peanuts causes a headache.)

But it isn't always cows' milk protein. Mothers will often volunteer a rationale for why one particular food is the problem: a major binge on eggs at four months into pregnancy; an overdose of milk which Mum didn't really like but made herself swallow because everyone said it was good for her and baby; a pregnancy craving for salicylate-rich peppermints and her constant use of peppermint tea …

So: if a woman discovers that her mother ate six raw lemons a day when gestating her, as one mother did, she could consider eliminating citrus or salicylate-laden food. If formula-fed and with suggestive symptoms to justify the effort, she might plan to go totally milk-free for at least three weeks and see what changes. If her mum describes what a beautiful baby

---

1844 Gerhardt S. *Why Love Matters: how affection shapes the baby's brain.* (Brunner Routledge 2005)
1845 Sunderland M. *The Science of Parenting.* (Dorling Kindersley 2008)

she was at first and how by ten to twenty-one days she had become a nightmare, hospital records might exist that show what brand of formula she was exposed to. (The mother should not need a Freedom of Information request to find out. Those assisting her should be prepared to go to these lengths, especially if this information will help with caring for future babies.) It is interesting that health professionals have noticed the emergence of symptoms in the first few weeks after birth without considering the possible role of milk exposure and reaction times.

It could be useful, but is currently impossible, to research the likely ingredients of any formula given. These have included wheat, potato (maltodextrin is made from potatoes or corn, and in Europe must *not* be made from wheat because of inevitable traces of gluten), corn, tapioca, sugar, soy, seaweed, egg, peanut, and much much more, including antigens from the diet of the cow who provided the milk. (Do you know what can be in stockfeed? See page 387.) Those ingredients are likely to be the problem foods. Wouldn't it be helpful to citizens' ability to take responsibility for their own health if it were to be made mandatory for companies to put on the public record the source of every formula ingredient and record every change in an accessible online database?

After settling on a candidate food, parents need to talk through *where* that suspect food will be found, *how* they will avoid it, and *what* food if any will replace it. It helps if fathers accept that they will not be eating that food at home while the trial withdrawal is underway. No-one ever died from giving up all white liquids for two or three weeks – except the very small ones depending on breastmilk for total nutrition. Humans can grow up healthy without animal milks: many cultures have never had access to them. Parents need to check thoroughly that all sources of the suspect food are known. Many parents are unaware that anything that says whey, casein, bovine or lacto- or caso- anything will be based on cows' milk, or that milk can be in sweets, in sausages, in bread, in sorbet, in cosmetics, in asthma sprays, in encapsulated algal oils, in paint ... so do what research you can. (But don't be put off by that list! It's better to try than to give up, for believe me, the only other options are all usually worse in the long run.)

## Eliminating the candidate food(s)

Busy sleep-deprived parents of young babies cannot manage multiple food eliminations without a huge amount of help. It is easier to take this just one step at a time. One chosen food needs to be completely eliminated for at least two, sometimes three weeks. Positive signs that parents chose the right food to eliminate are any change in the first week – for good *or* ill. Some people feel great within a few days, or symptoms abate in the baby, or both these things happen. If the person is addicted to the food, withdrawal symptoms can emerge around day four to five, sometimes shattering headaches, sometimes fever, sometimes just general fatigue and unwellness. This is the body adjusting, and usually means that after three weeks symptoms will disappear in both mother and child.

No new food should be introduced into the mother's diet as the suspect food is being withdrawn: don't replace bovine milk with soy milk, for example. This can confuse the issue: just as symptoms from cows' milk abate over two or three weeks,[1846] symptoms from equally gut-altering soy milk begin. Mothers can then conclude that diet change only seemed to help for a little while, when it would have solved the problem except for the excess soymilk put into a still disturbed gut.

In my experience, the younger the breastfed baby, and the less damaged the mother by her own artificial feeding, the quicker the baby seems to respond. And I am certainly not the only person to conclude that maternal diet changes 'may be beneficial for reducing symptoms of infant colic.'[1847] Gut distress or colic in babies can damp down in a couple of days. Skin symptoms will have taken longer to emerge and take longer to resolve, sometimes weeks, but a drop in irritability as the itch fades (as the histamine release gradually reduces) precedes the gradual clearance of eczema. And a child who loses eczema may emerge with a different 'temperament': cheerful and calm, not irritable and fretful and 'difficult'. Eczema has many serious effects on families.[1848]

Of course, changes in symptoms can happen in the right time frame but for different reasons. If the mother has been intensely stressed by not knowing what to do, getting on with a practical plan can bring a great sense of relief, lowering her stress levels. That in itself may mean some symptoms abate, as the body can manage the dietary stressors better. Conversely, if a mother finds the challenge of the new diet stressful,[1849] she may cope less well and be symptomatic. So a positive response in the first week of elimination, or a lack of response, proves nothing for certain. Time will tell.

## What next?

What if a single food elimination fails to make any difference? Think again. Go back into your history and look for clues, and try another likely suspect. This involves going back over everything afresh. *Don't* try a food just because someone else found it worked for them, if there seems to be no reason why it should affect you.

As long ago as 1984 the Royal College of Physicians of London stated in their then groundbreaking report *Food intolerance and food aversion*[1850] that it can take three weeks for symptoms to abate after one exposure, and three weeks for symptoms to appear after one exposure.

---

1846 Maternal CM avoidance was associated with lower levels of mucosal-specific IgA levels and the of CMA in infants: see Järvinen KM, Westfall JE, Seppo MS, James AK et al. Role of maternal elimination diets and human milk IgA in the development of cow's milk allergy in the infants. (PMID:24164317 *Clin Experim Allergy* 2014, 44(1):69-78. DOI: 10.1111/cea.12228

1847 Iacovou M, Ralston RA, Muir J, Walker KZ, Truby H. Dietary Management of Infantile Colic: A Systematic Review. *Matern Child Health J.* 2012;16(6):1319-1331

1848 Su JC, Kemp AS, Varigos GA, Nolan TM. Atopic eczema: its impact on the family and financial cost. (PMID:9068310) Free full text article *Arch Dis Child* 1997; 76(2):159-162.

1849 Hathaway MJ, Warner JO. Compliance problems in the dietary management of eczema. (PMID:6859943) *Arch Dis Child* 1983, 58(6):463-464. (PMID:6859943) Free online.

1850 Lessof MH. *Food Intolerance and Food Aversion.* Royal College of Physicians of London, with the British Nutrition Foundation. (Update Publications, 1984)

If after three weeks of complete elimination there is no change, I encourage mothers to take another look and try again. Single food eliminations are vastly preferable to going on elimination diets, or taking out six or sixty things at once. If that happens, because reaction times for foods can vary, reintroducing the foods and knowing which was the culprit can become impossible. Was a reaction on day six due to the food reintroduced that day? Or to the food reintroduced on day four that took forty-eight hours to trigger a response? Or did the total antigen load need to include both foods before symptoms emerged? Or was it all a coincidence anyway, and a virus has invaded?

Dieticians who suggest complicated multiple food eliminations to stressed breastfeeding mothers – or else the use of a supposedly hypoallergenic formula – simply undermine breastfeeding. Lactating mothers need to eat a wide, diverse good diet, not just because their milk may be affected, but for their own sake! Any such dietician has forgotten (or never knew) just how hard it is to make lifestyle changes when caring for a young baby, or else has too little respect for women's milk. As a first step, some mothers cut back to one small serve a day of the suspect food. Sometimes complete elimination is not necessary to end symptoms, though uncertainty about the cause of the problem will remain.

After a couple of single food eliminations, maybe six weeks has passed. If there is still a problem, parents should go back to their friendly and nutritionally-oriented doctor, tell her or him what's been done to date, and get the baby checked again. A few weeks have gone by and some more diagnostic symptoms may now be obvious which weren't previously. There could be a medical problem. Acid reflux is almost certainly present, although as a symptom of something else that needs to be identified. Any symptomatic relief for reflux needs to be carefully thought through (see Giving medications on page 647).

Conversely, in those few weeks baby has grown and the problem may have abated, while the parents' focus on doing something positive kept them sane and sympathetic. Babies' bodies are growing all the time, and 'tincture of time' remains a major healer. Healing, too, are all those wonderful pluripotent stem cells and growth factors and so on in the breastmilk baby has been getting throughout this journey. When a mother has an allergic older child and a breastfed baby, I often advise her to boost her supply so that she can give the older child some breastmilk in a glass or cup. Children in breastfeeding households do not know that some adults consider the udder product somehow nicer! Once again, those helping parents need to know about making and storing breastmilk, not just about allergies or disease.

Some fortunate mothers of distressed babies are able to get a complete package of help via their GP. There are doctors now in practice who take these concerns seriously, and recognise their importance to physical and mental health and family life. An innovative programme developed by a research-oriented GP has been shown to improve maternal wellbeing.[1851] Dealing with allergy is one small part of this Possums Clinic package.[1852]

Holistic treatment packages like this, preserving breastfeeding, are all too often overlooked because healthworkers don't really know where to begin. Referring parents to overcrowded allergy clinics is not practical, and dealing with the issues takes time that most general practitioners cannot give. Doctors whose practice includes too many 'long' consultations can be expected to suffer financially. Given everything that needs to be covered, an initial family consultation can take two hours, but a long GP consult is generally anything over fifteen minutes. We will never know the full extent of food allergy in the population until the day some company markets a quick test for it or a pill to treat it.

## The elimination diet

One last thing to try perhaps before heading down the difficult path of an elimination diet, if you have a willing doctor, is the use of oral sodium cromoglycate (SCG) by the baby and or mother. Professor John Gerrard in Canada found that in some cases this seemed to reduce gut absorption of antigens and symptoms in the breastfed baby, and prescribed it for both mother and baby with success.[1853] (Cromolyn, or sodium cromoglycate, is a mucosal mast cell stabiliser used as an inhalant by those with respiratory allergy.) Italian researchers studied ten children with cows' milk and/or egg IgE-mediated allergy.

> They were challenged with the offending food before and after a seven-day pre-treatment period with oral SCG (30 mg/kg b.w. per day). Full protection was achieved in six out of eight children with cow's milk allergy and in four of the five children with egg allergy.[1854]

Other researchers have come to different conclusions about oral cromoglycate,[1855] and it was never approved for oral use in some countries.

But not all problems resolve, and some babies are still very distressed, perhaps especially those who have been coping with repeated formula changes as mothers seek to find a brand that agrees with baby, sometimes after her milk supply has dwindled under the strain of coping with sleepless nights and little support. This is the point at which parents should insist on referral to specialist help. Surviving months with a desperately miserable baby

1851 Douglas PS, Hill PS *The crying baby: what approach?*(PMID:21799411) *Curr Opin Pediatr* 2011, 23(5):523-529. See also Douglas PS, Hill PS. Managing infants who cry excessively in the first few months of life. *BMJ* 2011; 343:d7772 doi: 10.1136/bmj.d7772

1852  Possums for Mothers and Babies: Home: possumsclinic.com.au/

1853 Gerrard JW. Oral cromoglycate: its value in the treatment of adverse reactions to **foods**. (PMID:106746) Ann **Allergy** 1979; 42(3):135-138. His book, *Food Allergy.: new perspectives* (CC Thomas 1980) was one of the few based on experience with any breastfeeding families.

1854 Businco L, Cantani A, Benincori N, Perlini R, Infussi R, De Angelis M, Businco E. Effectiveness of oral sodium cromoglycate (SCG) in preventing food allergy in children. (PMID:6408951) *Annals of Allergy* 1983, 51(1 Pt 1):47-50; Businco L, Meglio P, Amato G, Balsamo V etr al. Evaluation of the efficacy of **oral** cromolyn sodium or an oligoantigenic diet in children with atopic dermatitis: a multicenter study of 1085 patients. (PMID:8727267) *J Investig Allergol Clin Immunol* 1996; 6(2):103-109.

1855 Burks AW, Sampson HA. Double-blind placebo-controlled trial of oral cromolyn in children with atopic dermatitis and documented food hypersensitivity. (PMID:3123539) *J Allergy Clin Immunol* 1988, 81(2):417-423. DOI: 10.1016/0091-6749(88)90910-4

deserves a bravery award. If the mother is still breastfeeding, she will need to try out an elimination diet, and that is best done with professional support and guidance.

Yet I know many, many people who – for want of such support – have made an elimination diet work without professional help. Such help is not always available, in any case. I also have heard of a few who got themselves into a major muddle, confused and afraid to eat virtually anything, and whose life became almost impossible. Orthodox specialists report seeing such patients, which is one reason why they discourage self-help programmes. That doesn't mean DIY elimination diets won't work, just that there are problems to avoid, and it helps greatly to work with an experienced professional who understands the importance of human milk to infant development. Anyone attempting an elimination diet should try to find a reliable source of medical and nutritional supervision: perhaps a dietician who works with allergic patients in conjunction with a doctor who knows the problem is real.

Parents need help from people who appreciate and value breastfeeding as much as the baby does. Any health professional who asks breastfeeding mothers to wean, or gives the impression that the mother's milk is the problem (not what's in her diet), or that the hypoallergenic formulas they can prescribe are risk-free, and that there is no loss involved in ending breastfeeding, or who seeks to medicate a breastfeeding mother before enquiring about her diet: these should be totally shunned.

## Hospital-based allergy clinics

With a carefully chosen and supported food elimination diet, infant symptoms abate or disappear, usually quite rapidly. Some hospital allergy clinics can be marvellous places to get the help needed to make such changes work, but some are far less helpful to the breastfeeding mother. I have heard from mothers who were persuaded to stop breastfeeding by allergy clinics – on the distressing and unproven basis that her baby was allergic to the mother's milk itself (not what mother ate). It seemed to the mother that formulas were prescribed because they saved time for the overworked health professionals, not because they were better for the baby, though sometimes there had been an initial improvement, as you would expect with the removal of multiple antigens. (About two weeks later there may be new reactions developing.)

The loss of the comfort factor of breastfeeding is enormous, for both mother and baby, but seemed not to be thought important by some staff. And if the mother's food sensitivities are not discovered, allowing her to develop tolerance or remodel her diet, any subsequent baby is likely to be as much trouble as, or more than, the first.

What is more, being fed nasty-tasting formulas does affect acceptance of other foods, and if the mothers I have seen are typical, there can be ongoing problems with the child's food intake for years. Others say that the opposite can also be true, that children raised on elemental formulas accept bitter-tasting vegetables more readily than others fed bland sweet formulas. This may well be true, but overall there is good evidence that breastfed babies are best at eating the wide range of foods to which their mother's diet has exposed them.[1856]

While I acknowledge that the allergy-clinic mothers who contact me are a self-selected subset of the whole population, I do wonder what detailed independent auditing might reveal about outcomes, the more so as most of these once-breastfeeding mothers say that they have not told clinic staff what they tell me, although I always urge them to give feedback – politely but plainly.

What *good* allergy clinics can do is described in Susan Prescott's excellent book.[1857] The old approach of immunotherapy, inducing tolerance by carefully controlled doses of allergens under medical supervision, is making a global comeback. Oral immunotherapy to allergenic foods does seem to work, although long-term follow-up and outcomes need to be recorded,[1858] because throughout life – if the families I have dealt with are typical - it seems usual for sensitivity to change over time. There are also some suggestions that oral immunotherapy may result in a painful inflamed oesophagus, a condition known as EoE, eosinphilic oesophagitis,[1859] which would seem a likely outcome, and one of considerable concern if persistent. (Oesophageal inflammation might explain why allergic babies who seek the breast eagerly then pull off, as if scalded, as milk starts to flow.) In the early to mid twentieth century, child health nurses were expected to know about grading milk feeds and inducing tolerance. But now the significantly higher rate of anaphylaxis makes oral immunotherapy something only specialists can undertake: and there are simply not enough of such clinics and specialists to meet the need. Waiting times for appointments and treatment mean that only a few ever have this option. As noted earlier, in Australia waiting times can be 12 months: much too long a time for desperate families, and one which often ensures that symptoms are more severe by the time of admission, and family relationships under greater strains. Marital breakdown is one hazard of undiagnosed food allergy in children.

So one excellent aspect of the Finnish national response was the acknowledgement that self-management with input from allergy support groups was a needed part of a national strategy. Locally based allergy associations can also be a good source of information about allergy specialists who support breastfeeding and do more than prescribe infant formulas. Future children might well benefit if parents sought help with their own allergy problems, and modified their diet to reduce the levels of inflammation and allergy present both before conception, and during gestation and lactation.

---

1856 Beauchamp GK, Mennella JA. Flavor perception in human infants: development and functional significance. *Digestion* 2011; 83 Suppl 1:1-6. (PMID:21389721) Free full text article
1857 Prescott S. *The Allergy Epidemic.* Op. cit
1858 Savilahti EM, Savilahti E Development of natural tolerance and induced desensitization in cow's milk allergy. (PMID:22957704) *Pediatric Allergy and Immunology.* 2013; 24(2):114-121.
1859 Maggadottir SM, Hill D, Brown-Whitehorn TF, Spergel JM. Development Of Eosinophilic Esophagitis To Food After Development Of IgE Tolerance To The Same Food. *J Allergy Clin Immunol* 2014; 133: (2) Suppl p. AB 287.

Specialist help can take many forms in different countries and regions. Experienced paediatric dieticians with a knowledge of allergy, gastroenterologists, allergists, physicians: all can be of use. I have previously mentioned Dr Susan Prescottt's books as very helpful to understanding the issue and knowing the processes involved in hopsital-based care. There are also excellent (and appalling) parent resources on the web: retired dietician Joan Breakey[1860] has helped many families, for example, as has Sue Dengate, author of the "Fed Up" series of books. Again, allergy self-help groups like AESSRA, the Allergy and Environmental Sensitivity Support and Research Association, can often provide suggestions. Every western country has such groups. Not all are fully informed about breastfeeding, of course, and ongoing contact with breastfeeding groups is advisable.

Dr Doris Rapp's *Is this your child?*[1861] is a very valuable reference to own (even if –being American – there is not enough about the breastfed child) and can be ordered from online bookstores. It contains mountains of other useful information from someone who has worked in the field for decades as a paediatric specialist, and it is reassuring to read of the cases she has been able to deal with. She also wrote, and every teacher should read, *Is this your child's world?* available only secondhand at present. Similarly, Linda Gamlin's books,[1862] written with allergist Dr Jonathan Brostoff, provide practical and well-founded knowledge. Parents will also realise that they need to reduce other allergens and environmental challenges, and virtually every allergy clinic, group or specialist (like Dr Doris Rapp) gives guidance about this issue. The food-sensitive child is often affected by other environmental stressors.

Parents should always keep in mind that ultimately they are the ones who will have to judge the usefulness of any help they are offered. Anyone not living with the child will never know as much about their child and his or her problems, and how she or he reacts to environmental challenges or foods.

---

1860 *www.foodintolerancepro.com.* Joan's book, *Fussy Babies*, is very useful even though she has accepted the unproven theory that introducing allergenic foods as early as 4 months (rather than 6) may be beneficial, an idea I strongly disagree with as a general principle. See Chapter 7.5.

1861 Rapp DJ. *Is this Your Child?* op. cit., *Is This Your Child's World? how to fix schools and homes.* (Bantam USA1997)

1862 Gamlin L, Brostoff J. *The Allergy Bible.* (Quadrille Publishing 2005)

# 4.4  Beware the bandersnatch ...

We see families who become discouraged and decide to manage the condition without the guidance of medical providers or who turn to unproven alternative approaches. We have also seen a rise in unfounded Munchausen By Proxy claims against parents of children who are later diagnosed with FPIES [Food protein-induced enterocolitis syndrome]. We need an improved dialogue about the disorder and less dismissal of symptoms. As Philip E. Putnam posits in 'The mother of all food allergies', 'It is becoming increasingly clear that immunologic reactions to multiple foods can present in more subtle fashion than previously recognized and must be included in the broader differential diagnosis for a variety of symptoms'

Schultz F, Westcott-Chavez A (see below).

However, parents should be warned that some well-meaning, but seriously prejudiced, health professionals can threaten the whole family by inappropriate use of their extensive power. Those who don't believe in allergy as common have sometimes seen its symptoms as proof of parenting problems. They have been encouraged by the undoubted fact that in our sometimes bizarre and essentially selfish society,[1863] a few unbalanced, but very plausible, attention-seeking or vicious parents have medically maltreated their children. The diagnosis for such real maltreatment is Munchausen's Syndrome By Proxy (MSBP).

At times, parents who have persisted in seeking medical help and answers about their child's allergy problems have been suspected of inventing, or worse, creating those problems. Parents who have limited their children's diet to reduce symptoms, or who are giving supplements or digestive enzymes, or doing anything seen as odd or 'alternative,' have been suspected of harming their children. Two of the founding board members for the International Association for Food Protein Enterocolitis (IAFPE) have written that this is the experience of their members, in an article everyone working with allergic families should read. [1864] In extreme cases, this can cause the child to be taken into state care by ignorant social workers alerted by a disgruntled or anxious health or childcare worker.[1865] Some children have been taken into care on the grounds that they were fed only organic food![1866] The diagnosis for such behaviour was often MSBP. Many of these diagnoses have

---

1863 Gerhardt S. *The Selfish Society*. (Simon and Schuster 2011)
1864 (www.IAFFPE.org) is an advocacy group dedicated to bridging the gaps that exist between FPIES patients, families, and physicians. See Schultz F, Westcott-Chavez A. Food protein-induced enterocolitis syndrome from the parent perspective.(PMCID:PMC4011625 *Curr Opin Allergy Clin Immunol*. 2014; 14(3): 263–267. Published online Apr 30, 2014. doi:  10.1097/ACI.0000000000000059
1865 Read Megan's story in *The Age Good Weekend* magazine, October 13, 2012, pp. 15-18.
1866 Yet organic food reduces exposure to pesticides and antibiotic-resistant bacteria. See Smith-Spangler C, Brandeau ML, Hunter GE, Bavinger JC, Pearson M, Eschbach PJ, Sundaram V, Liu H, Schirmer P, Stave C, Olkin I, Bravata DM. Are organic foods safer or healthier than conventional alternatives?: a systematic review. (PMID:22944875) *Ann Intern Med* 2012; 157(5):348-366.

since been overturned by courts, but huge damage had been done meanwhile, with the child separated from family and fed inappropriately.[1867]

Protect yourself against this horrific possibility as much as you can. Create a good long-term relationship with a local doctor and other community authority figures who know and respect the family. Select only specialists who see nutrition as critically important, and allergies (or hypersensitivities) as common, and taking a huge variety of forms. Avoid those who are narrow-minded and dogmatic and ignorant of biomedicine and nutrition, any who always reach for drugs before taking careful histories, those who do not respect parental evidence or instincts, and any who expect instant compliance without question. Such people can be dangerous. (I am bitterly aware that the above implies that you are a parent with the personal and financial resources to make choices about health professional care. Many don't.)

At the same time, treat your doctors as you want them to treat you: with respect and politeness and awareness of the value of their knowledge and skills. A good doctor works with parents for their children, and brings extensive training to assist the parents to care for their children. A dangerous one doesn't listen, and expects blind obedience. Quietly find a better one, but don't badmouth the first: one of the great strengths (and weaknesses) of the medical profession is that doctors generally support one another, and are very wary of parents who criticise a colleague. Tell the doctor your story as objectively as you can; putting it on paper with dates and details is always a good idea.

As for using childcare centres, take care here too. Some may resent the idea that the standard of care they provide is not good enough for an individual child, and either ignore parental instructions about dietary or medical needs, or resent the problems these create. Look for a centre where difference is accepted, the individual nature of allergy is understood, and healthy food and drink are the norm. This is taken for granted in Finland, where a considerable proportion of childcare meals are low-allergen. It is getting easier as awareness grows, although it has taken injury and deaths of allergic children to create change.

The same applies to schools. Allergic children can be put at risk in school environments, as Doris Rapp makes very clear in her book on this subject,[1868] regrettably hard to find. Inhalant and chemical sensitivities as well as multiple food[1869] issues can cause difficulties, and the allergic child is often punished for being different from expected norms. Though that is not the focus of this book, it is worth mentioning.

## An aside for all those helping other parents

Meanwhile, if you, dear reader, have a role helping parents, use the questionnaire with both pregnant parents and postnatal ones, and contact me about its usefulness. Always allow

---

1867  Dr Helen Hayward-Brown. False and Highly Questionable Allegations of Münchausen syndrome by proxy – presented to the 7th Australasian Child Abuse and Neglect Conference in Perth 1999. See *http://www.pnc.com. au/~heleneli/paper.htm*

1868  Rapp D. *Is this your child's world?* Op cit.

1869  Host A, Halken S. Cow's milk allergy: where have we come from and where are we going? (PMID:24450456) *Endocrine Metabol Immun Disorders Drug Targets* 2014, 14(1):2-8. DOI: 10.2174/1871530314666140121142900

a couple of hours for talking things through, and if possible have both biological parents present. Both made the genome the child inherited. The expression of their genes has been affected by their own early diet, as well as the infant's. Involve partners or others who will be constantly caring for the child in the discussion as well.

A father who's just told you he can't sleep for scratching with eczema may even say to you, as one did to a colleague, that he can't understand why you're so bothered about formula: he was formula fed and he's normal. Let parents know that their *usual* can be very *abnormal*, physiologically speaking! And that their baby does not have to endure what they have. Help them to see that their practical and emotional support of one another and the baby is critical: *The science of parenting*[1870] is a good resource here. So too is Oliver James's *How not to f\*\*\* them up*. (see Bibliography)

It also helps if parents understand why our society has this problem. Figure 2-5-3 on page 100 is my attempt to compress one hundred years of poor infant nutrition and social change into a sketch that helps explain why some people and not others have severe problems. Have a look at that, along with the Nestlé infographic you can find at http://www.nestle. com/media/newsandfeatures/nestle-research-epigenetics. (Yes, I know some of my readers will think I should ignore Nestlé resources, but no one has yet created a better, universally accessible infographic. This one perhaps naturally ignores breastfeeding, depicting postnatal nutrition as a baby in a high chair, though by six months the key programming inputs are well underway. It should, of course, be amended if Nestlé is sincere in its claims to support breastfeeding. Critical reading of industry material is preferable to ignoring it, in my view.)

You can also map on to that confuseagram roughly where chemical contaminants (and motor cars and female smoking and radiation and plastics and even global warming's mould proliferation or any other factor) have increased their contribution to undermining health. Suggest that parents plot themselves and their parents into that history. Where do they fall in the intergenerational impact stakes? Because that's the problem, as I see it.

Why is this helpful? It helps parents to know first, that they alone have not created this problem, and second, that they can do something about it. There is often a lot of denial and subtle blame-shifting: 'I have no allergies but my partner and all their family have allergies ...' This is understandable because parents, especially mothers, don't want to feel they cause their baby's problems. Encourage parents to share this historical perspective with parents and grandparents as appropriate: it helps if all the support network are on side, and they are more likely to be on side if they understand that no *blame* is being attached to them, even if they share some *responsibility* for the problem, since their feeding decisions and actions had unforeseen consequences. But they did their best, and that's all we can do. In raising our children, we will always get some things wrong - I know I have!

The focus on understanding the past is to help us all do better in future. If it has taken three or more generations to create this degree of problem, we can expect that it will take time to remedy it – but we can make a start, and be proud of the legacy we're working to leave for future generations of our family.

---

1870 Sunderland M. op. cit.

# 4.5. Summary of how to proceed when allergy is suspected

## Dealing with the young breastfed baby:

### 1.  Exclude other feeding or medical issues as far as possible

If you are not confident to do this, take the baby to someone who is able to, such as your GP or maternal and child health nurse. If they say the baby is fine, believe them … unless you feel you have reason not to. Second and third opinions are always good if you're worried. Your instincts are sound, you know your baby. Talk to other experienced breastfeeding mothers.

### 2.  Optimise breastfeeding

Imagine you are on a desert island with nobody telling you what to do, and only your baby to indicate what needs doing. Respond to what your instincts tell you will make that baby happy. Forget clocks and rules, feed your baby whenever he or she wants to be fed, or is comforted by feeding, or you feel your breasts are full and you'd like them relieved. This little, early and often feeding is normal; it evolves over some weeks into lengthier intervals and an individual pattern, depending on your milk supply, your breast storage capacity, and your baby's energy and comfort needs.

Don't ignore discomfort. Be sure you are getting the baby well on, and your nipples don't look squashed or feel sore.or your breasts lumpy and painful, after or during feeding. Again, if you are not confident (and no one is, first time around) get an experienced breastfeeding counsellor or lactation consultant to help, at the first sign of trouble.

### 3.  Identify a possible culprit food

Think in detail about maternal and paternal infancy and childhood health, infant feeding, later dietary likes and dislikes, any previous children's history to date, what is known of wider family allergy history, maternal diet during pregnancy (changes, cravings, aversions, omega-3 intake), infancy diet to date and at present. What foods seem likely to have been a problem? One shortcut: if you were formula fed and your baby exposed to cows' milk in hospital via formula or fortifier, milk will almost certainly be part of the problem. While doing this research, document your baby's sleep, crying and feeding patterns so you can recognise any changes when on the avoidance diet. Don't rush into changes.

### 4.  Establish a baseline record

Once a suspect food is identified, find out where that food turns up in your daily intake. Read labels carefully. Common allergens will be in many foods, and before you begin you should identify replacements for these foods, or you may waste a lot of time! Cut back to one serve a day of high-intake suspect foods while you plan the next step.

## 5. Maternal avoidance diet

Only when you are organised and feel you can manage it, are you ready to avoid a single suspect food for up to three weeks, while still recording infant behaviour and also your own health and well-being. Feeling worse in the first week, usually days three to six, can be a sign that you have the right food: withdrawal symptoms are usual. Craving the food you have eliminated is also a suggestion that you've got it right! Your body is having to adjust to the absence of something it has become habituated to; it it wants that substance, which means that substance was having an effect.

## 6. What next?

If baby's crying lessened or stopped, and her/his growth continues to be satisfactory, continue the maternal avoidance diet plus exclusive breastfeeding to allow time for any needed repairs by breastmilk alone to six months. Don't worry about occasional accidental infant exposures via maternal diet: they are not likely to be disastrous, and may even be helpful in assessing tolerance levels. (A history of anaphylaxis would alter that advice, and any parent with that problem should have ready access to an Epi-pen.) Once the baby is settled and happy, if the foods do not provoke maternal symptoms, eat them in small quantities consistently, in the hope of inducing tolerance. Reduce the quantity if the baby reacts, and then build it up again, but while still breastfeeding, don't ever binge on foods that you know caused reactions.

If it didn't work, think through everything again from scratch. If no other likely suspect or group of foods emerges as significant, consult a dietician with extensive breastfeeding knowledge, or a nutritionally oriented doctor, or an allergy specialist who supports continued breastfeeding in practice, not just in theory.

# Dealing with the partially or wholly formula-fed baby (for lactation consultants and others)

*This is intended for any healthworker involved in helping parents. Many competent bottle-feeding parents may go ahead without such support, but I really can't recommend doing so by writing this in the same way as the advice for the breastfeeding mother. Artificially fed babies are always at greater risk than breastfed infants, and it is not a matter of a mother reviewing her own diet, feeling the internal consequences, but of parents reviewing their infant's diet. There is a narrower margin of safety involved. This means that there should always be a health professional in the equation, preferably one with experience of infant feeding problems, like a maternal and child health nurse or local equivalent, or a paediatric dietitian with experience in allergy.*

## 1. Exclude other medical issues as far as possible

Check child health growth records. Ask about minor and major illnesses, vaccination history, general health and development, sleep patterns. Enquire about stool colour and consistency – any constipation, diarrhoea, abnormal look, smell, frequency – and consider stool culture if appropriate, in conjunction with the family doctor. Consider probiotic use as well, but look for evidence of efficacy of the particular microbial strains available.

## 2. Optimise artificial feeding techniques

**Visit the home.**

- Check the infant formula. Is it age-appropriate? Where is it kept, how has it been used, does it look or smell abnormal, how long has this tin been open and in use? How warm is the place where it is stored? Ask about formula changes since birth: what, when, and why? Make a note of the brand and batch number of the product in current use. Later do an internet search to check for recalls.

- Check the bottles and teats and all equipment and their sterilisation and storage. Only gross contamination is visible, but even that can be overlooked.[1871]

- Check the water. Check the quality of water used for feeding, and avoidance of chlorine bleach sterilisation of feeding equipment. Is water no cooler than 70C used, to kill any bacteria in the powder? Water should be non-chlorinated, low in minerals, and not from tanks or ground water supplies.[1872] Smell and taste it yourself: some off flavours and musty smells can be noticeable. Are any filters used? Are they serviced regularly? Look carefully at any regular storage jug for algal growth or moulds in indentations.

- Check the mixing procedure. Ask the caregiving parent to make up a feed as she/he normally would, while you watch. Are hands washed with soap and water before beginning the task? What are they dried on? Check surrounds, scoop and use, bottle and teat used, rate of flow. What do the dishcloths and sponges look like, and how are they stored: will they air-dry or stay damp between uses? Do carers wash hands after using them to wipe a bench?

- If the parent insists on making up more than one bottle at a time, check that the extras are immediately refrigerated in the coolest part of a unit that keeps food at 5C or less. Is there a fridge thermometer? Where is it in the fridge and where are the bottles stored?

- Check that formula is cooled quickly and fed immediately, to reduce time for bacterial growth, and slow the formation of oxidative by-products..

- Check the feed. Observe a full feed and note baby's responses. Does the caregiver or parent facilitate infant self-regulation of intake by feeding with baby upright, not supine? Do they change the baby's position during the feed, to encourage bilateral development? Do parents recognise satiety cues and stop feeding, no matter how much is left in the bottle? What happens to any leftovers?

- Check that baby manages the teat effectively and feeds without signs of distress: clenched fists, frowning, pulling off and on, etc. Check for excessive air-

---

1871 During one hospital inspection, I noted substantial amounts of baked-on formula in Special Care Nursery bottles. Bacteria form biofilms on plastics, and some bacteria are heat -loving (thermophilic) or cope well with heat.

1872 Rogan WJ, Brady MT, Committee on Environmental Health, Committee on Infectious Diseases, Drinking water from private wells and risks to children.(PMID:19482772 *Pediatrics* 2009; 123(6):1599-1605.

swallowing, and for compression and constriction of any part of the baby's body during and after feeds. (A head tilted forward or chin on the chest or neck twisted sideways makes swallowing difficult or impossible; a squashed midriff makes for reflux.)

- Observe the feed-giver's communication with the baby during feeding. Is more attention being given to an electronic device than to the child? Does the carer look at and talk to the child, making the feed a social occasion and not just a refilling stop?

- Observe the feed-giver's posture and advise on any adjustments needed to prevent repetitive strain problems.

- Observe the furniture: do sofas and chairs pose a threat of suffocation if the parent dozes off while sitting on them to feed the baby? Are parents aware that co-sleeping deaths are frequently deaths on such surfaces, not on firm mattresses?

- Check that all sleep and travel surfaces do not slope backwards, and are firm and free of loose materials. A simple test to check the safety of the sleep surface can be found online at http://www.youtube.com/watch?v=9u-IUzGao2U&feature=shareSomers

- Educate about basic infant anatomy and simple sling use where relevant; make suggestions for inexpensive slings or carriers that can keep the baby upright after feeds or when complaining of indigestion.

## 3.   Review systematically, preferably with both biological parents

Ask both parents about:

- maternal and paternal infancy and childhood health, infant feeding, later dietary likes and dislikes; any previous children's history to date; what is known of wider family allergy history;

- this baby's pregnancy activity; maternal diet during pregnancy (changes, cravings, aversions); baby's birth; infancy diet to date, plus patterns of sleep and activity;

- stresses suffered by both mother and baby since conception; maternal diet; environmental stressors (exposure to chemicals, toxins, etc; intake of pharmacologically active substances);

- current stress levels and support networks of this family, so as to be able to assess possible options;

- help sought, tests done, advice given to date and any outcomes.

## 4.   Keep a baseline diary and note possible suspect foods

Various foods will be mentioned during the discussion – ask the caregiving parent to keep a diary of infant behaviour, sleep patterns, stools, any symptoms, the formula used, with batch number and brand name recorded. (Keep the tin and record the date when it was used.)

## 5. Check whether the infant's biological parents were artificially fed on cows' milk or soy formula, if this is or can be known

In my experience, this definitely increases the risk of milk or soy being a problem food for the infant. And it may help the parents to realise that their child's problem could well have its roots, not in what they themselves have done, but in what mothers or grandmothers did - with the best intentions, and even on medical advice. Where assisted fertility treatments have been involved, this information may not be available, and the parents' own history is not relevant unless the bottle-feeding mother is partially breastfeeding (as she may well be, of course).

## 6.    Discuss formula choice

Discuss formula choices with both parents, and ascertain practical and affordable options. Discuss the risks of all alternatives (low-lactose, HA, soy, etc.). If it is clear that allergy is already a problem, involve the family's medical adviser, as complex or serious problems like FPIES could emerge suddenly, and specialist advice about nutrition[1873] may well be necessary.

## 7.    Try an alternative formula

Swap the baby to an elemental formula for the duration of one or two tins as a washout period – if it can be afforded over the counter, or prescribed, and the baby accepts it. Some babies absolutely refuse.[1874] Perhaps donor breastmilk could be used for such a washout period, in the hope that some gut healing would allow a transition back to artificial feeds without distressing symptoms. However, no studies have been done of this possibility and its outcomes are therefore unknown, although in Leipzig in 1989 I was told that the milkbank did supply breastmilk for some (then rare) cases of cows' milk-allergic East German children. Otherwise extensively-hydrolysed formula (EHF) should be used at this stage, as the partially-hydrolysed (PHF, marketed as HA, or hypo-allergenic) are not recommended even by their makers in cases of allergy. Industry markets them for use as possible prevention, not for treatment. Cases of anaphylaxis are on record to all the varieties of infant formula (even the extensively-hydrolysed). If there are no severe reactions, keep the baby on the alternative formula for up to three weeks, recording infant behaviour, stools, sleep, etc.

Check in with the parents/caregivers at day three, five, seven and then at least weekly intervals to provide support, assess response and answer any questions. If you can't do this, set up some other reliable support structure among clients, as they need this for some time. In Australia, Dr Colin Little set up an allergy support group that has become AESSRA because he recognised this need. Other doctors employ a trained staff member to do this. Many of the problems parents run into can be avoided with such foresight.

---

1873  Venter C, Groetch M. Nutritional management of food protein-induced enterocolitis syndrome.
(PMID:24699338) *Opin Allergy Clin Immunol.* Jun 2014; 14(3): 255–262. Published online Apr 30, 2014. doi: 10.1097/ACI.0000000000000054
1874  Joneja JM. Infant Food Allergy: Where Are We Now? *J Parenter Enteral Nutr.* 2012; 36:49S-55S.

## 8. If baby settles well, advise avoidance of cows' milk formulas and milk foods

If baby settles well on the first alternative formula chosen by parents, and this was soy-based, advise them to continue avoiding cows' milk for their infant,[1875] and to use caution with other foodstuffs found in the initial formula, such as corn. Advise parents that sensitivity to soy formula may well develop after ten days or more, and that they will need specialist help if the young baby goes on to react to both cows' milk and soy formulas.

If the baby tolerates it with only minor symptoms, a partially hydrolysed cows' milk-based formula may be acceptable, and will certainly be less expensive and more palatable than the extensively hydrolysed.

## 9. If symptoms develop on a soy formula, inform parents about alternatives

Reactions to soy as well as bovine milk are not uncommon. Tell parents *again* about the existence of less allergenic formula brands, the extensively hydrolysed (EHF) types, how they differ from the so-called hypo-allergenic (HA) formulas, and how they can be accessed. Make sure they understand that each HA or EHF formula product is different, and some may not agree with their infant while others might, but there is no way of knowing ahead of time which will be acceptable. Check that they can afford various formulas and if not, try to source some for them. Inform parents that they may need to be quite assertive to be taken seriously, and write a supportive detailed referral to a paediatrician or paediatric dietician or allergy clinic. Advise parents of likely waiting times if they cannot afford private medicine. Suggest they find out what might be covered by any private health insurance they may have.

## 10. Consider probiotics and LC-PUFAs

Evidence is accumulating that some probiotic strains can be helpful in reducing the overall incidence of some allergy symptoms, when given for months as a preventive. This is a very new field and if the baby already is symptomatic, how the gut will react to added probiotics could be very different between babies. If this is suggested, close monitoring would seem like a good idea. But anecdotal reports sugges that it might help some not-breastfed infants, whose gut microbiome is abnormal by definition. Long-chain polyunsaturated fatty acids might also help.

## 11. Refer parents to existing local and online support services and groups

Stay in touch with the parents, as malnutrition is a risk for any allergic infant. Acknowledge their distress and the emotional power of this problem for all involved: guilt, anger, fear, denial, blame ...make sure they are not blaming themselves. Put them in touch with other

---

1875 There is some evidence that continuing exposure to milk even in the form of hydrolysed formulas results in a delay before functional tolerance is achieved: see Terracciano L, Bouygue GR, Sarratud T, Veglia F et al. Impact of dietary regimen on the duration of cow's milk allergy: a random allocation study. *Clin Exp Allergy* 2010,; 40(4):637-642. DOI: 10.1111/j.1365-2222.2009.03427.x

parents with similar problems where possible. Ensure that parents are in touch with a supportive doctor, whether general practitioner or physician.

## AN IMPORTANT REMINDER

Obviously, individual practitioners or parent helpers cannot do the tests or provide the treatments that allergy clinics should be able to do. It's important to realise that the role of the helper is to provide a framework for understanding, based on science and experience; to encourage and support the parents' search for specific causes; to help make sense of the information generated by their enquiries; to suggest practical symptomatic relief; and to provide access to community networks.

Above all, the helper's role is to counsel caution and refer to medical resources as appropriate, while reassuring the parents that the problem is real, common, and not of their making; and that their babies are in discomfort or pain, and need their loving care. To speak of allergic infants as "difficult" is to make life worse for everyone. I do not find it surprising that a follow-up study of infants with eczema found an excess of mental health problems by ten years of age.[1876]

Personally, I suspect that health professionals' treatment of this allergy reaction as a common, annoying, but not really serious, health problem has something to do with that finding. Some parents need to be helped to see just how dreadful a condition eczema can be for their children. It is horrible to feel itchy and irritable, but try not to scratch for fear of skin damage, to wake sweaty at night as histamine is liberated and body temperature rises, to feel scaly and unsightly and see people looking askance at you in public, to have headaches for no obvious reason, and to be treated as a problem, as if this is somehow your fault. If parents do not comfort you, but get annoyed, your world is horribly unfair, and as hostile as you may come to feel. Empathy and patience are needed from parents and doctors alike, not trivialisation.

In the 1980s, after *Food for Thought: a parent's guide to food intolerance* was published, the Australian College of Allergy (now ASCIA) invited me to join them "in recognition of your work educating the lay public about allergy." That was a rare honour that I couldn't afford to keep up for more than a few years, being a volunteer worker and (at the time) a clergy wife. If I live long enough, I'll revise and update *Food for Thought* and put it on the web, as it covered more than I can here. In this book I am attempting to do no more than cover the basics of the critical early stages with very young children, though of course I work with families.

Parents do often ask about older children and adults. They are right to: there is usually some continuity. We have one immune system, one body. Any part of that body can be affected by many different factors, including (but not limited to) allergens. Mental, cognitive, and behavioural effects can be more damaging than physical ones. Having many of the symptoms

---

1876  Schmitt J, Apfelbacher C, Chen CM, Romanos M, et al. Infant-onset eczema in relation to mental health problems at age 10 years: results from a prospective birth cohort study (PMID:20159252) *J Allergy Clin Immunol* 2010, 125(2):404-410.

listed earlier, or other ailments that are said to be psychosomatic, suggests that looking into allergy, especially food allergy, might be a very good idea for every reader. **Because while food is just one major source of allergens, it is the one which we can control, and can learn either to avoid or to tolerate.**

Dealing with allergy is hard, however you tackle it. But it is far better to diagnose allergy early, while the child is still fully breastfed, and the gut has a chance to heal and develop normally before other foods must be added to the diet. Continuing to breastfeed through the lengthy period when new foods are being explored[1877] seems sensible from many perspectives, not least the likelihood of reducing reactivity. A recent review on the link between coeliac disease and infant feeding found that being breastfed during the time of gluten introduction was protective,[1878] and some of the mechanisms to explain this protection are being elucidated.[1879]

All allergy bodies agree that *introducing other foods while still breastfeeding* is a good idea. Such bodies therefore ought actively encourage continued breastfeeding *well past six months*, so that the child can adjust to family food while still supported by breastmilk, and has an emergency fallback food in the event of severe reactions. Unfortunately, many such allergy groups and researchers and authors seem to accept as inevitable the status quo of short-duration breastfeeding, rather than supporting World Health Organization (WHO) recommendations of breastfeeding into the second year and beyond, as was once normal.

Many allergy families in fact do breastfeed for longer than usual, sometimes perforce as their children refuse many other foods. But most feel unsupported when they should be commended. No one wants to see a child subsisting on breastmilk alone past the age of nine months. Though some few have done just fine on such a diet (and analysis of their mothers' milk would be interesting), many will not get enough protein for their increasing growth needs. But if the parents have been frequently and persistently offering a wide variety of appropriate foods and the child refuses them all, it's just possible that the child knows best, and to have breastmilk as a backup is immensely helpful: real nutritional insurance in fact. However, professional support is needed to avoid problems developing after twelve months. The orofacial acts of managing non-milk foods help to shape the child's face, speech, and appetite. For both breastfed and formula-fed infants, extended delay in learning to eat such foods can have later negative consequences, even if physical growth monitoring (essential) is reassuring.

---

1877  That is, in the second six months or more, after 6 full months of exclusive breastfeeding, wherever possible.

1878  Henriksson C, Bostrom A, Wiklund IE (2012). What effect does breastfeeding have on coeliac disease? A systematic review update *Evid Based Med* published 4 August 2012, 10.1136/eb-2012-100607

1879  Palma GD, Capilla A, Nova E, Castillejo G, et al. Influence of milk-feeding type and genetic risk of developing coeliac disease on intestinal microbiota of infants: the PROFICEL study.(PMID:22319588)*PloS one* 2012; 7(2):e30791. DOI: 10.1371/journal.pone.003079[1]

# 4.6 Fourteen FAQs, Frequently Asked Questions

*These are the questions I often have to answer. Some of this repeats what has been said elsewhere, and more detailed information will be found in earlier chapters of the book under relevant headings.*

## Q1. Why is it so hard to work out what causes reactions?

### 1. The unpredictable nature of allergy

The problem with allergy is that there isn't always a neat and predictable 'eat x food, get y symptom' pattern. One day you may react badly, another day you may have no obvious problem, or not the same symptom, or not the same symptom as quickly as the last time. Even the IgE reactor, the classic allergic person, who usually reacts predictably, may not always react violently one day – and the next, react so strongly that it is fatal, especially if they are asthmatics. So the main reason it's hard to work out what caused a reaction is that you can expect many apparently inconsistent reactions.

Some key facts need to be understood. When you are sensitised, you are sensitised, but you need not be symptomatic. Whether or not you develop symptoms at a particular time depends on an ever-shifting balance between the total body load, i.e., everything the immune system is reacting to and coping with; and your current tolerance level, your ability to cope at that time. Both body load and tolerance level vary all the time, for different symptoms, and for different reasons, and in different environments. (See images from an early edition of *Food for thought*.) We have one body, one immune system, and how it deals with challenges -whether allergens, viruses, bacteria, moulds, pollens, chemicals, toxins, whatever – is affected by the sheer number and variety of what it has to deal with at any given moment.

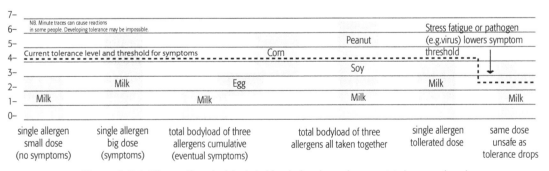

Figure 4-6-1 Allergy thresholds: total body loads and current tolerance levels

This helps explain why, tested in the very different low-dust, smoke-free, plant-free hospital environment, some people fail to respond to classic provocation tests - and are told that they are not allergic.

## 2. The role of stress

Whatever affects our hormones affects our ability to cope: so nutrition, menstrual cycle, puberty, pregnancy or menopause, work or family stress, lack of sleep, fatigue, pain, fear or grief – you name it, if it affects your body it affects *all* of your body, including your immune reactions.

So when you're on holiday and eating less of your usual allergens and you're relaxed and happy, your tolerance level is up. Rushing to work late, after a quarrel with your partner, worried about the children, eating junk food and tired? Your tolerance level is down. In hot dry climates you may react differently from when you're in humid or cold climates. In temperature controlled low-allergen environments away from house dust and cat dander your total body load is lower and your reaction less. Or the converse may be true: in clinics full of volatile chemicals – if you can smell them, your body is dealing with them - you may react more than at home. Changing hormones at puberty or pregnancy or menopause or stages of the menstrual cycle can mean symptoms change. A focussed stressful situation like studying for an exam may send your tolerance level down. The stress hormone cortisol does that to everyone, from babies to grannies.

So an exam, a serious quarrel, or a death, or relentless worry about money can mean that you manifest symptoms – break out in eczema you haven't had in years, for example. Or you may 'come down with a cold' which can be an opportunist rhinovirus strain taking advantage of your weakness while your immune system is overloaded dealing with allergens. (Or it may mean the symptoms of an allergic rhinitis are assumed to mean you're getting a cold.) Or you may take in a substance like aspirin or alcohol, (both of which increase the permeability of the gut lining, and so increase the amount of antigen absorption[1880]) and you then have a reaction to a food you normally tolerate without symptoms.

## 3. The uniqueness of every body and the value of awareness

No one can predict how anyone else's body will juggle all those issues. Or even predict how one's own body will over time. Scientists are showing that immune responses can vary with people's genetic patterns. The immune system's ability to rebalance the body (achieve homeostasis) after any challenge can also be undermined by both medication and poor nutrition, leading to worse immune function and serious disease, even autoimmune disease, over time.

So a viral infection may precede and trigger allergic reactions by overloading the immune system, which until then was coping. Or an allergic reaction may precede and facilitate a viral infection. Or the two may coexist. Or the presence of an environmental toxin such as mercury or some of the thousand chemicals in tobacco smoke may trigger a reaction.

Knowing your own allergens can be valuable, even if you choose not to avoid them, but to limit them to a tolerable level. I know many people who reduce the severity of infection

---

1880 Cant AJ, Gibson P, Dancy M. Food hypersensitivity made life threatening by ingestion of aspirin.
(PMID:6423064) *Br Med J (Clin Res Ed)* 1984, 288(6419):755-756.

612 |
Milk Matters: Infant feeding and immune disorder
Book Three: Crying out for attention

by cutting out their allergens much more strictly at the first sign of a cold or flu, or who curb an allergic pharyngitis that might result in a middle-ear infection (thanks to a blocked Eustachian tube) with a couple of mild antihistamines, or who eat carefully for the week before a long plane trip or exam or other stressful event. And yes, at other times all of these people get away with exposure to some allergen without too many serious side effects. This is particularly true when the problem is in fact a food intolerance rather than a strictly defined immune-mediated allergy: those with wheat protein allergy may react to the slightest trace. while those with gluten intolerance can sometimes cope perfectly well with small quantities.

It isn't always easy to know just what foods you react to, much less how you will react. But if people pay attention and notice their own body's response, over time a reasonable certainty emerges. You are unique, and only you will ever know all that affects you and when, and even you will get some surprises. You only have one body, and everything affects it. The fact that someone else refuses to believe your account of your problems usually means that they don't understand how unique and unpredictable allergy can be. (I'm assuming my readers are neither fools, nor liars nor hypochondriacs, of course. Doctors do see all three, so perhaps it's not surprising that they don't always believe a patient's account.)

Confused now? *Being allergic/hypersensitive* means *having the potential to react badly at times* to substances others tolerate with no problems. Sometimes, when not over-stressed in other ways, your body can deal with the allergen so quickly and effectively that the response produces no noticeable unpleasant symptoms. Over time, if this happens regularly, you may be told that you have (or your child has) 'grown out of allergy'. In fact, the person's tolerance level has risen. That's what we hope to achieve by feeding a wide diversity of foods to children while still breastfeeding: inducing tolerance, even if that may be a temporary reprieve, not a permanent state!

As well, your symptoms may not be the same as another person's reactions to the same food. It is not the case the milk always causes skin symptoms (though it commonly contributes to eczema and acne[1881]), or that wheat always causes gut or brain problems. Both do in many people; in others they cause different symptoms, probably relating to vulnerabilities in that person's genome: migraines, or arthritis, for example. And in some people they cause no reactions at all but are digested without incident. This depends on the person as much as on the food, as well as the age of first exposure and maternal factors.

One study discussed earlier showed that certain genetic variations increase the risk of food sensitisation in contemporary US breastfed children (predominantly African Americans, a group noted for a past history of artificial feeding, which might even explain the presence of the variation, though this is almost never considered).[1882] The authors were careful to

---

1881 Melnik BC. Evidence for Acne-Promoting Effects of Milk and Other Insulinotropic Dairy Products. (PMID:21335995) *Nestle Nutr Workshop Ser Pediatr Program* no 67 2011; 67:131-145; Melnik BC. Diet in acne: further evidence for the role of nutrient signalling in acne pathogenesis.(PMID:22419445) *Acta Derm Venereol* 2012; 92(3):228-23.

1882 Hong X, Wang G, Liu X, Kumar R, et al. Gene polymorphisms, breast-feeding, and development of food sensitization in early childhood. (PMID:21689850) *J Allerg Clin Immunol* 2011, 128(2):374-81.e2.

note that sensitisation can be part of a biological response to an allergen – the body deals with the threat the allergen poses without harmful symptoms – and not a clinical allergic reaction to a food: in short, *being sensitised* does not necessarily mean *being symptomatic*. Breastfeeding, like vaccination, sensitises the immune system, training it to recognise alien substances that should be speedily attacked and destroyed before they can do harm, and providing anti-inflammatory support to damp down any reactions that might become overactive. It's generally better to have an alert immune system than a sluggish non-responsive one.

Then too, as life goes on, the bodily systems in which you notice reactions can change. Your skin matures, or you live in a different climate, and eczema abates. Meanwhile, you develop premenstrual migraines, or as you get older you notice mouth ulcers after you have eaten certain foods. Maybe allergy, or the results of having had allergy in the past, maybe not. Maybe food, maybe not. It takes time and repetition to be sure. The process of monitoring dietary effects is lifelong and it becomes second nature to notice, sometimes to ignore, sometimes to act. Just don't talk about it too often to people who are oblivious to such things, as they will consider you the abnormal one! Keep a private record: over time this can be very helpful, because you will forget details if symptom-free for some time.

## 4. Inadequate labelling

Another obvious reason why it is hard to know what causes reactions is the fact that you cannot rely on food or drug labels to list everything in the food or drug.[1883] As noted earlier, if labelling regulations exist, they are geared to what regulators and industry can measure, not what may in fact be in the food. Human bodies can be exquisitely sensitive, and undeclared allergens can be detected below the current regulatory limits.[1884] As well, you may be allergic to flavourings and other food chemicals which everyone assumes are not a problem.[1885]

Allergen labelling varies from country to country, and it is non-existent for some drug ingredients, such as undeclared excipients (supposedly inert substances in tablets, capsules, etc., that help make the drug or vaccine work in a particular way, say releasing the active ingredient more slowly, or beyond the stomach, or stimulating the immune system to react). These can be a serious problem.[1886] Most are not labelled fully, even peanut oil.

And finally, there's no army of inspectors testing to see if labels are indeed accurate. If you react to some product but can find none of your known allergens on the label, *it doesn't*

1883 Frémont S, Kanny G, Bieber S, Nicolas JP et al. Identification of a masked allergen, alpha-lactalbumin, in baby-food cereal flour guaranteed free of cow's milk protein. (PMID:8905005) *Allergy* 1996; 51(10):749-754

1884 Spanjersberg MQ, Knulst AC, Kruizinga AG, Van Duijn G, Houben GF. Concentrations of undeclared allergens in food products can reach levels that are relevant for public health. *Food Addit Contam. Part A*, 2010, 27(2):169-74. PMID:20013443

1885 Kanny G, Hatahet R, Moneret-Vautrin DA, Kohler C, Bellut A. Allergy and intolerance to flavouring agents in atopic dermatitis in young children. (PMID:7945786) *Allergie et Immunologie* 1994; 26(6):204-6, 209-10

1886 Audicana Berasategui MT, Barasona Villarejo MJ, Corominas Sánchez M, De Barrio Fernández M, et al. Potential hypersensitivity due to the food or food additive content of medicinal products in Spain. (PMID:22312932) *J Investig Allergol & Clin Immunol* 2011, 21(7):496-506.

*mean that they aren't there,* even if labels are completely up to date. Take note of the product and your reaction, and check the product with relevant national authorities. I'm always seeing USFDA or FSANZ recall bulletins 'because of the presence of undeclared allergen.' In industrial-scale food production, mistakes do happen.

## 5.   The impact of the past

The  milk hypothesis, the old/new concept of intergenerational amplification of immune problems, or progressive degeneration of immune systems, also helps explain why allergy symptoms in a first generation allergic (say Grandma) may be very different from the results of the same exposure two generations on. A baby born from a breastfed healthy survivor's body starts life with a major advantage. 'I was bottle-fed and I'm OK' may be true, because the person was born easily (little stress) from the body of a well-nourished woman who had been breastfed as a baby (good *in utero* immune development, good microbiome) and then as a baby was given a mixed diet of home-prepared heavily heat-denatured milk-based formula, fresh orange juice, and cod liver oil, with solids introduced at three months. But that person, however OK he or she may or may not be, is *irrevocably different from what he or she would have been* if breastfed. (And what OK means is very dubious in a culture where cancer and cardiovascular disease and diabetes and irritable bowel and depression are commonplace.)

As well, a bottle-fed woman being OK tells us nothing about the consequences for any child she gestates, and then feeds a (substantially different) infant formula for six months. It may be in the second generation that the harms of the first become obvious. And the different formula fed to the second-generation baby may be a big factor in how any ill-health is manifested. Generation two might have been fed a low-iron casein-dominant formula and been constipated and iron deficient and prone to infection. Generation three, gestated by generation two, may be fed a whey-dominant high-protein formula, and have weight problems as well as allergy problems, morphing into autoimmune disorders.

If infant formula alters gene expression, and its effects are passed on, comparative studies of breastfed and artificially fed infants in two ethnic populations with different formula exposure over several generations, may return different and confusing results.

To put it plainly: it is possible that first-generation bottle-fed adopted Anna born from a breastfed African mother's body will have fewer obvious allergy problems than some children breastfed after being gestated by bottle-fed mother and grandmother, like those African Americans in the study referred to earlier, and like many other families in Western countries where bottle-feeding has been endemic since the 1960s. Yes, formula will alter gene expression for bottle-fed Anna, but perhaps the worst effects won't show until she produces her own children, or even until her grandchildren arrive. And meanwhile, Anna is healthy by comparison with breast-fed Belinda. (Everyone knows at least one highly allergic breastfed child, if community assertions are any guide.)

Why? Diana, Belinda's mother, was the product of three generations of bottle-feeding, and after good antenatal education, she decided to breastfeed despite her background, and her long history of smoking and agricultural pesticide exposure. The odds are that baby Belinda will undoubtedly do better if she breastfeeds than if she were bottle-fed, but even so, Belinda can be expected to have problems. Both mother's and baby's genes are expressed differently in every generation than they would have been had both been breastfed. The odds are, too, that baby Belinda will insist on being breastfed for a long period, if this is possible for Diana. In my experience, allergic babies are long-term breastfeeders by choice. It's often a choice their mothers are happy to go along with, because it's so hard to get reaction-free complementary foods (see Chapter 6.5 What are 'good quality complementary foods'?)

But if the Annas and Belindas are part of a study that measures symptoms of allergy, and correlates these with breastfeeding duration, the study may find a higher rate of allergy in long-term breastfeeders, with the duration of breastfeeding assumed to cause the allergy symptoms, when the allergy causes the long-term breastfeeding! This is called reverse causation, when the two are connected but in the opposite direction to that assumed. Most studies don't effectively eliminate this sort of confusion,. The idea of the baby as a passive agent and the mother being in complete control of his or her diet has become entrenched in bottle–feeding cultures. Breastfeeding women know that babies are in control of their feeding, and can steadfastly refuse to give up the breast for the bottle. Some women even dislike breastfeeding because it is a relationship in which they have no absolute control of the baby.

Belinda's problems stem from Diana's past. But as discussed earlier in this book, there may be another explanation for the rare hyperallergic breastfed child. Perhaps the worst thing for inducing allergy is giving a few early doses of alien proteins to the child of an allergic parent. Allergy studies rarely even mention, much less document, such 'comp' feeds. Classifying such comp-fed gut-disturbed babies as breastfed if they are being breastfed *at the time of the study*, or if the mother says she is *now* giving no formula, is absurd. Many have been exposed to probably ultra-sensitising traces of milk, soy, wheat and corn, some of it GM, maybe with added fungal or algal traces, maybe with peanut oil, in the formula given: mixed feeding indeed. And no one knows what protein traces in what amounts: few studies record the brand, much less the batch ,and what that batch was made of. As well, one study has detected and identified a soy protein component that cross-reacts with caseins from cows milk,[1887] so a rare breastfed child might react to soy protein on the assumed first exposure.

And as also discussed previously, some industry-supported allergy studies recruit infants after days, even three weeks of breastfeeding, to a 'formula feeding' group and then report on outcomes as though they were comparing children breastfed solely from birth with those formula-fed solely from birth. Given what we know about gut colonisation, that is just wrong; but it's beneficial to the marketing of multi-billion-dollar products, so it's no surprise that it keeps happening. This same confusion of groups is now happening in studies of new formulas for extreme preterms: and the results are claimed to show that these *may* be safe and beneficial. The formulas might then be used for infants never given

---

1887 Rozefeld F, Docena GH, Anon Mc, Fossati CA. Detection and identification of a soy protein component that cross-reacts with caseins from cows milk. *Clin Exp Immunol* 2002; 130: 49-58.

any breastmilk, with very different gut effects. Knowing if you or your children have been exposed to these sensitising early doses can help make sense of problems you now struggle with.

So to summarise:

- allergic people can be symptom-free and deemed to have 'grown out of allergy' for long periods, but many are still in fact allergic (in the sense that they have the potential lifelong to react adversely, and not always predictably, to allergens)
- allergic people can lose one symptom as a body system matures, but gain another (gut problems to mood changes; eczema to eosinophilic oesophagitis (inflamed oesophagus)
- they can learn to identify their own stressors and stay symptom free
- they may – or may not- be able to reduce the risk of passing on allergy problems to their children, and they should try to
- different family history means different genes and expression of genes with unknowable consequences.

## Q2. Should a mother stop breastfeeding and use formula?

Almost never. If any health care professional readily suggests as a first option that the very young baby will be better off on a formula, their knowledge of both lactation and infant formula is questionable, and parents need better informed support. I have known of some terrible outcomes after young allergic fully-breastfed babies were given formula. Mind you, as mentioned earlier, when a breastfed baby is changed to an elemental, or amino acid mix, formula there can be some marked improvement initially, if the baby is not already sensitised to any of the other ingredients of the formula. But such an alien mix in a disturbed gut can mean that two weeks later – as immune reactions are programmed and antibody formation in full swing – the baby is far worse than he ever was. And some babies go from bad to worse very quickly once mother's milk is no longer their sole feed, or breastfeeding ends abruptly.

(From admittedly limited experience, it seems to be at least two weeks before the full effect of total weaning kicks in. That is long enough for people to think that changing from breastfeeding had no bearing on the problems that then emerge – 'He was OK when I stopped breastfeeding but two weeks later he caught a virus.' Maybe. But it takes time for the gut flora to change, the immune system to develop antibodies, and obvious symptoms emerge.) And it takes time for breastmilk's protection to decline.

## Q3. Can babies be allergic to breastmilk?

There are similarities between mammalian milks, which mean that if a baby reacts to one, he/she may react to the other which is very like it in some way. This routinely happens with cows' and goats' milks, for example. Since this cross-reactivity can occur, it is possible that an initial sensitisation by cows' milk formula before birth or in hospital may result in the infant immune system reacting badly to a similar but human protein in breastmilk. Cross-reactivity is thought to be one of the causes of type 1 diabetes: antibodies sensitised to bovine protein attacking human pancreatic cells, which resemble the bovine protein.

For babies of a mammalian species to be allergic to their own mother's milk protein makes their survival to reproductive age very unlikely, and so this would have to be a rare or recent development. But nothing can be ruled out as impossible where allergy is concerned. And there is one study[1888] that suggests that at least in the laboratory a reaction to a human milk protein can occur. But in vitro tests with human milk are using a product quite different from the baby-specific mixture fresh from mother, in conditions that do not occur in real life. A human baby reacting to human milk proteins is so rare that despite decades of wide-ranging research and clinical work, I have yet to meet one, or read a convincing case history that could not have an alternative explanation So until we have proven real-life cases on record, mothers can safely be told that their baby is *not allergic to their milk itself, even when drinking it produces symptoms.*

When a breastfed baby does react to his mother's milk, it is a reaction to foreign proteins (like cows' milk or soy) in that breastmilk. Babies may well be allergic *to traces of foods eaten by the mother*, which the breast is designed to share with the baby in ways that should produce tolerance, *but can cause reactions*. This is why maternal diet change can be a useful strategy, and ideally donor breastmilk would be available. Given everything else that is in breastmilk and industrial formulas, it is highly unlikely that any breastfed baby would be better off on infant formula overall.

That said, there are breastfed babies for whom elemental or amino-acid based non-human formulas are needed, sometimes briefly, to resolve a serious and time-critical problem like gut bleeding.[1889] A case is on record where the infant was born with this condition, which proved in utero sensitisation to cows' milk was not only possible but seriously damaging.[1890] Of course such low-allergen products must be used, however reluctantly, and only after checking for unlabelled hazards. In these serious cases, parents have to be guided by the doctors caring for the child. The suggestions I offer here for investigating and treating the young colicky child may not work for a severely affected older child.

But there are no guarantees that even the most recent formula will not cause more problems than it eases for a particular baby. So if any mother stops breastfeeding abruptly, I always advise her to express her milk, if possible, so there is an option to relactate if things get worse on formula (as well as to reduce her risk of mastitis and depression from abrupt weaning). And of course, to try to identify what in her diet needs changing so that her milk does not cause such problems for the baby. Doctors need to consider returning babies to

1888 Järvinen KM, Geller L, Bencharitiwong R, Sampson HA Presence of functional, autoreactive human milk-specific IgE in infants with cow's milk allergy.(PMID:22092935) *Clin Exp Allergy* 2012, 42(2):238-247.
1889 Lucarelli S, Di Nardo G, Lastrucci G, D'Alfonso Y, et al. Allergic proctocolitis refractory to maternal hypoallergenic diet in exclusively breast-fed infants: a clinical observation. (MED:21762530). *BMC gastroenterology* 2011, 11:82.
1890 Alabsi HS, Reschak GL, Fustino NJ, Beltroy EP et al.Neonatal eosinophilic gastroenteritis: possible in utero sensitization to cow's milk protein.(PMID:23985469) *Neonatal Netw* 2013; 32(5):316-322.

breastmilk once serious symptoms abate or a new infant gut flora has been established or mothers have eliminated problem foods for long enough to eliminate reactive antigens in milk.

Many mothers who stopped breastfeeding on medical advice bitterly regret losing the one comfort food that really worked, the ability to put baby to breast. Some have relactated, but that can be hard work, is time-consuming, and there are no guarantees of success. It is indeed possible for some, as the WHO document *Induced lactation and relactation* made obvious. It is still current WHO policy to encourage relactation even in emergencies,[1891] and WHO states that the woman's 'confidence in her ability to produce adequate amounts of milk will largely determine the diligence and success of her efforts to do so'.[1892]

Of course helping women breastfeed and/or relactate and build up a full milk supply takes time. Sometimes a lot of time. I can't help feeling that advice from allergy clinics to stop breastfeeding proceeds from a desire to get the matter sorted as quickly as possible, by putting the baby on to an expensive elemental formula, often at taxpayer expense in Australia and the UK, and even the US for some Women Infants and Children (WIC) clients. This is understandable, if shortsighted, and not in the child's interest, because such clinics are seriously overworked with long waiting lists, at least in Australia. There also seems to be a perception that parents can't or won't manage the dietary changes that will be involved if the clinic goes down the path of trying to work out what in a mother's milk is causing reactions, and eliminating it. That has not been my experience.

Some parents do indeed find it all too much. Certainly working through these things can be a long and slow process, with mistakes along the way. But so too can be the process of getting a child to eat anything but an elemental formula once that path is chosen. I know of cases where children are still totally formula-dependent, unable to eat real food, years later, and the difficulties are enormous. As well, the loss of breastfeeding for both mother and child is incalculable.

## Q4. Other foods for infants: when?

*At this point in the book, the issue of introducing other foods is appropriate, with the focus being on children already manifesting symptoms of food sensitivities. The topic of foods other than breastmilk or formula is a book in itself, and not one I want to digress into at this stage. Later, in Chapter 7, the question of what foods and other practical suggestions are addressed, separately for the breastfed and the not-breastfed child. And Chapter 7 also covers several theoretical controversies that have influenced the practical advice parents hear about "introducing solids", that somewhat misleading phrase covering the widening the infant diet beyond breastmilk or formula. To include all these dimensions of the topic in this chapter of the book would be to take the allergy discussion way off track. However, this means there will be some overlap in what is covered in both places, though I'll keep it to a minimum.*

---

1891 http://www.who.int/nutrition/publications/guiding_principles_feedchildren_emergencies.pdf
1892 WHO *Induced Lactation and Relactation* (Geneva 1998) http://www.who.int/maternal_child_adolescent/
   documents/who chs_cah_98_14/en/index.html

## 1. Other foods for the breastfed allergic infant: when?

All babies need adequate amounts of tolerated food to thrive. WHO rightly and strongly advocates six months' exclusive breastfeeding[1893] for many reasons: it makes a positive difference to many diseases of mother and child, while giving other foods earlier reduces breastmilk's protective effects for mother and child, and alters nutritional bioavailability. To introduce solids at four months rather than around six months means doing so before the optimal age physiologically; it reduces breastmilk's protection against infection, and increases the risk of a shorter interbirth interval (without expensive contraception) along with poorer maternal health in the short and long term.[1894] And it is associated with increased risk of autism, among other problems.[1895] The scientific case for not giving *unnecessary* foods to breastfed infants as early as four months is strong, and parents do heed such guidelines: the number giving solids earlier than that has been dropping since 2000, as the official UK surveys document.

Some paediatricians and child health nurses are now suggesting introducing other foods in the period from four months on, while the mother is still breastfeeding, on the basis of studies showing that exposure to allergens during lactation results in tolerance.[1896] A recent study showed that infants who were diagnosed with <u>food allergy</u> by the time they were two had been introduced to solids earlier (at or under 4 months of age) than those not diagnosed, and had been less likely to be getting any breastmilk when cows' milk protein was first introduced into their diet. (That result was despite no intensive investigation of in-hospital comp feeds.)[1897]

To start giving other foods at four months makes sense only if you think mothers must stop breastfeeding at six months. While the mother is still breastfeeding, introduction of other foods between four and six months is *not* proven better than introducing allergens in the period six to twelve months, as many mothers of allergic children find themselves doing.

1893  Global Strategy on Infant and young child feeding, paragraph 10, p. 7. Online at http://whqlibdoc.who.int/publications/2003/9241562218.pdf?ua=1.
1894  Wiklund PK, Xu L, Wang Q, Mikkola T et al. Lactation is associated with greater maternal bone size and bone strength later in life. (PMID:21927916) *Osteoporos Int* 2012, 23(7):1939-1945; Wiklund P, Xu L, Lyytikäinen A, Saltevo J et al. Prolonged breast-feeding protects mothers from later-life obesity and related cardio-metabolic disorders. (PMID:21859508) *Public Health Nutr* 2011:1-8.
1895  Gallup GG Jr, Hobbs DR. Evolutionary medicine: bottle feeding, birth spacing, and autism. (PMID:21641730) *Medical Hypotheses* 2011; 77(3):345-346. DOI: 10.1016/j.mehy.2011.05.010
1896  Verhasselt V. Neonatal tolerance under breastfeeding influence: the presence of allergen and transforming growth factor-beta in breast milk protects the progeny from allergic asthma. *J Pediatr.* 2010 Feb;156(2 Suppl):S16-20. doi: 10.1016/j.jpeds.2009.11.015.; Prescott SL, Smith P, Tang M, Palmer DJ et al. The importance of early complementary feeding in the development of oral tolerance: concerns and controversies. (PMID:18266825) *Pediatric Allergy and Immunology* 2008, 19(5):375-380. DOI: 10.1111/j.1399-3038.2008.00718.x (PMID:20105659) *J Pediatr* 2010, 156(2 suppl):s16-20.. Nothing new in that idea, whether in mice or men!
1897  Grimshaw KEC, Maskell J, Oliver E, Morris RCG et al.  Introduction of Complementary Foods and the Relationship to Food Allergy.  *Pediatrics* 2013; 132 (6): e1529 -e1538. DOI: 10.1542/peds.2012-3692

Yet some health professionals have openly opposed the recommendations developed by WHO, and confused parents even further.[1898]

It is true, of course, that *at present in western countries* only a minority of women breastfeed past six months; in fact, only a minority breastfeed at all to six months, very few exclusively, perhaps 15% in Australia in 2010. That can and should be changed, along with the pressures that cause it.

As I've said before, and will doubtless say again, it *would* change if all health professionals and respected authorities spoke with one voice about the importance of the WHO/ NHMRC recommendation to breastfeed *solely to around six months and then breastfeed with appropriate complementary foods into the second year and beyond* (see Chapter 7.5 What are 'good quality complementary foods'?). Both the Talmud and the Koran advise breastfeeding as the child's birthright until twenty-four months, and now WHO has affirmed the wisdom of such traditional advice. A growing minority of educated women do breastfeed past six months; a majority of all women easily could if society supported such choices, and indeed once did so in almost every culture. Health professionals arguing for the universal widening of the infant diet beginning at four months or sixteen weeks are wrong to accept a damaging status quo rather than to advocate change enabling longer-term breastfeeding. Those who accept the status quo need to accept responsibility for its harms.

Interestingly, in the development of the Australian *Infant Feeding Guidelines* (published December 2012)[1899] there was strong pressure not to endorse the WHO position. Despite this, the Guidelines have reiterated that solids should be introduced 'around six months'. The Working Group reviewed the available evidence and was not swayed by unscientific considerations, like the inconvenience to babyfood manufacturers, who should be rebranding their products! As studies are done and compared across different generations, we might realise that introducing foods other than breastmilk earlier than six months produces different outcomes *according to the allergic status of the parents and grandparents*. This would help explain the confusion in the literature, especially in regard to the effects of neonatal introduction and those so-called 'comp feeds'. (See Chapter 2.5.)

The fact that many ill-informed voices are often heard so loudly does have something to do with industry's essential agenda. This surely has to be never to allow different recommendations for breastfed and formula fed infants, because that would make abundantly clear to parents that formula-fed infants are significantly different from what they would have been if breastfed. For more on this topic see Chapter 7.5.

---

1898 The 'standard' advice now can be found in the ASCIA (Australasian Society of Clinical Immunology and Allergy) position statement. ASCIA Infant Feeding Advice is 'intended to provide families in Australia and New Zealand with a summary of evidence based information on infant feeding, including an explanation as to why families may choose to introduce solid foods to their infants from 4-6 months (whilst breastfeeding) and not delay the introduction of potentially allergenic foods, to prevent allergy.' http://www.allergy.org.au/ health-professionals/papers/ascia-infant-feeding-advice

1899 Available online at http://www.nhmrc.gov.au/_files_nhmrc/publications/attachments/n56b_infant_feeding_ guideline_summary.pdf

Again, language is a big part of this problem. As lactation consultant and specialist dietician Joy Anderson has cogently remarked in commenting on this chapter, 'We might do better to reverse how this is expressed, i.e., "Breastfeeding is recommended for two years and beyond, with it being exclusive for the first six months". Otherwise many people just hear, "breastfeed until six months".' Spot on. But imagine the howls from infant formula advocates when that accurate wording of the WHO recommendation is used! Especially if the corollary were to be "The diet of the formula-fed infant should be widened from 4 months or 16 weeks, as body stores of essential nutrients might be exhausted and the formula might not be adequate." What government would be brave enough to speak those truths to parents?

## 2. Other foods for the formula-fed allergic baby: when?

We don't know. That giving new foods with breastmilk should lead to tolerance[1900] is obvious. It is also obviously irrelevant to formula-fed babies, already consuming a wide variety of foods in the formulas they swallow. The best age for giving new solid foods to the solely formula-fed infant (in relation to allergy induction) seems not to have been researched. I can see good reasons to widen the diet of the usual formula-fed baby from three to four months onwards, or even earlier, if he or she is not thriving on cows' milk infant formula. In theory at least, lowering the total load of cows' milk protein without eliminating it just might allow the infant to cope better and develop some tolerance. And if the whole diet is shifted away from cows' milk, consideration could be given to constructing a 'formula' based on less industrialised foods, such as a comminuted (pulverised) chicken diet used with success in some allergy clinics.[1901] (Mind you, I have seen no follow-up studies checking whether there are higher later childhood or adult rates of allergy to avian products.)

In fact, widening every artificially fed infant's diet as soon as practicable after three to four months seems prudent and in keeping with the most basic rules of dietary safety, which are *variety of foods* and *moderation of intake* of each. Giving other foods to formula-fed children at three to four months has been done in Western societies for most of the twentieth century, so this is not a new experiment, even if its outcomes remains largely unresearched. So working from first principles, and following the reasoning of the 1980 AAP directive (see Chapter 7.5) there seems to be very good reason to widen the diet of a four-month-old formula-fed baby. Just as there is good reason to give breastmilk alone till six months or more if baby is thriving on it. There is more about all this in Chapter 7.

## Q5. Should donor milk be considered for allergic babies?

Of course it should. People use donated milk wherever mothers know this to be possible. Now that we know the stem cells are incorporated into mammalian tissues, exploring the therapeutic use of donated breastmilk should become a priority. Like all other alternatives,

---

1900 Grimshaw KE, Maskell J, Oliver EM, Morris RC et al. Introduction of complementary foods and the relationship to food allergy. (PMID:24249826) *Pediatrics* 2013, 132(6):e1529-38] DOI: 10.1542/peds.2012-3692
1901 Dietetics texts contain recipes.

there are risks, and in most countries there is no commercial lobby to benefit from supplying the product while minimising risks.

I can't help wondering why those who see gut dysbiosis as a major cause of disease, and have even experimented with faecal transplants,[1902] have not begun to explore the use of human milk 'transplants'. The stem cells human milk contains are identical to fetal embryonic stem cells, and are intended for human ingestion.[1903] Milk is after all the food that routinely establishes a healthy gut flora! A complete washout, as for a colonoscopy, might possibly be the ideal precursor to a human milk lavage or feeding or diet for a few days or even weeks. Perhaps in some allergic children this could help resolve gut distress. In others, the lactose level of the breastmilk might first need to be lowered by incubation with lactase before ingestion (though this increases the concentration of solutes, or osmolarity[1904], of the milk[1905]) or by adding more cream from a second batch of breastmilk. Adding cream increases the caloric density of the milk, can be protein-sparing, and the increased fat slows gastric emptying, allowing more time for acid digestion of the milk. It has become routine care for very low birthweight infants at Baylor College of Medicine Hospital in Texas. ((See page 440.)

But lactose in human milk, fresh or donated, is not always a problem for damaged guts. When my son was almost four in 1980 he underwent surgery for a severe food reaction misdiagnosed as appendicitis. After removal of a healthy appendix, he developed repeated gut obstruction, relieved by repeat keyhole surgeries. A re-feeding diet began with chocolate-flavoured cows' milk, and orange juice. Painful gut spasms and even literally skin-blistering diarrhoea did not cause this to be amended. After three such episodes, I expressed breastmilk, added chocolate syrup to disguise it, and fed my son that mix instead, tipping out the cows' milk and drinking the juice. (I was breastfeeding my ten-week-old third child.) Lactose-rich and sugar-fortified, my chocolate-flavoured breastmilk helped his damaged gut: he promptly improved and recovered forthwith, and was able to be discharged two days later on this enriched breastmilk diet (looking like a famine victim with stick-thin arms, as he had lost so much condition in that period of semi-starvation and repeated surgery). On breastmilk plus a good diet at home, his catch-up growth was fantastic, putting back the muscle and condition he had lost. (He asked for and ate four boiled eggs, a high-quality protein source, each day for a week. He had and has no problems

1902 Not an attractive option, but it's logical and can work. Anderson JL, Edney RJ, Whelan K. Systematic review: faecal microbiota transplantation in the management of inflammatory bowel disease. (MED:22827693) *Alimentary pharmacology & therapeutics* 2012, 36(6):503-516. DOI: 10.1111/j.1365-2036.2012.05220.x; Guo B, Harstall C, Louie T, Veldhuyzen van Zanten S, Dieleman LA. Systematic review: faecal transplantation for the treatment of Clostridium difficile-associated disease. (MED:22360412) *Aliment pharm & ther* 2012, 35(8):865-875. DOI: 10.1111/j.1365-2036.2012.05033.x ! However, there are dangers in this as a DIY project!

1903 Unlike the stem cells sourced from a patient's nasal cavity and put into her damaged spine, which perhaps not surprisingly developed into a mass of nasal tissue that caused pressure, pain, and further surgery. See Dlouhy BJ, Awe O, Rao RC, Kirby PA et al. Autograft-derived spinal cord mass following olfactory mucosal cell transplantation in a spinal cord injury patient: Case report. (PMID:25002238) *J Neurosurg Spine* 2014, 21(4):618-622 DOI: 10.3171/2014.5.SPINE13992

1904 Basically the amount of dissolved matter that the kidney has to cope with

1905 Carlson SJ, Rogers RR, Lombard KA. Effect of a **lactase** preparation on lactose content and osmolality of preterm and term infant formulas. (PMID:1942472) *J Parenter Enteral Nutr* 1991; 15(5):564-566.

with eggs, which had been introduced as egg yolks mixed in mashed potato or in home-made soups at 6 months.)

A sample of one proves nothing, of course, but I have known of other cases where mothers have used their (undisguised and unadulterated) milk for older sick children. And human milk has been used to heal cases of colitis; it was routinely used as medicine in many societies, and has been used by cancer patients in Australia. Why not try this? Why wouldn't it work? There is a long multicultural tradition of using women's milk as medicine.[1906] And it has saved babies' lives and done much more: in 2009 a team of twenty local women organised to feed a Michigan baby whose mother died soon after birth. The story makes inspiring reading,[1907] but it is not exceptional.

So human milk may be an avenue to explore, preferably in concert with an open-minded physician. Donated milk will have its risks, but can be safer than any industrial product, if sensibly sourced. The Australian College of Midwives has recently endorsed the use of donor milk of known origin and is developing a position statement.[1908] *Donor Human Milk Banking in Australia - Issues and Background Paper*,[1909] was published by the Commonwealth Government in 2014, outlining the current legal and actual situation, but as usual in such documents, minimising by omission many potential harms of artificial formula as the alternative to donor milk. Risk benefit analysis is only useful if all the risks of both options are included.

Interestingly, such milk may not need to be from a donor mother on a diet free of the recipient's allergens. Obviously that would seem to be safer in terms of any immediate reaction. However, I remember, but cannot now locate, a UK study decades ago that showed that some allergic infants reacted to food antigen in their own mother's milk when she was consuming those foods, but not when drinking donated milk from a mother whose diet included the allergens.[1910] This raises interesting research questions as to how mothers' milks differ, and could be the subject of a lot more research. (And careful reporting of that research should not strengthen the old undermining belief that there is something wrong with many mothers' milk! Too many under-confident women still think industrial brews better than anything they can produce, which is emphatically not the case.) While so much research money goes into developing formulas, very little by comparison goes into researching breastmilk's peculiarities and uniqueness – except with an eye to commercialising it.

---

1906 Volume II of the remarkable 3 volume *Woman, an historical, gynaecological and anthropological compendium* op. cit., devotes a chapter to 'unusual uses of woman's milk.' pp 233-244, including its use as medicine and as food for toothless in-laws... but being German they failed to catalogue some of the more prominent Anglophone consumers, such as a Rockefeller and a Master of Caius College in Cambridge.

1907 seattletimes.com/html/living/2009579376_momsmilk01.html

1908 ttp://women.wcha.asn.au/system/files/news/13981/acm_draft_position_statement_on_the_use_of_donor_human_milk_consultation.pdf

1909 Go to http://www.health.gov.au/breastfeeding to locate and download this document.

1910 This was a study in the 1980s which I cannot now locate: but will before the next edition. I'd love someone to repeat it.

Women are taking control of their milk back into their own hands, a development not without some risks, but also with the promise of major benefits. The internet has made it possible to match women with milk to give, with those who are in need of it. This was reviewed in the free open access *International Breastfeeding Journal* in one of its most read articles, so I shan't repeat what was said there,[1911] but urge you to read it for yourselves. An online search for human milk for human babies, or HM4HB, will locate more information and resources.

Let me assure you, the medical profession at present has no idea how many babies are drinking donor breastmilk as well as their mother's own. It is a parent's right to choose this option for feeding their infant. The medical profession's conformist fear of acting outside accepted commercial practices is not a good enough reason to insist parents give a known-to-be–harmful substance – infant formula – instead of a possibly-risky one – donated human milk. An excellent study of comparative risks is available.[1912]

## Q6. Can allergy be prevented?

Parents who have survived one allergic baby want to know what can be done to prevent allergy in any future babies. The first baby is often the worst, for a wide variety of possible reasons, including a greater likelihood of being formula exposed and poorly breastfed. (Although if the allergic mother does not identify and manage her allergies, and goes on being increasingly depleted by short interbirth intervals, each subsequent baby may well be worse than the last. I have seen both patterns in families.)

Parents are usually said to be more relaxed with subsequent babies, but this is not true for those with allergic firstborns. Any mother who has survived a first allergic child is very tense indeed about the possibility that the crying and gut problems may start up with the second child and then not stop. Mothers – myself among them – who had been very relaxed about the first baby (and then stunned by the reality) did not relax until months had gone by with a placid happy second child. It almost seemed impossible that the changes made (guarding them night and day in hospital to try to prevent cows' milk exposure, for example) could make such a difference to the child. (It did, though.)

But is allergy prevention possible generally? The complexity of the problem's causes suggests that the answer will be 'possible for some, not for others'. But worth trying!

An Italian study says that allergy rates are significantly lower when women try an avoidance programme they outlined:[1913] breastfeeding for the first six months, mothers to consume no more than 200 ml bovine milk per day, no more than one egg per week, no foods to which

1911 Akre JE, Gribble KD, Minchin MK. Milk sharing: from private practice to public pursuit *International Breastfeeding Journal*, 2011; 6:8 . *http://www.internationalbreastfeedingjournal.com/content/6/1/8*

1912 Gribble K, Hausman BL. Milk sharing and formula feeding: Infant feeding risks in comparative perspective? *Australas Med J.* 2012; 5(5): 275–283. Published online 2012 May 31. doi: 10.4066/AMJ.2012.1222 (PMCID:PMC3395287)

1913 Bardare M, Vaccari A, Allievi E, Brunelli L et al.. Influence of dietary manipulation on incidence of atopic disease in infants at risk.(PMID:8214801) *Annals of Allergy* 1993, 71(4):366-371.

she was allergic, and/or no tomato, fish, shellfish or nuts. Avoidance of the mother's own allergens is significant. Ideally the creation of a healthy immune system or prevention of allergy begins in pregnancy, or perhaps even before.

The concept of pre-conceptual care is a good one: both parents optimise their health before conceiving. This involves sorting out allergies, eating well, not taking in excess dairy products, stopping smoking and alcohol, exercising, raising omega-3 levels by eating the right fish, good anti-oxidant intakes from fresh foods, all the good stuff we know about. This is for fathers as well as mothers: the quality of sperm does make a difference to fertility and infant health, just as the mother's contributions will. And refer again to what was said earlier about interbirth intervals if considering this.

Again, using my questionnaire gives an indication of whether the baby will be at high risk of allergy. If you feel after doing that questionnaire that you may have allergy problems, your baby may well be at higher risk. For if one or both parents are allergic, or siblings have suggestive symptoms, the next baby is always at increased risk.

If the baby is already hyperactive *in utero* (lots of kicking and hiccups and movement), it may already be sensitised, which makes a good birth andexclusive breastfeeding even more important.

If cord blood IgE levels are high at birth, there is definitely a much greater risk of allergy. You can ask for this test to be done if allergy is a family concern. I have been told that it is routine in some Scandinavian hospitals.

I can make no promises that allergy can be prevented, but in the geynerations and population I have worked with, many subsequent babies were dramatically easier to deal with when parents were aware of allergies and followed the suggestions made to reduce antigen exposure before, during and after the pregnancy. Not all, however. It would be unrealistic to hope that in one generation we could reverse damage done through multiple generations.

# Q7. Is a vaginal birth important?

Absolutely. As paediatric gastroenterologist Simon Murch said, '... the obstetrician who does a caesarean section may have a long-term impact on the immune development of a person'.[1914] I tell parents to avoid elective caesareans if humanly possible. They are usually done for other people's convenience, and mothers and babies pay a high price. No one should begin a career as a mother with an abdominal wound if this is at all avoidable. No sane man would begin any major life task by having needless abdominal surgery, or while recovering from it. Even late preterm birth can have significant effects on any baby's feeding readiness, while the stress hormones released don't help mother or child. Even when a good size, any preterm infant's neurological maturity is less.

---

1914  Murch S. Oral tolerance and gut maturation. In Isolauri E, Walker WA, op. cit, p.147.

The best way to avoid needless birth interventions is to labour somewhere safe and close to the hospital with an experienced midwife for company, who can ensure that you go into hospital *only when labour is fully established*. Before that time, if you leave your place of security, labour will stop (as though a predator threatened) as stress hormones kick in. Then, once in hospital, staff will want to get labour started again, especially if there is pressure on the birthing unit or labour wards, and the cascading intervention cycle will begin with membranes being ruptured or medication. If labour is well established before you go in, it's much more likely that nothing will stop the process, and you will give birth naturally. And your experienced midwife companion can usually stay with you, supporting your partner while hospital midwives help you birth, and giving you confidence that what you want will happen, whether that is skin contact or easy breastfeeding.

For some parents surgical delivery is medically necessary. They should discuss with medical staff how the baby can be exposed to normal vaginal flora immediately after delivery; having baby skin-to-skin; and facilitating early suckling and breast expression. All three measures are important, and early breast contact and care the most significant. Whatever the birth, breastfeeding is of course perfectly possible, and lactation capacity is not affected, though it is made much more awkward and painful, while the drugs used for pain relief can affect baby and mother alike, in some cases resulting in maternal addiction, and more often, ineffective infant suckling and drowsiness.

Other things to arrange include:

- *Calm and competent help with caring for baby by your bedside*. You will not be able to manage this by yourself if you have surgery, as not only the painful incisions, but the pain relief, handicap you.
- *Kangaroo care techniques* that keep baby skin-to-skin with either parent, especially the mother. This maximises infant exposure to family microbes that milk protects against, rather than institutional microbes. It also minimises infant stress and dysregulation, while helping restore normal hormonal balance in the mother.
- *Help with mundane housekeeping* after returning home, so you can be with the baby and rest, preferably for at least the 40 days traditionally set as a recovery from birth babymoon.
- *Do not let other people take over the baby* and leave parents the housework.
- *Do not let other people disrupt the baby's or mother's sleep and rest.*

Use of baby slings by both partners: simple ones that keep the newborn upright and close, ear against the adult chest, baby's head supported and not flexed down on to his or her chest, so that airways are free. There have been deaths when baby carriers or clothing or cushiony chests obstructed infant breathing. Learn about these things before your planned delivery date, and make sure that your birthing partners will calmly insist on them as much as humanly possible if you have an emergency caesarean birth. A well-informed lawyer grandparent or friend can be a great help if your wishes are not being respected by any hospital staff.

## Q8. Does pregnancy and lactation diet matter?

Short answer: yes, but *how* it matters varies, and whether or not the mother is herself allergic is one of the factors responsible. The official blanket medical advice these days, largely based on severe cases seen by doctors, is to eat normally and not exclude any particular food without specific reason. either in pregnancy or during lactation. Population studies show confusing results: some suggest avoidance in pregnancy may make for greater sensitivity on exposure, others say it helps reduce symptoms. Research studies are unclear: a systematic review reported that

> Prescription of an antigen avoidance diet to a high-risk woman during pregnancy is unlikely to reduce substantially her child's risk of atopic diseases, and such a diet may adversely affect maternal or fetal nutrition, or both.[1915]

But this report reviews studies based on aribitrary avoidance diets, not *individualised* avoidance diet based on history and understanding of the mother's own allergies. Other than the Italian study mentioned earlier, few such studies exist, so far as I could see, and they would be difficult. Given people's uniqueness and varying contextual and intergenerational burdens, as well as the different study methodologies, the results of studies of arbitrary antigen avoidance diets are likely to continue to be confusing. And when they are, because of the potential nutritional risks and the pressures it creates, experts will naturally advise against food avoidance. Only if avoidance could be proved to be generally helpful would they recommend it.

What does common sense and basic science suggest, at least to me? Evolutionary theory suggests not changing from any (good) foods the mother is accustomed to, so she can accustom her baby to them. It's likely that, as with lactation, the immunology of pregnancy is such that it develops protection in the child to foods consumed by the mother. So, no special food avoidance in pregnancy or lactation *for all women.* But equally, no fad binges or dietary excesses impossible in the millennia of human evolutionary history. Overall good nutrition gives a baby a well-stocked larder to grow from and optimises maternal health. When research is unclear, commonsense working from first principles *and taking the individual's history into account* is a reasonable guide.

***But what if the mother of a previous child is already affected by allergy and pregnant?*** In that case, avoiding during pregnancy (even good) foods *that trigger adverse reactions* in the mother may well be helpful, certainly for her, probably for her second baby. Of course, this means being careful to ensure her diet includes the nutrients in the foods being avoided.

---

1915 Kramer MS, Kakuma R. Maternal dietary antigen avoidance during pregnancy or lactation, or both, for preventing or treating atopic disease in the child. (PMID:22972039) *Cochrane Database Syst Rev* 2012; 9:cd000133

Where cows' milk allergy is involved, it may be worth also avoiding beef or other cow protein.[1916]

As noted earlier in Chapter 2, there are studies that support what many parents have found: that avoiding their allergens during pregnancy seemed to make a positive difference, reducing or preventing problems in the next child. (But of course we cannot know how that child, with a different genome, *might* have been; or whether the parents feeling less helpless was a critical variable.) However, if changing diet to avoid allergens makes a positive difference to the woman's own experience of pregnancy, for example ending even severe pregnancy vomiting, avoidance is certainly worthwhile. It reduces stress levels and improves nutrition, even if it does not reduce infant allergy (though my experience is that it does). So knowing whether Mum has a problem is important. And she may not know herself. This is true of first pregnancies as well: where there is a clear history of food allergy, the mother should minimise or avoid those foods, using her own bodily responses as a guide to the usefulness of this strategy.

For there is no doubt that pregnancy is important in the overall development of allergy or tolerance. Again, as noted in the earlier chapters, research is trying to discover the mechanisms. Maternal mitochondria (small structures within cells that we inherit from our mothers) may be involved, as they have been linked to a variety of diseases, including metabolic syndrome.[1917] The newly discovered placental microbiome may be involved, and that seems linked to the mother's oral microbiota (see page 87) Mice studies also suggest that prenatal exposure even to airborne particulates affects the infant immune system, for example.[1918] We just don't know enough to be dogmatic about what to advise about pregnancy diet.

Commonsense suggests the following dietary advice in pregnancy and lactation:

- *Variety and moderation of dietary intake.*
- *Avoid junk foods and diet drinks* laden with synthetic chemicals. They may even programme the baby's food habits.[1919]
- *Eat organic food,* especially meat and dairy, if you can afford it, to reduce exposure to pesticides and antibiotic-resistant bacteria. One study showed that even a week on organic food reduces pesticide residue levels.[1920]

1916 Allergies to bovine protein can include milk, meat and blood. See Martelli A, De Chiara A, Corvo M, Restani P et al. Beef allergy in children with cow's milk allergy; cow's milk allergy in children with beef allergy. *Annals of Allergy, Asthma & Immunology*: 2002, 89 (6 Suppl 1):38-43. (PMID:12487203); Wüthrich B, Stern A, Johansson SG Severe anaphylactic reaction to bovine serum albumin at the first attempt of artificial insemination. *Allergy*:1995, 50(2):179-183. (PMID:7604943)
1917 Wilson FH, Hariri A, Farhi A, Zhao H et al. A cluster of metabolic defects caused by mutation in a mitochondrial tRNA. *Science*. 2004;306(5699):1190-4. DOI: 10.1126/science.1102521
1918 Hong X, Liu C, Chen X, Song Y et al. Maternal Exposure to Airborne Particulate Matter Causes Postnatal Immunological Dysfunction in Mice Offspring. (PMID:23416701) *Toxicology* 2013, 306C:59-67
1919 http://www.scienceworldreport.com/articles/6546/20130430/pregnancy-junk-food-diet-can-cause-high-fat-high-sugar-addiction-in-baby.htm.
1920 Oates L, Cohen M, Braun L, Schembri A et al. Reduction in urinary organophosphate pesticide metabolites in adults after a week-long organic diet. *Environ Res* 2014; 132:105-111

- *Don't take single-mineral supplements* like iron tablets or excess calcium tablets, which can interfere with the absorption of other minerals. The mother who needs more iron may need more zinc as well, although this is hard to ascertain as most zinc is held in tissues and there is no easy reliable test. However, for what it's worth, one study showed that plasma zinc levels plummet within twenty-four hours of taking an unopposed iron supplement. And iron tablets swallowed with a cup of tea are chelated and so poorly absorbed. Inorganic iron in tablets is not as readily absorbed as haem iron in meats, while foods containing iron will also contain other minerals, so the body can balance its intake.

- *Don't eat huge amounts of any particular food*, especially if a mother 'just doesn't feel right' unless she does so, or craves that food intensely. Aversion and addiction seem to be the two sides of the same coin of food hypersensitivity. And in some people that addiction is as powerful as any other, affecting the same brain areas as heroin or cocaine. Addiction is capable of transferring from one substance to another.[1921] Some specialists now see addiction as 'a brain disease, not a character flaw'. Which would mean that some people will find it harder to make dietary changes than others, and should not be judged harshly for failure to comply with dietary suggestions. Remember, we don't know for certain what will or won't help! So they are suggestions, not diktats. And of course the problem here is how to distinguish between cravings that are bad for us, and cravings which mean our body knows more than we consciously do about what it needs!

- *Avoid margarine and other pro-inflammatory foodstuffs containing hydrogenated fats.* A German study of two-year-old children concluded that 'Children with predominant margarine consumption had an increased risk for eczema and allergic sensitisation, while butter intake was no predictor for allergic diseases ... [the researchers] could not determine whether margarine is a causal risk factor or whether other lifestyle factors have influenced this association.'[1922] The pro-inflammatory effects of too much intake of omega-6 fats and trans-fats, and too little omega-3, means that if margarines are part of the diet, omega-3 intake must be increased. (Perhaps this is so especially in America, where the production processes differ from those in Australia, resulting in higher trans-fat content.)[1923] Besides, butter tastes better and is far less processed, even if it is loaded with saturated fats! (Which are by no means as big a problem as the margarine industry made them out to be.)

- *Increase omega-3 fats from natural sources where possible.* At least two fish meals a week: salmon, tuna, sardines, scallops, mussels; egg yolks, walnuts, pumpkin seeds, flaxseed, dark green vegetables, and more: see http://www.bda.uk.com/foodfacts/omega3.pdf But be careful, tinned fish may have had its omega-3 extracted, or contain mercury.

---

1921 An interesting and accessible article in *New Scientist* outlines this developing issue in neuroscience. See Murphy S. Addictive personality. *New Scientist*, 8 Sept 2012, pp. 37-9.

1922 Sausenthaler S, Kompauer I, Borte M, Herbarth O et al. LISA Study Group. Margarine and butter consumption, eczema and allergic sensitization in children. The LISA birth cohort study. *Pediatr Allergy Immunol* 2006, 17(2):85-93. DOI: 10.1111/j.1399-3038.2005.00366.x

1923 Joy Anderson, personal communication 2013.

- *Consider probiotics in the last weeks of pregnancy, or if prescribed antibiotics during the pregnancy, and perhaps for the first weeks of lactation.* There is increasing evidence that this may be helpful; the difficulty is knowing what probiotics to choose! (There's more about this, and omega-3 fats, in the section on Supplements, below.)

- *Notice and respect bodily warning signals,* such as aversion or addiction. Record the foods involved. If a mother is nauseated by the smell of a food, forcing herself to eat it would be daft. A mother who as a child loathed milk products and had allergy symptoms may well be wise to reduce or eliminate all bovine protein whether milk or beef: this sometimes results in significant improvements in her sense of wellbeing, or ends persistent so-called pregnancy nausea and vomiting.

This last point is possibly the most important, and also the most difficult to advise about. In fact quite a bit of unconscious avoidance happens in pregnancy and lactation: mothers find they just can't stand certain foods. That may be a protective reflex kicking in. Our bodies sometimes know more than our rational minds do about what is good for us. All the items I found repellent or nauseating and instinctively avoided in early pregnancy turned out to be potentially harmful: alcohol and caffeine and paint chemicals among them. I already loathed cigarette smoke, but it made me violently ill in pregnancy.

All the same, we can't get away from the obvious fact that it is natural for infants to be exposed *in utero* and via breastmilk to the usual family diet, in order to create tolerance. So reduction to the point where the mother is symptom-free, but not total exclusion, may be the best compromise for the allergic mother of one already allergic child. Given how uncertain the evidence is, I suggest that mothers take responsibility here and go with their gut instincts: it's their bodies that monitor the effects, after all.

## Q9. Should breastfeeding mothers avoid common allergens?

As I've already said, the answer is in general *no, not unless there's a good reason to, arising from that mother's life experience: in which case it may help.*[1924] Food antigens will be in milk and should reach babies with milk, creating tolerance.[1925] And the fewer dietary restrictions a lactating mother has, the easier it is for her and her family. There have to be good grounds for avoiding any food, not simply following what a friend found worked for her, or someone else thinks is a good idea. We are unique individuals, and one woman's poison *can* be another's food.

That said, there are a substantial number of breastfeeding mothers who find that diet changes help their baby and themselves. And some studies have shown lower reactivity in children

---

1924 Kramer MS Kakuma R op. cit. 'Prescription of an antigen avoidance diet to a high-risk woman during lactation may reduce her child's risk of developing atopic eczema, but better trials are needed. Dietary antigen avoidance by lactating mothers of infants with atopic eczema may reduce the severity of the eczema, but larger trials are needed.' Personally, I think this works best on a case by case basis, not in arbitrary trials, which miss some allergens for some women.

1925 Palmer DJ, Makrides M. Diet of lactating women and allergic reactions in their infants. (PMID:16607130) *Curr Opin Clin Nutr Metab Care* 2006, 9(3):284-288.

of mothers who stick to an avoidance diet for three months of exclusive breastfeeding.[1926] So I always review and advise about maternal diet individually, and help parents identify alternative food sources of important nutrients, while steering them away from single-item supplements or doctrinaire avoidance of 'bad' foods. Food is just food; it's what we do with it that matters.

Literature searches throw up some amazing new ideas. Research funded by Nestlé Japan[1927] suggested that feeding *the breastfeeding mother* a new whey hydrolysate formula might result in fewer reactions in the baby! How ironic is that? Having created the problems for breastfeeding women by its products – which indeed were originally marketed as tonic foods for breastfeeding mothers as well as supplements for their babies – Nestlé Japan is now hoping that the 'long-term consumption' of a new hydrolysed milk product will reduce the amount of one allergen, beta-lactoglobulin, in maternal breastmilk. More is better! A whole new market opens up! And if the mother's own allergic symptoms get worse in the process? What then?

I have to confess that I have read only the abstract of this study: I did not search it out as the eagerly awaited breakthrough solution for any sensible woman with a family history of allergy and an at-risk baby ... I suspect it didn't work too well, as we've heard so little about it. What did follow-up reveal about allergy outcomes I wonder? Or was there no follow-up? I wouldn't advise any mother I know to be the experimental guinea pigs drinking whey-hydrolysate formula in pregnancy, even though there is a theoretical chance that this could work for some mothers. Remember, it is well documented that even extensively hydrolysed formulas can cause adverse reactions including anaphylaxis.[1928] But the mother drinking the stuff is preferable to the baby doing so!

One final caveat. Always remember that women from widely diverse cultures with very different diets, sometimes quite deficient, produce healthy babies. It was an industry strategy to suggest that breastmilk could be deficient unless it was "the milk of healthy well-nourished women." The baby's growth is influenced by far more than what a mother eats. Beware any message about " the milk of healthy mothers."

## Q10. Should mothers take supplements?

Possibly. There is no one answer that applies to everyone. In general, supplements are unnecessary during lactation. However, some mothers report health improvements when they increase their zinc and vitamin B intake. While that may be a placebo effect, it is also possible that some women are depleted and will benefit from targetted supplementation.

1926 Sigurs N, Hattevig G, Kjellman B. Maternal Avoidance of Eggs, Cow's Milk, and Fish During Lactation: Effect on Allergic Manifestations, Skin-Prick Tests, and Specific IgE Antibodies in Children at Age 4 Years. *Pediatrics* 1992; 89:4 735-739

1927 Fukushima Y, Kawata Y, Onda T, Kitagawa M. Long-term consumption of whey hydrolysate formula by lactating women reduces the transfer of beta-lactoglobulin into human milk. (PMID:9530619) J *Nutr Sci Vitaminol* 1997, 43(6):673-678.

1928 Hill DJ, Cameron DJ, Francis DE et al. Challenge confirmation of late-onset reactions to extensively hydrolyzed formulas in infants with multiple food protein intolerance. (PMID:7560641) *J Allergy Clin Immunol* 1995; 96(3):386-394.

Asking a qualified dietitian/nutritionist to assess this is sensible. Blood tests may show up deficiencies. Among the supplements suggested are probiotics and omega-3 sources.

When a mother takes antibiotics during pregnancy or lactation, I always suggest she takes a good source of some Lactobacillus species during the antibiotic course and for at least a week afterwards, in the hope that beneficial bacteria, rather than resilient pathogens, are re-established in her gut. Her gut flora is going to influence her baby's, after all, and so will her milk influence that infant gut flora. And there is some very preliminary evidence that probiotics consumed in pregnancy may favourably influence the development of allergy.[1929]

But which species of bug, which strains of which species of bug, how often, how much, for how long, we can't say as yet. Don't assume that because one strain works without apparent harms, another will have the same effect. Find out all you can about any bacteria you intend to swallow – before you begin. Know that it will be interacting with your unique microbiota, and don't assume that what worked well for someone else will be problem-free for you. You are unique. Remember that studies of probiotic consumption usually exclude allergic or unwell individuals, and 'long-term' can mean a few months, or at most a year or two. Record what you do and monitor any effects as best you can.

Depending on the mother's dietary intake, I often suggest added intake of omega-3 sources. The advice to increase maternal LCPUFA intake is given because so many mothers are being diagnosed with postnatal depression these days, and these fats seem to help with mood disorders.[1930] Such supplementation is being researched in relation to allergy prevention, but

> ... n-3 LCPUFA supplementation in pregnancy did not reduce the overall incidence of immunoglobulin E associated allergies in the first year of life, although atopic eczema and egg sensitisation were lower. Longer term follow-up is needed to determine if supplementation has an effect on respiratory allergic diseases and aeroallergen sensitisation in childhood.[1931]

In general, increasing LCPUFA intake from food sources is a very good idea, as standard Western diet has moved away from traditional fat balances, and some researchers think it helps.[1932] It sounds logical. But again, don't overdo a (probably) good thing.

---

1929 Böttcher MF, Abrahamsson TR, Fredriksson M, Jakobsson T et al.. Low breast milk TGF-beta2 is induced by Lactobacillus reuteri supplementation and associates with reduced risk of sensitization during infancy. (PMID:18221472) *Ped Allergy Immunol.* 2008, 19(6):497-504.

1930 Kendall-Tackett K. *Non-pharmacologic Treatments,* op.cit.

1931 D J Palmer, T Sullivan, M S Gold, S L Prescott, R Heddle et al.. Effect of n-3 long chain polyunsaturated fatty acid supplementation in pregnancy on infants' allergies in first year of life: randomised controlled trial *BMJ.* 2012; 344: e184.

1932 Furuhjelm C, Warstedt K, Larsson J, Fredriksson M et al.. Fish oil supplementation in pregnancy and lactation may decrease the risk of infant allergy.(PMID:19489765) *Acta Paediatrica* 2009, 98(9):1461-1467. DOI: 10.1111/j.1651-2227.2009.01355.x

# Q11. Does this approach to maternal diet work?

I find that it works more often than not, if the baby is still young enough to be fully and solely breastfed. A Dutch systematic review supports the idea that dietary treatment does work (though in my experience their suggested one-week trial is too short). Inter alia, they concluded that

> Dietary intervention should be combined with behavioural interventions: general advice, reassurance, reduction in stimuli, and sensitive differential responding (teaching parents to be more appropriately responsive to their infants with less overstimulation and more effective soothing) ... Anticholinergic drugs are not recommended because of their serious side effects.[1933]

Of course all those things are important, and part of what one does when working with allergic families. (I always have a simple sling in my car, as some techniques need to be taught hands-on to fathers as well as mothers, as soon as possible.[1934]) The real drawback of this approach is that it is individual and takes time. Only a group like the Possums Clinic for Mothers and Babies[1935] is really set up to provide such holistic evidence-based care. We need feedback about what works, from you as health professional or as parent, to the scientists researching these issues. The blogs in which parents share their problems may not be monitored, or may belong to industry which edits them: find more effective ways to express your experience.

We do need to be telling research scientists what this problem looks like at the milder community end of a very wide spectrum. I know that I see a biased sample – mostly parents who've seen many people before they reach me. I also know that the samples used in research studies are quite different, and just as biased, if not more so, but in different ways. And I know that the conviction and care and ongoing commitment I bring to helping parents is itself a factor in the apparent success that emerges when mothers take on the challenges of dietary change. But for whatever reason, it seems to work.

Intervening as early as possible is important, as there will never be another stage in their life when children can be solely fed on breastmilk. So we need to take parents seriously *as soon as* we hear that they are having problems. Mild problems either get better or worse. It would be many months before these distressed breastfed babies get to see a specialist. Those months can mean the difference between resolving the problem while the baby is still getting breastmilk, with its stem cells and other growth and repair factors, and trying to resolve it when much more damage has already been done, normal development has

1933 Lucassen PLBJ Assendelft WJJ, Gubbels JW, van Eijk JTM et al Effectiveness of treatments for infantile colic: systematic review. *BMJ*. 1998 May 23; 316(7144): 1563–1569. PMCID: PMC28556 See also *BMJ*. 1998 July 18; 317(7152): 17¹·

1934 Instructions for this sling can be found on my website. It costs almost nothing, and can be made from any suitable natural fabric, one that breathes and can withstand washing. More structured slings have their virtues, but this can work just as well especially for very young babies. So can very large wraps and strips of fabric, or scarves, or cotton elastane mix jumpers with a scarf bound around them....be ingenious. But make sure the baby's chin is not tucked down on his chest and nostrils are clear: easiest if the head is turned to one side. Babies have smothered in ample soft bosoms and heavy clothing!

1935 Check out http://www.possumsclinic.com.au

been skewed - and without the *only* food that provides a wide range of genuine proven immune support, mother's milk.

Once that milk is not available, problem solving becomes much more difficult. Dr Susan Prescott's book serves as a guide to what can then be expected if you find yourselves travelling to an allergy clinic, and I strongly recommend it to parents at all stages of this journey. Her forthcoming second book on allergy will also be worth reading. But don't expect to find such expertise everywhere, or to get help swiftly, unless ths problem seems life-threatening. This area is still hugely under-resourced.

## Q12. What else might help?

Having a baby is not something to do in isolation; all new mothers need a supportive network to help keep their own stress levels low. When dealing with mothers-to-be, or mothers of newborns, it is important to discuss the practicalities of creating a support team to ensure lots of skin-to-skin contact using simple slings, exclusive breastfeeding or breastmilk feeding, avoidance of nipple and breast problems, and (if possible) no antibiotics for either in the immediate post-partum period.

This simple recipe usually produces a calm and charming baby, who cries less and less as she comes to trust her world to supply her needs. The skin contact and breastfeeding are central to this sense of security, and biochemically improve maternal mood as well.

Parents with such babies consider themselves 'lucky' to have exceptionally 'good' babies. I tell them that their babies are normal, that normal breastfed babies really are such charming placid creatures, who cry to indicate needs or pain, and reward their caregivers. (Observing other naturally-fed baby mammals supports this idea.) Nomads on the margins of survival would not have succeeded in colonising the earth if their babies had been troublesome noisy creatures: predators would have found and eaten them!

As for the child who is at risk of allergy, I agree with the Europeans that

> A dietary regimen is effective in the prevention of allergic diseases in high-risk infants, particularly in early infancy regarding food allergy and eczema. The most effective dietary regimen is exclusively breastfeeding for at least 4–6 months or, in absence of breast milk, formulas with documented reduced allergenicity for at least the first 4 months, combined with avoidance of solid food and cow's milk for the first 4 months.[1936]

As noted earlier, western history suggests that 4-6 months could be around six to eight months exclusive breastfeeding for the thriving fully breastfed. The avoidance of early eczema is important to more than physical health: the happy nature of the child who no longer itches and scratches makes parenting a joy rather than a chore. After maternal dietary elimination has resulted in the reduction of eczema, some parents have commented that they did not know their own child, that he is a different child now he is no longer distressed.

---

1936 Høst A, Halken S, Muraro A, Dreborg S, et al Dietary prevention of allergic diseases in infants and small children. *Pediatric Allergy and Immunology* 2008, 19(1):1-4. DOI: 10.1111/j.1399-3038.2007.00680.x

As I mentioned earlier, one study showed higher rates of mental health problems in ten-year olds who had eczema in childhood.[1937] It would be interesting to have children whose eczema disappeared with diet changes in a repeat study of mental health at the age of 10: I am sure they would not differ from children who had never had eczema.

## Q13. Why go to this bother if children grow out of allergy?

As should be clear by now, I think it doubtful that children ever really grow out of allergy, in that broader sense of adverse reactions to things others find harmless. Yes, they can stop having some symptoms, yes, immune reactivity can decline to the point where it seems they are cured, because they can tolerate some exposure to foods or other substances which once caused their eczema to flare, or which triggered anaphylaxis or complete collapse. That is sometimes taken as proof that they have grown out of allergy, and at one level of understanding, that's accurate. Many children do become capable of handling, without apparent problems, foods which once caused particular symptoms. And it's great if children are no longer at risk of shock and death due to extreme reactions to common allergens such as peanuts or cows' milk.

But seeing families over the long term, as I have through connections within parent groups, I have yet to meet any child who was allergic as an infant, had no dietary changes or treatment other than anti-histamines and steroids and other drugs, and who never reacts to the environment, including foods. Sometimes this reaction is simply constipation[1938] or insomnia,[1939] problems that can have other causes and so are overlooked as potential allergy issues. Sometimes it is cognitive or behavioural problems which come and go with diet changes, but which are rarely thought of as related to allergy.

As I said earlier, symptoms can disappear or change, but the potential for reaction remains. Italian researchers recorded this in a study of 70 children with severe colic, 50 of whom lost symptoms on a cows' milk-free diet and proved positive on two challenges. Over an 18 months follow-up, 22 of the 50 developed overt gut intolerances.[1940]

And more serious problems can emerge as children get older, such as oesophagitis or exercise-induced asthma, which has been fatal for some. This is why it is so important to have a record of what children have reacted to in the past, and for them, the children themselves, not just the parents, to learn to monitor the overall balance in their lives between current tolerance levels and total body burden. For some, that means continuing avoidance, for others, exposure to small, even moderate amounts- which makes life a lot easier. But for none that I have met does it mean no long-term allergy.

---

1937 Schmitt J et al, op. cit.

1938 Duplantier JE. Lymphoid Nodular Hyperplasia and Cow's Milk Hypersensitivity in Children With Chronic Constipation. *Pediatrics* 2005; 116: Supplement 2, 547; doi:10.1542/peds.2005-0698Y

1939 Mozin MJ, Casimir G, Montauk L et al. Insomnia and Cow's Milk Allergy in Infants. *Pediatrics* 1985; 76:6 880-884.

1940 Iacono G, Carroccio A; Montalto G, Cavataio F et al. Severe Infantile Colic and Food Intolerance: A Long-Term Prospective Study. *J Pediatr Gastroent Nutr* 1991; 12 (3): 332-335.

## Q14. Isn't allergy a family – and individual – responsibility?

Where allergy is concerned, ultimately only the family can know their history and reactions in detail. Only they can assess the cost-benefit ratio of alternatives, and decide what to do, and when to do it. Sometimes a clear strategy is just not possible in the family's situation: after explaining what is involved, it may all seem to be impossible at that time. That's OK. I have supported mothers who simply can't manage to deal with this issue – without pretending that it is not an issue they will eventually need to deal with. At least the family can have some sense that there is a rational explanation for their problems, that this is not a matter of chance or some malicious fate afflicting them. Sooner or later, they will feel able to test the explanation and see if it helps. It usually does.

And if it makes a difference, all family members need to take responsibility for doing what they can. Each individual, even quite young children, must learn how to manage his or her unique body . I have been impressed by how well quite young children can understand and discipline themselves to avoid problem foods and chemicals, once the link with unpleasant symptoms has been made clear to them. Children do not like feeling ill or out of control any more than adults do. They can understand that actions have consequences if adults make that clear to them often enough, and kindly.

Of course, like adults, children will want to test the boundaries and try to get others to be responsible for negative outcomes. Parents need to be canny, and make sure they foster true autonomy of decision-making, not simply control what the child is exposed to. Control is possible for only a few short years. If children cared for outside the home have not learnt to take responsibility for their own diet, they will breach the rules when not policed, which could be dangerous.

If a child older than perhaps two or three – depending on their level of understanding - wants to eat known allergens, he or she should be told of the likely consequences, and told that the parent will provide the food if the child understands and accepts those consequences. (Obviously if anaphylaxis is likely, parental warnings and preparation will be much more extensive than for the child whose eczema will flare, or whose gut will hurt later that day, or who will toss and turn in a lather of sweat that night. In some cases, agreeing to provide the food needs to be in a medical setting where resuscitation is possible!)

But it is the child's body, so it is their decision, *just as soon as they are old enough* to understand what the decision involves and its consequences. That can be quite young, under school age. When the inevitable consequences arrive, parents can be comforting and offer suitable relief, but should also emphasise that this was the result of the child making a decision the parent strongly advised against; the suffering was what the child chose when deciding to break dietary bounds. The clever child will sometimes try to make it the parent's fault by saying that the parent should not have given them the food even though they asked for it. The message they get in return is along the lines of: 'It's your body, you have to decide what to eat, because we can't always be there; you need to know what this does to you. When it happens at home we can help you, but if you did this at Grandma's or daycare or school or camp we can't. So you have to decide not to eat things that make you ill. You have to control yourself, no one else can. We'll be here to help if you give in to temptation, but we'll remind you that you chose the pain it will cause you. It will hurt us to see you suffering, and we'll try to help you, but we won't stop you doing the wrong thing next time either. You have to be responsible: it's your body.' At the same time, the parent should take reasonable steps to ensure that home is a haven without multiple temptations to indulge in harmful foods: an addicted child will help himself to food from the fridge. Both parents need to model reasonable dietary habits, as children do learn what they live.

Allergy will shape the child's life in many ways, some of them beneficial, if my experience is any guide. Allergy can teach children valuable lessons about taking responsibility and accepting the consequences of their actions. Parents have often commented about the maturity that such illness can create, which is no bad thing. Understanding that even 'good' foods can have bad consequences can also make children wary of other substances parents would prefer them not to experiment with in their teens, such as smoking and alcohol. It can also give them a socially acceptable reason for refusing illicit drugs. That can be very useful!

Conversely, there can be real risks to mental health if allergy issues are not addressed, perhaps especially for adolescents. Many experienced parents and clinical allergy practitioners know that allergy can have both direct and indirect effects on mental functioning. Dr. Doris Rapp is just one such, and she catalogues many earlier physicians who came to the same conclusion in her book, Is this your child? Discovering and treating unrecognised allergies in children and adults (see Bibliography). In this she says

> I firmly believe that many allergic children and young adults need psychological counselling as well as recognition and treatment of their allergies. Most have had to withstand years of feeling unwell, rejection and reprimand. These children, and especially the teenagers, often have decimated self-images and no realisation of their true worth and unique personal gifts and abilities.

We'd all prefer our children never to have to suffer, but suffering can shape character in both positive and negative ways, to which parents need to be alert. Westerners experience very little suffering compared with the rest of humanity: let's never forget just how lucky we (and our children) are. I find it helpful to remember that, whenever I start wishing things had been different, as I often have. Without being Pollyanna-ish, it's better for one's mental health to count blessings whenever tempted to curse hospital systems influenced more by BigPharma than by science! And among those blessings in this free country is our ability to lobby for change to such systems.

# CHAPTER 5

# More about manifestations of infant intolerance

Some of the most common symptoms of infant food allergy are discussed at greater length in this chapter, along with some practical advice about relieving symptoms in ways that do not necessarily involve medication and its many side effect, which are also outlined where relevant. If you are confused about colic, or convinced the problem is lactose overload or intolerance, or gastric reflux, you need to read this chapter. And if you are using thickeners, or giving paracetamol or ibuprofen to your baby, make sure you do.

## 5.1 Colic and reflux: different names, same problem?

Many different gut-related problems produce the same or very similar symptoms, because they activate the central protective mechanism of humans: our immune system, whose varied lines of defence include inflammation. So it's easy to confuse one thing with another, and easy for vested interests of all kinds to shape medical and parental understanding in ways that suit their interpretation of the evidence. What follows is my interpretation of the evidence I've seen over more than three decades of helping families deal with the problems created by a healthcare system overly influenced by industry, and ignorant about women's milk. Every reader is perfectly free to reinterpret that evidence: but please take time to consider this alternate perspective.[1941]

---

1941 For a update on current medical thinking about infant colic, I suggest reading the entire Supplement to the December 2013 issue of the *Journal of Pediatric Gastroenterology and Nutrition*, entitled Infant Colic and Functional Gastrointestinal Disorders: Is There More Than a "Gut Feeling"? Online at http://journals.lww. com/jpgn/toc/2013/12001, all the articles are worth thinking about, while conscious of their different contexts.

# Is it classic colic?

When horses get colic – defined as 'the general term for a horse stomach ache' – it is taken seriously and the cause identified; if it cannot be resolved, such expensive animals may be killed – as an act of kindness. After experiencing the pain of colic (due to a virally triggered milk-protein allergy) eminent dairy scientist Dr Wattie Whittlestone of New Zealand commented at a LLLNZ conference in the 1980s that he no longer wondered why babies cried so powerfully with colic; he now knew just how painful such gut distress could be, and was astonished that they didn't cry even harder. Famously an advocate of dairy products, after that bout in Israel in his sixties, Dr Whittlestone had to avoid bovine milk protein totally or experience a recurrence: he chose to avoid milk, so severe was the pain..

I see no problem with parents using the term 'colic' to describe severe gut-related infant distress, or as a general term for an infant stomach ache. Why not? Parents have always thought crying was due to gut pain, even when told that the problem was parental handling skills, or the baby's temperament, or not a problem at all but normal behaviour. When you live with the baby, it looks and feels like baby's gut hurts. Yes, central nervous system immaturity may be involved, as may other factors. Yes, "Whether infantile colic is a normal developmental occurrence, a different central nervous system function, or a result of GI discomfort, it is a self-limiting condition that, when present without any other symptoms or alarming signs, should be looked at with empathy and reassurance."[1942] So what? Most painful conditions in adults are also self-limiting, but we take them seriously and offer treatments. Are babies any less human than adults? Let's rule out feeding issues before accepting that the crying can't be stopped within a few days! And much colic morphs into less acutely painful but still stressful symptoms, which still add up to years of disturbed nights and fatigue. As I well know.

So what causes colic, or gut distress, in normal healthy babies, especially breastfed ones? Classic colic, of the kind described in the pre-formula eras, and as described in old textbooks, seems to have consisted of

- crying and apparent gut discomfort,
- with babies drawing up their knees,
- typically mostly in the evening from say six to ten pm:
- with baby and mother sleeping relatively well after that, with some waking for feeds
- baby waking in the morning for a large feed from very full breasts
- baby then going back to sleep for around three to four hours, and cheerful most of the day, until the next evening bouts of crying – the arsenic hours.

That was colic as described to, but not as experienced by, me as a new mother in the 1970s. Classic colic, ten-week colic, evening colic which lasted three months, seemed to be very rare. Its memory may linger in texts and folklore, offering hope that babies will 'grow out

---

1942 Shamir R. Infant Colic and Functional Gastrointestinal Disorders: Is There More Than a "Gut Feeling"? *J Pediatr Gastroent Nutr* 2013; 57: S1–S2. doi: 10.1097/01.mpg.0000441923.90436.c7

of' any problem causing vociferous incessant crying. Occasionally I still come across such classic colic in fully breastfed infants of mothers with a good milk supply, and it does resolve rapidly with better management of milk supply.

Later definitions of colic were as arbitrary as they were unscientific. The rule of threes: crying for more than three hours a day for more than three days in a row … Research studies may make such arbitrary definitions necessary, but they are of little practical value. It seems to me, from reading the literature and living through the modern era of the Formula Invasion, that it was after neonatal exposure to the new 'humanised' formulas became routine and almost universal, that so many breastfed babies, like mine, cried savagely, unpredictably, inconsolably, day or night or both. Interestingly, the 1980s change to whey-dominant formulas may also have had some influence. As noted earlier, this change actually increased infant doses of some milk antigens which that industry is now reducing. (The older casein-based formulas had probably been less antigenic overall, though possibly more sedating because of their brain-affecting opioid peptides,[1943] and more obesogenic because of their higher protein levels.)

## Colic, lactose overload, lactose intolerance, and allergy

One theory that I thought possibly made some sense of classic/evening/ three-month colic was that it was due to the evening fermentation of the first morning feed's initial large lactose load that had gone into an overnight-emptied infant stomach. Gut transit time for lactose is about twelve hours, I am told, so fermentation would be well under way by evening. Experienced child health nurses (and older medical literature) once suggested practices that reduced the morning lactose load or increased the cream content of the milk: feed from only one breast and express the other; express from the first breast before you feed in the morning; even give some water before starting the morning feed (not a good idea), and more besides. By three months baby could have 'grown out of it', probably due to a larger, more distensible stomach, greater infant postural control, increased mobility, and a maternal milk supply adjusted to baby's needs in volume, content and delivery. I've written about the clinical dimensions of lactose overload in breastfed infants earlier. This is a relatively benign and asymptomatic problem, which resolves quickly and the infant happily continues to drink milk with 7 per cent lactose. So maybe lactose overload *was* classic colic in fully-breastfed infants.

It is true of course, only a minority of humans continue to be able to digest lactose after infancy: the persistence of lactase, the enzyme needed to do so, varies greatly, with, for example, approximately 100 per cent of all Native Americans, 90 per cent of Asian Americans, 80 per cent of African Americans, 53 per cent of Hispanic Americans, and 15 per cent of Anglo-Americans becoming lactose 'maldigesters'. [1944] Globally lactase persistence

---

1943  To my knowledge, whether those peptides blunt pain perception has not been researched.

1944  An excellent discussion of population variation in milk digestion and ramifications for dietary policy can be found in AS Wiley. *Re-Imagining Milk: Cultural and Biological perspectives.* (Routledge NY 2011). Ch. 2. Wiley sees the early-mid 20th century in the west as an unusual historical interlude in which fresh milk was drunk on a previously unheard of scale. Harvard School of Public Health no longer treats milk products as a separate dietary group: see www.hsph.harvard.edu.

after infancy drops even in communities that continue using milk in their diet. But it is also true, and has been taught in standard medical and gastroenterology textbooks forever, that *symptomatic* lactose intolerance is *usually secondary to gut damage* caused by some insult, whether antigen or microbe or hypoxia or physical trauma; milk protein or gluten are common causes of such gut damage, and we know now that partially-digested infant formula is another. (In Dr.Wattie Whittlestone's case, it was an Israeli virus, which damaged the gut into which he took his usual doses of milk.) So lactose intolerance can be – and usually is, in my experience – a symptom of cows' milk *protein* intolerance or allergy.

The 1980s to 1990s industry promotion of lactose intolerance as the common cause of colic or gut distress served industry well. Lactose intolerance is framed as a deficiency *in the baby*, who lacks enough of the enzymes needed for digestion. By contrast, cows' milk protein allergy is damage done *to the baby* by a foreign antigen that young humans are not accustomed to digesting. Diagnosing cases as lactose intolerance, not allergy, headed off the growing popular awareness of bovine protein 'allergy', which might have made more doctors question why such alien protein is used in formulas.

Portraying lactose intolerance as the issue did something else. It justified trying an alternative industrial formula on crying *breastfed* babies, since lactose is the sugar in breastmilk. Many babies were and are weaned off the breast on to the new products, to their detriment. (Or perhaps we should call that 'decreased benefit': the brilliant euphemism used in one paper that showed no advantage and possibly some risk for prems older than thirty-one weeks' gestation given a new preterm formula with probiotics.[1945] How can editors let such obfuscating language through?)

Just as some smokers refuse to believe that smoking is unhealthy, so some people prefer to deny the possibility of milk-protein allergy. Many adults nowadays talk about being 'lactose intolerant' when that symptom is due to an allergy they don't know they have ... or don't want to know, because they don't want to give up cheese or ice cream or beef. The 'lactose intolerant' can choose to continue to consume favourite cow products which would be ruled out if milk *protein* allergy were to be recognised as the cause. Reducing their fresh milk intake may be enough to get rid of a rumbling tummy, uncomfortable gut bloating and diarrhoea. Meanwhile, other symptoms of glue ears or sinus stuffiness or eczema or headaches are assumed to be irrelevant, though they were the more persistent symptoms of milk protein allergy.

Adults are free to choose denial over inconvenience. However, they should be aware that it is possible to be addicted to foods including milk, and what they think is their sensible free choice may reflect instinctive behaviour that is feeding an addiction. And, like all addictions, this one may keep ratcheting up as the body adapts to the level of intake. I described the mother who went from disliking milk to making cheese 'soup' on page 21.

---

1945 Modi N, Uthaya S, Fell J, Kulinskaya E. Randomized, double-blind, controlled trial of the effect of prebiotic oligosaccharides on enteral tolerance in preterm infants (ISRCTN77444690).(PMID:20639792) *Pediatr Res* 2010; 68(5):440-445.

The biological appropriateness of low-lactose infant formulas can be questioned, but low-lactose formulas (and milks for adults) will still sell. Because the lactose is not there to be fermented, some immediate symptoms like bloating will improve. But that says nothing about the *cause* of the gut damage that led to loss of the enzyme lactase in both breast- and bottle-fed babies. (That cause is often the alien proteins or maldigested fats in formula.)

As industry frames the issue, low-lactose formulas are needed because some babies are simply 'immature', or 'lactose maldigesters.' The problem can be solved by using a more expensive industrial formula with less lactose in it, or maybe added probiotics or prebiotics, or whatever is new in the market and can be portrayed as a plausible solution. Health professionals with no detailed knowledge of infant nutrition can generally be relied upon to follow their leader, the infant formula industry. That will only change when their education about infant nutrition does.

Genetically normal babies are not lactose maldigesters, or lactose would not be the main carbohydrate of breastmilk, involved in brain development. We don't know what (if any) harm is done by changing a bottle-fed child off a formula with lactose, to one without: nothing obvious has emerged, but perhaps the right questions have not been asked. However, considerable harm can be done by suggesting a low-lactose formula to a breastfeeding mother, especially one whose child is likely to be intolerant or allergic to cows' milk protein.

## Reflux, and the use of thickeners and less allergenic formulas

So far I've barely mentioned gastro-oesophageal reflux,[1946] another symptom made into a popular medical diagnosis by 1980–90s infant formula marketing. Gastro-oesophageal reflux describes gastric (stomach) contents coming back up into the oesophagus again. Sometimes this ends with regurgitation or vomiting, more often it doesn't. If swallowing an antacid has ended a burning sensation in your chest, you've experienced acid reflux, or heartburn as it's often called. It can be painful if it's acid enough, and unpleasant even if it isn't acutely painful. A baby can't know what is causing the pain, so she cries. If you're an adult you reach for antacids, which enjoy phenomenal sales in Western countries.

Most breastfed infant reflux is normal and protective, a matter of adjusting intake or relieving pressure. Some texts talk of the infant's 'inefficient' oesophageal sphincter, when that band of muscle at the junction of the oesophagus and the stomach seems to me to be perfectly adapted for the baby's age and needs. Why? An overfull baby needs to be able to bring up excess milk. Many breastfed babies guzzle away and look like bloated dumplings after a super-efficient breast ejects its milk in a rush. Some babies know when to stop, and come off looking dazed, even drunk. Some others want to keep sucking, so take in too much milk and later bring some back up again (and ask for a top up if too much came

---

1946 An important article on this subject is Dr Pamela Douglas's The Rise and Fall of Infant reflux: the limits of evidence-based medicine. *Griffith REVIEW* 2011, edition 32.. Other useful talks and articles can be found online at the Possums Clinic website.

back). Many bottle-fed babies are fed past the point where their behaviour indicates they have had enough: the carer looks at the amount still in the bottle, and pokes the teat right back into their mouth. A reclining baby finds milk once more at the back of his throat and swallows - the alternative is choking. Excess intake is later better sicked up than kept down, as dumping milk from the stomach into the bowel too rapidly can cause problems.

As well, babies (like us) always swallow air when feeding, and they can't actively burp, as adults do to relieve pressure. Some feed inefficiently and swallow too much air, which in the stomach turns into bubbles that will rise as burps. That adds to the pressure in the stomach: in fact some doctors think air swallowing is the real cause of the discomfort, while others have long since abandoned that idea. Babies need an efficient ring of muscle at the bottom of the oesophagus that allows some upward movement of air via burps, stomach contents via possets or 'spit up', when needed to relieve pressure. Too tight a muscle at the top of the stomach could hold everything in so that baby blows up like a balloon, or else dumps it all into the next section of the gastro-intestinal tract, which is also governed by a complex ring of muscle, the pylorus. Similarly, the pylorus has to allow stomach contents to move on into the intestine. If that muscle ring is damaged by inflammation and restricts movement of stomach contents, the baby will sick up, and even vomit forcefully, so forcefully sometimes that it is called projectile vomiting. Pyloric stenosis (narrowing of the bottom outlet from the stomach, resulting in projectile vomiting) has been much more common in formula-fed babies. I consider it likely to be yet another manifestation of damage from alien foods like cows' milk, when it occurs in breastfed babies. There is considerable evidence that this narrowing is not inborn, but develops after birth – presumably due to inflammation and its results.

Excess pressure anywhere in the gastro-intestinal tract can cause damage to the cells lining the area, and also affect the co-ordinated movement of food through the gut (gut motility). It seems to me that the ring of muscle, the oesophageal sphincter, at the top of the baby's stomach is not defective, or immature, or inefficient, as many describe it. It's beautifully evolved, and will go on changing to meet the child's needs as those needs change. Initally those needs include allowing the easy rejection (via regurgitation) of excess feed intake, which can do more harm further down the gut. Babies are not miniature adults. Normal infant deviations from an adult norm are not likely to be defects but adaptations. Once again, let's respect the normal as physiological and likely to be beneficial, and look carefully for reasons when normal functioning is problematic.

Reflux and regurgitation is common, and a symptom that says the baby's body wants to get rid of something that is either too much, or recognised as harmful. Thickening that something, in the baby's case infant formula, with yet *more* ingredients seems to me a daft enterprise, which has to affect the rate of transit of food through the gut, and its absorption. Constipation can be the result. A common problem in bottle-fed infants, constipation can have both simple and complex causes: too little water in feeds, or protein allergy, or damage to nerves, or congenital defects. Many cases both of intractable constipation or "toddler diarrhoea" resolve when allergens are removed from the diet: they affect gut motility, in ways that differ between individuals, and between products. Some bodies react by speeding up gut transit and diarrhoea results; others slow down gut transit; constipation can result from excess water absorption needed to flush the kidneys.

So thickening feeds  is not without risk: thickeners are food additives or foodstuffs that carry all the risks of industrial preparation, just as formula does. Usually these additives are assumed to be safe. But in 2012 'Simply Thick' was linked to the deaths of seven babies (most preterm, but not all) and at least twenty-two who developed NEC (necrotising enterocolitis).[1947] Its ingredients were water, xanthan gum, citric acid and potassium sorbate. It is still in use for adults and older infants and children. What does that mix do to gut flora, I wonder? Or to gastric emptying time?

Thickeners do indeed reduce the amount of food that gets out on to clothes and sheets. This is a benefit, but a small one. Taping the baby's mouth shut, as Dr Garland suggested (see page 234), would achieve the same effect, but neither can be recommended. The risks are obvious, and serious.

How unsafe have thickeners been? Obviously most children survive them. But because these thickeners have been made from foodstuffs that have been in general use, such as cornstarch, or (like peanut oil) are on that dubious FDA 'Generally Recognised As Safe' (GRAS) list, they have often been added to formula without any need for prior safety evaluation. Said the mother of one dead full-term baby: 'I was astounded how a hospital and manufacturer was gearing this toward newborns *when they never had to prove it would be safe for them*. Basically we just did a research trial for the manufacturer.'[1948] A trial with a disastrous outcome, like so many infant feeding experiments. There are still concerns about possible side effects of thickeners: see the table below.

| Thickening agents | Possible side effects |
| --- | --- |
| Locust bean gum | • lower *in vitro* availability of calcium, zinc, iron (not confirmed *in vivo*) |
| | • higher incidence of necrotizing enterocolitis in preterm infants |
| | • detection of one case of Immunoglobulin E-mediated allergic reaction |
| | • false-positive results at galactomannan test reactivity |
| Rice cereal | • increased energy density |
| | • increased coughing episodes |
| Cornstarch | • increased energy density |
| Xanthan gum | • higher incidence of necrotizing enterocolitis in preterm infants |
| Pectin | • reduced *in vitro* availability of calcium and iron (highly esterified pectin) |
| | • detection of one case of intestinal obstruction and enterocolitis |

Figure 5-1-1 Milk thickening: possible side effects[1949] © Wageningen Academic Publishers

1947 Baby Formula Thickener Recalled After Deaths, Illnesses. WKEF-TV ABC News report. Sept 20, 2012. www. abc22now.com/shared/news/top-stories/.../wkef_vid_8962.shtm...

1948 Catherine Saint Louis. Warning Too Late For Some Babies. *New York Times*, February 4, 2013 Online at well. blogs.nytimes.com/2013/02/04/warning-too-late-for-some-babies/

1949 Corvaglia LT, Martini S, Faldella G. *Thickening of infant formula*, in Preedy V, Watson RR,  Zibardi S (eds), op. cit., p. 335. © Wageningen Academic Publishers.

How useful have thickeners been? Recently Australia's National Health and Medical Research Council stated that 'Thickening of feeds (using a range of thickening agents) has some benefit in decreasing the amount regurgitated *[less comes up and out],* but is not effective in decreasing the number of episodes of gastro-oesophageal reflux (GOR) or acid exposure, *and thus has no real place in the management of complicated GOR.*'[1950] They didn't answer the question as to whether reducing regurgitation is always helpful for infants, when it keeps stuff down that their bodies want to bring up. What effects on the gut? In some cases I have seen or been told of by the mother, rapid expulsion via increased gut contractions, diarrhoea and even blood in the poo.

*No place at all,* real or imaginary, in complicated gastro-oesophageal reflux. I am not expecting to see much change in clinical practice, as the formula companies are now trying to develop and patent novel industrial products for those babies who experience reflux. Even for preterm infants, there are experiments with adding ingredients like pectins to the formula. One study suggests that there is no benefit in so doing.[1951] What are the risks? Read the processes involved in making these novel compounds, and see if you feel like trying them yourself. Would you eat such things rather than chuck up some food? (Sometimes nothing feels better than to have got rid of a dodgy food by vomiting, unpleasant though the experience is.) Search the FSANZ website for details of applications for use of ingredients classed as novel foods. The one I have footnoted was intended to assist with infant gut health and reflux.[1952] Or read the detailed section in the 2013 NHMRC Guidelines online.[1953]

Thickeners do not reduce reflux, just spitting up, so the stuff goes back down, probably only to rise again. How can we stop that happening? Do we change posture, give medication, or change diet?

## Changing positions and culture: where's the gas?

So all babies reflux, and some regurgitate stomach contents. Remember, reflux means stomach contents move up into and irritate the lower oesophagus; regurgitation means stomach contents get up to the mouth or out of it. Both reflux and regurgitation can be culturally induced. In the normal evolutionary context, babies are carried or otherwise upright and in motion with an adult body much of the day. This keeps swallowed air and gas at the top of their stomach so that a burp can escape whenever the muscle band at the top of the stomach relaxes, as it does periodically. Check out the two sketches on the next page.[1954] In the first sketch, the muscle band (sphincter) is initially tight and gases cannot easily escape. As the muscle relaxes this changes- as on the right - and gas can rise, baby burps. Burps happen normally when parents lift their baby to their shoulder, or keep him in

---

1950 NHMRC *Infant Feeding Guidelines* op. cit., p. 52

1951 Corvaglia L, Aceti A, Mariani E, Legnani E et al.. Lack of efficacy of a starch-thickened preterm formula on gastro-oesophageal reflux in preterm infants: a pilot study.(PMID:22725606) *J Matern Fetal Neonatal Med* 2012, 25(12):2735-2738.

1952 http://www.foodstandards.gov.au/foodstandards/applications/applicationa1059pect5162.cfm

1953 https://www.nhmrc.gov.au/_files_nhmrc/publications/attachments/n56_infant_feeding_guidelines.pdf

1954 Diagrams from Vartabedian, B. *Colic solved – your essential guide to infant reflux and the care of your crying, difficult to soothe baby* p. 148, p.165. © Random House; permission applied for.

an upright sling with legs hanging down, so that the infant torso stretches out and is not 'kinked' or compressed. If the baby is lying on her back, or her right side, stomach gases rise away from the sphincter, and stomach contents can reflux when the sphincter relaxes. Rotate the image and visualise what happens to the lighter gases and heavier stomach contents. Many adults find left-side sleeping more comfortable when suffering indigestion.

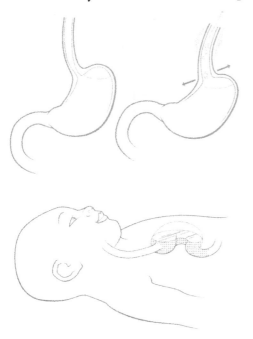

Figure 5-1-2 Bodies and burping. Illustrations by Briar Lee Mitchell; from *Colic Solved: The Essential Guide yo Infant Reflux and the Care Of Your Crying, Difficult-to-Soothe Baby* by Bryan Vartabedian, M.D., copyright © 2007 by Bryan Vartabedian, M.D.. Used by permission of Ballantine Books, an imprint of Random House, a division of Penguin Random House LLC. All rights reserved. Any third party use of this material, outside of this publication, is prohibited. Interested parties must apply directly to Penguin Random House LLC for permission.

In fact, humans of any age will be uncomfortable when lying down most of the day. That all dawned on me very painfully when confined to bed after surgery, with strict instructions to keep my feet up for a week. Without normal upright posture and movement, I experienced severe heartburn or reflux such as I hadn't known since being heavily pregnant and drinking lots of milk for calcium (another myth, of course). Along with the reflux came abdominal gas, bloating and flatulence. As I wriggled and shifted position to burp or fart, as discreetly as possible in a shared ward, I realised that unlike adults, babies cannot deliberately relieve any gut pressure building up due to immobility and posture. The gut pressure was painful. I soon chose to eat very little and munched calcium carbonate antacid tablets (not the aluminium- containing variety) to neutralise the painful acid burn I could feel at the lower end of my oesophagus. I lay on my back like a stranded beetle, pondering how horrible it must be for an infant to lie flat on her back for hours at a time, or to be left for hours in a pram, sometimes with head lower than feet, or be scrunched into a comma shape by a car seat or stroller. In all these places and positions babies are incapable of arching back, or stretching out, or deliberately burping or farting so that trapped wind can escape. Any normal young baby kept in these positions can be expected to become uncomfortable, to arch back and wriggle. Young ones don't even have the head control we use when burping. Just try to burp with your chin on your chest as though you had little forward-back head control![1955] Babies can only ask for breastmilk to neutralise acids, which is one reason why they want to feed often.

Reflux is inevitable – it happens mostly unnoticed in everybody – and posture-related. Heartburn in pregnancy – another name for painful reflux – is worse lying on the right

---

1955 Newborn babies do have some side to side head control from birth, as it may be important to be able to bobble across the mother's chest to get to the breast for food. Just watch them!

side, or with one's midriff compressed – pregnant women often lean back when seated, and sleep on their left side. Adults understand that heartburn can be very painful: the sale of antacids proves that!

Breastfed babies have evolved a low stomach pH, acid enough to kill moulds and bacteria, activate normal digestive enzymes, assist in absorption of minerals, and moderate ingested allergens. Yet that high acidity rarely causes problems for breastfed babies, unless something else is going on. I believe (but can't prove) that it is the damage done by allergic or infective inflammation that allows refluxing stomach contents to hurt the fully-breastfed baby. The bottle-fed baby's stomach pH is higher, less acid. Formula-fed babies have on occasion developed an 'auto brewery syndrome'[1956] in which yeasts ferment in the stomach and make alcohol. But bottle-fed babies also have unnaturally long inter-feed intervals, and different products of digestion to deal with; their different pH does not mean a lower likelihood of pain from acid reflux, probably because there are so many other differences in breastmilk's protection of the oesophageal mucosal surface. Breastmilk's anti-inflammatory and healing factors are absent for the formula-fed baby.

Young babies who cannot control their own body need to be supported in postures that facilitate keeping digesting milk down, burps possible, and milk moving through the gut, and they need to be fed small amounts easily when they wish. Slings are great if they allow for babies to be supported vertically with their necks supported, airways clear and gut not constricted: ABA's Meh Tai is brilliant for the young baby, and my variant of it costs almost nothing.[1957] Of course slings can also keep babies in awkward postures, and several babies have died in both slings and car seats that curl the baby's head down and obstruct breathing, so that suffocation was the stated cause of death.[1958] (Equally of course, some babies do die in every environment and posture. If all young babies were always carried in slings, then slings would always be associated with infant deaths: associations are not always causes. If they were, cots would have been banned long since, since that is where most Western babies have died! That is why unexpected infant death is commonly called cot death, after all.)

I suspect that the physical development of babies by three months explains why many crying babies ease off around then, as they develop the ability to roll over and move their bodies in response to internal stimuli. Perhaps this was why infant distress was called 'three-month colic', in the days before early formula comp-feeds ...Allergy-induced colic doesn't end at three months these days!

## Giving medications

Acid reflux is painful, as anyone suffering heartburn is aware. Suppressing gastric acid secretion, or neutralising its acidity by means of medication is another strategy sometimes

---

1956 Bivin WS, Heinen BN. Production of ethanol from infant food formulas by common yeasts. (PMID:3997687) *J Appl Bacteriol* 1985; 58(4):355-357.

1957 see *Breastfeeding Matters* p. 196-7 and run up your own version: I provide them for mothers of newborns that I deal with. I'll put a diagram on my website in 2015.

1958 Byard RW, Gilbert JG. Infant deaths associated with baby slings. *Med J Aust* 2011; 195 (6): 321. doi:10.5694/ mja11.10693 Google 'infant slings and death' for more information.

adopted. It is obvious that the use of drugs that suppress a normal body function that helps digest food and contributes to a normal gut microbiome could have side effects that may be harmful. Research has also shown that 'Treatment with GAS (gastric-acid-suppressing) medications is associated with the occurrence of food allergy'.[1959] Even simple antacids have risks, although an occasional small dose of those using calcium and magnesium carbonates (not aluminium) will have only a very temporary effect, and can be justifed as relieving the pain of acid contacting inflamed surfaces. Mothers may well remember how painful acid reflux was, and what a difference an antacid could make.

The so-called PPIs, the proton pump inhibitors, which reduce stomach acid secretion, have much more serious and longer–term potential side effects. Their use in infants has been off-label: manufacturers have not conducted research in infants, and do not stand behind their use for infants. Doctors prescribing them are taking risks. Parents for whose children they are being prescribed should read about this medication, and try to find a doctor who will look for causes rather than use such drugs in infants.

Reflux treatments have been marketed everywhere for the last few decades. Dr Bryan Vartabedian is a US gastroenterologist who has written a book called *Colic solved – your essential guide to infant reflux and the care of your crying, difficult to soothe baby*. Vartabedian argues that inconsolable babies are almost always either allergic to cows' milk or suffering from reflux or both. His book is useful for artificially fed infants, naturally most of his patients. However, I get a sense that Dr Vartabedian hasn't worked through these issues with many fully breastfeeding mothers who cope with oversupply issues and crying babies soon after birth, and who go on fully breastfeeding. America is not Australia, and I think that's manifest in his experience. The US is maybe two or more generations further down the formula road, and the population's infant mortality rates and general health reflect this.[1960]

*However, I agree with Vartabedian that truly inconsolable babies are almost always either allergic or suffering from reflux or both.* That's after weeding out all those whose problems resolve with better caregiving, via the process I outlined earlier. I'd only go looking for reflux as a stand-alone diagnosis *after* working through that process, and not being able to see any result of changes to the breastfeeding mother's diet, which usually end the crying. In my experience fully breastfed babies treated young lose their symptoms rapidly. Their stomachs no longer push back up and out what disagrees with them in mother's milk, once her diet changes and her system clears all residual antigen. That may take a while. Milk and egg antigens could be found in the milk of mothers on milk and egg avoidance diets for some time.[1961] See Figure 2-5-2 on page 98.

---

1959  Trikha A, Baillargeon JG, Kuo YF, Tan A et al. Development of food allergies in patients with gastroesophageal reflux disease treated with gastric acid suppressive medications.(PMID:23905907) *Pediatric Allergy and Immunology* 2013; 24(6):582-588.

1960  One of my pre-publication medical readers added here' 'I wonder if it's the explanation for so many young American actors sounding so adenoidal.' Could be, certainly!

1961  Kilshaw PJ, Cant AJ. The passage of maternal dietary proteins into human breast milk. (PMID:6746107) *Int Arch Allergy Appl Immunol 1984, 75(1):8-15*

# Changing diets: extensively-hydrolysed formula or human milk?

So I think it's not often necessary to try hypoallergenic formula *for breastfed babies* (as Vartabedian does). However, for one mother I have dealt with it was the only practical option. The problem had gone unaddressed for too long, and her hungry, distressed, and very lean baby clearly needed more food right away, although his very activity told me that his case was not yet extreme: lethargy and passivity is much more worrying! I informed this mother about less allergenic formula, as well as what would be involved in relactating while also altering her own diet. She realistically chose to introduce formula, a decision I supported. We discussed formula in detail, so she purchased at full retail price a tin of an extensively hydrolysed formula – and began the task of convincing her doctor that this was justified and should be prescribed, without the need to put her underweight baby through too many distressing challenges solely to convince the doctor. (Assertive educated mothers have some hope of doing this, as more and more doctors are seeing that the more expensive formulas make a difference.)

But this was to date the only case in which I have felt compelled to support a change to formula. Had I seen this mother perhaps even a week earlier, formula might not have been necessary. The mother's milk supply could possibly have been revived a week before. In her incredibly unsupported situation, doing so was unlikely to be a swift or easy process. And her baby was already clearly allergic and reacting to foods she ate, so that an elimination diet would have been necessary as well, and this can cause serious withdrawal symptoms for the mother. There are limits to what can be done when mothers have no help to call on, and the problem has gone on for weeks. Mothers should know to ask early and often for breastfeeding help.

Other mothers with an underweight allergic baby, but with better social connections and support, have been able to access safe-enough donor milk to feed the baby while building up their milk supply on an elimination diet. (Sometimes the mere fact of the mother no longer having to struggle with allergens in her diet means an immediate boost to well-being and milk supply, after the first difficult week of full avoidance.) Obviously human milk supplementation would be the better option where it is possible. The overall social situation determines what is possible, and it may not be what would be ideal.

Ideals are sometimes unattainable. But mothers still need to know what might be ideal: no one should influence their decisions by suppressing uncomfortable facts. Suggesting hypoallergenic formula is a big responsibility. Sometimes it can just be a stopgap, as mothers can continue to lactate and get baby back to the breast. Some damage to the baby's gut may already be done by then. No one really knows what the long-term consequences of short or long term substitution with such formulas might be. So I always try hard to make sure that a mother realises that she has not failed her baby: our health care system has failed her by not providing the support she needed to breastfeed more successfully.

That particular mother could afford to buy extensively hydrolysed infant formula. Until recently, most hypoallergenic brands have been simply too expensive for most families without a medical prescription, so it's been a last resort. Recently in Australia Nutricia has introduced a new product (Karicare Aptamil AllerPro), which is *said to be* equivalent to the prescription ones, but reasonably priced and available over the counter. That raises all sorts of questions: how can they produce it so much more cheaply? Are the others price-gouging? Are there real differences in quality? What comparative studies can parents access? Why does the website description say that 'AllerPro is not suitable for general use and should be used under medical supervision to ensure adequate infant growth and development', yet it is available over the counter? How will medical supervision ensure anything other than perhaps a change to another formula if the baby fails to thrive on this one? Is Australia a test market for a product not yet proven "to ensure adequate infant growth and development"?

Before continuing, I should point out that by hypoallergenic formulas in this context of the reactive child, I mean full-on extensively hydrolysed protein, whether whey or casein-based, or else amino acid based so-called 'elemental' formulas. Why are so many breastfed babies put onto such formula products, rather than maternal diet investigated and maternal supply managed better? Exactly who is that easier for? Not babies. Yet the baby is a person to whom health professionals have a duty of care, just as they do to its mother.

## What *do* we know about particular infant formulas and allergy?

Not a lot. What was known in 2008 is well summarised in Skypala and Venter's excellent book, *Food hypersensitivity*. They say:

> It is known that the immunogenicity of formulas will differ depending on the source of the protein (casein or whey), degree of hydrolyzation (partial or extensive), site of hydrolyzation, enzymes/chemicals used and filtration methodology [and that in research papers] results should be shown for each formula studied, rather than grouping results of partially hydrolyzed and extensively hydrolyzed.[1962]

A Danish study showed that one extensively hydrolysed casein formula was more effective in reducing allergic symptoms at eighteen months than an extensively hydrolysed whey formula.[1963] Which makes me wonder again, whether the global change to the first whey-predominant formulas affected allergy rates. Few long-term studies on the prevention of allergy compare extensively hydrolysed formulas with exclusive breastfeeding by mothers on individualised allergen avoidance diets. Too hard, or don't we want to know the answer? Prescribing a formula is certainly easier than helping a mother sort out her diet. But what about the hazards of those AGEs? (See page 251.)

---

1962 Skypala I, Venter A. *Food Hypersensitivity*. (Wily Blackwell 2009).
1963 Halken S, Høst A, Hansen LG, Osterballe O. Preventive effect of feeding high-risk infants a casein hydrolysate formula or an ultrafiltrated whey hydrolysate formula. A prospective, randomized, comparative clinical study. (PMID:8298708) *Pediatr Allergy Immunol* 1993; 4(4):173-181.

Paediatric gastroenterologists such as Bryan Vartabedian can prescribe hypoallergenic formulas and many drugs to patients. For me, all the expensive formulas and anti-reflux drugs and tests used by gastroenterologists and paediatricians are needed when the baby is clearly failing to thrive. Only a minority of affected babies get to that stage if parents take infant distress seriously in the early days. And they should: the longer damage goes on, the harder it can be to sort the problem. The anti-reflux drugs given are powerful and can have long-term side effects: suppressing gastric acid for example, may alter food processing and result in food intolerances[1964] – if these are not already the cause of the reflux, of course! They can also make for immediate problems in some infants: some babies cry even harder when on the drugs and improve when they are withdrawn!

When reading overseas books like Vartabedian's, parents need to keep in mind that the formulas he suggests are not necessarily the same as those available in Europe or Australia, *even if the brand name is the same.* Local doctors may suggest others, which they find work better. This may be because infant formulas are *not* all the same, and the range available in every country is different. There is very little independent research evidence to guide the choice of brand and type, so clinical experience is essential, as is regular parental feedback to doctors about outcomes in their child. And doctors need to be conscious that particular formulas may be risky for children who have certain problems, such as liver disorders. For example, hypoallergenic formulas, better for weight control, have been associated with Vitamin K deficiency bleeding (VKDB).[1965] There is a great deal more about formulas and allergy elsewhere in this book, so use the index to look into this further.

Some doctors still put breastfed babies on to partially hydrolysed or extensively hydrolysed infant formula apparently without any real appreciation of the extreme nature of such a change, and the losses and risks that it entails for mother and baby alike.

If this is because they don't know how to help with breastfeeding, or feel it all takes too much time, they should take stock of their deficiencies and learn what they need to know, or else employ someone who does. One very sought-after US paediatrician accepted as patients only parents who intended to breastfeed. He employed experienced lactation consultants to triage evening calls about young infants, as he was confident that competent help with feeding issues would save him from night call-outs. He reviewed their written reports first thing each morning, and found the system saved him much valuable time. He was always available in case of medical need but that was very rare, as his clients were mostly fully breastfeeding. Healthworkers should find and train suitable help, if they choose to remain ignorant about infant feeding, the single biggest influence on infant health.

---

1964 Trikha A, Baillargeon JG, Kuo YF, Tan A et al. Development of food allergies in patients with Gastroesophageal Reflux Disease treated with gastric acid suppressive medications.(PMID:23905907) *Pediatr Allergy Immunol* 2013; 24(6):582-588.

1965 van Hasselt PM, de Vries W, de Vries E, Kok K et al. Hydrolysed formula is a risk factor for vitamin K deficiency in infants with unrecognised cholestasis. *J Pediatr Gastroenterol Nutr* 2010; 51(6):773-776.

## The aftermath of infant colic and the hazards of wrong diagnoses

I agree with Vartabedian that as a diagnosis colic or gut distress is meaningless, if its cause is not understood. And thirty-eight years later, the infant gut that I knew best still hurts when inadvertently milk-exposed in the most unlikely ways, such as via green mango juice in Vietnam.[1966] I have to wonder how many current cases of adult inflammatory bowel disease, irritable bowel syndrome, Crohn's disease or coeliac disease began as colicky babies, whose parents were persuaded to ignore and accept those symptoms as normal infant behaviour.

> Extreme gut pain when my son was thirteen caused an emergency room visit in the dead of night .We waited for hours. By the time an abdominal X-ray was done, analgesics, anti-spasmodics and postural changes had improved matters and the pain had resolved, though discomfort remained. Reviewing the X-rays, a young resident doctor, as arrogant as he was ignorant, clearly suspected me of being a Munchausen by proxy case; he even invented and wrote into a hospital record 'facts' to support his theory. I roared with laughter (and rage) when I read his report, having obtained it under FOI legislation. My son was indignant: 'You never said any of that! He's made that up!'
>
> There can be deadly consequences from false public hospital records. School camps were a nightmare for me: what if my son had an acute attack of abdominal pain and was taken to a hospital and that false medical record accessed? Might a delay in accurate diagnosis lead to peritonitis and sepsis? So I found an eminent gastroenterologist at a major children's hospital and told him the whole story. This gastroenterologist set in place proper investigations and dealt with one more emergency admission with an 'acute abdomen' (suspected partial bowel obstruction) which resolved with anti-spasmodics and movement, without surgery.
>
> Then fortunately (!) just before he was sixteen, another hospital admission proved to be a complete bowel obstruction. The surgery revealed extensive previous damage, inflammation, scarring and adhesions constricting the bowel, with an almost necrotic area which the surgeon said he was gambling could recover, but might need to be cut out. The surgeon also commented that my son must have put up with a lot of pain over many years. He was startled when I wept on his shoulder in relief at this proof that I had been right to take my son's pain seriously - despite the medical psychobabble about psychosomatic gut pain and "abdominal migraine." Parents need to trust their gut feelings and daily knowledge, and stand up for their children! See Chapter 4.4.

That minority of 1980s parents who persisted in considering such crying behaviour unnatural, and trying to find remedies, were sometimes categorised as obsessive, neurotic, over-anxious, depressed, or just attention-seeking. These are the ongoing issues parents of

---

1966  He had walked a short distance before realising that he was feeling the early warning signs of a milk reaction. Going back to the street vendor, he asked if there was any cows' milk in the mango juice. Yes, sweetened condensed milk was part of the drink.

once-colicky babies may face. I know that it takes strength to persist in the face of medical obstinacy and obstruction, as that anecdote above illustrates.

I know other parents who have suffered similar indignity at the hands of arrogant doctors like those who called food intolerance "the muesli-belt syndrome"; they struggled to persuade healthworkers to take them seriously and investigate physical causes for a child's problems, not resort to dubious psychosocial explanations. I have no doubt that mental distress can affect the gut (and vice versa), or that there are a few loony parents. But physical causes should always be investigated thoroughly *before* psychological explanations are considered. And allergy is one of those overlooked physical causes.

There is now plenty of support in the scientific literature for allergy as a cause of gut distress of many kinds. One article worth reading is summarised as follows:

> Gastro-oesophageal reflux disease[1967], constipation and colic are among the most common disorders in infancy and early childhood. In at least a subset of infants with these functional disorders, improvement after dietary elimination of specific food proteins has been demonstrated. Gastrointestinal food allergy should therefore be considered in the differential diagnosis of infants presenting with persistent regurgitation, constipation or irritable behaviour, particularly if conventional treatment has not been beneficial. The diagnosis of food protein-induced gastrointestinal motility [alterations in the movement of food through the gut] disorders is hampered by the absence of specific clinical features or useful laboratory markers. Gastrointestinal biopsies [taking small samples of the gut tissue] before commencing a hypoallergenic diet may provide the most important diagnostic clues. Early recognition is essential for the optimal management of these patients to prevent nutritional sequelae or aversive feeding behaviours. Treatment relies on hypoallergenic formulae, as well as maternal elimination diets in breast-fed infants. Further research is required to better define the pathological mechanisms and diagnostic markers of paediatric allergic gastrointestinal motility disorders. The following article will present three instructive cases followed by discussion of the clinical presentation, diagnosis, treatment and natural history of food allergic motility disorders in infancy and early childhood.[1968]

So yes, cows' milk protein intolerance or cows' milk allergy can cause all these problems, and they can be hard to diagnose and treat. Read the whole article, and you will recognise the problems, if you have much experience of babies. What is more, children with colic are more likely to develop migraine in adolescence[1969] and adulthood,[1970] so some of these babies may be crying because they have a headache as well as a gut ache, but have no way of saying so. As Romanello et al said,

---

1967  Named and sold as a disease by those wanting a chunk of the massive antacid market that had developed due to western digestive problems.

1968  Heine RG Allergic gastrointestinal motility disorders in infancy and early childhood. (PMID:18713339) *Pediatric Allergy and Immunology* 2008, 19(5):383-391.

1969  Romanello S,Spiri D, Marcuzzi E, Zanin A, et al. Association Between Childhood Migraine and History of Infantile Colic. *JAMA* 2013; 309(15):1607-1612. epub 17 April 2013

1970  Grant EC. Food allergies and migraine. *Lancet* 1979;1(8123):966-9.

A study published today links migraine and colic [1]. In this research, children and adolescents aged 6–18 who suffered from migraine were much more likely to have had colic as infants compared to children without migraine (about 73 per cent versus 26 per cent). Statistics like these suggest that migraine and colic may have a common root.

Indeed they do, and food is the root of the problem for most, in my decades of experience. I could add to this cases of older children with severe constipation and encopresis (lack of bowel control) *at school*, children who continued to bed-wet into their teens, children with uncontrollable rages, children unable to sit still or to learn, children lost in day-dreams incapable of focussing for long. or maintaining a clear stream of thought or speech: all of whom lost those problems when allergy issues were identified and addressed. The social consequences of such anti-social behaviours were huge, and the whole family and its relationships suffered as a consequence of these problems being diagnosed as psychosomatic (mind influencing body) rather than somatopsychic (body affecting mind – and personality and self-esteem and relationships and social success ...). And the misery all began with infancy diet, and could have been ended there. One seven-year-old thought to be intellectually handicapped *caught up a whole year's learning in one term* after diet changes. Think about what that meant for his life trajectory.

If you are a health professional reading this book, but you don't recognise these problems as stemming from allergy all too often, please acknowledge with humility and remorse that you have not been helping some of the parents who may have come to you needing help. For this is now so common that any health professional dealing with young families should have dealt with many cases. You are the problem here, so learn what you need to know to help families, and listen to what mothers have to say. Please. You are fuelling the market for alternative medicine otherwise!

One mother, a physician, when first seen was aware that she was sensitive to milk, because drinking cow's milk had caused a persistent urticaria. The remainder of the parents did not know that they were in fact sensitive to milk. It was not therefore possible, when interviewing parents, to ask simply "Are either of you sensitive to milk?" and to take their answer at its face value... Those who appeared to have symptoms, for example a recurrent rhinorrhea, that might be referable to milk were asked to discontinue taking milk and dairy products for a trial period of a month, to make a note of any change in symptomatology, and then, a month later, to start drinking milk again in abundance. Those who were sensitive to milk were surprised to discover that what they had believed to be, for example, a smoker's cough, cleared completely in the course of two to three weeks on a milk-free regimen, and returned promptly when milk was taken again. Unexpected changes also occurred in bowel habits. For example, a father who thought that he had an "irritable" colon and who had had to visit the toilet three to five times a day and who experienced indigestion and pruritus ani, found that on a milk-free regimen his stools became formed and were passed only once daily and that his pruritus ani subsided. The studies on parents were time-consuming but rewarding.

Gerrard JW, Lubos M, Hardy LW et al Milk Allergy: Clinical Picture and Familial Incidence *Canad Med Ass J* 1967; 97: 780-785.

## 5.2 Pay attention to the baby, not the book

Implicit in everything I write is the need for responsible caregivers to be attentive and responsive to the young baby, and to use their common sense. If there is a problem, close observation will suggest what it is. And close observation is needed to assess the results of interventions. Babies are a full-time pre-occupation, not a hobby. I wish this was acknowledged, so that parents don't try to make any baby 'fit in' to an absurdly busy life. Parents and baby alike would enjoy life more if the societal norm was for them to be together with adequate support for the first couple of years – or to be assisted by substitute allo-parents[1971] whose continued presence in the child's life for at least three or more years is seen as important. Other work can fit around the baby: but the young baby's needs are immediate. Neither mother nor baby are mind-readers: it takes time and attention for both to learn what is needed for comfortable coexistence, and of course mothers have the advantage of an adult mind to analyse and verbalise their learning.

They also need other informed adults with whom to talk things through, and most cannot afford to pay professionals for every such discussion. Partners, fathers and other extended family members need to take an active interest and read and be informed about such issues, without attempting to dictate to any breastfeeding mother what she should do: that is for her to work out, as she is almost always the person best attuned to the baby and to her milk supply. (And yes, there have been small qualitative studies showing that not-breastfeeding mothers may not be so well-attuned, studies not followed up for the most part.)

When substitute care is needed for the young baby, the caregiver should also be an attentive, responsive person that the child can grow to love - and who will not inexplicably disappear from the child's life and be replaced by some other person. Like Penelope Leach before him, Oliver James is absolutely right to stress that group daycare is not the best option for a child under three. Nor is an au pair who will disappear in six months, or a nanny who makes sure that she does not bond with the child she will have to leave when the money for her wages runs out.

A young mother just commented to me that the infant formula companies must really think a notice important when they hide it is microscopic print at the bottom of the can or the back of a leaflet picked up in a paediatrician's office. I think this is so important that I am giving it a separate section. And I'd have it in bold type if that didn't seem a little over the top.

---

[1971] Blaffer Hrdy S. *Mothers and Others. The evolutionary origins of mutual understanding* (Belknap Press 2007) A marvellous book everyone should read. And Oliver James's book, *How not to f\*\*\* them up* (Vermilion 2011) is also worth reading

# 5.3 Dealing with immediate signals: fever and pain

Paying attention to the baby requires constant (though not uninterrrupted) adult presence. Two really important signals all caregivers need to notice in all children, especially young ones, are pain and fever. Both are indiscriminate responses to a wide range of problems that activate the immune system, among them allergy. And let it be said upfront, *both pain and fever are part of the solution, and only rarely problems that require instant or total suppression.*

## Hot and bothered: the fever response in allergic children

Allergic children will suddenly develop high temperatures, sometimes with no other symptoms, sometimes accompanying an obvious reaction. To feel your baby hot and flushed, especially for no apparent reason – no rash, no cough, no sniffle – can be very distressing for parents. It is a cause for concern, but not alarm. Some allergic infants and toddlers wake up at night drenched in sweat, and parents think they have to adjust bedclothes, then find the baby waking because too cool, seeking warmth. (Night is the time of greatest histamine release, and thus of immune response.) Temperature fluctuations, bed-wetting, complaints of headaches and joint pains (once they can talk) are all more common in children with food allergies,[1972] and Big Pharma is ready with remedies for symptoms, while obscuring causes.

Many parents are victims of what has been described as fever phobia.[1973] In the Western world, parents have been bombarded with drug company advertisements telling them to use drugs to relieve 'nasty pain and fever', and many use those drugs quite inappropriately. In my view, those symptoms are better described as lifesaving pain and fever, protective pain and fever. They are body signals that should not be suppressed arbitrarily or unnecessarily for up to eight hours. To do so is to cripple the immune response.

The fact that fever causes mother or child to feel awful, and so to rest, frees up bodily resources to deal with the immune challenge. That might be milk leaking into surrounding maternal breast tissue, or antigens causing mast cell breakdown and histamine release, or a virus, bacteria or parasites attempting to thrive in a new environment. We need to respect our body's signals, not reach for drugs to suppress those signals. A body fighting off disease with a normal or lower temperature is handicapped. The problem may get worse without a temperature rise (fever). Suppressing fever may make physical exertion possible - at a time when the body really needs to rest. Rest allows the body to use its resources for the primary task of defence, using protein to make antibodies, for example.

---

1972 Domínguez-Ortega G, Borrelli O, Meyer R, Dziubak R et al. Extraintestinal Manifestations in Children With Gastrointestinal Food Allergy. *J Pediatr Gastroent Nutr* 2014; 59 (2): 210-214. doi: 10.1097/MPG.0000000000000391. Other manifestations noted in this study include mouth ulcers, fatigue, and allergic shiners (pallor with panda eyes when tired).

1973 Crocetti M, Moghbeli N, Serwint J. Fever phobia revisited: have parental misconceptions about fever changed in 20 years? (PMID:11389237) *Pediatrics* 2001, 107(6):1241-1246.

Fever means something very important: that the immune system has been activated and is getting on with its job of restoring bodily order and balance. Inflammation is a *good thing*, an important defence mechanism. Fever allows immune cells faster passage to the area of the body where a battle is to be fought, as it does when a mother develops a fever with mastitis. It also makes life harder for any invading bugs, which can be quite sensitive to temperature changes. So we do *not* want to suppress all fever, though we want to keep it within reasonable bounds, as too high a temperature can sometimes trigger convulsions and may even cause brain damage.

Nor do we want to wait twenty to thirty minutes for a pill to take effect and bring excessive temperatures down. What helps relieve unpleasant fever symptoms in infancy immediately? Most fevers drop and lethargy disappears when we

- unwrap and sponge the baby,
- put the naked toddler to play in a tepid bath
- provide cool drinks of water or very dilute natural juices

Monitor the fever, and write down the temperatures. There may be no need for any liver-affecting, metabolism-altering medication if the temperature stabilises or drops. (If it continues to rise, or the child is sleepy or lethargic and does not respond, call for medical advice.) The fever may disappear as suddenly as it came, and the quiet or grizzling baby become active again, if a little clingy still, as their body recovers. Keep baby cool (but not shivering!), well-hydrated, and comforted, reducing all additional stress, and allow the clever body to rebalance itself.

When comforting includes body contact via a sling, don't overdress the baby: indoors, a short-sleeved T-shirt or singlet and nappy/diaper is the most babies need if feverish and in contact with an adult body. A warm core allows good circulation. Bare arms, legs and head can shed heat, and can be sponged with tepid water as needed. This and sweat both allow evaporative cooling.

Synthetic fabrics lock in heat and sweat, and so hinder temperature regulation. Fabrics are important for temperature control in children. Notice how cotton breathes, but can get cold when damp, while fine wool or silk/cotton mixes breathe, and even when damp don't feel cold or clammy, but stay skin temperature. This is why grandmas knitted soft woollen singlets and used red flannel pilchers for babies, for those readers young enough not to remember such things! Babies that sweat in cotton will wake as they cool down; wool keeping the body's core warm helps with uninterrupted sleep. Babies do like to be with a source of warmth at night, even if only a foot or hand is in touch, to help regulate their temperature.

Of course there can be times when conservative and local treatments don't reduce fever enough, and so systemic medication can be justified. The World Health Organization (WHO) recommends that fever in children be treated with paracetamol (acetaminophen) only if their temperature is higher than 38.5 °C (101.3°F). But medication doesn't start to take effect until after about ten to fifteen minutes, which may be too long to prevent seizures/fits in the baby. Questions are being raised about paracetamol, now known to result in gastrointestinal blood loss.[1974] So even with a high temperature, the simple measures like giving liquids and sponging with, or immersion in, tepid water should always be tried immediately, while waiting for medication to decrease the inflammatory response.

Fever can diminish rapidly when antibiotics are given. This is not because antibiotics have instantly killed all microbes. Antibiotics, like all drugs, can have a wide variety of effects on the body. As well as kill sensitive micro-organisms, some of them useful ones, they can help the body fight infection in other ways. Some antibiotics can initially enhance the normal process of white blood cells mopping up anything that oughtn't to be where it is (that's called phagocytic clearance in medical parlance.). But this stimulus to the natural immune system is temporary, and once the antibiotic is removed, phagocytic clearance is then less effective than it originally was. So symptoms may reoccur if the original problem that caused the fever has not been addressed by the time the antibiotic course ends.

Antibiotics may kill the pathogens responsible for the problem. But even if they don't, antibiotics can sometimes buy time to identify and fix the underlying problem. That problem might not even be bacterial infection, but might still improve, because of the effect of certain antibiotics on white blood cell clearance. On the other hand, if you can control the problem, not with systemic antibiotics, but with less drastic local means, do so. You are decreasing the risk of developing antibiotic resistance, as well as decreasing the risk of fungal overgrowth and infection, and not messing with the microbiome your breastmilk has created. Antibiotics are wonderful, and life-saving, and sometimes, but not always, needed to reduce fever.

As the problem of multiple antibiotic resistance grows, it is likely that we will come to see greater value in the body's fever response, which makes life very difficult for temperature-sensitive pathogens. Readers of Victorian literature will recall accounts of seriously ill heroes and careful nursing by devoted females, tepid sponging and feeding sips of fluids through long nights at the bedside, until with the dawn the fever breaks and the patient stirs back to life, weak but on the way back to health. Many died, the old and very young especially, from infectious diseases. But attentive nursing[1975] saved many very sick people too. And there were fever treatments in the early twentieth century that may have cured some cancers: the idea has been explored again recently.[1976] Totally suppressing the mechanism by which the body retards pathogenic growth and mobilises its defences to the invasion sites makes no sense at all to me. It may even be that suppression advantages cancer cells.[1977]

---

1974 O'Callaghan T. Cure-all no more. *New Scientist* 2014; 222(2971): 34-37. For ongoing pain, it may be time to start looking at alternatives. With any drug, there's a risk that side effects will outweigh benefits. For paracetamol, we need to decide which risks are still worth taking.

1975 Helping with temperature regulation and maintaining hydration, along with calming reassuring constant presence, seem to have been key components of personal nursing.

1976 Hobohm H-U. *Healing Heat: an essay on cancer immune defence.*(BOD, 2013) See also Hot, toxic and healing – summary article in *New Scientist* Jan 4, 2014, pp. 26-7.

1977 Ibid.

When fever strikes, most people think of infection with pathogens. In the allergic child there may be absolutely no infectious invasion, simply a rapid or more extreme response to an antigen, by an effective immune response, which needs to rebalance. Such temperature rises usually stabilise at tolerable levels then disappear as swiftly as they came, leaving the child a little grumpy and in need of nothing more than TLC and water. And the parents worried about what it all means, and assuming the cause was 'a virus', that catch-all diagnosis which usually means only that no obvious pathogen has been detected.

I started teaching this many years ago now, swimming vainly against the tide of marketing that engulfs parents. So it was with considerable interest that I read a very recent article indicating that needless chemical suppression of fever may be causing many thousands of deaths and illnesses worldwide.[1978] It causes deaths both by prolonging the illness in infected persons, and by providing symptomatic relief, which encourages infected persons to return to social settings such as the workplace, rather than staying at home to rest. 'Soldiering on' can mean both suffering the disease longer, and spreading it wider: just what any incipient pandemic needs humans to do, so that it can spread and become a global threat. So don't go out, leave the pills in the cupboard, and let that 'healing heat' do its work, while monitoring to ensure that dehydration and convulsions are not a threat, and that food intake is helpful. Don't spread the bug: catch any sneezes in tissues or soft toilet paper, and wash your hands often with soap and water. (And use your common sense!)[1979]

## Pain in allergic children: another symptom and signal

Many allergic symptoms are painful: the spasming gut, the headache, the glue ear, the aching joint, all cause children pain. Pain, like fever, is another signal from the body, indicating a problem and suggesting its location (sometimes misleadingly). Dealing sensibly with pain can save many tears for both parents and children. Pain is most scary when it is not understood and seems unlikely ever to end, so that anxiety and fear ratchet up stress hormone levels. Breastmilk and breastfeeding, cuddles, warmth, massage and distraction, explanations and reassurance, and teaching the toddler simple breathing techniques[1980] may be the only pain relief a healthy child needs in everyday life. Even when there is severe pain, such basic human interactions can help reduce pain.

Watching commercial television advertising, one would never think so, for we live in a society where we are told incessantly by the multi-billion-dollar drug industry[1981] that every trivial pain (or fever) must be instantly despatched by chemical means. It shouldn't be. Intolerable pain certainly needs some relief. But humans also need to learn to tolerate and monitor pain, as a way of knowing what's going on in our bodies and respecting what that tells us to do. And we need to teach our children that pain is a helpful signal, and usually can be endured and managed without pills, though drinking water is often a good

---

1978 MacKenzie D. A touch of flu? Hold the painkillers. *New Scientist* 25 Jan 2014, p. 12; citing Earn D. *Proc Roy Soc B*: DOI: 10.1098/rspb.2013.2570
1979 *Soap and Water and Common Sense: the definitive guide to viruses, bacteria, parasites and disease* is the title of an excellent book by Dr Bonnie Henry (House of Anansi Press 2009).
1980 This worked well post-abdominal surgery with my three year old son, so why not try it?
1981 An industry that grew out of selling infant foods, heroin, cocaine, and morphine, in some cases.

idea. (Many headaches arise from mild dehydration, and the water solves the problem, not the pill.) For a professional sportsman it may make sense to suppress all awareness of pain so as to participate in a match, but he knows there's a price to pay the next day. And without the daily medical care sports stars can access (and perhaps even with it), the price is likely to be long-lasting.

All drugs, whether used for fever or pain relief or anything else, put strain on some part of the human metabolism and bodily organs. For children with developing bodies, that is a risk. I am utterly appalled by the amount of liver-toxic paracetamol[1982] and anti-inflammatory ibuprofen many children today are swallowing, just as I was in the 1970s by the doses of anti-histamines and barbiturates that were then prescribed for sleepless babies. Like heroin and cocaine, once popular over-the-counter medicines, the alcohol that then accompanied many infant medications has largely gone now. These drugs were all an experiment no one monitored. Companies sold the products and kept the profits, healthworkers naively trusted them. It took decades before it was suggested (now disputed) that aspirin increased the risk of Reye's Syndrome, a rare condition leading to swelling of the brain and liver. This led to a huge increase in paracetamol/acetaminophen use – which if given in the first year of life is linked with a higher risk of later asthma.[1983] That discovery has led to an increased use of ibuprofen, which also has possible side effects including gut bleeding. ...

Paracetamol and ibuprofen and the like may well go the same way as barbiturates once people start looking seriously at how they are used. Paracetamol is, after all, not very good as an anti-inflammatory, and takes time to be absorbed and begin work anyway. I strongly suggest parents read current reports on these drugs before deciding to administer them to infants for any reason whatever, and pregnant women should be advised of their increased risk of miscarriage. As I wrote this, the FDA is moving to reduce the doses of paracetamol in compound pain relief tablets, from 500 mg to 325 mg.

Toxic as it is, that traditional smooth muscle relaxant, alcohol, was probably once the effective part of many paediatric medications, as it relieved gut spasms. Sugar is a pain-reliever, an analgesic that acts on the brain, and once was present in those paediatric mixtures as well. The old fashioned remedy of a *drop* of brandy on a small teaspoon of sugar thus possibly did less harm to a baby than the drug companies' current mixes. Certainly there were fewer artificial colours and flavours and coal tar derivatives and preservatives to swallow, which parent experts like Sue Dengate[1984] might see as a bonus, as these food chemicals are her chief concern. Of course nowadays some would consider even a tiny amount of alcohol unacceptable, thanks partly to industry advertising that their products are now alcohol-free. Personally, I still find small quantities of alcohol useful to relieve

---

1982 FDA Drug Safety Communication: Prescription Acetaminophen Products to be Limited to 325 mg Per Dosage Unit; Boxed Warning Will Highlight Potential for Severe Liver Failure". U. S. Food and Drug Administration (FDA). January 13, 2011. Retrieved January 13, 2011.

1983 Gonzalez-Barcala FJ, Pertega S, Castro TP, Sampedro M, et al. Exposure to paracetamol and asthma symptoms. (PMID:22645237) *Eur J Public Health* 2013; 23 (4): 706-10.

1984 Sue has done wonders in the areas of food intolerance and food chemicals. Her Food Intolerance Network has helped thousands of families whose problems are more complicated than those of breastfed babies who respond to maternal diet changes. Check out her website at www.fedup.com.au

cramps and relax, just as Grandma always said; red wine is good for many things. Massage and warmth and cuddles also help, or cold packs if the problem is inflammation. A natural fruit cordial heavily diluted, given with TLC, relieves most children's everyday pains. In summer dilute cordial or fruit juices can be frozen into ice-block treats. Such old-fashioned remedies do not disguise what the pain is doing – increasing or decreasing, changing location or staying the same –but they take the edge off and facilitate positive hormone responses that help make minor pain bearable. If the pain is serious, paracetamol and the like seem to make little difference to some people, and only some morphine derivative like codeine effectively blocks the perception of pain –at the price of addictive risk, sluggish digestion and constipation if there is not an increase in fluid intake and soluble carbohydrates in the diet. (Whole dates or prunes can be useful as a source both of sugar and fibre).

If the painful inflammation is due to allergy, significant levels of histamines are involved. In Australia since the 1970s one class of drug that is useful for the allergic young child has become much harder for poor people to access. Low dose, tiny, uncoloured unflavoured anti-histamine tablets were fifty for four dollars in the early 1980s. Many are now closer to $1 per tablet, as the drug companies have increased their margins. A very small dose of antihistamine given early in the allergic reaction cycle can help prevent the cascade of histamine release that causes many of the obvious symptoms.

A child or adult can learn to recognise the early signs of an inflammatory response that will progress to a more extensive reaction. An allergic sore throat can lead to a blocked eustachian tube, which in turn can facilitate middle-ear inflammation. One four-year-old child with a tendency to otitis media commented, 'Before I get an earache, my voice sounds different in my head.' When given a single dose of half an antihistamine tablet as soon as she reported this sound change, she never progressed to an earache. On one later occasion, travelling for some hours with no antihistamine available to take as soon as she first noticed the change, a middle ear infection developed, requiring antibiotics. Coincidence perhaps, but worth a try? Even if this were a placebo effect, it would be a good one to harness. So I advise having access to a suitable antihistamine and trying out a single small dose as part of the process of damping down, *but not extinguishing,* inflammatory responses that are the early warning of an allergic reaction. And I strongly advise against the use of artificially sweetened antihistamine syrups for anything, from sedation to allergy relief or coughs and colds. The overuse of sweetly flavoured antihistamine syrups has caused child deaths.[1985] This is part of my concern about the (true) association of migraine and colic becoming a (false) diagnosis of colic *as* migraine, and analgesics being used as a treatment.

Again, common sense is required in dealing with pain and fever. It is better for a first time parent to be thought over-anxious by going to see the doctor too often, than to be deemed negligent after harm has been done. And if a parent's gut instinct is that something is seriously wrong, it's always better to seek such help right away. But over time parents become confident in dealing with such problems without medication. Only a generation or so back in time, most western mothers would not have felt they needed to see a doctor for

---

1985  http://www.medsafe.govt.nz/profs/PUArticles/Mar2013ChildrenAndSedatingAntihistamines.htm; http:// pediatrics.aappublications.org/content/122/2/e318.abstract

every pain or fever their baby experienced- the doctor was reserved for serious damage or sickness. My mother (poor in the 1940s) once said that she could count on her fingers the number of times her four young children ever needed to see the doctor, even though we all had the usual infectious diseases: chickenpox, mumps, rashes and spots never formally diagnosed by any doctor. We all survived with rest, fluids and TLC. Well fed, watered, and loved children are tough little survivors.

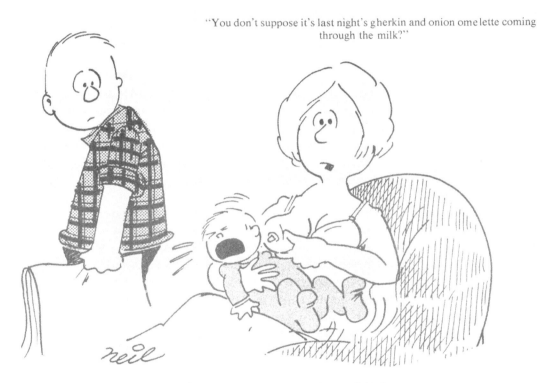

"You don't suppose it's last night's gherkin and onion omelette coming through the milk?"

Figure 5-3-1 Mothers recognise reactions. Image © Neil Matterson.
*Is he biting again?* (Marion Books, 1984) p. 54.

# CHAPTER 6

# Allergy, growth and other foods

Previous chapters have addressed more immediate and obvious aspects of allergy. Like any other physical challenge to normal bodily functioning, allergy will also affect growth. Sometimes food allergy is not taken seriously *until* it is affecting growth, so that the baby is failing to thrive. Failure to thrive is usually framed as breastmilk or breastfeeding being inadequate in quantity or quality, and one of the first solutions offered is often the early and unnecessary use of other foods, formula or solids of poorer nutritional value than breastmilk. As this book evolved, it seemed sensible to discuss a wider range of issues relating to allergy, continued breastfeeding, growth and current timing of introduction of other foods. Again, there is some overlap with other sections of the book, but I hope not too much needless repetition. After the first edition of the book, some sections may be removed to a website so they can be easily updated.

## 6.1  Food, growth, and the allergic infant

To begin with the obvious. Nutrients are needed for immune function, for maintaining body temperature and other functions, and for growth and development. In that sense, there is truth in the industry claim that formula provides nutrients to 'support the immune system'. What they don't say is that so does any food. Some parents may be misled by 'immuno' this or that labels into believing that that one 'unique blend' has been proven to make children's immune systems healthier than any other unique blend. So far as I can tell from the literature, that would be a mistake. Yes, the immune system needs nutrients. No, you don't need special products for it to work perfectly well in a normally well-nourished body. Nor does a baby need a mother who eats only a perfect diet. The human race would not have populated the globe if either myth were true.

But any sudden or excessive demand for nutrients for immune responses can affect growth: all skin damage, all infectious challenges, even vaccinations, can slow infant growth rates. Many mothers worry about their milk supply in the aftermath of vaccination producing a week or two of lower weight gain. They should be advised that this is normal. The immune system will use nutrients to make antibodies; protein and energy that might have been used in growth in length or weight gets directed elsewhere for a time. So long as there is plenty of both in the diet, any effect is fleeting and unimportant. When there is too little available, growth will suffer.

Long chain polyunsaturated fatty acids (LCPUFAs) and many other components of breastmilk help modulate the inflammatory processes generated by vaccination or infection or stress, tuning them up or down as the challenge requires. Increasing daily intake can help. Probiotics too, may help to relieve the symptoms of inflammation that result in eczema, although this possibility remains unproven to date. And it must always be remembered that not all probiotics have been tested – and they are not all the same![1986] Nor are all production and quality control processes equally reliable as has been described earlier.

So all bodily activity takes food (or body reserves) to power it. The universally rapid weight gain of the well-breastfed young solely-breastfed baby creates reserves that infection will plunder in poor communities. The baby who generates thick layers of cradle cap or eczematous lesions is wasting nutrients that could be used for growth and repair. Children with a history of severe eczema are often growth-retarded, and some have the pinched, stretched facial skin common in photographs of under-nourished slum children of the 1930s. Resolving allergy problems usually leads to an increase in growth rate as the baby catches up, then growth stabilises along his individual programmed trajectory. Allergy is evolutionarily counter-productive. But bodies can balance again, catching up lost growth, especially if the baby is still fully breastfed, or, if older, getting breastmilk plus adequate complementary foods (see Chapter 6.5 What are 'good quality complementary foods'?)

Breastfeeding mothers can expect that at times their allergic older baby or toddler will go off particular foods, or all food, for a few days, and increase breastfeeding frequency and duration. Where possible – that is, when the child is not seriously underweight or dehydrated, and is still active, not lethargic – this behaviour needs to be respected and accommodated. A child usually knows better than anyone else what he or she needs, and breastfed babies usually have ample bodily reserves, so there is no need to worry about this. With more frequent feeding and thorough breast drainage, the mother's milk supply will ramp up to higher levels of production, as about two days of more frequent suckling resets base-line levels of prolactin, a key hormone. This variability of infant appetite and maternal supply is the reason why breastfeeding women need to live in conditions that allow them to respond to the child's changing needs and suckling patterns. There are many breastfed babies who establish very predictable routines, but the more challenges the child has inherited or is exposed to, the more flexible the parents' responses need to be. A breastfeeding mother can't just hand her new baby and bottles of milk to someone else to deal with, except for short intervals.

Allergic children often refuse certain foods, and are often slow to start widening their diet, perhaps not wanting much by way of solids before nine to twelve months. Or they may eagerly dabble in new foods at six months only to go right off the idea for a month or so, as

1986 Murch, SH. Probiotics as mainstream allergy therapy? *Arch Dis Child* 2005;90:881–882. doi: 10.1136/
  adc.2005.073114

though it had adverse effects internally. Again, this is usual behaviour and nothing to worry about, simply a change to respond to calmly. A wide variety of interesting taste experiences in suitable forms should be on offer to the allergic infant from around six months, avoiding the most common allergens or those that the child reacted to in mother's milk. But the availability of a food is no guarantee that the infant will eat it, as experienced mothers know all too well: some infants seem determined not to, creating that reverse causal link between long-term exclusive breastfeeding and allergy. (Where it is the allergy that causes the long-term breastfeeding, not vice versa.)

So long as children's growth trajectory is appropriate on the recent WHO charts for breastfed babies (and they were not sick or extremely premature, with limited *in utero* stores) there is rarely any need to be concerned about thriving allergic children who don't want to take in other foods until later than six months in the first year of life, and who want to continue breastfeeding into the second year and beyond, as many do. Children of this age do not starve themselves. As will be discussed in Chapter 7.5, somewhere between nine and twelve months was once the normal time for widening western infant diet. Any industry-induced worries about the possibility of iron deficiency under nine months can be dealt with by getting a simple blood test done and taking appropriate action if there is need to. And addressing the allergy problem will free up resources for catch-up growth if that is needed.

But by twelve months, and in the second year where they morph from chubby babies into lean toddlers, breastfed children do need more protein than usual amounts of breastmilk alone can provide, and help should be sought if children steadfastly reject other suitable food. Children can become severely malnourished in the second year when no other foods are tolerated or available by twelve months. Too little fat and protein leads to protein-calorie malnutrition. This afflicts toddlers worldwide when a mother gets pregnant again and her milk supply drops, with no other fat and protein-rich food available to the toddler.

Protein-calorie malnutrition occurs even in affluent nations. It is worth describing because it can be misleading: the child can actually gain weight from retained fluid, but has match-stick upper arms, bloated belly, and general wasting. If the child is not being seen unclothed by a knowledgeable observer, or if weight alone is used as a guide, this can be missed, with devastating, even fatal results. At least one middle-class Australian child in my home town had been seen by a number of health professionals who failed to see just how severe the problem was. There was a similar case in Sydney around the same time, and I am sure that there have been more cases among children living in poverty. Mostly these were babies partly breastfed for a few months, then a deeply-deficient alternative formula – rice milk, say – was given. The dietary advice they followed meant that they offered only cereals and vegetables and fruit, with little fat or protein: the standard weaning diet since the 1980s. When the diet proved fatal, the alternative-leaning parents were blamed for their ignorance.

No one blamed the health professionals the parents had been consulting. Or the cutbacks that had reshaped the once open-house fully-staffed maternal and child health service into one which sees mothers by appointment only, for health surveillance purposes rather than wide-ranging unpressured conversation, and for weighing that involves experienced nurses undressing the baby. It is impossible to prosecute the architects of such cutbacks for the deaths they cause, so we prosecute the tragic parents, already suffering the worst of punishments for their ignorance. One simple diagram could have saved that Geelong child.

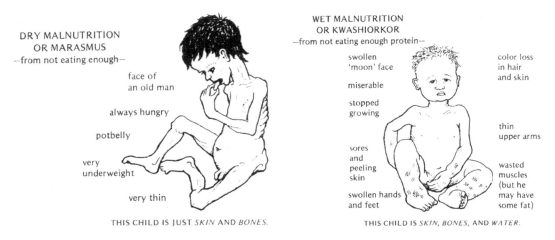

DRY MALNUTRITION
OR MARASMUS
—from not eating enough—

face of
an old man

always hungry

potbelly

very
underweight

very thin

THIS CHILD IS JUST *SKIN* AND *BONES*.

WET MALNUTRITION
OR KWASHIORKOR
—from not eating enough protein—

swollen
'moon' face

miserable

stopped
growing

sores
and
peeling
skin

swollen hands
and feet

color loss
in hair
and skin

thin
upper arms

wasted
muscles
(but he
may have
some fat)

THIS CHILD IS *SKIN, BONES,* AND *WATER.*

Figure 6-1-1 Two types of malnutrition. © Hesperian Health Guides.

As the images above show, serious malnutrition can look very different: the skin and bones wizened-old-man look of the underfed child, or the pot-bellied moon-faced child with matchstick upper arms and skin lesions, who can even gain weight as oedema increases. WIth clothes on, this latter malnutrition is not so obvious to the uneducated eye.

Infants even in Australia (see above) may develop that so-called 'wet' protein-calorie malnutrition which in Africa is called kwashiorkor. If the problem is identified and remedied in time to prevent death, it can still be damaging long term.

This diagram of the two kinds of malnutrition is from David Werner's excellent book, *Where there is no doctor* (Macmillan 2007 and still available).[1987] It is full of useful practical advice, such as "After one year of age, any child whose upper arm measurement is less than 13cm around is malnourished – no matter how "fat' his feet, face and hands may look. If the arm measures less than 12cm he is severely malnourished." The measurement is taken midway between the shoulder and the elbow.

Yet the information in this text for village healthworkers was both new and useful to some health professionals I have taught, especially those working in disadvantaged communities here in Australia and overseas. Protein-calorie malnutrition can happen anywhere in the world, with resultant stunting of infant growth. Appropriate growth monitoring is as important in Melbourne as in Mozambique. In doubtful cases, remember the arm circumference and always look for oedema! Take the time to really look at a baby, preferably bare.

---

[1987] Werner D. *Where There is no Doctor.* (Macmillan 2007). © Hesperian Health Guides. www.hesperian.org

# 6.2 Common causes of poor growth in infants under six months

Basically, poor growth will be due to:

- not enough nutrients going in
- too many nutrients not absorbed or coming out again, or
- not enough of what goes in being available for growth thanks to competing needs.

This chapter briefly outlines the most usual problems, but is no substitute for good ongoing professional oversight of your baby. Find a doctor and child health professional you like and trust, and monitor your child's growth and development along the global growth charts WHO has developed. Some babies are recognised as having been underfed only because when an underlying problem is corrected, they rapidly stack on weight as catch-up growth, and then go forward on a higher growth trajectory.

## 1. Not enough nutrients go into the breastfed baby

Almost all mothers, even those with only one breast, can make enough milk to feed a baby. The problem is more likely to be poor milk transfer than any basic inability to produce enough (rare when lactation is a survival mechanism).

Inadequate infant suckling – insufficient or inefficient, or both – is probably the most common cause of problems. Causes of poor suckling can include:

- poor positioning at the breast making efficient feeding difficult
- poor attachment to the breast (usually a result of poor positioning)
- pain or discomfort when feeding (most often due to poor attachment, but other causes less often)
- infant sedation (maternal or infant medication)
- physical anomalies (e.g., tongue-tie, muscle problems)
- neurological damage or under-development in the baby – prematurity, for example
- conditioned tongue use (in utero thumb-sucking, bottles, dummies), and of course, and most often,
- too little feeding time – limited or restricted access to the breast by mothers who think that babies should feed in a particular pattern or at regular intervals (both of which can result in low milk production and supply problems).

Both *insufficient* (not enough) suckling, or *inefficient* (not organised and productive) suckling, can result in an inadequate volume of milk being produced or consumed. That means a hungry baby, who wants the breast, may cry if not being fed or held, and may fuss when milk flow is low, but settles at the breast and never lets go voluntarily. Feeds are very protracted, as the baby cries and wants to go back to the breast if detached. This baby is getting too little milk. If this continues, the baby may conserve energy by becoming increasingly less energetic. This hungry baby will grow to look lean, and her weight will not be proportionate to her length. (Of course there are healthy long lean babies, and healthy short tubby babies: genetics influence how babies grow, so always check out the parents' body types before worrying about unusual length/weight ratios.)

Underweight babies need a greater volume or caloric density of milk, so the mother's supply must be boosted, or extra milk given. That means identifying the cause of the problem, whether physiological or behavioural or both. (It's most often simple positioning and attachment issues, as every health professional should know by now.) The lean and hungry breastfed baby who is active and otherwise well simply needs more food, preferably breastmilk, as soon as possible. Getting help from an experienced breastfeeding counsellor or lactation consultant turns this around in a couple of days, once the underlying cause of the problem is identified.

In very rare cases it may mean immediately addressing dehydration as a matter of urgency, using oral rehydration fluids, as the baby is becoming lethargic, or sleepier. Few breastfed babies reach this dangerous stage rapidly, but some do where parents do not have access to support. Parents would do well to have in the cupboard some oral rehydration tablets such as Gastrolyte that can be made up into a clear liquid to give to a feverish child or dehydrated infant. Look for products that contain no phenylalanine, or other synthetic chemicals or sweeteners or dyes. Simple solutions can also be made up at home for short-term use. Check out rehydrate.org. and take care with measurements.

## Signs of dehydration

All infant caregivers, young and old, need to know the signs of dehydration:

- loss of skin elasticity, so that skin feels slack, and can be pinched up, but doesn't spring back instantly when released

- dry mouth

- scanty or coloured urine

- sunken eyes or fontanelle (the soft spot on baby's skull)

- few and scanty stools

- increasing lethargy and sleepiness (loud alarm bells here)

Figure 6-2-1 Signs of dehydration

## Infrequent and inefficient suckling

Infrequent and inefficient suckling will both reduce available milk. This is reversible – frequent and efficient suckling will increase milk supply. This works in various ways:

- raising basal prolactin levels – perhaps the least important for most women

- removing from the breast an auto-control chemical known as FIL, the feedback inhibitor of lactation, and
- preventing the build-up of pressure within the breast, as this distorts the shape of the milk-making cells and makes them less efficient.

Without good drainage, milk is trapped in the breast and gives feedback to suppress production. A history of breast surgery means interference with breast drainage. While some mothers have managed to feed fully after such surgery, most have problems and many will fail to achieve complete breastfeeding, despite sometimes heroic efforts. These mothers need close and ongoing support both to maximise their milk production and to supplement appropriately. Many will need to formula feed, and if the baby is over three months, other foods may become part of the diet. Any donated milk is valuable.

## Very frequent but inefficient suckling, swapping breasts often

Both frequent *inefficient* suckling, or swapping breasts often, will raise hormone levels and stimulate milk *production*, but does not always allow good breast *drainage*. If the baby is constantly compressing the nipple (not the breast) the mother may develop fissures and extreme nipple pain, and come to dread feeding, which again, inhibits her letdown of milk. The mother's breasts can be constantly over-full, never well-drained, always leaking and heavy. The baby's growth may be less than optimal, although it can be within a normal range, and in some cases is tremendous.

The basic strategy is to enable the baby to feed more efficiently, then ensure the baby voluntarily finishes feeding on the first breast, before always offering the second. With a full breast ejecting milk, and a good oral vacuum drawing it into the baby's mouth, feeding at the first breast might be quite satisfying, so that the baby comes off looking full.

After burping, and maybe changing, he or she should in any case *be offered* the second breast. This by now will have a higher fat content than the first breast initially did. The baby may feed for a very short time on the second breast. If baby has taken enough for the breast to feel comfortable, there is no need to express any milk, but that second unmilked breast should be offered first next time. Top ups or mini-feeds can happen anytime : the baby is the guide to feeding frequency.

If the unmilked breast feels overfull or develops any flushed patch, it can be gently relieved of a little milk as many times as is necessary before the next feed. However, the high internal pressure of the unmilked breast is signalling to the mother's body to decrease production. As the day goes on and supply drops, even within twenty-four hours, the baby will feed for longer on the breast offered second. Usually the process ends two or three days later with the baby feeding roughly equal times on both sides, although many babies express a preference for one side and create a larger supply in that breast over time. This is a simple matter well dealt with by breastfeeding books and advisers. And it doesn't mean that one breast will always be larger after weaning!

Mothers with this problem will be more comfortable once they adjust their milk volume down and its cream content up. In the 1950s milkers were taught that to get the maximum amount of cream, they needed to 'strip' the cow, that is massage the udder and hand-milk after the machine milking had finished. Some babies may need help to get more cream! Gentle massage of the breast towards the nipple is thought to increase milk fat content, although the Hartmann team has shown that in fact each mother produces a fairly constant (for herself) fat amount each day, and this gets diluted into whatever volume of milk they are making – less in the milk when the breast is full and more when the breast is drained. But some oversupply or outflow-inhibited mothers never have anything but overfull breasts. Feeding as described above will reduce oversupply. At no stage in the process should either breasts be allowed to become too uncomfortable, as high pressure can cause milk leakage into tissue and trigger mastitis. (So can rough or bruising hand-expression: always be gentle with breasts.)

*There is no law or science about how many times or minutes to feed on either breast. Just don't keep swapping every few minutes; pay attention to the baby's behavioural cues. Feeds naturally space out as the baby gets bigger and the breast more efficient. Just go with the flow!*

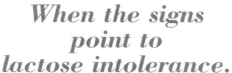

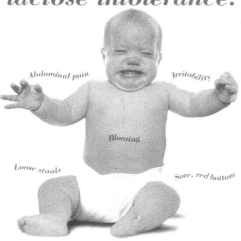

Figure 6-2-2 Misery: many diagnoses

## 2. Too many nutrients are not absorbed or come out again

Causes can include allergy, reflux, lactose intolerance, gut movement (or gut motility) disorders, infection, genetic disorders, or partial gut obstructions. But guess which industry wants you to think about first? I saw this image in many health facilities.

Those symptoms suggest many possible diagnoses indicating rapid gut transit and poor absorption, not just lactose intolerance. In many cases of poor absorption breastmilk is either vomited back up, or travels through the infant gut too fast for some reason, so that the baby has endless liquid green runny poo for days on end. (This can happen when the baby simply drinks too much milk, but baby's poo rapidly changes back to yellowish and more solid when the oversupply is reduced.) These liquid stools can be quite acid, and result in red bottoms that need immediate cleansing and protection via highly purified lanolin or zinc cream (without castor oil or nanoparticles). Too frequent loose stools –diarrhoea – can be triggered by allergies or pathogens at any age. Like vomiting, it is the body's natural reaction to the irritant causing problems. It is also the cause of innumerable deaths worldwide, mostly due to dehydration.

As noted above, in some babies, poor growth can be due to food intolerances or allergy, and growth improves when maternal or infant diet changes. When allergy is the cause, other symptoms usually emerge besides gut symptoms:

- patches of dry skin
- rashes
- night sweats
- loose stools and anal scald

- eczema
- cradle cap
- temperature rises
- urine scald despite colourless urine

- wheeze
- vomiting
- infections
- insomnia

A recent review of children with food allergy seen at London's prestigious Great Ormond Street Hospital found symptoms included "fatigue (53.0%), allergic shiners (49.1%), mouth ulcers (39.0%), joint pain/hypermobility (35.8%), poor sleep (34.4%), night sweats (34.4%), headache (22.7%), and bed-wetting (17.7%)."[1988]

The allergic young baby usually sleeps poorly and cries unpredictably, day or night; her or his night sleep is disturbed and often interrrupted by over-heating (sweats) then chilling as sweat evaporates; his or her skin quickly reacts with inflammation to antigens in saliva, urine or faeces, even breastmilk, and needs thorough cleansing and barrier creams to stay pale and feel comfortable.

The allergic breastfed baby may refuse the breast despite being hungry, arching after the first swallow, pulling off and screaming, then going back again and repeating the cycle. After feeding, these babies are most comfortable upright against a warm body.

But allergy is only one cause of poor growth in babies. Growth can also be limited by a deficiency of some specific nutrients: zinc, for example. Zinc deficiency can be caused by excesses of other competing nutrients, such as iron or copper, so that any baby being supplemented with just one of these may be affected. There are extremely rare cases of a condition in which mothers do not secrete sufficient zinc into breastmilk; a very characteristic rash develops in this case. (Check out a condition called *acrodermatitis enteropathica* to rule this out.)

The baby too, can lack one of many enzymes needed to metabolise some nutrients in mother's milk. In some cases this will show up in the early weeks; in others it can take months for this reason for an infant's failure to thrive to be identified as a rare metabolic disease. Medical causes can take time to diagnose. This is why doctors should always be consulted: to exclude (or identify) uncommon but serious problems. Never be shy about insisting on medical checks: medical input into persistent poor growth is important, and should not lead to weaning as doctors are learning more about breastmilk's unique qualities and infant formula's risks. (Get a second opinion if you run into a doctor who thinks infant

---

1988 Domínguez-Ortega G, Borrelli O, Meyer R, Dziubak R et al. Extraintestinal Manifestations in Children With Gastrointestinal Food Allergy. *J Pediatr Gastroent Nutr* 2014; 59 (2): 210-214. doi: 10.1097/MPG.0000000000000391

formula is the solution to breastfeeding problems. No matter how charming, such a doctor is a health hazard.)

Despite rare problems, all mothers can be confident that breastmilk is such a balanced and complete food that particular nutrient deficiencies or limiting excesses in breastmilk are much less common than they have historically been for artificially fed infants. In fact, giving other foods that interfere with breastmilk's bioactive absorption mechanisms, e.g., solids that chelate iron, have caused some deficiencies in infants for which their breastfeeding was blamed.

## 3. Not enough of what goes in can be used for growth

Growth comes second to survival. Where resources are chronically short for whole populations, it is growth that will be sacrificed, as various human groups attest over time. Better to be small and healthy than tall and sickly. Immune challenges (infection, allergy, vaccinations) cardiac defects, metabolic and congenital disorders can all increase the need for nutrients for purposes other than growth: the list is a long one.

One cause often overlooked is separation from another warm body. Contact assists the infant with breathing and temperature regulation, relieving the stress of the new environment, and preventing crying, a highly energetic activity. Skin to skin contact is calorie-sparing for the newborn, and those calories can be used for growth.

As previously noted, it seems common to see a brief slowing of growth after infant vaccinations, as the body ramps up its response using available nutrients. It is well understood that where there has been tissue destruction, as with burns, additional protein in excess of usual intakes is needed for rapid repair. The rapidly growing toddler is creating new tissue from food as he or she morphs from chubby baby to child. Similarly, sudden increases in physical activity burn calories that need to be replaced. And it takes nutrients to build those crusts of seborrhoeic or atopic dermatitis (cradle cap or eczema), nutrients that could have been used for growth.

Some babies, an infant with a cardiac problem for example, may need lower volumes of higher caloric milk than the mother usually supplies. Breastmilk can be 'engineered' to meet such needs. Dr Paula Meier's work in Chicago with mothers of premature infants shows how much could be achieved with lacto-engineering if anyone cared enough to try it. But formula is so much easier for change-resistant staff than learning new skills, and helping mothers. Even when shown how well it can work, some people refuse to believe it worth the effort. Not everyone learns from what they do not want to hear.

Some vociferously disapprove of any 'pressure' to breastfeed, even though this is a health behaviour of fundamental importance to a child and its descendants. There is absolutely no similar disapproval of the *almost universal and quite extreme* pressure to use infant formula in a thousand different situations, from the newborn to the toddler. I have never heard a health professional tell a bottle-feeding parent that their child will be brain-damaged if they do not give breastmilk, even though it is true their brain development will not be optimal. I have heard of many doctors and nurses telling breastfeeding parents that their baby will be brain-damaged if they do not give formula for what experts would see as mild jaundic, or refuse the Vitamin K injection. Some doctors say they will not be able to repair a heart condition unless the baby grows bigger faster with formula or fortifier. And I have never heard one apologise for scaremongering, or congratulate the mother for persisting with what was best for the baby, when she was proved right for thinking that formula was unnecessary. (Please email me - womensmilkmatters @gmail.com - to tell me about any exceptional health professional willing to admit their mistake on this topic.)

*One mother whose baby had a cardiac defect consulted me from a major children's hospital. She was being urged to give her breastfed baby a high-calorie formula, as his growth was very slow, and this was delaying surgery. Her milk supply was abundant, and she did not want to introduce formula. No other option was offered, and the pressure to use formula was intense, as it too often is – in some cases emotional blackmail and bullying best describe it. As this mother was expressing far more by volume than her baby could consume, I suggested she do the simplest of lacto-engineering: divide her expressed milk into two glasses, let it stand, skim the cream from one portion, add it to the other, and feed that to baby. She did, and from that first feed the baby's growth accelerated. She was very proud of herself, her baby thrived and the surgery was successful. Not at all surprisingly! While she was adding principally extra fats, the use of these for energy freed up her milk protein to be used for growth.*

*Sadly, when this mother rang me back to thank me for the suggestion, she told me of overhearing a nurse talking about her baby's spectacular improvement, saying something like 'the mother thinks it was what she did with her milk, but of course that was just a coincidence'. Had she adopted their suggestion to use formula and the baby had grown, would that have been a coincidence? For that nurse and doctor, it would have been coincidence for the baby to develop a serious infection soon after being fed infant formula. For me, that real possibility would have been no surprise!*

# 6.3 Survival and growth in babies born prematurely

Babies can be born prematurely, or growth retarded *in utero*, or with defects that make breastfeeding difficult. These immature and vulnerable populations require special care. It was understood until the 1970s that breastmilk was critical to their survival and growth. Then decades of artificial feeding ensued, until the very recent revival of breastmilk banking. Even today, in extremely low birthweight infants, mortality is four times greater when infants are not fully human milk fed.[1989]

There is another book to be written about infant formula and the preterm and 'abnormal' baby. That history too is one of progress and learning through triumph and disaster, but not a straightforward progress, as Book 2 illustrates. I have touched on the so-called 'human milk fortifiers' in Chapter 3.11. Much more could be said about the largely uncritical acceptance of commercial products and their use to adulterate breastmilk, instead of the use of appropriately modified human milk, if need be with less antigenic additives. Earlier research showed that premature babies could tolerate up to 4g/l of human milk protein and grow rapidly[1990] This is way in excess of what can be tolerated when foreign proteins like cow and soy are used.

Yet all formulas 'for medical purposes' were exempted from much of the early regulation of infant formula. One of the disappointments of the new Australian *Infant feeding guidelines* is that there is no critical or informed discussion of the very, very different regimes and treatments to which preterm or sick children can be subjected in Australian tertiary hospitals. The *Guidelines* simply reiterate a list of what is accepted practice – the use of infant formula along with breastmilk, as though this has no consequences other than nutritional. The way this is written serves only to validate the idea that formula is the solution for small or sick children, when in fact these are the children who are least able to cope with it, and educated paediatricians are beginning to go to great lengths to avoid giving such feeds.

In reality, between paediatric units there is sometimes very little agreement about specific artificial feeding regimens using infant formula or additives, with or without breastmilk: it depends on the paediatricians in charge, and varies over time and between neonatal units. There is even less accountability. Basic data such as how many mothers are enabled to express breastmilk and succeed in breastfeeding or take their babies home breastfed, is not always collected, and to my knowledge not publicly available. Yet with the right assistance, breastfeeding rates can be *higher* in this population of at-risk children than in normal babies, because their mothers are more motivated. Where mothers know that their milk can be the difference between life and death, there are few who fail to breastfeed. As Dr

1989 Abrams SA, Schanler RJ, Lee ML, Rechtman DJ. Greater mortality and morbidity in extremely preterm infants fed a diet containing cow milk protein products. (PMID:24867268) Free full text article *Breastfeed Med* 2014; 9:281-285.
1990 Williams AF, Baum JD. *Human Milk Banking*. (Raven Press/Nestlé 1984) NNI Workshop Series vol. 10.

Neil Campbell said repeatedly in the 1980s,[1991] whether or not preterm babies are breastfed depends more on the knowledge and attitudes of caregivers, than it does on the mother's lactational capacity.

But unless greater resources go into national milk banking schemes, and into *enabling* families to be involved in the daily care of their small sick children, that dependence on industry's formulas, and high-level endorsement of poor quality care will continue. There are much better world models – in Chicago, where Dr Paula Meier created her Milk Club for a predominantly disadvantaged population, in Sweden where whole new units have been built to facilitate Kangaroo Care of very small infants indeed, and many other places. It is no accident that for decades so few Scandinavian preterm infants died of NEC while the US rate was around 7 per cent of all preterm babies, with roughly 20 per cent of those dying. Even in Australia there are many differences in the availability and use of human milk for small or sick babies, and support for parents, and differences in outcomes. Breastfeeding at discharge rates for neonatal and maternity units should be mandated as what the bureaucrats inelegantly term "a key performance indicator," along with follow-up support for mothers after discharge. And the protocols for the use of human milk, and the rates of breastfeeding at discharge, should be made public on a government website. At present there is almost no accountability and babies suffer as a result.

Breastfeeding for intra-uterine growth restricted (IUGR) or small for gestational age (SGA) babies is just as important, if not more so, as breastfeeding for normal or preterm infants. Studies are showing that these growth-restricted children are at increased risk of adult metabolic disease, including diabetes. One study showed that by twelve months formula-fed babies had more adipose tissue and were hormonally different from those who were breastfed. Those fed a higher protein formula had even higher IgF-1 levels, known to be associated with childhood obesity.[1992] Yet protein levels for preterm infants are much higher than for term infants, and new post-discharge products for premature babies perpetuate a higher protein intake. Is this wise? Yes, with lower protein levels these babies may be smaller, but body-size is not everything.

Again, just like term infants, body composition differs if babies are not breastfed. Even brain composition differs.[1993] If you are gaining on food other than women's milk, gaining weight fast as a baby can shorten your life. Lucky babies getting only women's milk regulate their own intake and grow as suits them best. And if they are also fortunate enough to be

---

1991 Neonatologist at the Royal Children's Hospital in Melbourne, Dr Campbell gave an annual lecture in the course for health professionals I organsied from 1986 onwards. I regret that life has not allowed him to write a book about his experience as a paediatrician who was well ahead of his time – and his colleagues – and who suffered for it. But his lectures left a deep impression on the hundreds of students who went through this course. He deserves to be acknowledged by more than this footnote; I for one am deeply in his debt for the support he gave my work and the encouragement he always offered.

1992 de Zegher F, Sebastiani G, Diaz M, Gómez-Roig MD et al. Breast-feeding vs formula-feeding for infants born small-for-gestational-age: divergent effects on fat mass and on circulating IGF-I and high-molecular-weight adiponectin in late infancy. (PMID:23365126) *J Clin Endocrinol Metab* 2013; 98(3):1242-1247. DOI: 10.1210/jc.2012-3480.

1993 Farquharson J, Cockburn F, Patrick WA, et al: Infant cerebral cortex phospholipid fatty-acid composition and diet. *Lancet* 1992; 340(8823):810-813.

cared for skin to skin (see page 626), as well as given food absorbed and utilised without metabolic stress or gut disturbance, that growth can be remarkable. One such child has just grown from 2600grams at 36 weeks to 4700grams at 3 weeks post due date, having done little more than sleep peacefully, eat and cuddle for most of the time.

If your baby looks like being born preterm, it is important to know that evidence is emerging from *formula-fed* preterm infants (and most are, in Anglophone countries) that rapid post-partum growth (crossing centiles) can result in serious lifetime health risks. Aiming for *in utero* growth rates outside the womb seems to me to have little scientific justification. Small but healthy and smart children are preferable to large and damaged and stupid ones. Yes, I know there are social advantages to being tall, especially for men. But as I said to then-Dr. Alan Lucas in a Cambridge pub once, brains matter more than height! Soon after that conversation I was introduced to a doyen of Finnish paediatrics who had been born preterm in the early twentieth century, no bigger than a hand, they said; and they also said his first foods were brandy and sugar supplements and breastmilk. In his eighties, he was remarkably short, but had the bluest eyes and most acute intelligence; and he was still working. The Western obsession with size in babies and height in men has undoubtedly sacrificed brains to brawn.

There are babies with metabolic disorders that make breastfeeding or breastmilk feeding more difficult and sometimes impossible. However, this needs to be closely examined on an ongoing basis. The heel prick every baby painfully undergoes is to identify children with raised blood levels of the amino acid phenylalanine, who are at risk of PKU, or phenylketonuria. Infants with phenylketonuria lack enough of the enzyme to break down phenylalanine, and so are at risk of brain damage as it accumulates in tissue, and is excreted in urine. It was once orthodoxy that such children could not be breastfed and needed a phenylalanine-free infant formula and weaning diet. Children fed thus were rarely of above-normal, or even normal, intelligence, though this was blamed on their diet *after* formula feeding. They are doing much better cognitively, since it was realised that breastmilk is low in phenylalanine, and needs only to be supplemented with small quantities of formula, to achieve safe infant blood levels of phenylalanine. How much of the IQ loss in older cases of PKU was due to being formula-fed?

Other congenital metabolic disorders are incompatible with breastmilk feeding, but the base for making the specialised formulas they need to survive should be human milk, not bovine, if at all possible. If cows' milk can be rendered lactose-free for the galactosaemic, couldn't women's milk be? Now there's a new global niche market: specialty formulas from milk made by women, not GM cows!

# 6.4 A weighty issue: the next wave of mother-blaming

Mothers have always been blamed by society, and blamed themselves, for anything that adversely affects their children. Mothers should have known about it, they should have acted differently, and then maybe this harm would not have befallen their child. I fear that these new discoveries of how much babies are affected by their mother's life experience and her milk will result in yet another wave of mother-blaming. The new research about the considerable immunological and nutritional differences between women's unique tailor-made milks could be exploited – to bolster women's long-standing, common, and still-powerful anxiety and fear that however wonderful some ideal breastmilk might be, *my* breastmilk won't be good enough because I drank a glass of wine or enjoyed some chocolate or didn't eat enough fish or ate too much meat or not enough vegetables or was angry or upset.. Or won't be good enough, because my milk has been shown to have only 2% fat and someone else's has 13%. Or won't be good enough, because I was malnourished in childhood, or am one of the two million girls under fifteen bearing children, or I live in a community where females eat least and worst. Without extensive social marketing of the truth, how can women made to feel worthless or under-confident possibly think their fresh milk is worth more, or is better than, the expensive products rich women buy?

Or, and this is the new stick mothers will beat themselves with, my milk won't be good enough because I'm allergic and my milk contains more or less of some immune factor like TGFs (transforming growth factors)[1994] currently being explored as possibly significant to the development of allergy. Does such a mother blame herself for making her child allergic?

Sadly, some mothers will. While some may choose to stay in denial about their child's allergy, rather than accept what feels like blame for their child's problem. (Almost all mothers who realise the contribution their body makes to allergy in their child imediately ask me what the father's genes have contributed, and I am happy to be able to tell them that fathers do affect outcomes.[1995] Just not as much as mothers, since we do all the work of growing the baby.)

We need to give women clear messages that

- while breastmilk IS all different, and some is higher calorie than others, and some contains more of this or that, their own milk is still the best for their child, even if their diet isn't perfect, or even if their milk – or their breast storage capacity - dictates more frequent or longer feeding than their friend's milk might;

---

1994 Joseph CL, Havstad S, Bobbitt K, Woodcroft K et al. Transforming growth factor beta (TGFβ1 ) in breast milk and indicators of infant atopy in a birth cohort. (PMID:24520941) P*ediatr Allergy Immunol* 2014; DOI: 10.1111/pai.12205. This one of many growth factors was linked with a greater risk of atopy only in non-black, non-atopic (as defined by the study) mothers. See also Oddy WH in Zibadi (op. cit.)

1995 Mandhane PJ, Greene JM, Sears MR. Interactions between breast-feeding, specific parental atopy, and sex on development of asthma and atopy. (PMID:17353035) *JACI* 2007, 119(6):1359-1366. DOI: 10.1016/j. jaci.2007.01.043

- that all clean fresh breastmilk is better than any artificial substitute, and there is neither harm nor shame nor greater risk in sharing such milk from, or with, their friends and neighbours in case of scarcity, as women always have done
- that lactation is robust, resilient and reliable and that almost all problems can be resolved and supply restored, unless there are serious underlying conditions;
- that most problems that cause women to wean their babies too soon have a strong sociocultural basis, and say little about their body's lactation potential in better circumstances
- that they ought to be very angry about the society that lets them blame themselves rather than helps them

Not only breastfeeding advocates, but all who care about women, need to be aware that epigenetics could be made yet another rod for women's backs, taking us full circle to the bad old days when only *some* women's milk was considered fit for babies, and women were told by both industry and doctors that, while they might have plenty of milk, that milk might not be any good. That "women like that" – a phrase I heard about indigenous women in a major Melbourne hospital in the 1970s – shouldn't really breastfeed.

I've often heard mothers blame the quality or quantity of their milk for their swap to infant formula. The nineteenth and twentieth centuries saw a constant stream of mother-blaming for children's physical and mental problems, most since proven to have a definite physiological, even genetic basis. Not until educated assertive women insisted on being heard by the medical establishment did the stigma and blame for child development problems start to wear a little thinner.

Since the 1980s the number of women free to create and sustain voluntary support networks for mothers has plummeted, as pressures to return to paid work have become ever greater. I see the potential for new waves of mother blame and psychological oppression, in Western societies where there are now fewer women to challenge comfortable medical orthodoxies. I hope I will be proved wrong. But I wasn't wrong, when in *Breastfeeding matters* (1985) I predicted a growing backlash against breastfeeding promotion, spearheaded by vocal affluent women, in societies where breasts are sexual fetishes and women are preached at, but not enabled, to breastfeed. And after I'd written this chapter I found that I am not the only historian concerned about this possibility: an excellent article in *Nature* deserves wide reading. [1996]

How might epigenetic knowledge lead to more mother-blaming? Chief among those with good reason to fear how the science is presented are women whose weight does not meet local community perceptions of healthy. In one country, before marriage slim or underfed young women may be sent to a fat-*gain* farm to be made more desirable (and fertile) by gaining weight. In another country, young women of that same weight may be trying to slim at a fat-*loss* farm to fit a wedding dress a size smaller. Overweight and underweight are defined

1996 Richardson SS, Daniels CR, Gillman MW, Golden J et al. Society: Don't blame the mothers. *Nature* 2014; 512 (7513): 131-132. http://www.nature.com/polopoly_fs/1.15693!/menu/main/topColumns/topLeftColumn/pdf/512131a.pdf

differently in communities, but common to all is the woman's society-created perception that her weight is not ideal. In western communities, body fat has been demonised. Which can make problems for women bearing children, because the female body is programmed to set aside fat stores that can be used for breastfeeding. However, raised in an obesogenic environment, often having been formula-fed, long before pregnancy many women have already put on more weight than is ideal for their own health, and that of any future child. They are not to blame for that.

## Overweight mothers

Simplistic statements about the harms done to infants by their mother's pre-pregnancy weight and diet, and so on, are already circulating. One study is quoted as showing that infants did better if their obese mothers had bariatric surgery before becoming pregnant, by comparison with mothers who did not have such surgery or lose weight. That may indeed be a real effect of surgically induced weight loss. I would like to be sure, however, that any better outcomes were not largely due to the income and social advantage differences that permitted surgery as an option, as well as consequent and class differences in maternal confidence, mental well-being, and much more.

It seems likely that once the infant formula industry realises that society is beginning to see the harms infant formulas have done, there will be a concerted effort to shift any blame for poor outcomes in children. How convenient for everyone, that current maternal bodyweight and lifestyle habits like smoking and drinking, in pregnancy and by past generations, and even mother's genetic differences, can be shown to make a difference to child health!

Only the

- never-smoked,
- never-drank,
- non-allergic,
- breastfed-from-birth,
- perfect-bodyweight,
- mentally-healthy and optimistic,
- perfect-diet-and-moderately-exercising mother
- with an impeccable genome optimally-expressed (phew!) mother

would be in a position to allege that harm to her child was an outcome of formula feeding, not of her own life history. Who would risk a court case with a multi-billion-dollar company with a lot to lose if a precedent were to be set? Who could prove that their lifelong obesity stemmed from being programmed as a child by infant feeding, when there is evidence that maternal obesity may play a part in programming children for weight gain?

If we cannot blame the mother in this generation, we can blame past mothers. No, it wasn't the formula, but the obese mother and the careless way she used it. (We already allow companies to claim on formula cans, that only "improper" preparation or use can put a child at risk. ANY use of anything but breastmilk increases risks for any young infant.) More likely, it was an older formula that made the mother obese[1997] and the current lower-protein/wrong-fat formula had the same effect on the baby she gestated. But how to prove that?

One advantage of the milk hypothesis and its multiple-intergenerational perspective is that, rightly interpreted, it can reduce the possibility at least of *current* mother-blaming. What the mother is now is as much a result of her ancestors' lives (male and female) as her own. She, like her children's father (who also contributes immunologically, remember) is a victim of societal forces beyond her control – and of what they were both fed as infants. Since it is clear that infant nutrition is probably the biggest single determinant of post-partum programming, we need to realise that our children can indeed be victims of our childhood diet, or even their maternal grandmother's childhood diet. And in those childhoods, infant formula was present and a lot less sophisticated than it has since become; its harms, like obesity, may be echoing through generations.[1998] I hope this is how parents, especially mothers, hear what I have written. *It is not what parents have done, so much as what has been done to them, in a context where until recently the very fat baby was seen as the ideal.* Already I sense from some parents less resistance to the idea that maternal diet can affect their children, once they know that it is not only what the mother does, but what her body does *as a result of what others before her did*.

The good news from this epigenetic research is that reducing the effects of such earlier harms may become possible. If it is possible to identify affected genes, strategies to change how they are expressed will emerge in time.[1999] And breastfeeding will be part of the solution for childhood obesity. We do not have to wait for expensive gene therapy to prevent infant obesity. For the overweight mother in particular, breastfeeding is a strategy that, well managed, can help her reduce weight, and also help her child avoid obesity lifelong. As Nestlé scientist Professor Ferdinand Haschke says,

> If mothers are overweight or obese, their breastfed infants gain weight more quickly during the first six months in comparison to World Health Organization standards. On the other hand, infants from obese mothers gain less weight if breastfeeding continues beyond six months compared to infants that are fed formula, as defined by the Codex Alimentarius.

It is the latter part of this message that really matters, and that will be overlooked: *formula fed babies get fatter than babies breastfed for more than six months by overweight mothers.* Overweight mothers have additional reasons to breastfeed according to WHO suggestions: for a couple of years at least, with the first six months being completely unsupplemented so long as the baby grows well. It can be the most enjoyable form of weight loss activity for the mother!

---

1997  Take a look at Master Buck and Miss Dodson Figure 3-1-3 on page 207

1998  We have no hard proof that newer ones do less harm in this regard, of course.

1999  Kelley L. Baumgartel and Yvette P. Conley. The Utility of Breastmilk for Genetic or Genomic Studies: A Systematic Review. *Breastfeeding Medicine.* June 2013, 8(3): 249-256. doi:10.1089/bfm.2012.0054

And for those overweight mothers who cannot breastfeed or need to supplement, possibly the new low-protein partially hydrolysed formulas are preferable. This is implicit in that industry statement - Haschke has also said that

> 'Recent studies show that feeding formula with low protein content (whey-based, 1.65g protein/100kcal)[2000] to infants between three and twelve months by overweight/obese mothers results in weight gain similar to that observed in breastfed infants.'

Note that other foods were being given after four to six months, obviously just as important as what formula was used, or how "breastfed" was defined. But again, how similar is similar, and is it what each individual baby should be doing? Will some be underfed in the cause of not overfeeding?

Another group demonstrated that

> ... CMF-fed (normal cows' milk formulas) infants' weight gain was accelerated, whereas PHF-fed (protein-hydrolysate-formula) infants' weight gain was normative [that is, akin to the breastfed infant's growth profiles].

But as they also said,

> Whether such differences in growth are because of differences in the protein content or amino acid profile of the formulas and, in turn, metabolism is unknown. Research on the long-term consequences of these early growth differences is needed.[2001]

It would not be a benefit to infants simply to weigh less, but to be sick more often, for example. But if hydrolysed or lower-protein infant formulas prove to be significantly better for most children, can we hope any older more damaging ones will disappear altogether from infant feeding use? Or will cost be an insuperable barrier? Will we see infant formula becoming even more of a social class issue, with higher-protein cheaper formula being used by those already disadvantaged, and lower-protein, less obesogenic, but more expensive infant formula being the preserve of the already advantaged? Clearly the Babynes, with its capacity for exact dose formulation, is not going to be used by welfare recipients or homeless families. If governments do not take a keen interest in both breastfeeding support for disadvantaged groups, and infant formula marketing, market economics may well ensure that outcome, creating another invisible dimension to the poverty trap. Parents need to be enabled to improve outcomes for themselves and their children –without the mother driving herself into depression by thinking she is responsible for problems created by others, or by trying to be perfect in an imperfect world. Mother just need to do the best they can, and accept that they'll always wish they could do more. As Ned Kelly said, 'Such is life!'

---

2000 Just on 11g/L of a 67kcal formula. Less than half what was normal once. See Inostroza J, Haschke F, Steenhout P, Grathwohl D et al. Low-Protein Formula Slows Weight Gain in Infants of Overweight Mothers: A Randomized Trial. (PMID:24637965) Free full text article *J Pediatr Gastroenterol Nutr* 2014

2001 Mennella JA, Ventura AK, Beauchamp GK. Differential Growth Patterns Among Healthy Infants Fed Protein Hydrolysate or Cow-Milk Formulas. *Pediatrics* 2011; 127:110-118. DOI:10.1542/peds.2010-1675

## CHAPTER 7

# Widening the diet: more than white liquids

*This extends the earlier sketchy outline of when to introduce other foods to infants, in Chapter 4.6.*

As noted earlier, breastmilk is the *only* complete food for normal human growth and development. The breastfed infant's diet should not be widened before *six* months if the child is thriving on breastmilk alone, as allergic children usually do. Note that by contrast, for formula-fed infants, other suitable family foods can be, and have been, introduced from about three to *four* months of age.

There are many dimensions to the issue of widening the infant diet, and this chapter covers the practicalities first The timing of introduction of non-liquid foods has been very contentious, so a longer discussion of the issue and its historical context can be found at Chapter 7.5. Before that, I will simply summarise what seems to have emerged as relevant facts and sensible practical advice for parents. Read the politics and history at your leisure!

## 7.1 Introducing other foods to breastfed infants: what to do?

Babies are not tins to be filled at a parent-determined time with parent-determined foods. And general recommendations should never be applied obsessively, as though experts always know better than the individual child's body and the attentive mother's intuition. Expert knowledge is always based on generalities, averages, and clinical experience of other people, however valid and well-informed those things are. The child is the mother's responsibility. There is nothing sacred or magic about any particular moment in time, and babies are by definition individual. Some breastfed babies show they are ready to widen their diet earlier than six months, and cope quite well, while others are not ready until some months later. Some babies start eagerly at five months, then stop and refuse food other than breastmilk for two months or more.

It seems clear now that:

- Breastmilk exposes infants to manageable doses of other foods from maternal diet, along with immune factors to help regulate infant reactions to such foods. Breastmilk from different women, or from the same woman at different times, tastes and smells different, reflecting the family diet.

- Most mothers are physically capable of breastfeeding exclusively for six months post-partum given adequate support and time. A mother who feeds fully to four months has been making almost all a six-month-old baby needs: in fact average volume intake of around 750mL changes little from four to six months, while infant growth rates lessen and metabolic efficiency increases.

- Some mothers cannot make enough milk to feed their babies fully to six months. This is quite rare, and most often caused by factors beyond the mother's control and often, little to do with her lactation potential.

- Some mothers cannot spend the time with their babies that would allow for successful breastfeeding, and stop — or never try — because of social constraints. Any other feeding should be responsive and modelled on breastfeeding, with skin contact and changes of position as appropriate.

- Donor milk would be the optimal food for infants under six months if mother's milk supply is inadequate or non-existent; but other suitable food mixes can also be given if needed under six months. (Need can be social or physical.) Infant formula is one choice, but not the only or even necessarily the best choice as a supplement to breastfeeding. Careful consideration of the risks of all feeds, as well as their practicability, should determine the choice. (An excellent recent article reviews the relative risks of formula and donor breastmilk.[2002] Check out the Eats on Feets Four Pillars of Safe Breast Milk Sharing at http://www.eatsonfeets. org/#fourPillars.  For more on this see Chapter 4.6)

- Traditional wet-nursing and cross-nursing provides fresh environment-specific and unaltered human milk, which is rightly WHO's first option when maternal breastfeeding or breastmilk feeding are impossible.[2003]

- As with any fresh food, time from production, and temperature changes, both have effects on human milk nutrients and bioavailability, *so that no one should assume that it is safe to feed a very young baby for months solely on pasteurised or frozen donor breastmilk alone*. It is certainly safe for short periods, it may well be safe where feasible for longer periods, but it is another experiment requiring proper monitoring of the baby's growth and health. Recent studies about heat-processing effects on infant formula suggests that further research on the effects on processed breastmilk.

- Where other food is really needed under six months of age (due to intractable failure to thrive, inability to increase maternal milk supply, and absence of

---

2002 Gribble K, Hausman BL. Milk sharing and formula feeding: Infant feeding risks in comparative perspective? *Australas Med J.* 2012; 5(5): 275–283. Published online 2012 May 31. doi: *10.4066/AMJ.2012.1222* (PMCID:PMC3395287)

2003 http://www.who.int/nutrition/topics/global_strategy_iycf/en/index.html.

fresh donor breastmilk, for example) family foods can be introduced in suitable forms, such as energy- and protein-rich finely milled porridges and soups of a consistency young infants can handle. Widening the diet under six months may mean a greater likelihood of allergy. But malnutrition is worse immunologically and developmentally. Babies need food and water: breastmilk is the perfect combination, but other imperfect solutions are possible.

- Any amount of maternal breastmilk, however small, is better than none.

- From around six to seven months most normal (breastfed, non-allergic) infants will be interested in, and perhaps benefit from, other foods. But babies differ greatly, and stops and starts in acceptance of other foods are common, especially in allergic babies.

- In the six-to-nine-month period, all babies benefit from personally handling and learning to eat lumpy foods of a wide variety of tastes and textures, not simply sloppy purees and mashes.[2004] However, their intake needs to be monitored and parents need to ensure that over time, sufficient food gets eaten , not simply played with!  Babies should never be left alone with food.

- Up to nine months complete breastfeeding may meet infants' needs, but a minority will develop sub-clinical iron deficiency. Iron and zinc supplements can be used if this is clinically indicated for a baby, but a better choice of infant food sources may be more helpful. Iron-rich foods like red meat and egg yolks are usually good sources of other minerals as well. Commercial iron-fortified cereals may not be. And unopposed iron supplements can do harm. Excess iron can be damaging.

- Formula is never *necessary* for breastfed babies. It may be *convenient* as part of a mixed diet, and that can be useful. But formula should never replace quality family foods for older infants. For not-breastfed infants, intakes of 300-500ml by 12 months are more than adequate, and not necessary if  the child's diet of 3 meals and two snacks includes other dairy products such as yoghurt, cheese, and full-cream milk. (Low fat milk is unsuitable for children under two.)

- Parents should offer a wide variety of other foods in suitable forms, and not create aversions by force-feeding. Some would say that it is normal for babies to reject new foods (or formulas) initially and accept them after several attempts on different occasions. Others believe that if a baby persistently refuses a particular food, parents should respect that, as it may mean the baby will not tolerate it well. Only time will tell which is true for any individual baby.

- The smaller the baby, the smaller and more frequent the meals, and the more planned the total diet needs to be: at least three meals and two snacks (three+two).

- By twelve months babies ideally will be getting breastmilk freely, as well as being offered frequent (three meals plus  two snacks) small feeds of quality family

---

2004 Coulthard H, Harris G, Emmett P Delayed introduction of lumpy foods to children during the complementary feeding period affects child's food acceptance and feeding at 7 years of age. (PMID:19161546) *Maternal & Child Nutrition* 2009, 5(1):75-85.

Chapter 7: Widening the diet: more than white liquids
7.1 Introducing other foods to breastfed infants: what to do?

| 685

foods, with safe and palatable water offered as seems appropriate. A drop in infant interest in food around this time is common, and will be temporary if force-feeding is avoided.[2005]

- For optimal growth and health after twelve months, foods including high quality protein and fats are essential complements to continued breastfeeding. Animal protein such as egg and meat is not essential, especially while breastfeeding continues to provide some – but not enough – human protein; but constructing an adequate vegan infant diet requires detailed attention and care.[2006]

- If ill during the second year of life, babies will often refuse other foods and go back to the breast alone. This can cause transient oversupply problems as the baby first boosts the milk supply to increase daily intake, then lowers intake and begins eating other foods, leaving full breasts to down-regulate. Catch-up growth on breastmilk alone after bouts of illness can be amazingly rapid and self-limited.

- Spanish paediatrician Carlos Gonzalez has two sentences that cannot be over-emphasized. "Do not force your child to eat. Never make him eat in any way, under any circumstance, for any reason." Read his brilliantly reassuring book[2007] if things are not going well, however your baby is being fed.

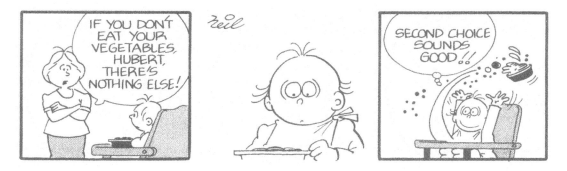

Figure 7-1-1 Infant autonomy in feeding. Image © Neil Matterson.
From *Sleepless Nights*. (Marion Books 1988)

---

2005 Gonzalez C. *My Child won't eat!* (Pinter & Martin 2011) is the best book for this issue.
2006 Hood S. *Feeding your vegan infant with confidence.* (Vegan Society UK 2005).
2007 Gonzalez C. op. cit. I know of no clearer, more sensible guide to dealing with young children and food than this book.

# 7.2  Introducing other foods to artificially fed infants: what to do?

There seems to be very little research evidence on which to base this chapter, other than the evidence of past practice and generally accepted nutritional advice. So what more can be said about introducing other foods to artificially fed infants, as distinct from the fully breastfed?

## Feeding formula and adding other foods: when and what

The World Health Organization studied exclusive breastfeeding in depth and different countries before changing its recommendation about exclusive breastfeeding to 6 months. I have been unable to find for any brand on the market some equivalent comprehensive post-1980 systematic study of the consequences of exclusive formula feeding for 6 months as compared with four months, whether partial or solely from birth. So formula-fed infants probably should be offered a wide variety of quality fresh and freshly-cooked foods from about sixteen to twenty weeks onwards, as their in utero body stores of nutrients may be depleted in some way by then.

That is not my idea. It was the stated rationale for the 1980s consensus about introducing other foods at four months. From the 1980s infant formula use typically was for three to six months, with other foods being introduced at three to four months, or by four completed months at the latest. That is what western society has experience of doing. *There is no well-documented twentieth century clinical experience of babies being fed solely on infant formula for six complete months: it is a new experiment seemingly based on a faulty assumption that if breastfeeding is safe for six months, so is infant formula.*

Until now very few infants have received only infant formula to six months of age (most got some breast milk initially). For formula fed babies only, it would therefore seem wise to continue widening the diet beginning at four months, until the results of multi-cultural experimental studies are on record. Judging by the labels on cans, many manufacturers of available formula products (first infant formulas or FIFs and follow-on formulas or FOFs) still suggest reliance on patent formulas should be absolute only until four months, even though they now promote formula use for as long as three to four years.

Such extended use of industrial products is another totally new experiment. We have NO proof of its safety. Worryingly, a recent study suggests that the risk of acute leukoblastic leukaemia increases with each additional month of artificial formula feeding.[2008] If this dose-response effect is confirmed by other studies, it raises many questions about the origin of other problems, such as autism, whose incidence has risen in parallel with this dramatic and unchallenged change in formula use and duration since 1980, when formula use had often ended by three to six months. I think that study suggests that getting babies off industrial

---

2008  Hsu C. The longer babies are fed formula, the greater their risk for pediatric acute lymphoblastic leukemia. Medical Daily.com October 18, 2012. See http://www.medicaldaily.com/articles/12766/20121018/longer-period-infant-formula-feeding-increase-leukemia.htm#iEBzCokEBoU3wCUW.99

synthetic milks by twelve months *at the latest,* and on to good quality fresh family foods, including cheese, yoghurt, and small quantities of fresh cows' milk if they tolerate milk protein, is a very good idea! Artificially fed babies need to go on drinking infant formula while the changeover to family diet occurs, but with amounts lessening. Forget all toddler milks: they do NOT act as nutritional insurance, but as a distraction from good diet for young children. As noted earlier, the fact that they are iron-fortified may damage already iron-replete children.

Infant formula is a child food. But all infant formula is made up of many different food sources: milk, wheat, soy, corn. In this sense artificially fed infants have already been exposed to a variety of foods via infant formula. The question arises as to whether parents should try to minimise or to expand even further the variety of different foods their formula-feeding child is exposed to under 6 months. And that includes asking whether a variety of infant formulas should be used, or whether parent should find one brand and stick to it.

I am unaware of any relevant research justifying persistence with a single brand of infant formula. Complete monotony of food intake breaches the basic dietary safety rules of variety and moderation of intake. Offering young artificially fed infants different brands of formula based on cows' milk in the first few months would reduce any risks of dependence on a single recipe. Which of course is why changing formulas regularly has been recommended by the parents of infants damaged by their reliance on a single brand, which proved to be chloride-deficient.[2009] But of course frequently changing brands also potentially introduces other damaging substances for the baby to deal with (or conversely reduces their exposure, if the brand they are changing from was more contaminated.) Parental reports of infant gut distress when changing brands are legion. So is varying formula brands good or bad? I don't know. Where are the studies showing microbiomic outcomes, to guide parents? Do we just go on assuming that it doesn't matter, without even recording how much brand-swapping occurs in reality?

One practical point to note: if babies have been fed a single formula for months, they may well reject a different tasting one. Parents should not purchase large tins of powder before trying out sachets for acceptability. And parents should be instructed repeatedly to taste any formula used for their child, so they know what it *should* smell and taste like, when not heavily contaminated or heat-affected.

If parents wish to use only one particular brand, buying one or two tins at a time or from different suppliers should mean sampling different production batches rather than being reliant on a single batch solely for months. (Batch number or production dates will be on most tins somewhere, and I think should be recorded in the child's health record.) As this book has made clear, infant formulas (even those with the same name) are not all the same; even the same brand can vary by batch.

Formula feeding should be done exactly as industry advises for the use of their individual branded product. But I would ignore any suggestions both to use the product exclusively

---

2009 Laskin C, Pilot L. in Moss, Sweet, Swift (eds) *Early Intervention Programs for Infants* (Haworth Press 1982.)

past four months, or to feed the child more than around 300-450 mL by twelve months. In the second half of the first year all babies, especially the formula-fed, need to learn to eat real food, and a good varied fresh food diet is better for them than a monotonous bland one.

## Introducing new foods to the formula fed infant

What new foods should be offered? Fresh and freshly cooked foods, as to this point all the infant's diet has been of heat-treated products. The 'tiny tastes of single foods' approach developed after 1980 was developed with formula-fed infants in mind. By six months infant formula should probably be just one of a variety of foods eaten, the main food still, but not the total diet of the artificially-fed infant. Young formula-fed infants absolutely should not simply move on to a sole diet of formula for older infants. The so-called follow on formulas (FOFs) are by definition *unsuitable as sole foods* for infants of any age. The Codex Standard for follow-up formula says so. Other quality preferably fresh foods *must* be provided if these are the infant's milk drink. The World Health Assembly [WHA] declared them unnecessary in 1988.[2010] They have not been proved better than Stage 1 formulas for older infants, who may consume a first, more complete, formula for the whole twelve months.

Toddler (stage three) formulas are totally unnecessary, and may displace real food in the second year of life, after twelve months. Can-label-suggested amounts of stage three formulas in Australia in 2011 ranged from 430 to 1250 ml/day. Even the low end of this range could interfere with infant appetite for family food, reinforcing the preference for bland sweet tastes over stronger ones. The new 2012 Australian NHMRC *Infant Feeding Guidelines* say clearly that these much-advertised sweet or bland drinks are not necessary for healthy children, and that by twelve months children should be eating a wide variety of good food and drinking water and some milk.

So by twelve months, and from then on, all babies ideally will be offered frequent (three meals + two snacks) small feeds of quality family foods, with palatable water offered as seems appropriate. Breastfeeding can continue as genuine nutritional insurance, but any industrial formula is unnecessary.

All infants should be allowed to learn to drink from a cup before twelve months, even if they are still breastfeeding. Bottles should be replaced by then. Habituation to solely bottle sucking can reduce acceptance of family foods, as well as increasing food-safety risks, and rates of orthodontic defect. There are no such risks from continued breastfeeding.

Other solid foods should never be added to bottles of formula or cows' milk. Arrowroot biscuits or gluten-containing baby cereals were once commonly used, as a way to add calories, and fatten babies. This still occurs: one doctor suggests adding cereal to the bottle to reduce reflux (instead of commercial thickeners). A child health nurse in one of my courses reported that she was present in a home where a cheeseburger was being blended for addition to the baby's bottle of formula. Needless to say, that was not ideal family food introduction, but the child had been getting it for some time.

---

2010  World Health Assembly Resolution WHA39.28, May 1988. Can be found in Shubber S, op cit.

Once other foods are introduced, all babies may need water to drink. Because of the higher solute load of infant formula, and the variability of its composition when made up from powder, some fully formula-fed young babies may need to be offered water in hot weather, or when they have lost water through sweating in synthetic fleece wraps, for example. Babies have very acute senses, and strong-smelling water may be rejected even if needed, though thirsty babies usually accept water. Some young children dislike the taste of chlorine from town supplies or equipment disinfectant. Strong plastic or chemical flavours and smells (from feeding equipment or town water supplies) can be noxious, causing infants to refuse to drink, and parents then to camouflage the taste with juices or cordials. Simple carbon filtration and storage in and drinking from glass or china (not plastic or latex) helps some children accept plain water as a normal drink. Again, the parent should taste and smell what the baby is being offered. Any filtration equipment must be maintained as the maker suggests, as filters can become a source of pathogens.

For optimal growth and health after four to six months, foods including high quality protein and fats are an essential part of artificial feeding. The current lowering of protein levels in first infant formulas makes other high quality protein such as egg and meat important to continued good growth, especially in the second year of life. Constructing an adequate vegan infant diet for any baby, especially one not being breastfed, is perfectly possible, but requires very detailed attention and care.[2011]

There are many studies still to be done about the microbiome, including the consequences of vegan diet. Some bigger questions also need to be answered. Has anyone conducted studies of the gut microbiome of children exclusively breastfed from birth as this ecosystem changes during the introduction (not of formula, or any processed babyfoods, but) of fresh family foods carefully prepared and home cooked? What effect does an organic foods diet have on child gut microbiomes when still breastfed or when formula fed? (Halving pesticide levels must have some effect, I suspect.) How does such a truly breastfed and family-food fed microbiome compare to the changes in the gut microbiome of the mixed-fed and the formula-fed-from birth as other foods are introduced? Do any differences persist even after the milk source has ended, if all other foods have been introduced while a mother still breastfeeds? Would there be less inflammatory gut disease (including appendicitis) in those fed a true family diet for the first year of life? A child of nine to twelve months needs to eat food and drink breastmilk and water, not subsist solely on industrially-processed foods, whatever they may be called. Yet it seems to me that nowadays many children are almost totally reliant on formulas of different kinds.

---

2011 *Feeding the Vegan Infant* Vegan Society UK.

# 7.3  What are 'good quality family foods'?

Not blended cheeseburgers. Whatever the culture, all basic recipes for a mixture of food for babies and toddlers will obey the dietary safety rules of variety and moderation of intake of any one food. Written as an equation the recipe would be:

**carbohydrate staple + high value protein + good fats + green/yellow vegetables + safe water + long-term breastfeeding = healthy growing child**

The image of the Food Square conveys this best: see below.

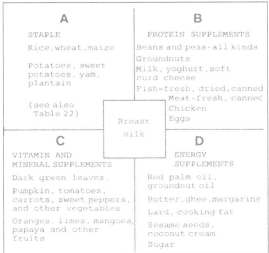

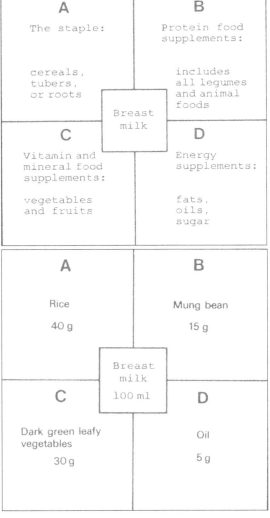

Figure 7-3-1 The food square: theory and one option (Cameron M, Hofvander Y. *Manual on Feeding Infants and Young Children* (1983) By permission of Oxford University Press.)

The best detailed guides in this area have been published by the World Health Organization. Complementary feeding was a special concern for Randa Saadeh of WHO Geneva's Department of Nutrition. A number of substantial publications preceded *Complementary feeding: family foods for breastfed children* (WHO/NHD/00.1), which works through basic information for local healthworkers. This can be accessed online and downloaded.[2012] The 1988 WHO

---

2012 *Complementary Feeding: family foods for breastfed children*, (WHO/NHD/00.1) http://www.who.int/
nutrition/publications/infantfeeding/WHO_NHD_00.1/en/

publication *Weaning: from breastmilk to family food* has been superseded, but still contains much useful practical information about how to create and feed suitable local food that truly complements breastmilk intake, without undermining breastfeeding. (After six months other foods are not competitive with, but complementary to, breastfeeding, and do not pose the risks of the earlier so-called "comp feeds" given to young babies.) Excellent materials are available online at First Steps Nutrition Trust (http://www.firststepsnutrition.org). There is also a classic text from the 1980s, available through secondhand-book websites such as abebooks.com, Cameron and Hofvander's *Manual on feeding infants and young children* (OUP 1983). This gives recipes using diverse, culturally appropriate, local staple carbohydrate foods. In multicultural societies like Australia, healthworkers should avoid foisting Western food habits and cows' milk intake on families from cultures that have evolved very different food habits over hundreds of years. Chinese babies do best on the foods their mothers eat, not solely on a western dairy-rich diet that their mothers would find very "heaty." (The traditional Asian concept of hot and cold foods seems to have been ignored where infant feeding is concerned.)

## Multi-mixes: porridges, soups, stews

Most traditional cultures have recipes for soups, porridges and stews that follow this WHO pattern as suitable foods for young children in environments where infant self-feeding is difficult or impossible. There are some important things to note about these mixes:

- Because newborn infants often do not receive all the placental blood they should (because the umbilical cord is clamped immediately, not two to three minutes after birth) such foods need to be good sources of minerals such as iron and zinc.[2013]

- Good quality protein and fat are an essential part of the diet after six to eight months of complete breastfeeding, or four to five months of formula feeding. Cereals and vegetables - mostly carbohydrates - alone can actually reduce the protein, fat, and total caloric value of the infant's diet, by displacing breastmilk. Equally, too much protein or fat can cause problems.

- Viscosity (thickness) and caloric density (richness) and texture (lumpiness or smoothness) are all important factors, and WHO gives guidance about these. Such foods should not run freely off a spoon, but be a soft paste that retains its shape until the infant mouth closes over it. If the mix seems a little stiff and dry, adding breastmilk is better than adding water.

- The most common mistake is to make infant food mixtures too watery or calorie poor. This can result in the protein-calorie malnutrition illustrated in Figure 7-3-2 on page 693. Because the child has a small stomach, at most around 200mL, good complementary foods need to be nutrient dense.

- Nutrient density can be increased by reducing the amount of water, or using breastmilk as liquid, and by the addition of some good fats and finely chopped or

---

2013 Upadhyay A, Gothwal S, Parihar R, Garg A et al.. Effect of umbilical cord milking in term and near term infants: randomized control trial.(PMID:23123382) *Am J Obstet Gynecol* 2013, 208(2):120.e1-6.; Andersson O, Hellström-Westas L, Andersson D, Domellöf M. Effect of delayed versus early umbilical cord clamping on neonatal outcomes and iron status at 4 months: a randomised controlled trial.(PMID:22089242) *BMJ* 2011, 343:d7157

ground protein sources. In the past, for example, an egg yolk might be added to the chicken and rice porridge, or some nut paste or ground fish or meat and cold-pressed oils or fresh butter or ghee or avocado to the vegetable porridges. Mixing with infant formula is not advised, as the sources of protein and fat need to be widened, not reliance on bovine protein increased.

- Obviously allergy concerns need to be addressed, but the principles are the same. And allergists now have reversed the advice to avoid exposure to nuts under twelve months,[2014] so that peanut butter, for example, might well be back on the menu after six months as a useful protein and fat booster to rice or mashed potatoes. (Babies can eat any foods in any combination, though they soon develop preferences)

- How much food is consumed at any time is the baby's business, not the parent's. Infant appetite should normally govern infant intake, provided the baby is not lethargic or sedated. If hungry, a well baby will lean forward and eat. If not, a baby will close his mouth and turn his head away. If parents are concerned about their child's food intake, a splendid book[2015] by a Spanish paediatrician, Carlos Gonzalez, will provide information and reassurance and prevent force-feeding and food aversions.

- Baby's growth, behaviour and stools all can be used to assess whether the mix, however constructed and fed, is right. A thriving, growing, active baby with normal stool output, neither constipated nor explosively liquid, is the outcome of good feeding. Weight loss will result if the amount the baby is eating is too little for his needs, or if the food needs to be richer in nutrients.

Of course these home-made multi-mixes were developed in the era when foods were being introduced from three to four months, while the baby's extrusion reflex is still active (the reflex which instinctively pushes solids out of their mouths before they can coordinate safe ingestion, protecting babies from choking.) Mixes had to be very smooth or they triggered a gag reflex. There is much less need for any such single-bowl mixtures after six months of age, when babies can learn to feed themselves. But multi-mixes are still the basic standby recipe, and an idea that can be adapted to cultural food choices.

## Commercial babyfoods tins, jars and pouches

From the 1920s onwards, tins of babyfoods became available, with preservatives added to extend their shelf-life. They then contained much more liquid – glued together with a variety of edible starches – and the first stages were completely smooth. The result was that in many cases they contained fewer calories or less usable protein than breastmilk, so that with their early introduction the child's total caloric intake dropped, as did his or

2014 Prescott S. *The Allergy Epidemic* op cit. There is also a video presentation of Dr. Prescott online at NNI: Early Life Nutritional Determinants of Allergic Diseases and Other Noncommunicable Diseases (NCDs) 2013 8th World Congress on Developmental Origins of Health and Disease. Go to http://www.nestlenutrition-institute. org/resources/online-conferences/Pages/OnlineConferences.aspx and search for Prescott. Open access.

2015 Gonzalez C. *My Child won't eat! How to enjoy mealtimes without worry.* (Pinter & Martin 2012) Available as an e-book.

her protein and fat intake. Lead-soldered tins of babyfoods gave way to glass jars, many vacuum-sealed with plastic lid linings that also leached chemicals into the babyfood.

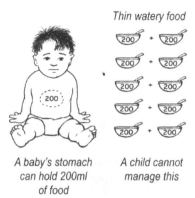

*Thin watery food*

A baby's stomach can hold 200ml of food

A child cannot manage this

With thin porridge or soup, a child needs to eat 2 bowls at each meal. This is impossible, so his needs are not met.

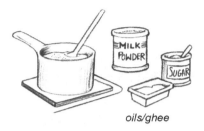

*oils/ghee*

Add extra energy and nutrients to enrich thick porridge.

Figure 7-3-2 Enriching low calorie multi-mixes with fats and protein. Saadeh R. *Complementary Feeding: family foods for breastfed children.* (WHO Geneva 2000) p. 11. Online at http://www.who.int/nutrition/publications/infantfeeding/WHO_NHD_00.1/en/

At present it seems that flexible pouches have supplanted the glass jar. To see young children feeding themselves by squeezing and sucking food from these pouches raises all sorts of questions about the possible facial and orthodontic impacts of foods extruded like toothpaste, and the materials the food and the baby are contacting so intimately for so long. Convenient they certainly are, but is there a price to be paid later? Do these materials also leach chemicals? If so, what? What safety standards exist for such foods?

This book cannot adequately discuss the pros and cons of convenience foods such as these. They certainly can be useful for travellers and families under time pressures. However, any readers who want to be thoroughly updated about commercial babyfoods should read more than the standard industry and dietetic literature which will assure them that such foods are as good as or better than home-prepared mixes. Those who read an online article called *The truth about baby food jars* are unlikely to rely solely or even heavily on these as the source of complementary foods for their child. http://www.thealphaparent.com/2013/02/the-truth-about-baby-food-jars.html Be warned: it is not for the faint-hearted. Don't go there if you don't want to know.

## The importance of appetite: offering is not forcing food intake

In general it can be said that whether breast or bottle fed, nutritional needs vary widely from birth, and even more as infants grow. And children's appetites vary, often decreasing when the child is not feeling well, increasing afterwards for a short time to catch up. Just like their parents, every normal baby should have the ability to decide what to eat and when.

The role of parents is to ensure that good quality food is available often, and to respect the baby's choices of how much to eat. *Keep offering food, at least five times a day for young children, whose small stomachs dictate that they must eat little and often.* But don't offer huge quantities unless baby signals that's what is wanted, and don't be upset if only a little is taken at times. It is the child's overall intake that counts, and how can you quantify what is being eaten while breastmilk is still being consumed?

## Finger foods and baby-led weaning

The overall composition of a suitable diet for a child will mirror the recipe for these multi-mixtures. The child can be offered and will consume (separately or mixed together) some variety of carbohydrate, high-quality protein, good fats, and a wide mix of coloured vegetables and fruit, along with access to clean palatable water. Most cultures also give babies finger foods, as much for entertainment as for nutritional learning. In a clean environment, where food is not scarce, babies can be allowed to self-feed messily from a range of good food choices. Their appetite can be respected and allowed to govern intakes so long as their growth remains good.

Despite the words, "baby-led feeding" must still be carer-determined and carer-led feeding; *it is not a licence to be casual or thoughtless about the introduction of complementary foods.* Babies cannot make decisions about what foods should be available for them to choose from. They cannot access those foods from refrigerators at suitable intervals during the day, so that they can choose small quantities five times a day (as well as breastfeed) by the time they are twelve months old. All parental feeding of babies, whether it is direct spoon-feeding of mixtures or simply supplying foods and implements on a suitable surface, should be attentive, responsive, culturally suitable, and flexible.

Those are very much the emphases found in the new buzzword of 'baby-led weaning',[2016] increasingly shortened to BLW. BLW would better be renamed BLCF – baby-led complementary feeding, since complete weaning from the breast – sevrage – is not intended. BLW encourages full confidence in old-fashioned responsive feeding with good family foods, once baby shows readiness and interest. The difference is that it emphasises allowing the baby to self-feed, even with a spoon or from a cup, although it does not rule out responsive spoon-feeding of mixtures such as the traditional porridges and soups and stews discussed above, where this is needed to facilitate good growth. Breastmilk has provided tastes, and developed tolerance, of family food. The baby is with the family at mealtimes, and given extra snacks in between meals to compensate for a small stomach and greater relative caloric need. The smaller the baby, the smaller and more frequent the meals, and the more considered the total diet needs to be. BLW does not mean offering haphazard bits of whatever's conveniently to hand, unless what is at hand has been thought about as suitable for the baby's needs. With breastfeeding freely as a backup, a casual totally unplanned approach can work quite well for some months, but after nine to twelve months

2016 Gill Rapley and Tracey Murlett. *Baby-led Weaning: helping your baby to love good food.* (Vermilion London 2008) *www.baby-led.com* is the website to check it out.

there is a risk of growth faltering, as the child's growth needs accelerate. This is why growth charting is essential.

However the baby is fed, it is the parents' responsibility to see that she or he is fed enough of the right foods, along with breastmilk as insurance, comfort and protection. Both WHO recommendations and baby-led weaning (BLW) are culturally adapted, and adaptable. Both

- stress variety and moderation of food intake
- advocate feeding little and often
- emphasise respect for infant appetite
- emphasise the importance of infant growth charts
- do not lead to obesity by overfeeding
- allow the child to eat family foods
- respect tradition and culturally diverse food

But BLW may not be practical in some circumstances, such as in severe poverty, where food cannot be wasted, or under poor living conditions where clean surfaces may be scarce and food would be quickly contaminated. The WHO approach is globally applicable, and is particularly useful for children who reject the chemical taste of industrially produced foods, or who need high density feeding in small doses.

That can include damaged children who are being fed via gastric tubes. At least one Australian paediatrician has been amazed at the progress of a little boy whose brain damage prevented him from swallowing and affected his breathing. His mother had expressed 900 ml of breastmilk and fed that via gastrostomy tube daily for many months. As he was nearly ten months, she was advised, but did not want, to add synthetic formulas, knowing that they could include, and would foster, pathogens. Once informed about the WHO approach she immediately began to use healthy family foods suitably liquidised and thinned to the right consistency with expressed breastmilk. The child's progress was remarkable, despite problems, and it was a pleasure to see him happily interacting with his siblings. How much of the cognitive damage in already congenitally damaged children has come from the poor diet inflicted on them by bottle and tube feeding?

## Industrially-produced foods for infants

By contrast with this flexible global multi-mix approach, the marketed twentieth-century industrial approach to infant feeding has been bland, sweet, infant formula too high in protein and energy supplemented by low-fat, low-protein, vegetable and fruit purees, with single foods introduced days apart in case of allergic reaction. The ongoing use of infant formula past nine months is often touted as 'nutritional insurance', yet its volume can displace family food, while its composition fosters a taste for bland and sweet foods. Children are being set up for long-term obesity and its consequences: hardly the insurance anyone wants! Sweetness overrides the baby's natural appetite controls, encouraging them to ignore their instinctive sateity cues.

It was to be expected that as these humane and scientifically based approaches to complementary foods became better known, parents would move away from industrially packaged weaning foods. Equally, it was to be expected that companies making these products would not watch their already diminishing market shrink further without fighting back. In the UK Cow & Gate (Nutricia-owned) have launched a new activity designed to promote weaning using their products. Says the website:

> Each session is led by an Ambassador Mum who's already weaned their *[sic]* own little ones. She's specially trainer [trained?] to show you: Ways to make weaning work for you, easy-to-remember baby nutrition, simple recipes for cooking at home, practical tips and spoon-feeding secrets, support and reassurance from someone who's been there!

Mothers with babies between seventeen weeks and seven months are recruited and weaning sessions take place either in mothers' homes or in community settings, with free baby feeding giveaways as inducements.[2017]

In my opinion, this is a gross promotional exercise which contravenes the International Code of Marketing of Breastmilk Substitutes. The company, a manufacturer of breastmilk substitutes, was clearly soliciting direct contact with mothers and using inducements. No doubt they argue that they are not affecting breastfeeding because the babies are being weaned. If the UK does nothing about this, I would expect to see such devious sidestepping of Code responsibilities happening in every other country. I see this as a test run for Nutricia/Danone globally, concealed behind a long-established UK brand name, Cow & Gate.[2018]

Equally clearly, though, there is an unmet need for families and carers to be educated about all aspects of infant feeding, including complementary feeding, the process of gradual weaning, and the ending of breastfeeding, as well as all dimensions of weaning an artificially fed child off its bland sweet diet. If awareness of this unmet need is what drives Cow & Gate/Nutricia, perhaps they would be willing to provide the funds they are spending on this, without strings, into an independent trust fund which could employ healthworkers, not sales people, to do this important work among those disadvantaged groups that have little access to such knowledge.

As for commercial baby foods like Cow & Gate's: WHO should have the last word.

> ... as WHO has pointed out on a number of occasions, industrially prepared food products, which are suitable as part of a mixed diet to complement breast milk in order to satisfy the nutritional requirements of the infant, might be a convenience under certain circumstances. They provide an option for some mothers who have both the means to buy them and the knowledge and facilities to prepare and feed them safely to their children. However, it is clear that when complementary feeding begins, *a balanced diet for the vast majority of the world's infants can and should be effectively and economically provided by using a variety of locally available foods in addition to breast milk. (my emphasis)*

---

2017  Check out the website for this Nutricia project. https://www.thefeedingclub.co.uk/

2018  Ironically, Cow and Gate was sold by Farley's after serious problems, long forgotten by most, and has been owned by other companies (Boots, Heinz) before being bought by Danone/Nutricia.

# 7.4 Supplementary foods in malnutrition and emergencies

I cannot discuss complementary feeding without referring to its use in the catastrophes becoming more common with global climate change. Many people unthinkingly assume that infant formula is necessary in disasters, and sometimes in bottle-feeding cultures like the USA, it is. However, the provision of infant formula is a two-edged sword that can do great harm, resulting in higher rates of infant sickness and death even long after the immediate disaster.[2019]

In many places malnutrition is endemic, and local food resources unavailable or of poor nutritional value. Provision of a high-quality low-allergy food may be needed around or after six months. This could be in the form of biscuits, or pastes, not powder to be added to water. Professor Roger Short has developed such biscuits as relief foods, which are intrinsically safer than drinks. Local peanut paste mixes have also been remarkably successful in rehabilitating malnourished children,[2020] obviously in communities with low rates of peanut allergy! While there are many controversies about how such foods should be sourced and fed, it is good to see that the international community is much more aware of the importance of protecting ongoing breastfeeding in emergency situations, restricting the use of infant formula. In the past emergency feeding programmes have been vehicles for cows' milk powder and infant formula promotion. A lot of recent work has been done to prevent this. To understand the scale of the problem and the sheer impossibility of safe formula feeding in emergencies, I strongly suggest reading the whole of this very detailed and practical open access article by Gribble and Berry.[2021]

To put the issue of complementary feeding into a global political context, read the slim volume *Complementary feeding: nutrition, culture and politics* by Gabrielle Palmer.[2022] It is not a practical how-to guide, but an impassioned overview of the difficulties that beset this area of policy making (and there are many useful snippets throughout). It encourages respect for multicultural and locally appropriate solutions to the weanling dilemma, as it has been called. It is an excellent book by an author who has done sterling work in alerting many to the wider dimensions of the infant formula issue.[2023]

2019 Hipgrave DB, Assefa F, Winoto A, Sukotjo S: Donated breast milk substitutes and incidence of diarrhoea among infants and young children after the May 2006 earthquake in Yogyakarta and Central Java. *Public Health Nutrition* 2012;15(2):307-315.DOI: 10.1017/S1368980010003423

2020 Manary M. Local production and provision of ready-to-use therapeutic food for the treatment of severe childhood malnutrition. See http://www.who.int/nutrition/topics/backgroundpapers_Local_production.pdf

2021 Gribble K, Berry N. Emergency preparedness for those who care for infants in developed country contexts. *Int Breastfeeding J* 2011, 6:16 doi:10.1186/1746-4358-6-16. Online at http://www.internationalbreastfeedingjournal.com/content/6/1/16 Gribble also has a chapter, Formula feeding in emergencies, in Preedy Watson & Zibadi, op. cit. It will eb eye opening and thought provoking for some.

2022 Palmer G. *Complementary feeding: nutrition, culture and politics*, Pinter and Martin, London 2011. Available from them or TALC.

2023 As it is, I was very touched when, over coffee in a Cambridge café many years ago, Gabrielle told me that reading *Breastfeeding Matters* (1985) had transformed her understanding and changed the nutrition book she had been working on, so that in 1988 *The Politics of Breastfeeding* emerged (a book which I think a must-read for anyone interested in this field, although some will not like its overt politics!) All authors are indebted to others, as I for one am glad to put on record. And authors are always glad to hear that their work has influenced those that follow them in the field: the work of serious writing has few other rewards, certainly not financial!

# 7.5  Four months or six? The debate over age

(*Note: This chapter was written as a stand-alone discussion of the issue in historical context, which may be removed to my website. This means there is some repetition of what has already been said elsewhere in the book.*)

Be clear about one thing. The World Health Organization (WHO) never gives detailed advice about the use of proprietary infant formulas, except for how to reduce their microbiological risks. Just as with any other industrial product, it's up to the formula makers to advise about their use.

So what do we know about the best time to widen the diet of either breastfed or formula-fed infants? In Breastfeeding matters (1985) I argued for 6 months exclusive breastfeeding, and four months formula feeding though WHO's 1978 policy was 'from four to six months" as the global population norm for the introduction of other foods to breastfed infants. Following a period in which extensive multi-national research was done to investigate the risks and benefits of introducing other foods to breastfed children, in 2001 WHO changed its policy. As the UK Department of Health summarised the process,

> Early in 2000, WHO commissioned a systematic review of the published scientific literature on breastfeeding; more than 3000 references were identified for independent review and evaluation. The outcome of this process was subject to a global peer review, after which all findings were submitted for technical scrutiny during an expert consultation. The WHO revised its guidance in 2001, to recommend exclusive breastfeeding for the first six months of an infant's life.

What WHO was doing was setting out general population-level guidance as to what research indicates as the optimum age, *for breastfed babies in general*. No such research has been done, or WHO guidance given, for formula-fed infants. This population guidance acknowledged that individual clinical care is  important for the best outcome for any individual baby. Which means that some babies may need to be given other food earlier than, and others may not want it till later than, six months, and doing so is still within the WHO guidelines. The recommendation was never an dictatorial inisistence than all babies must be solely breastfed until six months, though it is often misrepresented as that.

## The 20th century background

Ever-earlier use of commercial foods for babies became the trend from the 1920s onwards, once industry marketed babyfoods in cans and jars. In 1935 Marriott *revised downwards from twelve to six months* the recommended age for introduction of other foods. By 1978 most US infants were fed strained foods, mostly gluten-containing cereals, by six weeks of age.[2024] The 1975 UK survey found that 40 per cent of children had been given solids before six weeks of age, and 97 per cent before four months (Cow & Gate). Childhood obesity was

---

2024  Cone T. *A History of American Pediatrics.* (Little Brown and Co. 1979) p.257. Farex and rusks had both been wheat-based, though mixes including rice became more popular during 1970s – perhaps beginning the sequence of events that led to FPIES. (See p. 526 )

becoming evident by the 1970s, and the salt and sugar in commercial babyfoods was seen as a factor (which diverted attention from the infant formula they drank.) These concerns triggered discussion and research into the best age for introducing foods other than milk to the infant diet.

In 1980 both UK and US authorities raised the *earliest recommended age* to four months.[2025] This soon mutated into the *latest age* at which solids *must be* introduced to all infants. And that has somehow come to seem the traditional age for those whose memory goes back only a generation or two. In fact, it was very recent and not evidence–based so far as breastfeeding was concerned.

For experience with breastfed babies had always indicated that they were perfectly capable of thriving for much longer than four months on breastmilk alone. Sir Frederick Truby King was a New Zealand based doctor who became very influential throughout the British domains. He founded schools of mothercare which emphasised the importance of breastfeeding, while mandating dogmatic schedules that undermined its success; he created commercial baby foods under the Karitane label. Before the Second World War he was better-known than Dr Spock (the famous US paediatrician) among the educated elites who read baby books, and the nurses who advised all mothers. Standard advice from the Truby King camp, in books that circulated widely throughout the British Empire even after the Second World War, was as follows:

> Complete breastfeeding until the 12th month or longer may be carried out with great success, provided the mother's health is satisfactory. Baby should have been given a bone to chew from 6 months onwards; and at nine months ... some hard food such as twice-baked bread, hard crusts or crisp toast, should be gradually introduced into his diet.

'Complete breastfeeding' for this dominant British school of advice meant complete reliance on breastmilk for the nutrients baby needed. The bones and crusts were about tactile learning, not calories. When calories were needed, during the nine to twelve month weaning process for example, the Truby-King house brand of powdered milk, Karitane milk mixtures, were suggested. So some babies at nine and a half months consumed the following:

> 4 breastfeeds (6am, 2pm, 6pm and 10pm) + 1 Tblsp cereal jelly (starch and water) + 240ml Karitane recipe milk mixture + 1/4 tsp Kariol (fish oil emulsion) + a finger of baked wheaten bread (rusk).

The long intervals between breastfeeds would have ensured engorgement and assisted involution of breast glandular tissue, so milk supply would quickly drop. Two weeks later at ten months, the baby got only two breastfeeds (six am and ten pm) and the rest was 720 ml milk mixture plus the Kariol, rusk and cereal jelly. Orange juice was given to prevent scurvy: initially ½ tsp + ½ tsp water after three months, increasing to 2 Tblsp juice plus 2 Tblsp water at twelve months. Babies grew on such diets, though not all were happy. Babies

---

2025 Barness L. Reply to Ganelin letter. *Pediatrics* 1981; 67:165-6

had not read the Truby King manuals, and many mothers ignored the advice given in clinics under the influence of Truby King. It is easier to breastfeed than to listen to a baby cry.

But *not widening the diet of the breastfed child until twelve months* was not just a British idea. Vahlqvist said of Sweden:

> In the 1920s it was still customary for paediatricians to recommend semi-solids only at the end of the first year. It came almost as a shock when the renowned Swedish pediatrician Jundell proposed in 1921... that such food might and preferably should be introduced as early as 6 months of age ... today, this is usually recommended from 3 months and in practice is often introduced even earlier.[2026]

Spanish doctors had similar ideas. Gonzalez has an enlightening and amusing appendix which traces changes in dietary recommendations in hispanic medical writing. As he says,

> It seems that child feeding throughout the last century has changed almost as much as the length of skirts and the width of ties. Each new generation of doctors has recommended a totally different diet from the previous generation (in other words, different from what they learned in medical school, and different from what they ate as infants.) Each doctor also changed his recommendations as his career progressed.[2027]

Longer duration of breastfeeding was identified with poverty; women breastfed longer out of necessity. In Whitechapel, a London slum in 1910,

> A Jewish woman sits shamefaced before the doctor. '11 months on and baby still given the breast, mother?' The woman makes no reply and the interpreter whispers, 'Afraid of unemployment, so keeping one breast going as a safeguard.' They pass out, the wasting mother and the thriving child.[2028]

Note who suffers here. Not the child. Family income was and is always a factor in infant feeding realities. This visual and mental association of breastfeeding with poverty continues in many countries today, leaving poor mothers vulnerable to advertising that subtly positions 'Gold' formulas as proof of higher social status and affluence. (In 2013 "Platinum" formula emerged using milk from A2 herds: what comes next? Diamond?)

So: twelve months, six, or four? How can we know when a baby is ready to eat a wider variety of foods than breastmilk alone?

## Indicators of readiness for other foods

Not surprisingly, *the baby* indicates readiness, via behaviour and physiological markers of development that usually emerge between five and seven months of age. At this age babies may often be sitting nearby or on parental laps at mealtimes, and usually express interest in what their parents are eating.

---

2026 Vahlqvist B. The Evolution of Breastfeeding in Europe. *J Trop Ped Envir Child Hlth* 1975; 21:11.
2027 Gonzalez C, op.cit.
2028 Ross E. *Love and Toil. Motherhood in Outcast London 1870-1918.* (OUP 1993) p. 142.

Between five and seven months, most babies

- may have used up their in utero body stores of some nutrients
- have head control and better co-ordination
- can sit up, which facilitates swallowing of the new foods and reduces choking risks
- lose the extrusion reflex, which causes their tongue to push things out of their mouths.
- are interested in exploring new tastes and textures (if these are associated with pleasure, not made aversive by force-feeding)
- can grasp foods and transfer them to their mouths
- can indicate aversion or sateity by refusing food.
- have a more developed gut and immune system
- are developing teeth, the better to handle foods
- have more developed kidneys that are better able to handle a higher solute load

Some babies develop faster than others. Some will not want to do more than play with food (other than breastmilk) until well into the second half of their first year. This was obviously accepted as normal behaviour in the early 20th century. Regular growth monitoring will indicate if a child is under-fed, as the growth curve will falter and cross centile lines. Good growth monitoring can both reassure parents or indicate that there may be a problem. The most commonly cited risks of introducing other foods too late have not been growth concerns, but concerns about iron sufficiency, and food aversion.

Some babies will cope with absurdly early introduction of foods, at a few days or weeks rather than a few months, as had been proved by the 1970s. But as WHO rightly said in 1990, 'Of course the mere fact that the physiologically immature organism can adapt to a feeding mode that is nutritionally unnecessary hardly justifies its use.'[2029] The possible immediate problems of too early introduction of other foods include decreased milk production, decreased caloric intake, iron deficiency, infection, and allergy. The long-term risks include poor food habits, poor appetite control, obesity, hypertension, cardiovascular disease, kidney damage, food allergy and aversion.[2030]

## Patent baby foods: how safe?

Most mammals continue to suckle until they treble their birthweight, before eating other foods. During the 20th century, babyfood companies generally urged giving their products once a baby reached ten pounds (4.5kg) or 3 months, whichever came first. Giving foods to such very young babies requires them to be of an unnaturally fine consistency. This was the baby food companies' raison d'être, as they worked out ways to create products whose texture and consistency were tolerated by very young infants. (Similar results were achieved

2029  Akre J (ed) *Infant Feeding the Physiological Basis* op cit., ch.
2030  Ibid.

in human history only by maternal premastication and mouth feeding, not a practice likely to be revived, despite its utility and probable high immunological value!)

Industrial baby foods inevitably contain a good deal of water, but need to look like a food, not a drink, to justify their cost and facilitate spoon feeding. Something has to glue the fine solids together. Complex modified food starches were developed to stabilise and suspend the food particles, creating the desired consistency, texture, and shelf-life. Parents are generally unaware that in the scientific community there are still four concerns about such starches.

> The first relates to the bioavailability of the starch itself. The second is the potential that indigestible starch may have for producing diarrheal symptoms, malabsorption, and changes in gastrointestinal flora. The third is the possibility that modified food starches might be implicated in gastrointestinal disease like Crohn's ileocolitis. The fourth is the toxicological effect of the chemicals used to modify the starch and their possible mutagenic and carcinogenic properties.[2031]

Wow. So there are specific risks to widening the diet unnecessarily early, using industrially produced commercial baby foods. Those parents who keep breastfeeding till six months or so and then introduce suitable family foods need not worry about such things, as babies can handle other than super-smooth consistencies. Around six months is not an absolute upper limit for exclusive breastfeeding, as history tells us.

## Why then did the AAP in 1980 recommend four to six months?

The answer is surprising. *Pediatrics* records that AAP Committee Chair Professor Lewis Barness was challenged by a fellow paediatrician, Robert Ganelin, to explain why, when the physiological markers suggesting infant readiness - listed on the previous page - clearly emerge between five and seven months, not at three to four. His reply was startling in its honesty.

> Trying to convert from previous practices of feeding solids at 1 month of age to the present recommendations must be done step-wise. A compromise was felt to be necessary. For breastfed infants there seems no advantage and some disadvantage to early supplements. When one uses an artificial formula, no matter how good, one must beware of possible missing ingredients. Weighing advantages and disadvantages, the Committee on Nutrition felt that 4 to 6 months of age was reasonable with present evidence.[2032]

Implicit in Professor Barness's reply are two things.

---

2031 Lanciers S, Mehta DI, Blecker U, Lebenthal E. The role of modified food starches in baby food. (PMID:9188246) *Journal of the Louisiana State Medical Society* 1997; 149(6):211-214

2032 The Feeding of Solids debate. Barness LA reply to Ganelin RS, *Pediatrics* 1981; 67 (1) :166; cited in all editions of *Breastfeeding Matters* (p.356, 1998 edition). Barness also reported that he had received many 'bitter letters.. stating that solid feedings at one month have untold advantages.' Maybe they did for formula-fed children! they don't for the breastfed.

The first is a clear awareness that breastfed babies *can safely go longer* than four months, up to six months perhaps.

And secondly, that formula-fed infants may be at risk *if they go any longer than four months* on formula alone.

Note this well. *The basic reason for adopting four months, with its acknowledged 'disadvantage' to the breastfed infant, was the risk to the formula-fed infant of trusting fallible industrial mixes for any longer than that.* Barness and the AAP committee were worried about the artificially fed infant, rightly so given the recent damage. What was *not* mentioned in the reply was the elephant in the room in 1980: the Syntex CHO-Free/Neo Mull Soy formula problem (see page 407) in which babies who relied solely on one infant formula were the most damaged.

## Disadvantaging the breastfed (and women) to protect the artificially-fed

This 'four to six months' 1980 recommendation changed into "give other foods to all infants at no later than four months." But why disadvantage breastfed infants – who clearly could go longer on breastmilk alone – because of 'possible missing ingredients' [or added contaminants, or nutrient excesses, or antigen exposure] in formula? There simply was no credible evidence base to justify the application to breastfed infants.

There are other overlooked/ignored advantages to waiting until six months, and not just for the infants. Among the important reasons are health gains for lactating women, better able to recharge their body stores with another two months of lactational amenorrhoea, and further protection from hormone-linked cancers, as well as savings in time and money. Breastfeeding is not free, but it is certainly cheaper than its industrial competitors. And the foods that many mothers introduce at four months are time-consuming and less-nutritious infant formula or infant cereal, not a variety of carefully chosen and prepared complementary family foods.

Not until late in the twenty-first century was there a global effort to answer the question of the optimal age to widen the diet of fully-breastfed infants. After those global multi-centre studies, WHO, a notably conservative body, proposed six months as a population goal (for the breastfed, remember; they said nothing about the formula-fed) because high-quality research showed that this was best for both mothers and babies. Yet this overdue change would spark a storm of controversy globally. It is also sometimes misrepresented as pressure to breastfeed for doctrinaire reasons, not a scientific assessment of what would be best for most mothers and children.

## Health authorities' reactions

Astonishingly, however, some Western health authorities promptly translated the WHO evidence-based recommendation about *breastfed* infants into six months' exclusive *breast or formula* feeding. Once again Western society's underlying myth surfaced: that artificial formula is virtually the same as breastmilk, so what applies to one applies ot the other. What that implies is crystal clear: there is no need for experts to take decades to research an optimum age for exclusive formula feeding: if women's milk can be relied on for six months, how much more so can its artificial substitute be trusted? (The assumptions are breathtaking when you consider them.) *Too many people too often assume that whatever is said about breastfed infants applies to the artificially fed,* despite the biological differences that accumulate from birth.

## One recommendation or two?

Many interests disliked the idea of six months' exclusive breastfeeding, for a wide variety of reasons. Healthworkers long exposed to industry's subtle propaganda about the deficiencies of breastmilk were concerned that breastmilk could not be trusted that long: iron was needed. Some felt that they could not give different advice to mothers than they had in the past, and were uncomfortable about urging six months for formula-fed babies, having assumed – with no logical basis - that what WHO said about breastfeeding should be said to bottle-feeders. Few health authorities seemed to realise that what WHO implicitly demanded that industry fund research about the optimal age for introducing its foods to the formula fed, before changing from the accepted practice of four months for those infants. Some women felt six months to be unrealistic, an onerous burden that raised the bar for breastfeeding women.

The real issue that industry surely perceived was not articulated publicly. Having two different recommendations for the different feeding groups would begin to unravel the carefully crafted illusion of equivalence between infant formula and breastmilk. National health authorities would be saying clearly to parents, 'You can trust your own body to supply all your baby needs till six months, but formula is a fallible synthetic product, and no one can be sure that it will supply all your baby's nutritional needs. Since your bottle-fed baby's body stores of some nutrients will be depleted by around four months, it's sensible to widen their diet just in case formula has got something wrong: too much, too little.' True, sensible, not hard to do: but unacceptable to the powerful. Very little discussion took place about the ramifications of increasing the age for formula-fed infants beyond the point where in utero body stores of specific nutrients could be exhausted, *even though that had been the stated justification for the four months recommendation in 1980.*

## Resistance and controversy

Industry sought advice and support in the health community, and lobbied hard to keep the old single recommendation for all infants, preferably the (since 1980) usual four to six months. In the UK, a group titled INFORM was created by SMA Nutrition (then owned by Wyeth), Nutricia and HJ Heinz, all formula producers. INFORM's address was c/o IDFA, the Infant and Dietetic Foods Association. In 2005 a substantial INFORM report, *Infant Feeding in the UK,*[2033] was disseminated, an impressive-looking but error-riddled piece of

---

2033  The report is available as pdf download or searchable text @ *www.idfa.org.uk/inform* IDFA is also the acronym
for the International Dairy Foods Association, a global lobbying group.

special pleading targeted at health professionals. That particular document seems to have received little global coverage: the press was perhaps sceptical about a report created, funded and published by industry, however eminent the Expert Advisory Panel which endorsed it before publication.[2034]That Panel was chaired by Professor Alan Lucas, and included Professor Mary Fewtrell. The document argued for four to six months, not six, for all infants.

What really fed this controversy worldwide was a 2011 opinion piece in the *British Medical Journal*.[2035] Its lead author, Professor Mary Fewtrell, and her colleagues, have all done sterling work on infant feeding issues, and strongly support breastfeeding. However, they are UK-based academics, and very few UK women currently breastfeed at all, much less exclusively, for 6 months. Listening to a recent presentation, it seems to be empathy for women which underlies Fewtrell's determined resistance to the six months' guidance (or perhaps she just has a perversity gene from Irish ancestors, like me, and questions most things! Who can know another's motivations?) Fewtrell was also an author of the 2008 European Society for Paediatric Gastroenterology, Hepatology and Nutrition (ESPGHAN) statement[2036] which had supported the WHO 'exclusive breastfeeding to around six months' as 'a desirable goal', but was more widely quoted for its quite prescriptive 'not before seventeen, not after twenty-six weeks' variant on the WHO position.

Like their INFORM document, this Fewtrell et al *BMJ* article suggested that the evidence for six months exclusive breastfeeding was not sufficient, though it was better than the evidence had been for the four months' guidance in 1980. The article supported that once-controversial older four to six months range, that women adjusted to following because trusted health professionals told them to.

The *BMJ* article was initially described in press releases as research, or a review, when it was neither, just an opinion piece by people who seemed to think that because most women do not feed exclusively to six months (true), they could not do so (untrue, especially if health professionals spoke with one voice about the importance of exclusive breastfeeding). The article is still being cited as authoritative opinion, despite multiple errors of fact and assumption, and even internal contradiction.[2037] (Such is the power of the world press, when read uncritically, or by those who want to endorse a particular opinion as authoritative.) So the article needs to be critiqued in some detail.

The multiple industry connections of some of the article's high-profile authors and their previous work on this very topic, as industry consultants on the INFORM project in 2005,

---

2034 Who might have been some of the anonymity-requesting INFORM contributors thanked so profusely in the Report. Covert –paid?- assistance to industry makes it impossible to assess the impartiality of those contributing to public debate on this subject.

2035 Fewtrell M, Wilson DC, Booth I, Lucas A. Six months of exclusive breast feeding: how good is the evidence? (PMID:21233152) *BMJ* 2011, 342:c5955.. The answer to that question is: much better than the information, hypotheses, assumptions and interpretations found in this article!

2036 ESPGHAN Committee on Nutrition: Complementary Feeding: A Commentary by the ESPGHAN Committee on Nutrition. *J Pediatr Gastroenterol Nutr* 2008; 46: 99-110

2037 Appallingly, in perhaps the worst mistake of an otherwise generally useful document, the 2013 NHMRC *Infant Feeding Guidelines* for Healthworkers (op. cit) lent it credibility by describing it as 'a systematic review.'

was nowhere mentioned by the *BMJ*. It would have helped if *BMJ* had put this direct connection on record beneath the article, as those industry connections may also have helped explain the extraordinary global reach of this damaging opinion piece. Respect for the *BMJ* has been eroded by its willingness to publish and publicise such an article and then to follow it up with an ill-informed commentary[2038] that many in the lactation community – myself included – thought was both patronising and offensive. Many of the Rapid Responses to the article are worth reading,[2039] as are the letters which *BMJ* did publish.[2040]

But industry connections don't explain opinions held by reputable academics – though the connections can influence assumptions, and in rare cases, provide motives. There have to be other concerns and issues of substance involved for such researchers to contradict WHO. Two concerns often raised in connection with the age of introduction of other foods are the risk of iron deficiency, and the effects on acceptance of other foods.

## The iron furphy

As Wikipedia records, a "furphy is Australian slang for a rumour, or an erroneous or improbable story, but usually claimed to be absolute fact. Furphies are usually heard first or secondhand from reputable sources and until discounted, widely believed." No better word could be found to describe the concern about possible iron deficiency if breastfed babies are not given other foods at four months. Industry used this furphy globally as a marketing tool in the 1980s. The *BMJ* opinion piece talked of the catastrophic effects of iron deficiency anaemia, without providing any evidence that exclusive breastfeeding to six months posed a risk of clinical iron deficiency. What is more, the catastrophic effects cited were from anaemia of a different origin, not in breastfed children. The study referred to in the *BMJ* article was independently analysed by Adam of Dianthus Medical as follows:

> Chantry et al's study is described by Fewtrell et al as showing that 'US infants exclusively breast fed for six months, versus four to five months, were more likely to develop anaemia and low serum ferritin'. Did it? Chantry et al looked at two separate cohorts of children, and measured iron deficiency by three different measures: low serum ferritin, low haemoglobin, and a history of anaemia ...[the latter] based mainly on reports by the parents, with no medical verification ... the results were highly inconsistent...'

As Adam concluded,

> To cite that paper as evidence that exclusive breastfeeding for six months increases the risk of iron deficiency anaemia therefore strikes me as misleading.[2041]

Me too, Adam. How could that happen, when one of the *BMJ* article co-authors, Professor Alan Lucas, has previously expressed concern about iron deficiency only for *exclusively breastfed babies given low-iron solids after six months*, and small for gestational age (SGA) babies under six months? And of course, babies who have suffered any bleeding problems.

2038  Martyn C. Lactation wars Published 9 February 2011; BMJ 342 doi: 10.1136/bmj.d835
2039  http://www.bmj.com/content/342/bmj.c5955?page=1&tab=responses
2040  http://www.bmj.com/content/342/bmj.c5955?tab=related
2041  http://dianthus.co.uk/duration-of-exclusive-breastfeeding-and-risk-of-anaemia.

In healthy breastfed children given iron-poor weaning foods (which most are not in the UK) deficiency can emerge around nine months. Obviously that is not relevant to discussions about whether to introduce solids at four versus six months of age.

One problem factually linked to low iron levels in breastfed babies is the use of low iron solids that chelate breastmilk iron[2042] and make it unavailable. This is hardly a reason to introduce solids at four months rather than six! For as discussed elsewhere in this book, the young baby has a complex interactive metal transport uptake and system (copper, zinc, iron), which can be deranged by the addition of other foods, with unpredictable consequences.

The *quality* of complementary foods is important, and in the past only WHO multi-mix policies have properly addressed the issue of what to give. I am pleased to see that the Australian *Infant feeding guidelines* are now stressing the need for nutrient-dense iron-rich first foods, not the 1970s advice to give cereals and vegies with no fat and little protein. In the late twentieth century many young Western babies were given a virtual Pritikin weaning diet, and breastmilk (their sole source of quality protein and fat in some cases) was then blamed for any growth faltering or iron deficiency. I repeat: there has been no evidence of iron deficiency under six months in thriving breastfed infants, unless there has been significant infant blood loss post-partum. And new research now indicates that excess iron may foster gut pathogens, increase free radicals, and be as damaging to cognitive development as too little. (See page 359.)

## A question of taste?

The *BMJ* article also expressed concern about possible breastfed-infant refusal of different tastes if introduction of other foods was delayed until six months, rather than begun at four months. Perhaps the authors were unaware of those wildly differing patterns of solid food introduction over the twentieth century. Our parents and grandparents grew up to eat their vegies despite very different patterns of introducing beikost (mashed food).[2043] Until 1911, some US experts stated that green vegetables *absolutely* must not be given before thirty-six months; by 1929 this dropped to nine months. In 1935 Marriott suggested six months for solids, which was daringly early compared with UK and other recommendations of nine to twelve months. After that it was downhill all the way as manufacturers made products available in ever smoother gel or liquid forms. No one did comparative studies to check outcomes of such different patterns of introduction of 'weaning' foods other than milk. Taste aversion caused by infant feeding seems not to have been a problem that concerned doctors then.

However, research now suggests that there is indeed a sensitive early period *before four months of age* when infants need to be exposed to different flavours, or they resist them later. I have no reason to quarrel with that, *because breastmilk always exposes infants to*

---

2042 Oski F. op.cit.
2043 Fomon (1974) pp 16-17 summarises trends in feeding vegetables over the century.

*a huge variety of tastes*.[2044] That being the evolved norm, I would assume that all babies should experience a wide range of tastes from birth. This fact is yet another reason to vary infant formulas and give solids to formula fed children at 3-4 months, but it is irrelevant to breastfed children. It is a reason to encourage the breastfeeding mother to eat a diverse diet, and to persist with breastfeeding throughout the whole year or more that the child is exploring new tastes, and to share those foods with the baby.

The simple but salient fact that breastmilk flavour reflects the mother's diet is rarely noted in such discussions, and was not in the *BMJ article*. Yet babies exclusively breastfed for three or more months have been shown to eat more vegetables as preschoolers than formula-fed children.[2045] And recent research shows that eating vegetables is associated with lower rates of adult metabolic disease, also without commenting on whether breastfeeding might be the primary cause of *both* these desirable outcomes.[2046] Similarly, a national US study found that children fed new foods under six months were 2.5 times more likely to dislike new foods and to eat a narrower variety of foods; while children exclusively breastfed to six months were much less likely to become picky eaters.[2047]

As taste researchers said,

> 'The general principles observed are likely of broader significance, indicating a fundamental feature of mammalian development and reflecting the importance of familiarising infants with flavors that their mothers consume and transmit to breast milk.'[2048]

Research does indicate that there may be valid concerns about artificially fed infants and taste aversions, concerns not raised by the *BMJ* authors so concerned about exclusively breastfed children. Research shows that just experiencing tastes on the lips without eating the foods improves acceptance of new foods. That raises concerns about infants fed nothing but bland sweet formulas: how do they adjust to a wide range of flavours later? And what consequences arise from the bitter tastes of some denatured protein infant formula mixes – which smell and taste so vile[2049] that they can be used as sprays to protect crops from insect predation? (Another good reason to wash all fresh foods if you are milk-allergic. No one expects their tomatoes to be coated with casein, but they might be.) Common sense

2044 Mennella JA Mother's milk: a medium for early flavor experiences. (PMID:7748264) *Journal of Human Lactation* 1995, 11(1):39-45.

2045 Burnier D, Dubois L, Girard M Exclusive breastfeeding duration and later intake of vegetables in preschool children. (PMID:20978527 *Eur J Clin Nutr* 2011, 65(2):196-202.

2046 This is a typical example of unconscious bias: if breastfeeding is associated with a beneficial outcome, researchers often attribute this to socio-economic factors associated with breastfeeding; but fail to cross-link one known outcome of breastfeeding (vegetable eating) with yet another beneficial outcome, lower NCD rates.

2047 Shim JE, Kim J, Mathai RA. Associations of infant feeding practices and picky eating behaviours of preschool children. *J Amer Diet Ass* 2011; 111 (9): 1363-8.

2048 Hausner H, Nicklaus S, Issanchou S, Mølgaard C, et al. Breastfeeding facilitates acceptance of a novel dietary flavour compound. (PMID:19962799) *Clinical Nutrition* 2010, 29(1):141-148.

2049 Remember, a former industry scientist is on record as describing hydrolysate formulas as tasting 'like mud,' and 'horrible', saying that..'I mean, you would never drink it. But you would probably have a hard time when the formula bottle was open to be in the same room with it.' Transcript, FDA Food Advisory Committee meeting Nov 18, 2002. Op.cit.

suggests that continuing sweet and flavoured milk mixtures into the second year of life (via so-called toddler/growing up milks) could also be of concern in this regard. Human infants are simply not designed to have bovine milks and sugars as the dominant part of their diet until two years of age, but this is increasingly the case. And with that comes picky eaters, some stuffed full of formula and refusing other foods while their parents sigh and say, well, it's nutritional insurance, at least he drinks his formula.

## A question of textures?

Another concern often expressed in this discussion of when to introduce non-milk foods to infants, is that 'late' introduction of solids might lead to possible infant inability to handle other textures, lumps in food and so on. However, this concern is totally irrelevant to the discussion of four versus six months, or breastmilk versus formula, even though the INFORM report used it in that way. Six months is not late introduction. The study cited was of children not introduced to any lumpy food until *around ten months of age*, who are more likely to reject such foods *at fifteen months of age*.[2050]

That cited study also failed to explore why these particular babies were *not* given finger foods or some lumpy foods to explore before ten months of age. Was this a normal population of infants and mothers? If so, were mothers over-reliant on industry-packaged foods and formulas, all smooth and readily swallowed from 3 months on? Are packaged strained foods the direct cause of widespread aversions to real food? (Which they taste nothing like, if the ones I tried were typical.) Or were these lumpy-food-intolerant toddlers in fact hard-to-feed food-sensitive babies who rejected all efforts by mothers to get them to eat? Were they simply consuming too much white liquid to be hungry?

Different potential causes would emerge from careful consideration of the individuals in this population of babies. But there is no lesson here for those arguing about four versus six months for breastfed babies. Except perhaps that authors need to read cited literature studies for themselves, and not rely on others' interpretations. In fact, babies breastfed for longer are more likely to be eating a wider variety of foods at the age of two.[2051] As I'd expect given the basic science.

## Independent reviews

A systematic review is emphatically *not* what this *BMJ* article was. However, such professional systematic reviews have been published since then. Did genuinely objective reviewers support retention of four to six months as a universal recommendation for all infants, or suggest it was dangerous to breastfeed solely to six months? No.

---

2050 Northstone K, Emmett P, Nethersole F, The effect of age of introduction to lumpy solids on foods eaten and reported feeding difficulties at 6 and 15 months.(PMID:11301932) *J Hum Nutr Diet* 2001;14(1):43-54.

2051 Scott JA, Chih TY, Oddy WH. Food variety at 2 years of age is related to duration of breastfeeding. (PMID:23201765) Free full text article *Nutrients* 2012, 4(10):1464-1474

The Cochrane Collaboration is a database of reviews done according to strict criteria for assessing the quality of evidence provided, and strong disclosure requirements for contributors. There you can review the evidence that supports the conclusion that:

> although infants should be managed individually, the available evidence demonstrates no apparent risk in recommending, as a general policy, exclusive breastfeeding for the first six months of life in both developing and developed country settings.[2052]

That is *precisely* what WHO said. The European Food Safety Authority (EFSA) in 2009 and the UK Scientific Advisory Committee on Nutrition (SACN) in 2011 reached the same conclusion as the Cochrane Review and WHO. Breastfed babies in general can safely be fully breastfed till six months, and there is no advantage to introducing other foods before that time provided the individual baby's growth trajectory is satisfactory.

*All these reviews carefully refrained from suggesting when formula-fed infants might, could, or should have their diets widened; there is too little scientific evidence about artificially fed infants for it to be reviewed systematically. The real-world evidence we have since 1980 is for the results of feeding other foods beginning at four months, but how do we interpret what we see: as proof that children survive, certainly; but do they thrive normally or become obese too easily on the advice given everywhere since 1980? Where's the multi-centre growth reference study that includes details of the formulas fed, with protein at 1980s levels and 2010 levels to assess outcomes? Where's any guidance for bottle feeding parents?*

## Parents: too dumb to know what their babies eat?

As mentioned earlier, the ESPGHAN 2008 recommendation for the introduction of solid foods was 'not before seventeen weeks, not after twenty-six weeks'. There was no distinction between the breastfed and the not-breastfed infant. What was the justification for their support of the old position of four to six months, in a statement which has been thoroughly critiqued by other European experts with breastfeeding expertise?[2053] I think that the reason given absolutely undermines the credibility of the 2008 ESPGHAN Committee on Nutrition, Fewtrell included. As a parent I find it both amusing and insulting. The reason they gave in 2008 for not wholeheartedly endorsing the WHO position was not evidence-based or scientific. They had no further evidence than WHO. No, they simply said:

> devising and implementing separate recommendations for the introduction of solid foods for breast-fed infants and formula-fed infants may present practical problems and cause confusion among caregivers.

Basically, that's saying that parents would find two recommendations confusing. As though ESPGHAN isn't confusing them by saying six months is a 'desirable goal' but seventeen

2052 Kramer and Kakuma (2002, revised 2009; revised 2011) Optimal duration of exclusive breastfeeding. (PMID:22895934) *Cochrane Database of Systematic Reviews* (Online) 2012, 8:CD003517. DOI: 10.1002/14651858.CD003517.pub2

2053 This ESPGHAN expert opinion has been well critiqued by Cattaneo A, Williams C, Pallás-Alonso CR, Hernández-Aguilar MT et al. ESPGHAN's 2008 recommendation for early introduction of complementary foods: how good is the evidence? *Mat Child Nutr* (2011), 7: 335-343.

weeks on is OK! Yet separate recommendations are made for a variety of different groups of infants: former prems, the allergic, vegetarians, vegans,[2054] various religious communities ...

And Norwegian parents seem to manage: Norway is cited in a European Food Safety Authority (EFSA) document[2055] as having two recommendations: after six months for breastfed infants (though earlier if needed after four months), but between four and six months for all infants not breastfed. If Norway can make such recommendations, why not others? Are Norwegian parents so much smarter? They do seem to know whether their babies are exclusively breastfed or not. However, even in Norway the concern may be academic, as in 2006 less than half of Norwegian infants were in fact exclusively breastfed to even four months, and just 9 per cent were solely breastfed to six months.[2056] (Still, that's nine times the number in the UK!)

Do parents take notice of such recommendations? Yes they do. The UK's Scientific Advisory Committee on Nutrition published clear evidence of this.[2057] From 1990 to 2005 giving solids before three months dropped from roughly seventy percent to ten percent; and giving solids between four and six months rose from five percent to almost fifty percent. While in 2005 only a tiny number were already following the 2003 UK policy advice to feed solely to six months, SACN saw this as indicating the need to promote the message more widely, as parents did listen to professional advice. This has been made more difficult by the media's prominent reporting of dissenting opinions, which have left parents confused.

## The 2012 AAP statement

In 2012 the American Academy of Pediatrics, once divided on the subject, issued a strong statement supporting the WHO position. The 2012 Policy Statement on Breastfeeding reaffirmed the AAP recommendation of exclusive breastfeeding for about six months, 'followed by continued breastfeeding as complementary foods are introduced, with continuation of breastfeeding for one year or longer as mutually desired by mother and infant: and says that 'Because breast-feeding is immunoprotective, when such complementary foods are introduced, it is advised that this be done while the infant is feeding only breastmilk ... Mothers should be encouraged to continue breastfeeding through the first year and beyond as more and varied complementary foods are introduced.'[2058]

---

2054 ESPGHAN once expressed concern (*J Pediatr Gastroent Nutr* 2008; 46:99–110) about macrobiotic diets and vegans on the basis of a Dutch study showing poorer growth in infants. This was of 53 infants who had water-based, no-fat vegetable porridges given from around 4-5 months, displacing breastmilk fat and protein. Interestingly, low breastmilk output at 6 months (mean of 363ml) correlated with wasting in these children; BUT intakes at 6 months of an average of 824 mls did not. See Dagnelie PC, van Staveren WA. Macrobiotic nutrition and child health: results of a population-based, mixed-longitudinal cohort study in The Netherlands. *Am J Clin Nutr* 1994; 59(5 Suppl):1187S–1196S

2055 *EFSA Journal* 2009; 1423: 11-38

2056 Hörnell A, Lagström H, Lande B, Thorsdottir I. Breastfeeding, introduction of other foods and effects on health: a systematic literature review for the 5th Nordic Nutrition Recommendations. (PMCID:PMC3625706) *Food Nutr Res* 2013, 57:313-323.

2057 SACN Infant Feeding Survey 2005 op. cit.

2058 AAP Section on Breastfeeding. Breastfeeding and the Use of Human Milk. *Pediatrics* 2012; 129 (3): e827 -e841. (doi: 10.1542/peds.2011-3552. Online: http://pediatrics.aappublications.org/content/129/3/e827.full

Regrettably, however, the AAP, like ESPGHAN, has not yet dealt with the issue of complementary foods *for artificially fed infants*. They have to date ignored their own 1980 realisation that two different groups of children are involved, and have not affirmed the fact – obvious to them all in 1980 – that the diet of the formula-fed child should be widened before the exhaustion of body stores, which would be less than four months for some infants, and four for normal term babies.

In that 2012 AAP statement on breastfeeding they have said nothing to help the majority of American parents who are not solely and successfully breastfeeding to six months, much less those millions bottle-feeding from birth. As the European Food Safety Authority (EFSA) said, 'There are numerous publications which discuss the timing of initiating complementary feeding with regard to breast-fed infants, whilst the literature on non-breast-fed infants is limited.'[2059] Why this neglect of key questions for the still-dominant form of Western infant feeding? All too hard? No one wants to know the answers?

## Questions this raises

So let's do some critical thinking about why anyone might want to challenge WHO's goal of getting infants solely and well breastfed to six months (though given other food earlier if needed). Why might someone want four to six months left as the time of introduction of other foods for all children? In the world of realpolitik there are some impolite questions to ask.

Q. Who would have gained, or would gain, from the continuation of the 1980 four months recommendation? A. The commercial babyfood and infant formula industries, sometimes the same entities.

Q. Is there a major public health gain to telling parents that *all* babies should be offered solids at four months? A. None that I can see, though perhaps it possibly does protect the bottle-fed babies from deficiency.

Q. Does that gain outweigh the possible loss of breastfeeding, the loss of lactational amenorrhoea and its benefits for mothers, the increase in infections and cancer risk for mother and child, the poorer quality nutrition of the breastfed infant? A. Absolutely not.

*Or, if the single recommendation were to be six months for both sets of babies,*

*Q.* Does the public health gain of having one recommendation outweigh the unpredictable risk of harm to artificially fed babies after infant body stores are exhausted? Or the additional and increasing cost to parents? A. We can't know without proper research. If bottle-fed babies aren't given other food until six months, the deficiencies of formula might show up. But many nations, including Australia, have now adopted the WHO six months recommendation and applied it for all babies, not just breastfed ones. That's a whole new experiment which should be carefully monitored.

---

2059 EFSA Panel on Dietetic Products, Nutrition and Allergies (NDA): Scientific Opinion on the appropriate age for introduction of complementary feeding of infants. *EFSA Journal* (2009) 7(12):1423

Why *does* industry not want six months for both? Do they know that if bottle-fed babies weren't given other food until six months, deficiencies of formula would indeed show up? Or is it that a twofold approach to the issue of when to introduce other foods to infants makes plain to the simplest person that breastmilk and formula are not 'so close nowadays' as to make no difference? That myth has been the basis of their multi-billion dollar success.

# What I would like to know about widening the infant diet

Factually, breastfed and formula-fed infants are already different from one another by four months, because their diet is different over those four months. So some questions that occur to me are:

- Should a breastfed infant on a low- (but highly bioavailable) protein diet consume the same complementary foods as a formula-fed infant on a higher (but poorer quality) bovine milk-protein diet?

- Does the use of low calorie high-fibre cereals and vegetables that became common Western weaning advice suit the artificially fed infant, but not the breastfed one?

- Human milk nutrient bioavailability drops when other foods are added: eg, some solids reduce iron absorption. Doesn't that mean that nutrient-dense foods of good caloric, protein and mineral value are needed, not the low-calorie, low-iron vegies or fruit often suggested?

- When will there be research looking at weaning diets for infants known to be at greater risk – the mixed-fed and formula-fed?

- When will parents be given the information needed to devise suitable complementary foods from good family foods, not overloading the artificially fed child with protein, sugars, starches and fats, and not underfeeding the breastfed child with low calorie vegetables?

- Does the high-carbohydrate bland taste of many commercial infant formulas and baby foods cause later taste aversions and obesity?

- Do different infant formulas require different weaning diets? If lower-protein formula has been used for four solid months, should the weaning diet be richer in protein than if a higher-protein formula was used? Professor Alan Lucas (a co-author of the Fewtrell article, and chair of that 2005 INFORM Expert Advisory Panel, remember) has said clearly that infant formulas are *not* all the same, that even small differences may have *significant* effects.[2060] (My emphasis.) Each infant formula is a liquid mixed diet, not a single food.

- What about that seemingly inflexible *upper* limit of six months, or ESPGHAN's twenty-six weeks? Where is the research to say that this is an *absolute* upper limit? (I see it as essential *only* for artificially fed infants.) The fact that this is definitely a suitable age *to begin offering foods* does not mean that parents should panic if their fully breastfed and thriving baby shows no interest. Many babies do no more than

---

2060 Lucas A. *Infant Nutrition.* Op. cit p. 50.

play with other food initially, accidentally ingesting tastes as they explore. There is no need for concern while they continue to thrive on breastmilk alone, being charted on the appropriate WHO child development graphs. Yet much anxiety is generated by the breastfed baby who doesn't immediately guzzle down other foods as soon as they are offered. All sorts of suggestions are made to speed up the sometimes slow rate of acceptance by babies to whom food means breastmilk. Surely happily-thriving completely-breastfed babies under six months are the least of our concerns. So why has all the focus of media attention been on them, especially when they still constitute a tiny minority of all babies, even in Nordic countries? It makes very little sense that we worry so much about breastfed babes and so little about the artificially fed. But that works to sell products!

Science can't yet tell us what or when to give other foods to artificially fed infants (i.e., those babies consuming mixed-origin solids suspended in water, presenting as white liquids). Why? Because we don't know in detail either what they need, or what they're getting (see page 399). Loud-mouthed infant formula advocates are strangely silent on these issues of just when and what to give formula-fed babies as distinct from breastfed ones: in fact many seem to go on relying on formula, rather than focussing on transitioning the child to a life without formula by twelve months. WHO rightly considers breastfeeding the human norm for all populations, and simply cannot advise about proprietary products whose intimate details are commercial secrets. Thus where independent evidence-based advice for artificially feeding parents is needed, there is little other than dubious industry advice.

## What parents need to understand

There are two basic problems with the advice that all babies need to widen their diet by six months of age.

The first is the failure to appreciate past experience which says clearly that

- some –not all – children can be safely solely breastfed past six months, extending the period during which other foods can be gradually introduced, and reducing the pressure on mothers of thriving breastfed babies who refuse other foods until seven or eight months; and
- some – not all – formula-fed children really need to widen their diet by four to six months, as body stores may be depleted and formula is fallible.

The second and the most basic problem is the underlying attempt to create a single one-size-fits-all recommendation about the age of introduction of foods other than breastmilk or formula despite the differences between both infants and mothers' histories, exposures to allergens, and reactivity.

Solely breastfed children of solely breastfed mothers are not the same as children partially breastfed from birth or formula fed from birth; children gestated by allergic mothers are not the same as children born without such exposure.

Even within those categories each is child is genetically and epigenetically unique. Thus general advice needs to be tempered by knowledge of individual  history.  In general, it is best not to exclude any foods from the mother's diet, as breastfeeding is intended to create tolerance. In general, it is also best to exclude from the diet of the pregnant woman and breastfeeding mother foods to which she –and/or the biological father of the child - is clearly reactive.

Those two general statements are complementary, not contradictory. They simply imply that public health messages need to be more nuanced, and families need more detailed support and assistance, than is currently true.

If such support is not possible, at least public health officials and hospital-based specialists could acknowledge such important differences and not make matters worse by arbitrary diktats about the one best age for introduction of solids, ignoring the experience of breastfeeding families and of those who work with their relatively normal children as allergy problems emerge in infancy. Hospital-based specialists – and following them, most community-based doctors – still fail to see  the early end of the reactivity spectrum where these problems begin to manifest, and can be remedied more easily. Dietary intervention can lead to rapid improvement in young children – and others in the family, usually. Health policy should not be based on children sick enough to reach referral centres or meet strict criteria for existing allergy. Allergy is a wide spectrum, and the sooner it is identified and managed, the better chance there is of creating tolerance over time.

## Where to from here?

 WHO's population-level advice is to breastfeed exclusively to six months, and introduce other suitable foods while continuing to breastfeed 'into the second year and beyond'. WHO has always urged the use of appropriate individual growth monitoring to guide individual care. But it is not enough for WHO and other health authorities to tell us what is appropriate for breastfed babies. WHO also needs to spell out clearly that:

- what is true for breastfed babies *does not apply to* artificially fed babies; both science and commonsense suggest that it is unlikely to, given the differences between the fluids and their delivery mechanisms
- each company that creates artificial formulas needs to specify appropriate and safe complementary feeding suggestions for their products, as each formula is unique
- six months/26 weeks is not an absolute minimum *or maximum* for the introduction of other foods to breastfed babies
- widening the diet of artificially fed infants once body stores are exhausted is 'nutritional insurance'
- using toddler formulas is not nutritional insurance and can be nutritional risk
- population recommendations are just that – growth monitoring and parental care of *each* baby is essential to good individualised decision-making

- growth monitoring is about individual growth trajectories, weight for height, and proportionality, not simply gross body size and averages.

Of course the breastfed baby's growth should be plotted on the WHO growth charts, finalised in 2006, and based on breastfed children. Older charts have been based on US (almost all) bottle-fed children. The US CDC, the Centers for Disease Control and Prevention, has adopted the WHO charts for children up to the age of two, yet to date some countries have not. The WHO charts indicate substantial differences in normal child growth from those based on bottle-fed populations. It would greatly assist all families to know the normal growth curve of well-breastfed infants. Deviations could be uncovered sooner. The UK has not only adopted the WHO charts, but made available training materials in their use.[2061] Other countries are following suit. However, it may not be possible for formula-fed infants to follow the growth trajectory of breastfed infants without risking nutrient imbalances: greater intake and weight gain may be inevitable for the child to obtain necessary micronutrients less bioavailable in formula. There is still a great deal unresearched about both infant formulas and breastmilk. Every formula change creates a whole new experiment.

There are numerous salutary lessons to be drawn from the introduction of solids debacle, not least the power of industry and the media to shape and inform public opinion. With industry websites multiplying, more effective means of reaching parents with factual information about appropriate complementary foods are needed. Surely this should be the concern of national paediatric dietitian groups? And surely they need to critique what is reaching parents from industry-aligned sources?

For the present the only sites I can strongly recommend are:

First Steps Nutrition Trust (http://www.firststepsnutrition.org)

Saadeh R. *Complementary Feeding: family foods for breastfed children*. (WHO Geneva 2000) p. 11. Update recommendations to 6 months, but very practical. Online at http://www.who.int/nutrition/publications/infantfeeding/WHO_NHD_00.1/en/

Baby Led Weaning site, (www.babyledweaning.com/)

*My Child Won't Eat!* by Spanish paediatrician Carlos Gonzalez; you can read about him at http://www.theguardian.com/lifeandstyle/2012/may/28/carlos-gonzalez-doctor-parents-break-rules

Advice from reliable breastfeeding organisations such as LLLI (La Leche League International) – http://www.llli.org/ – and ABA (Australian Breastfeeding Association) – https://www.breastfeeding.asn.au/ to single output just two of many worldwide.

---

2061 These can be downloaded from the Dept of Health website: http://www.dh.gov.uk/prod_consum_dh/groups/dh_digitalassets/@dh/@en/@ps/@sta/@perf/documents/digitalasset/dh_127422.pdf

**CHAPTER 8**

# Thoughts, conclusions and beginnings

*This chapter tries to draw together some of the threads running through the book, and asks readers to step back and think about bigger issues than their own personal allergy or infant problems. As Al Gore said, "...inconvenient truths do not go away because they are not seen. Indeed, when they are not responded to, their significance doesn't diminish: it grows." (Introduction to his book, 'An Inconvenient Truth', (Rodale 2006).*

## 8.1 Where is allergy going globally?

Allergy authorities these days are realising that the extent of the problem is such that it simply cannot be dealt with by existing healthcare systems. Waiting lists of 12 months in a wealthy country like Australia make it clear that allergy clinics cannot cope even with the known serious cases, where lives may be at risk. Finland seems to be attempting to educate the whole population, and to prioritise the obviously serious cases for medical attention while providing guidance for self-management of lesser problems. Prevention has proved to be too difficult, and avoidance is thought to have resulted in greater sensitivity, so that the emphasis is on inducing tolerance by continued exposure. In general, that seems to be inevitable, although it fails to recognise the difficulties caused by allergy not serious enough to warrant health professional care. And if up to a third of Finnish parents consider that their child has allergy problems, I am certain that public education campaigns will not persuade them otherwise. From the 1970s parents persisted in recognising allergy problems long before doctors were willing to admit they were right to do so; they are not about to deny their own reality, and ignore connections with ill health that their close observation of themselves and their family convinces them are real. Nor are they about to deny the evidence they have seen that diet changes can bring relief to victims and that better pregnancy, birth and breastfeeding results in happier babies and families. Many parents now know, as I do, that allergy - or at least many of its painful manifestations - can be prevented by personalised dietary interventions and lifestyle changes. Population-level education about prevention wherever possible, and early intervention for infants, would

717

be better than the current trend towards refusing to recognise 'minor' allergy problems as requiring any intervention other than pills and creams.

And one important avenue for prevention (or at least amelioration) has been sadly neglected. No country has seriously tried the preventive package I am suggesting, of identifying and assisting allergic women before or during early pregnancy, reducing birthing stresses, ensuring and enabling exclusive breastfeeding or breastmilk feeding from birth to around six months, with dietary manipulation during prolonged maternal breastfeeding into the second year - and beyond if desired by mother and child. Even if pregnancy counselling and help is ignored, and the birth is a nightmare, the early identification of infants with minor problems while still fully breastfed is critical to success. Modification of infant and maternal diet to bring about symptomatic relief is important to both health and family functioning and relationships. A strategy of reintroducing reactive foods during prolonged lactation – that is, from about 6 months onwards but within the first year or two - makes sense (although the mother should continue to reduce or avoid foods that trigger her own symptoms) as breastmilk is **designed to induce tolerance.**

In my experience, symptoms that hospital-based allergists would dismiss as trivial always precede serious manifestations of allergy in infants. Severe distressing eczema begins with patches of rough dry skin or hectic red patches on cheeks: identify and resolve the problem at that point, and halt the allergic march before the brass band starts playing. Look for other subtle signs, both gut and extra-intestinal, skin and behavioural. Start from the premise that a well-fed breastfed baby should be happy, contented, and willing to sleep - albeit not in eight hour stretches. See crying as a sign of distress, and stress as a contributor to infant and family problems of all sorts, and vice versa. See fever as a sign of inflammation triggered as often by allergy as infection, and learn to respond appropriately before too many chemical mediators have been released for the immune system to bring inflammation back under control. Look for the clusters of minor problems which indicate that the body is not coping well, and if there is reason to consider allergy a likely contributor, don't wait till major problems emerge before suggesting ways of relieving the total body load and improving the current tolerance level. Those two concepts explain why many strategies and interventions can have an effect on an over-stressed body. And above all, address this as a physical problem before getting tied up in knots by the idea that it is all psychosomatic and proof of inadequacy or culpability as a parent or inherited temperament in a child. There will be psychological dimensions to most physical problems, as stress of any kind changes body hormones, but have confidence that physical and dietary changes can also be involved in both causing and helping fix psychological issues. We are embodied beings, and our bodies affect our minds, and our diet affects both. Believing that we are not powerless is important to health as WHO defines it.

I cannot believe that my experience is atypical. If, within days of a two hour discussion, I can have parents saying to me that they have a new child, that both sleep and behaviour are different, it is not because I have more charm or authority or conviction than the many other health professionals they have fruitlessly consulted. It is because this approach works. And if they tell me years later that their child copes well with formerly reactive foods except when under major stress, or that the allergy has persisted and avoidance is still necessary, it is not because either is what I predicted, it is because that is what they have observed. No one knows better than responsive attentive parents how allergy has changed in their children over time. I do counsel parents that if they want healthy grandchildren, they need to be sure their now adult child is aware of their past allergy, and is not sucked into arbitrary dietary patterns that might be prescribed as though everyone is tolerant of everything. It is the lack of such care before conception and during pregnancy which I believe is fuelling the ongoing damage, creating intergenerationally-communicated disease.

But maybe I'm wrong, and there is another explanation; and maybe Big Pharma will come up with a magic pill or gene-altering tool that actually solves the problems of those who can afford it. The record so far of modern medicine and infant formula does not inspire me to believe that likely to happen in reality, and certainly not to be available to everyone who needs it. Respecting and harnessing the power of women's milk seems to me likely to do much less harm (and more good) than trying to fiddle with intrinsically alien substances our bodies evolved to reject. Harnessing that power to make more profit for companies (with little or no proof of benefit to babies) is surely not the way to go. Yet that is why so many scientists are investigating human milk so intensively: many would not have jobs without infant formula industry funding, and few bite the hand that feeds them. Take away society's collective delusion that infant formula is good enough, and governments would soon see the wisdom of investing in women's milk. Because parents would demand access to supplies for their precious children. Any country that can support bloodbanking with all its problems can support milkbanking.

So even if I'm wrong, I'm more likely to do good than harm by sharing this information with other people who have less access to the literature and less time to read it and think. Let me know if you think I'm wrong about that!

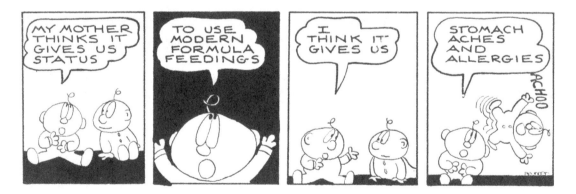

Figure 8-1-1 Infant feeding choice and outcomes. Image from *Protecting Infant Health: a healthworker's guide to the Internaitonal Code of Marketing of Breastmilk Substitutes.* (ICDC 1993 edition).

# 8.2 The underlying problem western society won't face

I'm almost seventy, an age when people tend to review their lives and think about issues that will affect their grandchildren. We all have light-bulb moments. One of mine was in 1985, when a charming senior FDA staffer patiently explained to me the rationale for what I saw as her biased and plagiarised[2062] *Pediatrics* article. Said she, 'You have to understand, after the CHO-Free disaster American parents were afraid of infant formula. We *[clearly meaning the FDA]* have to reassure American parents that infant formula is safe, because American society depends on bottle-feeding.' Do regulators exist to reassure parents and protect the current status quo? I didn't think so.

In fact not only America, but most modern Western societies are utterly dependent on artificial feeding. That is the problem. For, as I said in *Breastfeeding Matters* thirty years ago, without infant formula to allow mothers to be separated from their babies, radical social change is necessary.[2063] While such societal dependence does not excuse prejudice and falsehoods masquerading as science, we must acknowledge that reality.[2064]

I don't question that reality. My questions are simply:

- Must that dependence continue despite its risks and human and planetary costs?
- What can we all do to change it, so that future infants at least *begin* life with the ability to realise their full potential, no matter what epigenetic challenges and life difficulties they later face?
- And how soon will breastfeeding be seen as necessary for normalcy, and not a matter of personal preference? How soon will societies realise that artificial feeding is risky business in every country and every social class?

Well, what do you think now? Have you come to question any assumption that formula is safe enough as long as parents are careful and the water clean? That 'all baby milks come close' to breastmilk? Or are "top class nutrition off the shelf"?[2065] as an industry-linked dietitian asserts. That the perfect mix of science and love is available as a powder? As a new mother in 1976, I believed infant formula was completely safe. I did not arrive at my current position from any preconceived faith in nature or women's milk. What I read startled me, and so I kept reading. I came to believe that formula marketers have – perhaps unconsciously – followed Josef Goebbels's strategy: 'Tell big lies – because if the lie is big enough, some of it will be believed.' (And $30–$50 billion dollars are at stake, after all!) At

---

2062 Compare these articles: Anderson SA, Chinn HI, Fisher KD. History and current status of infant formulas. (PMID:7039294) *Am J Clin Nutr* 1982; 35(2):381-397 and Miller SA, Chopra JG. Problems with human milk and infant formulas. (PMID:6435088) *Pediatrics* 1984; 74(4 pt 2):639-647.

2063 Former WHO staffer James Akre outlines some of what is needed in Beyond 'Breast Is Best': Next Steps in the Counterrevolution. *Breastfeeding Review*, Vol. 18, No. 2, Aug 2010: 5-9... And of course in his book, The problem with breastfeeding. (Hale Publishing 2006)

2064 Hausman BL *Viral Mothers: breastfeeding in the age of HIV/AIDS.* (Uni of Michigan Press 2011) p. 96

2065 Hillis A. *Breast, Bottle, Bowl.* (Harper Collins 1998)

the very least, they continue to be guilty of wilful blindness – which will be no defence once the lawsuits start. In the trial of Enron's Chairman and CEO, Judge Simeon Lake stated that

> You may find that a defendant had knowledge of a fact if you find that the defendant deliberately closed his eyes to what would otherwise have been obvious to him. Knowledge can be inferred if the defendant deliberately blinded himself to the existence of a fact.[2066]

Overall, more than a million children still die every year for lack of breastfeeding, and not all of them are in developing nations with dirty water. Some of those who died were fed the latest formulas in Australia and Israel and America and the UK. Any senior neonatologist knows the names of children who died because they were formula-fed and not breastfed: though the words on the death certificate may be sepsis or NEC or respiratory failure or viral infection or SUDI or SIDS or pneumonia. Perhaps the United Nations could erect a tomb of the unknown baby to honour those whose deaths and disabilities have contributed to making a less dangerous infant feeding product. Parents like me, with adult children and/or grandchildren damaged by infant formula exposure, would probably be happy to chip in to help pay for it.

When so many previous infant formula products are now quietly discontinued as unsuitable, why would anyone believe that current man-made artificial substitutes for women's milk are totally safe? We need proof of safety in the short and long term, through the generations; safety from subtle accumulating harms, as well as overt toxicity or defect. No other fundamental challenge to normal infant development has been so little scrutinised, and so uncritically accepted, simply because it is so widespread, so socially convenient, and of course, so hugely profitable to the pharmaceutical and food multinational corporations who reap not only the direct profits from formula sales, but also the indirect profits from increasing needs for contraception, vaccination, medications, hospitalisations ... The facts say that formula sales are still growing fast, and growing fastest in countries where people can least afford both to feed artificially and to allow rapid population growth. Infant formula still feeds investors better than it feeds babies.

The burden of proof of safety for all children cannot be left with the men who make formulas. Industry scientists know perfectly well that such proof is impossible, and such absolute safety unattainable, however much care they take. So the formula corporations rely on clever marketing to persuade each generation of users and health professionals, while opening new markets when old ones decline where parental knowledge increases.

Despite all that spin, an accumulating body of proof says that infant formula reduces human potential and contributes to ill health. I have been appalled by what is in the scientific literature that never reaches parents. As Sandra Steingraber says in her wonderful book, *Raising Elijah*, 'As soon as you know, you can't not know.' (Her previous book, *Having Faith*, I also strongly recommend to all readers. Her perspective is one I share: where babies

---

2066 Heffernan, M. *Wilful Blindness: why we ignore the obvious.* Simon & Schuster, London 2011.

are concerned, and our fragile planet, we take precautions, not risks. Resources are finite, and I have grandchildren who may want to have children.)

Am I irresponsible to write this book when so many families absolutely depend on infant formula? It isn't me who is telling parents not to worry, that there are no real problems with artificial feeding, that it is a 'safe product', that their babies *will thrive* when not breastfed. Saying or writing that *would* be breathtakingly irresponsible; I shudder to think of the responsibility formula advocates undertake so blithely. Every child is a non-replicable experiment of one, with a unique and never-to-be-repeated genome – and of course, is an irreplaceable and beloved daughter or son. No one can predict the effects of artificial feeding, which for the unlucky range from possibly mild developmental distortion to death from infection or cancer. Every mother is unique and leaves an irreplaceable hole in her child's life if she dies young from reproductive cancers. Yet for one hundred and fifty years most doctors have been happy to reassure parents on the basis of their blind faith in industry and their monumental ignorance about women's milk. *All I want to do is let parents know what has been concealed from them about industrial products, in the hope that in future they can make informed choices, whether about infant feeding or legal redress for its harms.* Who is being irresponsible here?

But of course I assume that almost all parents who know enough to make a truly informed choice will be choosing to breastfeed *if they possibly can*. For I consider – who with a brain wouldn't? – that from the newborn baby's point of view, there is only one suitable food, and there will be consequences, almost certainly negative, if baby misses out on breastmilk and breastfeeding. And I take as a given that parents want to do their very best for their child (even though I know some don't). My perspective is that a baby has a right to be breastfed, just as the mother has a right to breastfeed, neither of which rights should be lightly thwarted or disregarded. I also think that society has an obligation to protect those rights, and to do so without demanding that mothers sacrifice other rights to exercise this one. To me, that is an obligation modern Western society is failing to honour, adopting the policy of wilful blindness.

Risk can be unavoidable, and risks sometimes have to be taken, including all too often the risk of formula feeding. Working out the balance of risk versus benefit of feeding choices can only be done by parents, and their choices have to be respected and supported. But I also believe that no parent has the right either to risk or harm a child *needlessly*, simply because they 'feel like' doing something other than what is known to be best for that baby, or doing so is difficult or inconvenient. No one can morally support a father's right to deprive his child of breastmilk, as some court orders have done by creating custody arrangements that interfere with breastfeeding. A woman has the right to choose to damage her own health by not breastfeeding, just as she can by smoking or drug use. But she has no right to damage another person, whether that is an adult or an infant. By this logic smoking, once a matter of personal choice, has rightly become a public health issue. So too with breastfeeding. As the American Academy of Pediatrics (AAP) said in its generally excellent 2012 policy,

> Breastfeeding and human milk are the normative standards for infant feeding and nutrition. Given the documented short- and long-term medical and neurodevelopmental advantages of breastfeeding, infant nutrition should be considered a public health issue and not only a lifestyle choice.[2067]

'Not only'? *Not* a 'lifestyle choice'. The lifestyle choice is whether to have a baby or not. Choose to have a baby, and there is a moral responsibility to put that helpless person's interests at the forefront of all relevant and important decision-making. Only rarely will that baby's best interests be served by artificial feeding. Yet a child who dies because *needlessly* formula-fed – and in every country there are some who do – is not seen as a case of culpable homicide. By contrast, an addicted breastfeeding mother has been jailed for six years after her six-week-old child died: because her addiction was seen as her lifestyle choice, so she was held responsible for her baby's death (though addiction experts might well debate her power to choose).

But most families do not make free and informed choices about infant feeding (and many, about having babies.) I hope that bottle-feeding parents can see from this history that they are in the position of needing to formula feed (or even of 'choosing to'), because of forces beyond their control. In fact they had little choice, and certainly not an informed one.

Many factors constrain infant feeding choice, as I made clear in *Breastfeeding Matters* as far back as 1985. Leslie Cannold writes well of the 'circumstantially childless', as very distinct from those 'childless by choice'.[2068] Most bottle-feeding parents likely to be reading this book would be circumstantial bottle-feeders, not bottle-feeders by choice from the baby's birth. That is a societal disgrace. It is *not* a reason to deny the increased risk for infants that those circumstances create over time – any more than road accidents are a reason not to publicly advocate the use of child restraints which reduce deaths, or the guilt potentially felt by smokers over their child's respiratory disease is a reason not to criticise smoking. Even 'bottle-feeders by choice' are rarely aware of what their choices mean to their own health and that of their children, and have little reason to feel guilty: ignorance is a valid excuse, provided that the ignorance is not wilful blindness. Refusing to learn is different – that is not ignorance but obduracy, and guilt might be quite appropriate. But I agree with Hausman that 'all the evidence in the world will not convince people *whose worldview depends on not seeing infant formula as a risk*'.[2069] And perhaps those whose income depends on it.

Some bottle-feeding parents reading this book may well realise with sinking hearts, as I did, that damage to their children has indeed been the result of early exposure to unnatural food. I hope they are honest enough, and brave enough, to resist the temptation both to deny the possibility and impugn my motives, in the uncouth language so often used by formula advocates. Truth is painful, but that is not a reason to conceal it. This book may help bottle-feeding parents both identify one powerful cause of their children's problems,

---

2067  *http://pediatrics.aappublications.org/content/129/3/e827.full.pdf*
2068  Cannold L. *What, no baby? How women are losing their reproductive freedom and how they can get it back.* (Fremantle Arts Centre Press 2005). I don't agree with all of this book, but it's a good read.
2069  Hausman B. op cit., p.

and also realise that those problems are not of their making. Guilt is pointless, and active rage appropriate.

I hope bottle-feeding parents become very angry, and support the many volunteers like myself who are trying to make a difference for the children of all parents. When well directed, and channelled by reason, anger is so much more productive of positive social change than self-indulgent name-calling about other people making you feel guilty. My rage has helped many, including my grandchildren. Parents, it's just *not about you and your emotions*. It's about the health of children and society. You're a grown-up. As an adult, your responsibility is not just to feel, but to act ethically on those feelings. Don't shoot the messenger. Get over your regrets – understandable as they are – and do something useful about the issue. You're needed, and you can help. And you may well find that doing something constructive about the issue is a powerful therapy for how you feel as well. It helps me to know my son's needless suffering has protected other children from harm – though it doesn't lessen his pain or make his life any easier, or his child less at risk of allergy!

I hope, above all, that when parents are distraught because of infant distress, they realise that they do not have 'naughty' or 'demanding' or 'difficult' children, but children with problems, possibly in pain, who need their care, so that they can find that extra strength to endure fatigue and comfort their children. Our children are small for such a short time; we cannot spoil them with love and hugs, but we can and do spoil them for life by denial of their pain and distress, physical or emotional, and diets that begin with formula and progress to other convenience foods less kindly classified as junk (even though they too provide nutrients, and almost all nutrients could be claimed to 'support the immune system.')

If there are parents whose children have no problems at all as a result of artificial feeding from birth, I am sincerely glad they were so lucky. However, I have yet to meet any, myself. Conversations along those lines almost always begin with a assertive challenge that *their* children have not suffered from bottle-feeding, and me responding, how do you know? Somehow, as we keep talking, problems emerge – often in the mother's own history as well as the child's – that may well be linked to the fact of artificial feeding. So if we meet, don't tell me you have a child unscathed by formula, if you really don't want to know how it may have affected that child!

If you are indeed a parent whose children have had no obvious health or development problems associated with bottle-feeding from birth, please do not assert that no such problems exist for others, or for your children's children in future. You do not know that. Becoming an outspoken advocate for such an unnatural activity as formula feeding is a huge moral responsibility, and in the case of health professionals, could rightly be judged as ignorance, negligence, wilful blindness, or even unprofessional conduct. Other families will not be so lucky as to avoid all the risks. And pray that your grandchildren will be free of related problems from such an unnatural diet fed to their parents.

Some writers actively advocate bottle-feeding as equal to breastfeeding or better, on the basis of their own, or others,' experience of painful or failed breastfeeding, or the difficulty women have blending breastfeeding with paid employment. That's understandable, but still wrong. (Yes, I do think in terms of right and wrong, however many shades of grey lie between.) Maybe that would have been me, if my mother had not breastfed in the 1940s, if I had not come across Gunther's book, if I had been forced to take paid work instead of volunteering... I identify strongly with some of those pro-bottle writers, and they have some important things to say. But, bluntly, I know a lot more than they do about how breastfeeding works, and how it fails, and the effects of the alternatives, as their writing makes crystal clear. Despite the best of motives and understandable passion, they are demonstrably wrong in important ways. So I think parents should deal with any such formula fans as an aspiring Olympian would with any promising athlete knocked out of competition in their first year by injury. Such athletes may well be helpful as empathetic companions when one has a similar injury; their experience, well-understood, may teach others how to avoid injury or deal with it; they deserve commiseration and understanding, and not condemnation or blame, if they tried their best and circumstances defeated them. Whether athlete or breastfeeder, they are not failures *as people or as parents* if they tried, but just could not overcome the obstacles they faced.

But are failed athletes (or breastfeeders) useful guides to the many skills the aspiring Olympian (or breastfeeder) needs? In what other area of life is *not* achieving a goal seen as conferring expertise? It is the successful athlete who is sought as a mentor, although their training regimes will not be slavishly copied but adapted to the learner. The coach who pays no attention to his athletes' unique physiology and circumstances, but rigidly prescribes the regime that worked for *his* body, is not likely to be very successful! So too, successful breastfeeders are useful mentors, along with those health professionals who have learned from them – but only if they are aware of the unique nature of each and every breastfeeding relationship, and capable of translating lactation science into *individualised* practice, finding a common language that doesn't alienate the mother. A big ask for busy mother volunteers, so it's no wonder some are less than perfect.

Constraints on successful breastfeeding are multiple, and begin even before hospital practices interfere with the initiation of lactation. An excellent collection of essays, *Beyond health, beyond choice*,[2070] should be required reading for policymakers. Pressure on women to breastfeed without freeing them from the structural constraints that prevent them from succeeding simply creates a backlash against the very idea, which seems to place mothers between a rock and a hard place, and promotes division between women over this fundamental and irreplaceable women's work. I pointed that out three decades ago in *Breastfeeding matters*, and wish that more of those who write in this area had read that book in the 1980s! There is a lot of ignorant writing about infant feeding; and unfortunately, as someone – I wish I could remember who - said recently, 'Ignorance is invisible to those who suffer from it.'

So if the mother of a tiny baby must work (for whatever reason) in an environment that does not support breastfeeding, *it is not the mother,* but society, that has caused breastfeeding

---

2070  Smith PH, Hausman BL and Labbok M. *Beyond Health, Beyond Choice; breastfeeding constraints and realities.* (Rutgers University Press 2012)

failure. If society valued breastfeeding, every mother would be supported to both breastfeed and have income security for the first two to three years after birth, with an assured return to work option, and backup supplies of breast milk available to women.

This has been done in various places. France used to pay breastfeeding mothers – taxpayers' money well spent, reducing healthcare costs. Remember those ninety-five paid donors in Leipzig who produced 10 000 litres of milk above their babies' needs over a year? This meant that all hospitalised children under twelve months, and all gastrointestinal surgery cases under five years of age, could be fed breastmilk, with excellent results. Finland has supported parents to be at home with children under three, providing quality childcare facilities only for the age when socialisation is more beneficial to the child and less of a health risk. Not long ago it would have been unthinkable to park babies in mass institutional daycare. It still should be, now we know how stress affects infant brains.

But now in most Western countries mothers are being rewarded for leaving their very young babies in the care of others, many under-qualified, overworked, and under-paid. The uniquely female act of breastfeeding for the first two years of life is almost completely devalued: mothers and fathers are seen as interchangeable 'parents', although only women can breastfeed (usually!).[2071] These shifts in societal attitudes and practices create profits for the few who own the commercial care facilities, and for those who exploit women workers along with men, but huge costs for the whole of society.

But having said all that, a baby is part of a family in the present, here and now. Each family has to work out what is best for the whole group, and only they can do that, in the social context they inhabit now. At present that often means that both baby and mother's rights are dishonoured. Surviving in any national economy can mean needing to ignore basic biology and infant rights in order to meet basic shelter and food needs. Many women have very little choice about infant feeding, although 'choice' is the flagship industry largely created and has pushed for so long, as if their product allows women to make choices. (Well, it does, just uninformed and bad choices for the most part!)

Did I know any such, I would feel very sorry for the baby of a woman who decided to artificially feed for totally frivolous or selfish reasons, like the myths about breast shape being affected by breastfeeding.[2072] I would always feel sorry for any child of any parent who puts their own *wishes* or appearance ahead of their child's basic *needs*. But I don't know any such parents. All the parents that I know seem to make the best decisions they can for

---

2071  Cases of male lactation and breastfeeding are on record. See Ploss, Bartels op cit., vol 3 pp. 213-216.

2072  Having introduced this red herring, it should be said that fat is mobilised from the breast in pregnancy as glandular tissue increases, and re-deposited there as the glandular tissue involutes gradually – provided of course that the mother's diet contains enough calories for fat to be re-deposited gradually over a gentle weaning process. Studies suggest that women who eat normally postpartum and during weaning regain much the same breast size they were before lactation. Gravity ensures that over time all tissues sag, and a Japanese study found that wearing bras did not prevent this. So tight little apples on the chest rarely survive unchanged regardless of infant feeding method: and in fact the gentle curve they assume during pregnancy facilitates breastfeeding. Meanwhile, many, male and female, rejoice in the increased mass of functional breast tissue, providing enviable cleavage and great delight!

their children in their own circumstances, and based on the information they have and the experience life provides.

I grieve for the many mothers whose breastfeeding experience was a disaster, and who turned to artificial feeding in desperation. I am glad when I hear that their baby tolerated formula well, perhaps because of the breastfed start they provided with such difficulty. I know many such women, almost all of whom could have breastfed successfully with the right help at the right time. I have provided that hands-on help to some, and know how much that can mean, and how grateful parents are for being rescued when it seemed artificial feeding was inevitable.

Equally, I have grieved with mothers for whom rescue came too late, and whose pain and loss was then being trivialised by those ignorant about breastfeeding. I am glad that infant formula was affordable for them, but wish that it could have been other women's milk! At least I was able to explain to them the origins of their breastfeeding failure, perhaps relieve or prevent undeserved guilt, acknowledge and endorse their pain as the appropriate human response to the loss of a fundamental human experience, and perhaps increase maternal confidence with another lactation. (I know how much that successful second lactation can mean to a woman's sense of self.[2073]) And because I did that, sometimes I was able to help them with the negative consequences of formula feeding in their children – not all babies go on to formula and thrive immediately!

And let's be clear: 'breastfeeding failure' is the absolutely accurate, factual term, if the baby did not get breastmilk for at least some months before other foods were needed. But to say that lactation or *breastfeeding failed* does not mean that breastfeeding *had* to fail, or even more, that *the mother failed*, or *was a failure as a mother*! Regrettably, that is how many women experience their inability to provide milk for their baby for as long as they know would be ideal.[2074] We live in a society that encourages women to be quick to assume that their bodies (and often they themselves) are 'inadequate' and even 'faulty', and even where women are able to resist these feelings, they will quite rightly be sensitive to implications that they *should* feel that way! Such women need to be helped to understand that the failure was not theirs, but society's, and especially those institutions and individuals that had particular responsibility for their infant's health, or particularly profited from the faulty arrangements, or both. Societies and institutions can be changed once enough people get angry about the status quo! And grandparents can do a lot to make change if they are educated.

I know some parents will be upset by much of what is written in this tome. So they should be. It upset me to discover it all. But I know that we will get the social support needed to prevent such needless breastfeeding failure only when society is convinced that

---

2073 Women should be told that glandular tissue growth continues with each pregnancy, so that the chance of success in a second lactation is greater, especially if the mother gets skilled help from birth.

2074 And this cuts very deep. Sensible grandmothers have wept when they recounted the story of their failed lactation and its consequences. No amount of glib reassurance that formula did no harm touches the deep sense of inadequacy that some feel, and their suspicion of the link with their children's health problems. Once they understand how their own bodily mechanisms were interfered with by usual practices of the time, these women can become tigers in the defence of their daughters' lactation.

breastfeeding does matter, that formula feeding is just not good enough, especially for poor and disadvantaged children, who are those most likely to be formula-fed in Western society, and so further disadvantaged. Awareness is growing, but resistance is widespread. One fact of that resistance is the emergence of those who try to make advantaged literate bottle feeding mothers feel good about themselves by rubbishing the science that shows the problems of infant formula. Breastfeeding deniers are harming other women, and slowing the pace of needed social change. (Breastfeeding deniers are those who say breastfeeding is good only if it is what the mother wants, but bottle feeding is equally good for the baby if the mother thinks it's better for her. It is almost never better for either, just sometimes unavoidable for mostly avoidable reasons.)

Change in this area can happen in a generation, if we reach the parents-to-be, and set in place the supports they need. Finland[2075] and Norway did it; any country could. Most women still develop breasts and still lactate after childbirth; possibly more women than ever before successfully induce lactation without giving birth. (Once normal in many societies, unthinkable in ours, this is now an option considered by adopting parents or lesbian partners.) Lactation, the human survival mechanism, is still reliable, robust and resilient. Mothers still care for their children. The problem is formula-friendly cultures and vested interests that profit from the status quo, at the expense of the least advantaged and most vulnerable.

There are always multiple contributory factors for any death. Acknowledged deaths due to formula feeding may be rare in the best of circumstances,where governments make sanitation and healthcare and affordable supplies of product available to people living with clean water and cheap energy. Proving that any particular death is due to the lack of breastfeeding, or the fact of formula feeding, is not easy. But *every* needless death is a profound tragedy. (So is needless disease and dysfunction, and the personal and social costs associated with it.) And the role modelling of affluent parents influences poorer parents, so that we should see the deaths of poor children as our responsibility. The world cannot afford the tunnel vision that says breastfeeding doesn't matter in conditions of affluence.

Am I being needlessly alarmist, as no doubt industry hacks will allege? How can we know? Current research can't yet prove or disprove my thesis about the compounding intergenerational damage having been done by infant formula. It simply hasn't asked the right questions or gathered the right data to this point. Although there are clues in many places, such as the peanut allergy studies that showed an increasing prevalence through three generations.

> Peanut allergy was reported by 0.1% (3/2409) of grandparents, 0.6% (7/1213) of aunts and uncles, 1.6% (19/1218) of parents, and 6.9% (42/610) of siblings.[2076]

---

2075  It may be relevant that women played a much larger presence in legislative assemblies: Australia's first female federal MP was elected about the time Finland had a majority of women in government!

2076  Hourihane JO, Dean TP, Warner JO. Peanut allergy in relation to heredity, maternal diet, and other atopic diseases: results of a questionnaire survey, skin prick testing, and food challenges. (PMID:8789975) *BMJ* 1996; 313(7056):518-521. Free full text article

The data we do have tend to support my hypothesis. (One –bottle-fed- medical reader of an early draft stated that she considered the case proven, and hypothesis the wrong word to use! But in science there are only ever hypotheses, never certainty.) It makes sense to many who have heard me talk about it over the last decade. It's true in other animals: ask any successful breeder. It fits the facts. It incorporates and addresses weaknesses in the case for the hygiene hypothesis, and the microbial deprivation hypothesis, and interlocks with that other credible hypothesis, that widespread industrial and agricultural pollution is undermining human health and immune systems. Common sense says that all these things must be synergistic, when they act on living bodies. In a society with ever-increasing rates of allergy and immunological disorders, what evidence is there that we have 'safe' substitutes for the uniquely human food that has evolved to support and develop normal human immune systems?

In any society more babies will be sicker without breastmilk. The UK Millennium Cohort studies are just some of many that prove it.[2077]

> By 8 months of age, 12% of infants had been hospitalised ... an estimated 53% of diarrhea hospitalisations could have been prevented each month by exclusive breastfeeding and 31% by partial breastfeeding. Similarly, 27% of lower respiratory tract infection hospitalisations could have been prevented each month by exclusive breastfeeding and 25% by partial breastfeeding.

Of course fewer artificially fed babies now die in any community where water is clean, and infectious disease constrained, and antibiotics affordable; possibly 'only' around 720–1000 each year in the United States.[2078] The infant formula companies diligently push the idea that it is only environmental factors and parental carelessness that make artificial feeding a risk, and then persuade parents that a few extra additives here and there will make up for any possible cognitive or visual or immune deficits. (Which their previous formulas without those additives never caused?)

But it is *not* true that only in poor communities do babies die. In every society some babies do still die because of formula-feeding. If it were made mandatory to note accurately on death certificates what infants had been fed from birth and were being fed at the time of death, analysis could make that very obvious. It's just that more babies die in poor communities. A recent online forum saw a persistent formula-fan assert repeatedly that babies in Australia do not die because of artificial feeding. I wish it were true! To name just one of the more obvious examples, necrotising enterocolitis still kills preterm and even term bottle-fed babies in the developed world; and in fully breastfed infants it is almost completely unknown.

But yes, if one looks only at externals, fully dressed children in park play areas, it can be hard to tell apart the child who was breastfed from the child who wasn't. This is boringly

---

2077 Quigley MA, Kelly YJ, Sacker A. Breastfeeding and hospitalization for diarrheal and respiratory infection in the United Kingdom Millennium Cohort Study. (PMID:17403827) *Pediatrics* 2007, 119(4):e837-42.
2078 Chen A, Rogan WJ. Breastfeeding and the risk of postneonatal death in the United States.(PMID:15121986) *Pediatrics* 2004; 113(5):e435-9

often said, as though it proves something important. It doesn't. Of course formula-fed children look superficially normal, with the usual bodily structures. Genes do their work in pregnancy to create bodies. Formula feeding allows bodily growth within wide ranges that were defined as normal – based on populations that had already been largely formula-fed. And formula feeding has created allergy through generations, so that the many visibly allergic children (and mothers) in the park may have been breastfed or not.

Bottle-feeding creates a wide variety of orthodontic defects, but even this more external impact is not always glaringly obvious, as inherited facial shapes are very varied. Most people can't even spot in an adult face the tongue tie which made breastfeeding difficult, and its dental consequences, and that can be very obvious once you know what to look and listen for.

However, especially in the early days of formula-feeding, experienced child health nurses could once tell a breastfed baby by the quality of their skin, just like the hide merchants of New Zealand who saw and graded solely-mother-fed calf hides much higher than the hides of bucket-fed calves drinking cows' milk.[2079] There were no calves fed another species' milk as a comparison, naturally. This fact suggests that the mother-fed animal got additional benefits from milk tailored to their own needs, or perhaps experienced less stress, with visible results in skin quality. Some child health nurses now say that the latest formulas have reduced this obvious difference, and add 'but there is still something different about the fully-breastfed baby's skin'. And they are right, the differences can now be measured![2080]

So external signs of formula damage may not be readily obvious to those who have grown up seeing the results as 'normal'. What does that prove? The uncomfortable facts remain. *The infant who is not breastfed is always subtly or profoundly altered from the infant he or she would have been if breastfed by his or her mother.* Artificially fed infants are physiologically abnormal. Boys lay down more adipose tissue and girls more lean muscle mass, four-month-old boys have less testicular tissue and girls more ovarian cysts. The very composition of their body fat is different, as are the levels of different neurotransmitters in their bodies: both facts have implications for all central nervous system function. They must cope with a higher metabolic load and are at greater risk of metabolic diseases and cancer.

Artificially fed infants are abnormal compared with the breastfed infant: that is, they have deviated, in greater or lesser degree, from the pattern of development in their genes that breastmilk and breastfeeding would have potentiated. Why would anyone think there won't be consequences, or assume that the consequences will be benign? We could excuse past generations who saw formula-feeding expand (along with refrigeration and sanitation) and assumed the dropping death rate was proof of safety. We can't excuse such a lack of awareness nowadays. We know how the subtle development of infants before and after birth can be warped by even traces of potent chemicals. So those who want to proclaim to parents that formula feeding is safe need to *prove* that there are no adverse consequences

2079 Montagu A. *Touching: the human significance of the skin.* (Harper and Row 1986 3rd edition) p.90
2080 Simon Klenovics K, Kollárová R, Hodosy J, Celec P et al.Reference values of skin autofluorescence as an estimation of tissue accumulation of advanced glycation end products in a general Slovak population. (PMID:24111899) *Diabet Med* 2013

of warped developmental trajectories. And let's start looking more closely for the evidence of chromosomal damage and epigenetic changes produced by artificial feeding, and their consequences. Why has there been so little interest in such important research, so few MRI scans of developing brains, so few studies which control carefully for all details of feeding?

There are cultural explanations for our blindness, and the role and status of women in history is involved. Artificial feeds literally were *man*-made products. As a feminist I cannot but wonder: if men lactated, and women created formula, would anyone have ever thought it possible to match either men's milk, or its effects? So much of what has happened and is happening to babies is tied up with how their mothers are regarded in any given society.

Given their benighted attitudes to women, it is understandable that nineteenth-century men assumed they could create substitutes that would be as good as the milk any woman could produce – especially poor and hungry and dirty women. Understandable, but wrong.

Given the status of women in twentieth-century Western societies, it is understandable that women believed what advertising sold them. Understandable, but lamentable.

Given the context in which feminism emerged in some of those societies, it is understandable that otherwise intelligent women considered breastfeeding to be a needless constraint on their freedom. Again, understandable, but desperately sad. Sad for the women themselves and their babies, and those who heed their polemic.

A recent *New Scientist* article[2081] asked, 'How can we test if breast is best?' That is simply the wrong question. We don't have to prove breast is best, any more than we need to prove healthy kidneys are better than dialysis machines, or intact limbs better than prostheses. The burden of proof of safety and efficacy lies with those who want to support the unphysiological, the unnatural, the deviation from the human normal – not with those who think that, over millions of years, breastfeeding has evolved as normal human behaviour and a natural bridge between the womb and the world, both as exposure to, and protection from, a hostile environment. I really don't even have to prove that artificial infant formula instead of breastmilk is risky: *highly* unsafe, even fatal for some, subtly damaging to others. I would like to see a *New Scientist* article headed "How can we test that formula is safe?" Because we never have.

All the indications that have accumulated from science and history say to me that formula-feeding is risky. Basic science says it distorts normal development. The fact that artificial blood replacers can keep some people alive for a time has not created a global belief that human blood can be replaced. Why has the fact that formula can grow babies created a belief that human milk can be replaced? The American Academy of Pediatrics (AAP) once summed up bluntly about cheap coffee whiteners, then being used for infant feeding: 'Popularity, extravagant claims, and special marketing practices cannot make white liquids nutritionally equivalent to infant formula.'[2082] Nor can popularity, extravagant claims, and

2081  Wilson C, de Lange C. *New Scientist* 8 March 2014, p.11.
2082  AAP Committee on Nutrition. Imitation and Substitute Milks. *Pediatrics* 1984; 73:6 876

special marketing practices make infant formula equivalent to breastmilk. Yet that is why formula *is thought to be* equivalent by too many people. It's time that all health authorities told the truth about infant feeding to parents, and just as bluntly as that AAP defence of infant formula against inferior competitors. The Royal College of Pediatrics and Child Health (RCPCH) has made a start: the NHS-funded e-Learning for Health (e-LfH) Healthy Child Programme overseen by the College and endorsed by many other organisations says categorically:

> The only accepted alternative to breast milk for infants up to 6 months of age is infant formula which supports bodily growth along parameters different from those of the breast-fed child, and provides no immunity against disease. Many of the health outcomes of breastfeeding compared to formula feeding are dose-related: that is, better outcomes are associated with longer duration and exclusive breastfeeding, or less exposure to infant formula.'[2083]

All bad choices have consequences. Rarely good ones. Yet in every generation most people, including most healthworkers, have expressed blind faith in all contemporary artificial feeding products – while simultaneously seeing previous versions as unsuitable for infant feeding! Without definitive proof, they have believed every new additive is important – and without wondering how much damage the prior absence of that additive must have caused if it is important. Most have seen no inherent contradiction in trusting so blindly, as others have trusted before, in fallible manufactured products produced by fallible human employees working in incredibly complex systems for companies making massive profits.

Most have also seen no ethical conflict in accepting freebies and subsidies and high salaries from formula manufacturers, and so increasing the absurdly high costs of formula for poor families. When malnourished infants present in clinics, such people do not connect the hungry baby and desperate family, or the obese toddler, or the wheezing schoolchild, with the lavish dinner industry paid for at their last professional conference or meeting. As I know all too well, we humans are very good at screening out inconvenient truths, facts that might make for personal inconvenience or serious reorganisation of the society we're doing quite nicely in.

Many of the minority aware of the defective nature of all substitutes keep quiet in the face of overwhelming concern about the societal impact of telling the truth, and sometimes, for fear of being thought 'extreme'. It will make mothers feel guilty or anxious, I am told, as though suppressing truth can be justified in those terms. What is being said there, is that it makes *us* feel uncomfortable, that we don't want to have to be the bearers of unpleasant truths, as we all know what happens to messengers bearing bad news.

Knowledge is power. It is also a burden that creates responsibilities. We are not caring about women when we deny them truth about what their milk can do for their children, and indeed their own long term health. We are complicit in — indeed, we bear more responsibility for — any harms that may result from their bad choices, whether that is more cases of breast cancer in mothers or lower IQ in children.

---

2083 Check out the URL http://www.e-lfh.org.uk/healthy-child

Yet many professional organisations which should be standing up for breastfeeding, and holding their members to account for the standard of care and support they provide to ensure breastfeeding succeeds – professional bodies for general practitioners, obstetricians, paediatricians, nurses and even midwives – are failing in this respect. Most do not even mandate adequate basic education about lactation. Most do not make and publicise unequivocal statements about the dangers of artificial feeding to members, policy-makers and the general public. Most do not see any connection between donations they accept from formula corporations and their willingness to accept the idea that, whatever the theoretical 'benefits' of breastmilk, in practice formula is an acceptable alternative, or even default, feeding method.

Even breastfeeding organisations in the past have concentrated on 'being positive rather than negative', as though highlighting breastmilk's advantages will have much effect while people presume that our modern formulas have become 'so close to breastmilk that it doesn't really matter what you feed the baby'. Organisations can be seduced by respectability. Sometimes this means wanting the good opinion of the powerful, whether medical men or politicians or media personalities. Sometimes it's just a failure of imagination to see that society could change, usually by those doing quite nicely as society is now ordered. Other times it means not wanting to upset vocal, intelligent formula advocates. And, as I know, it can mean the speaker distancing him or herself publicly from what has been said in private. Self-censorship takes many forms.

Similarly, those who wish to use the infant formula issue as a way of making multinational industry accountable seem to me not to have always paid enough attention to the realities of different infant formula products and the effect of their actions on market share[2084] and infant health. While infant formula remains necessary, it needs to be both affordable and adequate, or infants and families suffer. Discouraging the use of one brand over another without being sure of potential impacts on child health seems to me unethical, especially when there is little to choose between companies when it comes to marketing concerns, as this history demonstrates. Babies need to be given the best product available, even when we might dislike intensely its maker. And independent regulatory authorities making industry accountable for infant formula quality is at least as important as making it accountable for its unethical marketing.

I am glad to see that breastfeeding advocacy is finally getting some teeth, being willing to tell truths in ways that make them heard, despite the protests and slander this draws. It's overdue, even if many people still don't like it, and leap to the conclusion that it's those 'breastfeeding nazis' wanting to make them feel uncomfortable or guilty. (No, *it's just not about you at all*: it's about trying to stop the next generation being damaged. The world does not revolve around you.)

But I would be a rich woman if I had a dollar for every healthworker who has said to me that he or she cannot tell the truth about artificial feeding for fear of upsetting superiors, colleagues,

---

2084 Having said this for thirty years, I'm glad to see signs of improvement in this area over the last decade. But this still needs saying.

mothers, whoever. (I also know of some who have lost jobs they loved because they spoke truths unpalatable to the powerful.[2085]) I'd like a dollar for every director of an organisation who has said that his or her organisation cannot tell the truth because it would upset the members, or lead to reduced support for the organisation from funding bodies, or medical personnel, or government; or it would reduce their ability to raise money. I'd love a dollar for every breastfeeding book I have read which includes infant formula as the ultimate solution for persistent breastfeeding problems, without giving any warnings about how much worse things might become, and how careful mothers need to be about dealing with an intrinsically hazardous product. Then there's journalists writing without thinking critically about issues of women's so-called choice in infant feeding...More than one popular baby-care author has told me that it's good for *me* to tell the truth, and they love my writing, but they cannot write what they really think about formula feeding because their sales would suffer.

Truth does not make anyone popular when it is a deeply inconvenient truth. Which this is. I understand, but I really am very tired of such excuses. And at almost seventy years of age I have nothing to lose, and perhaps not much more time to make any difference. So I say, as I have said before:

Every person who behaves like that is part of the problem, and helps ensure the success of artificial feeding. Each person who fails to speak up plainly and clearly is making it that much harder for everyone else to speak up, the profound moral problem known as Bystander Effect, where everyone assumes someone else will fix things. (After all, if it were that bad, 'they' wouldn't let them sell it.)

If every member of the 'they' establishment is too ignorant or cowardly, too swayed by the comfort of their current non-controversial position, then those who are brave enough to tell the full, unvarnished truth will be attacked as extremists by well-resourced vested interests, and the truth will remain hidden or be ignored.

If anyone in a position of authority, such as a policymaker or health professional or journalist or public figure, stands by while this happens, rather than:

- audibly speaking the truth
- visibly supporting others who speak the truth
- and ensuring that any community to which she or he belongs is shaping its policy and behaviour around the truth

*then, in my view, that person bears some responsibility for the myth of formula as a 'safe alternative' and all the deaths and problems that causes.*

As a sign seen many years ago in Palmerston North bookshop put it, 'Taking paths of least resistance makes rivers – and people – crooked.'

---

2085 For an example, read Needleman HL (2008) The Case of Deborah Rice: Who Is the Environmental Protection Agency Protecting? *PLoS Biol* 6(5): e129. doi:10.1371/journal.pbio.0060129 I know of cases closer to home, and I salute those women for having the courage of their convictions.

It's time to be straight with parents.

We need plain speaking about the risks of infant formula or any substitute for women's milk, not just the 'benefits of breastfeeding'.

We need to insist that someone "feeling uncomfortable" seeing or hearing about breastfeeding is exactly why we must talk about it and see it in public, until it becomes normal and comfortable again. And that talk includes stating clearly, unambiguously, and unapologetically to society at large, and the young in particular, that giving babies formula is risky and alters normal development – and that it may have altered them, and their children to come.

Stop and think:

- How far would anti-obesity campaigns have come if policymakers had censored all discussion of the health hazards of excessive dietary fat, refused to do the research in crucial areas, and then run a campaign on the joys of eating low-fat foods, all the while assuring the public that high-fat foods were so close to low-fat as to not make much difference really, and after all, people must be free to make their own choices? Why weren't such campaigns worried about upsetting the many fat people? Wouldn't obese people like to know that the problem may stem from past actions of others, as much or more than from their own?

- How much good would road safety campaigns do if they chose to say only that 'driving sober is best', and not talk about the consequences of driving under the influence? If we knew of some rare few who genuinely *had* to drive while intoxicated – or if we knew that drink driving was common and people thought it safe – would concern about those people's feelings prevent us telling the truth about the proven risks of drink-driving?

- Can you seriously imagine a successful anti-smoking campaign that merely celebrated how great fresh air is for you and your unborn child, and downplayed all extreme talk of dangerous pollutants causing respiratory disease as being unproven? Acceptance of that dead-obvious truth came centuries after the commonsense concern, and some still dispute this as unproven. Why was it necessary to prove the bleeding obvious? Because vested interests refused to act responsibly.

Every new baby is a new beginning. Infant feeding is one of the few health-related variables that can be readily addressed and changed if there is political will to do so, as there was in Scandinavia in the 1970s. Again, from less than 30 per cent of mothers ever breastfeeding in 1968, Norway now has almost universal breastfeeding, and has mandated universal paid breastfeeding breaks. Why do so many scientists refuse to draw obvious conclusions and spell them out for politicians to hear and act on? Is this due to ignorance about the influence they could exert, fear of the personal consequences if employed by industry, or a belief that scientists have no such responsibility? Is it because they think adults are more important than babies? (If so, how many adults were never babies, or were unaffected by their infancy?) Was that how they arranged their own lives as parents, and do they not want to consider or admit any possible negative consequences? Is it because they believe that Western society cannot be changed, and so there is no point in telling truths that may upset women especially? Are they afraid of the vocal backlash from formula advocates?

I won't waste trees on a detailed critique of serious formula advocates. Their examination and understanding of the infant feeding evidence is poor, and they blithely defame those they disagree with, using deeply insulting language, so they find a welcome in populist mass media publications that support the status quo of profiteers in Western society. Is this because the corporations that sell formula also sell many other products, and buy advertising space for all of them, and give dividends to shareholders? Or just that controversy and rudeness sell papers in a culture foully debased by shock jocks and spin artists? Will the shock jocks seize on this book because controversial, or ignore it because it demands change to the comfortable status quo they inhabit?

Formula advocates who frame infant feeding as a matter of lifestyle choice have to believe that artificial feeding doesn't make any important difference to child health. They don't begin with the basic assumption that millions of years of mammalian evolution must have provided a safer food for infants than a hundred years of commercially-driven industrial science. That science has stumbled from discovery to discovery over the bodies of hapless infants and their mothers. Professor Jacqueline H Wolf has written a superb article[2086] summarising a feminist approach to this issue. Read some of it in Appendix 2 and be shocked. Did that scandal get worldwide airplay? Why not?

Just how much of this silence is due to vested interests, financial and emotional? Why do so many people fail to be open about their own experience, and how this affects their perception of these issues? I think it important for all participants in the infant feeding dialogue both to disclose their own infant feeding stories, and to make explicit any financial (including in-kind and institutional) interests they have that depend on artificial feeding. Parents need to be able to identify the pharmacist whose family income depends on selling infant formula, who has for years has assured mothers that current formulas are close to breastmilk, and who thus may feel a need to defend the product. When such a person writes in popular blogs, for example, their interests should be made very public, not concealed behind other, apparently impartial or authoritative, affiliations or memberships. [I am thinking of at least one I have come across online..For blog readers: always Google those who badmouth breastfeeding advocates – if you can spare the time, you may be surprised by what you discover. And ignore any cowards who hide behind anonymity.]

However, breastfeeding advocates need to be aware that adverse criticism is not always the result of emotional bias, vested financial interest, or interpretations of poorly defined research parameters. (Though there is a fascinating literature review waiting to be done examining exactly these factors and their relationship to research findings.) Many criticisms, including criticism of this book, may well be accurate and well-justified. But in a field with so much money and emotion at stake, and so much poorly defined research on record,

---

2086 Wolf, J. What Feminists Can Do for Breastfeeding and What Breastfeeding Can Do For Feminists. *Signs, Journal of Women in Culture and Society* 2006; 31 (2): 397-424

it is reasonable to ask everyone involved in the debate publicly to declare all the factors *other than empirical evidence and basic logic* that might give us incentives to draw particular conclusions. How else can parents judge our conflicting opinions?

This is why I have chosen to add an outline of my own lifetime of experience and independent and voluntary involvement, and its consequences for my children as Appendix 3. For anyone to think they are not affected by their own feeding history – both as babies and how they fed their babies – is laughable. We are human. Our thoughts and feelings interact. Of course we may instinctively reject the idea that any early exposure to infant formula is harmful if we now have children with problems of immune dysfunction or cognition. I was appalled to realise what my ignorance had allowed to happen to my child. It hurt me every time my son (and the whole family) suffered as a result. It takes effort, even courage, to get beyond feelings, to accept our mistakes and to try to prevent harm to *other* people's children.

AF Robertson wrote an excellent series of three articles reviewing some medical mistakes of the twentieth century. He concluded:

> Everyone will extract different lessons from these tales. Certainly, we should be more aware of neonatal physiology when we consider new treatments. We should not presume safety unless proven by adequate studies. We should be wary of all procedural changes. Hospital administration should ensure the education of ancillary personnel about the susceptibilities of infants so that no change in hospital procedure can occur without the consideration of its effect on babies. And we should be skeptical of authoritative opinions. This requirement is difficult since most of us are authoritarian by nature and experience. As Dr. Silverman states, 'Physicians depend, more than ever, on the judgments and opinions of authorities because of an exponential increase in scientific information and an increase in the complexity of medicine'
>
> For those of us who may be the educators, he continues, 'Authoritative lecturers should stimulate their listeners to responsible contemplation of incomplete evidence, instead of irresponsible, unrestrained action.'[2087]

I hope above all, that this book contributes to responsible contemplation of the (currently incomplete, but to me, damning) evidence that artificial feeding's inevitable damage is echoing and accumulating through populations and generations.

And I hope that impartial readers will conclude, as I have, that mothers' milk matters.

Matters now, and for the future.

As Cow & Gate once used to say, without challenge from health professionals:

> 'What we feed them now matters forever.'

As Australians once used to say, "Too bloody right it does."

---

2087 Robertson AF. Reflections on errors in neonatology III. The "experienced" years, 1970 to 2000. (PMID:12732863) *J Perinatol* 2003, 23(3):240-249

# Is this you? A story heard too often

*Read this and highlight the bits that resonate for you.*

All your life you have struggled with body issues, from a need to control your weight as a child, to anorexia in your teens. You conquered the anorexia, but could never 'let yourself go': the kilos just seemed to pile on at the first excuse. By contrast your younger sister always seemed fashionably thin and never put on weight (though she was later diagnosed with irritable bowel disease and then gluten intolerance). Diagnosed with depression in your twenties, you were prescribed psychiatric drugs, which left you feeling unsure what moods were you, and what side-effects of the drug. You eventually succeeded in getting off medication before getting pregnant at the age of thirty-eight, with the help of IVF technology.

The birth was a terrible shock, ending with an operative delivery, separation from your baby, and difficulty establishing breastfeeding. You found the help offered very confronting, confusing, and not always helpful. Fortunately one midwife was able to help you get your baby breastfeeding well. So lactation got underway and after four days you were discharged from hospital, an at-risk breastfeeding mother with an abdominal wound, and a baby who had been given small amounts of formula in the early days, when you were unable to get him latched on well, and staff were afraid that he needed 'something to prevent jaundice'.

The first few nights at home were scary. You hardly slept. Wound pain didn't help, and you were listening for noises from the baby swaddled in his cot. You got up to offer feeds or to check that he was still OK. You resented your partner who slept through it all, and thought breastfeeding a great idea because it meant there was no need for him to get up to the baby. At the end of that first week your mother came to stay, as you were exhausted. She was supportive of the idea of you breastfeeding, but disclosed to you that she had not been able to breastfeed, so you had been formula fed from three weeks with a new modern American formula that was so much better than the Lactogen she had been fed in 1946. She felt that perhaps you were trying too hard, that perhaps, like her, you could not make enough milk, that it would be better for baby if you were calmer and less distressed. And as you and she had both turned out perfectly fine, why not just let her get on with bottle-feeding baby while you recovered from that surgical wound?

This caring support created a lot of stress, as you were determined to breastfeed; you knew other women who had experienced worse starts and now were very happy they had not given up. After a week your mother left, as she had to get back to her doctor for a diabetes review; her long-standing eczema had suddenly flared from the stress of your situation and a lack of sleep, so she needed a new prescription for cortisone creams. And then in the third week, baby started to cry inconsolably and unpredictably for hours every single day, with what seemed like acute gut distress.

So you tried, but you failed to breastfeed for very long. It seemed pointless when your baby was crying inconsolably, obviously not thriving on your milk, despite frequent feeding. You wondered whether there was something wrong with your milk, or you couldn't produce enough. Sleepless nights made you depressed and exhausted. You tried supplementing with this and that formula, hoping to make baby grow, as he was hungry, you thought. All to no avail. You consulted a number of healthworkers, who told you different things, including that 'crying is normal and he will grow out of it', or that 'you need to relax as the baby can sense your distress and is reacting to that'. Your doctor told you it's reflux, and time will fix it. (Or you could try some thickened formula.) You could see that your baby was unhappy, and it made you feel desperate. Your partner repeated the suggestion that you were too tense and should relax, precipitating a major row.

When blood appeared in your baby's nappy, you were referred to a paediatrician. He told you that your baby might be allergic to your milk, and suggested a formula labelled HA for hypoallergenic. (Another might suggest rather arbitrary diet changes, difficult to implement when you are so sleep-deprived and disorganised. You might have tried this and found it did not work – although your baby seemed to improve for a few days, it all fell apart for some unknown reason.) Finally, when you kept coming back because the baby was still miserable, and now his eczema was worse, you were prescribed mood-altering medications once again, and your baby was prescribed an extensively hydrolysed infant formula. There was not much improvement, so the prescription was changed to an elemental formula, containing synthetic amino acids, and no natural protein. Success at last: no more blood in the nappy, eczema calming down, a calmer baby who gained weight and smiled, perhaps for the first time, at twenty weeks. But you were no longer breastfeeding, and felt very sad.

When you had rung your mother in tears at ten weeks to tell her how things were going, she disclosed that you had been just such a miserable baby, and suggested several old-fashioned remedies for dealing with wind and colic, saying that Phenergan had been a life-saver for her, although you were always grumpy next day. She learned to cope with only a few hours sleep each night, and reassured you that you would too. She suggested various creams to use if the small rough patches on baby's cheeks developed into eczema. You asked about the thickening cradle cap and the crusts behind baby's ears; the redness that seemed to arise everywhere that baby's drool settled on skin, and the inflammation on baby's rear end after every wee or poo. Zinc cream was suggested, but you wondered why baby's skin was so sensitive that it reacted that way. Obviously baby had inherited your partner's sensitive skin.

For he had been an eczematous bottle-fed baby: your mother-in-law recalled with pride that he had been 'a lovely big Similac/Lactogen/Cow & Gate baby'. He outgrew the eczema by the time he was five, and had been 'a typical boy': hyperactive and unwilling to sit still for any length of time, prone to tantrums and 'strong-willed'. He had been more than a bit of a handful at school, and left school early to work in a hands-on trade, where he did well, employing others to do the bookwork. He still has dry skin, which he's learned to live with, though it can get uncomfortable in cold weather, when it cracks, and affects his work. He wheezes a bit if he exercises too much, and has always been prone to bronchitis. But if asked, he would say that he is perfectly healthy, fit as a fiddle, as he has always played sport and generally eats well (though he too finds that weight gain is very rapid if his physical activity decreases). He does have some food fads, and won't drink plain milk as he thinks it smells awful, but can cope with cooked milk in foods. He also has a lot of sinus problems. But his mother assures you that he has never had any allergies.

You see your partner's bronchitis as asthma, and hope it won't get worse. His snoring and irritating little night cough don't help you sleep. Nor does your own 'tricky gut'. Stress seems to affect your innards, which are prone to both constipation and diarrhoea. You often feel bloated and fat, and this has always fed into your body-image problems. You've thought about investigations for inflammatory bowel disease. Your younger sister suggested limiting the amount of gluten in your diet. This improved the gut problems (though you still have them, especially before a period. Your once-regular premenstrual migraines disappeared with pregnancy, and you hope they won't return, as you just couldn't cope with a crying baby and a migraine. Now if only you had a bit more energy – you lost quite a bit of blood in surgery and post-partum and had no transfusion – you too would say you were healthy.

That could be you at twenty weeks post-partum. I could write another scenario months down the track, as you struggle to widen your allergic baby's diet, or years later as you cope with a child with eczema and ADHD or other learning disabilities. The scenario would be quite different if you were a poor mother with little English: there is almost no chance that you would have seen a paediatrician and had expensive formula prescribed, and you would still be struggling with a baby in distress, while perhaps being offered support in parenting skills ...

I haven't touched on your typical food cravings and aversions past and present, which have sometimes caused your mother to comment how you never liked that food as a child (but of course you were made to eat it). She tells you how she had made herself eat lots of good foods she didn't really like when carrying you. In that pregnancy she had to be ingenious in disguising the taste of some of those that the doctors and nurses told her she must eat: milk she couldn't bear plain, ever since being forced to drink the free school milk, but she could manage milk in cooking or as cheese, or with chocolate flavouring. She had sympathised with you over pregnancy nausea, and said it must run in the family, as both she and your grandma had experienced the same problem every pregnancy, but she was proud that she still got down the two pints of milk she was told to drink each day.

Your great-grandma could not afford to buy formula in the 1920s, so had breastfed your grandma for nine months, then weaned her on to milk from the local dairy. Grandma birthed your mum in 1946; your mum had kept crying for feeds every couple of hours, so she had to be given Lactogen to last four hours between feeds. (The clinic sister said she must wait, or baby would be spoiled, a rod for her mother's own back.) Grandma's milk dried up altogether by eight weeks, and she got pregnant again in the next couple of months with your auntie. (Who, like your mother, has recently developed diabetes.)

You were born in the early seventies, your mother's first child, in a hospital supplied with free infant formula. Your mum went home with a tin, which she started you on after two weeks of trying to breastfeed every three to four hours. Grandma had been there to help her, just as Mum was there for you, and Grandma reassured your mum that modern formulas were great, that she had grown big and strong on Lactogen and so would you. Your mum instead paid more to get the modern American brand the hospital had used, since she knew they chose that brand because it was the best. The clinic sister supported her choice, saying that the new products would cause fewer constipation problems.

Like you, great-grandma, grandma and your mum all made their choices based on what they thought was best for their babies. And the healthcare system failed every one of those mothers, yourself included. And subtle genetic changes were accumulating in each generation, so that your baby is more sensitive than you were.

## Do you recognise yourself in this history?

How much have you highlighted in the above? I know many people who would recognise more than a little of their own history, or their partner's, in this outline. This book is written in the hope that your children or grandchildren will have fewer problems than both our families have experienced to date, as a direct result of well-meaning but utterly misguided advice about infant feeding. The myth of the safety of artificial feeding may be almost universal, but alas, I have to agree with Bertrand Russell when he said,

'The fact that an idea has been widely held is no evidence that it isn't utterly absurd. Indeed, in view of the silliness of the majority of mankind, a widespread belief is more likely to be foolish than sensible.'

We are silly indeed if we think that laboratories can ever create an affordable, risk-free substitute for women's milk. A century of artificial feeding has taught us one thing: milk makes us, and we make our children, so milk matters.

# APPENDIX 2

# About guilt and responsibility

If any mother flippantly chooses to formula-feed, say for reasons of vanity, knowing all the real risks and possible harms, then for her to feel guilty would be the appropriate human emotion, and I'd be glad she felt it. Guilt might engender regret. Regret would be progress towards adult maturity: in future such a mother might think more of her baby's basic needs and less of her own wants, and so not have to deal with guilt feelings next time round – though still with regret.

However, the irony is that any such egocentric mother almost never would feel guilty, insulated by her selfishness. Those mothers who *do* feel guilty are those who have no reason to – all those hard-pressed mothers who try, who do their best, and fail to reach their goal despite pain and effort, or who choose the most expensive formula convinced that this would be better for their baby than any milk their imperfect body, on its imperfect diet, could produce.

For the capacity to feel guilt involves awareness of falling short, or of wrongdoing; it means the person has an ideal they aspire to, that of the best possible care for their baby. The truly self-centred don't feel guilty, because they assume that the world should revolve around them. Rather, the selfish get very annoyed that anyone has the temerity to raise questions about their conduct by thinking or speaking differently, or by not endorsing their decision as a good one for their baby. And they then accuse others of 'trying to make them feel guilty' – a judgment about other people's unknowable motives – when those others, breastfeeding advocates, may in fact be trying to help children for whom the decision is not yet made. (And breastfeeding advocates usually have helped countless others, often gratis.)

That sounds judgmental. It is. I don't apologise for it. I'm making a judgment; fallible, but mine. We shouldn't kid ourselves that we are never judgmental, or even accept the current truism that being so is wrong. Having brains and ethical values, we make judgments all the time. So we should. Some judgments are informed by compassion, reason, knowledge of the facts and understanding, and some are grossly unfair, irrational, ignorant and unkind; with some we get things right and some we get them wrong. (Yes, I think judgments and actions can be right or wrong, ever though reality is rarely black and white and we deal in shades of grey!) Every society and its members judges parents according to complex norms and criteria, for all the fashionable talk in Western society about being non-judgmental. Deciding with no evidence that someone's intention is to *make you feel guilty* is making an unfair judgment. Deciding that *you do feel guilty* is all your own work (and you might be right or wrong as to whether guilt is appropriate. Ask a brave friend!)

How we interact with any individual depends on the role we have, and our responsibilities. For a midwife to be boorishly insensitive and tactless when being paid to be supportive of a fragile new mother is utterly wrong. Equally, so is the midwife not telling the mother a truth the midwife suspects that the mother does not want to hear. 'She needed me to give her permission to wean' implies that health professionals can legitimately make a decision that is the mother's own. Supporting a mother is not the same as endorsing bad decisions – or creating them by withholding crucial, sensitive information, or treating a woman like a child and making decisions for her.

Health professionals need to state what is best for maternal and infant health and how to achieve it, where we know that: that's part of the job. And we do *know*, for a certainty, that in general breastfeeding is best for mother and baby alike, not to mention our society and our planet. It may not be possible for an individual mother, it may not make an obvious difference to an individual baby, but that doesn't alter the truth that breastfeeding is a critically important public health and environmental issue, and that the milk we feed our children matters into the next generations.

One person feels *guilty* when they recognise they did less than their best for a child; another feels *angry* because they did not know what the decision to formula-feed involved by way of risk. If speaking that truth makes the truly guilty feel bad, tough. If the innocent feel bad, they need support and de-briefing – and an understanding that regret is not guilt. It is true that no one can make another person feel guilty: how they *feel* is their own responsibility, and grown-ups do something about their feelings, not just wail or mope.

Despite any negative feedback, those who know the truth must go on telling it, and in plain language, because the stakes are too high to let *those already damaged and those with vested interest in the status quo* enforce a silence that will damage *yet more* mothers and children.

There are many vested interests that would prefer that this information about infant formula risks and realities is not widely known, some for financial reasons, other for more complex reasons. But all those who fail to communicate it clearly must take some responsibility for the continuing toll of death and damage that infant formula wreaks on hapless infants given no choice but to bottle-feed.

For example, for a group to list artificial feeding as a risk factor for SIDS may well make someone feel uncomfortable: formula-feeding parents are disproportionately represented in SIDS groups, precisely because it *is* a risk factor. The desire to say publicly 'no, feeding wouldn't have made any difference', is totally understandable. And in an individual case, it may –or may not- be true: how can we know?

But most parents who use formula do so after trying to breastfeed and not getting the help they need. They are *victims*; by definition they are not guilty, and rather than guilt should feel anger, that an avoidable failure to help them breastfeed might have been a factor in the death of their beloved children. Their acceptance of that truth, and their natural anger, might save another child.

It might be their own next child.

Some families have more than one SIDS death. That second child might have died *because* they believed those who told them that their feeding choice didn't make any difference to the risk of death, when it clearly does, and always did. Breastfeeding that second child might have prevented the death.

I know of one such case not far from where we lived in rural Australia. It was utterly devastating for that family, and if one or both deaths could have been prevented at the cost of making some people squirm, and others feel sad (until they realise that they are not to blame), a little social discomfort – for them or me – is a small price to pay.

Breastfeeding is a major health intervention, not a small difference. Artificial feeding *is* a risk factor for unexpected infant death. So how could we tolerate the statement 'Breastfeed if you can'? What subliminal message does that give? 'That breastfeeding is often not possible?' 'That it's not all that important?' 'That this recommendation matters less than the others in the list stated dogmatically?' All those subliminal messages are profoundly harmful and undermining of breastfeeding as a normal activity that women can succeed at, even if it does require some perseverance, like any other complex human activity.

Think about the wording. No SIDS group says 'Sleep baby on his back *if you can*'. (Lots of parents can't, or there'd be no market for all the restraints sold to keep babies tethered flat.) Or 'Don't smoke *if possible*' (and that's a major addiction which many people can't beat). 'Breastfeed if you can'? Well, without a double mastectomy, breast reduction surgery, or some rare disorder, there's a very good chance that you can, physically speaking. A better chance than that an addicted smoker will quit, or that babies will stop rolling onto their stomachs. Lactation is a basic survival mechanism, not some tricksy stunt that only the elite athlete can manage. It makes no sense in evolutionary terms to waste huge maternal resources creating a baby that will starve to death. As the baby grows, so does the mother's lactational capacity.

And if women can't breastfeed, for economic reasons, or because of discrimination or abuse they might face, or because the medical profession doesn't know enough about this vital biological process to give them the support they need, that's a bloody scandal, now we know how much breastfeeding matters. I use the great Australian adjective deliberately, as infant deaths result from the lack of breastfeeding.[2088]

Parents shouldn't just accept this status quo, but find out what the problem is. Demand that breastmilk be made available. Societies can arrange that. As I mentioned on page 117, I visited a bank where just ninety-five donors produced 10,000 litres a year above their own children's needs. It was seen as valuable by donors and recipients, and the women were paid for their milk, their own health and that of their child monitored and protected, and poor women had some extra income.

Society invests vast resources to supply human blood, semen, eggs, and tissue transplants. Human milk can be supplied far more easily, as women can readily increase production. (For some, it would be the perfect weight loss programme and stress buster!) That is, if vested interest groups (often representing those already harmed by or profiting from artificial feeding) don't keep undermining women's confidence in the possibility, or giving them excuses to not try, or to distrust those who can help them succeed.

Major campaigns have also changed parental awareness of the dangers of secondhand smoke to their children, and a smoke-free atmosphere in public places has become the sensible norm. That was inconceivable in the 1980s, when it could seem extreme to ask people not to smoke in your own home. Major campaigns have led to infants being put to sleep on their backs; to child car restraints being used; to seatbelt use by adults; to greater immunisation uptake. And in every single public health campaign involving parental care, risk and fear has been used as a motivating factor. Consider Australia's 'Never shake a baby' campaign: 'I only shook him for a few seconds, but he'll be blind for a lifetime ... every year thousands of babies suffer blindness, brain damage or even death.' *Why is talk of risks not acceptable as a strategy for reducing needless artificial feeding, which can cause harm not only for a lifetime but into the next generations? Why, when – as the advertisements in this book illustrate- the industry has always used and continues to use fear and other emotions to sell its inferior product to parents?*

Why? Because too much money is at stake, and governments and professional groups seem to be *afraid* to confront either the financially powerful or society's woefully ignorant formula fantasists. Consider what happened in the United States. Here I am publishing (with permission) an account written by Professor Jacqueline Wolf, whose book, *Don't Kill Your Baby,* should be required reading for health professionals, as should the whole of the article she wrote,[2089] from which this lengthy excerpt comes.

> In 2003 and 2004 ... an extraordinary public squabble occurred among infant formula companies, the U.S. Department of Health and Human Services (HHS), the American Academy of Pediatrics (AAP), and the Ad Council (McCullough 2003; Petersen 2003). The

---

2088  Chen and Rogan calculated at least 720 deaths each year in the USA alone. See Chen A, Rogan WJ. Breastfeeding and the risk of post-neonatal death in the United States. *Pediatrics* 2004; 113 (5) e: 435-439. DOI:

2089  Wolf JH. What feminists can do for breastfeeding and what breastfeeding can do for feminists. *Signs: Journal of Women in Culture and Society.* 2006; 31(2) pp. 398-424. ©University of Chicago Press; permission granted for reproduction.

disagreement should have been condemned as evidence of what U.S. scientists charge is the Bush administration's suppression and distortion of science to further its political agenda (Union of Concerned Scientists 2004). But while the scientific community has roundly criticized the refusal to fund stem cell research and the suppression of Environmental Protection Agency studies, the Bush administration's censorship of information about breastfeeding received relatively scant attention. Feminist involvement in breastfeeding advocacy might at least have gotten the matter the attention it deserved, in the same way that the media reported the refusal of the Food and Drug Administration to allow emergency contraception to be purchased over the counter despite overwhelming evidence of its safety. The uproar began when infant formula company representatives prevailed on the AAP leadership and Tommy Thompson, appointed secretary of HHS by George W. Bush, to quash a series of public service announcements (PSAs) about breastfeeding designed by the Ad Council, a consortium of the country's top advertising agencies that come together to offer personnel to design PSAs pro bono. Prompted by formula company concerns, HHS insisted that key elements be cut from the planned campaign. Feminist organizations never protested, although the editing of the ads undermined the right of U.S. women to get accurate medical information in order to make informed decisions about infant feeding. Although few think of formula as a public health threat, David Satcher, the U.S. Surgeon General under Bill Clinton, did. When he authored the HHS Blueprint for Action on Breastfeeding in 2000, he termed breastfeeding "one of the most important contributors to infant health," dubbed low breastfeeding rates in the United States "a public health challenge," and called for "national, culturally appropriate strategies to promote breastfeeding." Public service announcements were one of his proposed strategies (Department of Health and Human Services Office on Women's Health 2000, 3). Prompted by Satcher's call, the Ad Council announced in June 2002 that its next major campaign would publicize the importance of breastfeeding to health. As the instigator, HHS sanctioned and supervised the campaign. http://www.adcouncil.org/about/news061902.)

The breastfeeding community (including lactation consultants, LLL members, nurse-midwives, and select pediatricians, obstetricians, family physicians, and neonatal nurses) reacted to the Ad Council's announcement with enthusiasm. One Boston pediatrician recalled thinking, "Hallelujah, finally. You know, we're struggling here in the trenches. And to have the government get in and help us out is just going to be terrific" (Ross and Rackmill 2004a). Breastfeeding advocates like this physician had long made largely futile attempts to raise consciousness about the link between human milk and human health and so were particularly delighted that the Ad Council, renowned for its ability to change Americans' behaviors, would now be the conduit for this message. In the past, the Ad Council had altered national consciousness about an array of detrimental activities: the careless use of matches ("Only YOU can prevent forest fires"), seat belt use ("You can learn a lot from a dummy"), and drinking and driving ("Friends don't let friends drive drunk").

The anticipated PSAs on breastfeeding, however, were inexplicably delayed. Though they were first due to air in May 2003 in honor of Mothers' Day, they did not. Rescheduled to make their debut during World Breastfeeding Week in August, they failed to materialize again. Someone had leaked the ads to the formula companies, and formula company executives were not happy with what they saw. The Ad Council, as was its custom, had devised an atypical approach to an old topic. Instead of enumerating the familiar benefits of breastfeeding in its campaign, the Council highlighted the risks of not breastfeeding. This perspective, campaign developers believed, would prompt behavioral change because, while it is easy to dismiss a benefit, risks are hard to ignore. As lactation specialist Diane Wiessinger explains, "Our own experience tells us that optimal is not necessary. Normal is fine, and implied in this language is the absolute normalcy—and thus safety and adequacy—of artificial feeding." Long before the Ad Council decided to publicize the risks of not breastfeeding, Wiessinger advised a similar strategy. She observed, "Because breastfeeding is the biological norm, breastfed babies are not 'healthier'; artificially fed babies are ill more often and more seriously" (Wiessinger 1996, 1).

The three PSAs devised by the Ad Council and viewed covertly by formula company executives portrayed visibly pregnant women partaking in dangerous activities. One showed them participating in a logrolling contest, another showed them riding violently bucking mechanical broncos, and a third showed them bashing into each other in a roller derby. In all three spots a voice-over admonishes, "You wouldn't risk your baby's health before it's born. Why start after?" (See the Ad Council Web site at http://www.adcouncil. org.) Then statistics appear on-screen. Among babies who are fed formula, leukemia is up 30 per cent, ear infections are up 60 per cent, and insulin-dependent diabetes is up 40 per cent. The ads end with one of the Ad Council's trademark pithy slogans: "Babies were born to be breastfed" (Ross and Rackmill 2004a).

Formula company executives were horrified. Charging the campaign was "negative," they went directly to Joe Sanders and Carden Johnston, then the executive director and president (Sanders has since resigned), respectively, of the AAP, to seek support in denouncing the ads (Petersen 2003; Gartner n.d.). Sanders and Johnston proved a sympathetic audience. Johnston immediately wrote to HHS, now headed by Tommy Thompson, to repeat formula company concerns (Johnston 2003). Dismayed, Dr. Lawrence Gartner, chair of the AAP's Section on Breastfeeding, charged that AAP officials were simply appeasing the AAP's biggest donors—the formula companies. Ross Laboratories alone contributed $500,000 to the AAP in 2001. "There is a lot of money involved," Gartner told the New York Times (Petersen 2003, C1; Ross and Rackmill 2004a). Scrambling to keep the Ad Council campaign intact, Gartner wrote letters to both Thompson and Johnston explaining how the ads had been devised. The Ad Council, in conjunction with the country's foremost experts on breastfeeding and human milk, determined through focus groups that if the PSAs were to succeed in normalizing breastfeeding and undermining formula feeding in the collective American mind, the most convincing **strategy was to enumerate the risks of not breastfeeding.** Gartner pointed out that the Ad Council had used a similar ploy quite successfully in their seat belt campaign: "they provide[d] examples of what can happen when not wearing a seat belt" (Gartner 2003).

The battle continued. The International Formula Council hired Clayton Yeutter, U.S. Secretary of Agriculture under George H. W. Bush and former Republican Party chairman, to lobby the U.S. government. Yeutter wrote a letter to Thompson (bearing the salutation "Dear Tommy") complaining that the planned ads contained "egregious distortions... For our government to give all these mothers a guilt trip would just be appalling" (Yeutter 2004). Gartner countered, "The ad campaign is backed by scientific research... that has been reviewed now by two different panels." Yet with Yeutter's help, formula industry executives arranged a private meeting with Thompson to discuss the ads. Breastfeeding proponents were unable to arrange a similar meeting to defend the ads (Ross and Rackmill 2004a). Sanders and Johnston continued to ignore the exhortations of their own organization's breastfeeding experts to allow the ads to run intact. Instead, Sanders told the *New York Times* he was worried that if a mother saw the ads and still chose not to breastfeed she might feel guilty if her baby eventually developed leukemia or diabetes (Petersen 2003). Later that month, Johnston appeared on CBS's Early Show to explain that he wanted mothers to breastfeed for "positive reasons" rather than be persuaded by "scare tactics" (CBS Television 2003).

In early June 2004, the week before heavily edited breastfeeding PSAs began to appear in select markets, the ABC news show 20/20 aired a segment exposing the successful collusion of the nation's formula companies, the premier organization of American pediatricians, and HHS to hide the risks of not breastfeeding from mothers. Brian Ross, who narrated the segment, introduced the story by describing the planned breastfeeding campaign as having been "kept off the air by the Bush administration." Jay Gordon, a Santa Monica, California, pediatrician and a member of the AAP Section on Breastfeeding, explained why the 3-billion-dollar-a-year formula industry had worked so hard to alter the planned ads: "When you say 'not breastfeeding is risky,' what you're saying is 'using infant formula is risky,' and this is true and they know it." A befuddled Sanders, who clearly had never seen the ads he had worked so hard to suppress, told 20/20's Ross, "We saw the information from the Ad Council and there was something about a pregnant woman riding a bull. I don't think a pregnant woman belongs on a mechanical bull, do you?" (Ross and Rackmill 2004b).

The ads that began to air in mid-June 2004 in a few select areas (and then quickly disappeared) relayed a message so different from the campaign's original intent that the agency that developed the PSAs insisted its name be removed from the final product. The consequences of not breastfeeding and its obvious corollary—the ramifications of formula feeding—had disappeared. There was no mention of the 40 per cent increased incidence of diabetes, or the 30 percent increase in leukemia, or even the relatively well-known 60 percent increase in ear infections among formula-fed infants (Ross and Rackmill 2004a). **All reference to long-term diseases and the more obvious references to the health risks linked to not breastfeeding had disappeared.**[2090]

The National Breastfeeding Advertising Campaign (NBAC) lasted for two years and earned 30 million dollars in donated media—which is good for a public service advertising campaign.[2091] The coverage on TV, radio, billboard, and newspapers started a national discussion on breastfeeding, previously never talked about. But it could not have the impact it was designed to have. While it did increase breastfeeding initiation, a stronger and longer campaign could have made a difference to attitudes about infant formula, and so longer breastfeeding duration.

---

2090  Wolf J H. *Signs* article op cit. pp. 410-414

2091  Meanwhile, the infant formula industry spent $80million in paid advertising in 2004-2005. See the cached Evaluation of the campaign by Suzanne Haynes. http://www.iom.edu/~/media/Files/Activity%20Files/Nutrition/USDABreastfeeding/09_Haynes_Suzanne.pdf.

Once again, the US government and industry colluded to deny families the clear risk information they need to make intelligent choices about infant feeding. As Wolf concluded,

> "Women should indeed be free to choose between formula and human milk, but women also have the right to be fully informed when they make that decision. Feminists should be especially concerned when the nation's foremost health organizations use the concept of choice to deny women information."[2092]

As this Professor JH Wolf also says in a strongly critical review of another Professor Wolf's tendentious writing: '

> The fate of the NBAC... suggests that breastfeeding advocates are the ones who have been harangued and censored on a national scale, not formula-feeding mothers.'[2093]

However, this was an important American attempt to tell the truth clearly and powerfully. Very few such campaigns have been made in Western communities, certainly not in Australia. So all praise to those involved in the brave but doomed attempt. Perhaps the original advertisements could be up on YouTube? And it was not the end of the matter once the Obamas reached the White House. Michelle Obama is, after all, a mother who took her breastfed four month old with her to one job interview, and a mother who cares about nutrition.

And when will other countries' politicians be brave enough to tackle this issue and begin to undo the damage being done to the human race? Conservative governments are very strong on the value of motherhood; in reality they treat women and children as economic pawns and do not support women as mothers, merely as breeders.

A mother is more than a woman who births a baby, and breastfeeding has a huge effect on new mothers, for good or for ill. Yet infant formula is understood as equivalent to women's milk, or even better, despite the fact that it was, and is, the world's most damaging in vivo series of experiments on infants, creating incalculable collateral damage.

---

2092  Wolf JH. Op.cit
2093  Wolf J H, review in *Contemporary Sociology* 2012; 41 (2) 248-9.

# APPENDIX 3

# This is me: about the author

My parents were intelligent working-class Catholics of typically limited formal education, people with Irish-Australian roots and attitudes to authority. They escaped disadvantaged origins in the low-income western suburbs of Melbourne, thanks largely to the wages and conditions created by the Australian union movement, training in the permanent air force, and the postwar boom in the western world. Fortunately they were not part of the bottle-feeding middle class when I was born, just before the war ended, and my mother told me that she gave me nothing but breast milk for nine months, then other foods until by 12 months I was weaned and on a normal diet. Eldest girl in a family of four children, I attended seven different schools as my parents moved to find work or better prospects; I had three years on a pre-electric dairy farm in the bush in the 1950s, but they returned to regional towns after that. My secondary college, teacher training, and later university and postgraduate studies were possible only because of a variety of scholarships. Only two girls in my class would go on from school to university in the pre-Whitlam era of costly university fees. My most influential teachers were talented religious sisters, Australians with clear ideas about right and wrong, and a strong commitment to both natural justice and social justice, as well as to learning. A typical 1950s Catholic girl, I spent eight years from 1963 in a community of dedicated strong women of faith, rejoicing in the reforms that Vatican II initiated, studying psychology and theology and gaining teaching credentials. Formally educated (BA Hons, MA) and later employed by the excellent History Department of the University of Melbourne, I enjoyed two years (thanks to the Mannix Travelling Scholarship) at Oxford University, where I married a remarkable Anglican priest, Jim Minchin, in Oxford researching his outstanding study of Singapore's Lee Kuan Yew, *No Man is an Island* (Allen & Unwin 1986). Following the launch of my first book (*Revolutions and Rosewater: a history of the Victorian Nursing Council 1923-1973*) I returned to Australia in 1975 to have children, expecting to combine this with part-time academic work. I did not know that my life course was about to be dramatically re-routed by the 'modern formula' invasion of Australia.

I was "an elderly primip" in the 1970s, bombarded with free formula samples from hospital and clinic, having my children comp-fed without my consent. I suffered the agonies of the damned during my first three tortured months of breastfeeding with hospital-induced nipple fissures, until reading Dr Mavis Gunther's *Infant feeding*, and healing those 'cracks' in two days. (I cheered to read that Mavis thought 'cracks' "a slovenly term used only by those who have not troubled to see what the injury is.") I was sleep-deprived for years as a consequence of the allergy created in my firstborn by hospital comp feeding, which caused colic and night waking due to gut and joint pain.[2094]

Thanks to my mother, my son, my research background and Mavis Gunther, I learned how to breastfeed pain-free and joyfully – no thanks to either multiple medical personnel consulted, or timid self-help groups unwilling to offend doctors by giving "medical" advice. In fact, had my mother not empathised with my pain in those first three months, and assured me that 'When it gets better, it is marvellous, there's nothing like it,' I would certainly have joined all my educated middle-class friends of middle-class mothers, who had moved on to bottle- feeding. (Instead I evolved into a long-term breastfeeder, lactating for the best part of ten years with my three children. For which I am grateful as I approach seventy without osteoporosis or reproductive cancers!) So I feel nothing but empathy for those who experience the agony without the needed support and solutions. Been there, know it's hideous, but also know that women can survive it, *and that doing so is worth the effort it takes.*

So motivating was this ghastly experience, that ever since I have spent my time trying to provide needed support for other women, at many levels. As a new mother in 1976 I joined NMAA, the Nursing Mothers' Association of Australia (later ABA, the Australian Breastfeeding Association) and hosted new mothers' groups in my home in Fitzroy (Melbourne), and later in rural St Arnaud, where with a local midwife and part-time GP mum we set up an informal pregnancy education and support group called The Club. (St Arnaud in the late 1970s was not ready for an overtly-breastfeeding group: by reaching pregnant women we changed a rabidly bottle-feeding culture, in which one local health professional told me that breastfeeding a boy past three months is tantamount to incest. It was not coincidence that a NMAA group later grew there.)

I had been employed to write a history of the Victorian Nursing Council[2095] before having children, and knew my way around local medical libraries. Bad hospital practices and their consequences with my three children led me to write both *Food for thought: a parent's guide to food intolerance*, and *Breastfeeding matters: what we need to know about infant feeding*. Both were well received by those who read them, including many eminent medical and scientific figures: I have the incomparable (now Sir) Iain Chalmers to thank for Professor David Baum's introduction to *Breastfeeding Matters*, for example; and eminent US pediatrician Frank Oski even broke with tradition to recommend *Breastfeeding Matters* in the *1987 Yearbook of Pediatrics*. Both books went into multiple editions in Australia and overseas: OUP even sold *Food for Thought* to a Japanese publisher. They created new impetus for

---

2094 As is typical, this began in his third week of life, once antibodies had formed and were reacting to the milk I drank. The day we eliminated milk from his four-year-old diet, both I and his father woke during the night, sure that he had died, to find him sleeping silently – for the first time ever – in a bed not tossed about by his usual thrashing. Insomnia is a common problem for the allergic: "when no evident cause for sleeplessness can be found in an infant, the possibility of milk allergy should be given serious consideration." (Kahn A, op.cit.)

2095 *Revolutions and Rosewater: a history of the VNC 1923-1973.*

radical change, both among those who had ignored allergy in breastfeeding families, and among many, even healthworkers and corporate activists who had unthinkingly echoed industry's mantra that poverty and dirty water make infant feeding dangerous, inadvertently undermining breastfeeding promotion in their own societies. I was delighted when UNICEF bought 500 copies to put into medical libraries in India! (and amused later to discover South Asian doctors who really should have asked permission to quote what instead they claimed as their own work. I ignored this, because in male-dominant societies their names added greater weight to the message, and I record this here solely so that I can never be accused of plagiarising *them!)*

In the early 1980s I became an active participant in attempts to regulate infant formula marketing, initially as a member of IBFAN with Dr Kate Short. This collaboration resulted in the strong 1984 ICM statement on breastfeeding, which was the condition for our taking down an embarassing display headed "Breaches of the International Code at this ICM conference."[2096] I also urged IBFAN delegates in Thailand in 1986 to learn about lactation and actively support breastfeeding, rather than simply using the harms of infant formula as a weapon in the (much-needed) struggle for more ethical corporate behaviour. My national political activity had begun in 1981with lobbying the NHMRC about infant feeding and allergy, and continued through multiple inputs into the never-ending processes of infant formula regulation and International Code implementation in Australia. Subsequently I was co-creator of ACOIF, the Australian Coalition for Optimal Infant Feeding, with Greg Thompson of World Vision Australia; we helped create Australia's Advisory Panel on the Marketing in Australia of Infant Formula (APMAIF) which was formalised in 1992. Until 1996 I was the appointed APMAIF Community Alternate Representative, along with Ros Escott as the official Community Representative: she did an excellent job in that role, and like other former students of my Infant Feeding Matters course, her input into other areas of breastfeeding promotion and protection has been truly stellar.

It has always been my conviction that telling mothers that breastfeeding matters simply adds to their burdens, when they cannot find competent help with breastfeeding problems. Thus my principal goal was always, and remains, to educate health professionals and parents alike. In the later 1970s I was a member of NMAA's Editorial Panel, assisted outstanding NMAA Newsletter editor Lyn Lea, and acted as a NMAA Information Service resource officer while my children were young. Once the youngest was four, I began to travel overseas to try to remedy differences in the lactation knowledge base evident (to me, anyway) in literature written in the UK and USA. As a result of being in the right place at the right time, and thanks to the great vision and openness of the LLLI Board, I was able significantly to influence the creation of both the International Lactation Consultant Association (ILCA) and the

---

2096 Handouts from all the companies other than Nestlé Australia were represented there. Nestlé would have been, but they had no objectionable handouts to post up! Interestingly, the US companies said nothing to us directly, but went to ICM and complained. I was then asked by a Council member to take it down as we were "biting the hand that fed us." I replied not until we see ICM taking a strong stand about this issue, then we might. We were promised a strong statement that night, and knew that Dr Mary Renfrew would be involved in drafting it. We'd made our point, and knew that next time the companies would be more careful what they brought along, as Nestlé had been. So we took it down. Simple action, great result, you just need a thick skin to do politely and quietly, with a smile, something you know will not make you loved by organisers.

International Board of Lactation Consultant Examiners (IBLCE) in 1984–5, by ensuring ILCA had strong international representation on their US-based Boards of Directors, and by securing NMAA representation on the IBLCE Board, after arranging for midwife Sue Cox to come with me to their inaugural meeting in Washington in March 1985. Having turned down offers to come on Boards, I advised both ILCA and IBLCE behind the scenes as a founding member of ILCA's Professional Advisory Board, and in 1989-1991 was the ILCA Board's elected International Delegate, succeeding Helen Armstrong, whom I had persuaded to consider the role; similarly, I would persuade Dr Felicity Savage to succeed me, and the influence of both women on ILCA was profound. The lactation consultant profession always needs to draw on diverse influences and international experience, or it risks becoming just another US nursing specialty, or a gnostic cult.

Back in Australia I had set up in 1986 the first open access and affordable Australian Infant Feeding course, initially at Prahran College of TAFE thanks to the vision of lecturer Margaret Shepherd, and later independently. This would educate over a thousand health professionals in the next two decades, many going on to become lactation consultants after completing a two day ALMA seminar designed to assist them to do so. I have since been involved in developing or teaching many hospital, pharmacy college, and university-based lactation and infant-feeding courses, in Australia, America and Europe, my most recent input being into the University of York (UK) online modules, and the online e-learning for health package developed for NHS workers under the auspices of the Royal College of Paediatrics and Child Health (RCPCH).

In 1983, thanks to sales of *Food for Thought*, I had visited WHO in Geneva to urge action to change hospital practices undermining breastfeeding. This led to long-standing collaboration and friendships with some remarkable people. During the 1980s I worked with the Nutrition Unit of WHO Geneva in the process of developing better infant-feeding advice, and so had considerable input into the seminal text, *Infant feeding, the physiological basis*, which James Akré developed from a disparate series of essays commissioned by WHO, and which was eventually published in thirty-six languages. Consulted in the UNICEF New York/Wellstart development of the global Baby Friendly Hospital Initiative (BFHI) documents and the course for training BFHI assessors, I brought back to Australia in 1992 the Global BFHI documents (which had been faxed from Geneva to Lagos just in time for me to lead the pilot hospital assessments UNICEF New York was funding in Nigeria.) Then I persuaded the Director of Nursing at Royal Women's Hospital, Margaret Peters, President of the UNICEF Committee of Australia, to initiate BFHI in Australia, and created[2097]– and then handed over - the first Australian BFHI workshops to accredit BFHI assessors and educators. Acting as an educator and assessor until around 2010 gave me insight into the problems facing mothers, midwives and hospitals in creating change. The continuing need for better birthing and breastfeeding care was evident.

With NMAA's encouragement and my input a Melbourne-based group led by midwife April Blackwell created the Australian Lactation Consultants' Association (ALCA) in

[2097] With the assistance of remarkable midwife Janice Edwards, and Dr Pat Lewis (Director of the Lactation Resource Centre)

1986–7. I served on the Board of Directors of ALCA and other voluntary bodies for years. I spent months of each of several years collating and writing about the latest developments in infant feeding, to keep lactation consultants informed and motivated, as volunteer editor of *ALCA News*. Its radical perpective was appreciated by many, but upset some more conventional souls, who disappointingly chose to do a lot of needless damage to the cause of breastfeeding rather than abide by the canons of ethical organisational behaviour. As Seminar Co-ordinator for ALCA and member of countless conference committees, I and a small team of volunteers[2098] helped generate many thousands of dollars profit – from seminars and workshops and conferences – to support organisations working to protect, promote and support breastfeeding. We worked for the good of families everywhere, many of them more affluent than we volunteers.

Through the whole of this time my three children were growing up. The results of early exposure to infant formula and the stress generated by the health problems of my first-born have influenced their lives in many ways. They were raised by two workaholic cause-oriented parents who, perhaps too often, expected them to put important causes before their own perceived interests. All three are now wonderful caring adults loved and respected by both their parents, and we have four breastfed grandchildren, two in their teens and two under three months old. (One of those was an almost 36-weeker exclusively donor/mother milk fed, cared for skin to skin, and now fully breastfed and growing well: 700gms in two weeks post-discharge, and not yet at her due date. No other baby in that unit was so fortunate. The second has put on just over a kilogram in less than three weeks from birth. Both are blissful babies, eating and sleeping and giving their parents nothing but joy.) My perception is that breastfeeding my children taught me how to be a mother, and that the bonds breastfeeding creates are unbreakable.

From the 1970s onwards, I have worked with many families, some through known contacts (latterly my children's friends), others referred on as difficult cases by health professionals reluctant or unable to deal with suspected allergy in breastfeeding mothers. I have never billed families, as the ongoing contact needed for resolution of their problems could be compromised by any suspicion that I am 'in it for the money'. Any money I earned from education or book sales was spent on the work itself (regrettably, some being wasted on pointless legal action generated by those people who really should have behaved better). But most of my earnings went on travel to conferences, subscriptions, and a unique and irreplaceable library of works relating to infant feeding and lactation, for which I hope to find a good home before I die! In those travels I often made a point of meeting key researchers, both to learn from them, and often to challenge them about some aspect or other of their work: what I loved about meeting scientists was their interest in ideas, especially those they initially disagreed with! Interesting international trips included standing in for Professor Roger Short at a IAMANEH (International Association for Maternal and Neonatal Health) meeting in Lahore, speaking of how infant suckling affected fertility- and breastfeeding success; a USAID-sponsored meeting in Washington presenting a contracted report on

---

2098 Ev Vines, Philippa Thomson, Ann McNair, Lisa Amir notable among others  1984 A programme now abolished which paid an allowance for children's education.

breastmilk expression; a workshop in Malaysia with Randa Saadeh from WHO Geneva....
there were many more.

I was able to do volunteer work, although far from wealthy, because my husband (a lifelong
victim of 1940s Truby King bottle-feeding) shared my sense that this was uniquely important
work – and his job meant we did not have to worry about housing until retirement. Living on
a limited income, and dependence on op shops – decades before they became fashionable-
has been the family norm. Our children were educated via scholarships and Austudy[2099],
and so I never underestimate the struggle raising healthy children can be for those without
the resources of family, friendship, education, and welfare support which I have been lucky
enough to have all my life. (I am a classic case of social mobility through education, enabled
by those nine months of exclusive breastfeeding!)

Like many women of my age, I am also part of what has been called the Sandwich
Generation: from 1999 I spent almost a decade caring for my elderly parents – on a carer
pension after my mobility-limited mother went blind in 2002– while former students took
over the work of professional education in my home state. My father died of cancer at home
in 2004, and in mid-2009 I had a health crisis which meant that my sister Trish took over as
carer until Mum's death in June 2014.

Hence I was finally able to get on with completing this long-planned book, after two stints
in the UK in 2010 and 2011, possible thanks to paid work on University of York infant
feeding modules, and the online course overseen by the Royal College of Paediatrics and
Child Health for the UK National Health Service. That work, organised by Professor of
Midwifery Mary Renfrew, helped me recover from my decade as sole carer. During that
decade I had dropped out of most organisational and educational work, though I remained
a member of the Editorial Board of the important open access *International Breastfeeding
Journal* created by Dr Lisa Amir (who has done far more for breastfeeding nationally and
globally than has been publicly recognised, at least in Australia, to date). And during that
decade science finally caught up with this long-standing hypothesis, and the planned book
morphed into three books under one cover.

That is the background I bring to this work. I can honestly say that I have absolutely no
conflicting interests to declare. My family and I would have been far better off financially
had I returned to academia after having babies, rather than followed this life course. It has
had more than its share of challenging times and confrontation and frustration, due in part
to my inherited Irish incapacity to stay quiet about what I see as the abuse of power in
organisations or by individuals. There have been other downsides, too – leaving interesting
doctoral studies incomplete because educating healthworkers was more important than
another degree, while working in a medical milieu very prone to giving far too much weight
to such bits of paper. Which has meant that like many other parent advocates, I have had
to put up with a great deal of ignorance, patronising, and ill-informed judgmentalism for
being willing to speak the truth as I see it. Working as a volunteer has also meant zero
savings, while living on the carer (and now aged) pension has restricted my ability to travel

---

2099 A programme now abolished which paid an allowance for children's education.

in order to research this book internationally, so I am very grateful for the internet. I am also very grateful that the Gillard government increased the age pension, on which I depend. Publishing the book itself has meant going into serious debt, and as I will be giving away many copies in order to spread the word, it may be quite some time before the book has repaid what it has cost me. (Offers to help spread the word would be much appreciated!) Ultimately I want the book to be available free online: this has never been about fame or money, but about preventing the harms children have experienced needlessly.

The positives have been greater than the negatives. Had I stayed a teacher or academic, I would not have read so widely, and learned so much; and I would not have met the many hundreds of wonderful people around the world who work to empower women and protect children, and who have enriched my life. My children and grandchildren would not be as healthy as they are;in fact I'd be lucky not to have lost my son, as some mothers do, to unrecognised allergy, and my latest grandchildren could now be miserable with gut dysbiosis thanks to cows milk comp feeds. I would not have enjoyed the rewards of seeing women grow into responsive, confident mothers, and babies move from distress to delight, knowing that I have helped make that difference. Money can't buy a sense that one's life has been worthwhile. This book is a way of giving back some of what I have been given in life, by sharing my personal perspective on some of the knowledge that the scientific community has amassed in the era of what I see as the global formula catastrophe. I would love to be part of a global collaboration thoroughly documenting that GFC, more damaging to humanity than any financial crisis. But if that is not possible, at least I have made many resources available to kickstart the effort.

I hope that putting this information together helps others appreciate how little we modern westerners have understood and valued breastfeeding, possibly the most important survival and adaptation strategy in human evolutionary history. The book is obviously far from a perfect or complete account of what we need to know about infant feeding. However, I think that there is enough to stimulate more much-needed independent research about artificial feeding in every country.

As I said in the Preface, I know that I will have made mistakes in trying to cover and interpret so broad a canvas. I do not want to be unfair to anyone — even the infant formula industry — simply to put the truth on record as best I understand it. But don't let any errors, major or minor, distract you from seeing the big picture. Step back and consider it well. If I'm even half-right, this is one of the most important issues facing humanity in an age of more obvious great challenges. It doesn't matter much if I'm wrong. But if I'm right, a sea change in social support of women and children before, during and after birth is long overdue, to facilitating breastfeeding and reduce other stressors. Birthing units will function very differently, and so will NICUs; social security and childcare arrangements will change. Formula for infants under six months will be replaced by sources of human milk; women will again think it normal to breastfeed for nine to twelve months at least, and those who can do so will continue longer. New industries will emerge, and others will be radically changed.

If this book makes sense to you, see what you can do to change society so as to enable breastfeeding, protecting children from artificial feeding, the largest and most powerful of all the global plagues re-shaping human kind.

*And spread the word: please promote this book via social media. Review it. Give it as a present.\** Let me know key people who should be given a copy to consider – journalists, health ministers, whoever. Better yet, pay for a copy I can send on to them with your compliments, if you think it could do some good, or you have connections that will help make sure they read it.  In 2015 I hope to develop a web page, as I have registered a domain name, www. infantfeedingmatters.com. There I will post any needed corrections or modifications of what I have said in this first edition. There I can record your support if you would like to be part of the global process of persuading the world that indeed, Milk Matters.


Maureen Minchin

Email: womensmilkmatters@gmail.com

*\*It's expensive, I know, but I anticipate making maybe $20 profit per book sold via retailers, which would mean $10,000 from 500 copies, or $2000 a year since 2009. (Which does not even cover the cost of books I've needed to buy for research purposes: the last two were almost $400.) And  some of that 500 will not be sold but given away.  Authors are not the ones who make money out of books, as the tax man told me decades ago. Because I'll make more from those I sell directly, I will not charge postage and handling **within Australia** for any of this 500 that I mail out personally to people who cannot buy direct: I'd like it to cost no more for country readers, and expect postage to cost roughly $20. For subsequent editions, that may not be possible. And  remember that it is, after all, three books under one cover, and a limited edition that will have rarity value down the years. Overseas sales will be handled initially via Amazon, Book Depository and Bookpod, if people do not want to pay what will be horrendous postal costs from Australia. I would be happy to contract with breastfeeding support groups or serious publishers to handle sales of subsequent editions in a particular country or region or language.*

# Glossary

## Abbreviations and acronyms

| | | | |
|---|---|---|---|
| AAA | Allergy Awareness Association (UK) | COC | chemical of concern |
| AIA | Allergy-induced Autism (UK group) | COMA | Committee on Medical Aspects and Nutrition Policy (UK) |
| ABA | Australian Breastfeeding Association | | |
| ABM | Academy of Breastfeeding Medicine (US) | CON | Committee on Nutrition (of the AAP) |
| | | DCD | dicyandiamide |
| | Association of Breastfeeding Mothers (UK) | DHA | docosahexaenoic acid |
| | | DHSS | Department of Health and Social Security (UK) |
| AF | artificial feeding, artificially-fed | | |
| AAP | American Academy of Pediatrics | EBM | expressed breast milk |
| ACCC | Australian Competition and Consumer Commission | EFA | essential fatty acid |
| | | EFSA | European Food Safety Authority |
| ACOIF | Australian Coalition for Optimal Infant Feeding | IGF | epidermal growth factor |
| | | EHF or EH-F | extensively hydrolysed formula |
| ADHD | Attention Deficit Hyperactivity Disorder | EHF-C | extensively-hydrolysed-casein formula |
| | | EHF-W | extensively-hydrolysed-whey formula |
| AESSRA | Allergy and Environmental Sensitivity Support and Research Association | EM | evaporated milk |
| | | EPA | Environmental Protection Agency (US) |
| AGEs | advanced glycation end products | ESPGHAN | European Society for Paediatric Gastroenterology, Hepatology and Nutrition |
| AIA | Allergy Induced Autism (UK) | | |
| ALA | alpha-lactalbumin | | |
| ALCA | Australian Lactation Consultant Association | FAO | Food and Agriculture Organisation (UN) |
| | | FDA | (US) Food and Drug Administration |
| ANZFA | Australian and New Zealand Food Authority (precursor of FSANZ) | FFDCA | Federal Food, Drug, and Cosmetic Act (US) |
| AOAC | Association of Official Analytical Chemists | FIF | first infant formula |
| | | FODMAPS | fermentable oligosaccharides, disaccharides, monosaccharides and polyols |
| APMAIF | Advisory Panel on the Marketing in Australia of Infant Formula | | |
| AR | anti-reflux (supposedly, anyway) | FOF | follow-on formula |
| ARA | arachidonic acid | FOS | fructo-oligosaccharides |
| ART | antiretroviral therapy | FPIES | food protein-induced enterocolitis syndrome |
| ASCIA | Australasian Society of Allergy and Clinical Immunology | | |
| | | FSANZ | Food Standards Authority of Australia and New Zealand |
| BCM | beta-casomorphin | | |
| BFHI | Baby Friendly Hospital Initiative | FTC | Federal Trade Commission (US) |
| BFI | Baby Friendly Initiative (UK) | GALT | gut-associate lymphoid tissue |
| BFLG | Baby Feeding Law Group (UK) | GE | genetically engineered |
| BMAA | β-methylamino-L-alanine | GM/GMO | genetically modified organism |
| BMJ | British Medical Journal | GOR (D) | gastroesophageal reflux (disease) |
| BPA | Bisphenol A | GOS | galacto-oligosaccharides |
| BSSL | bile salt stimulated lipase | GRAS | generally recognised as safe |
| Codex | Codex Alimentarius Commission | GUL | guidance upper limit |
| CCNFSDU | Codex Committee on Nutrition and Foods for Special Dietary Uses | GUM | growing up milk (Toddler formula +) |
| | | HA | hypoallergenic, ie, less allergenic |
| CDC | Centers for Disease Control and Prevention (US) | HACSAG | Hyperactive Children's Support and Action Group (UK) |
| CGMPs | Current Good Manufacturing Practices | HFCS | High Fructose Corn Syrup |
| CJD | Creutzfeldt-Jacob Disease ('Mad Cow') | 4-HHE | hydroxyhenal (oxidation by-product) |
| CMF | cows' milk formula | 4-HNE | hydroxynonenal (oxidation by-product) |
| CNS | central nervous system | | |

| | | | |
|---|---|---|---|
| HHS | Department of Health and Human Services | NICE | National Institute of Clinical Excellence (UK) |
| HMO | human milk oligosaccharides | NICUs | neonatal intensive care nurseries |
| HTLV-1 | human lymphotrophic virus 1 | NIMA | non-inherited maternal antigens |
| IBCLC | International Board Certified Lactation Consultant | NIDDM | non-insulin dependent diabetes |
| | | NMAA | Nursing Mothers' Association of Australia |
| IBFAN | International Baby Food Action Network | NPN | non-protein nitrogen |
| IBLCE | International Board of Lactation Consultant Examiners | OFC | oral food challenge |
| | | PCB | polychlorinated biphenyl |
| ICAAC | International Congress of Antimicrobial Agents and Chemotherapy | PBB | polybrominated biphenyl |
| | | PCR | polymerase chain reaction |
| ICCR | Inter-Faith Center on Corporate Responsibility | PER | protein efficiency ratio |
| | | PFOA | perfluorooctanoic acid |
| ICDC | International Code Documentation Centre | PHF or PH-F | partially hydrolysed formula |
| | | PHF-C | patrially hydrolysed casein formula |
| IDFA | Infant and Dietetic Foods Association | PHF-W | partially hydrolysed whey formula |
| IF | infant formula | PSA | public service announcement |
| ICIFI | International Council of Infant Food Industries | rBST | recombinant bovine Somatotropin (growth hormone) |
| IGF-I | insulin-like growth factor-I | RCPL & BNF | Royal College of Physicians of London and British Nutrition Foundation |
| IgA | immunoglobulin A (or E, G, or M) | | |
| IL-1 | interleukin-1 (or other number) | RCTs | randomised controlled trials |
| ILCA | International Lactation Consultant Association | RDA | recommended daily allowance |
| | | RDI | recommended daily intake |
| INFORM | Wyeth-created UK industry group | rhBSSL | recombinant human bile salt stimulated lipase |
| IOMC | The Inter-Organization Programme for the Sound Management of Chemicals | RTF | ready to feed |
| | | RTU | ready to use |
| IPA | International Pediatric Association | SACN | Scientific Advisory Committee on Nutrition (UK) |
| ISRHML | International Society for Research into Human Milk and Lactation | | |
| | | SCFA | short chain fatty acids |
| LBW | low birth weight | SCID | Severe Combined Immune Deficiency |
| LCPUFAs | long-chain polyunsaturated fatty acids | SIDS | sudden infant death syndrome |
| LDL | low-density lipoprotein | SIgA | secretory immunoglobulin A |
| LF | lactose free | SIgM | secretory immunoglobulin M |
| LGBTQ | Lesbian, Gay, Bisexual, Transgender, Questioning | SF | soy formulas |
| | | UF | ultra-filtration |
| LLL | La Leche League | SUDI | sudden unexpected death in infancy |
| LSRO | Life Sciences Research Office (US) | TGF | transforming growth factor |
| MBD | Minimal Brain Damage | TLR | toll-like receptor |
| MCTs | medium chain triglycerides | TNF | tumor necrosis factor |
| MDA | malondialdehyde (oxidation by-product) | UHT | ultra heat treated |
| MF | micro filtration | UL | upper limit |
| MFGM | milk fat globule membrane | USDA | United States Department of Agriculture |
| MRSA | multiply resistant Staph aureus | | |
| MSBP | Munchausen's Syndrome By Proxy | USFDA | United States Food and Drug Administration |
| MTCT | mother-to-child transmission | | |
| MV | maximal values | VRE | Vancomycin-resistant Enterobacter |
| NABA | North American Breastfeeding Alliance | WAP | Weston A Price Foundation |
| NALT | nasal-associated lymphoid tissue | WHA | World Health Assembly |
| NBAC | National Breastfeeding Advertising Campaign (US) | WHO | World Health Organization |
| | | WIC | Women Infants and Children (USDA program) |
| NCI | National Cancer Institute (US) | | |
| NEC | necrotising enterocolitis | | |
| NFA | National Food Authority (precursor of ANZFA) | WMP | whole milk powder |
| | | WP | whey protein |
| NGF | nerve growth factor | WPC | whey protein concentrate |
| NHMRC | National Health and Medical Research Council (Australia) | | |

# Bibliography

*Some of the books and articles and reports and publications that have been referenced, or which have influenced this work, somewhat haphazardly collated and presented. There is no time, or space, for a Resources section but one may well emerge in mid to late 2015 on my website-to-be, infantfeedingmatters. com. And if you notice a few stars at the end of a book\*\*\*, it means I think everyone should read that title.*

## Books

Allain A. *Fighting an old battle in a new world: how IBFAN monitors the baby food market.* (2005); also IBFAN. *Protecting Infant Health: a health worker's guide to the International Code of Marketing of Breastmilk Substitutes.*

Angier N. *Woman. An intimate geography.* (Houghton Mifflin 1999)

Arrowsmith-Young B. *The Woman Who Changed Her Brain.* (Free Press 2012)

Ashton J, Laura R. *Perils of Progress. Health and Environment Hazards of Modern Technology, and What You can do About Them.* (UNSW Press 2007)

AOAC. *Production, Regulation and Analysis of Infant Formula.* 1985 Conference Proceedings.

AOAC. *Production, Regulation and Analysis of Infant Formula.* 1985 Conference Proceedings, Association of Official Analytical Chemists,

Atkinson S, Lonnerdal B. *Protein and Non-Protein Nitrogen in Human Milk* (CRC Press, 1989)

Bachmann C, Koletzko B (eds) *Genetic Expression and Nutrition.* (Lippincott, Williams and Wilkins/Nestec 2003) NNI Workshop Series vol. 50.

Baker R. *Quiet Killers. The Fall and Rise of Deadly Diseases.* (Sutton Publishing 2007)

Baker S. *Milk to Market: 40 years of milk marketing.* (Wm Heinemann 1973)

Ballabriga A (ed). *Feeding from Toddlers to Adolescence.*(Lippincott/Raven/Nestec 1996) NNI Workshop Series vol.37. Chapter on soft drinks.

Ballabriga A, Rey J (eds). *Weaning: why, what and when?* (Raven Press/Nestle 1987) NNI Workshop Series vol 10.

Barham-Floreani J. *Well Adjusted Babies.* (Vitality Productions, 2009)

Barnard J, Twigg K. *Nursing Mums: history of the Australian Breastfeeding Association 1964-2014.* (ABA Melbourne 2014)

Barston S. *Bottled Up.* ((University of California Press, 2012).

Baumslag N, Michels D. *Milk, Money, and Madness.* (Bergin and Garvey 1995)

Beasley A, Trlin A. (eds) *Breastfeeding in New Zealand: Practice, Problems and Policy.* (Dunmore Press, Palmerston North 1998)

Beeton I. *The Book of Household Management* (1861) facsimile published as *Mrs Beeton's Book of Household Management* (Chancellor Press 1982)

Bhatia J, Bhutta ZA, Kalhan Sc. *Maternal and Child Nutrition: the first 1000 days.* (Karger/Nestec 2013) NNI Workshop Series vol. 74.

Black RE, Michaelsen KF. (Ed) *Public Health Issues in Infant and Child Nutrition.* (Lippincott Williams and Wilkins/ Nestec 2002)        NNI Workshop Series vol. 48.

Blaffer Hrdy S. *Mother Nature: Natural Selection and the female of the species.* (Chatto & Windus 1999)

Blaffer Hrdy S. *Mothers and Others. The evolutionary origins of mutual understanding* (Belknap Press 2007) \*\*\*

Blair M, Stewart-Brown S, Waterston T, Crowther R (eds) et al, *Child Public Health* (OUP 2010)

Blaser MJ. *Missing microbes. How the overuse of antibiotics is fueling our modern plagues.* (Henry Holt 2014)

Bock, GR, Whelan J (eds) *The Childhood Environment and Adult Disease* (Wiley 1991). Ciba Symposium 156.

Bond JT, Filer LJ, Leveille GA et al (eds) *Infant and Child Feeding.* (Academic Press 1981)

Boswell-Penc M. *Tainted Milk: breastmilk, feminisms, and the politics of environmental degradation.* (State University of New York, 2006)

Brandtzaeg P, Isolauri E, Prescott SL (eds). *Microbial Host-Interaction: Tolerance versus Allergy.* NNI Workshop Series vol. 64, 2008.

Breggin P. *Your Drug may be Your Problem. How and Why to Stop taking psychiatric medications.* \*\*\*(da Capo Press 2007) Check out his website, www.breggin.com

Brostoff J, Challacombe *Food Allergy and Intolerance* (Saunders, 2002)

Bryan FL. *Hazard Analysis Critical Control Point Evaluation.* (WHO Geneva 1992)

Budin P. *The Nursling. The feeding and hygiene of premature and full-term infants.* (Paris; 1907 English translation) Online at http://www.neonatology.org/classics/nursling/nursling.html

Burgio GR, Hanson LA, Ugazio AG (eds) *Immunology of the Neonate.* (Springer-Verlag 1987)

Cameron M, Hofvander Y. *Manual on Feeding Infants and Young Children.* (OUP 1983)

Campbell K, Wilmot E. *A Guide to the Care of the Young Child. A textbook for workers in the field of maternal and child health.* (Dept of Health, Victoria 1978).

Cannold L. *What, no baby? How women are losing their reproductive freedom and how they can get it back.* (Fremantle Arts Centre Press 2005).

Chalmers I, Enkin M, Kierse MJNC (eds) *Effective care in pregnancy and childbirth.* (2 vols) (OUP 1987)

Chetley A. *The Politics of Baby Foods.* (Francis Pinter London 1986)

CIBA Foundation Symposium 169. *Aluminium in Biology and Medicine.* (John Wiley and Sons 1992)

CIBA Foundation Symposium 45 (new Series). *Breast-feeding and the Mother.* (Elsevier 1976)

CIBA Foundation Symposium 156. *The Childhood Environment and Adult Disease* (John Wiley & Sons 1991)

Clemens RA, Hernell O, Michaelsen KF (eds) *Milk and Milk Products in Human Nutrition.* NNI Workshop Series vol.67. (Karger/Nestec 2011)

Clements FW. *Infant Nutrition: its physiological basis.* (Bristol 1949)

Codex Alimentarius Commission. *Milk and Milk Products.* (WHO/FAO 2007)

Cohen R. *Milk the Deadly Poison.* (Argus Publishing, New Jersey 1997)

Colborn T, Dumanoski D, Myers JP. *Our Stolen Future. Are we threatening our fertility, intelligence and survival?* (Abacus 1997)

Cone T. A *History of American Pediatrics.* (Little Brown and Co. 1979)

Cook HL, Day GH. *The Dry Milk Industry.* (American Dry Milk Institute 1947)

Cook P. *Early Child Care. Infants and Nations at Risk.* (News Weekly Books 1996)

Crawley H, Westland S. *Infant Milks in the UK.* First Steps Nutrition Trust, 2013. Online version open access at www.firststepsnutrition.org

Cribb J. *The White Death.* (Angus & Robertson, 1996)

Crosse M. *The Premature Infant.* (Blackwell 1937)

Crowther SM, Reynolds LA, and Tansey EM (eds) *The Resurgence of Breastfeeding 1975-2000.* Wellcome Trust Witness Seminar no 35, 2009.

Crumpler D. *Chemical Crisis.* (Scribe Publications 1994)

Dadd DL. *Home Safe Home: Creating A Healthy Home Environment By Reducing Exposure To Toxic Household Products.* (Penguin London 2004)

Darnall B. *Less Pain, Fewer Pills: Avoid the dangers of prescription opioids and gain control over chronic pain,* 2014: Bull Publishing Company –http://www.bullpub.com The book comes with a free pain management CD and audiofile.

David TJ. *Food and Food Additive Intolerance in Childhood.* (Blackwell Scientific Publications 1993)

De la Peña C. *Empty Pleasures. The Story of Artificial Sweeteners from Saccharin to Splenda.* (University of North Carolina Press 2010.)

Dept of Health Working Group Report. *Weaning and the Weaning Diet.* (HMSO London 1994)

*Detection of Lead in the DC Drinking Water System.* Hearing before the Sub-Committee on Fisheries, Wildlife, and Water of the Committee on Environment and Public Works, US Senate 108th Congress, second session April 7 2004. Available online

Dex S, Joshi H (eds). *Children of the 21st Century. From birth to nine months.* (Policy Press, University of Bristol, 2005)

DHSS *Lead and Health.* (HMSO London 1980)

Diamond J. *The World Until Yesterday.* (Viking Penguin 2012)

Douglas P. *The Discontented Little Baby Book.* (University of Queensland Press 2014)

Duffy R (ed) *Enterobacter sakazakii and Salmonella in Powdered Infant Formula.* Meeting Report. (WHO/FAO 2006)

DuPuis EM. *Nature's Perfect Food. How milk became America's drink.* (New York University Press 2002.)

Dwork D. *War is good for babies and other young children: a history of the infant and child welfare movement in England 1898-1918.* (Tavistock Publication London 1987)

Dykes F. *Breastfeeding in hospital: mothers, midwives and the production line.* (Routledge 2006)

Dykes F, Moran VH. *Infant and Young Child Feeding: challenges to implementing a global strategy.* (Wiley

Ebrahim GJ. *Breastfeeding- the Biological Option.* (Macmillan 1978)

Eliot L. *What's Going On In There? How the brain and mind develop in the first five years of life.* (Allen Lane Penguin 1999)

Elkington J. *The Poisoned Womb. Human reproduction in a polluted world.* (Viking 1985)

Enig MG. *Know Your Fats: the complete primer for understanding the nutrition of fats, oils and cholesterol.* (Bethesda Press 2011)

Enkin M, Keirse MJ, Chalmers I. *A Guide to Effective Care in Pregnancy and Childbirth* (Oxford Medical Publications 1989)

Evans I, Thornton H, Iain Chalmers I. *Testing Treatments: Better Research for Better Healthcare.* (British Library Publishing 2006; Pinter and Martin 2011.)

Evans PR, McKeith R. *Infant Feeding and Feeding Difficulties.* (JA Churchill Ltd London 1958)

Falkner F. (ed). *Infant and Child Nutrition Worldwide: issues and perspectives.* (CRC Press inc., 1991)

Feinberg SM. *Allergy in Practice.* (Yearbook Publishers, Chicago 1946)

Fildes V. *Breasts Bottles and Babies.* (Edinburgh University Press 1986);

Fildes V. *Wet Nursing: a history from antiquity to the present.* (Blackwell 1988)

Fisher JC, Fisher C. *Food in the American Military.* (Macfarland & Co 2011)

Fomon SJ. *Infant Nutrition* (WB Saunders Philadelphia 1974)

Fomon SJ. *Nutrition of Normal Infants* (Mosby Year-Book Inc. 1993)

Frances A. *Saving Normal* (William Morrow, 2013)***

Fraser H. *The Peanut Allergy Epidemic.* (Skyhorse Publishing 2011)

Freed DLJ (ed) *Health Hazards of Milk.* (Bailliere-Tindall 1984)

Freinkel D. *Plastic: a toxic love story.* (Houghton Mifflin Harcourt 2011)

Gamlin L. *The Allergy Bible.* (Quadrille Publishing 2001)

Gandevia B. *Tears Often Shed. Child Health and Welfare in Australia from 1788.* (Pergamon Press 1978)

Garland J. *The Youngest in the Family* (Harvard University Press 1932)

Gerhardt S. *The Selfish Society. How We All Forgot to Love One Another and Made Money Instead* (Simon & Schuster 2011)***

Gerhardt S. *Why Love Matters: how affection shapes the baby's brain.* (Brunner Routledge 2005)***

Gethin A. Macgregor B. *Helping Your Baby to Sleep: why gentle techniques work best.* (Finch Publishing, Lane Cove 2007)

Gibson G. *It Takes a Genome.* (Pearson Education Inc. 2009)

Gilbert SF, Epel D. *Ecological Developmental Biology: integrating epigenetics, medicine and evolution* (Sinauer Associates 2009

Gillespie D. *Toxic Oil. Why vegetable oil will kill you and how to save yourself.* (Viking/Penguin 2012) (Warning: breastmilk references in this are outdated.)

Gobbetti M, Di Cagno R. *Bacterial Communication in Foods* (Springer 2013.)

Gold P. *Advertising politics and American culture, from salesmanship to therapy.* Paragon House (May 1987)

Goldacre B. *Bad Pharma. How drug companies mislead doctors and harm patients.* (Fourth Estate 2012) ***

Goldberg G, Prentice A, Prentice A, Filteau S. Simondon K (eds.) *Breast-feeding: Early Influences on Later Health.* (Springer 2009).

Golden J. *A Social History of Wet Nursing in America* (Cambridge University Press 1996)

Gonzalez C. *My child won't eat! How to enjoy mealtimes without worry.* (Pinter & Martin 2012)

Gordon J. *Preventing Autism: what you can do to protect your children.* (John Wiley 2013.)

Graetzer E, Sheffield HB. *Practical Pediatrics: a manual of the medical and surgical diseases of infancy and childhood.* (FA Davis Philadelphia 1905)

Graham G, Kesten D, Scherwitz. *Potttenger's Prophecy. How food resets genes for wellness or illness.* (White River Press 2011)

Frances A. *Saving Normal.* (Harper Collins 2013)

Groer M, Kendall-Tackett K. *How Breastfeeding Protects Women's Health Throughout the Lifespan: the Psychoneuroimmunology of Human Lactation.* (Hale Publishing 2011)

Gunther M. *Infant Feeding* (Methuen 1974; Penguin 1978)

Hale TW, Hartmann PEH. *Textbook of Human Lactation* (Hale Publishing 2007)

Halvorsen R. *Vaccines. A parent's guide.* (Gibson Square, London 3rd ed. 2013)

Hamburger RN (ed). *Food Intolerance in Infancy.* (Raven Press 1989)

Hansen K, Joshi H, Dex S. *Children of the 21st Century, The first five years.* (Policy Press, Uni of Bristol, 2010)

Hanson LA, Yolken RH (eds). *Probiotics, other Nutritional Factors, and Intestinal Microflora.* (Lippincott/Raven/Nestec 1999) NNI Workshop Series vol. 42.

Hanson LA. *Immunobiology of Human Milk: How Breastfeeding Protects Babies.* (Pharmasoft Publishing 2004)

Hardyment C. *Dream Babies: Childcare Advice from Locke to Spock* (Jonathan Cape Ltd London 1983); updated *Locke to Gina Ford* in the 2007 edition published by Frances Lincoln, London.

Hausfater G, Blaffer Hrdy S. (eds) *Infanticide: comparative and evolutionary perspectives.* (Aldine de Gruyter 1984)

Hausman B. *Viral Mothers.* (University of Michigan Press 2011)

Heffernan M. *Wilful Blindness: why we ignore the obvious at our peril.* (Simon and Schuster 2011).

Henderson JO, Collins SM, Muller LL, Harrap BS. *Bibliography of Infant Foods and Nutrition* 1938-1977. (CSIRO 1978)

Henry B. *Soap and Water and Common Sense. The Definitive Guide to Viruses, Bacteria, Parasites, and Disease.* (House of Anansi Press, 2009)\*\*\*

Hess JH. *Feeding and the Nutritional Disorders in Infancy and Childhood.* (FA Davis co, Philadelphia 4ᵗʰ ed 1925.)

Hess JH. *Infant Feeding. A Handbook for the Practitioner.* (AMA 1924)

Hewitt M. *Wives and Mothers in Victorian Industry* (Rockliff, London 1958)

Hilts PJ. *Protecting America's Health. The FDA, Business and 100 Years of Regulation.* (Alfred Knopf 2003).

Holt LE. *The Good Housekeeping Book of Baby and Child Care.* (Appleton Century Crofts 1957)

Anon. *Home Book, a Domestic Cyclopaedia forming a Companion Volume to Mrs Beeton's Book of Household Management.* (Ward Lock & Co, n.d.)

Horta BL, Bahl R, Martines JC, Victora CG. *Evidence on the long-term effects of breastfeeding: systematic reviews and meta-analyses.* Geneva: World Health Organization, 2007.

Howell RR, Morriss FH, Pickering LK. *Human Milk in Infant Nutrition and Health.* (CCThomas, Springfield IL. 1986)

Hoy S. *Chasing Dirt. The American Pursuit of Cleanliness.* (OUP 1995)

Hughes K. *The Short Life and Long Times of Mrs Beeton.* (Harper Perennial 2006.)

Hulbert A. *Raising America. Experts, parents and a century of advice about children.* (Vintage Books 2004).

Institute of Medicine, *Infant Formula: Evaluating the Safety of New Ingredients.* (National Academies Press, Washington DC, 2004)

Institute of Medicine. *Updating the USDA National Breastfeeding Campaign. Workshop summary.* (National Academies Press 2011)

Ip S, Chung M, Raman G, Chew P, Magila N, DeVine D et al. *Breastfeeding and maternal and infant health outcomes in developed countries.* AHRQ Publication No. 07-E007. Rockville, MD: Agency for Healthcare Research and Quality, 2007

Isolauri E, Walker WA (ed) *Allergic Diseases and the Environment.* (Karger/Nestec 2004) NNI Workshop Series vol. 53.

Jackson M. *The Mother Zone: love sex and laundry in the modern family.* (Henry Holt 1992)

James O. *How not to F\*\*\* Them Up.* (Vermilion Press 2010) In fact, read all his books.\*\*\*

Jelliffe DB Jelliffe EFP. *Advances in International Maternal and Child Health.* Vol. 3. (OUP 1983)

Jelliffe DB Jelliffe EFP. *Adverse Effects of Foods* (Plenum Press 1982)

Jelliffe DB, Jelliffe EFP. *Human Milk in the Modern World.* (OUP 1978)

Jelliffe EFP, Jelliffe DB. *Programmes to Promote Breastfeeding* (Oxford Medical Publications 1988)

Jensen RG (ed). *Handbook of Milk Composition.* (Academic Press London 1995)

Karen R. *Becoming Attached. First relationships and how they shape our capacity to love.* (OUP 1994)

Kendall Tackett K. *Non-pharmacologic Treatments for Depression in New Mothers.* (Thomas Hale Publishing 2001.)

Kendall-Tackett K. *Depression in New Mothers: causes, consequences and treatment options.* (Routledge Paul, London 2010).

Kent G. *Regulating Infant Formula.* (Hale Publishing 2011)

Kirkham M (ed.) *Exploring the dirty side of women's health.* (Routledge 2007)

Klaus A. *Every Child a Lion: the origins of maternal and infant health policy in the United States and France 1890-1920.* (Cornell University Press 1993)

Kleinman RE (ed) *Pediatric Nutrition Handbook* (AAP 5ᵗʰ ed. 2004)

Koerber A. *Breast or ? Contemporary controversies in infant feeding policy and practice.* (University of South Carolina 2013)

Koletzko B (ed) *Pediatric Nutrition in Practice.* (Karger/Nestlé 2008)

Koletzko B, Dodds P, Akerblom H, Ashwell M. (ed) *Early Nutrition and Its Later Consequences: Perinatal programming of Adult Health.* (Springer 2005)

Koletzko B, Koletzko S, Ruemmele F (eds.) *Drivers Of Innovation In Paediatric Nutrition.* NNI Workshop Series vol. 66, 2010.

Konner M. *The Evolution of Childhood.* (Harvard University Press 2010)

Kotsirilos V, Vitetta L, Sali A. *A Guide to Evidence-Based Integrative and Complementary Medicine.* (Churchill-Livingstone 2011)

Lawrence RA, Lawrence RM. *Breastfeeding: a guide for the medical profession.* (WB Saunders 2010)

Le Breton M. *Diet Intervention and Autism: Implementing the Gluten-free and Casein-free Diet for Autistic Children and Adults.* (Jessica Kingsley, London 2001)

Leach P. *Children First. What we must do - and are not doing- for our children today.* (Penguin 1994)

Lessof MH. *Food Intolerance and Food Aversion.* Royal College of Physicians of London, with the British Nutrition Foundation. (Update Publications, 1984)

Levenstein H. *Fear of Food: why we worry about what we eat.* (University of Chicago Press 2012.)

Levenstein H. *Paradox of Plenty: a social history of eating in modern America.* (Uni of California Press 2003)

Levenstein H. *Revolution at the Table. The Transformation of the American Diet.* (Uni of California Press 2003)

Lewis J. *The Politics of Motherhood.* Croom Helm London 1980

Loane S. *Who Cares? Guilt, hope and the child-care debate.* (Reed Books 1997)

Lovik M, Alexander J, Hastensen TS, Smith E. (eds) *Chemical Exposure and Food Allergy/Intolerance.* Special Issue of *Environmental Toxicology and Pharmacology*, 1997 Vol. 4 November. (Elsevier)

Lucas A, Zlotkin S. *Infant Nutrition.* (Health Press Oxford 2003)

Ludington Hoe SM, Golant SK. *Kangaroo Care: the best you can do to help your preterm infant* (Bantam Books 1993)

Maher V. (ed.) *The Anthropology of Breastfeeding. Natural Law or Social Construct?* (Berg, Oxford 1992)

Maier T. *Dr. Spock. An American Life.* (Harcourt Brace 1998)

Makrides M, Ochoa J, Szajewska H (eds). *The Importance of Immunonutrition* NNI Workshop vol 77, 2013

Manne A. *Motherhood. How should we care for our children?* (Allen & Unwin 2005)

McCalman J. *Struggletown: public and private life in Richmond 1900-1965* (MUP 1984)

McKay P. *100 Ways to Calm the Crying.* (Lothian Books 2002)

McKenna JJ. *Sleeping With Your Baby.* (Platypus Media 2007)***

MDAV. *Medicine and the Law. A practical guide for doctors.* (Medical Defence Association of Victoria, 2006)

Mein Smith P. *Mothers and King Baby: infant survival and welfare in an imperial world: Australia 1880-1950.* (Macmillan Press 1997

Mepham TB. *Physiology of Lactation.* (Open University Press 1987)

Mestecky J, Blair C, Ogra PL (eds) *Immunology of Milk and the Neonate.* (Plenum Press 1991)

Meyer HF. *Infant Foods and Feeding Practice. A reference text of practical infant feeding for physicians and nutritionists.* (CCThomas Springfield IL 1960)

Michaels D. *Doubt is Their Product: How Industry's Assault on Science Threatens Your Health* (OUP 2008)***

Michels D. (ed) *Breastfeeding Annual International 2001.* (Platypus Media Washington DC 2001)

Minchin MK. *Breastfeeding Matters: what we need to know about infant feeding.* (Alma Publications 1998; first edition 1985.)

Minchin MK. *Food for Thought: a parent's guide to food intolerance.* (Alma Publications 1982, '83; Allen & Unwin 1986; OUP 1986; Alma Publications 1992)

Minchin MK. *Towards Safer Artificial Feeding.* (booklet, Alma Publications, 2001)

Mitford J. *The American Way of Birth.* (Victor Gollancz 1992)

Moffat T, Prowse T. *Human Diet and Nutrition in Biocultural Perspective: Past Meets Present.* (Berghan Books Oxford, 2010)

Montagu A. *Touching: the human significance of the skin.* (Harper and Row )

More J. *Infant Child and Adolescent Nutrition.* (CRC Press 2013)

Morris M, Howard S. *Guilt-free Bottle Feeding.* (White Ladder Press 2014)

Morse JL, Talbot FB. *Diseases of nutrition and infant feeding.* (Macmillan 1922.)

Moss, Sweet, Swift (eds) *Early Intervention Programs for Infants* (Haworth Press 1982.) Contains the account of the CHO-Free disaster by Laskin and Pilot.

*Mothercraft: a selection from courses of lectures on infant care delivered under the auspices of the National Society for the Prevention of Infant Mortality.* Published by the National League for Physical Education and Improvement, London. Part 1, 1916.

*Mrs Beeton's Book of Household Management. (*Chancellor Press London 1982; Facsimile edition of the original published in 1861) p. 1035.

Murcott A. *Sociology of Food and Eating: Essays on the Sociological Significance of Food* (Gower International Library of Research & Practice,1983)

Murphy Y, Murphy RF. *Women of the Forest* (Columbia University Press NY 1985)

Narvaez D, Panksepp J, Schore AN, Gleason T (eds) *Evolution, Early Experience and Human Development.* (Oxford University Press 2012)

Nathoo T, Ostry A. *The One Best Way? Breastfeeding history, politics and policy in Canada.* (Wilfrid Laurier University Press 2009)

National Health and Medical Research Council (Australia). *Infant Feeding Guidelines.* (NHMRC 2012). Online

Nestle M. *Food Politics: how the food industry influences nutrition and health.* (Uni of California Press, 2007) ***

Nestle M. *Pet Food Politics.* (University of California Press, 2008)

Nicol P. *Sucking Eggs: what your wartime granny could teach you about diet, thrift and going green.* (Vintage Books London 2010.)

Nottingham S. *Eat Your Genes.* (Choice Books 1998)

Nylander G. *Becoming a Mother: birth to 6 months.* (Celestial Arts Press, 2002)

Oliviera et al. *WIC and the retail price of infant formula.* (USDA Economic Research Service 2004.)

Olmsted D, Blaxill M. *The Age of Autism. Mercury medicine and a man-made epidemic.* (Scribe Publications, 2010)

Oski FA. *Don't Drink Your Milk!* (Wyden Books, Chicago 1977)

Packard V. *Human Milk and Infant Formula.* (Academic Press 1982)

Paisseau G. *Le Lait Concentré Sucré: son emploi chez le nourrisson sain et le nourrisson malade.* (G. Doin et Cie Paris 1936.)

Palmer G. *Complementary Feeding: nutrition, culture and politics* (Pinter and Martin, London 2011.)

Palmer G. *The Politics of Breastfeeding.* (Pandora Press 1988; Pinter and Martin, London 2009.)

Park YW, Haenlein GFW (eds) *Milk and Dairy Products in Human Nutrition: Production, Composition and Health* (Wiley Blackwell 2013.)

Patton S. *Milk. Its Remarkable Contribution to Human Health and Well-being.* (Transaction Publishers, NJ. 2005)

Pennington H. *When Food Kills, BSE, E.coli and disaster science.* (OUP 2003)

Pepperall RA. *The Milk Marketing Board* (Clare, Son &Co Ltd, Somerset 1948).

Perman JA, Rey J. (ed) *Clinical Trials in Infant Nutrition* (Lippincott/Raven 1998) NNI Workshop Series vol. 40.

Pinchbeck I, Hewitt M. *Children in English Society: from the 18th century to the Children Act 1948.* (Routledge & Kegan Paul 1973.)

Ploss HH, Bartels M, Bartels P. *Woman, an historical, gynaecological and anthropological compendium* (Heinemann Medical Books London 1935, 3 vols.)

Pollan M, *The Omnivore's Dilemma* (Penguin 2006); *In Defence of Food* (Penguin 2008); *Cooked. A natural history of transformation.* (Penguin 2013)***

Pollard TM, Hyatt SB. *Sex, Gender and Health.* (Cambridge University Press 1999

Pottenger FM. *Pottenger's Cats: a study in nutrition.* (Pottenger-Price Nutrition Foundation 1983)

Potts M, Short RV. *Ever Since Adam and Eve: a history of human sexuality.* (Cambridge University Press 1998).***

Powell D, Leiss W. *Mad Cows and Mother's Milk. The perils of poor risk communication.* (McGill-Queens University Press Montreal 1997)

Prell MA. *An economic model of WIC, the infant formula rebate program, and the retail price of infant formula.* (USDA ERS 2004.)

Preedy VR, Watson RR, Zibadi S (eds.) *Handbook of dietary and nutritional aspects of bottle feeding.* (Wageningen Academic Publishers 2014) Highly recommended, as is its companion volume. Both should be on every serious infant feeding researcher's bookshelf.

Prescott, S. *The Allergy Epidemic.* (UWA Press 2011)***

Raiha NCR, Rubaltelli FF. (eds) *Infant Formula: Closer to the reference.* (Lippincott Williams and Wilkins/Nestec 2002) NNI Workshop v.47.

Raiha NCR.(ed) *Protein metabolism during Infancy.* (Raven/Nestle 1994) NNI Workshop Series 33.

Ransel DL. *Mothers of Misery: Child Abandonment in Russia (*Princeton University Press 1988)

Rapley G, Murlett T. *Baby-led Weaning.* (Vermilion London 2008)

Rapp D. *Is This Your Child's World?* (Bantam USA 1997)***

Rapp D. *Is This Your Child?* (Quill NY 1991)

Rees AR, Purcell HJ (eds). *Disease and the Environment.* ( John Wiley & Sons 1982)

Reiger KM. *Our Bodies, Our Babies. The forgotten women's movement.* (Melbourne Uni Press 2001)

Reiger KM. *The disenchantment of the home: modernizing the Australian family 1880-1940.* (OUP 1985)

Renfrew MJ, Woolridge MW, McGill HR. *Enabling Women to Breastfeed. A review of practices which promote or inhibit breastfeeding, with evidence–based guidelines for practice.* (HMSO London 2000)

Renner E. (ed) *Micronutrients in Milk and Milk-Based Food Products.* (Elsevier 1989)

Richter J. *Codes in context. TNC regulation in an era of dialogues and partnerships.* http://www.thecornerhouse.org.uk/resource/codes/context

Richter J. *Holding Corporations Accountable.* (Zed Books, London 2001)

Rigo J, Ziegler EE.(ed) *Protein and Energy Requirements in Infancy and Childhood.* (Karger/Nestlé 2006) NNI Workshop Series vol. 58.

Ross E. *Love and Toil. Motherhood in Outcast London 1870-1918.* (OUP 1993)

Royal College of Midwives *Successful Breastfeeding* (RCM London 1988; 1993; 2002)

SACN UK. *Infant Feeding Survey 2005: a commentary on infant feeding practices in the UK,* Position Statement by the Scientific Advisory Committee on Nutrition. (TSO London 2008)

Scantlebury V. *A Guide to Infant Feeding for the use of members of the medical and nursing professions.* (Public Health Department Victoria 1929 and all subsequent editions to 1976; from 1947 written by Dr Kate Campbell.)

Schmidl MK, Labuza TP (eds) *Essentials of Functional Foods.* (Aspen Publishers, 2000)

Schmid R. *The Untold Story of Milk. The history, politics and science of nature's perfect food: raw milk from pasture-fed cows.* (New Trends Publishing, Washington 2009)

Schmidt EHF, Hildebrandt AG. *Health Evaluation of Heavy Metals in Infant Formula and Junior Food.* (Springer-Verlag Berlin 1983)

Sears RW. *The Vaccine Book: Making the Right Decision for Your Child.* (Little Brown & Co. 2011)

Shaw IC. *Food Safety: the science of keeping food safe.* (Wiley Blackwell 2013)

Shaw R, Bartlett A. (ed) *Giving Breastmilk. Body Ethics and Contemporary Breastfeeding Practice.* (Demeter, Toronto 2010)

Short RV. *Lactation: the central control of reproduction.* Ciba Clinical Symposia 1976; 45: 73-86.

Shubber S. *The WHO International Code of Marketing of Breast-milk Substitutes: History and Analysis.* (Pinter and Martin 2011)

Sidel R. *Keeping Women and Children Last. America's War on the Poor.* (Penguin 1995)

Silverman WA. *Where's the Evidence?* Oxford: Oxford University Press; 1998.

Skypala I, Venter C. (ed) *Food Hypersensitivity.* (Wiley Blackwell 2009)

Small MF. *Our Babies, Ourselves. How biology and culture shape the way we parent.* (Anchor Books, 1998)

Smith DF (ed). *Nutrition in Britain. Science, scientists and politics in the 20th century.* (Routledge London 1997)

Smith FB. *The People's Health 1830-1910.* (ANU Press, Canberra 1979)

Smith JM. *Genetic Roulette. The documented health risks of genetically-engineered foods.* (Gene Ethics, Carlton 2007.)

Smith PH, Hausman BL, Labbok M (eds) *Beyond Health, Beyond Choice; breastfeeding constraints and realities.* (Rutgers University Press 2012)

Smith R, Lourie B. *Slow Death by Rubber Duck. How the toxic chemistry of everyday life affects our health.* (Knopf Canada 2009)

Soothill JF, Hayward AR, Wood CBS. *Paediatric Immunology.* (Blackwell 1983)

Steingraber S. *Having Faith. An ecologist's journey to motherhood.* (Berkely Books NY 2001)

Steingraber S. *Living Downstream. An ecologist looks at cancer and the environment.* (Virago 1998)

Steingraber S. *Raising Elijah: protecting our children in an age of environmental crisis.* (Da Capo Press, 2011)***

Still GF. *Common Disorders and Diseases of Childhood* (Oxford Medical Publications London 1910.)

Stuart-Macadam P, Dettwyler KA. (eds) *Breastfeeding: Biocultural Perspectives.* (Aldine de Gruyter 1995)

Sullivan D, Connolly M (ed) *Unbuttoned. Women open up about the pleasures, pains and politics of breastfeeding.* (Harvard Common Press 2009)

Sunderland M. *The Science of Parenting.* (Dorling Kindersley 2003)***

Sussman D. *Selling Mothers' Milk: the wet-nursing business in France 1715-1914.* (Uni of Illinois Press 1982)

Terman LM. *Genetic Studies of Genius.* (Stanford University Press 1926)

The Monopolies Commission. *Infant Milk Foods. A report on the supply of infant milk foods.* (HMSO London 1967)

Thompson A, Boland M, Singh H (eds) *Milk Proteins: From Expression to Food.* (Academic Press 2009)

Trager J. *The Food Chronology.* (Henry Holt &Co NY 1995)

Trevathan W, McKenna JJ, Smith EO. (eds) *Evolutionary Medicine.* (OUP 1999); *Evolutionary Medicine and Health* (OUP 2009)

Trevathan W. *Ancient Bodies, Modern Lives. How Evolution has shaped women's health.* (OUP 2010)***

Truby King F. *Feeding and Care of Baby.* (Whitcomb & Tombs 1913)

Truby King M. *Mothercraft.* (various editions)

Uvnas-Moberg K. *The Oxytocin Factor.* (da Capo Press 2003)

Valenze D. *Milk, a global and local history.* (Yale University Press 2011)

Valenze D. *The First Industrial Woman.* (OUP 1995)

Varnam AH and Sutherland, JP. *Milk and Milk Products: technology, chemistry and microbiology.* (Chapman & Hall, London 1994)

Vartabedian B. *Colic Solved: the essential guide to reflux and the care of your crying difficult-to-soothe baby.* (Ballantine Books 2007).

Walker H (ed) *Milk: Beyond the Dairy.* (Prospect Books, 2000)

Walker M. *Breastfeeding Management for the Clinician.* (Jones and Bartlett 2006)

Walker M. *Still selling out mothers and babies: marketing of breastmilk substitutes.* (NABA 2007)

Walker M. *Supplementation of the breastfed infant.* (Hale Publishing, 2014)

Waller H. *Clinical Studies in Lactation.* (WM Heinemann London nd.)

Waller H. *The Breasts and Breast Feeding.* (WM Heinemann London 1957)

Waring M. *Counting for nothing. What men value and what women are worth.* (Allen & Unwin 1988)***

Waring M. *Three Masquerades: essays on equality, work and human rights.* (Allen & Unwin 1996)

Wassenaar TM. *Bacteria: the benign, the bad and the beautiful.* (Wiley-Blackwell 2012.)

Welch RAS, Burns DJW, Davis SR, Popay AI, Prosser CG. *Milk Composition, Production and Technology.* (CAB International 1997)

Werner D. *Where There is no Doctor.* (Macmillan 2007).***

WHO Euro *PCBs, PCDDs and PCDFs in Breast Milk: Assessment of Health Risks.*

WHO *Induced Lactation and Relactation.* Online

Whorton JC. *The Arsenic Century: How Victorian Britain was Poisoned at Home, Work and Play.* (OUP 2010)

Wiley AS. *Re-Imagining Milk: Cultural and Biological perspectives.* (Routledge NY 2011).

Wilkinson AW. *The Immunology of Infant Feeding.* (Plenum Press 1981)

Wilkinson R, Pickett K. *The Spirit Level. Why equality is better for everyone.* (Allen Lane 2009)***

Williams AF, Baum JD. *Human Milk Banking.* (Raven Press/Nestlé 1984) NNI Workshop Series.

Williams F. *Breasts: a natural and unnatural history* (WW Norton Co NY 2012)

Wilson B. *Swindled. From Poison Sweets to Counterfeit Coffee- the Dark History of the Food Cheats.* (John Murray/ Hachette 2008)

Wilson D. *The Lead Scandal.* (Heinemannn 1983)

Winikoff B, Castle MA, Laukaran VH (eds) *Feeding Infants in Four Societies. Causes and Consequences of Mothers' Choices.* (Greenwood Press 1988)

Wolf JB. *Is Breast Best? Taking on the breastfeeding experts and the new high stakes of motherhood.* (NYU Press 2011) (Special pleading well critiqued by the next Professor JH Wolf.)

Wolf JH. *Don't Kill Your Baby: public health and the decline of breastfeeding in the 19th and 20th centuries.* (Ohio State University 2001)

Wolf N. *Misconceptions: truth, lies and the unexpected on the journey to motherhood.* (Vintage 2002)

Woodford K. *Devil in the Milk: illness health and politics. A1 and A2 milk.* (Craig Potton Publishing 2007)

Yalom M. *A History of the Breast.* (Alfred A Knopf NY 1997.)

Yeung DL *Infant Nutrition: a study of feeding practices and growth from birth to 18 months.* (Canadian Public Health Association 1983)

Zibadi S, Watson RR, Preedy VR (eds.) *Handbook of dietary and nutritional aspects of human breast milk.* (Wageningen Academic Publishers 2013) These two volumes (see Preedy) should be read by every nutrition researcher, allergist, paediatrician- and lactation consultant.

# Articles

*A note for the non-researcher: where a DOI is given, you can access the article or its abstract, by going to the following site in your browser and searching: http://dx.doi.org. Where a PMID is given, search for that in the online Pub Med sites.*

Aagaard K, Jun M, Antony KM, Radhika G et al. The Placenta Harbors a Unique Microbiome. *Sci Transl Med* 2014; 6:237. DOI: 10.1126/scitranslmed. 3008599

AAP Committee on Nutrition. Appraisal of nutritional adequacy of infant formulas used as cow milk substitutes. *Pediatrics* 1963; 31:2 329-338.

AAP Committee on Nutrition. Commentary on breastfeeding and infant formulas, including proposed standards for formulas. *Pediatrics* 1976; 57:278.

AAP Committee on Nutrition. Imitation and Substitute Milks. *Pediatrics* 1984; 73:6 876

AAP Committee on Nutrition. Proposed changes in FDA regulations concerning formula products and vitamin-mineral dietary supplements for infants. *Pediatrics* 1967; 40: 916

AAP Committee on Nutrition. Soy-protein formulas: recommendation for use in infant feeding. *Pediatrics* 1983; 72:359.

AAP Committee on Nutrition. The Use of Whole Cow's Milk in Infancy *Pediatrics* 1983; 72:2 253-255

AAP Section on Breastfeeding. Breastfeeding and the use of human milk. *Pediatrics* 2005; 115:496-506.

AAP Section on Breastfeeding. Policy statement: breastfeeding and the use of human milk. *Pediatrics.* 2012;129[3]:e827–e841. Available at: www.pediatrics.org/content/129/ 3/e827.full

Abrahamsson TR, Sandberg Abelius M, Forsberg A et al. A Th1/Th2-associated chemokine imbalance during infancy in children developing eczema, wheeze and sensitization. (PMID:21801246) *Clin Exp Allergy* 2011, 41(12):1729-1739

Abramovich M, Miller A, Yang H, Friel JK. Molybdenum content of Canadian and US infant formulas. (PMID:21279467) *Biological Trace Element Research* 2011; 143(2):844-853. DOI: 10.1007/s12011-010-8950-4

Abrams SA, Schanler RJ, Lee ML, Rechtman DJ. Greater mortality and morbidity in extremely preterm infants fed a diet containing cow milk protein products. (PMID:24867268) *Breastfeed Med* 2014; 9:281-285

ACA Aluminium in infant formula. *CHOICE* November 1990; pp. 27-30

Adab P, Jiang CQ, Rankin E, Tsang YW,et al. Breastfeeding practice, oral contraceptive use and risk of rheumatoid arthritis among Chinese women: the Guangzhou Biobank Cohort Study.(PMID:24395920) *Rheumatology* 2014; 53(5):860-866. DOI: 10.1093/rheumatology/ket456

Adgent MA, Daniels JL, Edwards LJ, Siega-Riz AM, Rogan WJ. Early-life Soy Exposure and Gender-role Play Behavior in Children. *Environ Health Perspect.* 2011;119(12):1811-1816.

Agostoni C, Axelsson I, Braegger C, Goulet O, et al. ESPGHAN Committee on Nutrition. Probiotic bacteria in dietetic products for infants: a commentary by the ESPGHAN Committee on Nutrition. (PMID:15085012) *J Pediatr Gastroenterol Nutr* 2004, 38(4):365-374.

Agriculture Department, Alberta Canada. Dessication or pre harvest glyphosate application: FAQ. See http:// www1.agric.gov.ab.ca/$department/deptdocs.nsf/all/faq7206Vajro P, Fontanella A, Avellino N. Breastfeeding enhances the clearance of HbsAG in infants wwith hep B virus infection. *Gastroenterology* 1985; 88:1702.

Akiyama H, Imai T, Ebisawa M. Japan food allergen labeling regulation-history and evaluation. (PMID:21504823) *Adv Food Nutr Res*2011; 62:139-71 DOI: 10.1016/B978-0-12-385989-1.00004-1

Akre J. Beyond 'Breast Is Best': Next Steps in the Counterrevolution. *Breastfeed Rev,* 2010; 18 (2): 5-9.

Akre JE, Gribble KD, Minchin MK. Milk sharing: from private practice to public pursuit. *Int Breastfeed J* 2011; 6:8. http://www.internationalbreastfeedingjournal.com/content/6/1/8

Aksit S, Caglayan S, Yaprak I, Kansoy S. Aflatoxin: is it a neglected threat for formula-fed infants? (PMID:9124050) *Acta Paediatr Jpn* 1997; 39(1):34-36

Al-Ahmed N, Alsowaidi S, Vadas P. Peanut Allergy: An Overview. *Allergy Asthma Clin Immunol.* 2008; 4(4): 139–143. doi: 10.1186/1710-1492-4-4-139

Al-Farsi YM, Al-Sharbati MM, Waly MI, Al-Farsi OA et al. Effect of suboptimal breast-feeding on occurrence of autism: a case-control study. (PMID:22541054) *Nutrition* 2012; 28(7-8):e27-32. DOI: 10.1016/j.nut.2012.01.007

Alabsi HS, Reschak GL, Fustino NJ, Beltroy EP et al.Neonatal eosinophilic gastroenteritis: possible in utero sensitization to cow's milk protein.(PMID:23985469) *Neonatal Netw* 2013; 32(5):316-322.

Allen KJ, Davidson GP, Day AS, Hill DJ, et al. Management of cow's milk protein allergy in infants and young children: an expert panel perspective. (PMID:19702611) *J Paediatr Child Health* 2009; 45(9):481-486.

Almgren M, Schlinzig T, Gomez-Cabrero D, Gunnar A et al. Cesarean section and hematopoietic stem cell epigenetics in the newborn infant - implications for future health? *Am J Obstet Gynecol* online 1 July 2014, DOI: http://dx.doi.org/10.1016/j.ajog.2014.05.014

Almond RJ, Flanagan BF, Antonopoulos A, Haslam SM et al. Differential immunogenicity and allergenicity of native and recombinant human lactoferrins: role of glycosylation. (PMID:23012214) *Eur J Immunol* 2013; 43(1):170-181.

Alvarez-Ordóñez A, Begley M, Clifford T, Deasy T,et al. Investigation of the Antimicrobial Activity of Bacillus licheniformis Strains Isolated from Retail Powdered Infant Milk Formulae.(PMID:24676765) *Probiotics Antimicrob Proteins s*2014, 6(1):32-40. DOI: 10.1007/s12602-013-9151-1

Amin SB, Merle KS, Orlando MS, Dalzell LE et al. Brainstem maturation in premature infants as a function of enteral feeding type. *Pediatrics* 2000; 106 (2) 318-322.

Amir LH, Ryan KM, Jordan SE. Avoiding risk at what cost? putting use of medicines for breastfeeding women into perspective. *Int Breastfeed J.* 2012; 7(1):14.

Anagnostou E, Soorya L, Chaplin W, Bartz J et al. Intranasal oxytocin versus placebo in the treatment of adults with autism spectrum disorders: a randomized controlled trial. *Molecular Autism* 2012; 3(1):16. (PMID:23216716)

Anderson J. Food-chemical intolerance in the breastfed infant. *Breastfeeding Rev* 2013; 21(1): 17-20. ( Joy refers to this book, then titled *Sacred Cows*, as she had read a draft. Apologies, Joy!)

Anderson JL, Edney RJ, Whelan K. Systematic review: faecal microbiota transplantation in the management of inflammatory bowel disease. (MED:22827693) *Aliment Pharmacol Ther* 2012, 36(6):503-516 DOI: 10.1111/j.1365-2036.2012.05220.x

Andersson Hellström-Westas L, Andersson D, Domellöf M. Effect of delayed versus early umbilical cord clamping on neonatal outcomes and iron status at 4 months: a randomised controlled trial.(PMID:22089242) *Br Med J* 2011; 343:d7157.

Andersson Y, Hammarström ML, Lönnerdal B, Graverholt G, et al. Formula feeding skews immune cell composition toward adaptive immunity compared to breastfeeding.(PMID:19734215) *J Immunol* 2009; 183(7):4322-4328

Andiran F, Dayl S, Mete E. Cows milk consumption and anal fissure in infants and young children. *J Pediatr Child Health* 2003; 39: 329-331

Ando Y, Ekuni Y, Matsumoto Y, Nakano S et al. Long-term serological outcome of infants who received frozen-thawed milk from human T-lymphotropic virus type-I positive mothers.(PMID:15566458) *J Obstet Gynaecol Res* 2004; 30(6):436-438

Andres A, Casey PH, Cleves MA, Badger TM. Body fat and bone mineral content of infants fed breast milk, cow's milk formula, or soy formula during the first year of life. (PMID:23375908) *J Pediatr 2013; 163(1):49-54*

Andrews T, Banks JR. Dietary baked milk accelerates the resolution of Cow's Milk Allergy in children. *Pediatrics* 2012; 130:Supplement 1 S13; doi:10.1542/peds.2012-2183R

Annand JC. Denatured bovine immunoglobulin pathogenic in atherosclerosis.(PMID:3964356) *Atherosclerosis* 1986; 59(3):347-351.

Anon If Queen Victoria had known about LAM. *Lancet* 1991; 337 i:703-4.

Anon. Baby's milk: soft sell success . *Marketing* 1980; May 14.

Anon. How evaporated and condensed milk is made - manufacture, making, history, used, processing, composition, steps, product, industry, History, Raw Materials, The Manufacturing Process of evaporated and condensed milk, Quality Control. http://www.madehow.com/Volume-6/Evaporated-and-Condensed-Milk.html#b#ixzz1oIC4KtMZ

Anthoni S, Savilahti E, Rautelin H, Kolho KL. Milk protein IgG and IgA: the association with milk-induced gastrointestinal symptoms in adults. *World J Gastroenterol* 2009; 15(39):4915-4918. (PMCID:PMC2764968)

Aoyama K, Matsuoka KI, Teshima T. Breast milk and transplantation tolerance.(PMID:21327152) Free resource *Chimerism* 2010; 1(1):19-20.

Apple RD. "Advertised by our loving friends": the infant formula industry and the creation of new pharmaceutical markets, 1870-1910. (PMID:3512689) *J Hist Med Allied Sci* 1986, 41(1):3-23

Apple RD. "To be used only under the direction of a physician": commercial infant feeding and medical practice, 1870-1940. (PMID:6998527) *Bull Hist Med* 1980, 54(3):402-417

Apple RD. The medicalization of infant feeding in the United States and New Zealand: two countries, one experience. (PMID:7619244) *J Hum Lact* 1994; 10(1):31-37

Arenz S, Rückerl R, Koletzko B, von Kries R. Breast-feeding and childhood obesity--a systematic review. *Int J Obes Relat Metab Disord.* 2004; 28(10):1247-56

Arnon SS, Damus K, Thompson B, Midura TF et al. Protective role of human milk against sudden death from infant botulism. (PMID:7038077) J Pediatr 1982; 100(4):568-573.

Asher P. The Incidence and Significance of Breast Feeding in Infants Admitted to Hospital. *Arch Dis Child.* 1952; 27(133): 270–272. PMCID: PMC1988521

Audicana Berasategui MT, Barasona Villarejo MJ, Corominas Sánchez M, De Barrio Fernández M, et al. Potential hypersensitivity due to the food or food additive content of medicinal products in Spain. (PMID:22312932) *J Investig Allergol Clin Immunol* 2011; 21(7):496-506.

Auerbach KG, Renfrew MJ, Minchin MK. Infant Feeding Comparisons: A Hazard to Infant Health. *J Hum Lact,* 1991; 7 (2): 63-71.

Azad MB, Bridgman SL, Becker AB, Kozyrskyj AL. Infant antibiotic exposure and the development of childhood overweight and central adiposity. *Int J Obes.* 2014 Jul 11. doi: 10.1038/ijo.2014.119.

Azad MB, Konya T, Maughan H, Guttman DS et al Gut microbiota of healthy Canadian infants: profiles by mode of delivery and infant diet at 4 months. *CMAJ* February 11, 2013 cmaj.121189, doi: 10.1503.

Badger TM, Gilchrist JM, Pivik RT, Andres A et al. The health implications of soy infant formula. . *Am J Clin Nutr.* 2009; 89(5):1668S-1672S.

Baghurst PA, McMichael AJ, Wigg NR, Vimpani GV et al. Environmental exposure to lead and children's intelligence at the age of seven years. The Port Pirie Cohort Study. (PMID:1383818) *NEJM* 1992, 327(18):1279-1284

Ball HL, Volpe LE. Sudden Infant Death Syndrome (SIDS) risk reduction and infant sleep location - moving the discussion forward. (PMID:22571891) *Soc Sci Med* 2013, 79:84-91. **DOI:** 10.1016/j.socscimed.2012.03.025

Ballard O, Morrow AL. Human milk composition: nutrients and bioactive factors. (PMCID:PMC3586783) *Pediatr Clin North Am* 2013, 60(1):49-74

Balmer SE, Harvey LS, Wharton BA Diet and faecal flora in the newborn: nucleotides. (PMID:2696432) *Arch Dis Child* 1994; 70: F137-140.

Balmer SE, Scott PH, Wharton BA Diet and faecal flora in the newborn: casein and whey proteins *Arch Dis Child* 1989; 64(12):1678-1684.

Balmer SE, Scott PH, Wharton BA Diet and faecal flora in the newborn: lactoferrin. *Arch Dis Child* 1989; 64(12):1685-1690.

Balmer SE, Wharton BA Diet and faecal flora in the newborn: breast milk and infant formula. (PMID:2696432) *Arch Dis Child* 1989; 64(12):1672-1677.

Barash JR, Hsia JK, Arnon SS. Presence of soil-dwelling clostridia in commercial powdered infant formulas. (PMID:20004414) *J Pediatr* 2010;156(3):402-408. DOI: 10.1016/j.jpeds.2009.09.072

Baratawidjaja IR, Baratawidjaja PP, Darwis A, Soo-Hwee L et al Prevalence of allergic sensitization to regional inhalants among allergic patients in Jakarta, Indonesia. (PMID:10403003) *Asian Pac J Allergy Immunol* 1999; 17(1): 9-12.

Barclay VC, Sim D, Chan BHK, Nell LA et al. (2012) The Evolutionary Consequences of Blood-Stage Vaccination on the Rodent Malaria Plasmodium chabaudi. *PLoS Biol* 2010(7): e1001368. doi:10.1371/journal.pbio.1001368.

Bardare M, Vaccari A, Allievi E, Brunelli L et al. Influence of dietary manipulation on incidence of atopic disease in infants at risk.(PMID:8214801) *Ann Allergy* 1993, 71(4):366-371.

Barker DJ, Gluckman PD, Godfrey KM, Harding JE et al. Fetal nutrition and cardiovascular disease in adult life. *Lancet* 1993;341(8850):938–941.

Barker DJ, Osmond C. Infant mortality, childhood nutrition, and ischaemic heart disease in England and Wales. *Lancet.* 1986;1(8489):1077–1081.

Barker DJ, Winter PD, Osmond C, Margetts B et al. Weight in infancy and death from ischaemic heart disease. *Lancet.* 1989;2(8663):577–580.

Barness LA. The Feeding of Solids debate. Reply to Ganelin RS, *Pediatrics* 1981; 67 (1):166.

Barthold JS, Hossain J, Olivant-Fisher A, Reilly A et al. Altered infant feeding patterns in boys with acquired nonsyndromic cryptorchidism. (PMID:23081935)*Birth Defects Research. Part A, Clinical and Molecular Teratology* 2012, 94(11):900-907.

Bartick M, Reinhold A. The burden of suboptimal breastfeeding in the United States: a pediatric cost analysis. *Pediatrics* 2010;125(5):e1048 –56

Bartick M. Breastfeeding and the U.S. economy. (PMID:22007819) *Breastfeed Med* 2011; 6:313-318.

Bartick M. The economic ramifications of improving maternity practices. (PMID:20942713) *Breastfeed Med 2010; 5(5):245.*

Bartick MC, Stuebe AM, Schwarz EB, Luongo C et al. Cost analysis of maternal disease associated with suboptimal breastfeeding. (PMID:23743465) *Obstet Gynecol* 2013; 122(1):111-119.

Baum CR, Shannon MW. The lead concentration of reconstituted infant formula.(PMID:9204097*) J Toxicol Clin Toxicol* 1997, 35(4):371-375

Becquet R, Marston M, Dabis F, Moulton LH, et al. Children who acquire HIV infection perinatally are at higher risk of early death than those acquiring infection through breastmilk: a meta-analysis. (PMID:22383946) *PLoS One* 2012; 7(2):e28510

Behrman D, Broadfoot M, Buchanan P et al.Early diet in preterm babies and later intelligence quotient. (PMID:10364137) BMJ 1999, 318(7198):1625. Surely study showed that breast milk is feed of choice for premature babies.

Bekelman JE, Li Y, Gross CP. Scope and impact of financial conflicts of interest in biomedical research: a systematic review. *JAMA* 2003; 289: 454-5.

Belderbos ME, Houben ML, Van Bleek GM, Schuliff L et al. Breastfeeding modulates neonatal innate immune responses: a prospective birth cohort study. *Ped Allergy Immunol* 2012; 23: 65-74

Belfort MB, Rifas-Shiman SL, Kleinman KP, Guthrie LB et al. Infant feeding and childhood cognition at ages 3 and 7 years: Effects of breastfeeding duration and exclusivity. (PMID:23896931) *JAMA Pediatr* 2013, 167(9):836-844.

Belfort MB, Rifas-Shiman SL, Rich-Edwards JW, Kleinman KP, Oken E, Gillman MW Infant growth and child cognition at 3 years of age. *Pediatrics* 2008, 122(3):e689-95. (PMID:18762504)

Bellinger DC, Stiles KM, Needleman HL. Low-level lead exposure, intelligence and academic achievement: a long-term follow-up study. (PMID:1437425) *Pediatrics* 1992, 90(6):855-861.

Bener A, Denic S, Galadri S. Longer breastfeeding and protection against childhood leukemia and lymphomas. *Eur J Cancer* 2001; 37: 234-238.

Bennett J, Gibson RA. Accuracy of infant formula preparation by Adelaide caregivers. *Breastfeeding Review* 1988 (November issue) pp.59-61.

Bent S, Böhm K. Copper-induced liver cirrhosis in a 13-month old boy(PMID:8527884) *Gesundheitswesen* 1995; 57(10):667-669. Benton D. Protein in the diet of neonates In Lebenthal E (ed) *Textbook of Gastroenterology and Nutrition* Vol 1 (Raven Press NY 1981) p. 388.

Bernard H, Ah-Leung S, Drumare MF, Feraudet-Tarisse C et al. Peanut allergens are rapidly transferred in human breast milk and can prevent sensitization in mice. (PMID:24773443) *Allergy* 2014, 69(7):888-897]DOI: 10.1111/all.12411

Bernbaum JC, Umbach DM, Ragan NB, Ballard JL, Archer JI, Schmidt-Davis H, Rogan WJ. Pilot studies of estrogen-related physical findings in infants. *Environ Health Perspect.* 2008 Mar;116(3):416-20.

Bernsen RM, Nagelkerke NJ, Thijs C, van der Wouden JC. Reported pertussis infection and risk of atopy in 8-to 12-yr-old vaccinated and non-vaccinated children. *Ped Allergy Immunol* 2008;19(1):46-52.

Berry NJ Jones SC, Iverson D. You're soaking in it: sources of information about infant formula. *Breastfeeding Review* 2011; 19(1): 9

Berry NJ, Jones S, Iversen D. It's all formula to me: women's understanding of toddler milk ads. *Breastfeeding Rev* 2010; 18 (1): 21-30.

Berry NJ, Jones SC, Iverson D. It's not the contents, it's the container: Australian parents' awareness and acceptance of infant and young child feeding recommendations. (PMID:22946149) *Breastfeed Rev* 2012, 20(2):31-35

Berry NJ, Jones SC, Iverson D. Toddler Milk Advertising in Australia: infant formula advertising in disguise? *Australasian Marketing Journal* 2012; 20 (1): 24-27

Betson D. Impact of the WIC Program on the Infant Formula Market. Final Report for Grant Award 43-3AEM-3-80107. Online at http://www3.nd.edu/~dbetson/research/documents/WICImpactonPrices.pdf

Beyerlein A, Hadders-Algra M, Kennedy K, Fewtrell M et al. Infant formula supplementation with long-chain polyunsaturated fatty acids has no effect on Bayley developmental scores at 18 months of age--IPD meta-analysis of 4 large clinical trials.. (PMID:19881391) *J Pediatr Gastroent Nutr* 2010; 50(1):79-84.

Snijders BE, Thijs C, Dagnelie PC, Stelma FF et al. Breast-Feeding Duration and Infant Atopic Manifestations, by Maternal Allergic Status, in the First 2 Years of Life (KOALA Study) *J Peds* 2007; 151 (4): 347-351.e2 DOI: 10.1016/j.jpeds.2007.03.022

Biasucci G, Rubini M, Riboni S, Morelli L, et al. Mode of delivery affects the bacterial community in the newborn gut.PMID:20133091) *Early Human Development* 2010; 86 Suppl 1:13-15.

Bier DM. Safety standards in infant nutrition: a US perspective. *Ann Nutr Metab* 2012; 60(3): 192-5.

Biesiekierski JR, Peters SL, Newnham ED, Rosella O, et al. No effects of gluten in patients with self-reported non-celiac gluten sensitivity after dietary reduction of fermentable, poorly absorbed, short-chain carbohydrates. (PMID:23648697) *Gastroenterology* 2013, 145(2):320-8.e1-3

Binns C, James J, Lee MK. Breastfeeding and the developing brain. *Breastfeed Rev.* 2013 Jul;21(2):11-3. PMID: 23957176

Binns CW, Lee MK. Exclusive breastfeeding for six months: the WHO six months recommendation in the Asia Pacific Region. (PMID:25164443) *Asian Pac J Cancer* Prev 2014; 23(3):344-350. DOI: 10.6133/apjcn.2014.23.3.21

Bird A, Epigenetics. New Scientist 5 January 2013 p. i-viii.

Bishop NJ, Dahlenburg SL, Fewtrell MS, Morley R et al. Early diet of preterm infants and bone mineralisation at age five years. *Acta Paediatr* 1996: 85:230-6.

Bivin WS, Heinen BN. Production of ethanol from infant food formulas by common yeasts. (PMID:3997687*) J Appl Bacteriol* 1985, 58(4):355-357.

Björkstén B. Pediatric Allergy Research – are we on the right track? *Pediatric Allergy and Immunology* 2014; 25(1): 4-6. DOI: 10.1111/pai.12184

Bjørnerem A, Ahmed LA, Jørgensen L, Størmer J et al.  Breastfeeding protects against hip fracture in postmenopausal women: the Tromsø study. (PMID:21898594) *J Bone Miner Res* 2011, 26(12):2843-2850. DOI: 10.1002/jbmr.496

Blake M. The Scary New Evidence on BPA-Free Plastics -And the Big Tobacco-style campaign to bury it. *Mother Jones* March/April 2014 Issue. Read at: http://motherjones.com/toc/2014/03

Blank D, Dotz V, Geyer R, Kunz C. Human milk oligosaccharides and Lewis blood group: individual high-throughput sample profiling to enhance conclusions from functional studies. (PMID:22585923) *Adv Nutr* 2012; 3(3):440s-449s

Blomqvist, Y., Ewald, U., Gradin, M., Nyqvist, K., Rubertsson, C. Initiation and extent of skin-to-skin care at two Swedish neonatal intensive care units. *Acta Paediatrica,* 2013; 102(1): 22-28.

Blum, D. On rice and arsenic. http://blogs.plos.org/speakeasyscience/2012/02/21, reprinted in *Sensitivity Matters* (AESSRA) 2012; 71 (March):12-13.

Blyton DM, Sullivan CE, Edwards N. Lactation is associated with an increase in slow wave sleep. *J Sleep Res* 2002; 11: 297-303.

Bollinger RR, Barbas AS, Bush EL, Lin SS, Parker W. Biofilms in the normal human large bowel: fact rather than fiction. *Gut* 2007, 56(10):1481-1482. (PMID:17872584)

Bollinger RR, Barbas AS, Bush EL, Lin SS, Parker W. Biofilms in the large bowel suggest an apparent function of the human vermiform appendix. (PMID:17936308) *J Theor Biol* 2007; 249(4):826-831.

Borgholtz P. Economic and business aspects of infant formula promotion: implications for health professionals. In Jelliffe DB, Jelliffe EFP (eds) *Advances in International Maternal and Child Health* volume 2. (OUP 1982)

Bornhorst J, Meyer S, Weber T, Böker C, et al. Molecular mechanisms of Mn induced neurotoxicity: RONS generation, genotoxicity, and DNA-damage response. Molecular Nutrition & Food Research 2013; 57(7):1255-1269] DOI: 10.1002/mnfr.201200758

Borschel MW, Baggs GE, Barrett-Reis B. Growth of Healthy Term Infants Fed Ready-to-Feed and Powdered Forms of an Extensively Hydrolyzed Casein-Based Infant Formula: A Randomized, Blinded, Controlled Trial. (PMID:24662422) *Clinical Pediatrics* 2014;

Böttcher MF, Abrahamsson TR, Fredriksson M, Jakobsson T et al. Low breast milk TGF-beta2 is induced by Lactobacillus reuteri supplementation and associates with reduced risk of sensitization during infancy. (PMID:18221472) *Ped Allergy Immunol.* 2008; 19(6):497-504

Bouhanick B, Ehlinger V, Delpierre C, Chamontin B et al. **Mode of delivery at birth and the metabolic syndrome in midlife: the role of the birth environment in a prospective birth cohort study.** *BMJ Open.* 2014;4(5):e005031. doi: 10.1136/bmjopen

Brady JP. Marketing breast milk substitutes: problems and perils throughout the world. *Arch Dis Child.* 2012; 97 (6): 529-32. PMID: 22419779. Free online

Brandtzaeg P. The mucosal immune system and its integration with the mammary glands. *J Peds* 2010; 156(2) S8-S15 DOI: 10/1016/lpeds.2009.11.2014

Braun-Fahrländer C, von Mutius E. Can farm milk consumption prevent allergic diseases? *Clinical and Experimental Allergy* 2011; 41(1):29-35 DOI: 10.1111/j.1365-2222.2010.03665.x

Brew BK, Marks GB, Almqvist C, Cistulli PA, et al. Breastfeeding and snoring: a birth cohort study. (PMCID:PMC3885662) *PloS one* 2014; 9(1):e84956 DOI: 10.1371/journal.pone.0084956

Britt K, Short R. The plight of nuns: hazards of nulliparity.(PMID:22153781) *Lancet* 2012; 379(9834):2322-2323.

Brooke OG, Wood C. Investigation of the 'satisfying' quality of infant formula milks. *Arch Dis Child* 1985; 60(6): 577-579.

Brooks M. Small shot, big impact. *New Scientist* 2013; 2930: 39

Brown A, Lee M. Breastfeeding during the first year promotes satiety responsiveness in children aged 18-24 months. (PMID:22911888) *Pediatric Obesity* 2012; 7(5):382-390

Brown C, Haringman N, Davies C, Gore C et al. High prevalence of food sensitisation in young children with liver disease: a clue to food allergy pathogenesis? *Pediatr Allergy Immunol* 2012 (PMID:23050587)

Brown K, DeCoffe D, Molcan E, Gibson DL. Diet-induced dysbiosis of the intestinal microbiota and the effects on immunity and disease. *Nutrients* 2012; 4(8):1095-1119. (PMCID:PMC3448089)

Brun JG, Nilsson S, Kvales G. Breastfeeding, other reproductive factors and rheumatoid arthritis: a prospective study. Br J Rheumatol 1995; 34: 542-6

Bu G, Luo Y, Chen F, Liu K, Zhu T. Milk processing as a tool to reduce cow's milk allergenicity: a mini-review. (PMCID:PMC3634986) Dairy Science & Technology 2013; 93(3):211-223.

Bucchini L, Goldman LR. Starlink Corn: A Risk Analysis *Environ Health Perspect* 2002; 110:5–13. Online 10 December 2001 http://ehpnet1.niehs.nih.gov/docs/2002/110p5-13bucchini/abstract.html

Buist A. Treating mental illness in lactating women. (PMID:11547266). *Medscape Womens Health* 2001; 6(2):3

Bullen CL, Tearle PV, Stewart MG The effect of "humanised" milks and supplemented breast feeding on the faecal flora of infants. (PMID:21296) *J Med Microbiol* 1977; 10(4): 403-413

Bullen CL, Tearle PV, Willis AT. Bifidobacteria in the intestinal tract of infants: an in-vivo study.*J Med Microbiol* 1976, 9(3):325-333 (PMID:8646)

Burd L, Fisher W, Kerbeshian J, Vesely B et al. A comparison of breastfeeding rates among children with pervasive developmental disorder, and controls. (PMID:3225319)*J Dev Behav Pediatr* 1988, 9(5):247-251/

Burkhardt MC, Beck AF, Kahn RS, Klein MD. Are our babies hungry? Food insecurity among infants in urban clinics. *Clin Pediatr (Phila)*. 2012; 51(3):238-43. doi: 10.1177/00099228

Burnier D, Dubois L, Girard M. Exclusive breastfeeding duration and later intake of vegetables in preschool children. (PMID:20978527 *Eur J Clin Nutr* 2011; 65(2):196-202

Burrell SA, Exley C. There is (still) too much aluminium in infant formulas. (MED:20807425) *BMC Pediatrics* 2010; 10:63 DOI: 10.1186/1471-2431-10-63

Businco L, Bruno G, Grandolfo ME, Novello F et al. Soy formula feeding and immunological response in babies of atopic families. (PMID:2570322) *Lancet* 1989; 2(8663):625-626

Businco L, Cantani A, Benincori N, Perlini R, et al. Effectiveness of oral sodium cromoglycate (SCG) in preventing food allergy in children. (PMID:6408951) *Ann Allergy* 1983; 51(1 Pt 1):47-50

Businco L, Meglio P, Amato G, Balsamo V etr al. Evaluation of the efficacy of oral cromolyn sodium or an oligoantigenic diet in children with atopic dermatitis: a multicenter study of 1085 patients.(PMID:8727267)*J Investig Allergol Clin Immunol* 1996; 6(2):103-109.

Butel JS. Simian Virus 40, poliovirus vaccines, and human cancer: research progress versus media and public interests. Bulletin of the World Health Organization, 2000, 78 (2) 195-197. http://www.who.int/bulletin/archives/78(2)195.pdf

Byard RW, Gilbert JG. Infant deaths associated with baby slings. *Med J Aust* 2011; 195 (6): 321. doi:10.5694/mja11.10693

Bygren LO, Kaati G, Edvinsson S. Longevity determined by paternal ancestors' nutrition during their slow growth period. (PMID:11368478) *Acta Biotheor* 2001, 49(1):53-59

Bystrova K, Matthiesen AS, Widström AM, Ransjö-Arvidson AB et al. The effect of Russian Maternity Home routines on breastfeeding and neonatal weight loss with special reference to swaddling. (PMID:16716541) *Early Hum Dev* 2007, 83(1):29-39

Cabrera-Rubio R, Collado MC, Laitinen K, Salminen S, et al. The human milk microbiome changes over lactation and is shaped by maternal weight and mode of delivery. *Am J Clin Nutr,* 2012; 96 (3): 544 DOI: 10.3945/ajcn.112.037382

Cahill SM, Wachsmuth IK, Costarrica Mde L, Ben Embarek PK. Powdered infant formula as a source of Salmonella infection in infants. (PMID:18171262) *Clin Infect Dis* 2008, 46(2):268-73

Campaign on Human Health and Industrial Farming. Avoiding Antibiotic Resistance: Denmark's Ban on Growth Promoting Antibiotics in Food Animals. Nov 1, 2010 Online at: http://www.pewtrusts.org/~/media/legacy/uploadedfiles/phg/content_level_pages/issue_briefs/DenmarkExperiencepdf.pdf

Canivet C, Jakobsson I, Hagander B. Infantile colic. Follow-up at four years of age: still more "emotional". *Acta Paed* 2000, 89(1):13-17 DOI: 10.1080/080352500750028988

Cant A, Marsden RA, Kilshaw PJ. Egg and cows' milk hypersensitivity in exclusively breast fed infants with eczema, and detection of egg protein in breast milk.(PMCID:PMC1417254) *Br Med J (Clin Res Ed)* 1985; 291(6500):932-935.

Cant AJ, Gibson P, Dancy M. Food hypersensitivity made life threatening by ingestion of aspirin.(PMID:6423064) *Br Med J (Clin Res Ed)* 1984, 288(6419):755-756.

Cantani A, Micera M. Neonatal cow milk sensitization in 143 case-reports: role of early exposure to cow's milk formula.. (PMID:16128043) *Eur Rev Med Pharmacol Sci* 2005; 9(4):227-230

Canterbury RJ, Haskins B, Kahn N, Saathoff G et al. Postpartum psychosis induced by bromocriptine. (PMID:3686155) *South Med J* 1987; 80(11):1463-1464.

Carl MA, Ndao IM, Springman AC, Manning SD et al. Sepsis From the Gut: The Enteric Habitat of Bacteria That Cause Late-Onset Neonatal Bloodstream Infections. (PMID:24647013) *Clin Infect Dis* 2014

Carlson SJ, Rogers RR, Lombard KA. Effect of a lactase preparation on lactose content and osmolality of preterm and term infant formulas. (PMID:1942472) *J Parenter Enteral Nutr* 1991; 15(5):564-566.

Carson DS, Guastella AJ, Taylor ER, McGregor IS. A brief history of oxytocin and its role in modulating psychostimulant effects. (PMID:23348754) *J Psychopharmacol* 2013; 27(3):231

Carter T. The Terror-Mob Crimes Link: Organized crime leaders and terrorists cross paths in cyberspace. *ABA Journal* January 1, 2014. http://www.abajournal.com/magazine/article/organized_crime_leaders_and_terrorists_cross_paths_in_cyberspace

Carver J. Advances in nutritional modifications of infant formula. *Am J Clin Nutr* 2003; 77 (6): 1550S-1554S

Casas R, Böttcher MF, Duchén K, Björkstén B. Detection of IgA antibodies to cat, beta-lactoglobulin, and ovalbumin allergens in human milk. (PMID:10856160) *J Allergy Clin Immunol* 2000; 105(6 pt 1):1236-1240.

Casey JA, Curriero FC, Cosgrove SE, Nachman KE et al. High-Density Livestock Operations, Crop Field Application of Manure, and Risk of Community-Associated Methicillin-Resistant Staphylococcus aureus Infection in Pennsylvania. JAMA Intern Med. 2013;():-. doi:10.1001/jamainternmed.2013.10408

Caspi A, Williams B, Kim-Cohen J, Craig IW, et al (2007). Moderation of breastfeeding effects on the IQ by genetic variation in fatty acid metabolism. *Proc Nat Acad Sci* 2007; 104 (47): 18860–5. doi:10.1073/pnas.0704292104. PMC 2141867. PMID 17984066.

Cattaneo A, Williams C, Pallás-Alonso CR, Hernández-Aguilar MT, et al. ESPGHAN's 2008 recommendation for early introduction of complementary foods: how good is the evidence? *MCN* (2011), 7: 335-343.

Cattaneo A. Infant and young child feeding: solid facts. *Breastfeed Rev*. 2013 Jul;21(2):7-9.

Cattaneo AG, Gornati R, Sabbioni E, Chiriva-Internati M, et al. Nanotechnology and human health: risks and benefits. (PMID:21117037) *J Appl Toxicol* 2010; 30(8):730-744.

Cattaneo A, Pani P, Carletti C, Guidetti M et al. Advertisements of follow-on formula and their perception by pregnant women and mothers in Italy. *Arch Dis Child* 2014. Published 22 December 2014, DOI: 10.1136/archdischild-2014-306996

Cavell B. Gastric emptying in infants fed human milk or infant formula. (PMID:7324911) *Acta Paediatr Scand* 1981; 70(5):639-641.

Center for Disease Control. Current trends recommendations for assisting in the prevention of perinatal transmission of human t-lymphotropic virus type III/lymphadenopathy-associated virus and acquired immunodeficiency syndrome. *Morbidity and Mortality Weekly Report* 1985;34:721-6,731-2.

Cetinkaya E, Joseph S, Ayhan K, Forsythe SJ Comparison of methods for the microbiological identification and profiling of Cronobacter species from ingredients used in the preparation of infant formula. (PMID:23089182) *Mol Cell Probes* 2012

Chaparro CM. Timing of umbilical cord clamping: effect on iron endowment of the newborn and later iron status. (PMID:22043880) *Nutr Rev* 2011, 69 Suppl 1:s30-6

Chapman DJ. Does breastfeeding resulting smarter children? A closer look. *J Hum Lact* 2013; 29 (4): 444-5.

Chappell JE, Clandinin MT, Kearney-Volpe C. Trans fatty acids in human milk lipids: influence of maternal diet and weight loss. *Am J Clin Nutr* 1985; 42(1):49-56. (PMID:4040321)

Chatelais L, JaminA, Gras-Le Guen C, Lallès J-P et al. The level of protein in milk formula modifies ileal sensitivity to LPS later in life in a piglet model. (PMCID:PMC3090415) *PLoS One*. 2011; 6(5): e19594. Published online 2011 May 9. doi: 10.1371/journal.pone.0019594

Chávez-Servín JL, Castellote A, Martín M, Chifré R, et al Stability during storage of LCPUFA-supplemented infant formula containing single cell oil or egg yolk *Food Chemistry* 2009; 113(2):484-492. DOI: 10.1016/j.foodchem.2008.07.082

Chávez-Servín JL, Castellote AI, Rivero M, López-Sabater MC. Analysis of vitamins A, E and C, iron and selenium contents in infant milk-based powdered formula during full shelf-life. *Food Chem* 2008; 107(3):1187-1197. DOI: 10.1016/j.foodchem.2007.09.048

Chen A, Rogan WJ. Breastfeeding and the risk of postneonatal death in the United States. (PMID:15121986) *Pediatrics* 2004; 113(5):e435-9.

Chen A, Rogan WJ. Isoflavones in soy infant formula: a review of evidence for endocrine and other activity in infants. (PMID:15189112) *Annu Rev Nutr* 2004, 24:33-54

Chen S, Binns CW, Zhao Y, Maycock B, Liu Y. Breastfeeding by Chinese mothers in Australia and China: the healthy migrant effect. (PMID:23468042) *J Hum Lact* 2013, 29(2):246-252. **DOI:** 10.1177/0890334413475838

Chen X, Chen J, Wen J, Xu. Breastfeeding is not a risk factor for mother-to-child transmission of hepatitis B virus. (PMID:23383145) *PLoS One* 2013; 8(1):e55303

Chen X, D'Souza R, Hong ST.The role of gut microbiota in the gut-brain axis: current challenges and perspectives. (PMID:23686721). *Protein & Cell* 2013; 4(6):403-414. DOI: 10.1007/s13238-013-3017-x

Chen Y. Synergistic effect of passive smoking and artificial feeding on hospitalization for respiratory illness in early childhood.(PMID:2785023) *Chest* 1989; 95(5):1004-1007; .

Chen ZY, Pelletier G, Hollywood R, Ratnayake WM. Trans fatty acid isomers in Canadian human milk. (PMID:7760684) Lipids 1995, 30(1):15-21

ChengKK, Chalmers I, Sheldon TA. Adding fluoride to water supplies. *BMJ* 2007; 335: 699-702.

Chesney RW. Taurine: its biological role and clinical implications. PMID:3909770 *Advances in Pediatrics* 1985; 32:1-42

Chiang WC, Huang CH, Llanora GV, Gerez I et al. Anaphylaxis to cow's milk formula containing short-chain galacto-oligosaccharide. (PMID:23102546) *J Allergy Clin Immunol* 2012; 130(6):1361-1367.

Chin KC,Tarlow MJ, Allfree NJ. Allergy to cows' milk presenting as chronic constipation. *BMJ* 1983; 287:405.

Chiu WC, Liao HF, Chang PJ, Chen PC et al. Duration of breast feeding and risk of developmental delay in Taiwanese children: a nationwide birth cohort study. *Paediatr Perinat Epidemiol.* 2011 Nov;25(6):519-27. doi: 10.1111/j.1365-3016.2011.01236.x. Epub 2011 Sep 15.

Chung CS, Yamini S, Trumbo PR. FDA's Health Claim Review: Whey-protein Partially Hydrolyzed Infant Formula and Atopic Dermatitis. (PMID:22778306) *Pediatrics* 2012, 130(2):e408-14

Church MW, Jen KL, Jackson DA, Adams BR, Hotra JW. Abnormal neurological responses in young adult offspring caused by excess omega-3 fatty acid (fish oil) consumption by the mother during pregnancy and lactation. (PMID:18834936) *Neurotoxicol Teratol* 2009; 31(1):26-33.

Clandinin MT, Larsen B, Van Aerde J. Reduced bone mineralization in infants fed palm olein-containing formula: a randomized, double-blinded, prospective trial. *Pediatrics.* 2004; 114(3):899-900; author reply 899-900. PubMed PMID: 15342879.

Clock, R. Intestinal Implantation of the Bacillus Lactis Bulgaricus in Certain Intestinal Conditions of Infants, with Report of Cases. *JAMA,* June 29, 1912

Cocchi P, Cocchi C, Weinbreack P, Loustad V. Postnatal transmission of HIV infection. *Lancet* 1988; 331 (8583) i: 482. doi:10.1016/S0140-6736(88)91284-6

Cocho JA, Cervilla JR, Rey-Goldar ML et al. Chromium content in human milk, cow's milk, and infant formulas. *Biol Trace Elem Re*s 1992; 32:105-107. (PMID:1375045)

Cohen R, Mrtek MB, Mrtek RG. Comparison of maternal absenteeism and infant illness rates among breast-feeding and formula-feeding women in two corporations. (PMID:10160049) Am J Health Promot 1995, 10(2):148-153.

Colen CG, Ramey DM. Is Breast Truly Best? Estimating the Effects of Breastfeeding on Long-term Child Health and Wellbeing in the United States Using Sibling Comparisons. *Soc Sci Med* (2014), doi: 10.1016/j.socscimed.2014.01.027.

Collaborative Group on Hormonal Factors in Breast Cancer. Breast cancer and breastfeeding: collaborative reanalysis of individual data from 47 epidemiological studies in 30 countries, including 50302 women with breast cancer and 96973 women without the disease. (PMID:12133652) Lancet 2002; 360(9328):187-195.

Collado MC, Laitinen K, Salminen S, Isolauri E. Maternal weight and excessive weight gain during pregnancy modify the immunomodulatory potential of breast milk. (PMID:22453296) *Pediatr Res* 2012; 72(1):77-85

Collins AM, Roberton DM, Hosking CS, Flannery GR. Bovine milk, including pasteurised milk, contains antibodies directed against allergens of clinical importance to man. (PMID:1809694) *Int Arch All App Immunol* 1991;96(4):362-7

Collins AM. Xenogeneic antibodies and atopic disease. *Lancet* 1988; 1(8588):734-737 DOI: 10.1016/S0140-6736(88)91539-5.

Collipp PJ, Chen SY, Maitinsky S. Manganese in infant formulas and learning disability. *Ann Nutr Metab* 1983; 27(6):488-494. (PMID:6651226)

Committee on Nutrition of the British Paediatric Association. Is breast feeding beneficial in the UK? *Arch Dis Child.* 1994; 71(4): 376–380. PMCID: PMC1030026

Comstock SS, Reznikov EA, Contractor N, Donovan SM. Dietary bovine lactoferrin alters mucosal and systemic immune cell responses in neonatal piglets. (PMID:24553692) J Nutr 2014; 144(4):525-532

Conway SP, Phillips RR, Panday S. Admission to hospital with gastroenteritis. *Arch Dis Child.* 1990; 65(6): 579–584.

Conway SP, Phillips RR. Morbidity in whooping cough and measles.(PMID:2817928) *Arch Dis Child* 1989; 64(10):1442-1445

Cooklin AR, Donath SM, Amir LH. Maternal employment and breastfeeding: results from the longitudinal study of Australian children. *Acta Paediatr.* 2008: 97(5):620-3.

Coombs RRA. Holgate ST. Allergy and cot death: with special focus on allergic sensitivity to cows' milk and anpahylaxis. *Clin Exper Allergy* 1990; 20: 259-366.

Cornblath M, Schwartz R, Aynsley-Green A , Lloyd JK. Hypoglycemia in infancy: the need for a rational definition. A Ciba Foundation discussion meeting. *Pediatrics* 1990; 85(5): 834-837. (PMID:2330247)

Corvaglia L, Aceti A, Mariani E, Legnani E et al Lack of efficacy of a starch-thickened preterm formula on gastro-oesophageal reflux in preterm infants: a pilot study. *J Matern Fetal Neonatal Med* 2012; 25(12):2735-2738

Cost TK, Lobell TD, Williams-Yee ZN, Henderson S et al. The effects of pregnancy, lactation, and primiparity on object-in-place memory of female rats. *Hormones and Behaviour.* 2014; 65, 32-39.

Coulthard H, Harris G, Emmett P. Delayed introduction of lumpy foods to children during the complementary feeding period affects child's food acceptance and feeding at 7 years of age. (PMID:19161546) *Matern Child Nutr* 2009, 5(1):75-85.

Couturier P, Basset-Stème D, Navette N, Sainte-Laudy J. A case of coconut oil allergy in an infant: responsibility of "maternalized" infant formulas (PMID:7702732) *Allergie et Immunologie* 1994; 26(10):386-7.

Cox LM, Yamanishi S, Sohn J, Alekseyenko AV et al. Altering the Intestinal Microbiota during a Critical Developmental Window Has Lasting Metabolic Consequences. *Cell* 2014. http://dx.doi.org/10.1016/j.cell.2014.05.052

Craven JA. Salmonella contamination of dried milk products. Vic Vet Proc. 1978; 36:56

Crawford MA. The elimination of child poverty and the pivotal significance of the mother. (PMID:19009739) *Nutrition and Health* 2008, 19(3):175-186.

Crevel RW, Kerkhoff MA, Koning MM. Allergenicity of refined vegetable oils. (PMID:10722892) *Food Chem Toxicol* 2000, 38(4):385-393 DOI: 10.1016/S0278-6915(99)00158-1

Crinella FM. Does soy-based infant formula cause ADHD? Update and public policy considerations. (PMID:22449212) *Expert Rev Neurother* 2012; 12(4):395-407.

Cristofalo EA, Schanler RJ, Blanco CL, Sullivan S et al. Randomized Trial of Exclusive Human Milk versus Preterm Formula Diets in Extremely Premature Infants. *J Pediatr* 2013; 163(6):1592-1595.

Crocetti M, Moghbeli N, Serwint J. Fever phobia revisited: have parental misconceptions about fever changed in 20 years? (PMID:11389237) *Pediatrics* 2001, 107(6):1241-6.

Cruse P, Yudkin P, Baum JD. Establishing demand feeding in hospital. (PMID:626524) Free resource *Arch Dis Child* 1978, 53(1):76-78

Cryn J, Dinan T. A light on psychobiotics. *New Scientist* 2014 Jan 25, p. 28-29

Cullen P. *Irish Times* July 7, 2008. http://www.irishtimes.com/news/ireland-criticised-over-controls-on-making-baby-food-1.943169

Currie D. Breastfeeding rates for black US women increase, but lag overall: Continuing disparity raises concerns. *The Nation's Health* 2013; 43 (3): 1-20. http://thenationshealth.aphapublications.org/content/43/3/1.3.full?sid=fd5bf00f-a218-43b0-9490-a40921f3b011

Curtin C. Don't make mums feel guilty. *Sunday Herald Sun* October 21, 2012 p. 68

D'Aloisio AA, Baird DD, DeRoo LA, Sandler DP. Association of intrauterine and early-life exposures with diagnosis of uterine leiomyomata by 35 years of age in the sister study. *Environ Health Perspect.* 2010 Mar;118(3):375-81. Erratum in: Environ Health Perspect. 2010 Mar;118(3):380.

D'Vaz N, Meldrum SJ, Dunstan JA, Martino D et al. Postnatal fish oil supplementation in high-risk infants to prevent allergy: RCT. (PMID:22945403) *Pediatrics* 2012;130(4):674-682.

Dabeka R, Fouquet A, Belisle S, Turcotte S. Lead, cadmium and aluminum in Canadian infant formulae, oral electrolytes and glucose solutions.*Food Addit Contam Part A Chem Anal Control Expo Risk Assess.* 2011; 28(6):744–753. doi: 10.1080/19393210.2011.571795

Dabeka RW, McKenzie AD. Lead and cadmium levels in commercial infant foods and dietary intake by infants 0-1 year old. (PMID:3396737) *Food Addit Contam* 1988, 5(3):333-342

Dabeka RW. Survey of lead, cadmium, cobalt and nickel in infant formulas and evaporated milks and estimation of dietary intakes of the elements by infants 0–12 months old. *Sci Total Environ.*1989; 89: 279–289.

Dagnelie PC, van Staveren WA, Roos AH et al. Nutrients and contaminants in milk from mothers on macrobiotic and omnivorous diets. *Eur J Clin Nutr* 1992; 46: 355-366.

Dagnelie PC, van Staveren WA. Macrobiotic nutrition and child health: results of a population-based, mixed-longitudinal cohort study in The Netherlands. *Am J Clin Nutr* 1994; 59(5 Suppl):1187S–1196S

Dairy Reporter.com is the site to sign up for a free industry newsletter - for anyone interested in milk products or issues, from regulation to asses' milk.

Dall'Erta A, Cirlini M, Dall'Asta M, Del Rio D et al. Masked mycotoxins are efficiently hydrolyzed by human colonic microbiota releasing their aglycones *Chem Res Toxicol* 2013; 26 (3): 305–312. DOI: 10.1021/tx300438c

Daniels L, Gibson RA, Simmer K, Van Dael P et al. Selenium status of term infants fed selenium-supplemented formula in a randomized dose-response trial. (PMID:18614726). *Am J Clin Nutr* 2008; 88(1):70-76.

Darling PB, Dunn M, Gilani GS, Ball RO, Pencharz PB. Phenylalanine kinetics differ between formula-fed and human milk-fed preterm infants.(PMID:15465744) *J Nutr* 2004; 134(10):2540-5.

Davanzo R, Giurici N, Demarini S. Hot Water and Preparation of Infant Formula: how hot does it have to be to be safe? *J Pediatr Gastroent Nutr* 2010; 50 (3):352–353. doi: 10.1097/MPG.0b013e31819f65b1

Davanzo R, Zauli G, Monasta L, Vecchi Brumatti L et al. Human colostrum and breast milk contain high levels of TNF-related apoptosis-inducing ligand (TRAIL). (PMID:22529245) *J Hum Lact* 201329(1):23-25]

David LA, Maurice CF, Carmody RN, Gootenberg DB et al Diet rapidly and reproducibly alters the human gut microbiome. (PMID:24336217) *Nature* 2014, 505(7484):559-563 DOI: 10.1038/nature12820

Davidson GP, Whyte PB, Daniels E, Franklin K, et al. Passive immunisation of children with bovine colostrum containing antibodies to human rotavirus. (PMID:2570959) *Lancet* 1989, 2(8665):709-712.

Davidson LA, Lönnerdal B. Persistence of human milk proteins in the breast-fed infant. (PMID:3661174) *Acta Paed Scand* 1987; 76(5):733-740. DOI: 10.1111/j.1651-2227.1987.tb10557.x

Davis MK, Savitz DA, Graubard DI. Infant feeding and childhood cancer. *Lancet* 1988; 8607, ii: 365-8.

Day JB, Sharma D, Siddique N, Hao YY, et al Survival of Salmonella Typhi and Shigella dysenteriae in dehydrated infant formula. (PMID:22417504*) J Food Sci* 2011, 76(6):m324-8

De Curtis M, Candusso M, Pieltain C, Rigo J Effect of fortification on the osmolality of human milk. Arch Dis Child 1999; 81:F141-3.

de Halleux V, Rigo J Variability in human milk composition: benefit of individualized fortification in very-low-birth-weight infants.(PMID:23824725) Am J Clin Nutr 2013, 98(2):529s-35s

de Halleux V, Rigo J. Variability in human milk composition: benefit of individualized fortification in very-low-birth-weight infants. Am J Clin Nutr 2013; 98(2):529s-35s.(PMID:23824725)

de Jong MH, Scharp V T M, van der Linden R, Aalberse R, et al. The effect of brief neonatal exposure to cows' milk on atopic symptoms up to age 5. Arch Dis Child 2002; 86:365–39

de Jong MH, Scharp VTM, van der Linden R, Aalberse RC. Randomised controlled trial of brief neonatal exposure to cows' milk on the development of atopy. Arch Dis Child 1998;79:126–30.

de Laffolie J, Turial S, Heckmann M, Zimmer KP et al. Decline in infantile hypertrophic pyloric stenosis in Germany 2000-2008. Pediatrics 2012, 129(4):e901-6. (PMID:22430445)

de Marco R, Pesce G, Girardi P, Marchetti P et al. Foetal exposure to maternal stressful events increases the risk of having asthma and atopic diseases in childhood. Pediatr Allergy Immunol 2012: 00

de Oliveira JE. Methionine supplementation of soy protein formulas. Am J Clin Nutr 1981; 34(4):605-606. (PMID:7194579)

de Onis M. Update on the Implementation of the WHO Child Growth Standards.World Rev Nutr Diet 2013; 106:75-82. (PMID:23428684)

de Regil LM, de la Barca AM. Nutritional and technological evaluation of an enzymatically methionine-enriched soy protein for infant enteral formulas. Int J Food Sci Nutr 2004; 55(2):91-99. (PMID:14985181)

de Zegher F, Sebastiani G, Diaz M, Gómez-Roig MD et al. Breast-feeding vs formula-feeding for infants born small-for-gestational-age: divergent effects on fat mass and on circulating IGF-I and high-molecular-weight adiponectin in late infancy. (PMID:23365126) J Clin Endocrinol Metab 2013, 98(3):1242-1247. DOI: 10.1210/jc.2012-3480

Dean TP, Adler BR, Ruge F, Warner JO. In vitro allergenicity of cows' milk substitutes. (PMID:8472190) Clin Exper Allergol 1993, 23(3):205-210 DOI: 10.1111/j.1365-2222.1993.tb00883.

Deelstra H, van Schoor O, Robberecht H, Clara R et al. Daily chromium intake by infants in Belgium. (PMID:3389133) Acta Paed Scand 1988; 77(3):402-407. DOI: 10.1111/j.1651-2227.1988.tb10667.x

Deoni S, DC, Piryatinksy I, O'Muircheartaigh J, et al. Breastfeeding and early white matter development: A cross-sectional study. NeuroImage, 2013; DOI: 10.1016/j.neuroimage.2013.05.090

Der G, Batty GD, Deary IJ. Effect of breast feeding on intelligence in children: Prospective study, sibling pairs analysis, and meta-analysis. BMJ 2006, 333, 945.

Deshpande GC, Rao SC, Keil AD, Patole SK. Evidence-based guidelines for use of probiotics in preterm neonates. (PMID:21806843) BMC Medicine 2011, 9:92.

Detection of Lead in the DC Drinking Water System. Hearing before the Sub-Committee on Fisheries, Wildlife, and Water of the Committee on Environment and Public Works, US Senate 108th Congress, second session April 7 2004. Available online

Dewey KG, Domellof M, Cohen RJ et al. Iron supplementation affects growth and morbidity of breastfed infants: results of a trial in Sweden and Honduras. J Nutr 2002; 132: 3249-55.

Di Prisco MC, Hagel I, Lynch NR, Barrios RM et al. Possible relationship between allergic disease and infection by G. lamblia. Annals of Allergy 1993, 70(3):210-3. (PMID:8452315)

Di Santis KI, Collins BN, Fisher Jo, Davey A. Do infants fed directly from the breast have improved appetite regulation and slower growth during early childhood compared with infants fed from a bottle? Int J Behav Nutr Phys Act 2011; 8:89

Diarrassouba F, Garrait G, Remondetto G, Alvarez P, et al. Increased stability and protease resistance of the β-lactoglobulin/vitamin D3 complex. Food Chem. 2014 Feb 15;145:646-52. doi: 10.1016/j.foodchem.2013.08.075. Epub 2013 Aug 28.

Dierselhuis MP, Blokland EC, Pool J, Schrama E, et al Transmaternal cell flow leads to antigen-experienced cord blood. PMID:22627770) Blood 2012, 120 (3): 505-510

Dieterich CM, Felice JP, O'Sullivan E, Rasmussen KM. Breastfeeding and health outcomes for the mother-infant dyad. (PMID:23178059) Pediatr Clin Nth Am 2013, 60(1):31-48 DOI: 10.1016/j.pcl.2012.09.010

Dixon D-L, Griggs KM, Forsyth KD, Bersten AD. Lower interleukin-8 levels in airway aspirates from breastfed infants with acute bronchiolitis. Paed Allerg immunol 2010: e691-6. DOI: 10.1111/j.199-3038.2010.01011.x

Dixon JJ, Burd DA, Roberts DG. Severe burns resulting from an exploding teat on a bottle of infant formula milk heated in a microwave oven. (PMID:9232290) Burns 1997, 23(3):268-269

Dlouhy BJ, Awe O, Rao RC, Kirby PA et al. Autograft-derived spinal cord mass following olfactory mucosal cell transplantation in a spinal cord injury patient: Case report. (PMID:25002238) J Neurosurg Spine 2014, 21(4):618-622.

Doan T, Gardiner A, Gay CL, Lee KA. Breast-feeding increases sleep duration of new parents. (PMID:17700096) J Perinat Neonat Nurs 2007; 21(3):200-206; doi: 10.4066/AMJ.2012.1222 (PMCID:PMC3395287)

Domestic use of infant formula: hearing before the Subcommittee on Oversight and Investigations of the Committee on Energy and Commerce, House of Representatives, Ninety-seventh Congress, first session, June 17, 1981. p. 24. Can be accessed from http://nla.gov.au/nla.cat-vn3853323

Domínguez-Ortega G, Borrelli O, Meyer R, Dziubak R et al. Extraintestinal Manifestations in Children With Gastrointestinal Food Allergy. *J Pediatr Gastroent Nutr* 2014; 59 (2): 210-214. doi: 10.1097/MPG.0000000000000391

Dórea JG, Marques RC. Infants' exposure to aluminum from vaccines and breast milk during the first 6 months. (PMID:20010978) *J Exp Sci Envir Epidemiol* 2010; 20(7):598-601. DOI: 10.1038/jes.2009.64

Dorfman B. Baby, look at Mead Johnson now. http://uk.reuters.com/article/2010/03/01/us

Dörner G, Bewer G, Lubs H. Changes of the plasma tryptophan to neutral amino acids ratio in formula-fed infants: possible effects on brain development.(PMID:6686152) *Exper Clin Endocrinol* 1983; 82(3): 368-71.

Dörner G, Grychtolik H. Long-lasting ill-effects of neonatal qualitative and/or quantitative dysnutrition in the human. *Endokrinologie* 1978, 71(1):81-88

Dorner K, Schneider K, Sievers E et al. Selenium balances in young infants fed or breastmilk or adapted formula. *J Trace Elem Electrolytes Health* 1990; 4: 37-40

Dosch H-M, Becker DJ. Infant feeding and auto-immune diabetes. Chapter in Davis et al. *Integrating Population Outcomes, Biological Mechanisms And Research Methods In The Study Of Human Milk And Lactation.* (Kluwer Academic/Plenum Publishers 2002)

Douglas P. The Rise and Fall of Infant reflux: the limits of evidence-based medicine. *Griffith REVIEW* 2011, edition 32.

Douglas PS, Hill PS. Managing infants who cry excessively in the first few months of life. *Br Med J* 2011; 343:d7772 doi: 10.1136/bmj.d7772

Douglas PS, Hill PS. The crying baby: what approach? (PMID:21799411) *Curr Opin Pediatr* 2011, 23(5):523-529.

Dowling DA, Meier PP, DiFiore JM, Blatz MA et al. Cup-Feeding for Preterm Infants: Mechanics and Safety. *J Hum Lact* 2002; 18(1): 3-210.

Drane DL, Logemann JA. A critical evaluation of the evidence on the association between type of infant feeding and cognitive development.(PMID:11101022) *Paediatr Perinat Epidemiol* 2000; 14(4):349-56.

Dufault R, LeBlanc B, Schnoll R, Cornett C et al. Mercury from chlor-alkali plants: measured concentrations in food product sugar. *Environ Health.* 2009; 8:2.

Dugdale AE. Evolution and infant feeding. (PMID:2869357) *Lancet* 1986, 1(8482):670-3

Duintjer Tebbens RJ, Pallansch MA, Kim JH, Burns CC et al. Oral poliovirus vaccine evolution and insights relevant to modeling the risks of circulating vaccine-derived polioviruses (cVDPVs). (PMID:23470192) *Risk Anal* 2013; 33(4):680-702 (1) e164 -e169. doi: 10.1542/peds.2008-2189

Dündaröz R, Aydin H, Ulucan H, Baltaci V et al. Preliminary study on DNA damage in non breast-fed infants. Pediatr Internat 2002; 44 (2): 127–130. PMID:11896867)

Dündaröz R, Ulucan H, Aydin HI, Güngör Tet al. Analysis of DNA damage using the comet assay in infants fed cow's milk. (PMID:12907847) *Biol Neonate* 2003, 84(2):135-141

Dunlop RA, Cox PA, Banack SA, Rodgers KJ (2013) The Non-Protein Amino Acid BMAA is misincorporated into human proteins in place of l-Serine causing protein misfolding and aggregation. *PLoS One* 8(9): e75376. doi:10.1371/journal.pone.0075376

Dunsmore DG, Wheeler SM. Iodophors and Iodine in Dairy Products 8: The Total Industry Situation. *Aust J Dairy Tech* 1992; 32 (4)

Duplantier JE. Lymphoid Nodular hyperplasia and cow's milk hypersensitivity in children with chronic constipation. *Pediatrics* 2005; 116: Supplement 2 547; doi:10.1542/peds.2005-0698Y

Edwards AM. Oral sodium cromoglycate: its use in the management of food allergy. (PMID:8542460) *Clin Exp Allergy* 1995; 25 Suppl 1:31-33.

Edwards EA, Grant CC, Huang QS, Powell KF, Croxson MC. A case of vaccine-associated paralytic poliomyelitis. (PMID:10940185) *J Paediatr Child Health* 2000; 36(4):408-411.DOI: 10.1046/j.1440-1754.2000.00514.x

EFSA NDAS http://www.efsa.europa.eu/en/consultations/call/140424.pdf Essential composition of infant and follow-on formula – draft for public consultation. EFSA Panel on Dietetic Products, Nutrition and Allergies. doi 10.2903/j.efsa.20xx.NNNN

EFSA Panel on Dietetic Products, Nutrition and Allergies (NDA): Scientific Opinion on the appropriate age for introduction of complementary feeding of infants. *EFSA Journal* (2009) 7(12)1423: 11-38

Egger J, Carter CH, Soothill JF, Wilson J. Effect of diet treatment on enuresis in children with migraine or hyperkinetic behavior. (PMID:1582098) Clin Pediatr 1992, 31(5):302-307

Egger J, Carter CM, Wilson J, Turner MW, Soothill JF. Is migraine food allergy? A double-blind controlled trial of oligoantigenic diet treatment. (PMID:6137694) *Lancet* 1983, 2(8355):865-869 DOI: 10.1016/S0140-6736(83)90866-8

Ekstrand J, Boreus LO, de Chateau P. No evidence of transfer of fluoride from plasma to breast milk. (PMCID:PMC1506856) Free full text article *BMJ* 1981; 283(6294):761-762

El-Merhibi A, Lymn K, Kanter I, Penttila IA. Early oral ovalbumin exposure during maternal milk feeding prevents spontaneous allergic sensitization in allergy-prone rat pups. (PMCID:PMC3235444) *Clin Dev Immunol* 2012:396232 DOI: 10.1155/2012/396232

Elliot, MM. *Infant Care*. Children's Bureau Publication no 8, 1945. (Social Security Commission, Federal Security Agency.)

Ellsworth WL. Injection-Induced Earthquakes. *Science* 12 July 2013: 1225942 DOI:10.1126/science.1225942

Elton C. Hard to Swallow: the truth about infant formula. *Consumer's Digest* June 2011 www.consumersdigest.com/health/hard-to-swallow

Engel S, Tronhjem KM, Hellgren LI, Michaelsen KF et al. Docosahexaenoic acid status at 9 months is inversely associated with communicative skills in 3-year-old girls. (PMID:22642227) *Matern Child Nutr* 2013; 9(4):499-510

Ergun M, Soysal Y, Kismet E, Akay C et al. Investigating the in vitro effect of taurine on the infant lymphocytes by sister chromatid exchange. *Pediatrics International* (2006) 48, 284–286 doi: 10.1111/j.1442-200X.2006.02205.x

Erikson KM, Thompson K, Aschner J et al. Manganese neurotoxicity: a focus on the neonate. (PMID:17084903) *Pharmacol Ther* 2007; 113(2):369-377.

Escribano J, Luque V, Ferre N, Zaragiza-Jordana M et al. Increased protein intake augments kidney volume and function in healthy infants. *Kidney International* 2011; 79: 783-790

ESPGHAN Committee on Nutrition, Agostoni C, Axelsson I, Goulet O, Koletzko Bet al Soy protein infant formulae and follow-on formulae: a commentary by the ESPGHAN Committee on Nutrition. (PMID:16641572) *J Pediatr Gastroenterol Nutr* 2006; 42(4):352-361.

ESPGHAN Committee on Nutrition: Arslanoglu S, Corpeleijn W, Moro G, Braegger C et al. Donor Human Milk for Preterm Infants: Current Evidence and Research Directions *J Pediatr Gastroent Nutr* 2013; 57 (4) 535-542. doi: 10.1097/MPG.0b013e3182a3af0a

ESPGHAN Committee on Nutrition: Complementary Feeding: A Commentary. *J Pediatr Gastroent Nutr* 2008; 46 (1): 99–110. doi: 10.1097/01.mpg.0000304464.60788.bd

ESPGHAN Committee on Nutrition. Supplementation of Infant Formula With Probiotics and/or Prebiotics: A Systematic Review and Comment. *JPGN* 2011;52: 238–250. Online.

EU Food and Veterinary Commission Annual Report 2007. http://ec.europa.eu/food/fvo/annualreports/ann_rep_2007_en.pdf

Evenhouse E, Reilly S. Improved Estimates of the Benefits of Breastfeeding Using Sibling Comparisons to Reduce Selection Bias. *Health Serv Res.* 2005; 40(6 Pt 1): 1781–1802. PMCID: PMC1361236 doi: 10.1111/j.1475-6773.2004.00453.x

Everstine K, Spink J, Kennedy S. Economically Motivated Adulteration (EMA) of Food: Common Characteristics of EMA Incidents. *J Food Prot.* 2013;76(4):723-35. doi: 10.4315/0362-028X.JFP-12-399.

Eysink PE, De Jong MH, Bindels PJ, Scharp-Van Der Linden VT et al. Relation between IgG antibodies to foods and IgE antibodies to milk, egg, cat, dog and/or mite in a cross-sectional study. *Clinical and Experimental Allergy* 1999; 29(5):604-610.

Farrington P, Pugh s, Colville A, Flower A et al. A new method for active surveillance of adverse events from diphtheria/tetanus/pertussis and measles/mumps/rubella vaccines.(PMID:7619183) *Lancet* 1995; 345(8949):567-569.

Farrow C, Blissett J Maternal mind-mindedness during infancy, general parenting sensitivity and observed child feeding behavior: a longitudinal study. (PMID:24684543) *Attachment & Human Development* 2014

Feehley T, Stefka AT, Cao S, Nagler CR. Microbial regulation of allergic responses to food. (PMID:22941410) *Semin Immunopathol* 2012; 34(5):671-688

Fein SB, Falci CD. Infant formula preparation, handling, and related practices in the United States. (PMID:10524388) *J Am Diet Assoc* 1999, 99(10):1234-1240 DOI: 10.1016/S0002-8223(99)00304-

Feldman R, Gordon I, Influs M, Gutbir T, Ebstein RP. Parental Oxytocin and Early Caregiving Jointly Shape Children's Oxytocin Response and Social Reciprocity. *Neuropsychopharmacology (PMID:23325323)*

Feldman-Winter L, Douglass-Bright A, Bartick MC, Matranga J. The new mandate from the Joint Commission on the perinatal core measure of exclusive breastfeeding: implications for practice and implementation in the United States. *J Hum Lact* 2013; 29(3);: 291-295.

Fewtrell M, Wilson DC, Booth I, Lucas A. Six months of exclusive breast feeding: how good is the evidence? (PMID:21233152) *BR MED J* 2011, 342:c5955 .

Fewtrell M. The long-term benefits of having been breastfed. *Currrent Pediatrics* 2004; 14: 97-103

Fewtrell MS, Williams JE, Singhal A, Murgatroyd PR et al. Early diet and peak bone mass: 20 year follow-up of a randomized trial of early diet in infants born preterm. (PMID:19306955) *Bone* 2009; 45(1):142-149. DOI: 10.1016/j.bone.2009.03.657

Field T, Diego M, Hernandez-Reif M, Figueiredo B et al. Depressed mothers and infants are more relaxed during breastfeeding versus bottlefeeding interactions. (PMCID:PMC2844930) *Infant Behav Dev.* 2010 April; 33(2): 241–244.

Findlay L, Renfree MB. Growth, development and secretion of the mammary gland of macropodid marsupials. *Symp Zool Soc Lond* 1984; **51**: 403-432.

Findlay LC, Janz TA. The health of Inuit children under age 6 in Canada. (PMCID:PMC3417691) *Int J Circumpolar Health* 2012, 71:537-542

Finegold SM Therapy and epidemiology of autism--clostridial spores as key elements. (PMID:17904761) *Med Hypotheses* 2008, 70(3):508-511

Finegold SM, Downes J, Summanen PH. Microbiology of regressive autism. (PMID:22202440) *Anaerobe* 2012; 18(2):260-262

Finger JW Jr, Gogal RM Jr. Endocrine-disrupting chemical exposure and the American alligator: a review of the potential role of environmental estrogens on the immune system of a top trophic carnivore. (PMID:24051988) *Arch Environ Contam Toxicol* 2013, 65(4):704-714

Finn R, Newman Cohen H. "Food Allergy": fact or fiction? *Lancet* 1978; 1(8061): 426-428.

Fiocchi A, Brozek J, Schünemann H, Bahna SL, et al. World Allergy Organization (WAO) Diagnosis and Rationale for Action against Cow's Milk Allergy (DRACMA) Guidelines. *World Allergy Organ J* 2010; 3(4):57-161. (PMCID:PMC3488907) doi: 10.1097/WOX.0b013e3181defeb9

Flaherman VJ, Aby J, Burgos AE, Lee KA, Cabana MD, Newman TB. Effect of Early Limited Formula on Duration and Exclusivity of Breastfeeding in At-Risk Infants: An RCT. *Pediatrics*; originally published online May 13, 2013; DOI: 10.1542/peds.2012-2809.

Flohr C, Perkin M, Logan K, Marrs T et al. Atopic dermatitis and disease severity are the main risk factors for food sensitization in exclusively breastfed infants. (PMID:23867897) *J Invest Dermatol.* Feb 2014; 134(2): 345–350. DOI: 10.1038/jid.2013.298

Flohr C, Perkin M, Logan K, Marrs T et al. Atopic dermatitis and disease severity are the main risk factors for food sensitization in exclusively breastfed infants. (PMID:23867897) *J Invest Dermatol* 2014, 134(2):345-350

Flöistrup H, Swartz J, Bergström A, Alm JS, et al. Parsifal Study Group. Allergic disease and sensitization in Steiner school children. (PMID:16387585) *J Allergy Clin Immunol* 2006; 117(1):59-66

Florey CD, Leech AM, Blackhall A. Infant feeding and mental and motor development at 18 months of age in first born singletons. *Int J Epidemiol* 1995; 24 (3): S21-S26.

Fomon SJ. A pediatrician looks at early nutrition. *Bull NY Acad Med* 1971; 47(6): 569-578

Fomon SJ. Breast-feeding and evolution. (PMID:3950274) *J Am Diet Assoc* 1986; 86(3):317-318.

Fomon SJ. Reflections on infant feeding in the 1970s and 1980s. *Am J Clin Nutr* 1987 46: 171-182.

Fomon SJ, Ekstrand J, Ziegler EE. Fluoride intake and prevalence of dental fluorosis: trends in fluoride intake with special attention to infants. (PMID:11109209) *J Pub Health Dent* 2000, 60(3):131-139 DOI: 10.1111/j.1752-7325.2000.tb03318.x

Fomon SJ, Ziegler EE, Filer LJ Jr, Nelson SE et al. Methionine fortification of a soy protein formula fed to infants. *Am J Clin Nutr* 1979; 32(12):2460-2471. (PMID:574352);

Fomon SJ. Infant Feeding in the 20th century: formula and beikost. *J Nutr* 2001; 131(2):409s-20s

Forbes AL, Miller SA. FDA's perspectives on infant formula. Association of Official Analytical Chemists. *Production, Regulation and Analysis of Infant Formula.* Proceedings of a Topical Conference, Virginia, May 14-16 1985.

Forsyth JR, Bennett NM, Hogben S, Hutchinson EM, Rouch G, Tan A, Taplin J. The year of the Salmonella seekers--1977. (PMID:14705299) *Aust N Z J Public Health* 2003, 27(4):385-389

Fort P, Moses N, Fasano M, Goldberg T, Lifshitz F. Breast and soy-formula feedings in early infancy and the prevalence of autoimmune thyroid disease in children. (PMID:2338464) *J Am Coll Nutr* 1990, 9(2):164-167

Fouda GG, Amos JD, Wilks AB, Pollara J, et al. Mucosal immunization of lactating female rhesus monkeys with a transmitted/founder HIV-1 envelope induces strong Env-specific IgA antibody responses in breast milk. (PMID:23596289) *J Virol* 2013, 87(12):6986-6999.

Fourreau D, Peretti N, Hengy B, Gillet Y et al. [Pediatric nutrition: Severe deficiency complications by using vegetable beverages, four cases report]. (PMID:23021957) *Presse Medicale* (Paris, France : 1983) 2013; 42(2):e37-43. DOI: 10.1016/j.lpm.2012.05.029

Franck P, Moneret-Vautrin DA, Morisset M, Kanny G, et al. Anaphylactic reaction to inulin: first identification of specific IgEs to an inulin protein compound. (PMID:15650313) *Int Arch Allergy Immunol* 2005; 136(2):155-158

Frazier AL, Camargo CA, Malspeis S, Willett WC et al. Prospective Study of Peripregnancy Consumption of Peanuts or Tree Nuts by Mothers and the Risk of Peanut or Tree Nut Allergy in Their Offspring *JAMA Pediatr.* Published online Dec 23, 2013. doi:10.1001/jamapediatrics.2013.4139

Freitas RG, Nogueira RJ, Antonio MA, Barros-Filho Ade A, et al.Selenium deficiency and the effects of supplementation on preterm infants.(PMID:24676200) *Revista Paulista de Pediatria* 2014; 32(1):126-135

Frémont S, Kanny G, Bieber S, Nicolas JP, Moneret-Vautrin DA. Identification of a masked allergen, alpha-lactalbumin, in baby-food cereal flour guaranteed free of cow's milk protein. (PMID:8905005) Allergy 1996; 51(10):749-754

Frey MR, Brent Polk D. ErbB receptors and their growth factor ligands in pediatric intestinal inflammation. (PMID:24402051) *Ped Res* 2014, 75(1-2):127-32]

Friedman NJ, Zeiger RS. The role of breast-feeding in the development of allergies and asthma. (PMID:15940141) *J Allergy Clin Immunol* 2005; 115(6):1238-1248 DOI: 10.1016/j.jaci.2005.01.069

Friel JK, Andrews WL, Edgecombe C, McCloy UR et al. Eighteen-month follow-up of infants fed evaporated milk formula. (PMID:10489720) *Can J Public Hlth* 1999; 90(4):240-3.

Fukagawa NK. Protein requirements: methodologic controversy amid a call for change. (PMID:24572564) Am J Clin Nutr 2014, 99(4):761-762

Fukushima Y, Kawata Y, Onda T, Kitagawa M. Long-term consumption of whey hydrolysate formula by lactating women reduces the transfer of beta-lactoglobulin into human milk. (PMID:9530619) *J Nutr Sci Vit* 1997; 43(6):673-678

Furuhjelm C, Warstedt K, Larsson J, Fredriksson M et al. Fish oil supplementation in pregnancy and lactation may decrease the risk of infant allergy.(PMID:19489765) *Acta Paediatrica* 2009, 98(9):1461-1467 DOI: 10.1111/j.1651-2227.2009.01355.x

Gale C, Logan KM, Santhakumaran S, Parkinson JR et al. Effect of breastfeeding compared with formula feeding on infant body composition: a systematic review and meta-analysis. (PMID:22301930) *Am J Clin Nutr* 2012; 95(3):656-669. DOI: 10.3945/ajcn.111.027284

Gale C, Thomas EL, Jeffries S, Durighel G et al. Adiposity and hepatic lipid in healthy full-term, breastfed, and formula-fed human infants: a prospective short-term longitudinal cohort study. (PMID:24572562) *Am J Clin Nutr* 2014, 99(5):1034-1040 DOI: 10.3945/ajcn.113.080200.

Gallup GG Jr, Hobbs DR. Evolutionary medicine: bottle feeding, birth spacing, and autism. (PMID:21641730) *Medical Hypotheses* 2011; 77(3):345-346. DOI: 10.1016/j.mehy.2011.05.010

Galtry J. Punching above its weight: does New Zealand's responsibility for protecting, promoting, and supporting breastfeeding extend beyond its own borders? (PMID:23592421) *J Hum Lact* 2013; 29(2):128-131

Galtry J. The impact on breastfeeding of labour market policy and practice in Ireland, Sweden, and the USA. (PMID:12753825) *Soc Sci Med* 2003, 57(1):167-177

Gammill HS, Adams Waldorf KM, Aydelotte TM, Lucas J, Leisenring WM, Lambert NC, Nelson JL. Pregnancy, microchimerism, and the maternal grandmother. (PMID:21912617) Free resource *PLoS One* 2011, 6(8):e24101

Gammill HS, Nelson JL Naturally acquired microchimerism. (PMID:19924635) *Internatl J Dev Biol* 2010;54(2-3):531-43 .

Ganapathy V, Hay JW, Kim JH. Costs of necrotizing enterocolitis and cost-effectiveness of exclusively human milk-based products in feeding extremely premature infants. (PMID:21718117) *Breastfeed Med* 2012, 7(1):29-37

García-Ara C, Pedrosa M, Belver MT, Martín-Muñoz MF et al. Efficacy and safety of oral desensitization in children with cow's milk allergy according to their serum specific IgE level. Ann Allergy Asthma Immunol 2013; 110(4):290-294

Gardarsdottir O . The dramatic decline of infant mortality in Iceland 1770-1930. http://www.rhd.uit.no/kvinnforsk/papers/Olof_Gardarsdottir.pdf

Gartner L.M. On the Question of the Relationship between Breastfeeding and Jaundice in the First 5 Days of Life. *Sem Perinatol* 1994; 18 (502): 508-9.

Gartner LM, Herschel M. Jaundice and Breastfeeding. *Ped Clin N Am* 2001; 48: 389-99 See also the chapter in Hale & Hartmann. text above.

Geddes, DT, Kent JC, Mitoulas LR, Hartmann, PEH. Tongue Movement and intra-oral vacuum in breastfeeding infants. *Early Hum Dev* 2008; 84: 471 – 477.

Gerrard JW, "Cows' milk and breastmilk" in Brostoff and Challacombe's mammoth volume *Food Allergy and Intolerance* (Saunders, 2nd edition 2002)

Gerrard JW, Lubos MC, Hardy LW, Holmlund BA et al. Milk allergy: clinical picture and familial incidence. *Can Med Assoc J.* Sep 23, 1967; 97(13): 780–785. PMCID: PMC192331

Gerrard JW. Oral cromoglycate: its value in the treatment of adverse reactions to foods. (PMID:106746) *Ann Allergy* 1979; 42(3):135-138.

Ghandehari H, Lee ML, Rechtman DJ, H2MF Study Group. An exclusive human milk-based diet in extremely premature infants reduces the probability of remaining on total parenteral nutrition: a reanalysis of the data. (PMID:22534258) *BMC Res Notes* 2012; 5:188.

Ghebremeskel K, Crawford MA. Nutrition and health in relation to food production and processing. (PMID:8065663) *Nutr Health* 1994, 9(4):237-253.

Giannì ML, Roggero P, Morlacchi L, Garavaglia E et al. Formula-fed infants have significantly higher fat free mass content in their bodies than breastfed babies. (PMID:24673117) *Acta Paediatrica* 2014; DOI: 10.1111/apa.12643

Gibbs BG, Forste R. Socioeconomic status, infant feeding practices and early childhood obesity. (PMID:23554385) *Pediatric Obesity* 2013. DOI: 10.1111/j.2047-6310.2013.00155.x

Gilbert R, Salanti G, Harden M, See S. Infant sleeping position and the sudden infant death syndrome: systematic review of observational studies and historical review of recommendations from 1940 to 2002 *Int. J. Epidemiol.* first published online April 20, 2005 doi:10.1093/ije/dyi088

Gilchrist JM, Moore MB, Andres A, Estroff JA, Badger TM. Ultrasonographic patterns of reproductive organs in infants fed soy formula: comparisons to infants fed breast milk and milk formula. *J Pediatr.* 2010 Feb;156(2):215-20.

Gillespie B, d'Arcy H, Schwartz K, Bobo J, Foxman B. Recall of age of weaning and other breastfeeding variables. *Internat Breastfeeding J* 2006, 1:4

Ginty M. Infant-Formula Companies Milk U.S. Food Program. *WeNews* Monday, November 7, 2011 Source URL (retrieved on 2012-05-11 19:26): http://womensenews.org/story/reproductive-health/111106/infant-formula-companies-milk-us-food-program

Gladen BC, Rogan WJ, Hardy P, Thullen J et al. Development after exposure to polychlorinated biphenyls and dichlorodiphenyl dichloroethene transplacentally and through human milk. *J Pediatr* 1988; 113(6):991-995. DOI: 10.1016/S0022-3476(88)80569-9

Glassman MS, Newman LJ, Berezin S, Gryboski JD. Cow's milk protein sensitivity during infancy in patients with inflammatory bowel disease. (PMID:2371984) *Am J Gastroenterol* 1990; 85(7):838-840.

Goldie F. Farley Health Products: a case history *Brit Food Journal,* 1988; 90 (1) : 20 - 1

Goldman AS. Evolution of immune functions of the mammary gland and protection of the infant. (PMID:22577734) *Breastfeed Med* 2012, 7(3):132-142

Gonzalez-Barcala FJ, Pertega S, Castro TP, Sampedro M et al. Exposure to paracetamol and asthma symptoms. (PMID:22645237) *Eur J Public Health* 2012

Gottlieb S. Early exposure to cows' milk raises risk of diabetes in high risk children PMCID: PMC1173447 *BR MED J.* 2000 October 28; 321(7268): 1040.

Graef JW, Shannon M. (letter) *Pediatrics* 1992; 90 (1):132

Grant EC. Food allergies and migraine. *Lancet* 1979;1(8123):966-9.

Greer FR, Apple RD. Physicians, formula companies, and advertising. A historical perspective. (PMID:1781817) *Am J Dis Child* 1991, 145(3):282-286

Greer FR, Kleinman RE. An infant formula with decreased weight gain and higher IQ: are we there yet? (PMID:24598153) Am J Clin Nutr 2014; 99(4):757-758 DOI: 10.3945/ajcn.114.084798

Greer FR.Vitamin K the basics--what's new? (PMID:20116943) *Early Hum Dev* 2010; 86 Suppl1:43-47

Gribble K, Hausman BL. Milk sharing and formula feeding: Infant feeding risks in comparative perspective? *Australas Med J.* 2012; 5(5): 275–283. Published online 2012 May 31. doi: 10.4066/AMJ.2012.1222 (PMCID:PMC3395287)

Gribble K. 'A better alternative': why women use peer-to-peer shared milk. *Breastfeeding Review* 2014; 22 (1): 11-21

Grimshaw KE, Maskell J, Oliver EM, Morris RC et al. Introduction of complementary foods and the relationship to food allergy. (PMID:24249826) *Pediatrics* 2013, 132(6):e1529-38] DOI: 10.1542/peds.2012-3692

Groer MW, Davis MW. Cytokines, infections, stress, and dysphoric moods in breastfeeders and formula feeders. *Obstet Gynecol Neonat Nurs.* 2006; 35:599–607.

Groppe SE, Gossen A, Rademacher L, Hahn A et al. Oxytocin influences processing of socially relevant cues in the ventral tegmental area of the human brain. *Biol Psychiatry* 2013. (PMID:23419544)

Grulee CG, Hanford HN. The influence of breast and artificial feeding on infantile eczema. J Pediatr 1936; 8: 223-5.

Gubbels JS, Thijs C , Stafleu A, Van Buuren S et al. Association of breast-feeding and feeding on demand with child weight status up to 4 years. *Internat J Pediatr Obes,* 2011; 6: e515–e522

Geueke B1, Wagner CC, Muncke J. Food contact substances and chemicals of concern: a comparison of inventories. *Food Addit Contam Part A Chem Anal Control Expo Risk Assess.* 2014;31(8):1438-50. doi: 10.1080/19440049.2014.931600. Epub 2014 Jul 7.

Guilloteau P, Zabielski R, Hammon HM, Metges CC. Nutritional programming of gastrointestinal tract development. Is the pig a good model for man? *Nutr Res Rev* 2010, 23(1):4-22. PMID:20500926

Gulson BL, James M, Giblin AM, Sheehan A, Mitchell P. Maintenance of elevated lead levels in drinking water from occasional use and potential impact on blood leads in children. (PMID:9372633) *Sci Tot Envir* 1997, 205(2-3):271-275 DOI: 10.1016/S0048-9697(97)00198-8.

Gunther M. The neonate's immunity gap, breast feeding and cot death. (PMID:48624) *Lancet* 1975, 1(7904):441-442.

Guo B, Harstall C, Louie T et al. Systematic review: faecal transplantation for the treatment of Clostridium difficile-associated disease. (MED:22360412) *Aliment Pharm Ther* 2012, 35(8):865-875 DOI: 10.1111/j.1365-2036.2012.05033.x

Gupta R, Sheikh A, Strachan DP, Anderson HR. Time trends in allergic disorders in the UK. (PMID:16950836) *Thorax* 2007, 62(1):91-96

Gustafsson D, Lowhagen T, Andersson K. Risk of developing atopic disease after early feeding with cows'milk-based formula. *Arch Dis Child* 1992; 67: 1008-10.

Gutiérrez-Castrellón P1, Mora-Magaña I, Díaz-García L, Jiménez-Gutiérrez C, et al. Immune response to nucleotide-supplemented infant formulae: systematic review and meta-analysis. *Br J Nutr.* 2007; 98 Suppl 1:S64-7.

Haahtela T. What is needed for allergic children. *Pediatr Allergy Immunol* 2014; 25: 21-24. DOI:10.1111/pai.12189

Haahtela T, Holgate ST, Pawankar R, et al. The biodiversity hypothesis and allergic disease: World Allergy Organization position statement. *World Allergy Organ J* 2013: 6: 3.

Haahtela T, Valovirta E, Kauppi P, Tommila E, et al.The Finnish Allergy Programme 2008-2018 - scientific rationale and practical implementation.(PMID:23130334) *Asia Pac Allergy* 2012, 2(4):275-279

Haahtela T, Von Hertzen L, Mäkelä M, Hannuksela M and the Allergy Programme Working Group Finnish Allergy Programme 2008–2018 – time to act and change the course *Allergy* 2008; 63:4634-4563| DOI: 10.1111/j.1398-9995.2008.01712.x

Hack L. ASD prevalence in kids continues to increase. *Contemporary Pediatrics* April 3, 2014

Haenlein O. Conference calls for responsible use of livestock antibiotics *Global Meat News*. Oct 3, 2014. http://www.globalmeatnews.com/Industry-Markets/Conference-calls-for-responsible-use-of-livestock-antibiotics

Hagelberg S, Lindblad BS, Lundsjo A et al. The protein tolerance of VLBW infants fed human milk protein-enriched mothers' milk. *Acta Paediatr Scand* 1982; 71 (4):597-601.

Hakansson AP, Roche-Hakansson H, Mossberg AK, Svanborg C. Apoptosis-like death in bacteria induced by HAMLET, a human milk lipid-protein complex. *PLoS One* 2011, 6(3):e17717 (PMID:21423701)

Halken S, Høst A, Hansen LG, Osterballe O. Preventive effect of feeding high-risk infants a casein hydrolysate formula or an ultrafiltrated whey hydrolysate formula. A prospective, randomized, comparative clinical study. (PMID:8298708) *Pediatr Allergy Immunol* 1993; 4(4):173-181.

Hallgren O, Aits S, Brest P, Gustafsson L et al. Apoptosis and tumor cell death in response to HAMLET (human alpha-lactalbumin made lethal to tumor cells). *Adv Exp Med Biol* 2008, 606:217-240

Hambraeus L. Proprietary milk versus human milk in infant feeding. *Ped Clin N Am* 1977; 24(1): 17-36.

Hamosh M. Breastfeeding: Unraveling the Mysteries of Mother's Milk. (PMID:9746642) *Medscape Womens Health* 1996, 1(9):4

Hamosh M. Bioactive factors in human milk. *Ped Clin N America* 2001; 48 (1): 69-

Hampton SM. Prematurity, immune function and infant feeding practices. (PMID:10343343) Proc Nutr Soc 1999, 58(1):75-78

Hansen LG, Host A, Halken S, Holmskov A, Husby S et al. Cord blood IgE. III. Prediction of IgE high-response and allergy. A follow-up at the age of 18 months. *Allergy* 1992; 47 (4 pt 2): 404-410.

Hanski I, von Hertzen L, Fyhrquistc N, et al. Environmental biodiversity, human microbiota, and allergy are interrelated. Proc Natl Acad Sci USA 2012: 109: 8334–9.

Hanson LA, Silferdahl SA. The infant's immune system is a balanced threat to the foetus, turning to protection of the neonate. *Acta Paediatr* 2009; 98:221-228. DOI: 10.1111/j.1651-2227.2008.01143.x

Hanson LÅ, Telemo E, Wiedermann U, et al. Immunological mechanisms of the gut. *Pediatr Allergy Immunol.* 1995;6(Suppl 8):7–12

Hanson LA. The mother-offspring dyad and the immune system. (PMID:10772267) *Acta Paediatr* 2000, 89(3):252-258

Harari F, Ronco AM, Concha G, Llanos M, Grandér M, Castro F, Palm B, Nermell B, Vahter M. Early-life exposure to lithium and boron from drinking water. (PMID:23017911) *Reproductive Toxicology.* 2012, 34(4):552-560

Harbord MG, Finn JP, Hall-Craggs. Myelination patterns on magnetic resonsance of children with developmental delay. *Dev Med Child Neurol* 1990; 32: 295-303.

Hariharan K, Kurien S, Rao SV Effect of supplementation of milk fat with peanut oil on blood lipids and lipoproteins in infants. (PMID:8574857) *Int J Food Sci Nutr* 1995; 46(4):309-17

Hariharan K, Rao SV. Influence of partial replacement of butter fat with peanut oil (in infant formula) on erythrocyte fatty acids in infants. (PMID:9475076) *Indian J Exp Biol* 1997, 35(9):957-963

Harney A. How big formula bought China. Reuters Special report, November 7, 2013. http://www.reuters.com/article/2013/11/08/us-china-milkpowder-specialreport-idUSBRE9A700820131108

Harrington R. Abbott infant formula recall to cost US $100m. 29-9-2010

Harrison GE, Sutton A, Shepherd H, Widdowson EM. Strontium Balance In Breast-Fed Babies. (PMID:14275943) *Br J Nutr* 1965, 19:111-117

Hassiotou F, Beltran A, Chetwynd E, Stuebe AM, et al. Breastmilk is a novel source of stem cells with multilineage differentiation potential. (PMID:22865647) Stem Cells [2012, 30(10):2164-2174]

Hassiotou F, Geddes DT, Hartmann PE. Cells in Human Milk: State of the Science. PMID:23515088. *J Hum Lact.* 2013 Mar 20. [Epub ahead of print]

Hassiotou F, Geddes DT. Programming of appetite control during breastfeeding as a preventative strategy against the obesity epidemic. (PMID:24646683) J Hum Lact [2014, 30(2):136-142]

Hassiotou, F, Beltran, A, Chetwynd, E. Stuebe, AM et al (2012), Breastmilk Is a Novel Source of Stem Cells with Multilineage Differentiation Potential. *Stem Cells* 2012; 30: 2164–2174. doi: 10.1002/stem.1188

Hastrup K. A Question of Reason: Breast-Feeding Patterns in 17th and 18th century Iceland. in Maher V (ed.) *The Anthropology of Breastfeeding: Natural Law or Social Contract*? (Berg Publishers Oxford 1992)

Hathaway MJ, Warner JO. Compliance problems in the dietary management of eczema. (PMID:6859943) *Arch Dis Child* 1983, 58(6):463-464.

Hauser M, Roulias A, Ferreira F, Egger M. Panallergens and their impact on the allergic patient. Allergy Asthma Clin Immunol. 2010; 6(1): 1. Published online 2010 January 18. doi: 10.1186/1710-1492-6-1. PMCID: PMC2830198

Hausner H, Nicklaus S, Issanchou S, Mølgaard C, et al. Breastfeeding facilitates acceptance of a novel dietary flavour compound. (PMID:19962799) *Clinical Nutrition* 2010, 29(1):141-148.

Heacock HJ, Jeffery HE, Baker JL, Page M Influence of breast versus formula milk on physiological gastroesophageal reflux in healthy, newborn infants. (PMID:1573512) *J Ped Gastroent Nutr* 1992, 14(1):41-6.

Heikkilä K, Kelly Y, Renfrew MJ, Sacker A, Quigley MA. Breastfeeding and educational achievement at age 5. (PMID:22462489) *Maternal & Child Nutrition* 2012; 10(1):92-101. DOI: 10.1111/j.1740-8709.2012.00402.x

Heikkilä K, Sacker A, Kelly Y, Renfrew MJ, Quigley MA. Breast feeding and child behaviour in the Millennium Cohort Study. (PMID:21555784) *Arch Dis Child* 2011, 96(7):635-642. DOI: 10.1136/adc.2010.201970

Heine RG Allergic gastrointestinal motility disorders in infancy and early childhood. (PMID:18713339) *Pediatr Allergy Immunol* 2008, 19(5):383-391

Heinz-Erian P, Gassner I, Klein-Franke A, Jud V et al. Gastric lactobezoar - a rare disorder? (PMID:22216886) *Orphanet Journal of Rare Diseases* 2012, 7:3 DOI: 10.1186/1750-1172-7-3

Heird, WC. Taurine in neonatal nutrition – revisited. *Arch Dis Child Fetal Neonatal Ed* 2004; 89, 473–474.

Heisler EJ. U.S. Infant Mortality Rate 2012 www.fas.org/sgp/crs/misc/R41378.pdf.

Helsing E. Women's liberation and breastfeeding. *J Trop Paediatr Environ Child* Health 1975; 21 (5) 290-4.

Henrick BM, Nag K, Yao XD, Drannik AG et al. Milk matters: soluble Toll-like receptor 2 (sTLR2) in breast milk significantly inhibits HIV-1 infection and inflammation. *PLoS One* 2012, 7(7):e40138 (PMID:22792230)

Henriksson C, Bostrom A, Wiklund IE. What effect does breastfeeding have on coeliac disease? A systematic review update *Evid. Based Med 2102;* published 4 August 2012, 10.1136/eb-2012-100607

Heppell UM, Sissons JW, Pedersen HE. A comparison of the antigenicity of soya-bean based infant formulas. *Br J Nutr.* 1987; 58: 393-403.

Herman-Giddens ME, Steffes J, Harris D, Slora E et al. Secondary sexual characteristics in boys: data from the pediatric research in office settings network. (PMID:23085608) *Pediatrics* 2012, 130(5):e1058-68

Hesselmar B, Sjöberg F, Saalman R, Aberg N et al.. Pacifier cleaning practices and risk of allergy development. (PMID:23650304) *Pediatrics* 2013; 131(6):e1829-37. DOI: 10.1542/peds.2012-3345

Hettiarachchi CA, Melton LD, Gerrard JA, Loveday SM Formation of ?-lactoglobulin nanofibrils by microwave heating gives a peptide composition different from conventional heating.(PMID:22877308) *Biomacromolecules* 2012, 13(9):2868-2880

Hill CM, Ball HL. Parental manipulation of postnatal survival and wellbeing: are parental sex preferences adaptive? In Pollard TM, Hyatt SB. *Sex , Gender and Health.* (Cambridge University Press 1999).

Hill DJ, Cameron DJ, Francis DE et al. Challenge confirmation of late-onset reactions to extensively hydrolyzed formulas in infants with multiple food protein intolerance. (PMID:7560641) *J Allergy Clin Immunol* 1995; 96(3):386-394.

Hinde K. Night milk. *Splash* July 2014. http://milkgenomics.org/article/night-milk/ Subscribe to Splash online for fascinating updates.

Hipgrave DB, Assefa F, Winoto A, Sukotjo S: Donated breast milk substitutes and incidence of diarrhoea among infants and young children after the May 2006 earthquake in Yogyakarta and Central Java. Public Health Nutrition 2012;15(2):307

Hoarau G, Pelloux I, Gayot A, Wroblewski I, Popoff MR, Mazuet C, Maurin M, Croizé J. Two cases of type A infant botulism in Grenoble, France: no honey for infants. (PMID:22159905) *Eur J Pediatr* 2012, 171(3):589-591 DOI: 10.1007/s00431-011-1649-5

Hobsbawm EJ. *The Present as History: Writing the History of One's Own Times.* 1993 Creighton lecture. (University of London 1993)

Hoefer A, Hardy MC. Later development of breast and artificially fed infants. Comparison of physical and mental growth. *JAMA* 1929; 92: 615-19.

Holgerson PL, Vestman NR, Claesson R, Ohman C, et al. Oral microbial profile discriminates breast-fed from formula-fed infants. *J Pediatr Gastroenterol Nutr* 2013, 56(2):127-136. (PMID:22955450)

Holick MF, Shao Q, Liu WW, Chen TC. The vitamin D content of fortified milk and infant formula. (PMID:1313548) *N Engl J Med* 1992; 326(18):1178-1181.

Holt WL. Medical milk commissions and the importance of a pure milk supply. *Cal State J Med.* 1909 April; 7(4): 136. 1

Hong X, Liu C, Chen X, Song Y et al. Maternal Exposure to Airborne Particulate Matter Causes Postnatal Immunological Dysfunction in Mice Offspring. (PMID:23416701) *Toxicology* 2013, 306C:59-67

Hong X, Wang G, Liu X, Kumar R, et al. Gene polymorphisms, breast-feeding, and development of food sensitization in early childhood. (PMID:21689850) *J Allergy Clin Immunol.* 2011; 128(2):374-81.e2

Hörnell A, Lagström H, Lande B, Thorsdottir I. Breastfeeding, introduction of other foods and effects on health: a systematic literature review for the 5th Nordic Nutrition Recommendations. (PMID: 23589711) *Food & Nutrition Research* 2013; 57:313-323 DOI: 10.3402/fnr.v57i0.20823

Høst A, Halken S, Muraro A, Dreborg S et al.. Dietary prevention of allergic diseases in infants and small children. *Pediatr Allergy Immunol* 2008, 19(1):1-4. DOI: 10.1111/j.1399-3038.2007.00680.x

Host A, Halken S. Cow's milk allergy: where have we come from and where are we going? (PMID:24450456) Endocrine, Metabolic & Immune Disorders Drug Targets 2014, 14(1):2-8.

Høst A, Husby S, Osterballe O A prospective study of cow's milk allergy in exclusively breast-fed infants. Incidence, pathogenetic role of early inadvertent exposure to cow's milk formula, and characterization of bovine milk protein in human milk. (PMID:3201972) *Acta Paediatrica Scandinavica* 1988, 77(5):663-670

Høst A. Importance of the first meal on the development of cow's milk allergy and intolerance. (PMID:1936970) *Allergy Proceedings* 1991, 12(4):227-232

Houdebine LM. Transgenic animal bioreactors. (PMID:11131009) *Transgenic Res* 2000; 9(4-5):305-320

Hourihane JO, Dean TP, Warner JO. Peanut allergy in relation to heredity, maternal diet, and other atopic diseases: results of a questionnaire survey, skin prick testing, and food challenges. (PMID:8789975) *BMJ* 1996; 313(7056):518-521.

Houghteling PD, Walker WA. Why is Initial Bacterial Colonization of the Intestine Important to the Infant's and Child's Health? (PMID:25313849) *J Pediatr Gastroenterol Nutr* 2014 e-pub ahead of print DOI: 10.1097/MPG.0000000000000597

Howie PW, Forsyth JS, Ogston SA, Clark A et al. Protective effect of breastfeeding against infection. BMJ 1990; 300: 11-16.

Hrboticky N, MacKinnon MJ, Innis SM. Effect of a vegetable oil formula rich in linoleic acid on tissue fatty acid accretion in the brain, liver, plasma, and erythrocytes of infant piglets. (PMID:2305703) *Am J Clin Nutr* 1990; 51(2):173-182

Hreschyshyn MM, Hopkins A, Zylstra S et al. Associations of parity, breastfeeding, and birth control pills with lumbar spine and femoral neck bone densities. Am J Obstet Gynecol 1988; 159: 318-22.

Hsu C. The longer babies are fed formula, the greater their risk for pediatric acute lymphoblastic leukemia. *Medical Daily.com* OCT 18, 2012 12:13 PM EDT http://www.medicaldaily.com/articles/12766/20121018/longer-period-infant-formula-feeding-increase-leukemia.htm#iEBzCokEBoU3wCUW.99

Hsu NY, Wu PC, Bornehag CG, Sundell J, Su HJ Feeding bottles usage and the prevalence of childhood allergy and asthma. (PMID:22291844) *Clin Dev Immunol* 2012; 2012:158248 doi: 10.1155/2012/158248

Humenick SS, Howell OS. Perinatal Experiences: The Association of Stress, Childbearing, Breastfeeding, and Early Mothering. *J Perinat Educ.* 2003; 12(3): 16–41. doi: 10.1624/105812403X106937. PMCID: PMC1595161

Humphrey JH. The risks of not breastfeeding. *J Acquir Immune Defic Syndrome* 2010; 53 (1):1-4.

Hurley WL, Theil PK. Perspectives on immunoglobulins in colostrum and milk. *Nutrients* 2011; 3(4):442-474. (PMCID:PMC3257684) .

Hvatum M, Kanerud L, Hällgren R, Brandtzaeg P. The gut-joint axis: cross reactive food antibodies in rheumatoid arthritis. (PMID:16484508) *Gut* 2006, 55(9):1240-1247

Hyde MJ, Mostyn A, Modi N, Kemp PR. **The health implications of birth by Caesarean section.** *Biol Rev Camb Philos Soc.* 2012;87(1):229-43. doi: 10.1111/j.1469-185X.2011.00195.x. PMID: 21815988

Iacono G, di Prima L, D'Amico D et al. The "red umbilicus": a diagnostic sign of cows' milk protein intolerance. *JPGN* 2006; 42: 531-534.

Iacovou M, Ralston RA, Muir J, Walker KZ, Truby H. Dietary Management of Infantile Colic: Systematic Review. *Matern Child Health J.* 2012;16(6):1319-1331.

Iacovou M, Sevilla A. Infant feeding: the effects of scheduled vs. on-demand feeding on mothers' wellbeing and children's cognitive development. (PMID:22420982) *Eur Journal of Public Health* 2012

Iffy L, Lindenthal J, Szodi Z, Griffin W. Puerperal psychosis following ablaction with bromocriptine. (PMID:2516595) *Med Law* 1989; 8(2):171-174.

Illingworth RS, Stone DG, Jowett GH. Self-demand feeding in a maternity unit. *Lancet* 1952; i: 683-7.

Indumathi S, Dhanasekaran M, Rajkumar JS, Sudarsanam D Exploring the stem cell and non-stem cell constituents of human breast milk. (PMID:22940915) *Cytotechnology* 2012

Infant Feeding Literature Review 2009 available online at https://www.nhmrc.gov.au/_files_nhmrc/publications/attachments/n56a_infant_feeding_literature_review.pdf

Innis SM, Hamilton JJ. Effects of developmental changes and early nutrition on cholesterol metabolism in infancy. *J Am Coll Nutr* 1992; 11 (S1) 63S-68S.

Inostroza J, Haschke F, Steenhout P, Grathwohl D et al. Low-Protein Formula Slows Weight Gain in Infants of Overweight Mothers: A Randomized Trial. (PMID:24637965)  *J Pediatr Gastroenterol Nutr* 2014

Institute of Medicine (U.S.) (2004). Defining Safety for Infants. In *Infant Formula: Evaluating the Safety of New Ingredients* (National Academic Press) pp. 22–42, Retrieved on November 15, 2009.

Irmak MK, Oztas Y, Oztas E Integration of maternal genome into the neonate genome through breast milk mRNA transcripts and reverse transcriptase. PMID:22676860 *Theoretical Biology & Medical Modelling* 2012, 9:20.

Isaacs EB, Fischl BR, Quinn BT, Chong WKET AL. Impact of breast milk on intelligence quotient, brain size, and white matter development. (PMID:20035247) *Pediatr Res* 2010; 67(4):357-362.

Isaacs EB, Morley R, Lucas A. Early diet and general cognitive outcome at adolescence in children born at or below 30 weeks gestation. *J Pediatrics* 2009; 155(2):229-234.(PMID:19446846)

Issue dedicated to Professor Günter Dörner on the occasion of his 60th birthday. (PMID:2689188) *Exp Clin Endocrinol* 1989, 94(1-2):1-225

Jackson BP, Taylor VF, Punshon T, Cottingham KL Arsenic concentration and speciation in infant formulas and first foods. (PMID:22701232) *Pure and Applied Chemistry*, 2012; 84(2):215-223

Jacobsen K. Diagnostic politics: the curious case of Kanner's syndrome. (PMID:21877421) *History of Psychiatry* 2010, 21(84 Pt 4):436-454

Jacobson JL, Jacobson SW, Humphrey HE. Effects of in utero exposure to polychlorinated biphenyls and related contaminants on cognitive functioning in young children. (PMID:2104928) *J Pediatr* 1990, 116(1):38-45

Jain N, Walker WA. Diet and host-microbial crosstalk in postnatal intestinal immune homeostasis. (PMID:25201040) Nat Rev Gastroenterol Hepatol [2014] DOI: 10.1038/nrgastro.2014.153 Exceptionally good summary, a must-read.

Jakobsson I, Lindberg T, Benediktsson B, Hansson BG. Dietary bovine beta-lactoglobulin is transferred to human milk. (PMID:4003058) *Acta Paediatr Scand* 1985, 74(3):342-345

Jakobsson I, Lindberg T. Cow's milk as a cause of infantile colic in breast-fed infants. (PMID:79803) *Lancet* 1978, 2(8087):437-439

Jakobsson I. Unusual presentation of adverse reactions to cow's milk proteins. (PMID:4046494) *Klin Padiatr* 1985, 197(4):360-362

Janas LM, Picciano MF, Hatch TF. Indices of protein metabolism in term infants fed either human milk or formulas with reduced protein concentration and various whey/casein ratios. (PMID:3495653) *J Pediatr* 1987, 110(6):838-848

Jarvenpaa AL, Raiha NCR, Rassin DK, Gaull GE. Preterm infants attain intrauterine weight gain. *Acta Paed Scand* 1983 72 (2) 239-243.

Järvinen KM, Geller L, Bencharitiwong R, Sampson HA Presence of functional, autoreactive human milk-specific IgE in infants with cow's milk allergy. (PMID:22092935) *Clin Exp Allergy* 2012, 42(2):238-247

Järvinen KM, Westfall JE, Seppo MS, James AK et al. Role of maternal elimination diets and human milk IgA in the development of cow's milk allergy in the infants. (PMID:24164317 *Clin Experim Allergy* 2014, 44(1):69-78. DOI: 10.1111/cea.12228

Jason J. Prevention of invasive Cronobacter infections in young infants fed powdered infant formulas. (PMID:23045556) *Pediatrics* 2012, 130(5):e1076-84

Jayachandran S, Kuziemko I. Why do mothers breastfeed girls less than boys? Evidence and implications for child health in India. (PMID:22148132) *Quart J Econom* 2011; 126(3):1485-1538.

Jelinek CF. Levels of lead in the United States food supply. (PMID:7118801) *J Association of Official Analytical Chemists* 1982; 65(4):942-946.

Jenkins HR, Pincott JR, Soothill JF, Milla PJ, Harries JT. Food allergy: the major cause of infantile colitis. Arch Dis Child 1984; 59: 326-9.

Jensen RG, Ferris AM, Lammi-Keefe CJ, Henderson RA et al. Possible alleviation of atopic eczema in a breastfed infant by maternal supplementation with a fish oil concentrate.(PMID:1517955) *J Pediatr Gastroenterol Nutr* 1992; 14(4):474-475.

Jiménez E, Marín ML. Martín R, Odriozola J et al. Is meconium from healthy newborns actually sterile? *Research in Microbiology* 2008; 159 (3):187–193. http://dx.doi.org/10.1016/j.resmic.2007.12.007.

Jing H, Gilchrist JM, et al . A longitudinal study of differences in electroencephalographic activity among breastfed, milk-fed, and soy formula-fed infants during the first year of life. *Early Hum Dev.* 2010 Feb;86(2):119-25

Jirapinyo P, Densupsoontorn N, Kangwanpornsiri C, Limlikhit T. Lower prevalence of atopic dermatitis in breast-fed infants whose allergic mothers restrict dairy products.*J Med Assoc Thai.* 2013; 96(2):192-5. PMID: 23936985

Jirapinyo P; Densupsoontorn N; Kangwanpornsiri C; Wongarn R. Chicken-based formula is better tolerated than extensively hydrolyzed casein formula for the management of cow milk protein allergy in infants. *Asia Pac J Clin Nutr.* 2012; 21(2):209-14.

Joneja JM. Infant food allergy: where are we now? (PMID:22237876) *JPEN.* 2012, 36(1 Suppl):49S-55S

Jongenburger I, Reij MW, Boer EP, Gorris LG, Zwietering MH Actual distribution of Cronobacter spp. in industrial batches of powdered infant formula and consequences for performance of sampling strategies. (PMID:21893361) *Int J Food Microbiol* 2011, 151(1):62-9

Joseph CL, Havstad S, Bobbitt K, Woodcroft K et al. Transforming growth factor beta (TGFβ1 ) in breast milk and indicators of infant atopy in a birth cohort. (PMID:24520941) *Pediatr Allergy Immunol* 2014; DOI: 10.1111/pai.12205

Jost T, Lacroix C, Braegger CP, Chassard C. New insights in gut microbiota establishment in healthy breast fed neonates. (PMID:22957008) *PLoS One* 2012; 7(8):e44595. doi:10.1371/journal.p one.04495

Judge D. Switching to food-grade lubricants provides safety solution. *Machinery Lubrication* July 2005

Juvonen P, Månsson M, Kjellman NI, Björkstén B, Jakobsson I. Development of immunoglobulin G and immunoglobulin E antibodies to cow's milk proteins and ovalbumin after a temporary neonatal exposure to hydrolyzed and whole cow's milk proteins. (PMID:10565560) *Pediatr Allergy Immunol* 1999, 10(3):191-198

Kaati G, Bygren LO, Edvinsson S. Cardiovascular and diabetes mortality determined by nutrition during parents' and grandparents' slow growth period.(PMID:12404098) *Eur J Hum Genet* 2002, 10(11):682-8

Kaati G, Bygren LO, Pembrey M, Sjöström M. Transgenerational response to nutrition, early life circumstances and longevity. (PMID:17457370) *Eur J Hum Genet* 2007, 15(7):784-790

Kahn A, Mozin MJ, Casimir G, Montauk L et al. Insomnia and Cow's Milk Allergy in Infants. *Pediatrics* 1985; 76:6 880-884

Kahn A, Rebuffat E, Blum D et al. Milk intolerance in children with persistent sleeplessness: a double blind crossover study. *Pediatrics* 1989; 84: 595-603.

Kainonen E, Rautava S, Isolauri E. Immunological programming by breast milk creates an anti-inflammatory cytokine milieu in breast-fed infants compared to formula-fed infants. (PMID:23110822) Br J Nutr 2013; 109(11):1962-1970

Kaleita TA, Kinsbourne M, Menkes JH. A neurobehavioral syndrome after failure to thrive on chloride-deficient formula. *Dev Med Child Neurol* 1991; 33:626-635.

Kaminis M. A Growing Boost for Baby Formula. *BusinessWeek,* January 11, 2005 http://www.businessweek.com/stories/2005-01-10/a-growing-boost-for-baby-formula

Kanny G, Hatahet R, Moneret-Vautrin DA, Kohler C, Bellut A. Allergy and intolerance to flavouring agents in atopic dermatitis in young children. (PMID:7945786) *Allergie et Immunologie* 1994; 26(6):204-6, 209-10

Karlsson H, Blomström A, Wicks S, Yang S, Yolken RH, Dalman C. Maternal antibodies to dietary antigens and risk for nonaffective psychosis in offspring. (MED:22535227) *Am J Psychiatr* 2012, 169(6):625-632

Kary T. Colgate Total Ingredient Linked to Hormones, Cancer Spotlights FDA Process. *Bloomberg News* Aug 12, 2014. http://www.bloomberg.com/news/2014-08-11/in-35-pages-buried-at-fda-worries-over-colgate-s-total.html

Katz Y, Rajuan N, Goldberg MR, Eisenberg E, Heyman E, Cohen A, Leshno M. Early exposure to cow's milk protein is protective against IgE-mediated cow's milk protein allergy. (PMID:20541249) *J All Clin Immunol 2010*, 126(1):77-82.e1 DOI: 10.1016/j.jaci.2010.04.020

Kawase K, Katamine S, Moriuchi R, Miyamoto T et al. Maternal transmission of HTLV-1 other than through breast milk: discrepancy between the PCR positivity of cord blood samples for HTLV-1 and the subsequent seropositivity of individuals. (PMID:1429208) *Jpn J Cancer Res* 1992, 83(9):968-977.

Keating JP, Schears GJ, Dodge PR. Oral water intoxication in infants. An American epidemic. (PMID:1877579) *Am J Dis Child* 1991; 145(9):985-990.

Kember RL, Dempster EL, Lee TH, Schalkwyk LC et al. Maternal separation is associated with strain-specific responses to stress and epigenetic alterations to Nr3c1, Avp, and Nr4a1 in mouse. (PMCID:PMC3432968) *Brain and Behavior* 2012, 2(4):455-467

Kemp AS, Van Asperen PP, Douglas J. Anaphylaxis caused by inhaled pavlova mix in egg-sensitive children. (PMID:3200200) *Med J Aust* 1988; 149(11-12):712-713.

Kendall-Tackett K. A new paradigm for depression in new mothers: the central role of inflammation and how breastfeeding and anti-inflammatory treatments protect maternal mental health. (PMID:17397549) *Int Breastfeed J* 2007; 2:6.

Kennedy K, Ross S, Isaacs EB, Weaver LT et al. The 10-year follow-up of a RCT of LCPUFA supplementation in preterm infants: effects on growth and blood pressure. (PMID:20515959) *Arch Dis Child* 2010, 95(8):588-595

Kent G. Regulating fatty acids in infant formula: critical assessment of U.S. policies and practices. *International Breastfeeding Journal* 2014, 9:2 doi:10.1186/1746-4358-9-2

Kent G. WIC's promotion of infant formula in the US. *Int Breastfeed J* 2006, 1:8. doi:10.1186/1746-4358-1-8.

Kessler R. Food: Picky Eaters. *Nature* (Outlook) 2011; 479: S8

Kilshaw PJ, Cant AJ. The passage of maternal dietary proteins into human breast milk. *Int Arch Allergy Appl Immunol* 1984; 75(1):8-15. (PMID:6746107)

Kim P, Feldman R, Mayes LC, Eicher V, et al. Breastfeeding, brain activation to own infant cry, and maternal sensitivity. *J Child Psychol Psychiatr,* 2011; DOI: 10.1111/j.1469-7610.2011.02406.x

Kimata H. Latex allergy in infants younger than 1 year. (PMID:15663567) *Clin Exp Allergy* 2004; 34(12):1910-1915

Kimura C, Matsuoka M. Changes in breast skin temperature during the course of breastfeeding. (PMID:17293552) *J Hum Lact* 2007;23(1):60-69.

Kinsley CH, Bardi M, Karelina K, Rima B et al. Motherhood induces and maintains behavioral and neural plasticity across the lifespan in the rat.(PMID:18074214) *Arch Sex Behav* 2008; 37 (1): 43-56. DOI: 10.1007/s10508-007-9277-x

Kinsley CH, Lambert KG. The maternal brain. *Scientific American* 2006; 294 (1): 72-79. (PMID:16468436)

Kliegman RM. Neonatal necrotizing enterocolitis: bridging the basic science with the clinical disease. (PMID:2231220) *J Pediatr* 1990; 117(5):833-835

Koetting CA; Wardlaw GM. Wrist, spine, and hip bone density in women with variable histories of lactation. *Am J Clin Nutr* 1988; 48: 1479-81.

Kois WE, Campbell DA Jr, Lorber MI, Sweeton JC et al. Influence of breast feeding on subsequent reactivity to a related renal allograft. (PMID:6379295*) J Surg Res* 1984; 37(2):89-93 DOI: 10.1016/0022-4804(84)90166-5

Koletzko B, Tangermann R, von Kries R et al. Intestinal milk-bolus obstruction in formula-fed premature infants given high doses of calcium. *J Pediatr. Gastroent Nutr* 1988; 7: 548-53.

Koletzko B. Standards for infant formula milk. Commercial interests may be strongest driver of what goes into formula milk *BMJ*. 2006; 332: 621–622. PMCID:1403284 doi: 10.1136/bmj.332.7542.621

Korecka A, Arulampalam V. The gut microbiome: scourge, sentinel or spectator? *J Oral Microbiol*. 2012; 4: 10.3402/jom.v4i0.9367. Published online 2012 February 21. doi: 10.3402/jom.v4i0.9367

Kosaka N, Izumi H, Sekine K, Ochiya T microRNA as a new immune-regulatory agent in breast milk. (PMCID:PMC2847997) *Silence* 2010; 1(1):7

Kramer M, Kakuma . Optimal duration of exclusive breastfeeding. (PMID:22895934) (2002, revised 2009; revised 2011) *Cochrane Database Syst Rev* (Online) 2012, 8:CD003517 DOI: 10.1002/14651858.CD003517.pub2

Kramer MS, Aboud F, Mironova E, Vanilovich I et al. Breastfeeding and child cognitive development. New evidence from a large randomized trial. *Arch Gen Psychiatry*. 2008;65(5):578-584 DOI: 10.1001/archpsyc.65.5.578

Kramer MS, Kakuma R. Maternal dietary antigen avoidance during pregnancy or lactation, or both, for preventing or treating atopic disease in the child. (PMID:22972039) *Cochrane Database Syst Rev* 2012; 9:cd000133

Kramer MS, Kakuma R. Maternal dietary antigen avoidance during pregnancy or lactation, or both, for preventing or treating atopic disease in the child. (PMID:16855951) *Cochrane Database Syst Rev* 2006(3):cd000133

Kramer MS. "Breast is best": The evidence. (PMID:20846797) *Early Hum Dev* 2010, 86(11):729-732

Kramer MS. Do breast-feeding and delayed introduction of solid foods protect against subsequent obesity? *J Pediatr*. 1981; 98(6):883-7.

Krawinkel MB. Benefits from longer breastfeeding: do we need to revise the recommendations? (PMID:21939907) *Curr Probl Pediatr Adolesc Health Care* 2011, 41(9):240-243

Kremer W. The brave new world of DIY faecal transplant http://www.bbc.com/news/magazine 27503660

Krewski D, Yokel RA, Nieboer E, Borchelt D et al. Human health risk assessment for aluminium, aluminium oxide, and aluminium hydroxide. *J Toxicol Environ Health B Crit Rev* 2007; 10 Suppl 1:1-269. (PMCID:PMC2782734)

Krogh C, Biggar RJ, Fischer TK, Lindholm M et al. Bottle-feeding and the Risk of Pyloric Stenosis. (PMID:22945411) *Pediatrics* 2012, 130(4):e943-9

Ku M-S, Sun H-L, Sheu J-N, Lee H-S et al. Neonatal jaundice is a risk factor for childhood asthma: a retrospective cohort study. *Pediatr Allergy Immunol* 2012: 00.

Kuitunen M, Kukkonen K, Jutunen-Backman K, *et al.* Probiotics prevent IgE-associated allergy until age 5 years in cesarean-delivered children but not in the total cohort. *J Allergy Clin Immunol* 2009; 123:335–341.

Kuitunen M. Probiotics and prebiotics in preventing food allergy and eczema. *Curr Opin Allergy Clin Immunol*. 2013;13(3):280-286.

Kukkonen AK, Savilahti EM, Haahtela T, Savilahti E, et al. Ovalbumin-specific immunoglobulins A and G levels at age 2 years are associated with the occurrence of atopic disorders.(PMID:21771118) *Clin Exper Allergy* 2011, 41(10):1414-1421.

Kumpulainen J, Salmenperä L, Siimes MA, Koivistoinen P et al. Formula feeding results in lower selenium status than breast-feeding or selenium supplemented formula feeding: a longitudinal study. *Am J Clin Nutr* 1987; 45(1):49-53. (PMID:3799503)

Kunz C. Historical aspects of human milk oligosaccharides. (PMID:22585922) *Adv Nutr*. 2012, 3(3):430S-9S] DOI: 10.3945/an.111.001776

Labayen I, Ruiz JR, Ortega FB, Loit HM et al. Exclusive breastfeeding duration and cardiorespiratory fitness in children and adolescents. (PMID:22237059) *Am J Clin Nutr* 2012, 95(2):498-505

Labbok M, Marinelli KA, Bartick M, Calnen G et al. Regulatory monitoring of feeding during the birth hospitalization. (PMID:22167859) *Pediatrics* 2011; 128(5):e1311-4; author reply e1317-9.

Labbok M; Bobrow KL, Quigley MA, Green J et al (2012). Persistent effects of women's parity and breastfeeding patterns on their body mass index: results from the Million Women Study. *International Journal of Obesity* advance online publication, 10 July 2012; doi:10.1038/ijo.2012.76

Labbok MH, Hendershot GE Does breast-feeding protect against malocclusion? An analysis of the 1981 Child Health Supplement to the National Health Interview Survey. (PMID:3452360) *Am J Prev Med* 1987, 3(4):227-232

Labiner-Wolfe J, Fein SB, Shealy KR. Infant formula-handling education and safety. (PMID:18829836) *Pediatrics* 2008; 122 Suppl 2:s85-90.

Lack G, Fox D, Northstone K, Golding J. Factors associated with the development of peanut allergy in childhood. (PMID:12637607) *NEJM* 2003, 348(11):977-985 DOI: 10.1056/NEJMoa013536

Laguerre JC, Pascale GW, David M, Evelyne O et al. The impact of microwave heating of infant formula model on neo-formed contaminant formation, nutrient degradation, and spore destruction. *J Food Engineering* 2011; 107(2):208-213

Lakati AS, Makokha OA, Binns CW, Kombe Y. The effect of pre-lacteal feeding on full breastfeeding in Nairobi, Kenya. (PMID:21516965) *East African Journal of Public Health* 2010, 7(3):258-262.

Lanciers S, Mehta DI, Blecker U, Lebenthal E. The role of modified food starches in baby food. (PMID:9188246) *J Louisiana State Medical Society* 1997; 149(6):211-214

Lange FT, Scheurer M, Brauch HJ. Artificial sweeteners-a recently recognized class of emerging environmental contaminants: a review. (PMID:22543693) *Analytical and Bioanalytical Chemistry* 2012, 403(9):2503-2518

Langellier BA, Pia Chaparro M, Whaley SE. Social and institutional factors that affect breastfeeding duration among WIC participants in Los Angeles County, California. (PMID:22205423) *Matern Child Health J* 2012; 16(9):1887-1895

Langley-Evans SC. Nutrition in early life and the programming of adult disease: a review. (PMID:24479490) *J Hum Nutr Diet* 2014

Lanting CI, Fidler V, Huisman M, Touwen BCL et al. Neurological differences between 9-year-old children fed breast-milk or formula milk as babies. *Lancet* 1994; 344: 1319-1322.

Lawrence RM, Lawrence RA. Breast milk and infection. *Clin Perinatol* 31 (3): 501–28. PMID 15325535. doi:10.1016/j.clp.2004.03.019.

Le Page M. A brief history of the genome. *New Scientist* 215 (2882); 30-35.

Lequin MH, Vewrmeulen JR, van Elburg RM, Barkhof F et al. Bacillus cereus meningoencephalitis in preterm infants: neuroimaging characteristics. *AJNR* 2005 26: 2137-2143.

Leung C, Chang WC, Yeh SJ Hypernatremic dehydration due to concentrated infant formula: report of two cases. (PMID:19453082) *Pediatrics and Neonatology* 2009, 50(2):70-3

Levander OA. Upper limit of selenium in infant formulas.(PMID:2693651) *J Nutr* 1989; 119(12 Suppl):1869-72; discussion 1873.

Levin ME, Motala C, Lopata AL. Anaphylaxis in a milk-allergic child after ingestion of soy formula cross-contaminated with cow's milk protein. *Pediatrics* 2005, 116(5):1223-12251 (PMID:16264012) doi:10.1542/peds.2005-0020

Levy S. Reduced antibiotic use in livestock: how Denmark tackled resistance. *Environ Health Perspect.* 2014;122(6)

Li DP, Du C, Zhang ZM, Li GX et al. Breastfeeding and ovarian cancer risk: a systematic review and meta-analysis of 40 epidemiological studies. (PMID:24998548) *Asian Pac J Cancer Prev* 2014; 15(12):4829-4837 DOI: 10.1177/0890334413475838

Li J, Wang Y, Tang L, de Villiers WJ et al. Dietary medium-chain triglycerides promote oral allergic sensitization and orally induced anaphylaxis to peanut protein in mice. *J Allergy Clin Immunol.* 2013;131(2):442-50. doi: 10.1016/j.jaci.2012.10.011. Epub 2012 Nov 22.

Li R, Fein SB, and Grummer-Strawn LM. Do infants fed from bottles lack self-regulation of milk intake compared with directly breastfed infants? *Pediatrics* 2010; 125(6): e1386-93.

Li R, Magadia J, Fein SB, Grummer-Strawn LM. Risk of bottle-feeding for rapid weight gain during the first year of life.. (PMID:22566543) *Arch Pediatr Adolesc* Med 2012, 166(5):431-436

Lien EL. Infant formulas with increased concentrations of alpha-lactalbumin. (PMID:12812154) *Am J Clin Nutr* 2003, 77(6):1555S-1558S

Lilburne AM, Oates RK, Thompson S, Tong L. Infant feeding in Sydney: a survey of mothers who bottle feed. (PMID:3355446) *Aust Paediatr J* 1988, 24(1):49-54

Lillycrop KA, Burdge GC.The effect of nutrition during early life on the epigenetic regulation of transcription and implications for human diseases. (PMID:22353662) *J Nutrigenet Nutrigenomics* 2011; 4(5):248-260.

Linnamaa P, Nieminen K, Koulu L, Tuomasjukka S, et al. Black currant seed oil supplementation of mothers enhances IFN-γ and suppresses IL-4 production in breast milk. (PMID:23980846) *Pediatr Allergy Immunol* 2013; 24(6):562-566.

Lipkie TE, Banavara D, Shah B, Morrow AL, et al. Caco-2 accumulation of lutein is greater from human milk than from infant formula despite similar bioaccessibility. (PMID:24975441) *Mol Nutr Food Res* 2014;

Litmanovitz I, Davidson K, Eliakim A, Regev RH et al. High Beta-palmitate formula and bone strength in term infants: a randomized, double-blind, controlled trial. (PMCID:PMC3528957) *Calcif Tissue Int* 2013; 92(1):35-41

Liu B, Beral V, Balkwill A et al, Childbearing, breastfeeding, other reproductive factors and the subsequent risk of hospitalization for gallbladder disease. *Int J Epidemiol*, 2009; 38(1): 312-318.

Lodato P. Mead Johnson & Company. *International Directory of Company Histories*. 2007. Encyclopedia.com. (May 31, 2014). http://www.encyclopedia.com/doc/1G2-3480000067.html

Lombeck I, Kasperek K, Bonnermann B, Feinendegen LE et al. Selenium content of human milk, cow's mild and cow's milk infant formulas. *Eur J Pediatr* 1978; 129(3):139-145. (PMID:699919)

Lönnerdal B Bioactive proteins in breastmilk. *J Paediatr Child Health* 2013; 49(Suppl 1):1-7. DOI: 10.1111/jpc.12104

Lönnerdal B, Keen CL, Ohtake M, Tamura T. Iron, zinc, copper, and manganese in infant formulas. *Am J Dis Child* 1983; 137(5):433-437. (PMID:6846270)

Lönnerdal B, Kelleher SL. Iron metabolism in infants and children. *Food and Nutrition Bulletin* 2007; 28 (3), S491-499.

Lönnerdal B. Effects of milk and milk components on calcium, magnesium, and trace element absorption during infancy. *Physiol Rev* 1997; 77(3):643-669. (PMID:9234961)

Lönnerdal B. Human milk proteins: key components for the biological activity of human milk. (PMID:15384564) *Adv Exper Med Biol* 2004; 554:11-25.

Lönnerdal B. Infant formula and infant nutrition: bioactive proteins of human milk and implications for composition of infant formulas. (PMID:24452231) *Am J Clin Nutr* 2014, 99(3):712s-7s DOI: 10.3945/ajcn.113.071993

Lönnerdal B. Novel Insights into Human Lactation as a Driver of Infant Formula Development, in Koletzko B, Koletzko S, Ruemmele F (eds.) *Drivers Of Innovation In Paediatric Nutrition.* Nestle Nutrition Workshop Series, vol 66. (2010) Online.

Lönnerdal B. Nutritional aspects of soy formula. *Acta Paediatrica* Supplement 1994, 402:105-108

Lönnerdal B. Recombinant human milk proteins.(PMID:16902336) Nestle Nutrition Workshop Series. Paediatric Programme 2006, 58:207-15; discussion 215-7 DOI: 10.1159/000095064

Lönnerdal B. Trace element absorption in infants as a foundation to setting upper limits for trace elements in infant formulas. *J Nutr* 1989; 119(12 suppl):1839-44; discussion 1845] (PMID:2693645) These limits have altered!

Lönnerdal B., Hernell O. (1998). Effects of feeding ultrahigh-temperature (UHT)-treated infant formula with different protein concentrations or powdered formula, as compared with breast-feeding, on plasma amino acids, hematology, and trace element status. *Am. J. Clin. Nutr.* 68: 350–6.

Looker C, Kelly H. No-fault compensation following adverse events attributed to vaccination: a review of international programmes. *Bulletin of the World Health Organization* 2011;89:371-378. doi: 10.2471/BLT.10.081901

Lothe L, Lindberg T, Jakobsson I. Cow's Milk Formula as a Cause of Infantile Colic: A Double-Blind Study. *Pediatrics* 1982; 70:1 7-10

Lothe L. Lindberg T. Cow's Milk Whey Protein Elicits Symptoms of Infantile Colic in Colicky Formula-Fed Infants: A Double-Blind Crossover Study. *Pediatrics* 1989; 83:2 262-266

Lozoff B, Castillo M, Clark KM, Smith JB Iron-fortified vs low-iron infant formula: developmental outcome at 10 years *Archives of Pediatrics & Adolescent Medicine* 2012, 166(3):208-15 http://www.medscape.org/viewarticle/574363

Lubec G, Wolf C, Bartosh B. Amino acid isomerisation and microwave exposure. *Lancet* 1989; 2(8676): 1392-1393.

Lucarelli S, Di Nardo G, Lastrucci G, D'Alfonso Y et al. Allergic proctocolitis refractory to maternal hypoallergenic diet in exclusively breast-fed infants. *BMC Gastroenterol* 2011, 11:82

Lucas A, Blackburn AM, Aynsley-Green A, Sarson DL et al. Breast vs bottle: endocrine responses are different with formula feeding. *Lancet* 1980; I 1267-1269.

Lucas A, Cole TJ, Morley R, Lucas PJ et al. Factors associated with maternal choice to provide breast milk for low birthweight infants.(PMID:3348648) *Arch Dis Child* 1988; 63(1):48-52.

Lucas A, Cole TJ. Breast milk and neonatal necrotising enterocolitis. (PMID:1979363) *Lancet* 1990; 336(8730):1519-1523.

Lucas A, et al., Multicentre Trial on Feeding of Low Birthweight Infants: Effects of Diet on Early Growth. *Arch Dis Child* 1984; 59: 722-30. DOI: 10.1136/adc.59.8.722

Lucas A, Fewtrell MS, Morley R, Lucas PJ et al.Randomized outcome trial of human milk fortification and developmental outcome in preterm infants.(PMID:8694013) *Am J Clin Nutr* 1996, 64(2):142-151.

Lucas A, Lockton S, Davies PS. Randomised trial of a ready-to-feed compared with powdered formula. (PMID:1519960) *Arch Dis Child* 1992; 67(7):935-939.

Lucas A, Morley R, Cole TJ, Gore SM et al. Early diet in preterm babies and developmental status in infancy. *Arch Dis Child* 1989; 64: 1570-1578.

Lucas A, Morley R, Cole TJ, Gore SM. A randomised multicentre study of human milk versus formula and later development in preterm infants.(PMID:8154907) *Arch Dis Child Fetal Neonatal Ed* 1994; 70(2):f141-6.

Lucas A, Morley R, Cole TJ, Lister G et al.. Breast milk and subsequent intelligence quotient in children born preterm. (PMID:1346280) *Lancet* 1992, 339(8788):261-264] DOI: 10.1016/0140-6736(92)91329-7.

Lucas A, Morley R, Cole TJ. Randomised trial of early diet in preterm babies and later IQ. (PMID:9831573) *BMJ* 1998, 317(7171):1481-1487.

Lucas A, Morley R, Isaacs E. Nutrition and mental development. *Nutr Rev* 2001; 59 (8): S24-S33

Lucassen PLBJ Assendelft WJJ, Gubbels JW, van Eijk JTM, van Geldrop WJ et al Effectiveness of treatments for infantile colic: systematic review. *BR MED J.* 1998 May 23; 316(7144): 1563–1569. PMCID: PMC28556 See also Br Med J 1998; 317(7152): 171.

Lunney KM, Iliff P, Mutasa K, Ntozini R. Associations between breast milk viral load, mastitis, exclusive breast-feeding, and postnatal transmission of HIV. (PMID:20121424) *Clin Infect Dis* 2010; 50(5):762-769.

Mabuka J, Nduati R, Odem-Davis K, Peterson D et al. HIV-specific antibodies capable of ADCC are common in breastmilk and are associated with reduced risk of transmission in women with high viral loads. (PMID:22719248) *PLoS Pathog* 2012; 8(6):e1002739

Macdougall CF, Cant AJ, Colver AF. How dangerous is food allergy in childhood? The incidence of severe and fatal allergic reactions across the UK and Ireland. (PMID:11919093) *Arch Dis Child* 2002, 86(4):236-239 DOI: 10.1136/adc.86.4.236

Macé K, Steenhout P, Klassen P, Donnet A. Protein quality and quantity in cow's milk-based formula for healthy term infants: past, present and future. (PMID:16902335) Nestle Nutr Workshop Ser Pediatr Program 2006, 58:189-203; discussion 203-5

MacLean WC, Van Dael P, Clemens R, Davies J et al. Upper levels of nutrients in infant formulas: Comparison of analytical data with the revised Codex infant formula standard. *J Food Comp Anal* 2010, 23(1):44-53 DOI:10.1016/j.jfca.2009.07.008

Madan JC, Salari RC, Saxena D, Davidson L, et al. Gut microbial colonisation in premature neonates predicts neonatal sepsis. (PMID:22562869) *Arch Dis Child Fetal Neonatal Ed* 2012; 97(6):f456-62.

MAFF UK. *Food Standards Committee Report on Infant Formulae (*Artificial Feeds for the Young Infant) (HMSO 1981)

Maggadottir SM, Hill D, Brown-Whitehorn TF, Spergel JM. Development Of Eosinophilic Esophagitis To Food After Development Of IgE Tolerance To The Same Food. *J Allergy Clin Immunol* 2014; 133: (2) Suppl P. AB 287.

Magnuson B, Munro I, Abbot P, Baldwin N,et al. Review of the regulation and safety assessment of food substances in various countries and jurisdictions *Food Addit Contam Part A* 2013; 30(7): 1147–1220. PMCID: PMC3725665 doi: 10.1080/19440049.2013.795293

Maher TJ, Wurtman RJ. Possible neurologic effects of aspartame, a widely used food additive. (PMID:3319565) *Envir Health Persp* 1987, 75:53-57

Mahurin-Smith J, Ambrose NG. Breastfeeding may protect against persistent stuttering. *J Commun Disord* 2013. (PMID:23849886)

Makrides M. DHA supplementation during the perinatal period and neurodevelopment: do some babies benefit more than others?(PMID:22698951) *Prostagland Leukot Essent Fatty Acids* 2013, 88(1):87-90

Manary M. Local production and provision of ready-to-use therapeutic food for the treatment of severe childhood malnutrition. http://www.who.int/nutrition/topics/backgroundpapers_Local_production.pdf

Mandhane PJ, Greene JM, Sears MR. Interactions between breast-feeding, specific parental atopy, and sex on development of asthma and atopy. (PMID:17353035) *JACI* 2007, 119(6):1359-1366] DOI: 10.1016/j.jaci.2007.01.043

Manzoni P, Rinaldi M, Cattani S, Pugni L et al Bovine lactoferrin supplementation for prevention of late-onset sepsis in very low-birth-weight neonates: a randomized trial. (PMID:19809023) *JAMA* 2009, 302(13):1421-1428

Marks LR, Clementi EA, Hakansson AP. Sensitization of Staphylococcus aureus to methicillin and other antibiotics in vitro and in vivo in the presence of HAMLET. (PMID:23650551) *PloS One* 2013, 8(5):e63158. DOI: 10.1371/journal.pone.0063158

Martelli A, De Chiara A, Corvo M, Restani P, Fiocchi A. Beef allergy in children with cow's milk allergy; cow's milk allergy in children with beef allergy. *Ann Allergy Immunol* 2002; 89 (6 Suppl 1):38-43. (PMID:12487203)

Martin NW, B. Benyamin, N. K. Hansell, G. W. Montgomery et al. Cognitive function in adolescence: testing for interactions between breast-feeding & FADS2 polymorphisms. *J Am Acad Child Adol Psychiatr* 2010; 50, 55-62 e4. 10.1016/j.jaac.2010.10.010

Martín V, Maldonado-Barragán A, Moles L, Rodriguez-Baños M et al. Sharing of bacterial strains between breast milk and infant feces. *J Hum Lact* 2012 28: 36-44, doi:10.1177/0890334411424729

Martin-Calama J, Buñuel J, Valero MT, Labay M, et al. The effect of feeding glucose water to breastfeeding newborns on weight, body temperature, blood glucose, and breastfeeding duration. (PMID:9341413) *J Hum Lact* 1997, 13(3):209-213.

Martín-Muñoz MF, Fortuni M, Caminoa M, Belver T et al. Anaphylactic reaction to probiotics: Cow's milk and hen's egg allergens in probiotic compounds. *Pediatr Allergy Immunol* 2012: 23(8):778-784

Martín-Muñoz MF, Pereira MJ, Posadas S, Sánchez-Sabaté E et al. Anaphylactic reaction to diphtheria-tetanus vaccine in a child: specific IgE/IgG determinations and cross-reactivity studies. *Vaccine* 2002; 20(27-28):3409-3412

Martineau A, Jolliffe D. *Vitamin D and Human Health: from the Gamete to the Grave*: Report on a meeting held at Queen Mary University of London, 23rd–25th April 2014. (PMCID:PMC4113768) *Nutrients.* 2014; 6(7): 2759–2919. Published online Jul 22, 2014. doi: 10.3390/nu6072759

Martyn C. Lactation wars. Published 9 February 2011; *Br Med J* 342 doi: 10.1136/bmj.d835

Mason T, Rabinovich CE, Fredrickson DD et al. Breastfeeding and the development of juvenile rheumatoid arthritis. J Rheumatol. 1995; 22:1166-70.

Matturri L, Ottaviani G, Corti G, Lavezzi AM Pathogenesis of early atherosclerotic lesions in infants. (PMID:15239349) *Pathology, Research and Practice* 2004; 200(5):403-410

Mayor S. Three quarters of babies consume too much energy, finds UK survey. (PMID:23503190) *BMJ* 2013; 346:f1740.

Mazumdar M, Bellinger DC, Gregas M, Abanilla K et al. Low-level environmental lead exposure in childhood and adult intellectual function: a follow-up study. (PMID:21450073) *Envir Hlth* 2011; 10:24. DOI: 10.1186/1476-069X-10-24

McCarver G, Bhatia J, Chambers C, Clarke R et al. NTP-CERHR expert panel report on the developmental toxicity of soy infant formula. (PMID:21948615) *Birth Defects Research. Part B, Developmental and Reproductive Toxicology* 2011, 92(5):421-68

McDonald K, Amir LH, Davey MA. Maternal bodies and medicines: a commentary on risk and decision-making of pregnant and breastfeeding women and...(PMID:22168473) *BMC Public Health* 2011, 11 Suppl 5:S5

McElroy SJ, Castle SL, Bernard JK, Almohazey D et al. The ErbB4 ligand neuregulin-4 protects against experimental necrotizing enterocolitis. (PMID:25216938) Am J Pathol 2014, 184(10):2768-2778. DOI: 10.1016/j.ajpath.2014.06.015.

McFadden JP, White JM, Basketter DA, Kimber I. Does hapten exposure predispose to atopic disease? The hapten-atopy hypothesis. *Trends in Immunology* 2009, 30(2):67-74 (PMID:19138566)

**McGilligan** KM, Thomas DW, Eckhert CD. Alpha-1-antitrypsin concentration in human milk. *Pediatr Res* 1987; 22(3):268-70. (PMID:3498927)

McGuire L. Ruth goes home: an adult's use of breastmilk. *Breastfeeding Review* 2012; 20 (3) 44-48.

McMillan JA, Landaw SA, Oski FA. Iron sufficiency in breast-fed infants and the availability of iron from human milk. (PMID:989894) *Pediatrics* 1976, 58(5):686-691

McTiernan A, Thomas DB. Evidence for a protective effect of lactation on risk of breast cancer in young women. *Am J Epidemiol* 1986; 124: 353-8.

Mehr SS, Kakakios AM, Kemp AS. Rice: a common and severe cause of food protein-induced enterocolitis syndrome.(PMID:18957470) *Arch Dis Child* 2009;94(3):220-223.

Meier P, Engstrom JL, Patel AL, Jegier B et al. Improving the use of human milk before and after the NICU stay. *Clin Perinatol* 2010; 37 (1) 217-245. doi 10.1016/j.clp.2010.01.013

Melnik BC, John SM, Schmitz G. Milk is not just food but most likely a genetic transfection system activating mTORC1 signaling for postnatal growth. (PMID:23883112) *Nutr J* 2013; 12:103.

Melnik BC, John SM, Schmitz G. Milk: an exosomal microRNA transmitter promoting thymic regulatory T cell maturation preventing the development of atopy? (PMID:24521175) *J Transl Med* 2014; 12:43

Melnik BC. Diet in acne: further evidence for the role of nutrient signalling in acne pathogenesis.(PMID:22419445) *Acta Derm Venereol* 2012, 92(3):228-231

Melnik BC. Evidence for Acne-Promoting Effects of Milk and Other Insulinotropic Dairy Products (PMID:21335995) *Nestle Nutr Workshop Ser Pediatr Program* 2011; 67:131-145

Melnik BC. Excessive Leucine-mTORC1-Signalling of Cow Milk-Based Infant Formula: The Missing Link to Understand Early Childhood Obesity. *J Obes.* 2012; 2012: 197653. Published online 2012 March 19. doi: 10.1155/2012/197653

Mendez MA, Anthony MS, Arab L. Soy-based formulae and infant growth and development: a review. (PMID:12163650) *J Nutr* 2002; 132(8):2127-2130.

Mennella JA, Ventura AK, Beauchamp GK. Differential Growth Patterns Among Healthy Infants Fed Protein Hydrolysate or Cow-Milk Formula. *Pediatrics* 2011; 127:110-118. doi:10.1542/peds.2010-1675

Mennella JA. Mother's milk: a medium for early flavor experiences. *J Hum Lact* 1995, 11(1):39-45. (PMID:7748264)

Menzies BR, Shaw G, Fletcher TP, Renfree MB. Perturbed growth and development in marsupial young after reciprocal cross-fostering between species. (PMID:18076830) *Reprod Fertil Dev* 2007, 19(8):976-983.

Mepham TB. Humanizing milk: the formulation of artificial feeds for infants, 1850-1910. *Medical History* 1993; 37: 225-249.

Mepham TB. Science and the politics of breastfeeding: birthright or birth rite? *Science and Public Policy* 1989; 16(3): 189-191.

Metcalf R, Dilena B, Gibson R, Marshall P et al. How appropriate are commercially available human milk fortifiers? *J Pediatr Child Health* 1994; 30: 350-5.

Meucci V, Razzuoli E, Soldani G, Massart F. Mycotoxin detection in infant formula milks in Italy.(PMID:19787514) *Food Additives & Contaminants. Part A, Chemistry, Analysis, Control, Exposure & Risk Assessment* 2010, 27(1):64-71

Meulenbroek LA, Oliveira S, den Hartog Jager CF et al. The degree of whey hydrolysis does not uniformly affect in vitro basophil and T cell responses of cow's milk allergic patients.(PMID:24330309) *Clin Exp Allergy* 2013

Michaelsen KF, Larnkjær A, Mølgaard C. Amount and quality of dietary proteins during the first two years of life in relation to NCD risk in adulthood. (PMID:22770749) *Nutr Metab Cardiovasc Dis* 2012; 22(10):781-786

Mihatsch WA, Braegger CP, Decsi T, Kolacek S et al. Critical systematic review of the level of evidence for routine use of probiotics for reduction of mortality and prevention of necrotizing enterocolitis and sepsis in preterm infants. (PMID:21996513) *Clinical Nutrition* 2012, 31(1):6-15.

Minchin MK. Artificial feeding and risk: the last taboo. The Practising Midwife 2000

Minchin MK. Colic and other manifestations of food intolerance in normal breastfed infants and their families. Proceedings ICM 1984

Minchin MK. Infant formula: a mass, uncontrolled trial in perinatal care. *Birth.* 1987;14:25-35.

Minchin MK. Smoking and breastfeeding: an overview. J Hum Lact 1991; 7(4): 183-188

Minchin MK. Towards Safer Artifical Feeding. (Alma Publications, 2001) (booklet)

Minor P. Vaccine-derived poliovirus (VDPV): Impact on poliomyelitis eradication. (PMID:19428874) *Vaccine* 2009; 27(20):2649-2652.

Modi N, Uthaya S, Fell J, Kulinskaya E. A randomized, double-blind, controlled trial of the effect of prebiotic oligosaccharides on enteral tolerance in preterm infants. *Pediatr Res* 2010, 68(5):440-445 . (ISRCTN77444690). (PMID:20639792)

Modi N. Ethical pitfalls in neonatal comparative effectiveness trials. (PMID:24931328) *Neonatology* 2014;105(4):350-351. DOI: 10.1159/000360650

Molska A, Gutowska I, Baranowska-Bosiacka I, Noceń I et al. The Content of Elements in Infant Formulas and Drinks Against Mineral Requirements of Children. (PMID:24706326) Biological Trace Element Research [2014]

Moneret-Vautrin DA, Hatahet R, Kanny G, Ait-Djafer Z. Allergenic peanut oil in milk formulas. (PMID:1682569) *Lancet* 1991; 338(8775):1149

Moneret-Vautrin DA, Hatahet R, Kanny G. Risks of milk formulas containing peanut oil contaminated with peanut allergens in infants with atopic dermatitis. *Pediatr Allergy Immunol* 1994; 5(3):184-8. (PMID:7951761) DOI: 10.1111/j.1399-3038.1994.tb00236.x

Montgomery-Downs HE, Clawges HM, Santy EE. Infant feeding methods and maternal sleep and daytime functioning. (PMID:21059713) *Pediatrics* 2010, 126(6):e1562-8

Moore JC, Spink J, Lipp M. Development and application of a database of food ingredient fraud and economically motivated adulteration from1980 to 2010. *J Food Sci* 2012; 77(4): R118-126.

Morgenstern V, Zutavern A, Cyrys J, Brockow I et al. Atopic diseases, allergic sensitization, and exposure to traffic-related air pollution in children. (PMID:18337595)*Am J Respir Crit Care Med* 2008, 177(12):1331-1337

Morin S, Fischer R, Przybylski-Nicaise L, Bernard H et al. Delayed bacterial colonization of the gut alters the host immune response to oral sensitization against cow's milk proteins. *Mol Nutr Food Res* 2012; 56(12):1838-1847. (PMID:23065810)

Morley R, Cole TJ, Powell R, Lucas A. Mother's choice to provide breast milk and developmental outcome. (PMID:3202647)  Arch Dis Child 1988; 63(11): 1382-1385

Morley R, Lucas A. Randomized diet in the neonatal period and growth performance until 7.5-8 y of age in preterm children. PMID:10702179) *Am J Clin Nutr* 2000; 71(3):822-828.

Moro G, Arslanoglu S, Stahl B, Jelinek J et al. A mixture of prebiotic oligosaccharides reduces the incidence of atopic dermatitis during the first 6 months of age. *Arch Dis Child* 2006; 91: 814-819. Doi: 10.1136/adc.2006.098251

Morris S, Simmer K, Gibson R. Utilization of docosahexaenoic acid from intravenous egg yolk phospholipid. (PMID:10858022) *Lipids* 2000, 35(4):383-388 DOI: 10.1007/s11745-000-535-9

Morrison P, Israel-Ballard K, Greiner T. Informed choice in infant feeding decisions can be supported for HIV-infected women even in industrialized countries. *AIDS* 2011, 25:1807–1811.

Morrow M. Breastfeeding in Vietnam: poverty, tradition, and economic transition. (PMID:8932039) *J Hum Lact* 1996, 12(2):97-103

Mortenson EL, Michaelsen KF, Sanders SA, Reinisch JM. The association between duration of breastfeeding and adult intelligence, *JAMA* 2002;287:2365-2371.

Mott GE, Lewis DS, McGill HC Jr. Programming of cholesterol metabolism by breast or formula feeding.Ciba Foundation Symposium 1991, 156:56-66; discussion 66-76. (PMID:1855416)

Moussa S, Jenabian MA, Gody JC, Léal J, et al. Adaptive HIV-Specific B Cell-Derived Humoral Immune Defenses of the Intestinal Mucosa in Children Exposed to HIV via Breast-Feeding. (PMCID:PMC3660449) *PLoS One* 2013; 8(5):e63408. http://www.ncbi.nlm.nih.gov/pmc/articles/PMC3660449/pdf/pone.0063408.pdf

Mpairwe H, Webb EL, Muhangi L, Ndibazza J et al. Anthelminthic treatment during pregnancy is associated with increased risk of infantile eczema: RCT results. (PMCID:PMC3130136) *Pediatric Allergy and Immunology* 2011, 22(3):305-312 DOI: 10.1111/j.1399-3038.2010.01122.x

Muir JG, Gibson PR. The low FODMAP diet for treatment of Irritable Bowel Syndrome and other gastrointestinal disorders. (PMID:23935555)  *Gastroenterol Hepatol* 2013; 9(7):450-452.

Murch, SH. Probiotics as mainstream allergy therapy? *Arch Dis Child* 2005;90:881–882. doi: 10.1136/adc.2005.073114

Murphy S. Addictive personality. *New Scientist*, 8 Sept 2012, pp. 37-9.

Muytjens HL, Roelofs-Willemse H, Jaspar GH. Quality of powdered substitutes for breast milk with regard to members of the family Enterobacteriaceae. *J Clin Microbiol* 1988, 26(4):743-746 (PMID:3284901)

Najnin N, Forbes A, Sinclair M, Leder K. Risk factors for community-based reports of gastrointestinal, respiratory, and dermal symptoms: findings from a cohort study in Australia. (PMID:24240632) J Epidemiol 2014, 24(1):39-46 DOI: 10.2188/jea.JE20130082;

Nakatsuji T, Chiang H-I, Jiang SB, Nagarajan H, Zengler K, Gallo RL. The microbiome extends to subepidermal compartments of normal skin. *Nat Commun* 2013: 4: 1431

Nath DC, Goswami G. Determinants of breast-feeding patterns in an urban society of India. (PMID:9198314) *Human Biology* 1997; 69(4):557-573.

National Center for Toxicological Research, Jefferson Arkansas 72079. Final Report: Chronic Toxicity and Carcinogenicity Studies of Gentian Violet in Mice. September 1984. (National Technical Information Service, US department of Commerce. Springfield VA. 22161)

Nauta AJ, Kaouther BA, Knol J, Garssen J et al. Relevance of pre- and postnatal nutrition to development and interplay between the microbiota and metabolic and immune systems. *Am J Clin Nutr* 2013; 98 (2): 586S-593S. doi: 10.3945/ ajcn.112.039644

Navarro-Blasco I, Alvarez-Galindo JI. Selenium content of Spanish infant formulae and human milk: influence of protein matrix, interactions with other trace elements and estimation of dietary intake by infants. (PMID:15139390) *J Trace Elem Med Biol* 2004; 17(4):277-289DOI: 10.1016/S0946-672X(04)80030-0

Needleman HL, Bellinger D. The health effects of low level lead exposure. *Ann Rev Publ Hlth* 1991; 12: 111-40

Needleman HL. (2008) The Case of Deborah Rice: Who Is the Environmental Protection Agency Protecting? *PLoS Biol* 6(5): e129. doi:10.1371/journal.pbio.0060129

Needleman HL. The persistent threat of lead: a singular opportunity. (PMID:2650573) *Am J Public Health* 1989; 79(5):643-645.

Neville MC, Anderson SM, McManaman JL, Badger TM, et al. Lactation and neonatal nutrition: defining and refining the critical questions. (PMID:22752723) *Journal of Mammary Gland Biology and Neoplasia* 2012, 17(2):167-188

Newburg DS, Woo JG, Morrow AL. Characteristics and potential functions of human milk adiponectin. In Makrides M, Ochoa J, Szajewska H (eds). *The Importance of Immunonutrition* NNI Workshop Series vol 77, 2013http://dx.doi.org/10.1016/j.jpeds.2009.11.020

Ng R, Martin DJ. Lead poisoning from lead-soldered electric kettles. (PMID:837317) Canadian Medical Association Journal [1977, 116(5):508-9, 512.

Ngoma M, Raha A, Elong A, Pilon R et al. Interim Results of HIV Transmission Rates Using a Lopinavir/Ritonavir based regimen and the New WHO Breast Feeding Guidelines for PMTCT of HIV. International Congress of Antimicrobial Agents and Chemotherapy (ICAAC) Chicago Il, 2011. Available at http://www.icaac.org/index.php/component/content/article/9-newsroom/169-preliminary-results-of-hiv-transmission-rates-using-a-lopinavirritonavir-lpvr-aluvia-based-regimen-and-the-new-who-breast-feeding-guidelines-for-pmtct-of-hiv-

NHMRC 2013. Infant Feeding Guidelines for Healthworkers. 2013 Online.

NHMRC Clinical Trials Centre University of Sydney. *An international comparison study into the implementation of the WHO code and other breastfeeding initiatives.* Final Report. http://www.health.gov.au/internet/main/publishing.nsf/Content/1C29E44FE6BB3C4DCA257BF0001BDBC5/$File/111027%20Final%20Report.pdf

Nielsen H. Hen age and fatty acid composition of egg yolk lipid. (PMID:9568299) *British Poultry Science* 1998, 39(1):53-56 DOI:10.1080/00071669889394

Nikitiuk NF. The antimeasles immunity in infants in the 1st year of life. (PMID:10876898) Zhurnal Mikrobiologii, Epidemiologii, i Immunobiologii [2000(1):63-65.

Nobili V, Bedogni G, Alisi A, Pietrobattista A, et al. A protective effect of breastfeeding on the progression of non-alcoholic fatty liver disease. *Arch Dis Child* 2009, 94(10):801-805. (PMID:19556219)

Nobili V, Day C. Childhood NAFLD: a ticking time-bomb? *Gut* 2009, 58(11):1442 (PMID:19834114

Noel-Weiss j, Boersma S, Kujawa-Myles S. Questioning current definitions for breastfeeding research. *Int Breastfeeding J.* 2012, 7:9. 10.1186/1746-4358-7-

Noel-Weiss J, Courant G, Woodend AK. Physiological weight loss in the breastfed neonate: a systematic review. *Open Med* 2008, 2(4):e99-e110 (PMID: 21602959)

Noel-Weiss J, Woodend AK, Groll DL. Iatrogenic newborn weight loss: knowledge translation using a study protocol for your maternity setting. (PMID:21843331) *Int Breastfeed J* 2011, 6(1):10 ;

Noel-Weiss J, Woodend AK, Peterson WE, Gibb W, Groll DL. An observational study of associations among maternal fluids during parturition, neonatal output, and breastfed newborn weight loss. (PMID: 21843338) *Int Breastfeed J* 2011, 6:9

Northstone K, Emmett P, Nethersole F, The effect of age of introduction to lumpy solids on foods eaten and reported feeding difficulties at 6 and 15 months. (PMID:11301932) *J Hum Nutr Diet* 2001; 14(1):43-54.

Nyqvist KH, Anderson GC, Bergman N, Cattaneo A et al. Towards universal Kangaroo Mother Care: recommendations and report from the First European conference and Seventh International Workshop on Kangaroo Mother Care. (PMID:20219044) *Acta Paediatr* 2010, 99(6):820-826

Nyqvist KH, Häggkvist AP, Hansen MN, Kylberg E et al. Expansion of the ten steps to successful breastfeeding into neonatal intensive care: expert group recommendations for three guiding principles. *J Hum Lact* 2012;28(3):289-96

Nyqvist KH, Häggkvist AP, Hansen MN, Kylberg E et al. Expansion of the Baby-Friendly Hospital Initiative ten steps to successful breastfeeding into neonatal intensive care: Expert group recommendations. *J Hum Lact* 2013; 29(3):300-9.

O'Callaghan T. Cure-all no more. *New Scientist* 2014; 222(2971): 34-37

Oates L, Cohen M, Braun L, Schembri A et al. Reduction in urinary organophosphate pesticide metabolites in adults after a week-long organic diet. *Environmental Research* 2014; 132:105-111

Oddy WH, Holt PG, Sly PD, et al. Association between breast feeding and asthma in 6 year old children: findings of a prospective birth cohort study. *Br Med J* 1999; 319:815–819.

Oddy WH, Kendall GE, Li J, Jacoby P et al. The Long-Term Effects of Breastfeeding on Child and Adolescent Mental Health: A Pregnancy Cohort Study Followed for 14 Years, *J Pediatrics* 2010, 156(4):568-574

Oddy WH, Li J, Whitehouse AJ, Zubrick SR, Malacova E. Breastfeeding duration and academic achievement at 10 years. (PMID:21172993) *Pediatrics* 2011; 127(1):e137-45

Oddy WH, Li J,Robinson M, Whitehouse AJO. The Long-Term Effects of Breastfeeding on Development in Özdemir O (ed), *Contemporary Pediatrics* 2012. ISBN 978-953-51-0154-3 DOI: 10.5772/34422 Open access. Available at http://www.intechopen.com/books/contemporary-pediatrics/the-long-term-effects-of-breastfeeding-on-development

Oddy WH, McMahon RJ. Milk-derived or recombinant transforming growth factor-beta has effects on immunological outcomes: a review of evidence from animal experimental studies. (PMID:21492269) *Clin Exp Allergy* 2011; 41(6):783-79

Oddy WH. Infant feeding and obesity risk in the child. *Breastfeeding Review* 2012; 20 (2): 7-12.

Offit PA, Moser CA. The Problem With Dr Bob's Alternative Vaccine Schedule. Pediatrics 2009; 123 (1) e164 -e169. doi: 10.1542/peds.2008-2189. http://pediatrics.aappublications.org/content/123/1/e164

Oftedal OT. Lactation in the dog: milk composition and intake by puppies. *J Nutr* 1984, 114(5):803-812. PMID:6726450 See http://jn.nutrition.org/content/114/5/803.full.pdf

Ogg SW, Hudson MM, Randolph ME, Klosky JL. Protective effects of breastfeeding for mothers surviving childhood cancer. *Journal of Cancer Survivorship.* 2011; DOI 10.1007/s11764-010-0169-z

Oh Se-Wook, Chen Pei-Chun, Kang Dong-Hyun. Biofilm formation by Enterobacter sakazakii grown in artificial broth and infant milk formula on plastic surface (Agr:Ind43982644) *J Rapid Method Autom Microbiol.* 2007; 15(4):311-319.

Olejnik M, Szprengier-Juszkiewicz T, Jedziniak P. Semduramicin in eggs - incompatibility of feed and food maximum levels. *Food Chem.* 2014 Apr 15;149:178-82. doi: 10.1016/j.foodchem.2013.10.091. Epub 2013 Nov 1.

Oliveira V, Frazão E, Smallwood D. *Rising Infant Formula Costs to the WIC Program: Recent Trends in Rebates and Wholesale Prices,* ERR-93, U.S. Department of Agriculture, Economic Research Service, February 2010

Oliveira V, Frazão E. *The WIC Program: Background, Trends, and Economic Issues*, U.S. Department of Agriculture, Economic Research Service, 2009.

Oliviera V. Winner takes (almost) all. How WIC affects the infant formula market. Downloaded from httpwww.ers. usda.gov/AmberWaves/September 11/Features/InfantFormulaMarket.htm

Olson DT, Financing Terror. *Law Enforcement Bulletin* 2007; 76 (2); 1-5.

Ortega-García JA, Ferrís-Tortajada J, Torres-Cantero AM, Soldin OP et al. Full breastfeeding and paediatric cancer. *J Paediatr Child Health* 2008; 44(1-2):10-13. (PMID:17999666(

Osaili T, Forsythe S. Desiccation resistance and persistence of Cronobacter species in infant formula. (PMID:19720413) *Internat J Food Microbiol* 2009, 136(2):214-220

Osborn GR. Aetiology of coronary artery disease.(PMID:5131544) *Med J Aust* 1971, 2(20):1039-40.

Oski FA, Landaw SA. Inhibition of iron absorption from human milk by baby food. (PMID:7377151) Am J Dis Child 1980; 134(5):459-460

Oski FA, Paige DM. Cow's milk is a good food for some and a poor choice for others: eliminating the hyperbole. (PMID:8143001) *Arch Pediatr Adolesc Med* 1994, 148(1):104-107

Oski FA. Health Hazards of Cow's Milk. *Pediatrics* 1985; 76:6 1022-1023

Oski, FA. Heating Up the Bottle Battle. *The Nation* 1989; 249 (19)

Palma GD, Capilla A, Nova E, Castillejo G et al. Influence of milk-feeding type and genetic risk of developing coeliac disease on intestinal microbiota of infants: the PROFICEL study. *PLoS One* 2012; 7(2):e30791 (PMID:22319588) DOI: 10.1371/journal.pone.0030791

Palmer DJ, Makrides M. Diet of lactating women and allergic reactions in their infants. (PMID:16607130) *Curr Opin Clin Nutr Metab Care* 2006, 9(3):284-8

Palmer DJ, Sullivan T, Gold MS, Prescott SL et al. Effect of n-3 long chain polyunsaturated fatty acid supplementation in pregnancy on infants' allergies in first year of life: randomised controlled trial *Br Med J* 2012; 344: e184.

Pandelova M, Lopez WL, Michalke B, Schramm KW. Ca, Cd, Cu, Fe, Hg, Mn, Ni, Pb, Se, and Zn contents in baby foods from the EU market: Comparison of assessed infant intakes with the present safety limits for minerals and trace elements. *J Food Comp Anal* 2012; 27(2):120-127

Patki S, Kadam S, Chandra V, Bhonde R. Human breast milk is a rich source of multipotent mesenchymal stem cells. (PMID:20712706) *Hum Cell* 2010; 23(2):35-40

Paton LM. Pregnancy and lactation have no long-term deleterious effect on measures of bone mineral in healthy women: a twin study. *Am J Clin Nutr.* 2003; 77:707-714.

Pearson F, Johnson MJ, Leaf AA. Milk osmolality: does it matter? (PMID:21930688) *Arch Dis Child* 2013; 98(2):F166-9. DOI: 10.1136/adc.2011.300492

Pedersen, K M; Laurberg, P et al. Iodine in drinking water varies by more than 100-fold in Denmark. Importance for iodine content of infant formulas. *Eur J Endocrinol, 1999*;140 (5):400-3

Pembrey ME, Bygren LO, Kaati G, Edvinsson S et al. ALSPAC Study Team. Sex-specific, male-line transgenerational responses in humans.(PMID:16391557) *Eur J Hum Genet 2006*, 14(2):159-166.

Pérez-Hernández AI, Catalán V, Gómez-Ambrosi J, Rodríguez A et al. Mechanisms Linking Excess Adiposity and Carcinogenesis Promotion Endocrinol (Lausanne). 2014; 5: 65. doi: 10.3389/fendo.2014.00065

Perkkiö M, Savilahti E. Time of appearance of immunoglobulin-containing cells in the mucosa of the neonatal intestine. (PMID:7191555) *Pediatric Research* 1980, 14(8):953-955

Pettit DJ, Forman MR, Hanson RL, Knowles WC et et al BF and incidence of NIDDM in Pima Indians. *Lancet* 1997; 350: 166-168.

Pfaender S, Heyden J, Friesland M, Ciesek S et al. Inactivation of hepatitis C virus infectivity by human breast milk. (PMID:24068703) *J Infect Dis* 2013, 208(12):1943-1952

Phillips CM. Nutrigenetics and metabolic disease: current status and implications for personalised nutrition. *Nutrients* 2013; 5(1):32

Pickering LK, Granoff DM, Erickson JR, Masor ML, et al. Modulation of the immune system by human milk and infant formula containing nucleotides. *Pediatrics.* 1998; 101(2):242-9.

Pikwer W, Bergstrom U, Nilsson JA et al. Breastfeeding but not use of oral contraceptives is associated with a reduced risk of RA. *Ann Rheum Dis* 2009; 68:526-530.

Pisarik P, Kai D. Vestibulocochlear toxicity in a pair of siblings 15 years apart secondary to aspartame: two case reports.(PMID:20126318) *Cases Journal* 2009, 2:9237

Pischetsrieder M, Henle T. Glycation products in infant formulas: chemical, analytical and physiological aspects. *Amino Acids* 2012, 42(4):1111-1118 DOI: 10.1007/s00726-010-0775-0

Pittard WB, Anderson DM, Cerutti ER, Boxerbaum B. Bacteriostatic qualities of human milk. *J. Pediatr.* 1985; 107(2) 240-243.

Pivik RT, Andres A, Badger TM. Effects of diet on early stage cortical perception and discrimination of syllables differing in voice-onset time: a longitudinal ERP study in 3 and 6 month old infants. *Brain and Language* 2012, 120(1):27-41 DOI: 10.1016/j.bandl.2011.08.004

Plagemann A, Heidrich I, Götz F, Rohde W, Dörner G. Lifelong enhanced diabetes susceptibility and obesity after temporary intrahypothalamic hyperinsulinism during brain organization.(PMID:1639125) *Exp Clin Endocrinol* 1992, 99(2):91-95

Pokhrel S, Quigley MA, Fox-Rushby J, McCormick F et al.Potential economic impacts from improving breastfeeding rates in the UK. (PMID:25477310) Arch Dis Child 2014;  DOI: 10.1136/archdischild-2014-306701

Pollock I, Young E, Stoneham M, Slater N et al. Survey of colourings and preservatives in drugs. (PMID:2508849) *BMJ* 1989; 299(6700):649-651.

Polte T, Hansen G. Maternal tolerance achieved during pregnancy is transferred to the offspring via breast milk and persistently protects the offspring from allergic asthma.(PMID:18778271) *Clin Exp Allergy* 2008, 38(12):1950-1958

Polte T, Hennig C, Hansen G. Allergy prevention starts before conception: maternofetal transfer of tolerance protects against the development of asthma.(PMID:19000583) *J Allergy Clin Immunol* 2008, 122(5):1022-1030.e5

Pop M. We are what we eat: how the diet of infants affects their gut microbiome. (PMID:22546514) *Genome Biol* 2012, 13(4):152.

Popp A, Cleenwerck I, Iversen C, De Vos P et al. Pantoea gaviniae sp. nov. and Pantoea calida sp. nov. isolated from infant formula and an infant formula production environment. (PMID:20061487 *International Journal of Systematic and Evolutionary Microbiology* 2010, 60(Pt 12):2786-92

Post GB, Cohn PD, Cooper KR. Perfluorooctanoic acid (PFOA), an emerging drinking water contaminant: A critical review of recent literature. (PMID:22560884 *Environmental Research* 2012, 116:93-117

Potter PC, Warner JO, Pawankar R, Kaliner MA,  et al. Recommendations for competency in allergy training for undergraduates qualifying as medical practitioners: a position paper of the world allergy organization. World Allergy Organ J 2009, 2(8):150-154.doi: 10.1186/1939-4551-2-8-150

Prell M. *An Economic Model of WIC, the Infant Formula Rebate Program, and the Retail Price of Infant Formula.* U.S. Department of Agriculture, Economic Research Service, available online.

Prescott SL, Smith P, Tang M, Palmer DJ et al. The importance of early complementary feeding in the development of oral tolerance: concerns and controversies. *Pediatric Allergy and Immunology* 2008, 19(5):375-380 (PMID:18266825) DOI: 10.1111/j.1399-3038.2008.00718.x (PMID:20105659)

Prescott SL, Wiltschut J, Taylor A, *et al.* Early markers of allergic disease in a primary prevention study using probiotics: 2.5-year follow-up phase. *Allergy* 2008; 63:1481–1490.

Prescott. JW. Nurturant versus non-nurturant environments and the failure of the environment of evolutionary adaptedness, in Narvaez D, Panksepp J, Schore AN, Gleason T (eds) *Evolution, Early Experience and Human Development.* (Oxford Uni Press 2012)

Promar International. Strategic development Plan for the Irish Dairy Processing Sector. (2003) Online at http://www.agriculture.gov.ie/publications/2000-2003/dairyindustryprospectusreport2003/

Qawasmi A, Landeros-Weisenberger A, Leckman JF, Bloch MH. Meta-analysis of Long-Chain Polyunsaturated Fatty Acid Supplementation of Formula and Infant Cognition. (PMID:22641753) *Pediatrics* 2012; 129(6):1141-9

Quigley MA, Hockley C, Carson C, Kelly Y et al. Breastfeeding is associated with improved child cognitive development: a population-based cohort. (PMID:21839469) *J Pediatr* 2012; 160(1):25-32

Quigley MA, Kelly YJ, Sacker A. Breastfeeding and hospitalization for diarrheal and respiratory infection in the UK Millennium Cohort Study. (PMID:17403827) *Pediatrics* 2007, 119(4):e837-42

Quinello C, Quintilio W, Carneiro-Sampaio M, Palmeira P. Passive acquisition of protective antibodies reactive with Bordetella pertussis in newborns via placental transfer and breast-feeding. (PMID:20591078) Scand J Immunol. 2010; 72(1):66-73. DOI: 10.1111/j.1365-3083.2010.02410.x

Quinlan PT, Lockton S, Irwin J, Lucas AL. The relationship between stool hardness and stool composition in breast- and formula-fed infants. (PMID:7884622) *J Pediatr Gastroenterol Nutr* 1995; 20(1):81-90.

Quinn EA. Too much of a good thing: evolutionary perspectives on infant formula fortification in the United States and its effects on infant health. (PMID:24142500) *Am J Hum Biol* 2014; 26(1):10-17. DOI: 10.1002/ajhb.22476

Raiha NCR. Milk Protein quantity and quality in human milk and infant formulae. *Acta Pediatr Scand.*1994; S402: 57-8.

Raiten DJ, Talbot JM, Waters JH. Assessment of nutrient requirements for infant formulas. *J Nutr* 1998; 128:2059S–293S.

Ramezani Tehrani F, Momenan AA, Khomami MB & Azizi F. Does lactation protect mothers against metabolic syndrome? Findings from the Tehran Lipid and Glucose Study. *J Obstet Gynaecol Res* 2014; 40(3):736–742.

Rammer P, Groth-Pedersen L, Kirkegaard T, Daugaard M et al. BAMLET activates a lysosomal cell death program in cancer cells.(PMID:20053771) *Molecular Cancer Therapeutics* 2010, 9(1):24-32 DOI: 10.1158/1535-7163.MCT-09-0559

Rancé F, Brondeau V, Abbal M. Utilite des prick-tests dans le "screening" de l'allergie immédiate aux proteines: 156 cas. *Allergie et Immunologie* 2002; 34 (3): 71-3.

Randall BB, Paterson DS, Haas EA, Broadbelt KG et al. Potential asphyxia and brainstem abnormalities in sudden and unexpected death in infants. (PMID:24218471) *Pediatrics* 2013; 132(6):e1616-25.

Rautava S, Walker WA. Breastfeeding--an extrauterine link between mother and child.(PMID:19292608) Free resource *Breastfeed Med* 2009, 4(1):3-10.

Reeves RR, Pinkofsky HB. Postpartum psychosis induced by bromocriptine and pseudoephedrine. (PMID:9267376) *J Fam Pract* 1997; 45(2):164-166.

Reilly, PM. Play It Again, Bach! New Mothers to Get Classical Music CDs—Mead Johnson to Hand Out Tunes, as Well as Formula, So Infants Drink It All In. *Wall Street Journal*, May 11, 1999, p. 1.

Reinhart GA, Simmen FA, Mahan DC, White ME, Roehrig KL. Intestinal development and fatty acid binding protein activity of newborn pigs fed colostrum or milk. *Biol Neonate* 1992; 62(2-3):155-163. (PMID:1420614)

Remer T, van Eyll B, Tölle HG, Manz F. Contents and batch-dependent variations of mineral substances in milk formula for premature infants and possible effects on renal acid burden. (PMID:2079941) *Monatsschr Kinderheilkd* 1990, 138(10):658-663

Renfrew MJ, Ansell P, Macleod KL. Formula feed preparation: helping reduce the risks; a systematic review. *Arch Dis Child* 2003; 88: 855-8. Doi: 10.1136/adc.88.10.855

Renfrew MJ, McLoughlin M, McFadden A. Cleaning and sterilisation of infant feeding equipment: a systematic review. (PMID:18298883) *Public Health Nutr* 2008, 11(11):1188-1199

Report on Health and Social Subjects 47. *Guidelines on the Nutritional Assessment of Infant Formulas*. Report of a Working Group of the Committee on Medical Aspects (COMA) of Food and Nutrition Policy.(HMSO 1996)

Riedijk MA, van Beek RH, Voortman G, de Bie HM et al. Cysteine: a conditionally essential amino acid in low-birth-weight preterm infants? *Am J Clin Nutr* [2007; 86(4):1120-1125. (PMID:17921391)

Rintala EM, Ekholm P, Koivisto P, Peltonen K et al. The intake of inorganic arsenic from long grain rice and rice-based baby food in Finland - Low safety margin warrants follow up. *Food Chem.* 2014 May 1;150:199-205. doi: 10.1016/j.foodchem.2013.10.155. Epub 2013 Nov 4.

Rippe JM, Angelopoulos TJ. Sucrose, high-fructose corn syrup, and fructose, their metabolism and potential health effects: what do we really know? (PMID:23493540) *Adv Nutr* 2013; 4(2):236-245. DOI: 10.3945/an.112.002824

Rishel PE, Sweeney P. Comparison of breastfeeding rates among women delivering infants in military treatment facilities with and without lactation consultants. *Military Medicine* 2005; 170(5):435

Riskin A, Almog M, Peri R, Halasz K et al.Changes in immunomodulatory constituents of human milk in response to active infection in the nursing infant. (PMID:22258136) *Pediatr Res* 2012, 71(2):220-225

Riva E, Agostini C, Biasucci G et al. Early breastfeeding is linked to higher intelligence quotient scores in dietary-treated phenylketonuric children. *Acta Paediatr* 1996; 85: 56-8

Roberts JR, Karr CJ, Health CoE. Pesticide exposure in children. *Pediatrics* 2012; 130 (6) e1757 -e1763. doi: 10.1542/peds.2012-1757

Roberts TJ, Carnahan E, Gakidou E. Can breastfeeding promote child health equity? A comprehensive analysis of breastfeeding patterns across the developing world and what we can learn from them.(PMID:24305597) *BMC Med* 2013, 11:254

Roberts SA, Soothill JF. Provocation of allergic response by supplementary feeds of cows' milk. (PMID:7065708) 1982, 57(2):127-130 **DOI:** 10.1136/adc.57.2.127

Robertson AF. Reflections on errors in neonatology: I. The "Hands-Off" years, 1920 to 1950. (PMID:12556927) *J Perinatol* 2003, 23(1):48-55

Robertson AF. Reflections on errors in neonatology: II. The "Heroic" years, 1950 to 1970. (PMID:12673267) *J Perinatol* 2003, 23(2):154-161

Robertson AF. Reflections on errors in neonatology: III. The "experienced" years, 1970 to 2000. (PMID:12732863) *J Perinatol* 2003, 23(3):240-249

Robinson M. A review of twenty years of breast feeding in Liverpool. *Arch Dis Child.* 1939; 14(79): 259–264. PMCID: PMC1975624

Robinson S, Fall C. Infant Nutrition and Later Health: A Review of Current Evidence. *Nutrients* 2012, *4*, 859-874; doi:10.3390/nu4080859

Rodriguez B, Prioult G, Bibiloni R, Nicolis I et al. Germ-free status and altered caecal subdominant microbiota are associated with a high susceptibility to cow's milk allergy in mice. *FEMS Microbiology Ecology* 2011, 76(1):133-44 DOI: 10.1111/j.1574-6941.2010.01035.

Rodriguez-Garcia R, Frazier L. Cultural Paradoxes Relating to Sexuality and Breastfeeding *J Hum Lact* 1995; 11(2): 111-115.

Rogers MF. Breastfeeding and HIV infection. *Lancet* 1987; ii: 1278

Rollins N, Coovadia HM. Breastfeeding and HIV transmission in the developing world: past, present, future. (PMID:23756997) *Curr Opin HIV AIDS* 2013, 8(5):467-473

Romanello S,Spiri D, Marcuzzi E, Zanin A, et al. Association Between Childhood Migraine and History of Infantile Colic. *JAMA* 2013; 309(15):1607-1612. epub 17 April 2013

Rook GA, Raison CL, Lowry CA. Microbiota, immunoregulatory old friends and psychiatric disorders. (PMID:24997041) Adv Experimental Med Biol 2014; 817:319-356. **DOI:** 10.1007/978-1-4939-0897-4_15

Rosegger H. Maltodextrin in a 13% solution as a supplement in the first 4 days of life in breast-fed mature newborn infants. Effect on drinking behavior, weight curve, blood picture, blood glucose and bilirubin (MED:3727591) *Wiener Klinische Wochenschrift* 1986, 98(10):310-315

Rosenfeld E, Beyerlein A, Hadders-Algra M, Kennedy K, et al. PD meta-analysis shows no effect of LC-PUFA supplementation on infant growth at 18 months. *Acta Paediatr* 2009, 98(1):91-97. (PMID:18691337)

Rosenthal HL, Austin S, O'Neill S, Takeuchi K et al. Incorporation of fallout Strontium 90 in deciduous incisors and fetal bone. *Nature* 1964; 203: 615.

Rossignol DA, Genuis SJ, Frye RE. Environmental toxicants and autism spectrum disorders: a systematic review. (PMCID:PMC3944636) *Translational Psychiatry* 2014, 4:e360 DOI: 10.1038/tp.2014.4

Rozenfeld F, Docena GH, Anon Mc, Fossati CA. Detection and identification of a soy protein component that cross-reacts with caseins from cows milk. *Clin Exp Immunol* 2002; 130: 49-58.

Ruemmle F, Garnier-Lengliné H. Transforming Growth Factor and Intestinal Inflammation: The Role of Nutrition. Nestle Nutr Inst Workshop Ser 2013, 77:91-98

Rundall P. Milk for babies and children. *BMJ* 1991; 302(6769): 177

Ryan JJ, Shewchuk C, Lau BPY, Sun WF. Polychlorinated dibenzo-p-dioxins and polychlorinated dibenzofurans in Canadian bleached paperboard milk containers (1988-1989) and their transfer to fluid milk. (AGR:IND93016105) *J Agric Food Chem* 1992, 40(5):919-923 DOI: 10.1021/jf00017a045

Rzehak P, Sausenthaler S, Koletzko S, Reinhardt D et al. Long-term effects of hydrolyzed protein infant formulas on growth--extended follow-up to 10 y of age: results from the German Infant Nutritional Intervention (GINI) study. (PMID:21849601) *Am J Clin Nutr* 2011, 94(6 suppl):1803s-1807s

Saadeh R. *Complementary Feeding: family foods for breastfed children.* (WHO Geneva 2000) p. 11. Online at http://www.who.int/nutrition/publications/infantfeeding/WHO_NHD_00.1/en/

Saarinen KM, Juntunen-Backman K, Järvenpää AL, Kuitunen P et al. Supplementary feeding in maternity hospitals and the risk of cow's milk allergy: prospective study of 6209 infants. (PMID:10452771) *J Allergy Clin Immunol* 1999, 104(2 Pt 1):457-461

Saarinen UM, Kajosaari M. Breastfeeding as prophylaxis against atopic disease: prospective follow-up study until 17 years old. (PMID:7564787)? *Lancet* 1995, 346(8982):1065-1069 DOI: 10.1016/S0140-6736(95)91742-X

Saavedra JM, Abi-Hanna A, Moore N, Yolken RH. Long-term consumption of infant formulas containing live probiotic bacteria: tolerance and safety. (PMID:14749232) *Am J Clin Nutr* 2004; 79(2):261-267.

Saavedra MA, da Costa JS, Garcias G, Horta BL, et al. [Infantile colic incidence and associated risk factors: a cohort study].(PMID:14502331) *Jornal de Pediatria* 2003, 79(2):115-122. DOI: 10.1590/S0021-75572003000200005

Saavedra-Rodríguez L, Feig LA. Chronic social instability induces anxiety and defective social interactions across generations. (PMID:22906514) *Biol Psychiatr* 2013, 73(1):44-53.

Sacker A, Kelly Y, Iacovou M, et al. Breast feeding and intergenerational social mobility: what are the mechanisms? *Arch Dis Child* 2013; 98(9):666-671 doi:10.1136/ archdischild-2012-303199.

Sacker A, Quigley MA, Kelly YJ. Breastfeeding and developmental delay: findings from the millennium cohort study. *Pediatrics.* 2006 Sep;118(3):e682-9.

SACN. (Scientific Advisory Committee on Nutrition) and COT (Committee on Toxicity) Joint Statgement. Timing of introduction of gluten into the infant diet. March 2011. https://www.gov.uk/government/publications/sacn-statement-on-the-introduction-of-gluten-to-the-infant-diet

SACN. The influence of maternal, fetal and child nutrition on the development of chronic disease in later life. Both downloadable at http://www.sacn.gov.uk/reports_position_statements/index.html

Sacri AS, De Serres G, Quach C, Boulianne N et al. Transmission of acute gastroenteritis and respiratory illness from children to parents. (PMID:24476955) *Pediatr Infect Dis J* 2014, 33(6):583-588 **DOI:** 10.1097/INF.0000000000000220

Sadauskaite-Kuehne V, Ludvigsson J, Padaiga Z, Jasinskiene E, et al. Longer breastfeeding is an independent protective factor against development of type 1 diabetes mellitus in childhood. *Diabetes Metab. Res. Rev.* 2004; 20 (2): 150–7. doi:10.1002/dmrr.425. PMID 15037991.

Sala-Vila A, Campoy C, Castellote AI, Garrido FJ et al. Influence of dietary source of docosahexaenoic and arachidonic acids on their incorporation into membrane phospholipids of red blood cells in term infants. (PMID:16326086) *Prostaglandins, Leukotrienes, and Essential Fatty Acids* 2006, 74(2):143-8

Salariya EM, Easton PM, Cater JI. Duration of breast-feeding after early initiation and frequent feeding. (PMID:82695) *Lancet* 1978, 2(8100):1141-1143

Salisbury l, Blackwell A. Public Advocates Inc. Petition to Alleviate Domestic Infant Formula Misuse and Provide informed Infant Feeding Choice. June 1981. In Orloff LE (ed) Citizen Petitioning of Federal Administrative Agencies - Domestic Infant Formula Misuse: A Case Study, *Golden Gate University Law Review*. (1982). http://digitalcommons.law.ggu.edu/ggulrev/vol12/iss3/4

Salpietro CD, Gangemi S, Briuglia S, Meo A, et al. The almond milk: a new approach to the management of cow-milk allergy/intolerance in infants. (PMID:16172596) *Minerva Pediatr* 2005; 57(4):173-180.

Salvatore S, Vandenplas Y. Gastroesophageal Reflux and Cow Milk Allergy: Is There a Link? *Pediatrics* 2002; 110:5 972-984; doi:10.1542/peds.110.5.972

Samsel A, Seneff S. Glyphosate, pathways to modern diseases II: Celiac sprue and gluten intolerance. *Interdiscip Toxicol.* 2013; Vol. 6(4): 159–184. doi: 10.2478/intox-2013-0026 Published online in: www.intertox.sav.sk & www.versita.com/it

Sausenthaler S, Kompauer I, Borte M, Herbarth O et al. Margarine and butter consumption, eczema and allergic sensitization in children: LISA birth cohort study. *Pediatric Allergy and Immunology*2006, 17(2):85-93 DOI: 10.1111/j.1399-3038.2005.00366.x

Savilahti E, Kuitunen M. Allergenicity of cow milk proteins. (PMID:1447629) *The Journal of Pediatrics* 1992, 121(5 Pt 2):S12-20

Savilahti E, Kukkonen K, Kuitunen M. Probiotics in the treatment and prevention of allergy in children. *World Allergy Organ J* 2009; 2(5):69-76. (PMCID:PMC3651021)

Savilahti E, Siltanen M, Pekkanen J, Kajosaari M. Mothers of very low birth weight infants have less atopy than mothers of full-term infants. (PMID:15663558) *Clin Exp Allergy* 2004; 34(12):1851-4

Savilahti EM, Savilahti E Development of natural tolerance and induced desensitization in cow's milk allergy. (PMID:22957704) *Pediatr Allergy Immunol.* 2013; 24(2):114-121.

Sawatzki G, Georgi G, Kohn G. Pitfalls in the design and manufacture of infant formulae. (PMID:7841620) *Acta Paediatr* Suppl 1994, 402:40-45.

Saylor J D, Bahna SL 45.Saylor J D, Bahna SL: Anaphylaxis to casein hydrolysate formula. *J Pediatr* 1991;118:71-73.

Scariati PD, Grummer-Strawn LM, Fein SB. A longitudinal analysis of infant morbidity and the extent of breastfeeding in the United States. (PMID:9164801) *Pediatrics* 1997; 99(6):e5

Schaefer O. Otitis media and bottle-feeding. An epidemiological study of infant feeding habits and incidence of recurrent and chronic middle ear disease in Canadian Eskimos. (PMID:5133823) *Can J Public Health* 1971; 62(6):478-489

Schaller JP, Kuchan MJ, Thomas DL, Cordle CT et al. Effect of dietary ribonucleotides on infant immune status. Part 1: Humoral responses. (PMID:15496604) Pediatr Res 2004, 56(6):883-890. DOI: 10.1203/01.PDR.0000145576.42115.5C

Schanler RJ and the AAP Section on Breastfeeding. Concerns with universal iron supplementation of breastfeeding infants. *Pediatrics* 2011; 127:e1097.

Schanler RJ,Burns PA, Abrams SA, Garza C. Bone mineralisation outcomes in human-milk fed preterm infants. *Pediatr Res* 1992; 31: 583-586

Schier JG, Wolkin AF, Valentin-Blasini L, Belson MG et al. Perchlorate exposure from infant formula and comparisons with the perchlorate reference dose. (PMID:19293845)*J Expo Sci Environ Epidemiol* 2010; 20(3):281-287.

Schlinzig T, Johansson S, Gunnar A, Ekström TJ, et al. **Epigenetic modulation at birth - altered DNA-methylation in white blood cells after Caesarean section. Acta Paediatr 2009, 98(7):1096-1099. DOI: 10.1111/j.1651-2227.2009.01371.x**

Schmidt CW. Questions persist: environmental factors in auto-immune disease. *Envir Health Perspect* 2011; 119: a248-253. Doi: 1289/ehp.119-a248

Schmidt IM, Damgaard In, Boisen KA, Mau C et al. Increased kidney growth in formula-fed versus breastfed infants. *Pediatr. Nephrol* 2004; 19: 1137-1144.

Schmitt J, Apfelbacher C, Chen CM, Romanos M, et al. Infant-onset eczema in relation to mental health problems at age 10 years: results from a prospective birth cohort study (PMID:20159252) *J Allergy Clin Immunol* 2010, 125(2):404-410.

Schultz ST, Klonoff-Cohen HS, Wingard DL, Akshoomoff N et al. Breastfeeding, infant formula supplementation, and Autistic Disorder: the results of a parent survey. (PMID:16978397) *Int Breastfeed J* 2006, 1:16

Schwart S, Iddo Friedberg I, Ivanov IV, et al. A metagenomic study of diet-dependent interaction between gut microbiota and host in infants reveals differences in immune response. *Genome Biology* 2012, 13:r32 doi:10.1186/gb-2012-13-4-r32

Schwartz RH, Amonette MS 46. Schwartz RH, Amonette MS: Cow milk protein hydrolysate infant formulas not always "hypoallergenic." *J Pediatr* 1991; 118:839-840.

Schwarz EB, McClure CK, Tepper PG, Thurston R et al. Lactation and maternal measures of subclinical cardiovascular disease. (PMID:20027032) *Obstet Gynecol* 2010; 115(1):41-48

Schwarz EB. Infant feeding in America: enough to break a mother's heart? (PMID:24112066) *Breastfeed* Med 2013; 8:454-457

Schwarz PJ, Amnon SS: Botulism immune globulin for infant botulism arrives - one year and a Gulf War later. *West J Med* 1991;156:197-198.

Scott JA, Aitkin I, Binns CW, Aroni RA. Factors associated with the duration of breastfeeding amongst women in Perth, Australia. (PMID:10342541) *Acta Paediatrica* 1999; 88(4):416-421. DOI: 10.1080/080352599

Scott JA, Binns CW, Graham KI, Oddy WH. Temporal changes in the determinants of breastfeeding initiation. *Birth* 2006; 33(1):37-45. DOI: 10.1111/j.0730-7659.2006.00072.x

Scott JA, Chih TY, Oddy WH. Food variety at 2 years of age is related to duration of breastfeeding. (PMID:23201765) *Nutrients* 2012, 4(10):1464-1474

Scott JA. The relationship between breastfeeding and weight status in a national sample of Australian children and adolescents. (PMID:22314050) *BMC Public Health* 2012, 12:107

Semple JL, Lugowski SJ, Baines CJ, Smith DC et al. Breast milk contamination and silicone implants: preliminary results using silicon as a proxy measurement for silicone. (PMID:9703094) *Plast Reconstr Surg* 1998, 102(2):528-533

Serpero LD, Frigiola A, Gazzolo D. Human milk and formulae: neurotrophic and new biological factors. (PMID:22261291) *Early Human Development* 2012, 88 Suppl 1:S9-12 DOI: 10.1016/j.earlhumdev.2011.12.021

Shafai T. Presentation, The Impact of infant feeding methods; breastfeeding, breast-milk or formula-feeding on the prevalence of autism spectrum disorders at the Global Online Lactation (GOLD) conference, May 1, 2012.

Shah PE, Fonagy P, Strathearn L. Is attachment transmitted across generations? The plot thickens. (PMID:20603421) *Clin Child Psychol Psychiatry* 2010, 15(3):329-345

Shamir R, Shehadeh N. Insulin in human milk and the use of hormones in infant formula. In Makrides M, Ochoa J, Szajewska H (eds). *The Importance of Immunonutrition* NNI Workshop Series v. 77, 2013

Shamir R. Infant Colic and Functional Gastrointestinal Disorders: Is There More Than a "Gut Feeling"? *JPGN* 2013; 57 Supplement. doi: 10.1097/01.mpg.0000441923.90436.c7

Shamir R. Thiamine-deficient infant formula: what happened and what have we learned? *Annals of Nutrition & Metabolism* 2012, 60(3):185-7 .

Shanahan F. A commentary on the safety of probiotics. (PMID:23101692) *Gastroenterology Clinics of North America* 2012, 41(4):869-876.

Shannon MW, Graf JW: Lead intoxication from lead contaminated water used to reconstitute infant formula. *Clin Pediatr* 1989; 28: 380-382. 50169800

Shaw JC, Jones A, Gunther M. Mineral content of brands of milk for infant feeding.(PMID:4739637) *Br Med J* 1973, 2(5857):12-5

Shim JE, Kim J, Mathai RA. Association of infant feeding practices and picky eating behaviours of preschool children. *J Amer Diet Ass* 2011; 111 (9):1363-8.

Shoji H, Oguchi S, Shimizu T, Yamashiro Y. Effect of human breast milk on urinary 8-hydroxy-2'-deoxyguanosine excretion in infants. *Pediatr Res* 2003, 53(5):850-852 (PMID:12621121)

Shoji H, Shimizu T, Shinohara K, Oguchi S et al (2004). Suppressive effects of breast milk on oxidative DNA damage in very low birthweight infants. *Arch Dis Child Fetal Neonatal Ed* 2004; 89(2):f136-8. *Free online*

Short RV, Lewis PR, Renfree MB, Shaw G. Contraceptive effects of extended lactational amenorrhoea: beyond the Bellagio Consensus. (PMID:1672186) *Lancet* 1991; 337(8743):715-717.

Sicherer SH. The Natural History of IgE-Mediated Cow's Milk Allergy. *Pediatrics* 2008; 122: Supplement 4 S186; doi:10.1542/peds.2008-2139X

Sigurs N, Hattevig G, Kjellman B. Maternal Avoidance of Eggs, Cow's Milk, and Fish During Lactation: Effect on Allergic Manifestations, Skin-Prick Tests, and Specific IgE Antibodies in Children at Age 4 Years. *Pediatrics* 1992; 89:4 735-739

Sigusch V, Schorsch E, Dannecker M, Schmidt G. Official statement by the German Society for Sex Research (Deutsche Gesellschaft für Sexualforschung e.V.) on the research of Prof. Dr. Günter Dörner on the subject of homosexuality. (PMID:7181651) *Arch Sex Behav* 1982, 11(5):445-449

Siimes MA, Salmenpera L, Perheentupa J. Exclusive breastfeeding for 9 months: risk of iron deficiency. *J Pediatr* 1984; 104 (2): 196-199

Silfverdal SA, Ehlin A, Montgomery SM. Breast-feeding and a subsequent diagnosis of measles. (PMID:19133867) Acta Paediatrica 2009, 98(4):715-719. DOI: 10.1111/j.1651-2227.2008.01180.x

Siltanen M, Kajosaari M, Poussa T, Saarinen KM, Savilahti E. A dual long-term effect of breastfeeding on atopy in relation to heredity in children at 4 years of age. *Allergy* 2003, 58(6):524-530.

Siltanen M, Wehkalampi K, Hovi P, Eriksson JG, et al. Preterm birth reduces the incidence of atopy in adulthood. (PMID:21333345) *J Allergy Clin Immunol* 2011, 127(4):935-942

Simon Klenovics K, Kollárová R, Hodosy J, Celec P et al.Reference values of skin autofluorescence as an estimation of tissue accumulation of advanced glycation end products in a general Slovak population. (PMID:24111899) *Diabet Med* 2013

Sinatra FR, Merritt RJ. Iatrogenic kwashiorkor in infants. *Am J Dis Child* 1981; 135: 21-23

Singh GK, Kogan MD, Dee DL.Nativity/immigrant status, race/ethnicity, and socioeconomic determinants of breastfeeding initiation and duration in the United States, 2003. *Pediatrics*. 2007 Feb;119 Suppl 1:S38-46.

Singhal A, Kennedy K, Lanigan J, Fewtrell M, et al. Nutrition in infancy and long-term risk of obesity: evidence from 2 randomized controlled trials. (PMID:20881062) *Am J Clin Nutr* 2010; 92(5):1133-1144. DOI: 10.3945/ajcn.2010.29302

Singhal A, Morley R, Cole TJ, Kennedy K et al. Infant nutrition and stereoacuity at age 4-6 y. (PMID:17209191) *Am J Clin Nutr* 2007; 85(1):152-159.

Singhania RU, Bansal A, Sharma JN. Fortified high calorie milk for optimal growth of VLBW babies. *J Trop Pediatr* 1989; 35: 77-81.

Sleator RD, Banville N, Hill C. Carnitine enhances the growth of Listeria monocytogenes in infant formula at 7 degrees C. (PMID:19610343) *J Food Protect* 2009, 72(6):1293-5

Smith AM, Picciano MF, Milner JA. Selenium intakes and status of human milk and formula fed infants. *Am J Clin Nutr* 1982;35(3):521-526. (PMID:7064903);

Smith GD, Kuh D. Does early nutrition affect later health? Views from the 1930s and 1940s. Chapter in Smith DF (ed) *Nutrition in Britain: Science, Scientists and Politics in the Twentieth Century.* (Routledge, London 1997)

Smith HA. Formula supplementation and the risk of cow's milk allergy. *Brit J Midwifery,* 2012; 20 (5) 345-350.

Smith JP, Blake M. Infant food marketing strategies undermine effective regulation of breast-milk substitutes: trends in print advertising in Australia, 1950-2010. *ANZ J Publ Hlth* 2013; 37(4): 337-344.

Smith JP, Dunstone MD, Elliott-Rudde ME . 'Voldemort' And Health Professional Knowledge Of Breastfeeding - Do Journal Titles And Abstracts Accurately Convey Findings On Differential Health Outcomes For Formula Fed Infants? *ACERH Working Paper Number 4* December 2008. Online .acerh.edu.au/publications/ACERH_WP4.pdf

Smith JP, Ingham , Dunstone MD. The Economic Value of Breastfeeding in Australia. http://nceph.anu.edu.au/Publications/Working_Papers/WP40.pdf

Smith JP. "Lost Milk?" Counting the economic value of breast milk in gross domestic product. *J Hum Lact* 2013; 29 (4): 537-546.

Smith-Spangler C, Brandeau ML, Hunter GE, Bavinger JC et al. Are organic foods safer or healthier than conventional alternatives?: a systematic review.(PMID:22944875) *Ann Intern Med* 2012, 157(5):348-366

Smith, JP, and Harvey PJ. Chronic Disease and Infant Nutrition: Is It Significant to Public Health? *Public Health Nutrition* 2011; 14 (2): 279-89.

Smith, JP, Thompson J, Ellwood DA. Hospital System Costs of Artificial Infant Feeding: Estimates for the Australian Capital Territory." *ANZ J Public Health* 2002; 26: 543-51

Sokolowski M, Boyce WT, McEwen BS. Scarred for Life? *New Scientist* 2013;

Sola-Larrañaga C, Navarro-Blasco I. Chromium content in different kinds of Spanish infant formulae and estimation of dietary intake by infants fed on reconstituted powder formulae. (PMID:17071518) *Food Addit Contam.* 2006, 23(11):1157-1168. DOI: 10.1080/02652030600812956

Sonne C, Letcher RJ, Bechsheft T, Riget FF et al. Two decades of biomonitoring polar bear health in Greenland: a review. (PMCID:PMC3305763) *Acta Vet Scand* 2012, 54(suppl 1):s15-s15

Soto NE, Lutwick LI. Poliovirus immunizations. What goes around, comes around. PMID:10198803) *Infect Dis Clin North Am* 1999; 13(1):265-78, ix.

Spanjersberg MQ, Knulst AC, Kruizinga AG, Van Duijn G et al. Concentrations of undeclared allergens in food products can reach levels that are relevant for public health. *Food Additives & Contaminants. Part A, Chemistry, Analysis, Control, Exposure & Risk Assessment* 2010, 27(2):169-74. PMID:20013443

Sripada CS, Phan KL, Labuschagne I, Welsh R et al. Oxytocin enhances resting-state connectivity between amygdala and medial frontal cortex. *Int J Neuropsychopharmacol* 2013; 16(2):255-260. (PMID:22647521)

Stahlberg MR. Infantile colic: occurrence and risk factors. *Eur J Pediatr.* 1984; 143(2): 108-111.

Stanger J, Zwicker K, Albersheim S, Murphy JJ 3rd. Human milk fortifier: an occult cause of bowel obstruction in extremely premature neonates. (PMID:24851756) J Pediatr Surg 2014; 49(5):724-726

Stastny D, Vogel RS, Picciano MF. Manganese intake and serum manganese concentration of human milk-fed and formula-fed infants. *Am J Clin Nutr* 1984; 39(6):872-878. (PMID:6539060)

Steer CD, Davey Smith G, Emmett PM, Hibbeln JR et al. FADS2 polymorphisms modify the effect of breastfeeding on child IQ. *PLoS One* 2010; 5 (7): e11570. doi:10.1371/journal.pone.0011570. PMC 2903485. PMID 20644632.

Steinwender G, Schimpl G, Sixl B, Wenzl HH. Gut-derived bone infection in the neonatal rat. (PMID:11726738) *Pediatric Research* 2001, 50(6):767-771.

Steube A. http://bfmed.wordpress.com/2010/05/03/why-we-still-need-to-watch-our-language/

Steube A. The risks of not breastfeeding. *Rev Obstet Gynecol* 2009; 2(4): 222-231. PMCID: PMC2812877.

Stevens EE, Patrick TE, Pickler R. A history of infant feeding. (PMCID:PMC2684040) J Perinat Educ 2009;18(2):32-39.

Stewart, GJ, Cunningham, AL, Driscoll, GL et al. Transmission of human T-cell lymphotropic virus type III (HTLV-III) by artifical insemination by donor. *Lancet*. 1985; 2: 581–584.

Stoner R, Chow ML, Boyle MP, Sunkin SM et al. Patches of Disorganization in the Neocortex of Children with Autism. *N Engl J Med* 2014; 370:1209-1219. DOI: 10.1056/NEJMoa1307491

Storm P, Klausen TK, Trulsson M, Ho C S J, et al. A unifying mechanism for cancer cell death through ion channel activation by HAMLET.(PMID:23505537) PLoS One 2013; 8(3):e58578. Free online.

Straarup EM, Lauritzen L, Faerk J et al. The stereospecific triacylglycerol structures and fatty acid profiles of human milk and infant formulas. (PMID:16540799) *J Pediatr Gastroenterol Nutr* 2006; 42(3):293-9

Strathearn L, Mamun AA, Najman JM, O'Callaghan MJ Does breastfeeding protect against substantiated child abuse and neglect? A 15-year cohort study. *Pediatrics* 2009; 123 (2): 483 -493 (doi: 10.1542/peds.2007-3546)

Strathearn L. Maternal neglect: oxytocin, dopamine and the neurobiology of attachment. (PMID:21951160) *J Neuroendocrinol* 2011, 23(11):1054-1065

Straub CP, Murthy GK. A comparison of SR90 component of human and cows' milk. *Pediatrics* 1965; 36:5 732-735

Strom BL, Schinnar R, Ziegler EE, Barnhart KT et al. Exposure to soy-based formula in infancy and endocrinological and reproductive outcomes in young adulthood. *JAMA* 2001; 286(7):807-814 (PMID:11497534) DOI: 10.1001/jama.286.7.807

Sturman JA, Gaulle G, Raiha NC. Absence of cystathionase in human fetal liver: is cystine essential? *Science.* 1970;169:74–76.

Su JC, Kemp AS, Varigos GA, Nolan TM. Atopic eczema: its impact on the family and financial cost. (PMID:9068310) *Arch Dis Child* 1997; 76(2):159-162.

Sullivan JL. Cognitive Development: Breast-Milk Benefit vs Infant Formula Hazard. *Arch Gen Psychiatry* 2008; 65( 12): 1456. Downloaded from www.archgenpsychiatry.com April 24, 2012

Sullivan S, Schanler RJ, Kim JH, Patel AL et al. An exclusively human milk-based diet is associated with a lower rate of necrotizing enterocolitis than a diet of human milk and bovine milk-based products. (PMID:20036378)*J Pediatr* 2010, 156(4):562-7.e1

Szajewska H. Supplementation of infant formula with probiotics/prebiotics: lessons learned with regard to documenting outcomes. (PMID:22955362)*J Clin Gastroent* 2012, 46 Suppl:S67-8. DOI: 10.1097/ MCG.0b013e3182647a49

Szépfalusi Z, Nentwich I, Gerstmayr M, Jost E, et al. Prenatal allergen contact with milk proteins. (PMID:9117877) Clinical and *Experimental Allergy* 1997, 27(1):28-35 DOI: 10.1046/j.1365-2222.1997.d01-417.x

Tachibana M, Kagitani-Shimono K, Mohri I, Yamamoto T et al. Long-term administration of intranasal oxytocin is a safe and promising therapy for early adolescent boys with autism spectrum disorders. *J Child Adolesc Psychopharm* 2013; 23(2):123-127. (PMID:23480321)

Takezaki T, Tajima K, Ito M, Ito S et al. Short-term breast-feeding may reduce the risk of vertical transmission of HTLV-I. (PMID:9209298). *Leukemia* 1997, 11 Suppl 3:60-62

Tang ML, Lahtinen SJ, Boyle RJ. Probiotics and prebiotics: clinical effects in allergic disease. *Curr Opin Pediatr* 2010; 22:626–634.

Tanoue Y, Oda S. Weaning time of children with infantile autism. (PMID:2793787) J *Autism Dev Disord* 1989, 19(3):425-434.

Tarrant M, Kwok MK, Lam TH, Leung GM, Schooling CM. Breast-feeding and childhood hospitalizations for infections. (PMID:20864890) *Epidemiology* 2010, 21(6):847-854

Tawia S. Iron and exclusive breastfeeding. *Breastfeeding Review*, 2012; 20(1) 35-47.

Tay M, Fang G, Chia PL, Li SF.Rapid screening for detection and differentiation of detergent powder adulteration in infant milk formula by LC-MS. *Forensic Sci Int.* 2013;232(1-3):32-9. doi: 10.1016/j.forsciint.2013.06.013. Epub 2013 Jul 27

Taylor AL, Dunstan JA, Prescott SL. Probiotic supplementation for the first 6 months of life fails to reduce the risk of atopic dermatitis and increases the risk of allergen sensitization in high-risk children: a randomized controlled trial. *J Allergy Clin Immunol* 2007; 119:184–191.

Terhune TD, Deth RC. How aluminum adjuvants could promote and enhance non-target IgE synthesis in a genetically-vulnerable sub-population. (PMID:22967010) *Journal of Immunotoxicology* 2012

Terracciano L, Bouygue GR, Sarratud T, Veglia F et al. Impact of dietary regimen on the duration of cow's milk allergy: a random allocation study. *Clin Exp Allergy* 2010,; 40(4):637-642 DOI: 10.1111/j.1365-2222.2009.03427.x

Tharner A, Luijk MP, Raat H, Ijzendoorn MH et al. Breastfeeding and its relation to maternal sensitivity and infant attachment. (PMID:22580735) *J Dev Behav Pediatr* 2012, 33(5):396-404

The NS, Richardson AS, Gordon-Larsen P. Timing and Duration of Obesity in Relation to Diabetes: Findings From Ethnically Diverse, Nationally Representative Sample *Diabetes Care.* 2013; 36:865-72.

Thijs C, Mu¨ ller A, Rist L, Kummeling I et al. Fatty acids in breast milk and development of atopic eczema and allergic sensitisation in infancy. *Allergy* 2011; 66: 58–67.

Thomas DW, Greer FR. Probiotics and Prebiotics. *Pediatrics* 2010; 126 (6);1217 -1231. (doi: 10.1542/peds.2010-2548); See http://pediatrics.aappublications.org/content/126/6/1217.

Thorkelsson T, Mimouni F, Namgung R, Fernandez-Ulloa M et al. Similar gastric emptying rates for casein- and whey-predominant formulas in preterm infants. (MED:7808829) *Pediatric Research* 1994, 36(3):329-333. DOI: 10.1203/00006450-199409000-00010

Thorsdottir I, Birgisdottir BE, Johannsdottir IM, Harris DP et al. Different β-Casein Fractions in Icelandic Versus Scandinavian Cow's Milk May Influence Diabetogenicity of Cow's Milk in Infancy and Explain Low Incidence of Insulin-Dependent Diabetes Mellitus in Iceland. *Pediatrics* 2000; 106:4 719-724

Threlfall EJ, Ward LR, Hampton MD, Ridley AM et al. Molecular fingerprinting defines a strain of Salmonella enterica serotype Anatum responsible for an international outbreak associated with formula-dried milk. (PMID:9825779) *Epidemiol Infect* 1998, 121(2):289-293

Thum C, Cookson AL, Otter DE, McNabb WC, et al. Can nutritional modulation of maternal intestinal microbiota influence the development of the infant gastrointestinal tract? (PMID:22990463) *J Nutr* 2012; 142(11):1921-1928.

Tillisch K. The effects of gut microbiota on CNS function in humans. (PMID:24838095) *Gut Microbes* 2014, 5(3)

Timby N, Domellöf E, Hernell O, Lönnerdal B, Domellöf M. Neurodevelopment, nutrition, and growth until 12 mo of age in infants fed a low-energy, low-protein formula supplemented with bovine milk fat globule membranes: a randomized controlled trial. (PMID:24500150) *Am J Clin Nutr* 2014; 99(4):860-868. DOI: 10.3945/ajcn.113.064295

Tolle HG, Manz F, Diekmann L et al. Effect on renal net acid excretion of various mineral contents in three lots of a common preterm formula. *J Trace Elem Electrol Hlth Dis* 1991; 5:235-8.

Tomicić S, Johansson G, Voor T, Björkstén B, et al. Breast milk cytokine and IgA composition differ in Estonian and Swedish mothers-relationship to microbial pressure and infant allergy. (PMID:20581738) *Pediatr Res* 2010, 68(4):330-334 DOI: 10.1203/00006450-201011001-00646

Tørris C1, Thune I, Emaus A, Finstad SE et al. Duration of lactation, maternal metabolic profile, and body composition in the Norwegian EBBA I-study. *Breastfeed Med* 2013; 8(1):8-15. doi: 10.1089/bfm.2012.0048. Epub 2012 Oct 11.

Tow J. Heal the Mother, heal the baby: epigenetics, breastfeeding and the human microbiome. *Breastfeeding Rev* 2014; 22 (1): 7-9.

Trabulsi JC, Mennella JA. Diet, sensitive periods in flavour learning, and growth. (PMID:22724643) *Int* Rev Psychiatry 2012; 24(3):219-230.

Trikha A, Baillargeon JG, Kuo YF, Tan A et al. Development of food allergies in patients with gastroesophageal reflux disease treated with gastric acid suppressive medications.(PMID:23905907) *Pediatr Allergy Immunol* 2013; 24(6):582-588.

Trivedi B. Eat your way to dementia. *New Scientist* 1 Sept 2012, pp. 32-37.

Trott JF, Simpson KJ, Moyle RL, Hearn CM, Shaw G, Nicholas KR, Renfree MB. Maternal regulation of milk composition, milk production, and pouch young development in the tammar wallaby (*Macropus eugenii*). *Biology of Reproduction* 2003; **68**:929-936.

Troy SB, Ferreyra-Reyes L, Huang C, Mahmud N, et al. Use of a novel real-time PCR assay to detect oral polio vaccine shedding and reversion in stool and sewage samples after a Mexican national immunization day. (PMID:21411577). *Journal of Clinical Microbiology* 2011; 49(5):1777-1783.

Tully KP, Ball HL. Maternal accounts of their breast-feeding intent and early challenges after caesarean childbirth. (PMID:24252711) *Midwifery* 2014, 30(6):712-719 DOI: 10.1016/j.midw.2013.10.014

Tully KP, Ball HL. Trade-offs underlying maternal breastfeeding decisions: a conceptual model. (PMID:22188564) Free full text article *Matern Child Nutr* 2013, 9(1):90-98

Turan D, Yeşilçubuk NS, Akoh CC. Production of Human Milk Fat Analogue Containing Docosahexaenoic and Arachidonic Acids. J Agricult Food Chemistry, 2012; 60 (17): 4402 DOI: 10.1021/jf3012272

Twigger AJ, Hodgetts S, Filgueira L, Hartmann PE, Hassiotou F. From breast milk to brains: the potential of stem cells in human milk. (PMID:23515086) *J Hum Lact* 2013; 29(2):136-9.

Tyler JP, Dobler KJ, Driscoll GL, Stewart GJ. The impact of AIDS on artificial insemination by donor. (PMID:3542178) *Clin Reprod Fertil* 1986, 4(5):305-317

U.S. Department of Health and Human Services, Centers for Disease Control and Prevention. *CDC National Survey of Maternity Care Practices in Infant Nutrition and Care (mPINC),* 2009.

Udall J. Gastrointestinal host defence and NEC. *J Pediatr.* 1990; 117 (1):S33-S43.

Udall JN Jr, Dixon M, Newman AP, Wright JA et al. Liver disease in alpha 1-antitrypsin deficiency. A retrospective analysis of the influence of early breast- vs bottle-feeding. (PMID:3872949) *JAMA* 1985; 253(18):2679-2682

Upadhyay A, Gothwal S, Parihar R, Garg A et al. Effect of umbilical cord milking in term and near term infants: randomized control trial.(PMID:23123382) *Am J Obstet Gynecol* 2013, 208(2):120.e1-6

Urbaniak C, Burton JP, Reid G. Breast, milk and microbes: a complex relationship that does not end with lactation. (PMID:22757730) *Women's Health* 2012; 8(4):385-398. DOI: 10.2217/whe.12.23

USDA Food Advisory Committee on Infant Formula Transcripts of the November 18-19 2002 meeting. Go to http://www.fda.gov/ohrms/dockets/ac/cfsan02.htm; http://www.fda.gov/ohrms/dockets/ac/02/transcripts/3903T1.htm Regrettably the government stopped putting such transcripts on the public record.

U.S. General Accounting Office. Food assistance potential to serve more WIC infants by reducing formula cost. 2003. www.gao.gov/products/GAO-03-331

Usowicz AG, Dab SB, Emery JR, McCann EM et al. Does gastric acid protect the preterm infant from bacteria in unheated human milk? (PMID:3345705) *Early Hum Dev* 1988, 16(1):27-33

Utrera Torres MI, Lopez CM, Roman SV, Diaz CA et al. Does opening a milk bank in a neonatal unit change infant feeding practices. A before and after study. *Internat Breastfeed J* 2010; 5:4 http://www.internationalbreastfeedingjournal.com/content/5/1/4

Vadas P, Wai Y, Burks W, Perelman B. Detection of peanut allergens in breast milk of lactating women. (PMID:11277829) *JAMA* 2001: 285(13):1746-1748. Immediately rehashed as Stock S. Peanut allergy can be carried in breastmilk. *Weekend Australian* April 21, 2001, p. 7.

Vahabnezhad E, Mochon AB, Wozniak LJ, Ziring DA. Lactobacillus bacteremia associated with probiotic use in a pediatric patient with ulcerative colitis. (PMID:23426446) *J Clin Gastroenterol* 2013; 47(5):437-439.

Vajro P, Fontanella A. Breastfeeding and Hepatitis B. J Pediatr Gastroeneterol Nutr 1991;12(1):141

Van den Eeden SK, Koepsell TD, Longstreth WT Jr, van Belle G, et al. Aspartame ingestion and headaches: a randomized crossover trial. (PMID:7936222) *Neurology* 1994, 44(10):1787-1793.

van den Hazel P, Zuurbier M, Babisch W, Bartonova A et al. Today's epidemics in children: possible relations to environmental pollution and suggested preventive measures. (PMID:17000565) *Acta Paediatrica Supplement* 2006; 95(453):18-25.

van Hasselt PM, de Vries W, de Vries E, Kok K et al. Hydrolysed formula is a risk factor for vitamin K deficiency in infants with unrecognised cholestasis. *J Pediatr Gastroenterol Nutr* 2010; 51(6):773-776.

Vance GH, Grimshaw KE, Briggs R, Lewis SA et al. Serum ovalbumin-specific immunoglobulin G responses during pregnancy reflect maternal intake of dietary egg and relate to the development of allergy in early infancy. (PMID:15663559) *Clin Exp Allergy* 2004; 34(12):1855-1861.

Verd S, García M, Gutiérrez A, Moliner E et al. Blood biochemical profile of very preterm infants before and after trophic feeding with exclusive human milk or with formula milk. (PMID:24576499) *Clin Biochem* 2014, 47(7-8):584-587

Verhasselt V. Neonatal tolerance under breastfeeding influence: the presence of allergen and transforming growth factor-beta in breast milk protects the progeny from allergic asthma. *J Pediatr* 2010;156(2 Suppl):S16-20. doi: 10.1016/j.jpeds.2009.11.015.

Victora GD, Bilate AM, Socorro-Silva A, Caldas C et al. Mother-child immunological interactions in early life affect long-term humoral autoreactivity to heat shock protein 60 at age 18 years. *J Autoimmunity* 2007, 29(1):38-43 DOI: 10.1016/j.jaut.2007.02.018

Vissing NH, Chawes BL, Bisgaard H. Increased risk of pneumonia and bronchiolitis after bacterial colonization of the airways as neonates. (PMID:24090102) *Am J Respir Crit Care Med* 2013; 188(10):1246-1252

Vohr BR, Poindexter BB, Dusick AM, McKinley L et al. Beneficial effects of breast milk in the NICU on the developmental outcome of ELBW infants at 18 months of age. *Pediatrics* 2006; 118 (1) e115 -e123. DOI: 10.1542/peds.2005-2382) doi 10.1542/peds.2005-2382

Volpe LE, Ball HL, McKenna JJ. Nighttime parenting strategies and sleep-related risks to infants. (PMID:22818487) Free full text article *Soc Sci Med* 2013, 79:92-100.

von Hertzen l, Mäkelä MJ, Petäys T, Jousilahti P et al. Growing disparities in atopy between the Finns and the Russians: A comparison of 2 generations. *J Allergy Clin Immunol* 2006; 117 (1): 151-157, DOI: 10.1016/j.jaci.2005.07.028

Von Kries R, Koletzko B, Sauerwald T, et al. Breast feeding and obesity: cross sectional study. *BR MED J* 1999;318(7203):147–150.

von Mutius E. The environmental predictors of allergic disease. *J Allergy Clin Immunol.* 2000;105:9–19

Vuillermin PJ, Ponsonby AL, Kemp AS, Allen KJ. Potential links between the emerging risk factors for food allergy and vitamin D status.(PMID:23711121) *Clin Exp Allergy* 2013; 43(6):599-607.

WABA. HIV and breastfeeding, available online from WABA at http://waba.org.my/whatwedo/hcp/ihiv.htm#kit

Wafula SW, Ikamari LD, K'Oyugi BO. In search for an explanation to the upsurge in infant mortality in Kenya during the 1988-2003 period. (PMID:22708542) *BMC Public Health* 2012, 12:441

Wales JK, Milford D, Okorie NM. Milk bolus obstruction secondary to the early introduction of a premature baby milk formula: an old syndrome re-emerging in a new population. *Eur J Pediatr* 1989; 148: 676-8.

Walker A. Breastmilk as the gold standard for protective nutrients. *J Pediatrics* 2010; 156, I56 (2), Supplement, S3–S7 http://dx.doi.org/10.1016/j.jpeds.2009.11.021

Walker WA, Shuba Iyengar R. Breastmilk, Microbiota and Intestinal Immune Homeostasis. (PMID:25310762) *Pediatr Res* 2014. DOI:10.1038/pr.2014.160.

Walker B. Lead content of milk and infant formula. *J Food Prot* 1980; 43 (30 178-179; see also the September 1980 issue of *Food Chemical News.*

Walker, WA. Initial intestinal colonization in the human infant and immune homeostasis. Annals of Nutrition & Metabolism 2013; 63 Suppl 2:8-15.

Walker WA, Shuba Iyengar R. Breastmilk, Microbiota and Intestinal Immune Homeostasis. (PMID:25310762) *Pediatr Res* [2014] DOI:10.1038/pr.2014.160.

Walsh P, Elsabbagh M, Bolton P, Singh I. In search of biomarkers for autism: scientific, social and ethical challenges. (PMID:21931335) *Nature Reviews. Neuroscience* 2011, 12(10):603-612 DOI: 10.1038/nrn3113

Walton RG, Hudak R, Green-Waite RJ. Adverse reactions to aspartame: double-blind challenge in patients from a vulnerable population.(PMID:8373935) *Biological Psychiatry* 1993, 34(1-2):13-17

Wang T, Xu RJ. Effects of colostrum feeding on intestinal development in newborn pigs. *Biol Neonate* [1996, 70(6):339-348. (PMID:9001695)

Wang X, Meng J, Zhang J, Zhou T et al. Characterization of Staphylococcus aureus isolated from powdered infant formula milk and infant rice cereal in China. Internat J Food Microbiol, 2012;153(1–20: 142-147. http://dx.doi.org/10.1016/j.ijfoodmicro.2011.10.030.

Ward TL, Hosid S, Ioshikhes I, Altosaar I. Human milk metagenome: a functional capacity analysis. (PMID:23705844) BMC Microbiol 2013; 13:116

Warner JA, Jones CA, Jones AC, Miles EA et al. Immune responses during pregnancy and the development of allergic disease. (PMID:9455773) *Pediatr Allergy Immunol* 1997; 8(10 suppl):5-10.

Warner JO. Breast is best: is research for the next best ethically acceptable? (PMID:16771776) *Pediatr Allergy Immunol* 2006; 17(4):239-240.

Warner JO. Genetic polymorphisms and their association with various allergic diseases. (PMID:19832745) *Pediatr Allergy Immunol* 2009; 20(7):612-613.

Warner JO. Peanut allergy: a major public health issue. (PMID:10410912) *Pediatr Allergy Immunol* 1999; 10(1):14-20.

Watchko JF, Oski FA. Bilirubin 20 mg/dL = vigintiphobia. (PMID:6682217) *Pediatrics* 1983, 71(4):660-663

Watchko JF. Vigintiphobia revisited. *Pediatrics* 2005; 115(6):1747-1753. (PMID:15930239)

Weaver L T. Relationships between paediatricians and infant milk formula companies. *Arch Dis Child* 2006. 91386–387.387

Wegienka G, Joseph CL, Havstad S, Zoratti E et al. Sensitization and allergic histories differ between black and white pregnant women.(PMID:22857795) *J Allergy Clin Immunol* 2012;130(3):657-662.e2 DOI: 10.1016/j.jaci.2012.06.024

Weiner ML. Food additive carrageenan: Part II: A critical review of carrageenan in vivo safety studies. (PMID:24467586) *Crit Rev Toxicol* 2014; 44(3):244-269. DOI: 10.3109/10408444.2013.861798

Weisselberg B, Dayal Y, Thompson JF, Doyle MS et al. A lamb-meat-based formula for infants allergic to casein hydrolysate formulas.(PMID:8902326) *Clin Pediatr* (Phila) 1996, 35(10):491-495.

Weizman Z, Ursacha C, Leader D et al. Whey deionization method of infant formula affects plasma lipids. *J Pediatr Gastroent Nutr* 1997; 25: 529-532.

Wells JC. The evolution of human adiposity and obesity: where did it all go wrong? *Dis Model Mech* 2012; 5(5):595-607. (PMCID:PMC3424456) .

Weng SF, Redsell SA, Swift JA, Yang M et al. Systematic review and meta-analysis of risk factors for childhood overweight identifiable during infancy. (PMID:23109090) *Arch Dis Child* 2012, 97(12):1019-1026 doi: 10.1136/archdischild-2012-302263

West CE, Gothefors L, Granström M, Käyhty H et al. Effects of feeding probiotics during weaning on infections and antibody responses to diphtheria, tetanus and Hib vaccines. (PMID:18086218) *Pediatr Allergy Immunol* 2008, 19(1):53-60

Weyermann M, Rothenbacher D, Brenner H. Duration of breastfeeding and risk of overweight in childhood: a prospective birth cohort study from Germany. *Int J Obes* 2006;30:1281–7.

Wharton B. Bottle-feeding. *BMJ* 1976; 1: 1326-1331.

Wharton B. Nutrition in the 1980s.(PMID:3444564) *Nutr Health* 1987; 5(3-4):211- 220.

Wharton BA, Marley R, Isaacs EB, et al. Low plasma taurine and infant development. *Arch Dis Child Fetal Neonatal Ed* 2004;89.

Wharton BA. Food for the suckling: revolution and development. (PMID:6963542) *Acta Paediatr Scand* Suppl 1982; 299:5-10.

Whitehouse AJ, Robinson M, Li J, Oddy WH. Duration of breast feeding and language ability in middle childhood. *Paediatr Perinatal Epidemiol* 2011; 25(1):44-52 (MED:21133968) DOI: 10.1111/j.1365-3016.2010.01161.x (PMID:21133968)

Whitten DO, Whitten B (eds). *Handbook of American business history: extractives manufacturing and services.* (Greenwood Press NY 1990) vol 2

Whittle S, Yücel M, Lorenzetti V, Byrne ML et al. Pituitary volume mediates the relationship between pubertal timing and depressive symptoms during adolescence. (PMID:22071452) *Psychoneuroendocrinology 2012,* 37(7):881-891

WHO. PMTCT and strategic visions 2010-2015 http://www.who.int/hiv/pub/mtct/strategic_vision.pdf )

WHO. Guidelines on HIV and infant feeding. 2010. Principles and recommendations for infant feeding in the context of HIV and a summary of evidence, ISBN 978 92 4 159953 5 http://www.who.int/child_adolescent_health/documents/9789241599535/en/index.html (online)

WHO. Programmatic Update: Use of antiretroviral drugs for treating pregnant women and preventing HIV in infants, Executive Summary, April 2012, available at http://whqlibdoc.who.int/hq/2012/WHO_HIV_2012.8_eng.pdf

Wickham S (2010). Antibiotics for Group B Strep: are they effective? *Essentially MIDIRS* 1(1): 27-30; http://www.sarawickham.com/research-updates/whether-and-how-to-treat-group-b-strep-the-continuing-gulf-between-evidence-and-practice/

Widdowson EM, McCance RA, Harrison GE, Sutton A. Effect Of Giving Phosphate Supplements To Breast-Fed Babies On Absorption And Excretion Of Calcium, Strontium, Magnesium, And Phosphorus. (PMID:14066845) *Lancet* 1963, 2:73

Widström AM, Lilja G, Aaltomaa-Michalias P, Dahllöf A et al. Newborn behaviour to locate the breast when skin-to-skin: a possible method for enabling early self-regulation. (PMID:20712833) *Acta Paediatr* 2011; 100(1):79-85

Wiessinger D. Watch Your Language! *J Hum Lact* 1996; 12: 1-4. doi:10.1177/089033449601200102. Available online at http://www.motherchronicle.com/watchyourlanguage.html

Wiklund P, Xu L, Lyytikäinen A, Saltevo J et al. Prolonged breast-feeding protects mothers from later-life obesity and related cardio-metabolic disorders. *Pub Health Nutr* 2011:1-8 (PMID:21859508)

Wiklund PK, Xu L, Wang Q, Mikkola T et al. Lactation is associated with greater maternal bone size and bone strength later in life. (PMID:21927916) *Osteoporos Int* 2012, 23(7): 1939-1945

Wilce R. Spinning suspect ingredients in baby formula. Feruary 22, 2012. http://www.cornucopia.org/2012/02/spinning-suspect-ingredients-in-baby-formula/

Willis AT, Bullen CL, Williams K, Fagg CG et al. Breast milk substitute: a bacteriological study. (PMID:4583181) *Br Med J* 1973, 4(5884):67-72

Willis E , Pearce M, Tom Jenkin T, Wadham B et al. Indigenous Engagement with Modernity: Domestic Water Supply, Risk and Reflexive Modernization. *TASA Conference, University of Western Australia & Murdoch University, 4-7 December 2006.* Online

Wilson C. Breast milk stem cells build baby. *New Scientist,* 2014; 2994: . Online at http://www.newscientist.com/article/dn26492

Wilson FH, Hariri A, Farhi A, Zhao H et al. A cluster of metabolic defects caused by mutation in a mitochondrial tRNA. *Science.* 2004;306(5699):1190-4. DOI: 10.1126/science.1102521

Winkler B, Aulenbach J, Meyer T, Wiegering A et al. Formula-feeding is associated with shift towards Th1 cytokines. (PMID:24691724) *Eur J Nutr* 2014

Wolf J H, *Contemporary Sociology* 2012; 41 (2) 248-9.

Wolf JH. What feminists can do for breastfeeding and what breastfeeding can do for feminists. *Signs.* 2006; 31(2) pp. 398-424.

Wolff JJ, Gu H, Gerig G, Elison JT et al. IBIS Network. Differences in white matter fiber tract development present from 6 to 24 months in infants with autism. *Am J Psychiatry* 2012, 169(6):589-600. (PMID:22362397)

Wright C M, Waterston A J R. Relationships between paediatricians and infant formula milk companies. *Arch Dis Child* 2006. 91383–385.385

Wright RJ. Moving towards making social toxins mainstream in children's environmental health. *Curr Opin Pediatr* 2009; 21(2):222-229 (MED:19300262) DOI: 10.1097/MOP.0b013e3283292629

Wu FM, Beuchat LR, Doyle MP, Mintz ED. Survival and growth of Shigella flexneri, Salmonella enterica serovar enteritidis, and Vibrio cholerae O1 in reconstituted infant formula. (PMID:12224592) *Am J Trop Med Hyg* 2002, 66(6):782-786

Wurtman RJ. Synapse formation and cognitive brain development: effect of docosahexaenoic acid and other dietary constituents. (PMID:18803968) *Metabolism: Clinical and Experimental* 2008, 57 Suppl 2:S6-10

Wüthrich B, Stern A, Johansson SG. Severe anaphylactic reaction to bovine serum albumin at the first attempt of artificial insemination. *Allergy*:1995, 50(2):179-183. (PMID:7604943)

Xu F, Qiu L, Binns CW, Liu X. Breastfeeding in China: a review. (PMID:19531253)*Internat Breastfeed J* 2009, 4:6. doi: 10.1186/1746-4358-4-6

Yamamoto T, Tsubota Y, Kodama T, Kageyama-Yahara N et al. Oral tolerance induced by transfer of food antigens via breast milk of allergic mothers prevents offspring from developing allergic symptoms in a mouse food allergy model. *Clin Dev Immunol.* 2012; 2012: 721085. Published online 27/3/2012. doi: 10.1155/2012/721085 PMCID:PMC3310277)

Yan QQ, Condell O, Power K, Butler F et al. Cronobacter species (formerly known as Enterobacter sakazakii) in powdered infant formula: a review of our current understanding of the biology of this bacterium. (PMID:22420458) *J Appl Microbiol* 2012, 113(1):1-15

Yang Q. Gain weight by going diet? Artificial sweeteners and the neurobiology of sugar cravings. *Yale J Biol Med* 2010; 83: 101-8.

Ye M, Mandhane PJ, Senthilselvan A. Association of breastfeeding with asthma in young Aboriginal children in Canada. (PMID:23248799) *Canad Respirat J* 2012, 19(6):361-366

Yilmaz G, Hizli S, Karacan C, Yurdakök K. Effect of passive smoking on growth and infection rates of breast-fed and non-breast-fed infants. (PMID:19400822) *Pediatrics International* 2009, 51(3):352-358 DOI: 10.1111/j.1442-200X.2008.02757.x

Yorifuji T, Kubo T, Yamakawa M, Kato T et al. Breastfeeding and behavioral development: a nationwide longitudinal survey in Japan. (PMID:24529622) *J Pediatr* 2014

Young J, Watson K, Ellis L, Raven L. Responding to evidence: breastfeed baby if you can--the sixth public health recommendation to reduce the risk of sudden and unexpected death in infancy. (PMID:22724308) *Breastfeed Rev* 2012, 20 (1):7-15

Youngster I, Russell GH, Pindar C, Ziv-Baran T et al. **Oral, capsulized, frozen fecal microbiota transplantation for relapsing *Clostridium difficile* infection.** *JAMA.* Published online October 11, 2014. doi:10.1001/jama.2014.13875

Zachariassen G, Fenger-Gron J . Preterm dietary study: meal frequency, regurgitation and the surprisingly high use of laxatives among formula-fed infants following discharge. (PMID:24286180) *Acta Paediatrica* 2014, 103(3):e116-22

Zeiger RS, Friedman NJ. The relationship of breastfeeding to the development of atopic disorders. (PMID:16632962) *Nestle Nutr Workshop Ser Pediatr Program* 2006; 57:93-105; discussion 105-8.

Zelman NE. The Nestle Infant formula controversy:restricting the marketing practices of multinational corporations in the Third World. *Transnational Lawyer* 1990; 3 (2) 697-758.

Ziegler EE. Consumption of cow's milk as a cause of iron deficiency in infants and toddlers. *Nutr Rev* 2011, 69 Suppl 1:s37-42. (PMID:22043881)

Ziegler JB, Cooper DA, Johnson RO, Gold J. Postnatal transmission of AIDS-associated retrovirus from mother to infant. (PMID:2858746) *Lancet* 1985, 1(8434):896-898.

Zivkovic AM, German JB, Lebrilla CB, Mills DA Human milk glycobiome and its impact on the infant gastrointestinal microbiota. (PMID:20679197) *Proc Nat Acad Sci* 2011, 108 Suppl 1:4653-4658.

Zoppi G, Mantovanelli F, Pittschieler K, Delem A et al. Response to RIT 4237 oral rotavirus vaccine in human milk, adapted-and soy-formula fed infants. (PMID:2556883) *Acta Paediatr Scand* 1989, 78(5):759-762.

Zung A, Glaser T, Kerem Z, Zadik Z. Breast development in the first 2 years of life: an association with soy-based infant formulas. *J Pediatr Gastroenterol Nutr.* 2008 Feb;46(2):191-5.

Zutavern A, Hirsch T, Leupold W, Weiland S et al. Atopic dermatitis, extrinsic atopic dermatitis and the hygiene hypothesis: results from a cross-sectional study. *Clin Exp Allergy* 2005; 35(10):1301-1308 DOI: 10.1111/j.1365-

Zutavern A, von Mutius E, Harris J, Mills P et al. The introduction of solids in relation to asthma and eczema. *Arch Dis Child* 1998; 79:126–130.

## Copyright acknowledgements

A note about using industry sources

Among these books and articles are many useful volumes from workshops organised by Nestle Nutrition Institute, as it now is. They are included for two very good reasons:

- they contain some of the best uncensored scientific discussion publicly available on the subject of infant feeding, and
- any information cited from them –and there is a lot in this book, deliberately so- can hardly be deemed to be unfairly prejudiced against artificial feeding!

I would not insult scientists willing to work with and for industry by suggesting that this fact alone means their research is dubious. I am told that some people refuse to read what industry produces. On the contrary, I think it critical to read *as much as possible of what* industry produces, and not just the marketing puffery and emotional propaganda. I have bought most of these books as they appeared. The entire series is now among the many excellent resources that Nestlé freely makes available online to those willing to sign in to their information service, the Nestlé Nutrition Institute, or NNI. I listen to their videos and read their press releases. This is extremely useful, so long as it is not the *only* source of one's information about infant feeding, and one is capable fo recognising assumptions that colour presentations. (The underlying ones being that society cannot be changed so that breastfeeding would be possible for women without severe penalty, and that many women cannot breastfeed so formula is necessary.) However, others may see using industry resources as consorting with their enemy, and would feel compromised: to each her or his own conscience, but it's difficult to be fully informed if ignoring such industry sources! And I believe that my chief enemy is societal ignorance, not industry.

Readers of this book will know that I am critical of industry, Nestle included - just as I am of other powerful forces preventing babies being breastfed. But readers need to realise that Nestle has earned respect among many health professionals and world-leading scientists by being open and professional about so much research information. I have found no comparable open-access industry site elsewhere. (Let me know if you have.) Yes, this is subtle marketing strategy. Personally, I am glad that some of the profits provided by bottle-feeding parents are put to such use. I would prefer that governments and international agencies were providing such a resource, having taxed the industry to make this possible. Being a pragmatist, I know that won't happen in my lifetime! But knowledge is powerful: so I find it wherever I can.

If anyone thinks that this tangential connection with industry has modified my views, I'd suggest they go back and read the first edition of *Breastfeeding Matters*, and compare that with what I am saying in *Milk Matters*. My perspective has not changed, and I work from the same basic assumptions now as then. These are not the assumptions industry has managed to inculcate in so many intelligent people, including many who see themselves as breastfeeding advocates or supporters of informed choice. The problem of artificial feeding is not restricted to poor people in underdeveloped communities. Babies are universal, and their basic needs and rights are identical wherever they are born. None of them will realise their full potential without being breastfed. I hope my work will continue to get rid of some of the blinkers so subtly constructed by the interplay between the powerful and their profits, whether those profits arise from the exploitation of women as workers, or children as consumers. When babies cannot be breastfed, everyone loses. We are only just beginning to realise that the losses are intergenerational. I hope they are reversible over generations.

Maureent Minchin, 2015

# Index

Lightning Source UK Ltd.
Milton Keynes UK
UKHW03n0254161018
330602UK00011B/115/P